PEDIATRIC TRAUMA

*Prevention, Acute Care,
Rehabilitation*

PEDIATRIC TRAUMA

Prevention, Acute Care, Rehabilitation

MARTIN R. EICHELBERGER, M.D.,
F.A.C.S., F.A.A.P.
Professor of Surgery and of Pediatrics
George Washington University School of Medicine
Washington, District of Columbia
Director of Emergency Trauma Services
Children's National Medical Center
Washington, District of Columbia

with 399 illustrations

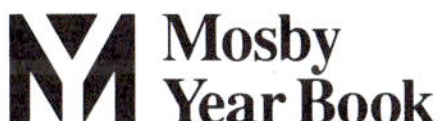

St. Louis Baltimore Boston Chicago London Philadelphia Sydney Toronto

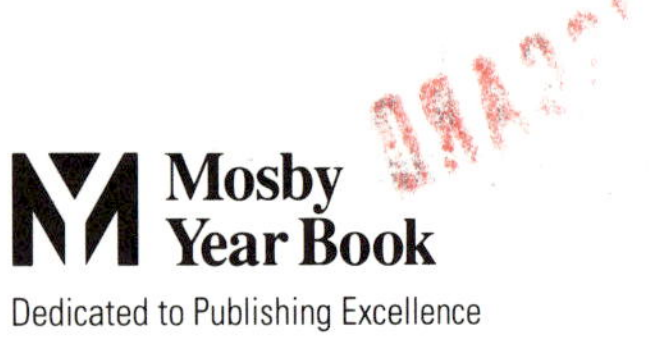

Editor: Laurel Craven
Developmental Editor: Leslie Fenton
Project Manager: Linda J. Daly

Printed in the United States of America

Mosby–Year Book, Inc.
11830 Westline Industrial Drive
St. Louis, Missouri 63146

Library of Congress Cataloging in Publication Data

Pediatric trauma : prevention, acute care, rehabilitation/[edited by] Martin R. Eichelberger.
   p.   cm.
     Includes bibliographical references and index.
     ISBN 1-55664-242-3
     1. Children—Wounds and injuries—Prevention. 2. Children—Wounds and injuries—Treatment. 3. Wounds and injuries—Patients—Rehabilitation. I. Eichelberger, Martin.
     [DNLM: 1. Wounds and Injuries—in infancy & childhood. 2. Wounds and Injuries—prevention & control. 3. Wounds and Injuries—therapy. WO 700 P37135]
     RD93.5.C4P459 1993
     617.1'0083—dc20
     DNLM/DLC   92-19170
     for Library of Congress   CIP

92 93 94 95 96 GW/MY 9 8 7 6 5 4 3 2 1

To the families who entrust us
with our greatest resource—children

Contributors

MICHAEL A. ALEXANDER, M.D., F.A.A.P.
Associate Professor of Physical Medicine and Pediatrics, Jefferson Medical College of Thomas Jefferson University, Philadelphia, Pennsylvania; Chief of Rehabilitation, Alfred I. duPont Institute, Wilmington, Delaware

WILLIAM E. ALISON, Jr., M.D.
Instructor, Department of Surgery, Tulane University School of Medicine, New Orleans, Louisiana; Surgical Research Fellow, University of Texas Medical School at Galveston and Shriners Burns Institute, Galveston, Texas

MICHAEL J. ALLSHOUSE, D.O.
Assistant Clinical Professor of Surgery, University of California Davis–East Bay School of Medicine, Oakland, California; Trauma Fellow, Children's National Medical Center, Washington, District of Columbia

RICHARD J. ANDRASSY, M.D., F.A.C.S., F.A.A.P.
A.G. McNeese Professor of Surgery and Pediatrics, University of Texas Medical School at Houston; Surgeon-in-Chief, Hermann Children's Hospital and Chief, Pediatric Surgery, M.D. Anderson Cancer Center and Lyndon B. Johnson General Hospital, Houston, Texas

ROBERT M. ARENSMAN, M.D.
Professor of Surgery and Pediatrics, University of Chicago Pritzker School of Medicine; Surgeon-in-Chief, Wyler Children's Hospital, Chicago, Illinois

JANE W. BALL, R.N., DrPH
Program Director, Pediatric Emergency Education and Research Center for Trauma Service, Children's National Medical Center, Washington, District of Columbia

JAMES M. BETTS, M.D., F.A.A.P., F.A.C.S.
Assistant Clinical Professor of Surgery, University of California Davis–East Bay School of Medicine; Chief of Pediatric Surgery, Director of Trauma Services, Children's Hospital, Oakland, California

ESHA BHATIA, M.A.
Program Assistant, National SAFE KIDS Campaign, Children's National Medical Center, Washington, District of Columbia

SHELDON J. BOND, M.D.
Assistant Professor of Surgery, University of Louisville School of Medicine; Attending Surgeon, Kosair Children's Hospital, Louisville, Kentucky

MICHAEL J. BOYAJIAN, M.D.
Assistant Professor, Surgery and Pediatrics, George Washington University School of Medicine and Health Sciences; Chairman, Plastic Surgery, Children's National Medical Center, Washington, District of Columbia

SHERYL BRISSETT-CHAPMAN, Ed.D., LICSW, ACSW
Baptist Home for Children and Families, Bethesda, Maryland

JOHN T. BRITTON, M.D.
Assistant Professor of Anesthesiology and Pediatrics, George Washington University School of Medicine and Health Sciences and Children's National Medical Center, Washington, District of Columbia

DEREK A. BRUCE, M.B., Ch.B.
Clinical Associate Professor, Department of Neurosurgery, University of Texas Southwestern Medical Center at Dallas Southwestern Medical School; Director of Pediatric Neurosurgical Institute, Humana Advanced Surgical Institute, Humana Hospital, Medical City, Dallas, Texas

DOROTHY I. BULAS, M.D.
Assistant Professor, Departments of Diagnostic Imaging and Radiology and Pediatrics, George Washington University School of Medicine and Health Sciences and Children's National Medical Center, Washington, District of Columbia

JOAN M. BURG, M.D., F.A.A.P., F.A.C.E.P.
Instructor in Pediatrics, Harvard Medical School; Attending Physician, Division of Emergency Medicine, Children's Hospital, Boston, Massachusetts

JAMES M. CHAMBERLAIN, M.D.
Assistant Professor of Pediatrics, George Washington University School of Medicine and Health Sciences; Assistant Medical Director, Emergency Medical Trauma Center, Children's National Medical Center, Washington, District of Columbia

GAIL F. COOPER
Chief, Emergency Medical Services, San Diego County Department of Health Services, San Diego, California

WAYNE S. COPES, Ph.D.
Tri-Analytics Incorporated, Bel Air, Maryland

CHARLES S. COX, Jr., M.D.
Surgical Research Fellow, University of Texas Medical School at Galveston, Shriners Burns Institute, Galveston; Resident in Surgery, University of Texas Health Science Center at Houston, Houston, Texas

JANE A. CROWLEY, Psy.D.
Clinical Co-Director, Brain Injury Unit, Alfred I. duPont Institute, Wilmington, Delaware

CURTIS A. DICKMAN, M.D.
Attending Neurosurgeon, Barrow Neurological Institute, Phoenix, Arizona

ANN-CHRISTINE DUHAIME, M.D.
Assistant Professor of Neurosurgery, University of Pennsylvania School of Medicine; Associate Neurosurgeon, Children's Hospital of Philadelphia, Philadelphia, Pennsylvania

MARTIN R. EICHELBERGER, M.D.
Professor of Surgery and of Pediatrics, George Washington University School of Medicine and Health Sciences, Washington, District of Columbia

MARY E. FALLAT, M.D.
Assistant Professor of Surgery, University of Louisville School of Medicine; Director of Trauma Services and Attending Surgeon, Kosair Children's Hospital, Louisville, Kentucky

HERTA B. FEELY, B.A.
Executive Director, National SAFE KIDS Campaign, Children's National Medical Center, Washington, District of Columbia

GEOFFREY C. FENNER, M.D.
Chief Resident, Department in General Surgery, University of Chicago Pritzker School of Medicine, Chicago, Illinois

ALAN I. FIELDS, M.D.
Professor of Anesthesiology and Associate Professor of Pediatrics, George Washington University School of Medicine and Health Sciences; Associate Director, Department of Critical Care Medicine, Children's National Medical Center, Washington, District of Columbia

GARY R. FLEISHER, M.D., F.A.A.P., F.A.C.E.P.
Associate Professor of Pediatrics, Harvard Medical School; Chief, Emergency Medicine, Children's Hospital, Boston, Massachusetts

DONALD J. FORRESTER, D.D.S., M.S.D.
Professor, Department of Pediatrics, George Washington University School of Medicine and Health Sciences; Chairman, Department of Pediatric Dentistry, Children's National Medical Center, Washington, District of Columbia

DAVID S. FRIENDLY, M.D.
Professor of Ophthalmology, George Washington University School of Medicine and Health Sciences; Chairman, Department of Ophthalmology, Children's National Medical Center, Washington, District of Columbia

VICTOR F. GARCIA, M.D.
Department of Surgery, Children's Hospital of Cincinnati, Cincinnati, Ohio

CATHERINE S. GOTSCHALL, Ph.D.
Trauma Services, Children's National Medical Center, Washington, District of Columbia

JAY L. GROSFELD, M.D.
Lafayette Page Professor and Chairman, Department of Surgery, Indiana University School of Medicine; Surgeon-in-Chief, James Whitcomb Riley Hospital for Children, Indianapolis, Indiana

PHILIP C. GUZZETTA, M.D.
Professor of Surgery and of Pediatrics, George Washington University School of Medicine and Health Sciences; Attending Surgeon, Children's National Medical Center, Washington, District of Columbia

J. ALEX HALLER, Jr., M.D.
Robert Garrett Professor of Pediatric Surgery and Professor of Emergency Medicine and of Pediatrics, Johns Hopkins University School of Medicine; Director, Division of Pediatric Surgery, Johns Hopkins Hospital, Baltimore, Maryland

ROBYN M. HATLEY, M.D.
Associate Professor of Surgery and Pediatrics, and Pediatric Surgeon, Medical College of Georgia School of Medicine, Augusta, Georgia

DAVID E. HEPPEL, M.D.
Director, Division of Maternal, Infant, Child, and Adolescent Health, Maternal and Child Health Bureau, Rockville, Maryland

DAVID N. HERNDON, M.D.
Jesse H. Jones Professor of Burn Surgery, University of Texas Medical School at Galveston; Chief of Staff, Shriners Burns Institute, Galveston, Texas

CHARLES G. HOWELL, Jr., M.D.
Professor of Pediatric Surgery and Pediatrics, and Pediatric Surgeon, Medical College of Georgia School of Medicine, Augusta, Georgia

MOHAMAD S. JAAFAR, M.D.
Assistant Professor of Ophthalmology and Pediatrics, George Washington University School of Medicine and Health Sciences; Associate in Ophthalmology, Children's National Medical Center, Washington, District of Columbia

DENNIS L. JOHNSON, M.D.
Associate Professor, George Washington University School of Medicine and Health Sciences, Washington, District of Columbia

MIREILLE B. KANDA, M.D.
Assistant Professor of Pediatrics, George Washington University School of Medicine and Health Sciences; Director, Division of Child Protection, Children's National Medical Center, Washington, District of Columbia

M. MARGARET KNUDSON, M.D.
Assistant Professor of Surgery, University of California, San Francisco, School of Medicine; Attending Trauma Surgeon, San Francisco General Hospital, San Francisco, California

TOBEY S. LAWSON, J.D.
Miller and Martin Attorneys at Law, Chattanooga, Tennessee

DANIEL J. LEDBETTER, M.D.
Assistant Professor of Surgery and Pediatrics, University of Chicago Pritzker School of Medicine; Attending Surgeon, Wyler Children's Hospital, University of Chicago Hospitals, Chicago, Illinois

WILLIAM A. LOE, Jr., M.D.
Assistant Professor of Surgery and Pediatrics, University of Chicago Pritzker School of Medicine; Director, Trauma Service, University of Chicago Hospitals and Chicago Safe Kids Coalition, Chicago, Illinois

JOHN M. LOISELLE, M.D.
Instructor in Pediatrics, University of Pennsylvania School of Medicine; Fellow, Pediatric Emergency Medicine, Children's Hospital of Philadelphia, Philadelphia, Pennsylvania

STEPHEN LUDWIG, M.D.
Professor of Pediatrics, University of Pennsylvania School of Medicine; Division Chief, General Pediatrics, Children's Hospital of Philadelphia, Philadelphia, Pennsylvania

THOMAS G. LUERSSEN, M.D.
Associate Professor of Surgery, Indiana University School of Medicine; Director, Pediatric Neurosurgery, James Whitcomb Riley Hospital for Children, Indianapolis, Indiana

DAVID K. MAGNUSON, M.D.
Acting Instructor, Department of Surgery, University of Washington School of Medicine; Pediatric Surgical Fellow, Children's Hospital and Medical Center, Seattle, Washington

RONALD V. MAIER, M.D., F.A.C.S.
Professor of Surgery, University of Washington School of Medicine; Director, Northwest Regional Trauma Center and Surgical Intensive Care Unit, and Co-director, Harborview Injury Prevention and Research Center, Harborview Medical Center, Seattle, Washington

MAUREEN S. McARDLE, R.N.
Emergency Medical Services Coordinator and Trauma Program Manager, Emergency Medical Services, San Diego County Department of Health Services, San Diego, California

WILLIS A. McGILL, M.D.
Professor of Anesthesiology, George Washington University School of Medicine and Health Sciences; Chairman, Department of Anesthesiology, Children's National Medical Center, Washington, District of Columbia

BARBARA A. McHUGH, R.N., M.P.H.
Administrative Director, Division of Rehabilitation Medicine, Alfred I. duPont Institute, Children's Hospital, Wilmington, Delaware

LEZLEY P. McILVEEN, B.D.S., M.S.
Assistant Professor, Department of Pediatrics, George Washington University School of Medicine and Health Sciences; Clinical Director, Department of Pediatric Dentistry, Children's National Medical Center, Washington, District of Columbia

GREGORY MILMOE, M.D.
Associate Professor of Surgery, Department of Otolaryngology, George Washington University School of Medicine and Health Sciences; Associate, Department of Otolaryngology, Children's National Medical Center, Washington, District of Columbia

MELINDA G. MURRAY, J.D.
Associate Counsel for Litigation and Risk Management, Children's National Medical Center, Washington, District of Columbia

CATHERINE A. MUSEMECHE, M.D.
Assistant Professor of Surgery, University of Texas Medical School at Houston; Chief of Pediatric Surgery, Lyndon B. Johnson General Hospital, Houston, Texas

KURT D. NEWMAN, M.D.
Associate Professor of Surgery and of Pediatrics, George Washington University School of Medicine and Health Sciences; Attending Surgeon, Children's National Medical Center, Washington, District of Columbia

LESLIE M. O'BRIEN, R.N., B.S.N.
Trauma Coordinator, Children's National Medical Center, Washington, District of Columbia

LAVDENA A. ORR, M.D.
Division of Child Protection, Children's National Medical Center, Washington, District of Columbia

RAMESH I. PATEL, M.D.
Associate Professor of Anesthesiology and of Pediatrics, George Washington University School of Medicine and Health Sciences; Attending Anesthesiologist, Children's National Medical Center, Washington, District of Columbia

LYNN E. PATTEN, R.N.C., M.S.N.
Pediatric Nurse Practitioner, Traumatic Brain Injury Unit, Alfred I. duPont Institute, Wilmington, Delaware

SHARON L. PILMER, M.D.
Assistant Professor of Anesthesiology and Pediatrics, University of Pennsylvania School of Medicine; Assistant Anesthesiologist, Children's Hospital of Philadelphia, Philadelphia, Pennsylvania

LAURENCE J. PLATT, M.D., M.P.H.
Visiting Scholar, Institute for Health Policy Studies, University of California School of Medicine, San Francisco, California; Assistant Director for Clinical Health Policy, Division of Maternal, Infant, Child, and Adolescent Health, Maternal and Child Health Bureau, Rockville, Maryland

MURRAY M. POLLACK, M.D.
Professor, Anesthesiology and Pediatrics, George Washington University School of Medicine and Health Sciences; Associate Director, Pediatric Intensive Care Unit, Children's National Medical Center, Washington, District of Columbia

GERALDINE S. PRATSCH, R.N., M.P.H.
Pediatric Emergency Education Coordinator, Emergency Trauma Service, Children's National Medical Center, Washington, District of Columbia

RUSSELL C. RAPHAELY, M.D.
Professor of Anesthesiology and Pediatrics, University of Pennsylvania School of Medicine; Senior Anesthesiologist, Chief, Division of Critical Care Medicine, and Medical Director, Pediatric Intensive Care Complex, Children's Hospital of Philadelphia, Philadelphia, Pennsylvania

HAROLD L. REKATE, M.D., F.A.C.S.
Clinical Professor of Surgery, University of Arizona College of Medicine, Tucson; Chairman, Section of Pediatric Neurosurgery and Director, Pediatric Neurosurgical Research Laboratory, Phoenix, Arizona

FREDERICK J. RESCORLA, M.D.
Assistant Professor of Surgery, Indiana University School of Medicine, James Whitcomb Riley Hospital for Children, Indianapolis, Indiana

LINDA JO RICE, M.D.
Associate Professor of Anesthesiology and Assistant Professor of Pediatrics, George Washington University School of Medicine and Health Sciences and Children's National Medical Center, Washington, District of Columbia

FREDERICK P. RIVARA, M.D., M.P.H.
Professor of Pediatrics, Adjunct Professor of Epidemiology, and Medical Doctor of Pediatrics, University of Washington School of Medicine, Seattle, Washington

WILLIAM W. ROBERTSON, Jr., M.D.
Professor of Orthopaedic Surgery and Pediatrics, George Washington University School of Medicine and Health Sciences; Chairman, Department of Pediatric Orthopaedic Surgery, Children's National Medical Center, Washington, District of Columbia

WILLIAM J. RODRIGUEZ, M.D., Ph.D.
Professor, Child Health and Development, George Washington University School of Medicine and Health Sciences; Chairman, Microbiology Research and Infectious Diseases Departments, Children's National Medical Center, Washington, District of Columbia

THOMAS M. ROUSE, M.D.
Assistant Professor of Surgery and of Pediatrics, George Washington University School of Medicine and Health Sciences; Attending Surgeon, Children's National Medical Center, Washington, District of Columbia

RANDI L. RUTAN, R.N., B.S.N.
Clinical Data Coordinator and Research Nurse, University of Texas Medical Branch and Shriners Burns Institute, Galveston, Texas

WILLIAM J. SACCO, Ph.D.
Visiting Professor of Neurosurgery, University of Virginia School of Medicine, Charlottesville, Virginia; President, Tri-Analytics Incorporated, Bel Air, Maryland

RONALD J. SCORPIO, M.D.
Research Fellow, Department of Surgery, University of Toronto Faculty of Medicine; Research Fellow, Department of Surgery, Hospital for Sick Children, Toronto, Ontario, Canada

MARGARET J. SCHAEFFER, R.N., C.P.T.C.
Registered Nurse, Certified Procurement Transplant Coordinator, and Director of Recovery Services, Washington Regional Transplant Consortium; Member, American Association of Critical Care Nurses, North American Transplant Coordinators Organization, and Association Organ Procurement Organizations, Washington, District of Columbia

CARLOS J. SIVIT, M.D.
Assistant Professor of Radiology and Pediatrics, George Washington University School of Medicine and Health Sciences; Staff Radiologist, Children's National Medical Center, Washington, District of Columbia

AMY R. TEMPLETON, J.D.
Associate Counsel, Legal Department, Children's National Medical Center, Washington, District of Columbia

JOHN M. TEMPLETON, Jr., M.D.
Associate Professor, Pediatric Surgery, University of Pennsylvania School of Medicine; Associate Surgeon, Children's Hospital of Philadelphia, Philadelphia, Pennsylvania

MICHAEL D. THOMAS, M.D.
Assistant Professor of Orthopedic Surgery and of Pediatrics, George Washington University School of Medicine and Health Sciences and Children's National Medical Center; Staff Orthopedic Surgeon, Children's National Medical Center and Orthopedic Consultant, Health Services for Children with Special Needs, Washington, District of Columbia

W. RALEIGH THOMPSON, M.D.
Staff, Department of Surgery, Naval Hospital, San Diego, California

A. MARGARITA TORRES, M.D.
Pediatric Surgery Fellow, Cincinnati Children's Hospital, Cincinnati, Ohio

ORRAWIN TROCKI, M.S., R.D., C.N.S.D.
Clinical Dietitian, Children's National Medical Center, Washington, District of Columbia

RAPHAEL UDASSIN, M.D.
Senior Lecturer in Surgery, and Head, Department of Pediatric Surgery, Hadassah University Hospital Mount Scopus, The Hebrew University Medical School, Jerusalem, Israel

DENNIS W. VANE, M.D., F.A.C.S., F.A.A.P.
Chairman, Section of Pediatric Surgery and Associate Professor of Surgery and Pediatrics, University of Vermont College of Medicine, Burlington, Vermont

ITZHAK VINOGRAD, M.D.
Senior Lecturer in Surgery, Sackler School of Medicine, Tel-Aviv University, Tel-Aviv; Head and Surgeon-in-Chief, Department of Pediatric Surgery, Assaf-Harofeh Medical Center, Zerifin, Israel

YEHESKEL WAISMAN, M.D.
Assistant Medical Director, Emergency Medical Trauma Center, Children's National Medical Center, Washington, District of Columbia

THOMAS L. WALSH, M.D.
Associate Professor of Psychiatry and Pediatrics, George Washington University School of Medicine and Health Sciences; Director of Psychiatric Consultation–Liaison Services, Children's National Medical Center, Washington, District of Columbia

DAVID E. WESSON, M.D.
Associate Professor of Surgery, University of Toronto Faculty of Medicine; Staff Surgeon and Director of Trauma Program, Hospital for Sick Children, Toronto, Ontario, Canada

BERNHARD L. WIEDERMANN, M.D.
Associate Professor of Pediatrics, George Washington University School of Medicine and Health Sciences; Attending in Infectious Diseases and Director, Pediatric Residency Training Program, Children's National Medical Center, Washington, District of Columbia

CYNTHIA J. WRIGHT, M.S.N., R.N.C., C.R.R.N.
Trauma Rehabilitation Coordinator, Emergency Medical Service, Children's National Medical Center, Washington, District of Columbia

ARNO L. ZARITSKY, M.D.
Associate Professor of Pediatrics, University of North Carolina at Chapel Hill School of Medicine; Director, Pediatric Intensive Care Unit, North Carolina Children's Hospital, Chapel Hill, North Carolina

Foreword

For more than half a century, pediatricians and surgeons have stood in the doorways of emergency rooms across the land receiving injured children and reacting to injuries with the methodology and principles of the moment. As hard data on the national carnage of head trauma surfaced, it became ever more evident that disability, disfigurement, and death far exceeded the sum total of infections, malignancy, and other more celebrated causes of childhood illness. It began to be apparent that our increasingly complex and crowded societal enclaves had spawned an epidemic—a torrent of death and destruction of our children more devastating than the plagues of the Dark Ages or publicized infections of the present day. For children's hospitals and pediatric units, the question loomed: "Are we doing all we can to treat childhood victims of trauma?" We believed we were doing well in the operating rooms and in the increasingly sophisticated pediatric intensive care units. What, however, of transport of the injured child? What of the environment spawning these accidents: bicycles ridden without helmets, hot water faucets without temperature regulators, playgrounds without adult supervision, and gun and knife stores without restrictions? What of the responsibility of parents, schools, police and fire departments, health planning centers, clinics, hospitals, nurses, and physicians? It was all sort of an amorphous mass—a myriad of well-intentioned but disconnected, unfocused efforts.

Twelve years ago, at the Children's National Medical Center in Washington, D.C., I watched a trauma center for children come alive. We had a solid department of pediatrics, a good outpatient program, and some very skilled surgeons and specialty surgeons. We could plug gunshot wounds, straighten fractures, and treat burns on a par with any children's facility. Then, in came Dr. Martin Eichelberger, who proposed tackling all phases of children's trauma with the same vigor and drive that he put to opposing ball carriers as a defensive halfback.

The first part of Dr. Eichelberger's game plan involved overhaul of our in-house trauma response. Designated players were assigned specific positions around the trauma bed. All persons who were to serve with first hospital response unit were drilled, timed, and graded on every conceivable reaction. Overnight the trauma receiving unit became an orderly, efficient haven with no distractions, no snags, and no onlookers. Chaos vanished and was replaced by quiet effective treatment. The second arduous step involved all departments and people throughout the hospital. Next, the Eichelberger program spread to envelope the city-wide services for recovery of accident victims. Our city ambulances did not even have child-size oxygen masks or neck collars. Even intravenous containers, needles, and arm boards had to be down-sized. This led naturally to regular education sessions for all existing emergency medical technicians, paramedics, police, firefighters, and those in training. Then, logically, came a new ambulance reception area, then a heliport, then a communication center with experts at a console to enhance doctor-to-ambulance and doctor-to-helicopter interaction. All of this led, in turn, to parent education and community education through meetings and through television and radio messages explaining how to childproof the home and how to set up neighborhood safety strategies.

Over the past 10 years I have watched the children's trauma team in Washington grow to a sophisticated comprehensive program capable of searching out trouble spots in the system and collecting valid outcome data. Now in the Children's National Medical Center, as in others, there exists a region-wide awareness of and response to injured children. Now young people move through the system, from the moment of injury to successful rehabilitation, via a smoothly functioning process that utilizes all of the necessary strengths of a modern pediatric hospital.

It's all here in this book. Many experts, including key players from Children's National Medical Center, have brought their contributions to this volume. I can attest that Dr. Eichelberger's system works for the betterment of the injured child. The reader can learn how to create such a unit in his or her setting, or if yours is in place, to measure it against a yardstick of success.

Judson Randolph

Preface

Pediatric trauma is a disease entity that challenges our capacity for teamwork. The concept "continuum of care" facilitates understanding childhood injury as a disease that encompasses prevention, acute care, and rehabilitation. In the past, treatment of injury was a preoccupation. After considerable experience, evidence demonstrates that the needs of injured children necessitate a systematic approach that begins with prevention and includes rehabilitation.

Pediatric Trauma: Prevention, Acute Care, Rehabilitation addresses the components necessary to control injury as a disease entity. The field of prevention is population based and requires a multifaceted strategy to curtail entry of children into the acute care system. This text links the basic tenets outlined by Haddon, who delineates a framework to understand the role of prevention in the continuum of care, with acute care and with rehabilitation. When primary or secondary prevention fails to control injury of children, a tertiary phase of acute care becomes imperative. With the enhanced capability to reverse injury mortality, many children live with disability, necessitating a long-term commitment to rehabilitation of the child and family. Reconstitution of the injured family is the most difficult challenge for the team that provides successful acute care.

Other essential components that contribute to the continuum of care are education, research, and outcome analysis. These provide an opportunity to categorize injury in childhood and to develop an understanding of the patterns of injury. Analysis of outcome permits improvement of care, since evaluation of specific cases permits a variety of opportunities for improvement.

Pediatric Trauma: Prevention, Acute Care, Rehabilitation is a useful reference textbook for all professionals who contribute to a coordinated continuum of care. The epidemiologist who is interested in injury prevention must understand how failed strategies result in injured children who require a commitment to long-term rehabilitation. Effective injury control strategies are now linked in sequence with acute care and rehabilitation. Any individual committed to injury control will benefit from the superb information presented by the authors who expand the perspective of the field of injury.

The textbook focuses upon the needs of children and their families. Each author provides a unique perspective on a particular area of expertise; the textbook is meant to be a "how-to" manual. The authors provide you, the reader, with their best judgment and reference additional material that will enhance understanding of the basic principles forming their personal approaches. This information is a dedicated effort to reduce mortality and morbidity of a preventable disease—childhood injury. Many of the ideas expressed will benefit children and their families.

I would like to express my sincere appreciation to Ceil Hendrickson, RN, who is the reason this textbook exists. I am deeply indebted to Ceil for her personal encouragement, enthusiasm, grace, and commitment to excellence. She is a caring soul and a mother who understands the heavy burden of individuals who care for injured children and their families. All of the authors, as well as myself, recognize her keen sense of humor and delicate touch. This textbook is her contribution to injury control for children; I admire her professionalism and good common sense. Many children are in her debt.

I would like to thank Mary Mansor, former Medical Editor at Mosby–Year Book, for offering us the opportunity to develop this textbook for children. Her unique editorial skills and commitment to excellence are evident throughout this book. Leslie Fenton demonstrated great patience with all of us and provided constant encouragement. She attended to a thousand editorial details, for which we will always be grateful. Linda Daly contributed to the final stages of the book and encouraged us with her enthusiasm.

Also, my friend and mentor Judson G. Randolph, MD, provided me the opportunity to learn about injured children and develop a system of care to test many thoughts. His enthusiasm, encouragement, friendship, and guidance stimulated a sense of direction for me to pursue an understanding of children and of injury control. I am one of the fortunate to benefit from daily contact with "JR," who always found the best in his colleagues and students. He provided me a track upon which to run and a chance to improve the lives of children.

Finally, I found the opportunity to develop this textbook a challenge. It is a privilege to learn from my patients and to possess the goodwill of colleagues who function as a team. I hope that each of you will find a new perspective and encouragement to improve the quality of care we provide to children and to their families. Their young lives depend upon us.

Martin R. Eichelberger

Contents

xvii

PEDIATRIC TRAUMA

Prevention, Acute Care,
Rehabilitation

PART ONE

Injury to Children

The disease

1 Public Health of Children

David E. Heppel and Laurence J. Platt

As in many of the health problems that children suffer, many factors influence the occurrence of childhood injury. Some have to do with the individual child, but a number of others relate to the child's environment: for example, the family, the house, the school. Still other factors relate to society: the development of technology at a faster pace than our ability to relate to it safely, the way a particular culture views time, and the social network within a community. The complex interaction of factors means that it is difficult to understand why an injury has occurred; but it also means that there are many opportunities for its prevention. And prevention is the traditional work of public health.

Medical practice defines and intervenes in a problem in terms of an individual and the individual's parts and systems. In the field of injury, the individual-based approach means research and progress in treatment of head trauma, of respiratory insufficiency, and of skeletal fractures. Because of the complexity of the problem, however, injury lends itself well to community-based interventions aimed at *groups* of individuals, the traditional target of public health.

MISSION OF PUBLIC HEALTH

In its 1988 report, *The Future of Public Health,* the Institute of Medicine defines the mission of public health as fulfilling society's interest in ensuring conditions in which people can be healthy. Carrying out this mission has involved interventions directed at both individuals and populations. Examples include control measures to ensure safe food and water, disposal of toxic waste, immunizations against disease, epidemiologic control measures to prevent the spread of communicable diseases, and provision of individual health care services to those unable to procure such services on their own. Individuals and organizations, both public and private, have responsibility to fulfill this mission.

Although each citizen has some responsibility for public health, government has a particular role to play. The Institute of Medicine perceives all levels of government to have responsibility for assessment of need, for policy development, and for assurance.

Assessment requires the systematic and recurrent collection, analysis, and dissemination of information concerning the overall health status of the community, state, or nation. This knowledge is crucial to the development of appropriate and effective interventions. As Leon Robertson has said, "You don't prevent falls out of windows by putting abrasive strips on bathtubs." Communities must determine the existing health problems in their midst, as well as the contributing factors. Government, as the agent for all, must be certain that this information is available.

Policy development is the means by which problem identification, technical knowledge of possible solutions, and societal values join to set a course of action. The Institute of Medicine views government, in general, and health departments, in particular, as playing an important role in facilitating this process.

The final responsibility is that of *assurance* that services required to carry out the policies of the community relating to health are in fact provided. This responsibility involves encouraging actions by other organizations or individuals, regulation of activities, or providing services directly. Although most of these services are population-based, the report emphasizes the responsibility of public health agencies to assure provision of individual health care for those unable to afford it. It is in this context of assessment, policy development, and assurance that the relationship of public health to children and adolescents will be considered.

HISTORY OF PUBLIC HEALTH SERVICES FOR CHILDREN AND ADOLESCENTS

The history of health care specifically for children is surprisingly short; the history of *public* health care for children is even shorter. Because it is easier to see and relate to a single hurt child, approaches to the individual have understandably preceded and predominated over public health approaches. It is harder to perceive an affected community and there is a generally a lack of rigorous and regular attempts at such diagnoses.

It was only at the start of the century that the idea of public responsibility, of government responsibility for health, generally, and maternal and child health (MCH), in particular, emerged, in part, because children began to be viewed as a "public resource" and not just as members of a family.

The opposing view, which persists, is that responsibility for health is the family's. To the extent that government should be involved, the feeling is that the state government, not the federal government, should lead. At the turn of the twentieth century, however, most state governments were not doing anything in the area of health services or MCH.

Nevertheless, there are interventions that can prevent injury, help to assure access to services, and determine and respond to community need. Only a social institution can perform these tasks. Unfortunately, the social philosophy of individualism is so strong in the United States that its citizens are still ambivalent about supporting such interventions.

In the latter 1800s, increased knowledge of communicable diseases stimulated an expanded view of the role of public health in prevention of childhood illness. In 1892 in New York City, the first milk station opened to provide uncontaminated milk for children. During this time also the use of silver nitrate to prevent gonorrheal ophthalmia neonatorum was adopted. Both of these actions were quite effective in reducing mortality and morbidity among children, but it is interesting to note that although the scientific knowledge existed for decades, government took no immediate active role.

In 1910 a national conference was held, the first White House Conference on Children, of which one outcome was the creation in 1912 of the first national agency for children, the Children's Bureau. Federal responsibility for health of mothers and children was thereby established for the first time. The Children's Bureau was directed to "investigate and report . . . upon all matters pertaining to the welfare of children and child life among all classes of our people and shall especially investigate the questions of infant mortality, the birth rate, orphanage, juvenile courts, desertion, dangerous occupations, accidents and diseases of children . . . and legislation affecting children in the several states and territories."[2] The reports issued by the Children's Bureau provided the basis for the passage of the Sheppard-Towner (Maternal and Infancy) Act in 1921. This legislation provided for grants to states to develop services for mothers and children.

In the 1920s, almost all states had a maternal and child health agency, and most large cities had programs for children. Schools of public health were organized at about this time, as health scientists appreciated more and more the value of community-based research and interventions, particularly in relation to infectious diseases and nutrition.

The Sheppard-Towner Act lapsed in 1929 under accusations of being "socialist"; when the American Medical Association refused to support its continuation, pediatricians formed the American Academy of Pediatrics in 1930 and lobbied for a maternal and child health program. Their efforts were successful when, in the midst of the economic depression, the Social Security Act was passed in 1935. Although most benefits provided by this law were for the elderly, it included a few child-related provisions. One of these was Title V, creating the federal Maternal and Child Health program.

Title V revitalized the Sheppard-Towner program, providing federal funds to states to assure access to child and maternity services. It also provided support for demonstration projects. Finally, the original law created what was then called the Crippled Children's Services program. These three types of programs persist to this day: all states, even with tremendous variability in their respective programs, have an agency related to children with special health care needs and another related to preventive primary care and public health services for mothers and children. The third line of demonstration projects has evolved into a program called Special Projects of Regional and National Significance (SPRANS).

The 1960s was the time of a prevailing social philosophy that distrusted government. It was the era of civil rights. Children were seen as having rights, independent of the family and beyond their value as social resource, allowing us for the first time to recognize and define child abuse, which had been present for centuries, as a health problem of legitimate concern.

In this context, a number of community-based health programs were created. The Office of Economic Opportunity (OEO) was established outside the traditional suspect bureaucracy, in the Office of the President, to "wage a war on poverty." Some of the health-related programs developed under the aegis of OEO included the Neighborhood Health Centers (which were the model for the current Community and Migrant Health Centers), Family Planning (the model for Title X programs), the Women, Infants and Children program (WIC, a nutritional program), Legal Aid, and Head Start. As a general rule, funding for these programs went from the federal government directly to a community organization.

The Children's Bureau likewise supported community-based projects, bypassing states for the first time. These included the Maternal and Infant Care (M + I) and Children and Youth Projects (C + Y). These programs defined new models of service delivery emphasizing comprehensiveness, a multidisciplinary approach, humanistic improvements in the delivery of services, and a willingness to pay for primary care services, to be a complete medical home for children.

The federalist philosophy reemerged in the early 1970s. Title V's Program of Projects transferred management of the M + I and C + Y projects to the states in 1974, although they still operated under federal guidelines defining the programs and how money was to be spent.

The Omnibus Budget Reconciliation Act (OBRA) of 1981 amended Title V to establish the MCH block grant; there were to be no more federal guidelines or oversight for the funds going to states for MCH programs. Whereas federal programming with input from the states only at federal discretion was emphasized in the 1960s, the block grant defined a state MCH program with federal input only at the states' discretion.

Concerned about accountability, as well as disquieting trends in infant mortality, immunization levels, and lack of significant progress in maternal and child health, Congress in 1989 once again amended Title V as part of the Omnibus Budget Reconciliation Act (OBRA 89). These amendments defined both federal and state roles in reporting on maternal and child health; it left definition and management of programs to the states, but called for national leadership in defining general objectives and reporting requirements.

The major emphases in OBRA 89 were on accountability, national direction, developing *systems* of health services, and universal access of children to primary care. It represented the end of the block grant, no-federal-regulations, state-wisdom era, and the start of the accountability, specific-requirements, state-federal-partnership era.

OBRA 89 for the first time called for national objectives related to maternal and child health, and the U.S. Public Health Service has published a set of health objectives for the nation to reach by the year 2000. The national MCH objectives are consistent with those overall national objectives. The Year 2000 Objectives related to childhood injury are listed in Table 1-1.[1]

PUBLIC HEALTH RESPONSIBILITIES AND FUNCTIONS

Of the total money appropriated by Congress for Title V, 85% of the funds is given on a formula basis as a "block grant" to all states submitting an acceptable application. The program of each state is different; but since 1990 all have objectives consistent with the national MCH objectives, all have common reporting requirements, and all are required to spend 30% of federal allotment on *assuring access to primary and preventive services for all children and adolescents in the state*, and 30% on *developing family-centered, coordinated, community-based, culturally competent systems of care for children with special health care needs.*

Fifteen percent of the funds appropriated by Congress is given out as discretionary grants that public and nonprofit agencies compete for: Special Projects of Regional and National Significance. These grants support *training of MCH public health workers; demonstrations related to improved services* for mothers, children, and children with special health care needs; and *research on MCH service issues.* From time to time, Congress earmarks a separate, specific appropriation to meet a particular categorical service-related problem (for example, improved pediatric emergency medical services).

Throughout all the changes in philosophy regarding social responsibility for health and in the view of federal, as opposed to state, responsibilities, it should be understood that most of the health dollars, including government dollars, that are spent in the United States are spent in medical care through private providers, *not* through government or public agencies. The responsiblity left to public health agenices, ambivalent as our society is about this, is to provide care for groups that the private sector does not want to serve: the poor, the uninsured, the chronically ill, the mentally ill, and the handicapped. And these groups, with the greatest health care needs, are allotted the fewest financial resources.

Federal, state and local governments also address other public health responsibilities, such as *data collection and reporting.* The collection of data has many public health purposes. *Surveillance* allows health departments to know which diseases are occurring to enable appropriate intervention and control. Among the sources of surveillance data are case reports, including mandated reporting for some diseases, laboratory reports, emergency room visits, hospital discharge summaries, case follow-ups, death certificates, and surveys. All health departments include fatal injuries as part of the vital statistics function; some may also conduct routine surveillance of morbidity related to injury. Massachusetts, for example, builds surveillance into its statewide Childhood Injury Prevention Program.

Data are also the fodder of *epidemiology,* the basic science of public health. Epidemiology seeks to find out how and why a disease process occurs by looking at its distribution within a population. A basic methodology of epidemiology is the col-

Table 1–1 Year 2000 national objectives related to childhood injury

Health status objectives

Reduce deaths caused by motor vehicle crashes to no more than 1.9 per 100 million vehicle miles traveled and 16.8 per 100,000 people. (Baseline: 2.4 per 100 million vehicle miles traveled (VMT) and 18.8 per 100,000 people (age adjusted) in 1987.)

Deaths caused by motor vehicle crashes (per 100,000)	*1987 Baseline*	*2000 Target*
Children aged 14 and younger	6.2	5.5
Youth aged 15 to 24	36.9	33

Reduce deaths from falls and fall-related injuries to no more than 2.3 per 100,000 people. (Age-adjusted baseline: 2.7 per 100,000 in 1987.)

Reduce drowning deaths to no more than 1.3 per 100,000 people. (Age-adjusted baseline: 2.1 per 100,000 in 1987.)

Drowning deaths (per 100,000)	*1987 Baseline*	*2000 Target*
Children aged 4 and younger	4.2	2.3
Men aged 15 to 34	4.5	2.5
Black males	6.6	3.6

Reduce fire deaths to no more than 1.2 per 100,000 people. (Age-adjusted baseline: 1.5 per 100,000 in 1987.)

Residential fire deaths (per 100,000)	*1987 Baseline*	*2000 Target*
Children aged 4 and younger	4.4	3.3

Reduce nonfatal poisoning to no more than 88 emergency department treatments per 100,000 people. (Baseline: 103 per 100,000 in 1986.)

Nonfatal poisoning (per 100,000)	*1986 Baseline*	*2000 Target*
Among children aged 4 and younger	650	520

Reduce nonfatal head injuries so that hospitalizations for this condition are no more than 106 per 100,000 people. (Baseline: 125 per 100,000 in 1988.)

Reduce nonfatal spinal cord injuries so that hospitalizations for this condition are no more than 5 per 100,000 people. (Baseline: 5.9 per 100,000 people in 1988.)

Nonfatal spinal cord injuries (per 100,000)	*1986 Baseline*	*2000 Target*
Males	8.9	7.1

Reduce the incidence of secondary disabilities associated with injuries of the head and spinal cord to no more than 16 and 2.6 per 100,000 people, respectively. (Baseline: 20 per 100,000 for serious head injuries and 3.2 per 100,000 for spinal cord injuries in 1986.)

Risk reduction objectives

Increase use of occupant protection systems, such as safety belts, inflatable safety restraints, and child safety seats, to at least 85% of motor vehicle occupants. (Baseline: 42 percent in 1988.)

Use of occupant protection systems	*1988 Baseline*	*2000 Target*
Children aged 4 and younger	84%	95%

Increase use of helmets to at least 80% of motorcyclists and at least 50% of bicyclists. (Baseline: 60% of motorcyclists in 1988 and an estimated 8% of bicyclists in 1984.)

Services and protection objectives

Extend to 50 states laws requiring safety-belt and motorcycle helmet use for all ages. (Baseline: 33 states and District of Columbia in 1989 for automobiles; 22 states, District of Columbia, and Puerto Rico for motorcycles.)

Enact in 50 states laws requiring that new handguns be designed to minimize the likelihood of discharge by children. (Baseline: 0 states in 1989.)

Extend to 2000 local jurisdictions the number whose codes address the installation of fire-suppression sprinkler systems in those residences at highest risk for fires. (Baseline data not yet available.)

Increase the presence of functional smoke detectors to at least one on each habitable floor of all inhabited residential dwellings. (Baseline: 81% of residential dwellings in 1989.)

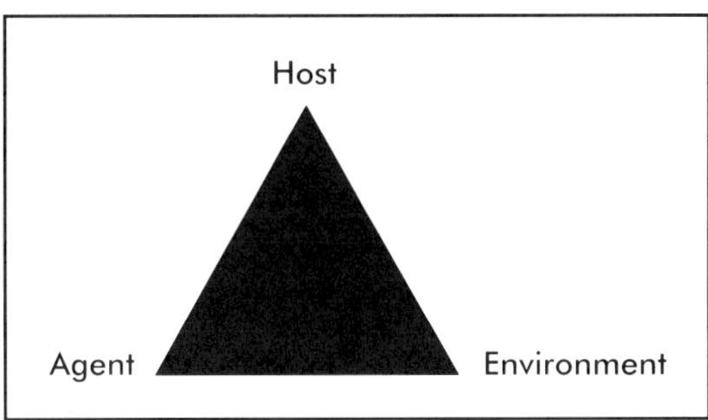

Figure 1–1 Epidemiologic triangle. Interactions between host, agent, and environment are represented by the sides of the triangle.

lection of mortality data and morbidity data on *incidence*—the number of cases of a problem that occur for the first time in a population over a given period of time; on *prevalence*—the total number of cases, old and new, that exists in a population at a given point in time; and about the *distribution* of health problems, such as injuries, over time and location. Although an epidemiologic approach is traditional to public health, its application to noninfectious problems such as injuries is relatively recent and still not routine.

Mortality data show that injuries are the leading cause of death in people from age 1 to 44, accounting for more than half of all deaths occurring between ages 1 and 32. Homicide, not even in the top 10 in the middle of this century, is now the fourth leading cause of death in *children* in the United States. It is the second leading cause of death in young adolescents, except for black male teenagers, in whom it is the leading cause of death.

Both black and white male youth die from homicide more often than from all natural causes of death—the diseases on which we spend so much time and money—combined.

Adolescent white males have replaced the elderly as the group with the highest suicide rate. Suicide is now the second leading cause of death for older adolescents, just nosing out homicide.

The annual incidence of injury in the United States is approximately 310 per 1000. Injury prevalence is reflected in the rate of 3570 days of restricted activity per 1000 people. Another public health measure of injury is *years of potential life lost* (YPLL), a measure of premature death. It is the difference between the age at death and a given age of expected longevity, or loss of economic productivity, usually 65 or 70 years. At 3.5 million YPLL (relative to age 65), injuries are the leading cause of YPLL, an indication of their greater impact on young people.

Another way to "measure" injury is in terms of utilization: physician's office visits, emergency room visits, hospitalizations, and hospital days.

Injuries account for 8% of physician visits (the fourth leading cause), for 25% of emergency room visits, and for 9% of hospital discharges, with an average stay of 6.8 days.

Public health responsibility also includes monitoring and analysis of the resources used and required for a particular problem, and, perhaps, where indicated, efforts to measure and influence the distribution of resources so that it more closely follows the pattern of need than that produced by the free market. An estimated $90 billion a year in resources are currently used to deal with injuries in the United States.

The *epidemiologic triangle* consists of host, agent, environment, and the interactions among them, which are represented by the sides of the triangle (Fig. 1-1).

The triangle is part of the concept of an "epidemiological web," which sees a disease or outcome as the result of a combination of events. The outcome can be blocked by intersecting the triangle at any of the three of its sides. This concept lends itself particularly well to the epidemiology of injury. The *host* is the individual who is at risk for being injured. Host factors include age, sex, race, existing medical conditions, and so on. The *environment* includes the location at which an injury occurs, the *physical environment,* and such things as the culture, laws, and education that constitute the *social environment.* The *agent* is that which immediately causes the injury, a form of energy and the vector or vehicle of injury.

The public health challenges to childhood injury include *primary prevention,* ways to change communities so that fewer children are hurt in the first place (such as building fences around swimming pools); *secondary prevention,* ways in which a community can assure that any injury that does occur is as minimal as possible (such as the use of helmets and installation of guard rails); and *tertiary prevention,* mechanisms for reducing the disability that results from injury (for example, making sure resources such as those that are part of a pediatric

	Agent/vector	Host	Environment	
			Physical	Social
Primary prevention/pre-event strategy	Child-proof bottle caps	Swimming lessons	Swimming pool fence	Child abuse prevention programs
Secondary prevention/event strategy	Soft-surface playgrounds	Bicycle and motorcycle helmets	Breakaway roadside poles	Gun control laws that decrease the availability of handguns at time of disputes
Tertiary prevention/post-event strategy	Mechanism for opening refrigerator doors from the inside	Teaching child about 911 service	Pediatric emergency medical service program	Universal insurance coverage for medical and rehabilitative services

Figure 1–2 The Haddon Matrix.

emergency medical system, are available, distributed, and accessible so that any child who is hurt is treated quickly and well).

The Haddon Matrix (Fig. 1-2) combines the various kinds of prevention with the framework provided by the epidemiologic triangle to suggest various public health intervention strategies.

Community-based interventions, such as placement of a stop sign, a crossing guard, a fence around a swimming area, and designing soft-surface playgrounds may do more to address childhood injuries than a host of services aimed at the individual child. Public agencies can provide consultation to schools, to day-care centers, and to institutions. Public health personnel can visit homes and schools to inspect and advise regarding safety and injury prevention. Funding of these public health interventions and services is variable from state to state and community to community, and uncertain from year to year. Nevertheless, specific noteworthy approaches and programs related to childhood injury have emerged.

EXAMPLES OF PUBLIC HEALTH PROGRAMS

A historical analogy is often drawn between injury today and infectious disease in the nineteenth century. In the last century, the major cause of death among children and youth was contagious disease. Today it is injury. Before the causes of disease were understood, illness was viewed either fatalistically or moralistically, as the result of individual moral failings. Accidents and violence are generally viewed the same way today. Progress in preventing disease began with recognition that pre-

vention required multifaceted strategies at primary, secondary, and tertiary levels. Progress in preventing injury occurs today to the extent that these same methods are employed. Public health agencies, which focus on identifying risk through epidemiology and on designing interventions based on these findings, have the tools, the mandate, and the responsibility to prevent injury.

Activities of both the government and the private sector in the last few years have led to certain improvements in child safety and in the ability of states and localities to respond to injury as a public health problem. Several federal agencies are working to develop knowledge and implement interventions to reduce the toll of injury on the child and adolescent population. For example, the National Highway Traffic Safety Administration (NHTSA) conducts research and provides funds for demonstration projects focused on a variety of traffic-related issues. Infant car seat loan programs and pedestrian and bicycle safety campaigns are examples of NHTSA activities. Youth Safety Officers were established by NHTSA in every state in 1991 to better assist states to decrease child and adolescent traffic-related injuries.

The Centers for Disease Control (CDC) has in recent years developed a major program of injury prevention through its center for Environmental Health and Injury Control. Funded projects have encompassed surveillance, state system development, and research. Several of the currently funded CDC grants address child and adolescent populations and issues, including the Harborview Injury Prevention Research Center in Seattle. Examples of funded CDC injury research addressing children's issues include studies of suicide risk assessment in adolescents and of injury hazards in family day-care homes. Other federal agencies that address injury include the National Institute of Child Health and Human Development, which supports research on unintentional injuries; the Alcohol, Drug Abuse and Mental Health Administration, which funds research on violence, traumatic stress, suicide, and the relationship of alcohol to injury; the Consumer Product Safety Commission, which evaluates the safety of products sold to the public, including children's furniture and toys; the Department of Agriculture, which emphasizes safety issues for youth through its extensive network of 4-H clubs; and the Indian Health Service, which conducts training on injury prevention for Native American populations and operates a fellowship program with a focus on injury prevention.

The activities of the Maternal and Child Health Bureau (MCHB) have been designed to demonstrate and test specific interventions to prevent child and adolescent injury, to assist in the development of state health infrastructures to address local problems of child and adolescent injury, and to disseminate effectively the information and knowledge gained to a broad audience of federal, state, and local policymakers, service providers, and private citizens. Since 1979 the MCHB has given demonstration grants to states, universities, and local agencies to assist them in the development of targeted activities related to injury prevention, and 27 grants to increase the pediatric capabilities of state Emergency Medical Services systems. In addition to the service demonstration grants, the MCHB has also awarded Implementation Incentive grants for the purpose of establishing state-based infrastructures to work on child injury prevention. Such grants are sometimes referred to as "capacity building" because they are designed to provide assistance to states to plan, to gather epidemiologic data, to develop an ongoing state structure, and to build constituencies for injury prevention activities. The most recent MCHB grants were funded in 1990 as "state-local partnerships," two of which focused on violence prevention. In addition to federal agencies, there are many private organizations and groups that work to prevent childhood injury. One is the American Academy of Pediatrics (AAP), which has been a major force in promoting childhood injury prevention for several years. The AAP has authorized a policy statement, developed educational materials for pediatricians and parents, and lobbied Congress for additional funding for injury prevention activities. Another important group is SAFE KIDS, an advocacy organization that works to help local communities to implement strategies to prevent injuries. SAFE KIDS produces a newsletter for injury prevention activists, tracks legislation, functions as a lobby for children's safety, develops educational materials that address a variety of audiences, and sponsors conferences and a national awareness week. It is noteworthy that today there are many federal agencies and private groups working on various aspects of the problem of child and adolescent injury.

Findings that have emerged from these programs include the following:

1. Injury prevention programs should not be developed separately from other public health activities. In fact, a "systems approach" is the most effective manner of organizing an injury prevention program in a state public health department. This involves assessment of local needs by collecting and analyzing epidemiological data, developing interagency ties with other governmental entities, formulating focused objectives with clearly specified target audiences, and identifying an intervention that is based on a comprehensive understanding of possible countermeasures at preevent, event, and postevent phases.

2. Local epidemiological injury data is much more powerful in garnering support for community injury prevention programs than national data and should form the basis for developing programmatic goals and objectives.

3. Coalition building in which a broad base of support is generated for a particular injury prevention strategy is critical to the long-term success of any program.

4. Ultimately, outcome data is the strongest indicator of the success or failure of an intervention program and should be collected whenever feasible. The relatively low incidence of certain events on a local level, however, frequently means that a more useful evaluation will be one that assesses "proxy" measures of program success; for example, the percent increase in seat belt use, as opposed to the percent decrease in car-related injuries.

5. Injury prevention is more likely to be effective when it is integrated within other programs (such as Head Start) and fully "institutionalized," that is, accorded full status for funding and for staffing within an agency.

A major conclusion drawn from these findings is that injury prevention activists need to be politically astute, to continually sharpen their skills at constituency building, while retaining a scientific capacity to translate epidemiology and program evaluation into terms that can generate action for children's health. Over the past decade, interest has been generated among state maternal and child health agencies in addressing injury prevention. Some state health departments have established an infrastructure. A study of state health departments published in 1988 found that 29 states used the Maternal and Child Health block grant funds more frequently than any other source of funds to support injury prevention activities (Harrington, Gallaher, Burgess, and Guyer, 1988).

While a few states have developed relatively impressive programs in unintentional injury, violence prevention is a particularly complex problem, and few state agencies have yet to come to fully address it. The 1988 health department study found 11 state health departments with suicide prevention programs and only 2 with homicide prevention, although 23 states did have child abuse prevention programs.

CONCLUSION

A variety of organizations, both public and private, are dedicated to preventing child and adolescent injury and reducing the impact of trauma when it occurs. The magnitude of the problem is such, however, that these resources are scarcely commensurate with the need. Injury continues to be the major preventable child and adolescent health problem that is inadequately addressed by services, research, and training. It is of critical importance to move forward in preventing many of the unnecessary deaths and serious disabilities caused by injury each year. To do so successfully will require a multidisciplinary and multiagency approach. Public health agencies must collaborate with environmental, law enforcement, traffic safety, educational, social service, and other agencies, as well as with coalitions of private groups. A problem of this magnitude demands the talents of many dedicated individuals representing diverse fields, all working together for a common goal.

REFERENCES

1. Healthy children 2000, national health promotion and disease prevention objectives related to mothers, infants, children, adolescents, and youth. Adapted from *Healthy people 2000; national promotion and disease prevention objectives*, US Department of Health and Human Services, Public Health Service, Health Resources and Services Administration, Maternal and Child Health Bureau, DHHS Publ No HRSA-MCH 91-2, Washington, DC, 1991. (Note that the numbers of the objectives relate to the numbers in *Healthy people 2000*.)
2. US Statutes, 62nd Congress, 2nd Session (1911-1912) Pt 1, Ch 73, pp 79-80.

2 Control of Childhood Injury

Science of prevention

Frederick P. Rivara

The problem of childhood injuries has always been with us. With advances in public health and medical care, however, death and disability caused by other diseases have declined whereas those resulting from injury have scarcely decreased. As a result, trauma is the leading cause of death and disability of children and adolescents. This chapter discusses a scientific approach to prevention and demonstrates some successful methods of combating the problem.

UNDERSTANDING THE PROBLEM

Perhaps the best way to approach the problem of injury prevention is to use the model developed by Haddon[1] for understanding injury causation (Fig. 1). His framework is based on a number of tenets. First, the circumstances or event surrounding the injury should be distinguished from the injury itself. A fall from a bike is an event separate from the injury that may or may not result. Second, factors that increase the risk of injury can influence either the likelihood that the event occurs or, once the event occurs, the risk of injury. Finally, to these dimensions should be added the response to injury, both immediate and long term. The likelihood of death or disability from injury is affected by the accessibility and quality of the emergency medical service (EMS), trauma care, and appropriate rehabilitation services.

Within each phase are aspects of the host, agent, and environment: the classic epidemiologic triad. Consideration of this second dimension creates a matrix of categories for the systematic study of injuries. Each component in the matrix can be examined for its role in controlling injury occurrence and reducing injury loss.

GUIDELINES FOR CHOOSING A PROBLEM

Given the myriad of injury problems among children and the many interventions that might be possible, how does one choose which injury problem to address with a prevention program? Three criteria are important: the problem must be frequent, it must be severe, and an effective intervention must be available or worth trying as an experiment.

The problem must be frequent. Problems that have an extensive impact on public health and are therefore appropriate targets for intervention must occur frequently. Many problems do not meet this

	Host	Vector	Physical environment	Social environment
Pre-event	Alcohol abuse	Antilock brakes	Road surfacing	DWI laws
	Age	Speed of travel	Highway design	
	Cognitive impairment	Ease of control	Lighting	
Event	Seat belt use	Air bags	Guard rails	Legislation/regulation
	Osteoporosis	Side impact protec-	Breakaway poles	on car design
	Age	tion		Seat Belt Laws
Post-event	Trauma services	Fuel system integrity	EMS systems	Job retraining
	Rehab care			Provision of trauma
				care
				EMS regionalization

Figure 2–1 Haddon matrix: the model developed by Haddon for understanding injury causation.

criterion and, thus, should have lower priority than those that are more common. Injury to school bus occupants is one example that comes readily to mind. In 1987 the National Highway Traffic Safety Administration reported only four fatal injuries to child occupants of school buses. In contrast, 10 times that number were killed when they were struck by cars while getting on or off a bus.

The problem must be severe. Many injuries are frequent but not severe; thus, they are probably not appropriate targets for intervention programs. At one end of the spectrum are injuries that result in death; the other end is represented by those injuries that do not require medical attention. Given the current scarcity of resources available for prevention, the greatest amount of attention should be directed to those injuries that result in death, hospitalization, or serious disability. Burns and head trauma come readily to mind as injuries that are both frequent and likely to lead to prolonged medical care and permanent sequelae. In contrast, injuries caused by toys, although frequent, are rarely severe or fatal.

Effective prevention strategies should be available. Many injury problems meet the criteria outlined above, as shown in Table 2-1, but currently there is a lack of effective programs for their prevention. Only those prevention programs that have been shown to be effective should be implemented. All too often, prevention programs are developed and implemented at great expense before any evaluation; when finally evaluated, many are shown to be ineffective or, worse, harmful. Driver's education is one program that has been widely incorporated in high schools throughout the country. Although its aim is to teach safe driving skills to adolescents, evaluations indicate that students are no better drivers after taking the course than those who have never taken it.[7] In fact, the net impact of driver's education is to increase the crash and fatality rate in young drivers because it allows adolescents to be licensed at younger ages without making them safer drivers.

Clearly, new prevention programs should be tried. Initial attempts at new interventions, however, should be made only in conjunction with rigorous evaluations of their effectiveness. Only in this way will scarce resources be best utilized and the field of injury control move forward.

EDUCATION AND PERSUASION

Efforts to persuade individuals, particularly parents, to change their behaviors have constituted the greater part of injury control efforts in this country. Unfortunately, many of these efforts have had little effect on either changing behavior or reducing injuries. For too long health professionals have been telling parents to "be careful," "supervise their children," and "child-proof" their homes. Educational efforts are much more likely to be successful if they are focused on specific problems and offer specific solutions rather than general advice. In addition, programs that persuade individuals to adopt passive prevention measures, that is, protection that works automatically, are more likely to prevent injuries than those that require repeated behavior change on the part of the parent or child. This guideline must be tempered by the recognition that for some types of injury problems, effective passive interventions are not available or feasible, and thus some interventions must rely heavily on attempts to change the behavior of individuals.

Some examples illustrate these points well. A common problem among children and adolescents is bicycling injuries, which account for more than 400,000 emergency room (ER) visits and 500 to 600 deaths each year in the United States. Most bicycle-related hospital admissions and deaths are from injuries to the skull and brain, and almost one fourth of all significant brain injuries in children 14 years of age or younger are bicycle-related. A case-control study in Seattle, Washington, of injuries among bicycle riders experiencing a crash showed that safety helmets reduce the risk of head injury by 85% and brain injury by 88%.[8]

Spearheaded by the Harborview Injury Prevention and Research Center, a coalition was organized to persuade parents to purchase bicycle helmets and children to wear them. The coalition consisted of various community agencies in the Seattle area, including state and local health departments, a large Health Maintenance Organization (HMO), the bicycling community, and private businesses. The coalition used three strategies to promote helmet use: increase parent awareness through use of the media, lower the price of helmets through a discount coupon, and provide incentives for children to wear helmets.

The campaign was accompanied by a rigorous evaluation of its effectiveness. Observations of helmet use were conducted in Seattle and in Portland, Oregon, as a control community.[1] Helmet use in Seattle increased from 5% to 16% over a 2-year

Table 2–1 Injury problems that are frequent and severe

Pedestrian injuries	Suicides
Drowning	Assaults
Bicycle-related injuries	Asphyxiation/choking
Falls from heights	in infants
Scald burns	Smoke inhalation
Flame burns	

period, whereas in Portland use remained steady, at 1% to 3%. Use has continued to increase in Seattle; by September 1991, 38% of Seattle school-aged children wore bicycle helmets.

Another outstanding success in persuading parents to change their behavior has been the field of child-occupant protection. Within a 10-year period, safety seat use by infants has climbed from less than 15% to more than 80%, and mandatory use laws have been passed in all 50 states. A number of lessons can be learned from this effort. The specific problem of child-occupant injuries was addressed with a specific solution: child safety seats. Community intervention programs with broad grass roots support were effective in educating parents about the importance of using safety seats. This broad support, combined with local physician support, persistence, and skillful use of facts resulted in the cascade of legislation mandating use of restraints. Loaner and donor programs to provide car safety seats to low-income families were developed to help overcome the barriers to their use in lower-income families. The effort demonstrated that primary care physicians can play a major role in the success of educational, legislative, and community efforts to persuade parents to use safety seats.

One area in which education has played, and will continue to play, a central role is that of child-pedestrian injuries. For 5- to 9-year-old children, pedestrian injuries are the single most common cause of traumatic death. Many environmental changes are either economically unfeasible or unlikely to result in a reduction of injuries to children.[6] Few injuries occur to children at night; most happen during the day, their frequency peaking in the after-school period. Improved lighting or retroreflective clothing cannot, therefore, be expected to prevent injuries. Most injuries occur on major roads, indicating that speed bumps on residential streets are not the answer. Surprisingly, 30% of pedestrian injuries occur while the individual is in a marked crosswalk. It appears that children in particular feel a false sense of security when in a crosswalk, whereas few drivers routinely stop and look for children when approaching such crosswalks.

Education of young school-aged children appears to be a necessary part of any comprehensive program; however, the effectiveness of such programs in producing behavior change is not overwhelming.[6] Lead by a special teacher, a six-session training program in Seattle produced a twofold to threefold improvement in child-pedestrian behavior; yet even after the training approximately half of the children still displayed unsafe street-crossing behavior.

CHANGES IN PRODUCTS

The most successful injury prevention programs are those involving changes in product design. These interventions protect all individuals in the population, regardless of cooperation or level of skill. Many of the most notable of such interventions have been specifically beneficial to children.

One of the first successful injury prevention interventions involved flammable fabrics. Flame burns resulting from the ignition of clothing were common serious injuries to small children, especially in young girls. At least one third of these injuries were associated with infant sleepwear. The burns were usually extensive, involving, on average, more than 30% of the body surface with full thickness burns and requiring hospitalization for an average of 70 days. In 1967 the federal Flammable Fabrics Act was passed, requiring children's sleepwear to be flame retardant. As a result of this and similar state legislation, clothing ignition burns now account for only a small fraction of burns in children.

Another example of product modification resulting in substantial reduction in injury losses involves tap water scalds. Scald burns account for 40% of the burn injuries in children requiring hospitalization, at least 25% of which involve tap water. A study in Seattle showed that 80% of residences surveyed had hot tap water temperatures greater than 130° F.[2] The risk of full thickness burns increases exponentially at temperatures above 130° F; at 150° F, full thickness burns occur in less than 2 seconds. A simple and effective preventive maneuver is simply to turn down the water heater temperature to 125° F. At this setting, dishwashers and washing machines will still operate effectively, and the risk of serious scald injury is greatly reduced. Legislation in Washington State in 1983 required new water heaters to be preset at 120° F. Five years later, as a result of the law and a public education campaign, 77% of homes had tap water temperatures below 130° F, as compared with 80% of homes with tap water temperatures greater than 130° F in 1977. The number of tap water scald burn victims admitted to the hospital was decreased by more than half; there has also been a decrease in the total body surface area burned, the proportion of patients needing grafting, and the average length of hospital stay.

Potentially, one of the greatest impacts on burn prevention will be the passage of legislation requiring a fire-safe cigarette. Of the more than 6000 fire deaths each year in the United States, 25% to 50% are secondary to cigarettes. Cigarettes are by far the single leading cause of residential fire deaths. In most cases, cigarettes ignite upholstered furniture or mattresses, and three fourths of the deaths occur between 6:00 P.M. and 6:00 A.M. Cigarettes that self-extinguish in less than 10 minutes are far less likely to cause ignition of these substances than are presently designed cigarettes, which burn continuously even without being puffed. Fire-safe, self-extinguishing cigarettes are feasible; more than 100 patents have been issued in the United States and other countries for such cigarettes. At this writing, mandatory manufacture of self-extinguishing cigarettes appears to be at hand.

In yet another arena, product modification has resulted in a marked reduction in the poisoning deaths of children, particularly those under 5 years of age. There were 226 deaths from poisoning in this age group in 1970, but only 55 in 1985. Poisoning prevention is one of the success stories of pediatrics, representing the effectiveness of passive strategies: child-resistant packaging and dose limits per container. The Poison Prevention Packaging Act presently includes 16 categories of household products, including nearly all prescription drugs. This law has been remarkably effective in reducing poisoning deaths and hospitalizations.[9] However, compliance with the law by pharmacists is only 70% to 75% at present. An additional and significant cause of poisoning in young children today is the difficulty of some older adults in using child-resistant containers. A survey by the Centers for Disease Control found that in 18.5% of households in which poisoning had occurred to children less than 5 years of age the child-resistant closure had been replaced with a non-child-resistant cap, and that 65% of those used did not work properly. Nearly one fifth of harmful ingestions are of drugs owned by grandparents, a group that has difficulty using traditional child-resistant closures. There is a need for better child-resistant closures that do not require manual dexterity or strength beyond the capabilities of older adults.

Other poisoning interventions, such as "Mr. Yuk" stickers, are far less effective. These stickers do not deter young children from ingesting labeled medications and may, in fact, be attractive to children less than 3 years old.[3]

CHANGES IN THE ENVIRONMENT: PHYSICAL AND SOCIAL

For many years, much injury research has focused on attempts to pinpoint the accident prone child. Most serious scientists involved with injury research have now discounted the theory of accident proneness. The concept is, in fact, counterproductive in that it shifts attention away from potentially more modifiable factors such as a product or the environment.

Although some children do have an increased risk of injury, this increased risk is not from innate characteristics of the child but the child's environment—physical, cultural, and social. Changes in the environment to eliminate these hazards can be quite effective in decreasing the risk of injury or lessening its severity.

The majority of residential fire deaths in the United States are not caused by flame burns but by smoke inhalation. The highest death rates, which are in poor urban areas, correlate inversely with the prevalence of smoke detectors in homes. A smoke detector is clearly one of the most cost-effective devices for preventing death and injury in a residential fire. A number of programs have been successful in increasing the number of homes that use smoke detectors. Miller and colleagues demonstrated that a 1-minute educational message by pediatricians in their offices, combined with making detectors readily available, can cut the number of homes without smoke detectors in half.[5] Giveaway programs targeted at low-income families in Baltimore and Philadelphia were successful in increasing smoke detector use in these high-risk homes to 85% to 90%. Countywide legislation that required retrofitting all homes with smoke detectors significantly decreased the number of homes without detectors and was associated with a decrease in residential fire deaths.

Drowning is the third leading cause of injury death for children between birth and 4 years of age, and is second only to motor vehicle crashes as a cause of death in older children. Drowning is unique among injury problems in its extremely high rate of mortality. Of children requiring hospital care for immersion incidents, nearly 50% die. Children under the age of 5 account for more than one third of all childhood drowning deaths. Medical care, including all interventions available in the intensive care unit, appears to have little impact on the outcome of drowning victims.

An important subset in children's drownings are those occurring in pools. In the birth-to-4-year age group, 60% to 90% of drownings occur in residential swimming pools.[10] A recent CPSC study found that 69% of children in this age group who drowned were supervised by parents. Typically, there was a lapse of supervision lasting only a few minutes, during which the child was immersed and drowned.

Environmental modification in the form of pool fencing can be very effective in eliminating these deaths. In Australia, comparison of areas that require pool fencing with those that do not reveals a 3.6-fold higher rate of drowing deaths in the areas without mandatory fencing. A number of estimates predict that the widespread use of pool fencing would prevent 50% to 90% of childhood swimming pool drownings and near-drownings. The fencing must completely enclose the pool, rather than using the house as the fourth side of the fence, should have self-latching gates, and be at least 5 feet high. Unfortunately, few jurisdictions in the United States require appropriate pool fencing; in a recent survey nearly one half of pool owners did not support such a requirement.

Falls from heights are a major cause of traumatic death and serious disability, particularly brain injury, in urban children. In Chicago, they account for 6% of all trauma deaths, and 12% of deaths in children up to 4 years of age. In a study in New York City, falls were found to be responsible for 20% of all unintentional traumatic deaths. One of the first efforts at environmental modification for injury prevention was directed at falls. In 1967 the New York City Health Department conducted a simple epidemiologic study of children's falls from heights. It demonstrated a clear relationship between falls from windows and warm weather; the intervention was simple and effective: install window guards (bars) for the windows of apartments housing young children. Under the "Children Can't Fly" program, the city designed and obtained several thousand inexpensive window guards and assigned Model Cities workers to install them. The city also revised the New York City Health Code in 1977 to require guards on all windows of apartments in which a child under the age of 11 resided. Deaths caused by falls decreased markedly following institution of the program.

The environment of the child includes not only the physical world, but the legal and social spheres in which the child lives as well. Legislation has proven to be an effective method of injury control. An example is seat belt legislation. As of June 1990, 36 states and the District of Columbia had enacted seat belt–use laws. Safety belt laws in most states cover front seat occupants only, although the laws in five states cover both front and rear seat occupants. As mentioned earlier, all 50 states have laws requiring children, generally under the age of 4, to be restrained in an appropriate seat restraint device when riding in the parent's vehicle.

These laws have been effective, although their effect on use is much greater when combined with an active enforcement and publicity program. Prior to legislation, belts are generally used by approximately 8% to 20% of drivers. Usage increases to as much as 80% immediately following passage of the laws and then drops down to the range of approximately 50%. Even among teenage drivers belt use increases substantially. Special enforcement and publicity campaigns can keep belt use at 60% to 70%.

This type of legislation can be improved. Only eight states allow police to issue tickets for belt law violations alone, so-called primary laws. In other states, drivers can be cited only if they are stopped for another offense. Primary laws have proven to be more effective in increasing belt use than secondary laws. Increasing coverage to include rear seat passengers could result in a further decrease in motor vehicle deaths and injuries, as could extending coverage to other vehicles such as light trucks and vans.

CONCLUSION

The most important step in preventing injuries is overcoming a sense of fatalism, that injuries are "accidents," "acts of God," or random events that cannot be predicted. Injuries must be viewed as diseases that can be prevented by using the principles of epidemiology, engineering, biomechanics, and health education. Only in this way can the epidemic of pediatric trauma in this country be successfully addressed.

REFERENCES

1. Diguiseppi CG, Rivara FP, Koepsell TD et al: Bicycle helmet use by children: evaluation of a community-wide helmet campaign, *JAMA* 262:2256-2261, 1989.
2. Feldman KW, Schaller RT, Feldman JA et al: Tap water scald burns in children, *Pediatrics* 62:1-7, 1978.
3. Fergusson DM, Horwood LJ, Beautris AL et al: A controlled field trial of a poisoning prevention method. *Pediatrics* 69:515-520, 1982.
4. Haddon W: A logical framework for categorizing highway safety phenomena and activity. *J Trauma* 12:193-207, 1972.
5. Miller RE, Reisinger KS, Blatter MM et al: Pediatric counseling and subsequent use of smoke detectors, *Am J Public Health* 72:392-393, 1982.
6. Rivara FP: Child pedestrian injuries in the United States: current status of the problem, potential interventions, and future research needs, *Am J Dis Child* 144:692-696, 1990.
7. Robertson LS, Zador PL: Driver education and fatal crash involvement of teenaged drivers, *Am J Public Health* 68:959-965, 1978.
8. Thompson RS, Rivara FP, Thompson DC: A case-control study of the effectiveness of bicycle safety helmets, *New Engl J Med* 320:1361-1367, 1989.
9. Walton W: An evaluation of the Poison Packaging Prevention Act, *Pediatrics* 69:363-370, 1982.
10. Wintemute GJ: Childhood drowning and near-drowning in the United States, *Am J Dis Child* 144:6663-6669, 1990.

3 Epidemiology of Childhood Injury

Catherine S. Gotschall

Injuries are not random events, the tragic confluence of fate and misfortune. Rather, they are the often predictable results of the intersection of potentially dangerous environments and human behavior. Thus, distinct patterns of childhood injury can be identified, based on the season, the time of day, the geographic locale, and the age and sex of the child involved.

The application of the epidemiologic model of host, agent, and environment to the study of injury has advanced our understanding of the distribution of injury among populations and has become the backbone of successful injury control and prevention strategies. Accurate and available data are the basis of sound epidemiology. This chapter discusses the conceptual framework of injury epidemiology, the patterns of injury in children, and the use of trauma registry and other data for the study of the epidemiology of pediatric trauma.

MAGNITUDE OF THE PROBLEM

Injury is the most important threat to the health of American children and the leading cause of death in children after the first year of life.[2] In fact, injuries cause more deaths from ages 1 to 19 than all other causes combined. In 1988 more than 22,400 children in the United States aged 19 and younger died as the result of injuries.[6] Nearly 75% of all childhood injury deaths are due to unintentional injuries, and the rest are due to violence.[6]

Mortality, however, is only a small part of the picture; acute morbidity and disability resulting from injury are additional burdens on the health of the nation's children. Each year nearly 16 million children under the age of 20 visit emergency departments in the United States, approximately 600,000 are hospitalized, and 30,000 suffer permanent disability.[10] Each year nearly one child in four receives medical treatment for an injury.

The financial burden of childhood injury is staggering. The estimated lifetime costs for children injured in 1985 amount to more than $13 billion. Direct medical costs for treating injuries to children under 15 years of age were nearly $6 million in 1985; indirect costs for these injuries exceeded $14 million.[26] Hospital charges for injury admissions vary greatly according to the type of injury. Burns and child abuse result in the highest mean charge for hospital admission; falls and poisoning are associated with considerably lower costs.[25]

Traffic-related injuries are the greatest killers of children and adolescents in the United States today, accounting for 47% of injury deaths.[10] Injuries to pedestrians and occupants of motor vehicles represent approximatley a third of all cases treated at pediatric trauma centers.[9] These injuries are the major cause of paraplegia, quadriplegia, severe brain injury, and severe facial laceration.[19]

In 1986 there were more than 640,000 nonfatal injuries and 7400 deaths in motor vehicle occupants below the age of 19.[10] Injuries to young occupants of motor vehicles take their greatest toll among adolescents. Approximately 28 children and youth are killed daily on American streets, nearly 75% of whom are aged 10 or older.[6] Nearly two thirds of teenage occupant deaths occur when another teenager is driving.[12]

More than 1700 children and adolescents died as a result of pedestrian injuries in 1988.[6] Pedestrian injuries are of greatest risk to elementary school–aged children, in whom these injuries are the leading cause of death. Toddlers and preschoolers are at greatest risk of fatal injury while playing in driveways and parking lots,[3] whereas older children are more often injured in midblock "dart outs" and "intersection dashes."[27]

Violent injury is increasing in America. Homicide, the second leading cause of death by injury among children and adolescents, resulted in 3290 deaths in 1988. Children in the United States are 15 times more likely than English children to be victims of homicide.[6] Two distinct patterns of childhood homicide have emerged: deaths in children under the age of 5 are most frequently the result of parental abuse and neglect, whereas adolescent deaths result from firearms injuries following disputes among peers.[8]

Submersion injuries kill nearly 2000 children each year,[11] and in 18 states are the leading cause of injury death for children aged 1 to 4 years. In addition to these deaths, near drownings account for considerable disability and resource utilization. It has been estimated that for every drowning death there are approximately 2 to 10 children hospitalized and between 8 and 40 treated in hospital emergency departments.[30] Severe, permanent brain damage results in 5% to 20% of children hospitalized for near drownings.[24]

Each year nearly 1200 children under the age of 15 die in house fires, 65% of whom are 4 years old or younger.[5] Although house fires are the cause of most burn-related deaths, scald burns cause the greatest morbidity. According to data from the National Health Interview Survey, approximately 440,000 children either received medical treatment for burns or had at least 1 day of restricted activity because of burns in 1985. In 1989 there were approximately 21,000 hospital admissions for burn injuries to children under 20 years old.

Although the injuries just discussed result in the greatest childhood mortality, injury morbidity is an important consideration in regard to many injuries with low mortality rates. According to a Massachusetts study, children between the ages of 13 and 19 years visit hospital emergency departments for athletic trauma more than for any other type of injury.[21] In a related study, the authors found that each year 1 child in 14 visits a hospital emergency department for an injury resulting from participation in sports and recreational activities.[16] An estimated 100,000 children are treated in emergency departments annually for playground-related falls.[32] Although falls are associated with low mortality rates, they account for the highest proportion of costs in the treatment of injured children under the age of 15.[22]

CONCEPTUAL FRAMEWORK

The classic epidemiological model "agent-host-environment" was first applied to the study of injury by Gordon in 1949.[13] It was Haddon who pioneered the application of this model to the development of interventions to prevent and control injuries.[17,18] The Haddon Matrix has become the standard tool for the development of comprehensive strategies for injury control (see Chapter 2). It unites the agent-host-environment triad with the preevent, event, and postevent phases of an occurrence of injury.

HOST RISK FACTORS FOR CHILDHOOD INJURY

The individual and combined factors of a child's age, sex, and behavior result in distinct patterns of injury. Understanding these host factors is important to the development of effective injury-control interventions.

Age

Age is the single most important factor affecting the patterns of childhood injury. The milestones of child development—crawling, walking, riding a bicycle—are mirrored by developmentally related risks of injury.

As early as the first year of life, differences can be seen in the patterns of childhood injury. For toddlers and preschoolers (ages 1 to 4 years), mortality rates are highest for children injured by fires and burns (667 per 100,000) and by drowning (620 per 100,000).[6]

It is during adolescence that injury takes the greatest toll. Nearly 80% of all adolescent deaths result from injury. Although adolescent mortality rates from natural causes have fallen dramatically in the last half century, death rates from injury have increased.

Sex

Sex differences in injury rates among children are apparent as early as the first year of life. Although injury rates for boys and girls are similar during the first 5 months of life, differences emerge at about the time a child learns to crawl[14] and are pronounced by the time the child celebrates a first birthday.[28] These differences become more pronounced with age; adolescent boys experience more than two times the injury rate of girls of the same age.

For children under the age of 20, the risk of mortality resulting from injury is higher for males than for females. These differences are most dramatic in suicide, for which males are at a 4 times greater risk than females, drowning (3 times greater risk), homicide (2.5 times greater risk), and motor vehicle–related deaths (2 times greater risk).[6] Sex differences in childhood injury rates have been attributed to differences in both exposure and behavior. Several studies of high school athletes, in which exposure time was controlled for, have shown no difference in injury rates for sports of comparable risk. Even correcting for differences in exposure, however, boys have been shown to have higher rates in playground injuries,[28] bicycle injuries,[7] and pedestrian injuries,[29] indicating an important behavioral component of injury risk.

AGENTS AND VECTORS OF INJURY

The causative agent of injury is the acute transfer of kinetic, thermal, radiation, or chemical energy, resulting in tissue failure or damage. The vectors of this energy, for example, automobiles, carry and transfer the energy to the human host. Some of the most effective means of injury control function at the level of the energy vectors (see Chapter 2).

ENVIRONMENTAL FACTORS

The single most important environmental factor affecting childhood injury rates is poverty. A study of childhood mortality in Maine found that economically disadvantaged children were 2.6 times more likely to die from trauma than other children.[23]

Children living in poverty are exposed to many injury risk factors: their homes often do not have working smoke detectors, those in public housing frequently lack control over hot water temperatures, and they are less likely to be properly restrained in automobiles. Other socioeconomic variables, such as teenage motherhood, the single-parent family, and poor maternal education, which have been associated with higher rates of childhood injury, are more common among children living in poverty. Modification of children's environments at home and in their neighborhoods offers many opportunities for intervention to prevent injury.

DATA NEEDS FOR PEDIATRIC INJURY CONTROL

To identify childhood injury problems of local or national importance, accurate and available sources of data on pediatric trauma are needed. This information is needed not only to identify problems and target populations, but to plan realistic goals and objectives for injury control strategies and to evaluate success in meeting such goals. Unfortunately, accurate data on childhood injury are often difficult to obtain.

SOURCES OF INJURY DATA

Accurate surveillance data are the underpinning of epidemiologic research. There is no single source for injury surveillance data. Mortality records are maintained at both the national and state levels and are aggregated annually. These records can be used to enumerate the number of deaths according to various mechanisms of injury. Studies have shown that death certificates, on which these data are based, however, may contain inaccurate information on the cause of death for pediatric trauma victims.[20]

Information on deaths resulting from motor vehicle crashes is included in the Fatal Accident Reporting System (FARS) operated by the National Highway Traffic Safety Administration of the U.S. Department of Transportation. Vital records and the FARS are important sources of injury data, but they have one important limitation: they provide no information on the more numerous and more costly nonfatal injuries.

A good source of injury morbidity data is the uniform hospital discharge data summary. These data include the ICD-9 N codes describing the nature of the injury (for example, pulmonary contusion) and may also contain the E codes documenting the external cause of injury, (for example, scald burn). E codes provide the more useful epidemiologic data, but are not mandated to be included in the discharge summaries of all states.

Trauma registries maintained by regional trauma centers are an important source of both morbidity and mortality information on childhood injury. These data bases typically contain much more detailed information on the circumstances surrounding the injury than hospital discharge summaries.[4,15] Perhaps the most important information they contain, in addition to etiologic data, is that on the outcome of specific injuries. A limitation of hospital-based trauma registries is their lack of population-based data; they do not provide any data on uninjured children or on those treated at other facilities.

Several states have undertaken the establishment of state trauma registries. These data bases contain information on a subset of trauma admissions, usually encompassing the most severe injuries. Participant hospitals submit data periodically to the state registries. The limitations of individual trauma registries are amplified by the aggregation of data from multiple hospitals, each with its individual problems of data control. As a result, statewide registries are of limited use for epidemiologic purposes.

An important gap in injury data is the lack of follow-up information on recovery and disability in victims of childhood injury. The ultimate mission of acute trauma care is to ensure that injured children and their families recover from their injuries as fully as possible. Little is known, however, about children's long-term disability following injury. Better data systems and research methodologies must be developed to measure the cognitive, psychological, and physical disabilities resulting from childhood injury.

The goal of pediatric trauma care is to minimize the burden of injury on the nation's children. The weapons to combat childhood injury must include not only the surgeon's scalpel, but epidemiologic research as well. A unified approach to the continuum of care is needed, combining the primary and secondary preventive efforts of injury prevention and control with the tertiary prevention offered by acute care and rehabilitative services. To provide optimal trauma care without addressing the problems of primary and secondary prevention is like collecting water from an overflowing dam with golden buckets.

REFERENCES

1. Baker S, Waller A: *Childhood injury state-by-state mortality facts,* Baltimore, Md, 1989, Johns Hopkins Injury Prevention Center.
2. Baker SP, O'Neill B, Ginsburg M, et al: *The injury fact book,* New York, 1991, Oxford University Press.
3. Brison R, Wickland K, Mueller B: Fatal pedestrian injuries to young children: A different pattern of injury, *Am J Public Health* 78:793-795, 1988.
4. Cales RH, Bietz S, Heilig RW: The trauma registry: a method for providing regional system audit using the microcomputer. *J Trauma* 25:181-187, 1985.
5. Centers for Disease Control: *1986 mortality data.* Atlanta, Ga, 1987, The Centers.
6. Children's Safety Network: *A data book of child and adolescent injury,* Washington, DC, 1991, National Center for Education in Maternal and Child Health.
7. Chlapeck TW, Schupack S, Planek TW et al: *Bicycle accidents and usage among elementary school children in the United States,* Chicago, 1975, National Safety Council.
8. Christoffel K: Violent death and injury in U.S. children and adolescents, *Am J Dis Child* 144:697-706, 1990.
9. DiScala C: *National Institute on Disability and Rehabilitation Research pediatric trauma registry: Phase 2.* Boston, Mass, March 1991, New England Medical Center.
10. Divison of Injury Control, Centers for Disease Control: Childhood injuries in the United States, *Am J Dis Child* 144:627-652, 1990.
11. Fingerhut L, Kleinman J: Trends and current status in childhood mortality, United States 1900-1985, *Vital Health Stat 3* (26):1-44, January 1989.
12. Fleming A, editor: Facts: 1990 edition, Arlington, Va, 1991, Insurance Institute for Highway Safety.
13. Gordon JE: The epidemiology of accidents, *Am J Public Health* 39:504-515, 1949.
14. Gotschall CS, Hamberger D, Newman KD et al: *Injuries during the first year of life.* Paper presented at the annual meeting of the American Trauma Society, Arlington, Va, 1991.
15. Graitcer P: The development of state and local injury surveillance systems, *J Safety Res* 18:191-198, 1987.
16. Guyer B, Gallagher SS: An approach to the epidemiology of childhood injuries, *Pediatr Clin N Am* 32:5-15, 1985.
17. Haddon, W: A note concerning accident theory and research with special reference to motor vehicle accidents, *Annal NY Acad Sci* 107:635-646, 1963.
18. Haddon W: The changing approach to the epidemiology, prevention, and amelioration of trauma: the transition to approaches etiologically rather than descriptively based, *Am J Public Health* 58:1431-1438, 1968.
19. Holden JA, Christoffel T: *A course on motor vehicle trauma: instructor's guide—final report [users manual],* Pub No (DOT HS)807 245, Washington, DC, 1986, US Department of Transportation.
20. Lapidus GD, Gregorio DI, Hansen H: Misclassification of childhood homicide on death certificates, *Am J Public Health* 80:213-214, 1990.
21. Listernick D, Finison K, Gallagher S et al: the problem of sports and recreational injuries, *SCIPP Reports, Massachusetts Department of Health* 4:1-8, 1983.
22. Malek M, Chang B, Gallagher S et al: the cost of medical care for injuries to children, *Ann Emerg Med* 20:997-1005, 1991.
23. Nersesian WS, Petit MR, Shaper R et al: Childhood death and poverty: a study of all childhood deaths in Maine, 1976 to 1980, *Pediatrics* 75:41-50, 1985.
24. Pearn J, Wong RYK, Brown J et al: Drowning and near drowning in children: a five-year total population study from the city and county of Honolulu, *Am J Public Health* 69:450-454, 1979.
25. Peclet M, Newman KD, Eichelberger MR et al: Patterns of injury in children, *J Pediatr Surg* 25:85-91, 1990.
26. Rice DP, MacKenzie EJ, et al: *Cost of injury in the United States: a report to Congress,* San Francisco, Institute for Health and Aging, University of California, and Baltimore, Injury Prevention Center, Johns Hopkins University.
27. Rivara FP, Barber M: Demographic analysis of childhood pedestrian injuries, *Pediatrics* 76:375-381, 1985.
28. Rivara FP, Bergman AB, LoGerfo J et al: Epidemiology of childhood injuries. II. Sex differences in injury rates, *Am J Dis Child* 136:502-506, 1982.
29. Routledge DA, Repetto-Wright R, Howarth CI: The exposure of young children to accident risk as pedestrians, *Ergonomics* 17:456-480, 1974.
30. Spyker DA: Submersion injury, *Pediatr Clin N Am* 32:113-125, 1985.
31. Starfield B. Morbidity in childhood—a longitudinal view, *N Engl J Med* 310:824-829, 1984.
32. United States Consumer Product Safety Commission (CPSC): *Playground surfacing: technical information guide,* Washington, DC, 1990, US Government Printing Office.

4   Mechanism of Injury: Biomechanics

John M. Templeton, Jr.

Acute injury occurs when there is a transfer of external energy that exceeds the ability of one or more body tissues to absorb that energy without loss of cellular or structural integrity.[19,22,31] Kinetic energy, and the dissipation of that energy, is the most common element in acute traumatic injuries. Chemical, thermal, electrical, and radiation energy primarily produce injury in the form of direct cellular damage and anatomic disruption. Secondary injury occurs as a result of impaired physiology and metabolism. Examples of secondary injury include deprivation of oxygen,[22] loss of body heat, impaired perfusion, and systemic toxicity from abnormal metabolites in the presence of infection and inflammation.

This chapter concentrates on kinetic energy and the related concepts of force and momentum as the principal agents in childhood trauma injury. The special susceptibility of children to trauma and specific mechanisms of trauma are also addressed.

NATURE OF PHYSICAL FORCES PRODUCING INJURY

Three formulae define the physical properties specific to trauma[19]:

$$\text{Kinetic energy} = \frac{\text{mass} \times \text{velocity}^2}{2}$$

$$\text{Force} = \text{mass} \times \text{acceleration (or deceleration)}$$

$$\text{Momentum} = \text{velocity} \times \text{mass}$$

In every case, the potential for injury is directly proportional to (1) mass (of the victim and/or the colliding object), (2) the speed or velocity of the victim and/or the colliding object,[19] (3) the rate of change in the velocity, (4) the focality or diffusion of the transfer of kinetic energy to body tissue.

To understand injury one must assess the response of body tissue to trauma. Wiegelt[31] has identified three inherent features of body tissue that enable it to resist the effects of kinetic energy. The ability to resist trauma varies from one tissue to another, depending on the presence or absence of these features: (1) tensile strength, the amount of tension a tissue can withstand and its ability to resist stretching forces; (2) elasticity, the ability of a tissue to resume its original shape and size after being stretched; and (3) compressive strength, the tissue's ability to resist squeezing forces or inward pressure. Injury occurs when the force applied against a tissue is sufficient to overcome one or more of these resistance features.

In children, the elasticity of tissue is often greater than that of adults. In contrast, the tensile strength and compressive strength may be less. Many traumatic injuries in children, therefore, are shearing injuries in which adjacent structures slip relative to each other. This is a major component of serious brain injury in children. Subdural hemorrhages are relatively rare, presumably because of improved elasticity. Axonal shearing injuries, however, are common and often devastating. In general, many organs, such as the diaphragm, visceral pleura, serosal surfaces of liver and spleen, pericardium, and skin are under a constant biaxial tension. Hence, they are more vulnerable to injury when sudden blunt force is applied than in the case of relaxed skeletal muscle.[22]

Elasticity has other limits. Whereas the relative elasticity of the chest wall of a child may result in less frequent bony injury, such as rib fractures, it can allow kinetic energy to be more readily transmitted to internal organs, particularly the lungs and the mediastinum. As a result, lung contusion is quite common in children with significant blunt chest injury. Transfer of kinetic energy to internal organs can produce injury in three ways: (1) by exceeding the longitudinal tensile strength of structures, such as mobile blood vessels; (2) by exceeding the vertical tensile strength of fixed structures, as in shearing of bowel and vessels at their points of fixation; and (3) by exceeding the compressive strength of structures such as bone and solid viscera.[31] The extent of specific injury typically encompasses a spectrum from a localized tear or a contusion to a complete tear or disruption. This spectrum, once again, is directly proportional to the mass effect producing compression and to the velocity of compression.

PATTERNS OF INJURY IN CHILDREN

Excluding burns, poisonings, and foreign bodies, trauma in children is either blunt trauma or penetrating trauma. Knowledge of specific mechanisms of trauma helps to determine the potential transfer of kinetic energy and the resultant injury. In a study at the Children's National Medical Center (CNMC), falls accounted for the largest number of injuries and yet produced the lowest injury severity score (ISS) and lowest mortality. In order of increasing ISS, the following mechanisms of trauma were shown to reflect increasing severity of injury (mean ISS/mortality rate): falls (6.5: 0.6%), motor vehicle accident, cyclist or pedestrian (9.0:2.8%), motor vehicle accident, occupant (12.2:4.4%), stab or gunshot (12.5:11.6%), and abuse (16.1:15.8%). In these categories, penetrating trauma and abuse accounted for only 6% of hospital admissions, but 30% of deaths.[26]

Blunt trauma continues to be the predominant cause of injuries in children. In Pennsylvania, where population is evenly distributed between metropolitan and rural, 90% of trauma admissions and 90% of trauma deaths in children are due to blunt trauma. The incidence of penetrating trauma in children correlates with the availability of weapons, particularly guns, in the home and in the environment of violence outside the home in certain inner-city areas of major cities in the United States.

Blunt trauma

Blunt trauma produces injury, first to the outer shell of the body and then to its contents. On the surface, these injuries are due to concussive forces that produce lacerations when the tensile strength of the integument is exceeded. Internally, the danger of blunt trauma is that injury to one or more internal organs may initially be obscure. Diagnosis and treatment of blunt trauma require a high level of suspicion and selective diagnostic evaluation. In blunt trauma the depth of deformation and the speed of deformation determine the extent of injury. Deformation and, therefore, injury, are much greater when a person hits or is hit by an unyielding object, as happens when falling out of a window and hitting concrete. By contrast, in contact sports the hitting object or person often yields to some extent, allowing for dissipation of kinetic energy and lowering the potential for injury.[31]

In regard to the speed of deformation, rapid deceleration can be just as harmful as rapid acceleration. Optimally, in blunt trauma, kinetic energy is dissipated slowly and diffused. The greatest danger arises when energy transfer is both rapid and focal. Figure 4-1 shows the pattern of tissue or organ injury when assessed for the percent

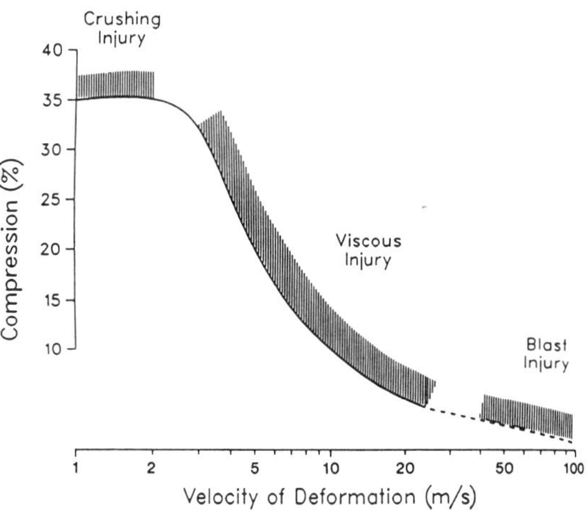

Figure 4–1 The range of validity for viscous injury (3 to 30 m/s) *(middle shaded area),* crushing injury *(left shaded area),* and blast injury *(right shaded area).* (From Miller MA: The biomechanical response of the lower abdomen to belt restraint loading, *J Trauma* 29:1582, 1989. Copyright by Williams & Wilkins, 1989.)

compression or depth of deformation versus the velocity of deformation in the presence of focal loading.[20] When the rate of compression is high in association with low velocity, trauma is primarily effected by crushing. Such injuries are due to tissue displacement and shearing forces exerted on the organs involved.

In contrast, when the percent of compression is low in association with high velocity, the resultant injuries are characterized as blast injuries. At intermediate levels of compression and velocity, a variety of viscous injuries can occur. For example, severe hepatic injury occurs at a forced compression of 16% when velocity exceeds 12 m per second. In trauma to the lung, no pulmonary lesions are seen when the impact velocity is below 5 m per second, even when chest deflections exceed 50%. A transition to severe pulmonary injury, however, occurs at a forced compression of only 16% when velocity is 10 m per second.[20] The Theory of Viscous Tolerance states that injury can occur at lower levels of compression as the rate of deformation increases; hence the power of a karate chop in which speed is such a factor. The mechanism begins to be a significant factor for deformation rates at about 3 m per second.

Figure 4-2 shows the relationship of the product of forced compression and velocity of deformation and the extent of the resultant injury in blunt abdominal trauma.[27] There is a linear relationship between the product of velocity and forced

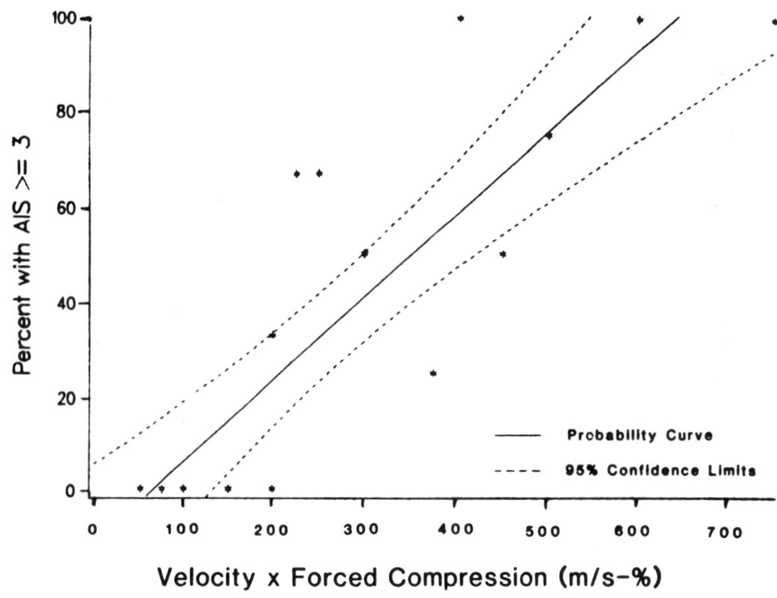

Figure 4–2 Risk of serious abdominal injury from *left*-side impacts versus (velocity × forced compression) (R^2 = 0.72). (From Rouhana SW, Lau IV, Ridella SA: Influence of velocity and forced compression on the severity of abdominal injury, *J Trauma* 25:496, 1985. Copyright by Williams & Wilkins, 1985.)

compression and the percentage of subjects with an adjusted injury severity score of greater than 3.

In some cases secondary injury can occur following blunt trauma, which can be more severe than an initial primary injury. This is particularly the case in children with head trauma. Compromise of the central nervous system, yielding a low Glasgow Coma Scale score, can occur with or without skull fracture. This injury is often associated with mechanical loss of the airway, hypoventilation, or apnea.[22] Failure to manage the airway successfully in a seriously injured child is a common problem in the prehospital setting, and even in the emergency department. Secondary anoxic brain damage can result, which can be more severe than the original insult to the brain. Another cause of secondary injury is lack of proper immobilization of the spine or extremities in cases of dislocation and/or fracture.

Penetrating trauma

Penetrating trauma, although less common in young children, is becoming an increasing problem in adolescents, particularly in the inner city. Penetrating trauma is caused by the entry of foreign objects through the skin into the body. The foreign object, such as a knife or a bullet, is usually in motion. In some cases, however, the penetration occurs when the victim falls onto a stationary object. The severity of injury is directly proportional to the size, speed, and trajectory of the penetrating

object. These factors determine the number of organs hit, the extent of injury to each organ, and how ciritically each organ is injured relative to other organs. Thus, a 4 cm–long stab wound in the neck perforating the carotid artery and esophagus can be more critical than a 10 cm–long stab wound to the liver.

Stab wounds. Stab wounds can be simple or complex. The size of the entry wound can be deceptive. For example, an aggressive stab wound can be associated with multiple vectors of injury with only one entry site. Two factors can help determine the potential seriousness of a stab wound: (1) the anatomic vulnerability of the area (for example, neurovascular bundles are relatively superficial at joint areas such as the groin, axilla, or popliteal regions); (2) the vulnerability of certain specific anatomic zones (for example, deep stab wounds in the lateral torso between the nipple level and the lower costal margin can produce simultaneous chest and abdominal injuries, plus occult lacerations of the diaphragm). In the precordial or xiphoid area, even shallow lacerations can produce potentially fatal cardiac tamponade.[5] There are several aids to predicting the trajectory and potential for internal organ injury. First, knowledge of the sex of the assailant is helpful; males tend to stab upward and females downward. Second, when the knife or impaling object is still in place, if the trajectory and depth of the penetrating weapon warrant exploration, the object is best left in place until

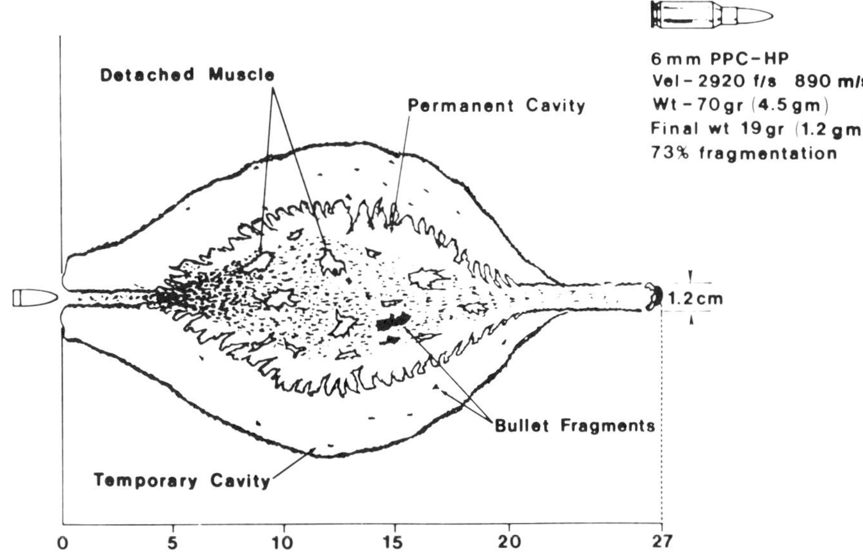

Figure 4–3 Wound profile of 6-mm PPC (this is a cartridge developed especially for "bench rest" shooting when maximum accuracy is required) hollow-point bullet. Free detached pieces of muscle are found in the permanent cavity. (From Fackler ML, Malinowski JA: The wound profile: a visual method for quantifying gunshot wound components, *J Trauma* 25:525, 1985. Copyright by Williams & Wilkins, 1985.)

it can be removed in a controlled fashion during surgical exploration.[31]

Gunshot wounds. There is an increasingly high frequency of penetrating trauma in children resulting from gunshot wounds. The potential for injury depends on the size or caliber of the bullet, its velocity, alteration in the trajectory of the bullet within the body, and distance of the victim from the weapon. The kinetic energy of the missile is expressed in this modified formula[25]:

$$\text{Kinetic energy} = \frac{\text{mass } (v_1^2 - v_2^2)}{2 \times g}$$

In this formula, v_1 is the missile velocity at impact, and v_2 is the velocity of the missile when it exits the body. If the bullet does not exit the body, then all of the kinetic energy is dissipated in the body, increasing the severity of injury. A principal factor in the potential for injury is missile velocity, inasmuch as kinetic energy is proportional to the square of that velocity. Because of air friction, velocity is affected by the distance of the weapon from the victim. The size of the missile and what happens to it after penetration can determine the amount of tissue damage. A large caliber missile produces a larger direct crush of tissue, called the *permanent cavity*. Larger missiles also increase the stretch of surrounding tissue, called the *temporary cavity*.

Of greater importance are changes in the character of the bullet after it enters the body. Bullets of higher velocity are often light in weight and therefore more likely to tumble or oscillate, thus increasing the size of the permanent cavity.[19,25,31] Some bullets have altered tips, such as a hollow point. These bullets begin to deform or to fragment as they pass through the body. With fragmentation, tissue damage is more widespread, resulting in an increase of both the permanent cavity and the temporary cavity (Fig. 4-3).[9] Bullets of this latter type are characteristic of hunting and military assault rifles. Hunting rifle bullets tend to fragment early. The maximum permanent cavity, therefore, is usually produced within the first 5 to 10 cm of penetration. In contrast, the maximal permanent cavity caused by military assault rifles is produced between 10 and 20 cm after penetration.[19,25] Hence, a child shot through the thigh muscle by a military assault rifle bullet may have a relatively small permanent cavity in contrast one wounded by the same missile traversing from one flank to the other. Pistol bullets and low-velocity rifle bullets do not fragment as readily, causing less tissue damage.[19,31]

There are several clinical guidelines that can help in determining the extent of injury from a gunshot wound. Elastic tissue such as skin and muscle tolerate stretch in the temporary cavity of the missile trajectory relatively well. This is exemplified in wounds caused by low-velocity bullets that do not fragment. Therefore, unless frankly devitalized fragments of muscle are seen, as in the case of a fragmenting bullet, excision of missile tracts through muscle is usually not indicated. In most cases, if the exit site has split and viable skin has fragmented, wound edges can be folded together with the expectation of satisfactory healing by secondary intention.[19] Nonelastic tissue, such as liver and spleen, do not tolerate stretch and are therefore more prone to massive disruption as a consequence of the temporary cavity produced by the bullet. In general, irregular movement of a bullet, such as its tumbling or fragmentation as it passes through the tissue, results in an exit wound larger than the entry wound. In wounds produced by high-velocity missiles, however, the area of unseen internal injury may greatly exceed that of the exit wound.[19] Knowing the nature of the gun, such as a .22 or .38 caliber versus a 9 mm gun, may thus determine the extent of debridement and drainage.

It is axiomatic that even with x-rays and other studies to help, the trajectory of a penetrating bullet cannot always be determined. For example, the position of the victim at the time he or she was shot may be unknown. In addition, because of the wide excursion of the diaphragm between inspiration and expiration, a gunshot wound to one body cavity may unexpectedly be found to have penetrated another cavity. This phenomenon played a role in President Reagan's case, when he was shot in the left chest. Prior to thoracotomy, the president underwent diagnostic peritoneal lavage to help rule out an occult penetration of the abdomen.

Shotgun injuries at close range also cause massive tissue destruction, but the severity of injury starts at the surface of the body. When a shotgun is fired within 3 feet of the victim, its muzzle blast can inject hot gas and powder directly into the wound, creating an internal explosion and burns. Fired within 6 feet, the pellets hit the skin in a dense, tight pattern, producing a cavity of destruction 1½ to 2 inches wide. Depending on the part of the body hit, most of the kinetic energy of the blast effect and pellets is expended within the first 15 cm and, usually, entirely within 20 cm.[31] At close range, the amount of kinetic energy released can be enough to amputate an adult's upper extremity. A blast in the flank of a child can pulverize the kidney and puncture structures such as the bowel and the inferior vena cava. Even when pellets do not reach the spinal cord, paralysis can result from the concussive forces released. Extensive debridement is required because of contamination from shotgun wadding, clothing, and powder burns of adjacent skin. A full load of small lead pellets retained in a small child can produce significant lead poisoning within a few weeks after injury.[28]

The kinetic energy imparted to the body of a victim of a shotgun wound is directly proportional to the size and number of the shotgun pellets striking the body and inversely proportional to the distance of the gun from the victim. Shotgun gauge (the bore of the gun) and the size of each missile are numbered inversely. For example, in shotgun gauges of 10, 12, 16, and 20, a larger numbered gauge denotes a smaller bore. Common shotgun pellets range from sizes 2 to 9; their pellet diameters range from 0.15 to 0.08 inches, respectively. Buckshot sizes are designated in order of increasing size: 4, 3, 2, 1, 0, and 00. Each 00 buckshot is 0.328 inches in diameter.[31] Compared with rifle bullets, shotgun missiles have initial lower velocity, the velocity more rapidly decreasing with increasing distance from the victim. In contrast, at close range, when the entire mass of pellets and wadding hit the victim, the kinetic energy imparted by a shotgun can be greater than that of a high-velocity rifle bullet (1900 ft-lb for a 12-gauge shotgun with no. 6 pellets versus 1248 ft-lb for an M-16 assault rifle).[10,31] The penetrating force of each shotgun missile varies, therefore, with distance from the victim. These various consequences allow a classification of injury: Type 1, penetration only of subcutaneous tissue and deep fascia (long range); Type 2, penetration of structure beneath the deep fascia (close range); Type 3, extensive destruction of tissue and organs (point blank).[7]

SPECIAL VULNERABILITY OF CHILDREN
Psychological

Childhood and adolesence is a time of exploration and risk taking. Children are inclined to sudden, unexpected movements and may not be fully aware of their environment. In addition, youngsters often have a sense of invulnerability. Their knowledge base is often limited, which handicaps them in regard to assessing risk and the consequence of injury.[1] Finally, because of peer pressure, children who hope to gain recognition and approval may not be able to resist a dare that actually involves an appreciable risk.

Environment of injury

Key factors in the environment of injury include dangerous streets and play areas, dangerous home situations, failure in properly securing motor vehicle passengers, lack of protection in recreational vehicle crashes, and the easy availability of guns. A California study found that 21% of all deaths of children up to age 18 in the city of Los Angeles were due to violence. Death resulting from violence in children typically had a bimodal curve, with peaks between birth to 3 years (child abuse) and 12 to 18 years (assault). In rural counties in California, however, only 8.9% of deaths in children were due to violence. Clearly, urban children

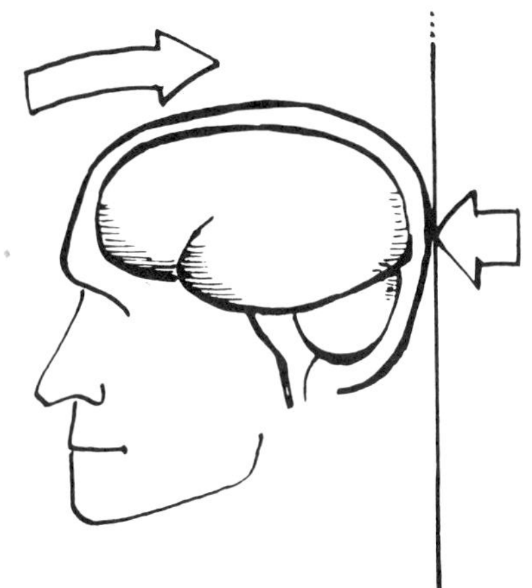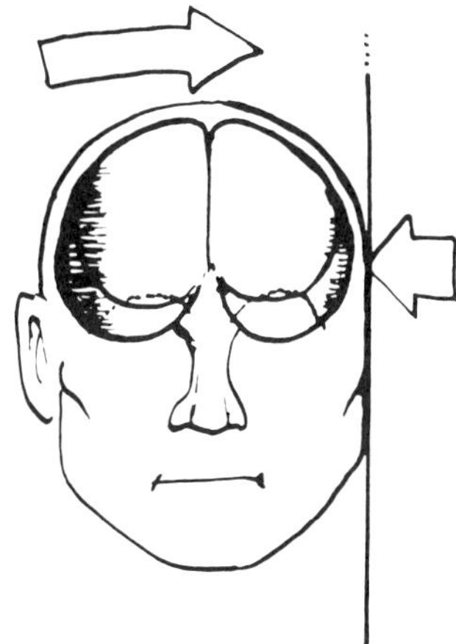

Figure 4–4 Contusion-type brain injuries that are generally more severe on the side opposite the point of impact are called coup-contrecoup contusions. (From Raasch FO: Forensic analysis of trauma. In Nahum AM, Melvin J, editors: *The biomechanics of trauma*. Norwalk, Conn, 1985, Appleton Century Crofts, p 173.)

were at greater risk because of the environment in which they lived. In the urban setting, availability of firearms is a major contributor to the environment of trauma. From 1962 to 1982, homicides caused by firearms increased dramatically. This increased incidence directly paralleled the availability, production, and sale of new firearms.[32] In the urban setting, 92% of firearm deaths in 1982 were intentional. Moreover, in the 10 years from 1972 to 1982, the most rapid increase in firearm homicides occurred in children between 5 and 9 years of age.

Of all unintentional deaths caused by firearms, 65% to 85% were found to occur in the victim's own home. In more than 85% of unintentional firearm deaths the shooter is known to the victim.[33] The smaller size of a child is also a factor. That a child is in the way may not be noticed when an altercation develops. Likewise, in urban traffic situations children are usually not seen by drivers who hit them.

Head injuries

The three most common mechanisms of head injury in children are falls, motor vehicle crashes, and assaults. In younger children the size of the head is a significant factor. Until the age of 10 years, the head of a child is larger in relation to the body than a teenager's or an adult's.[1] In motor vehicle crashes, therefore, children who are not properly restrained hurtle about the car like missiles. Typically, the head is the leading part of the body to come in contact with an unyielding part of the car.

A small child's scalp is much thinner than that of an older child or adult and is, therefore, less able to absorb the kinetic energy of a blow to the head. Children who incur blunt head trauma are more susceptible to epidural hemorrhage than adults. Fortunately, most epidural hemorrhages in children are small venous hemorrhages that do not require surgical intervention. Subdural hemorrhage is relatively rare in children. In contrast to an adult's, the brain of a young child has less myelin, making the brain softer. The unfused sutures and softness of the calvarium provide more room for movement of the brain during periods of rapid acceleration and deceleration. When a direct blow occurs to the head, a positive pressure develops at the interface of the brain and the skull on the side that is hit. A simultaneous negative pressure develops on the opposite side (inertial loading),[22] which produces a transient cavitation (Fig. 4-4). This factor, plus the sliding of the brain within the skull, contributes to the phenomenon of contrecoup injuries on the side of the brain opposite from the direct blow.[19,31]

Direct trauma on one side, contrecoup injuries on the opposite side of the brain, and the addition of rotational[22] forces are major findings in children with shaken baby syndrome. In virtually every such case, the head of the child has been banged against a hard object, such as a table, in the course of being shaken violently back and forth. In addition to direct trauma on the side of a blow and contrecoup injuries, the brain of the child develops diffuse axonal shearing injuries, particularly of the corpus callosum and brainstem.[22] These shearing injuries affect the microvasculature of the brain and the attachment of the cranial nerves. They are also the cause of the characteristic retinal hemorrhages seen in children who sustain head trauma as a result of child abuse.

The incidence of facial fractures in children is low compared with that in adults. The most common causative factor is vehicular trauma. Excluding fractures of the nose, the most common facial bone fracture in children is a mandibular fracture.[14] Because of the presence of primary and unerupted permanent teeth, children have a high tooth-to-bone ratio in the mandible. There are areas of weakness, therefore, in the developing tooth crypt. The weakest portions of the mandible are either at the condyle or in these crypts.[22] Sixty-six percent of mandible fractures in children less than 10 years of age involve the condyle, whereas 76% of mandible fractures in patients over 15 years of age involve the angle or body of the mandible. Mandible fractures in children are often initially overlooked. In a child who has sustained a blow to the head, the constellation of a chin laceration, hemotympanum, or blood in the external auditory canal in addition to malocclusion should suggest the presence of a mandibular fracture or temporomandibular joint disruption. Hemotympanum in this setting does not necessarily signify a basilar skull fracture. Fracture of either the condyle or ramus of the mandible can tear the eardrum without concomitant skull fracture.[14]

Spine injuries

The physical properties of the spine of a child, especially a young child, increase its vulnerability to injury. First, the cervical spine is less protected than an adult's, owing to the relatively weak muscles of the neck; second, in a young child, the facets in the upper cervical spine are flatter; third, the ligaments are more lax; fourth, the vertebral bodies are wedged anteriorly and have a tendency to slide forward with flexion.[11] The result is an increased risk of dislocation injuries which, in many cases, may not be accompanied by any apparent changes, such as fractures, upon x-ray examination.

Trauma to the spine can have single or multiple components. Axial loading injury can occur when the head is hit at its apex. The force is transmitted through the vertebral column, producing a burst fracture of the vertebral body or extrusion of the disk.[19] In flexion injuries, the spine is flexed forward beyond its normal range. This typically occurs when the head is flexed forward violently on the cervical spine.[22] When there is acute rotation plus flexion, the resultant injury can be more severe.[31] For example, when the head is in rotation, a blow to the head from the opposite side can cause the lateral mass of C2 to act as a hammer, striking the odontoid and causing a shearing-type fracture of the odontoid.[21] In severe flexion injuries the vertebral body is thrown forward, compressing the

cord. Risk of injury to the cord is increased with associated disruptions of longitudinal and articular ligaments.

Hyperextension injuries occur primarily in the neck. These injuries produce compression of the vertebral bodies and fractures of the pedicles or lamina. Posterior dislocation of the upper vertebrae on the lower vertebrae increases the chance of cord injury. Sudden acceleration can produce the form of hyperextension injury known as whiplash.[19] Torn ligaments can result in displacement of the vertebral body, thus causing stress in the center of the cord. This can produce the syndrome of acute central cervical cord injury, in which there is greater motor impairment of the upper extremities than of the lower extremities.[31]

The potential for irreversible cord injury is directly proportional to the amount of cord compression and the velocity at which it occurs; in other words, directly porportional to the rate at which kinetic energy is absorbed by the cord. In children with cervical spine injury, the primary mechanism of trauma is flexion in 79% and extension in 19%. In contrast, almost all thoracic and lumbar injuries are due to a flexion mechanism. Most spine injuries in children occur in the cervical and upper throacic area. In children less than 8 years old, cervical spine injuries are confined almost entirely to the C1-2 area. In children older than 8 years, 62% of cervical spine injuries occur at some point below C2.[2]

Airway

The airway of a child is at risk because of its intrinsic anatomy and because of increased risk factors. First, the tongue of a small child is relatively large in relation to the overall size of the pharynx. In a child who is lethargic or unconscious as a result of trauma, the tongue may collapse to the back of the pharynx, producing airway obstruction. In addition, the larynx of a small child is relatively more superior and anterior. When trauma produces bleeding in the pharynx, there may be increased difficulty in successfully intubating a traumatized child who needs good oxygenation and ventilation.[1] Second, the thin, weak tissues around a child's trachea increase the hazard of direct trauma to the trachea and larynx. Added to these factors are the types of activities children engage in. For example, a child riding a bicycle may not see the clothesline that suddenly hits him in the middle of the trachea. The result can be varying degrees of partial or complete disruption of the trachea. Such a patient will have a marked pneumatosis of the neck, face, and chest.[5] Urgent identification of this injury is key to successful preservation of an adequate airway.

Thorax

The chest wall of a child is much more compliant than an adult's. As a result, kinetic energy is transmitted more readily to structures within the thorax. A child with significant blunt trauma to the chest may have relatively few rib fractures and yet have an increased risk of life-threatening contusion to the lungs or heart.[1,22] When rib fracture does occur, the biomechanics at the site of the fracture depend on whether the transmission of kinetic energy is direct or indirect. Direct transmission of kinetic energy results in the inward displacement of the rib and a fracture of the rib on its inner surface. In a more diffuse crushing injury, such as a blow to the sternum, the ribs may bend laterally outward, resulting in a fracture on the outer surface.[5] In cases of child abuse, rib fractures can result from a forceful crushing of the lateral chest wall by the squeezing hand of an adult perpetrator. The result is a series of adjacent rib fractures, with the fracture on the inner surface.

In general, the presence of rib fractures in a young child suggests a great magnitude of kinetic energy applied focally or globally against the child's body. The mortality rate of children with multiple rib fractures is approximately 20 times higher than that of injured children without rib fractures. In one study[11] rib fractures were present in nearly 25% of trauma-related deaths, and 42% of children with rib fractures died. The characteristics of rib fractures in children that correlate most frequently with death are young age (less than 6 years), two or more rib fractures, the presence of head trauma, and child abuse or motor-vehicle occupant crash as the mechanism of trauma. When the forces exerted in child abuse or a motor vehicle crash are sufficient to fracture ribs, associated injuries to the head and torso are frequent and severe.

Compared with the ribs, certain structures in the thoracic wall are naturally better protected, such as the scapula and transverse processes of the thoracic vertebrae. Because the amount of kinetic energy required to fracture one of these structures is relatively great, the clinician must be alert, in the presence of such fractures, to associated internal injuries to the lung and heart.

The biomechanics of a traumatic pneumothorax resulting from blunt trauma to the chest are associated with two mechanisms. Penetration of a fractured rib through the visceral pleura with laceration of the lung is responsible for some instances of pneumothorax. More commonly, pneumothorax occurs when external compression produces a sudden, marked increase in the internal pressures within the lung, resulting in rupture of distal bronchioles with leaking from the visceral pleura. This is particularly likely when the victim inspires and then closes the glottis, trapping air within the lung.[19] Because the mediastinum of a child has increased elasticity and mobility, a tension pneumothorax in a child is poorly tolerated.[1]

In traumatic events with high kinetic energy, more devastating injuries to the contents of the chest can occur. Typical of such events are motor-vehicle and pedestrian crashes, in which a child is hit by a motor vehicle at a high rate of speed. In this case, rupture of the heart or severe myocardial contusion can occur. A common site for cardiac rupture is the right atrium, when it is forcefully compressed during diastole.[22] Although less common in children than in adults, events of high kinetic energy can produce aortic rupture. In its rare instances of appearance in children, it occurs typically at the ligamentum arteriosum where the aorta is held in a relatively fixed position. The aorta distal to this point is relatively fixed to the chest wall. Proximally, the aorta is more mobile, allowing the possible development of a shearing injury at the site of the ligamentum arteriosum.[19,22,31] When the mechanism of trauma involves a high transfer of kinetic energy, suspicion of injury to the aorta may be confirmed by recognition of a widened mediastinum and an apical cap sign on a chest radiograph. These findings suggest the accumulation of blood in the mediastinum.

Abdomen and retroperitoneum

The contents of the abdomen and retroperitoneum of a child are more vulnerable to blunt trauma than those of an adult. The lower rib cage of a younger child does not extend as far downward over the organs of the upper abdomen. In addition, the ribs are less ossified. As a result, the kidneys, spleen, and liver are more vulnerable to trauma. In children, the most commonly injured organs as a result of blunt abdominal trauma are, in order of frequency, the kidneys, spleen, liver, pancreas, and bowel.

Because 80% to 90% of abdominal and retroperitoneal injuries in children are due to blunt trauma, the nature of the injuries that result depends on whether an injury itself is focal or diffuse. Focal injuries can be best understood by dividing the abdomen into four anatomic areas: a left and a right lateral segment extending from above the costal margin down to the level of the iliac crest, a central portion extending from the xyphoid down to the level of the iliac crest, and a lower abdominal portion including all contents below the level of the iliac crest (Fig. 4-5).[15] Focal blunt trauma, such as a blow by a hockey stick or bicycle handle, may result in injuries confined to one particular segment. Examples include an isolated splenic fracture from a focal blow to the left side and an isolated

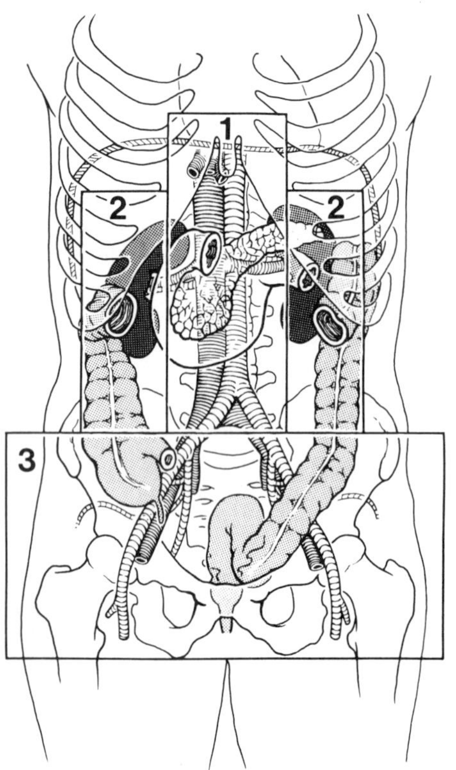

Figure 4–5 Relation of anatomic zones to indication for exploration of retroperitoneal hematomas, correlating the retroperitoneal anatomy with indications for operative management. (From Kudsk KA, Sheldon GF: Retroperitoneal trauma. In Blaisdell FW, Trunkey DD, editors: *Abdominal trauma*, New York, 1982, Thieme-Stratton, p 281. Reprinted by permission.)

pancreatic or duodenal injury from a blow in the mid-upper abdomen. Diffuse blunt trauma applied forcefully and suddenly over the entire abdomen and lower thorax can produce contusion and laceration to multiple solid viscera or shearing injuries involving the blood supply of the liver, spleen, and bowel.[31] When there is a sudden, massive increase of intraabdominal pressure owing to diffuse abdominal trauma, there can also be indirect trauma in the form of a rupture of the diaphragm. This rupture usually occurs on the left side.[19,22] The biomechanics of such a bursting injury to the diaphragm relate to the fact that the left diaphragm is largely unprotected. In contrast, on the right side the liver may absorb most of the kinetic energy, with the result that rupture of the right diaphragm owing to blunt trauma is uncommon.[5]

Most kidney injuries in children are self-limited contusions. Their susceptibility to contusion is increased because they have relatively little perinephric fat and, therefore, a reduced buffer to

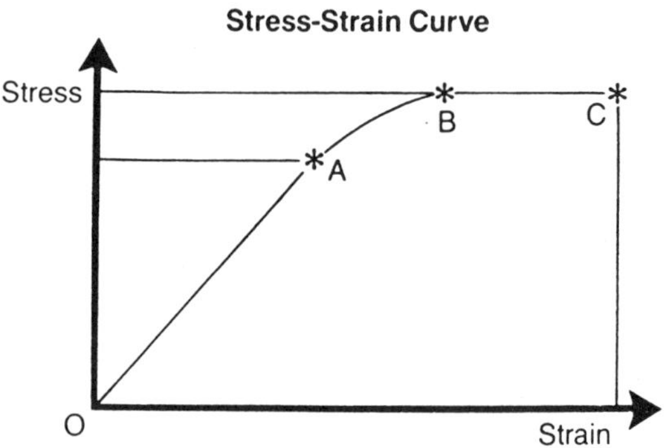

Figure 4–6 Stress-strain curve. Strain increases proportionately with stress to point *A*. From point *A* to point *B*, the strain is greater than the stress. Point *A* is called the yield point, or limit of proportionality, and Point *B* represents the ultimate tensile strength. Point *C* is the break point, or breaking strain, of the material. At *C* the material remains permanently deformed and does not recover its original shape. (From Weigelt JA, McCormack A: Mechanism of injury. In Cardona V et al, editors: *Trauma nursing from resuscitation through rehabilitation*, Philadelphia, WB Saunders, 1988, p 113.)

trauma. Moreover, because of the relatively thin abdominal wall of the child, organs that lie over the spinal column are less well protected; in particular, the pancreas, duodenum, and transverse column.

Musculoskeletal system

Two biomechanical factors help to determine the potential for musculoskeletal injury and, in particular, for fractures. The first factor is *strain*, defined as a change in length divided by initial length. The major types of strain are tensile, shear, and compressive. The second biomechanical factor is *stress,* defined as the internal resistance to deformation or the internal force generated from the application of a load.[31] Specifically, stress is directly proportional to the load placed on an object, and inversely proportional to the area on which the load acts. When kinetic energy is applied against a bone, the potential for fracture grows with increasing stress and strain. Stress-strain curves (Fig. 4-6)[31] for individual bones demonstrate that as stress increases, the strain increases proportionally until the bone reaches the *yield point.*[22] Then, as stress further increases, strain increases to the point of ultimate tensile strength. At that point, any slight increase in stress results in a break-point occurring for that bone at the site of maximal strain. With fracture, the bone is permanently deformed and will not recover its original shape.

Intrinsic features of their bones contribute to the biomechanics of fractures in children. The haversian systems, which are the primary mechanisms by which cortical bone resists stress, are reduced in number in children. In addition, a child's bone has a lower modulus of elasticity, lower bending strength, lower mineral content, and a thicker periosteum. "Compact adult bone principally fails in tension, whereas the more porous nature of the child's bone, particularly in the metaphysis, allows failure in compression as well, especially in those bones that go into greenstick failure or simple plastic deformation.[24]

Bone fracture also depends on the size and shape of the individual bone. A large bone resists fracture because any forces exerted on it are distributed over a larger volume of bone material. A tubular structure, such as the diaphysis of a long bone, more evenly distributes stresses caused by bending and torsional load than it could if it were a solid cylinder.[22] Other tissues such as ligaments and tendons also display near-linear stress-strain reactions. These tissues, for example, have little elastin or glycosaminoglycans (noncollagenous macromolecules). Their resistance to sudden or sustained stretch is, therefore, limited.[22]

The force applied to a bone can be both direct and indirect (Fig. 4-7).[12] In blunt trauma the two direct forces resulting in fractures are tapping forces and crush forces. There are a wider number of indirect forces that also produce fracture. These include traction, which involves tendons pulling pieces of bone away from their attachments, and angulation, in which the convex surface of the bending bone is under tension stress and the concave surface is under compression stress. Vertical compression produces fractures that usually occur at an angle of approximately 45°. Such fractures are usually seen as T- or Y-shaped fractures at the lower end of the bone. Axial loading usually involves long bones and occurs in association with angulation, or torsion plus angulation, resulting in a midshaft fracture.[31] When a bone is exposed to very rapid axial loading, the presence of only moderate lateral force is enough to fracture it.[22] A common example of such a fracture is that sustained by an unrestrained front-seat passenger in a motor vehicle crash hurtling forward and striking his knees against the dashboard.

Femoral fractures in children and adolescents occur primarily as a result of falls and traffic crashes. The incidence pattern of femoral fractures is different for falls than for traffic incidents. Falls are the predominant cause of femoral fractures in children from the age of 2 to 6 years. The incidence of falls as a cause of femoral fracture then steadily diminishes after the age of 7. In the case of traffic incidents involving children, especially, boys, there is a bimodal incidence pattern with an early peak between 4 and 7 years and a later peak between 14 and 18 years. The first peak correlates predominantly with pedestrian injuries and pedal-cyclist injuries. The second peak correlates with injuries to motorcyclists or motor vehicle occupants.[13] In contrast, femoral fractures in children less than 2 years of age should raise the possibility of child abuse when the mechanism of trauma is not clear cut.

One of the most common isolated fractures in children is a supracondylar humeral fracture. The anterior capsule and collateral ligaments of a child's elbow are stronger than the adjacent bone. Where the tensile strength of the ligaments is stronger than the adjacent bone, avulsion fractures can occur.[22] Therefore, when the elbow is locked in extension, as in a child falling backward, the force applied to the elbow causes supracondylar bone to fracture. These fractures can be displaced or nondisplaced. In either case, delay in treatment can result in tense swelling around the elbow with progressive vascular compromise to the forearm and hand.[31] The earliest sign of such injury is paresthesia or sensory abnormality of the hand. Surgical intervention in such a situation is a relative emergency in order to prevent the development of an irreversible Volkmann's ischemic contracture.

Children's pelvic bones are weaker than adults', and the ligaments more lax. As a result, there is an increased danger of vascular disruption in certain types of blunt trauma to the pelvis. Injuries to the pelvis are indirect or direct. In a motor vehicle crash in which the passenger is unrestrained, a frontal impact may produce indirect shearing injuries of the pelvis, often in the form of a posterior dislocation of the hip or an acetabular fracture.[19,31] These injuries typically occur when the hip is flexed and abducted at the moment of impact. More severe pelvic fractures occur when kinetic energy is applied directly to the pelvis, as in the case of a pedestrian injured in a motor vehicle crash. If the blow is lateral, the result is a direct compression of the lateral pelvis. Because of the rapid and focal transfer of kinetic energy to the pelvis, the resultant injuries are more severe, usually in the form of multiple, comminuted fractures with varying degrees of pelvic disruption. A particularly severe form of pelvic fracture occurs with a direct anterior or posterior blow against the pelvis, resulting in a Malgaigne fracture in which there is fracture through both the sacroiliac joint and the pubic ramus on the same side.[22] This cleavage plane is comparable to a hemipelvectomy. The resultant sudden stretch of associated nerve and vascular structures can cause avulsion of nerves to the leg and shearing of the iliac vessels with massive bleeding. Because of the significant amount of in-

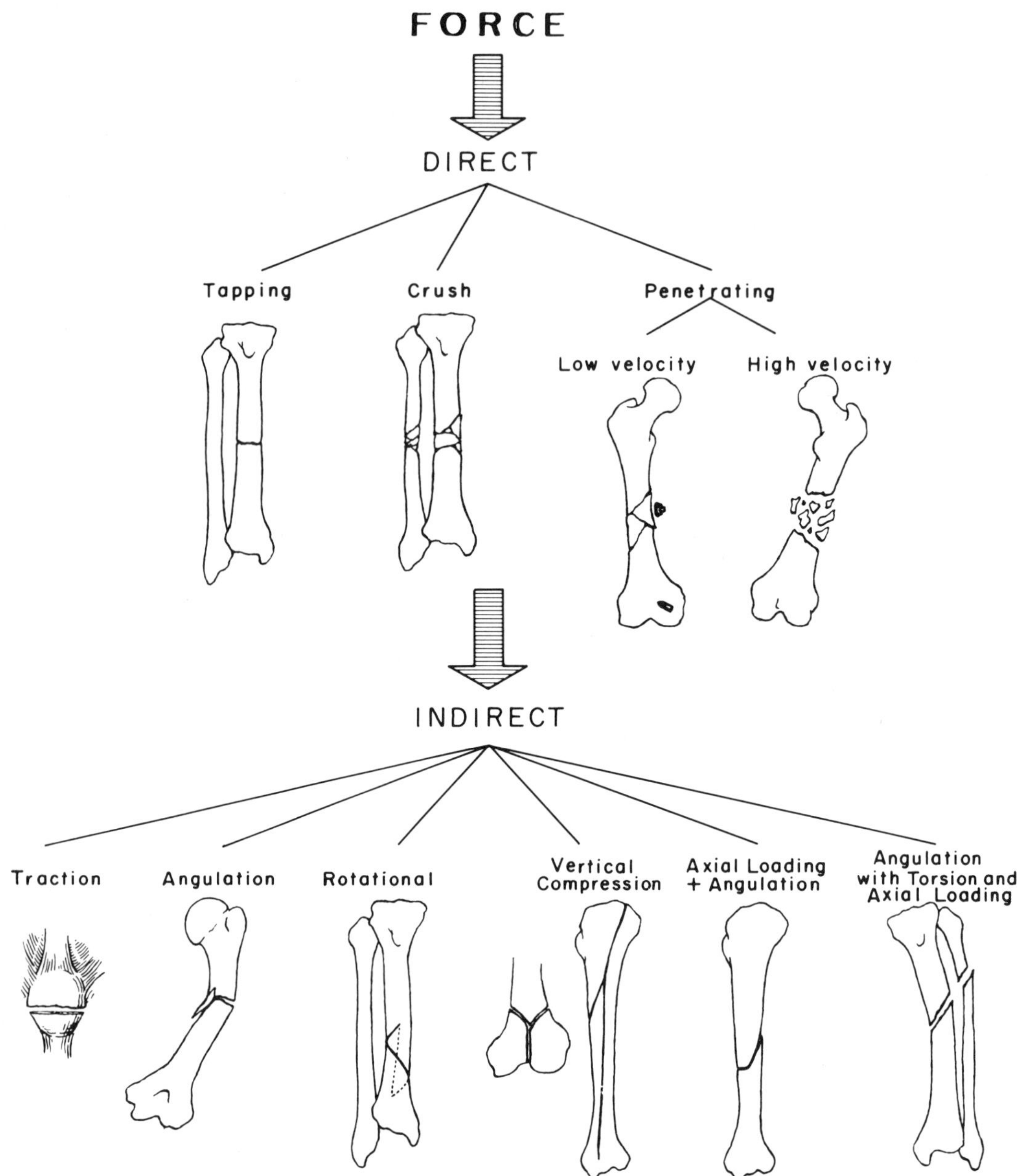

Figure 4–7 Classification of fractures according to the mechanism of injury. (From Harkness JW, Ramsey WC, Ahmadi B: Principles of fractures and dislocations, vol 1. In Rockwood CA, Green DP, editors: Fractures, ed 2, Philadelphia, 1984, JB Lippincott, p 10.)

ternal bleeding that occurs with more severe pelvic fractures, open pelvic fractures do not permit tamponade of internal bleeding to occur. As a result, open pelvic fractures can have a mortality rate four times that of closed fractures.[31]

MECHANISM OF INJURY

Except in some cases of child abuse, the mechanism of trauma in injured children is usually known at the time of admission. A knowledge of biome-chanics pertaining to that mechanism can provide valuable information about potential underlying injuries. A heightened level of suspicion can direct the trauma team in their diagnostic evaluation and reduce delay in definitive treatment.

Motor vehicle crashes

Of 165,000 trauma deaths each year, 45,000 are due to motor vehicle crashes. Motor vehicle crashes are the leading cause of permanent brain damage and new cases of epilepsy, as well as the leading cause of death and serious injury in children. In 1985, in the age group from birth to 14 years, there were 4000 deaths and 145,000 injuries caused by motor vehicle crashes. Motor vehicle crashes were the mechanisms of injury in 72% of all deaths of persons 15 to 24 years of age.

In assessing the injury of an occupant involved in a motor vehicle crash, it is essential to get certain information pertaining to the vehicle: speed of the vehicle at the time of crash; type of collision (frontal, rear, side, spin, roll-over); type of secondary collision against other object (pole, tree, building); vehicle damage (focal intrusion, buckled frame, interior damage); displacement of the object hit by the primary vehicle (such as a stationary car at the side of the road). In addition, it is necessary to determine specific occupant information: the use or non-use of restraints, including passive restraints such as air bags; evidence regarding proper or improper use of restraints (for example, infant car seat not secured by vehicle safety belts); displacement of the occupant; location of the occupant relative to the site of primary collision and any secondary collisions (for instance, an unrestrained child in the back seat of a vehicle involved in a front-end crash); ejection of the occupant; death of another occupant.

In a motor vehicle crash the vehicle and occupant are traveling at the same rate of speed. The deceleration forces transmitted to the body are measured according to gravity (g-forces)[8]:

$$\text{Gravity} = \frac{\text{mph}^2}{30 \times \text{stopping distance (ft)}}$$

The g-forces of a vehicle at the time of a crash vary considerably depending on the stopping distance. For example, for a vehicle traveling at 70 mph, sharp braking over a distance of 50 meters produces 1 g. In contrast, a vehicle hitting a tree with a braking distance of only a half meter produces a deceleration force of 100 g.[5] The g-forces experienced by an unrestrained occupant approximate those of the motor vehicle. In other words, the momentum of the occupant is maintained.[19,22] In a collision at 45 mph the deceleration force equals 40 g.[8] Even at moderate or high speeds g-forces are greatly ameliorated by passive and active restraints, which have the effect of distributing the forces over a broad area of the body. In that regard, three-point restraints are more effective than two-point restraints. Loose-fitting restraints, however, present a risk. The g-forces experienced by a loosely restrained subject are twice those experienced by a tightly restrained subject. Studies by Volvo in Sweden showed that among properly belted front-seat occupants there were no deaths in vehicular crashes associated with speeds up to 60 mph. For unbelted front-seat occupants, death occurred in crashes associated with speeds as low as 17 mph.[31] In a frontal collision, the most effective dissipation of g-forces occurs when the occupant strikes an air bag.

In any motor vehicle crash, three collisions occur.[31] The first is the collision of the vehicle itself. The second is the collision of the occupant with the interior of the vehicle, including a seatbelt, an air bag, or the dashboard. An unrestrained child involved in a front-end crash at 30 mph hits the dashboard with the same force as in a three-story fall. The third collision occurs when internal organs collide with rigid or unyielding body wall structures.[19] Tissues such as the lung, brain, liver, and spleen are particularly vulnerable to this trauma. Sudden deceleration of the head of an unrestrained occupant when it hits the dashboard can produce both direct trauma at the site of impact and contrecoup or shearing injuries on the opposite side. The second and third collisions are magnified when an occupant is ejected from a motor vehicle. The potential for death of ejected occupants is 25 times greater than that for occupants who remain within the vehicle.[19] For occupants remaining within a vehicle, the potential g-forces and, therefore, the potential for death are greatest in side impacts followed by impact with the steering wheel and dashboard.[8] The transfer of kinetic energy and, thus, the potential for injury, are greatest when an intrusion into the vehicle results in direct trauma to the occupant. For this reason, side crashes that involve the weakest portion of a vehicle are associated with the highest mortality rates.

Head and chest injuries. The leading cause of death in unbelted motor vehicle occupants involved in fatal crashes is head injury. Chest injury, particularly severe in passengers who are ejected from a motor vehicle, is the second most frequent cause of death. Severe injuries to the chest wall include sternal fracture and multiple bilateral rib fractures. Fracture of the lower ribs can result in puncture of the diaphragm and of the spleen or liver, resulting in continued bleeding into the chest. Mediastinal injuries can include cardiac rupture and rupture of the ascending aorta.[22] In unrestrained passengers, rupture of the aorta usually occurs in the ascending portion, whereas in restrained passengers the vulnerable portion of the aorta is distal to the subclavian artery on the left side. Because of the deceleration forces involved, a high proportion of the latter passengers also sustain thoracic vertebral fractures.

Maxillofacial injuries. Maxillofacial injuries are also affected by the use or non-use of restraints. Facial lacerations are significantly increased in unrestrained passengers, particularly those in the front seat. In addition, the number of complex injuries such as lacerations plus fractures is three times higher in unrestrained passengers; midface fractures, such as LeFort II and LeFort III fractures, are characteristic injuries. Such fractures are most likely to result when the load forces occur focally, as when the face hits a part of the steering wheel. Failure to restrain back-seat passengers is a problem particularly with children, who often ride in the back seat. In a study in England, 3% of restrained back-seat passengers involved in a crash required hospital admission, in contrast to 16% of unrestrained passengers who required admission. The 11 deaths reported all involved unrestrained occupants. All occupants who were ejected had been unrestrained; 9 of the 11 deaths belonged to this group.[6]

Car seats. With the passage of legislation in most states mandating the use of car seats for infants and toddlers, there has been a significant increase in the use of these restraints. However, biomechanical analysis of how car seats are used has demonstrated the hazards of their improper use or positioning. For example, in the first year of life a child's head represents 19% of the surface area of the body. As a result, the child has a higher center of gravity. The fulcrum of cervical spine movement is higher, generally at C2, as opposed to that of adults', which is at C5-6. In a forward crash the head is propelled forward like a missile. Even if the child is properly restrained, the neck will crack like a whip. Because of this biomechanical factor, there are a growing number of reports of infants and toddlers who, while facing forward in a car seat, incurred a cervical fracture at the level of C1-3. Proper restraint of infants and children in rear-facing seats can largely overcome this hazard. Studies have demonstrated that the risk of injury in restrained children is 1.2% when they are secured in a rear-facing restraint. Injury frequency increases to 6.9% with use of a forward-facing restraint, to 8.9% when a child is placed in an adult seat belt and to 15.6% when the child is unrestrained.[30]

Seat belts. With the wider use of seat belts, certain patterns of seat-belt injuries have been noted. Because most seat belts are fairly narrow and unpadded, the *g*-forces associated with the vehicle crash can be transmitted focally to the point at which the belt touches the body. With the use of three-point restraints, for example, soft tissue injuries in the cervical spine area are relatively common. The injuries are usually mild, associated with pain and tenderness and restricted cervical motion because of muscle strain. Occasional neurologic deficits may occur, but usually no cervical

fractures or dislocations. On rare occasions there have been isolated fractures of the clavicle with injury to the underlying subclavian artery.

Improper use or loose fitting of a seat belt can result in a "submarine" effect in which the body forcefully slides beneath the seat belt and the belt impinges on the abdomen and the lumbar spine.[22,23] Injuries to the abdominal wall can result, including hematoma in the rectus sheath or even avulsion and necrosis of the rectus muscle. Rupture of the stomach or bowel may occur in the form of shearing injuries, particularly at points of fixation such as the ligament of Treitz. The direct crushing effect of the belt can also produce injury to the bowel mesentery, pancreas, gall bladder, aorta, or inferior vena cava.[4] With direct injury to the abdominal aorta, for example, the intima may be torn, resulting in partial or complete obstruction. Most of these injuries are distal to the inferior mesenteric artery. When aortic occlusion occurs acutely there is frank distal arterial insufficiency, with or without neurologic deficit, and an acute abdomen.

The use of lap-belt devices alone has resulted in a phenomenon known as the *seat-belt syndrome*.[22,23] Characteristic of this syndrome, the kinetic energy imparted by the seat belt not only produces injuries to the bowel and other structures in front of the spine, but is also associated with major lumbar fracture and dislocation as a result of a hyperflexion of the torso over the lap belt. The biomechanics of such an injury are due to the fact that the axis of flexion is shifted from the center of the spinal column at the nucleus pulposus to the point of contact of the belt on the abdominal wall. This produces a flexion-distraction stress, usually associated with absence of rotation. The injury patterns involve osseous or ligamentous disruption of the posterior elements of the spine, or both, and either a compression fracture or a transverse fracture of one or more lumbar vertebral bodies.[19] When a fracture dislocation is severe there may also be partial or complete cord injury resulting from subluxation dislocation to the spine.[23] Failure to recognize the injury complex associated with seat belt syndrome has resulted in delay in diagnosis of common duct avulsion, duodenal perforation, and small and larger bowel perforation.[4]

MOTOR VEHICLE/PEDESTRIAN CRASHES

Pedestrian injury involving motor vehicles can be a particularly lethal form of trauma in children. In urban settings with limited playground facilities, children more commonly sustain trauma as pedestrians than as occupants in motor vehicles. The biomechanics of resultant injuries depend on the speed and size of the colliding vehicle and the age and height of the victim. Left-sided injuries are more common in the United States because of the practice of driving on the right side of the road. Not surprisingly, multiple injuries are also quite common, including injuries to the central nervous system, spine, musculoskeletal system, and various internal organs.

Depending on the size of the child, the nature of injury is determined by two forms of trauma. The first injury is the result of the initial, direct impact of a motor vehicle against a child. The second injury occurs as a result of what happens to the child after the initial blow. For example, a child may be thrown through the air and then hit the ground or another object.[31] In an older or taller child, a catapult-type injury may occur in which the upper part of the body forcefully flexes over the hood of the car. The force involved in such a catapult phenomenon can leave the impression of the child's head on the hood or on the windshield; primary and contrecoup injuries to the head are common in this situation. Secondary information can be helpful in predicting the extent of injury, including evidence of damage to the colliding vehicle (which may tell whether the blow was direct or glancing), the amount of displacement of the victim as a result of being hit, and whether or not the child was separated from his shoes. The velocity of a motor vehicle need only be 40 mph for the force of impact to knock a child out of his shoes.

RECREATIONAL VEHICLE CRASHES

Recreational vehicles that can cause injury in children include motorbikes, bicycles, skateboards, and all-terrain vehicles (ATV's). Most recreational vehicle crashes do not involve another vehicle. Nevertheless, because the child rider is largely unprotected, collision with a fixed structure such as a tree, wall, or clothesline can be fatal. There are 700 deaths owing to bicycle trauma in children 15 years old and younger in the United States each year. For children less than 10 years of age, deaths resulting from bicycle injuries exceed those resulting from falls, poisonings, suffocation, and firearms. In adolescents, the toll is even greater— 64% of all bicycling deaths occur in adolescents. More than 85% of deaths resulting from bicycle injuries are associated with irreversible brain injury. The threat to a child is even greater when the rider's bicycle or other recreational vehicle collides with a motor vehicle. In this case, the kinetic energy imparted to the body of the child reflects both the velocity of the child and the velocity of the motor vehicle at the time of the collision. In such cases, most of the victims sustain global injuries.

Two such injuries, for example, reflect different biomechanics. Rupture of the heart or of the septum between the right and left ventricles can result from sudden compression of the heart between the sternum and vertebral bodies. These injuries are particularly likely to occur if the heart is in late diastole or early systole when the ventricles are full and the valves are closed. Second, when the rider of a recreational vehicle is catapulted forward through the air, he or she typically lands on the back of the thoracic spine. As a result, thoracic spine injuries are more common than cervical spine injuries. The most common site of injury in this mechanism of trauma is between T4 and T7 (Fig. 4-8).[16] This is an especially hazardous site for injury to occur, as the blood supply to this area is particularly tenuous. In addition, the thoracic spine at this level has a relatively narrow canal.[22] The thoracic spinal cord, therefore, is more susceptible to impingement. The biomechanics of this type of catapult injury explains why 70% to 80% of its victims develop cord injury with complete paraplegia.

Nevertheless, head injury remains the single most important determinant of outcome in victims of recreational vehicle crashes. Studies involving head injuries and bicyclists show that in 70% of cases the head hit the road first; in 17%, a flat surface, such as a car body; and in 8%, an angled or projecting structure.[34] The potential for serious head injury is almost entirely a factor of the presence or absence of a proper helmet. In general, motorcycle riders are traveling faster when involved in a crash than are bicycle riders. Yet, in a study in Australia, 59% of injured bicycle riders were reported to have sustained head injury, as compared with only 26% of motorcycle riders. This difference reflects the nearly universal use of helmets by motorcyclists and the very low incidence of bicycle helmet use in that country at the time of the study.[18] In a carefully controlled study in Seattle, it has been shown that bicycle riders who wear helmets have an 88% reduction in the risk of brain injury as a result of being involved in a bicycle crash.[29] The biomechanics of helmet use reflect the fact that much of the kinetic energy of a blow to the head is diffused across the surface of the helmet and dissipated in the underlying padding.

FALLS

Falls are the single most common cause of injury in children. Fortunately, serious injury or death resulting from truly accidental falls is relatively uncommon. Factors involved in the biomechanics of injuries caused by falls are the height from which the child fell, the velocity of the child during the fall, the mass of the child, and whether the child was in free fall as opposed to a bouncing fall. These

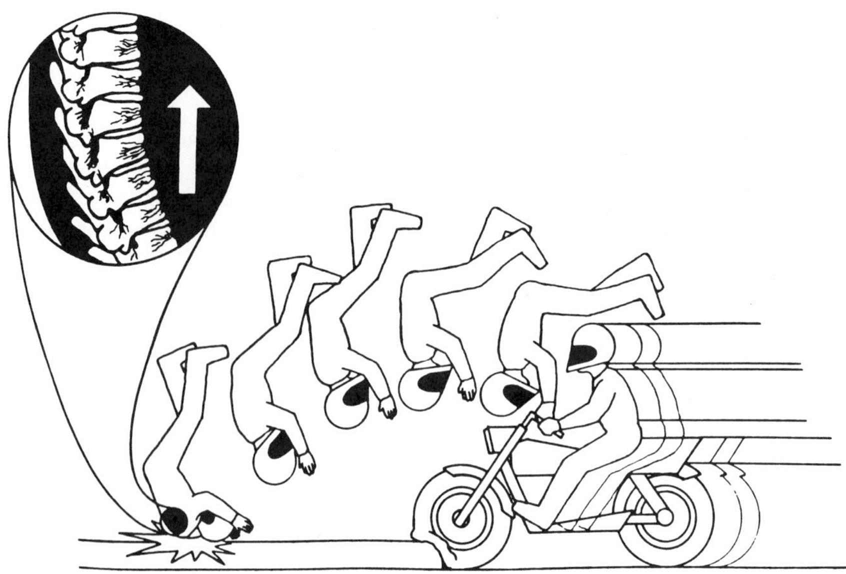

Figure 4–8 A catapulting injury to a motorcyclist is depicted. The *arrow* in the inset depicts the force vector directed caudal along the axial skeleton. The area between T3 and T9 is shown, highlighting multiple anterior compression fractures and the resulting strain pattern placed along the posterior elements. (From Kupferschmidt JP, Weaver ML, Raves JJ et al: Thoracic spine injuries in victims in motorcycle accidents. *J Trauma* 29:595, 1989. Copyright by Williams & Wilkins, 1989.)

factors determine the severity of direct impact injuries and of secondary deceleration injuries.

Maull[17] described the biomechanics of injuries resulting from falls: "The injury producing potential of a body in motion is a function of the dissipation of kinetic energy and the tendency upon impact to displace the tissues in the direction of the motion, while the movement of the body itself is arrested." In effect, when dissipation of kinetic energy is slow, injuries are slight. When dissipation is rapid, injuries are severe. The forces at impact are expressed as *g*-forces. A formula presented by Maull delineates the factors involved in such injuries[17]:

$$W = \frac{KE}{T \times A} \times K$$

The extent of wounding (W) is directly related to the kinetic energy (KE) but inversely related to the time of deceleration (T), and the area through which the energy is dissipated (A). K represents biomechanical factors of the injured subject. Forces of compression, stretching, and shearing can produce critical injuries when the point of impact (A) is focal, such as to the head or feet. In such impacts, all the kinetic energy may be transmitted to vulnerable structures such as the brain, spinal column, and spinal cord. Associated injuries include combined bony injuries of the lower body, including the pelvis, lower extremity, and calcaneus.[17,31]

In most falls, the victim travels at an accelerating speed (32 ft/sec); hence the kinetic energy is magnified by the square of the velocity at the time of impact. Other factors, such as mass, can modify the potential for injury. Mass was a factor in the case of a 3-year-old child who fell from a ninth-floor window. The child landed on his left side, sustaining on that side a fractured humerus, two fractured ribs, a small hemopneumothorax, and a renal contusion. The child's small mass and the fact that he hit soft, rain-soaked ground contributed to his relatively mild injuries. The soft ground, for example, contributed to an increased time of deceleration. Because the child landed on his side, the area through which the energy was absorbed (A), was increased.

VIOLENCE

Although progress continues in reducing death and serious injury resulting from most forms of trauma, such as motor vehicle crashes, statistics show that violence as a cause of trauma is increasing in frequency and severity. Violence takes a particularly heavy toll on young persons. When calculated in terms of years of potential life lost, homicide ranks as the fourth leading cause of death, and suicide as the fifth leading cause. The vast majority of homicide and suicide deaths are caused by gunshot wounds and stabbings. The biomechanics for these injuries have been discussed previously. However, because of today's social and political climates, the biomechanics of two forms of blunt trauma warrant review.

Blunt trauma is the most common cause of injury resulting from the abuse of young children. This typically involves direct blows to the head and body. A forceful punch by an adult can produce a velocity of impact of 8.9 m per second. The force on impact of such a punch is 0.4 tons on soft tissue, and on the head and face, because of the proximity of bone, a force of 0.63 tons. The result of such a punch to the head is a sudden, backward acceleration of the head at 520 m per second, squared.[3] Extremity fractures and rib fractures are also common in child abuse. The biomechanics involve a sudden, violent twisting of an extremity or a crushing squeeze of the chest wall. In child abuse cases, 80% of extremity fractures occur in the age range from birth to 18 months. No extremity fractures resulting from abuse occur in children over 5 years of age. In contrast, truly accidental causes of extremity fracture are very rare (only about 2% of cases) in children less than 18 months old. Instead, 85% of truly accidental causes of extremity fractures occur in children 5 to 12 years of age, as might be expected by their increased activity level. Overall, 55% of child abuse victims have three or more fractures at the time of diagnosis.

Because of the growing threat of indiscriminate terrorism in today's world, children may be the victims of explosions. The biomechanics of traumatic injury in an explosion are determined by three components of a blast's shock wave: a positive phase, a negative phase, and mass movement of air. In the positive phase there is a sudden increase in environmental pressure. The force of this increased pressure is directly related to the size of the explosion and inversely related to the distance of the victim from the explosion. During the positive pressure phase, injury can be inflicted by shrapnel and other debris hitting the victim, as well as by displacement of the victim against a hard object, which produces typical impact and deceleration injuries.[31]

Immediately after the positive pressure phase there is a negative phase that can last 10 times as long as the positive phase. Air that is displaced by the positive pressure phase enters behind the blast wave. This mass movement of air can cause extensive injuries, including amputation and evisceration. The organs most vulnerable are those that contain gas or that contain gas and water. Therefore, the organs most commonly injured in a blast injury are the eardrums, the lungs, and the bowel.

The amount of force necessary to cause lung contusion is 3 times the amount of force necessary to rupture eardrums. The wave speed in the lung, for example, is 30 to 45 m per second. Hence, much of the energy from a shock wave traveling at 450 m per second will be expended within the lung tissue.[22] Two circumstances increase the effect of the blast shock wave. First, blast injuries in water may be more severe because the greater density of water allows the blast wave to travel farther and more rapidly. Second, explosions in closed areas do not permit dissipation of the blast shock wave. In addition, survivors of such explosions are exposed to toxic gases and smoke.[31]

In summary, knowledge of the biomechanics of trauma in children can greatly assist the clinician in early identification and treatment of significant underlying injuries that may not be apparent on initial assessment. Of equal importance is the role that an understanding of biomechanics can play in injury prevention. Trauma specialists must take an active and continuing role in trauma prevention if they are to make an impact on the needless toll of death and serious injury in children. Their knowledge of the anatomy and physiology of injury in children is important to designers of improved motor vehicle restraints for children. Active involvement of health professionals is likewise essential in social and legal intervention to achieve gun control, universal bicycle helmet use, and a safer play environment for children. A revolution in society's awareness of the hazards of smoking has been achieved. A similar revolution and commitment to injury prevention can save billions of dollars and the needless suffering of children and their families.

REFERENCES

1. Advanced Trauma Life Support Program, Chicago, 1989, American College of Surgeons, pp 217-230.
2. Apple JS, Kirks DR, Merten DF, et al: Cervical spine fractures and dislocations in children, *Pediatr Radiol* 17:45-49, 1987.
3. Atha J, Yeadon MR, Sandover J et al: The damaging punch, *Brit Med J (Clin Res)* 191:1756-1757, 1985.
4. Banerjee A: Seat belts and injury patterns: evolution and present perspectives, *Postgrad Med J* 65:199-204, 1989.
5. Besson A, Saegesser F: Chest trauma and associated injuries, Oradell NJ, 1989, Medical Economics Books, pp 90-121.
6. Christian MS, Bullimore DW: Reduction in accident injury severity in rear seat passengers using restraints, *Injury* 20:262-264, 1989.
7. Deitch EA, Grimes WR: Experience with 112 shotgun wounds of the extremities, *J Trauma* 24:600-603, 1984.
8. Dolan WD et al: Automobile-related injuries, *JAMA* 249:3216-3222, 1983.
9. Fackler ML, Malinowski JA: The wound profile: a visual method for quantifying gunshot wound components, *J Trauma* 2:522-529, 1985.
10. Flint LM, Cryer HM, Howard DA et al: Approaches to

management of shotgun injuries, *J Trauma* 24:415-419, 1984.

11. Garcia VF, Gotschall CS, Eichelberger MR et al: Rib fractures in children: a marker of severe trauma, *J Trauma* 30:695-700, 1990.

12. Harkness JW, Ramsey WC, Ahmadi B: Principles of fractures and dislocations, vol 1. In Rockwood CA, Green DP, editors: *Fractures,* Philadelphia, 1984, JB Lippincott, p 10.

13. Hedlund R, Lindgren U: The incidence of femoral shaft fractures in children and adolescents, *J Pediatr Orthop* 6:47-50, 1986.

14. Hurt TL, Fisher B, Peterson BM et al: Mandibular fractures in association with chin trauma in pediatric patients, *Pediatr Emerg Care* 4:121-123, 1988.

15. Kudsk KA, Sheldon GF: Retroperitoneal trauma. In Blaisdell FW, Trunkey DD, editors: *Abdominal trauma.* New York, 1989, Thieme-Stratton, pp 279-293.

16. Kupferschmidt JP, Weaver ML, Raves JJ et al: Thoracic spine injuries in victims of motorcycle accidents, *J Trauma* 29:593-596, 1989.

17. Maull KI, Whitley RE, Cardea JA: Vertical deceleration injuries, *Surg Gynecol Obstet* 153:233-236, 1981.

18. McDermott FT, Klug GL: Injury profile of pedal and motor cyclist casualties in Victoria, *Aust NZ J Surg* 55:477-483, 1985.

19. McSwain NE, Kerstein MD, editors: *Evaluation and management of trauma,* Norwalk, Conn, 1988, Appleton Century Crofts, pp 1-41.

20. Miller MA: The biomechanical response of the lower abdomen to belt restraint loading, *J Trauma* 29:1571-1584, 1989.

21. Mouradian WH, Felti VG, Cochran GV et al: Fractures of the odontoid: a laboratory and clinical study of mechanism, *Orthop Clin North Am* 9:985-1001, 1978.

22. Nahum AM, Melvin J, editors: *The biomechanics of trauma,* Norwalk, Conn, 1985, Appleton Century Crofts.

23. Newman KD, Bowan LM, Eichelberger MR et al: The lap belt complex: intestinal and lumbar spine injury in children, *J Trauma* 30:1133-1140, 1990.

24. Ogden JA: The uniqueness of growing bones. In Rockwood CA, Wilkins KE, King RE, editors: *Fractures in children,* Philadelphia, 1984, JB Lippincott, pp 1-71.

25. Ordog GJ: Wound ballistics: theory and practice, *Ann Emerg Med* 13:1113-1122, 1984.

26. Peclet MH, Newman KD, Eichelberger MR et al: Patterns of injury in children, *J Pediatr Surg* 25:85-91, 1990.

27. Rouhana SW, Lau IV, Ridella SA: Influence of velocity and forced compression on the severity of abdominal injury in blunt, non-penetrating lateral trauma, *J Trauma* 25:490-500, 1985.

28. Selbst SM, Henretig F, Fee MA et al: Lead poisoning in a child with a gunshot wound, *Pediatrics* 77:413-416, 1986.

29. Thompson RS, Rivara FP, Thompson DC: A case-control study of the effectiveness of bicycle safety helmets, *N Engl J Med* 320:1361-1367, 1989.

30. Tingvall C: *Children in cars: some aspects of the safety of children as passengers in road traffic accidents,* Stockholm, 1987, Almquist & Wiksell.

31. Weigelt JA, McCormack A: Mechanism of trauma. In Cardona V et al, editors: *Trauma nursing from resuscitation through rehabilitation,* Philadelphia, 1988, WB Saunders, 105-128.

32. Wintemute GJ: Firearms as a cause of death in the United States, 1920-1982, *J Trauma* 27:532-536, 1987.

33. Wintemute GJ, Kraus JF, Teret SP et al: Unintentional firearm deaths in California, *J Trauma* 29:457-461, 1989.

34. Worrell J: Head injuries in pedal cyclists, *Injury* 18:5-6, 1987.

PART TWO

The Child

Unique features

5 Anatomy, Growth, and Development

Impact on injury

Stephen Ludwig and John Loiselle

The goal of pediatrics is to enable children to reach their maximum physical and intellectual potential. Injuries are the leading cause of morbidity and mortality in the pediatric age group and, therefore, pose the greatest threat to this goal. Because of differences in anatomy, growth, and development, children are more at risk than adults for certain injuries. Although developmental changes are unique for each child and do not exactly follow chronologic age, each child does pass through a regular sequential progression of anatomic, physiologic, and neurodevelopmental stages. At each stage, a child is at risk for specific injuries and will experience certain predictable responses to these traumatic forces. In addition, an injury and its treatment may influence subsequent growth and development. It is important to know and recognize these differences in growth and development for the optimal evaluation and management of pediatric trauma victims.

ANATOMICAL DIFFERENCES: GROWTH AND DEVELOPMENT
Size

Children, as pediatricians are fond of pointing out, are not just smaller versions of adults. The most obvious differences between adults and children are in size and body proportion. Growth potential varies with each individual and is affected by multiple factors including genetics, nutrition, and illness. Most children, however, grow in a predictable manner, as illustrated by standardized growth curves. These growth curves have been generated for various tissue components (Fig. 5-1). In general, weight gain is rapid during the first 3 years of life, then levels off for several years until it increases rapidly again with the adolescent growth spurt. Height follows a similar curve, although it increases less dramatically than weight during the second year of life. This rate differential contributes to the trim appearance of most toddlers and is

often referred to as the "losing of baby fat." In subsequent years, children gain weight faster than height. Thus, preadolescents are generally stocky.

Fat, which provides some protection from injury, is the most variable component of body tissue. Fat and subcutaneous tissue accumulate rapidly during the third trimester of gestation, which explains the emaciated appearance of premature infants. Fat accumulation continues after birth, subcutaneous tissue reaching a maximum thickness in children 9 months of age. This fact is reflected in the difficulty of placing peripheral intravenous lines at this age. The subcutaneous tissue gradually diminishes until children are 6 years of age, when fat accumulates again before adolescence. During adolescence, sex differences in body fat composition appear. In females the percentage of body fat increases through the late teens and eventually composes 24% of adult total body weight. In males the percentage of body fat actually falls during puberty, eventually making up only 12% of the total body weight. A newborn thus has less protective soft tissue than a 9-month-old, and the preschool child less than the adolescent.

Skeletal muscle growth follows a growth curve similar to that for weight. Muscle mass makes up about 25% of birth weight. Boys, however, subsequently have greater muscle development than girls through all ages, the difference becoming more pronounced during adolescence. Muscle mass accounts for 50% of adult male weight, as opposed to only 40% of adult female weight.

Although children have minimal lymphoid tissue at birth, this tissue grows rapidly until a child reaches 11 years of age and then atrophies in the older adolescent and adult. As a result, in an 11-year-old the mass of the lymphoid tissue is nearly double that of the lymphoid tissue in an adult. This has practical importance in management of the pediatric airway, especially in children of preschool age, in whom the tonsils and adenoids occupy a

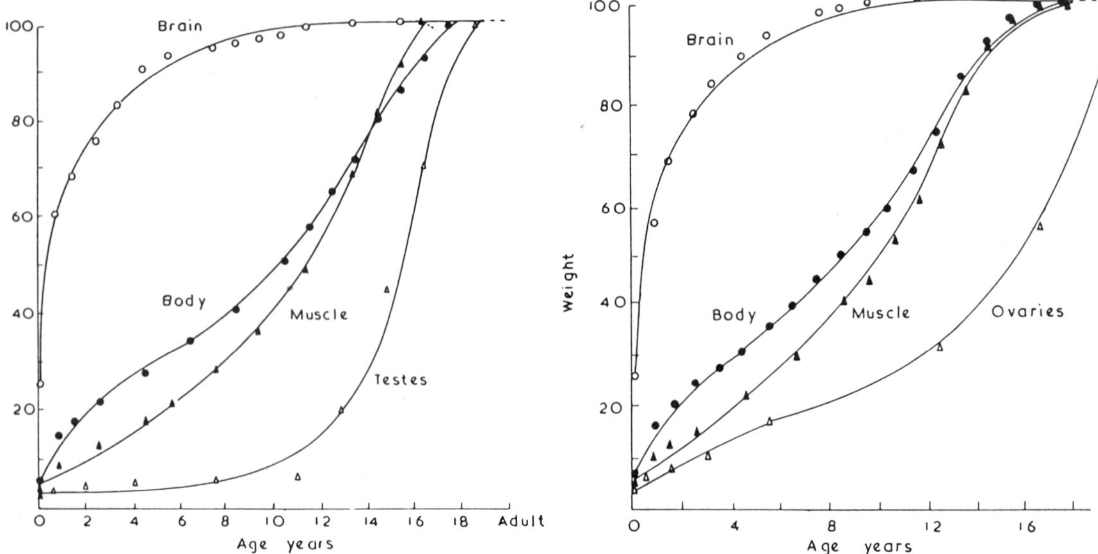

Figure 5–1 Weights of muscle, fat, and brain as the percent of body weight in males *(left)* and females *(right)*. (From Widdowson, EM: Growth of the body and its components and the influence of nutrition. In Ritzen M, et al, editors: *The biology of normal human growth*, New York, 1981, Raven Press, p 257.)

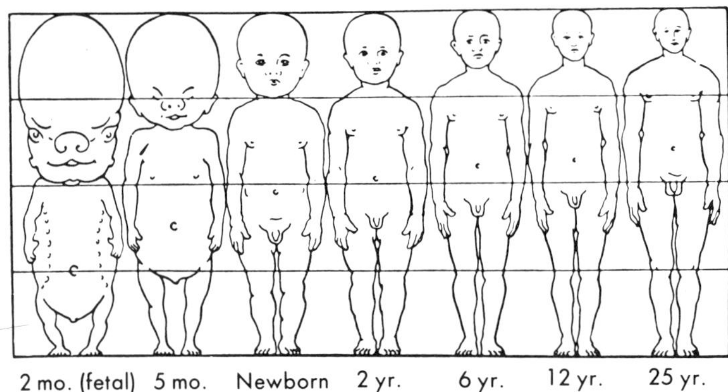

Figure 5–2 Change in relative body proportions from fetus to adult. (From Robbins et al: *Growth*, New Haven, 1928, Yale University Press.)

larger proportion of the airway than in any other age group.

Apart from changes in actual size, body proportions constantly change in the developing child (Fig. 5-2). The most obvious example is the comparatively large size of the head and the short extremities in infants. The midpoint in the height of an infant is the umbilicus, whereas the midpoint of an adult occurs at the symphysis pubis. Younger children are at increased risk of head injuries from falls and motor vehicle accidents as a result of this higher center of gravity. Because of their short stature, children are more likely to suffer abdominal, chest, or head trauma when struck by a car, whereas an adult is more likely to receive injuries of the lower extremities. Children also suffer a higher incidence of multiple organ injury from trauma than adults, because kinetic energy is dissipated into a smaller mass.

Although rapid weight increases during infancy and childhood make estimates of weight difficult, accurate estimates are essential for appropriate drug and fluid therapy. Accordingly, several methods are used to make a quick estimation of the weight of a child. The Broselow Pediatric Resuscitation Tape provides an estimate of weight based on a child's length.[8] Endotracheal tube sizes, as well as drug and fluid doses, are printed next to each length marker on the tape (Fig. 5-3). In addition, there are several rules of thumb for approximating

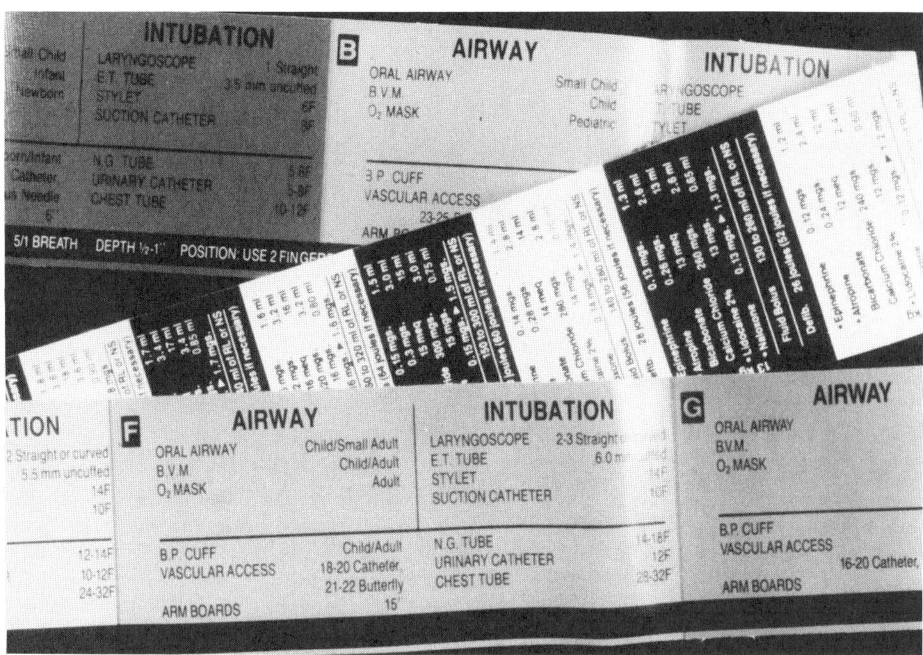

Figure 5–3 The Broselow Pediatric Resuscitation Tape.

Table 5–1 Change in relative body surface area with age

Area	Birth 1 Yr	1–4 Yr	5–9 Yr	10–14 Yr	15 Yr	Adult
Head	19	17	13	11	9	7
Neck	2	2	2	2	2	2
Ant trunk	13	13	13	13	13	13
Post trunk	13	13	13	13	13	13
R buttock	2½	2½	2½	2½	2½	2½
L buttock	2½	2½	2½	2½	2½	2½
Genitalia	1	1	1	1	1	1
R U arm	4	4	4	4	4	4
L U arm	4	4	4	4	4	4
R L arm	3	3	3	3	3	3
L L arm	3	3	3	3	3	3
R hand	2½	2½	2½	2½	2½	2½
L hand	2½	2½	2½	2½	2½	2½
R thigh	5½	6½	8	8½	9	9½
L thigh	5½	6½	8	8½	9	9½
R leg	5	5	5½	6	6½	7
L leg	5	5	5½	6	6½	7
R foot	3½	3½	3½	3½	3½	3½
L foot	3½	3½	3½	3½	3½	3½

From Fleisher G, Ludwig S, eds. Textbook of pediatric emergency medicine, ed 2. Baltimore: Williams & Wilkins, 1986, p 1056.

weights based on age. For example, the average child's birth weight will double by 5 months of age and triple by 1 year. Assuming a birth weight of 3.5 kg, 7 times the birth weight, or 25 kg, is an appropriate estimate for the average 7-year-old, and 14 times birth weight, or 50 kg, is accurate for a 14-year-old. Ten kg is also an accurate weight estimate for a 1-year-old; 15 kg, or 30 lb, for a 3-year-old; and 20 kg for a 6-year-old. Estimated weights may be interpolated for other ages.

The relative body surface area is much larger in children than in adults. This has important consequences in thermoregulation and in the evaluation and treatment of burns (Table 5-1). The commonly

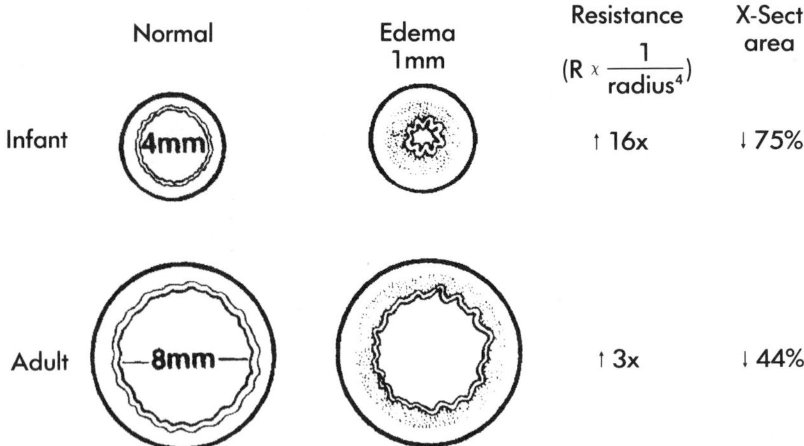

Figure 5–4 Relative effects of 1 mm of edema on airway resistance in the infant as compared with the adult. Cross-sectional area is reduced 75% in the infant airway vs 44% in the adult, resulting in a 16-fold increase in resistance in the infant vs a 3-fold increase in the adult. (From Cote CJ, Todres ID: The pediatric airway. In Ryan JF, Todres ID, Cotes CJ, et al, editors: *A practice of anesthesia for infants and children*, New York, 1986, Grune & Stratton, p 39.)

applied rule of 9s for assessing the percentage of burns in adults is accurate only in those children over 15 years of age. In infants and children, the head represents more of the total body surface area, and the lower extremities account for less of the total body surface area. A rapid estimate of the percentage of burn in a child can be obtained by using the patient's palm size as representative of 1% of the body surface area. The larger relative body surface area predisposes the child to increased heat loss through radiation, convection, and conduction. Hypothermia is poorly tolerated, especially by a critically injured child. Extreme heat loss, often found in drowning or exposure victims, can result in hypoxia, arrhythmias, progressive metabolic acidosis, and failure to respond to medications.

Airway

There are multiple anatomic differences between the pediatric and adult airways besides their respective sizes. These differences make the pediatric and infant airways more difficult to evaluate and manage, in addition to placing the child at a higher risk of airway obstruction. Minimal degrees of airway edema result in disproportionately higher resistance to flow in the child than in the adult, as demonstrated in Fig. 5-4. The mouth, pharynx, and trachea form a more acute angle in the infant and young child. The "sniffing position" provides for optimal airflow through the alignment of these structures (Fig. 5-5). The relatively large occiput tends to produce flexion of the neck in the supine child, which can subsequently obstruct the airway. Overzealous hyperextension using the head tilt maneuver will also obstruct the compliant pediatric trachea.

Endotracheal intubation is a challenging procedure in the pediatric age group for several reasons. First, the position of the larynx in the child is both more anterior and cephalad than in the adult. Second, where the adult's vocal cords are perpendicular to the trachea, the child's vocal cords are angled higher posteriorly, which makes it more difficult to pass an endotracheal tube through the cords. Third, soft tissues in this region are highly compliant and form a potential space for edema formation. Fourth, a child's epiglottis is longer and narrower and protrudes farther into the pharynx than an adult's (Fig. 5-6). Obtaining optimal exposure of the vocal cords during laryngoscopy of an infant or young child requires a lifting maneuver, with placement of the blade below the epiglottis as opposed to placement of the blade in the vallecula of adolescents and adults. A straight laryngoscope blade allows a clearer view of the airway in infants and young children, whereas a curved blade more effectively controls the tongue in older children and adults. Finally, an infant's relatively large tongue and a preschooler's hypertrophied tonsils also impede visual examination of the vocal cords.

In children under 8 years of age, the acute angle of the nasopharynx, the anterior position of the vocal cords, and the highly vascularized adenoidal tissue with its risk of bleeding combine to make nasotracheal intubation a prohibitively difficult emergency procedure that is not recommended.

The variation in airway size and structure in children of different ages necessitates a large selection

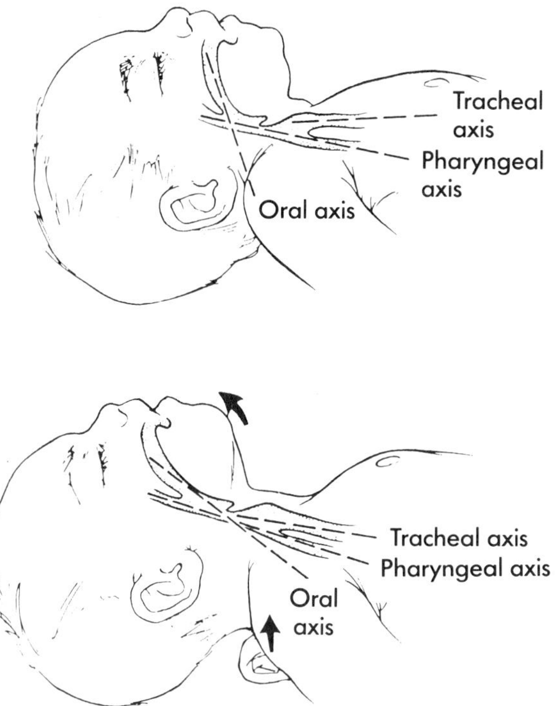

Figure 5–5 Alignment of the mouth, pharynx, and trachea in the infant. (From Chameides L, editor: *Textbook of pediatric advanced life support,* Dallas, 1988, 1990, Dallas American Heart Association, p 29. Copyright American Heart Association.)

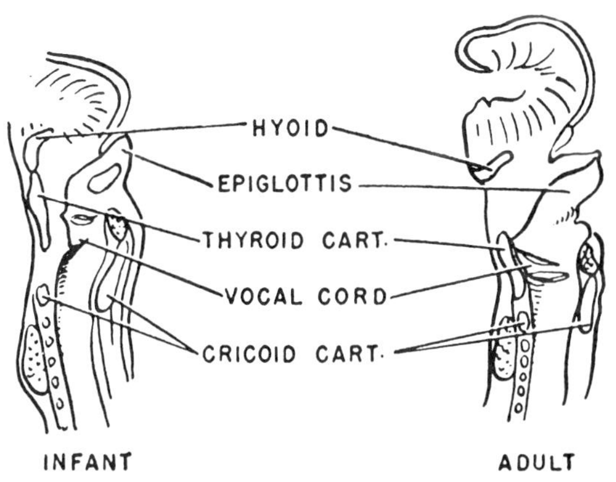

Figure 5–6 Comparison of anatomic differences between the adult and infant larynx. (From Eckenhoff J: Some anatomic considerations of the infant larynx influencing endotracheal anesthesia, *Anesthesiology.* 12(4):403, 1951.)

of airway equipment. A rapid method for estimating airway size is to use a formula (internal diameter of the endotracheal tube in millimeters equals: $\dfrac{16 + \text{age in yr}}{4}$ or to approximate the airway diameter, using the width of the small finger of the patient. Because of the shorter distance from the mouth to the carina, physicians who are more accustomed to the adult airway frequency intubate the right mainstem bronchus.

In children under the age of 8, there is an area of subglottic narrowing formed by the developing cricoid cartilage, which is the narrowest point in the airway. In older children and adults, the narrowest point in the airway occurs at the level of the vocal cords. For this reason, cuffed endotracheal tubes are rarely used in patients less than 8 years of age.

Cervical spine

Before the age of 8 there are multiple anatomic differences between the pediatric and adult spine that have an impact on the type, evaluation, and management of pediatric spinal injuries. By the time a child has reached 8 years of age, the cervical spine has essentially assumed adult characteristics.

In a young child or infant, the larger relative mass of the head provides increased momentum in acceleration-deceleration injuries such as those caused by motor vehicle accidents or seen in the shaken baby syndrome resulting from child abuse. Combined with the lack of muscle strength in the

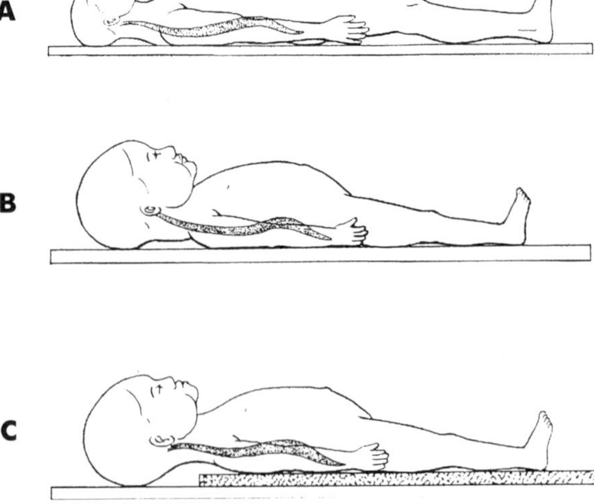

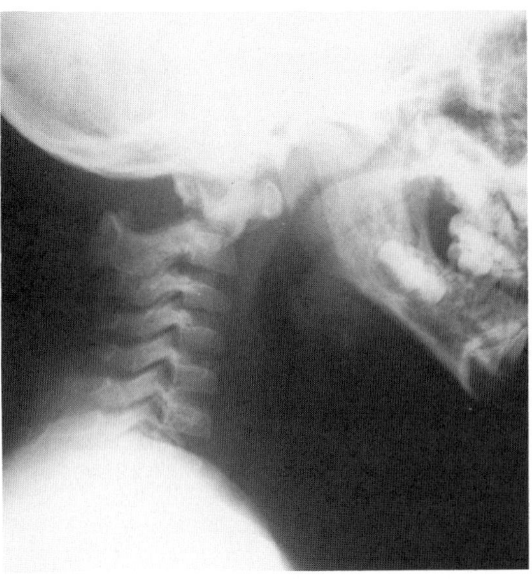

Figure 5–7 Adult (**A**) and young child (**B**), immobilized on standard backboard; **C**, young child immobilized on modified backboard demonstrating improved cervical alignment. (From Herzenberg JE et al: Emergency transport and positioning of young children who have an injury of the cervical spine, *J Bone Joint Surg* 71-A:16, 21, 1989.)

Figure 5–8 Fracture of the odontoid process with anterior angulation in a 3½-year-old child.

neck of a small child, such momentum results in greater stress to the cervical spine region. This stress also occurs at a higher level of the pediatric spine. The fulcrum of cervical mobility in the infant or young child is at the C2-3 level, whereas in the adult it occurs between C5-6 and C6-7. This is demonstrated by the fact that 60% to 70% of pediatric fractures occur in C1 or C2, as opposed to only 16% of adult cervical spine fractures.[5]

In the clinical evaluation of adults with suspected cervical injuries, the coherent patient with an unstable spinal injury generally will not permit a passive range of motion, which would jeopardize neurologic function. The inadequate muscle strength in the neck of an infant or young child makes this form of evaluation particularly hazardous. The examiner must be sure to avoid exacerbating injuries as a result of the examination. Consequently, immobilization is imperative before radiologic diagnosis of younger children. A rigid pediatric or infant collar appropriate to the size of the child provides the best immobilization.

Motion can be further limited by anchoring the forehead, maxilla, and body to a full or half spine board with tape. The standard backboard may need to be modified for infants and children. The pronounced occiput and small chest diameter in children of these ages results in excessive flexion while they are in the supine position.[6] A roll beneath the shoulders or an additional pad supporting the trunk provides a more neutral alignment of the cervical spine (Fig. 5-7).

The ligamentous laxity of the pediatric spine may partially account for the fact that cervical spine fractures are less common in infants and young children than in adolescents and adults. Unstable fractures in pediatric patients are associated with severe trauma. The most common etiologies are motor vehicle crashes, falls, and sports injuries. Additional causes include obstetric complications and child abuse.

The two most common cervical injuries seen in pediatrics are fractures of the odontoid process with atlanto-axial dislocation and subluxation (Fig. 5-8), and fracture of the neural arch of the axis, which is commonly known as a "hangman's fracture." Predisposition of the pediatric spine to these fractures can be attributed to the higher fulcrum and the inherent weakness of the growth plate at the base of the dens.

Reliance on roentgenograms for the diagnosis of cervical spine injuries in children entails certain hazards. Of greatest concern is that ligamentous laxity and excessive spinal mobility can predispose a child to significant spinal cord injury, including transection, without x-ray evidence of cervical spine fractures or dislocation.

Several anatomic variants in the pediatric cervical spine may be misinterpreted as actual injuries. A phenomenon known as pseudosubluxation often causes confusion. Pseudosubluxation refers to the anterior displacement of C2 onto C3 with flexion (Fig. 5-9). This finding on a lateral x-ray suggests a fracture or ligamentous tear in the adult, but can be seen as a normal variant in up to 20% of young children.[1] The anatomic correlation is based on three findings. First, the intervertebral ligamentous

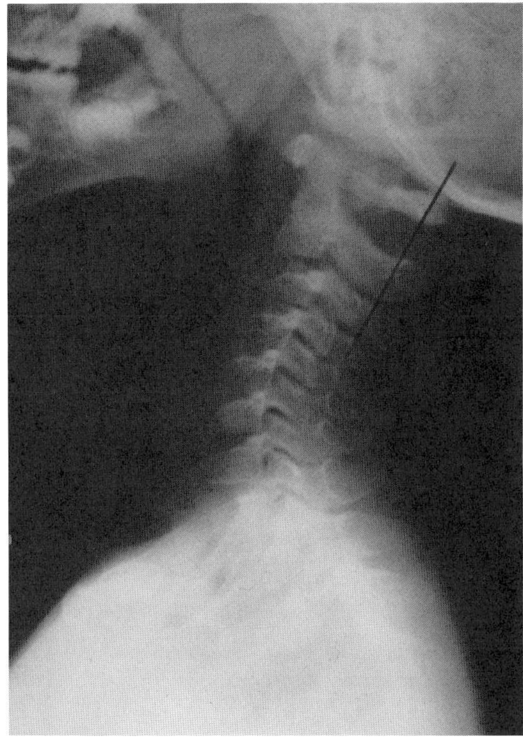

Figure 5–9 Pseudosubluxation of the cervical spine with anterior displacement of the body of C2 on C3 with flexion. Posterior cervical line passes throughout anterior cortex of C2, confirming this as a normal physiologic variant.

Table 5–2 Upper normal limits of cervical spine measurements in adults and children

	Adults	Children
Predental space	2.5 mm	4–5 mm
C2-3 override (flexion)	3 mm	4–5 mm
Prevertebral space (extension)	7 mm	½–⅔ AP distance vertebral body

laxity allows a certain degree of hypermobility of the spine. Second, the vertebrae are wedged anteriorly, allowing one vertebrae to slide onto another. Third, the articular facets are more horizontal. Altogether, this allows as much as 4 mm of override of C2 onto C3 with flexion and, to a lesser degree, of C3 onto C4. Although pseudosubluxation often corrects with a normal degree of lordosis, this position can be difficult to achieve in a young child because of immature musculature, lack of cooperation, muscle spasm, or distortion by the cervical collar. The flattened facets may also predispose a child to actual subluxation in minor trauma. Rotary subluxation can occur in the toddler through a forceful rotation of the head to one side.

The anterior wedging of pediatric vertebral bodies is often mistaken for a compression fracture. Several synchondroses visible on pediatric cervical spine films may simulate fractures. The growth plate at the base of the odontoid process is present at birth and closes between 3 and 6 years of age. It is frequently visible on a lateral x-ray and commonly misinterpreted as a fracture. Four additional synchondroses are present in the axis, any one of which may be mistaken for a fracture. When seen together in an oblique view, these may appear as a Jefferson fracture. Superior and inferior annular ring epiphyses of the vertebral bodies develop during puberty and fuse by 25 years of age. These can resemble avulsion or teardrop fractures.

Enlargement of the prevertebral space beyond 2.5 mm in the adult suggests injury to the anterior spinal ligament or vertebral body with subsequent edema or hematoma formation. It is more difficult to accurately assess this space in a child than in an adult because of the variability of its size. In a child the maximum normal prevertebral space is 7 mm, or one half to two thirds the antero-posterior diameter of a vertebral body above the glottis, 14 mm being within the normal range for the space below the glottis (Table 5-2).[9] The prevertebral space increases further with crying, exhalation, or the presence of adenoidal tissue. True injury commonly has clinical correlation and evidence of airway compression.

The distance of the anterior arch of the atlas to the odontoid process, or the "predental space," is commonly used to evaluate suspected injuries of the odontoid process. The laxity of the atlanto-axial and the transverse ligament of the axis can result in an increased predental space in children under 8 years old (Fig. 5-10). This distance is further exaggerated with flexion and can extend to 5 mm in normal children, as compared with only 2.5 mm in uninjured adults.[9]

A conservative management approach is essential when dealing with a suspected cervical injury in a pediatric trauma victim, given (1) the difficulty of clinically evaluating young children and (2) the problems inherent in interpreting radiologic findings that suggest fractures at sites of normal anatomic variants.

Head

Head injury is the most common cause of death in the pediatric trauma victim. Anatomic differences affect the response of the child to the injury, as well as the type of injury likely to be inflicted.

Head injuries are common in the types of accident to which children are prone. The relatively large size of the head in a child makes it an obvious target for injury.

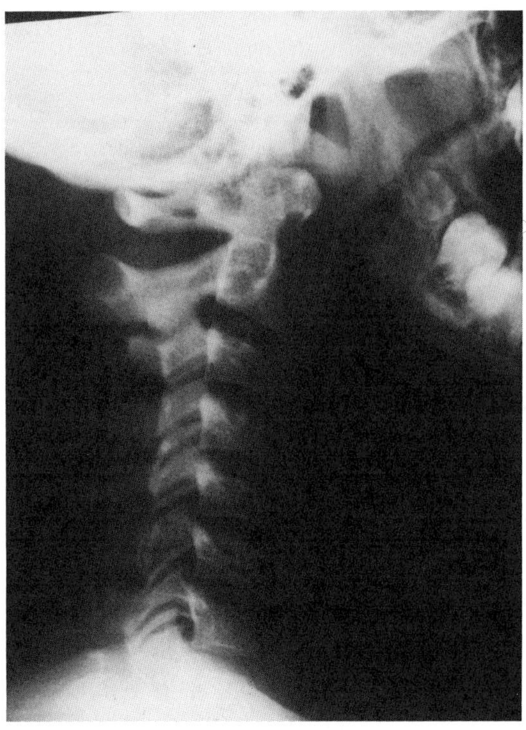

Figure 5–10 Normal cervical spine film of a 7-year-old child with a predental space of 4 mm.

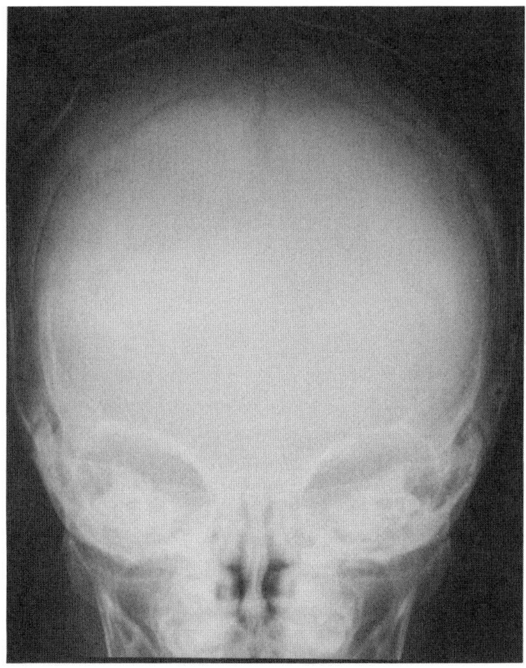

Figure 5–11 Ping-Pong fracture of the skull in a newborn.

The soft tissues, skull, and brain are significantly more compliant in children than in adults. The remarkable pliability of the infant skull is demonstrated by the "Ping-Pong" fracture in the newborn (Fig. 5-11) and the low incidence of skull fractures as compared with adults. Fontanelles and sutures remain open until an average age of 16 months, adding to the compliance and providing a natural escape valve for elevations in intracranial pressure. As a result, infants initially may be more tolerant of an increase in intracranial pressure and can have delayed signs.

The severity of head trauma is more difficult to assess in pediatric patients than in adult patients. The Glasgow Coma Score is inadequate for the infant who has yet to develop verbal skills and certain motor abilities. A modified infant version has been produced, but this, too, remains less accurate and results are less reproducible than in the adult version (Table 5-3).

Serious intracranial hemorrhage is less common in pediatric patients with head trauma than in adults and, when present, suggests an increased severity of brain injury. This may be caused, in part, by the fact that the middle meningeal artery in young children does not fit tightly into a groove of the skull as it does in adults. As a result, the artery is more mobile and less susceptible to shearing forces. When epidural hemorrhage occurs in children, it often is not accompanied by skull fracture. X-rays are, therefore, not helpful in detecting such injuries.

A subdural bleeding portends a worse prognosis in children than in adults, not on the basis of the bleed, but rather because the bleed suggests increased severity of brain injury. Although not a common cause of shock, a subdural bleed in an infant can result in anemia, and even hypotension, as the result of the compliance of the cranial vault and the lower total body blood volume.

The thinner and more compliant cranial bones provide less protection in the child, allowing more of an impact to be transmitted to the brain. Acute diffuse brain swelling as a result of head injury is more common in children. Intracranial hypertension and its sequelae are more likely to develop despite the initial protection provided by the compliant skull.

Skeletal system

Properties of the developing skeletal system predispose the child to unique injuries in response to trauma. The two major anatomic features accounting for these properties are the presence of growth plates and a cortex more porous than that of the adult.

Lengthwise growth of long bones in children occurs at the growth plate or physis, which may

Table 5–3 Glasgow Coma Scale, modified for infants

Glasgow Coma Scale			Modified coma score for infants		
Activity	**Best response**	**Score**	**Activity**	**Best response**	**Score**
Eye opening	Spontaneous	4	Eye opening	Spontaneous	4
	To verbal stimuli	3		To speech	3
	To pain*	2		To pain	2
	None	1		None	1
Verbal	Oriented	5	Verbal	Coos, babbles	5
	Confused	4		Irritable cries	4
	Inappropriate words	3		Cries to pain	3
	Nonspecific sounds	2		Moans to pain	2
	None	1		None	1
Motor	Follows commands	6	Motor	Normal spontaneous movements	6
	Localizes pain	5		Withdraws to touch	5
	Withdraws to pain	4		Withdraws to pain	4
	Flexion to pain	3		Abnormal flexion	3
	Extension to pain	2		Abnormal extension	2
	None	1		None	1

*Indicates response to painful stimulus applied to child.

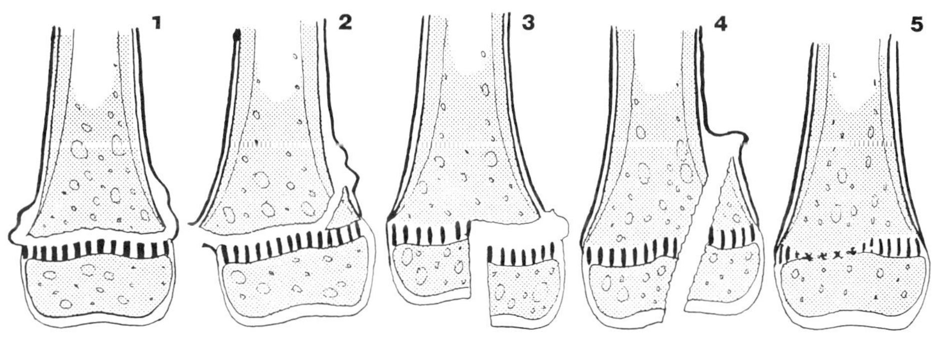

Figure 5–12 The Salter-Harris classification of pediatric growth plate fractures. (From Salter RB, Harris WR: Injuries involving the epiphyseal plate, *J Bone Joint Surg* 45-A:587, 1963.)

be located at one or both ends of the bone. The physis is composed of cartilaginous elements separating the diaphysis from the epiphysis. The periosteum continues past the physis and forms a tough perichondrial ring, which stabilizes the epiphysis on the diaphysis. Without careful clinical evaluation, use of comparison views of opposite extremities, and use of references of normal radiologic variants, the physis can be mistaken for a fracture. Alternatively, true fractures at normal growth centers are often overlooked. The physis is the weakest point in the bone and the most likely to be injured. The surrounding ligaments, joint capsules, and tendons are stronger than the physis and, as a result, a child with an open physis is more likely to sustain a fracture through the growth plate than a sprain or dislocation.

Fractures through the growth plate are categorized according to the Salter-Harris classification, as illustrated in Fig. 5-12. In a Salter I fracture the perichondral ring remains intact and displacement is not commonly seen on x-ray. Whereas stress views to accentuate the fracture or comparison views may be helpful, the diagnosis is based on the finding of point tenderness over the growth plate. A Salter II fracture is the result of a tear of the perichondral ring on one side with the avulsion of a piece of the metaphysis on the opposite side. Salter IV and V fractures have the worst prognosis. They can cause growth arrest, which results in a disparity of limb length in a growing child and, in turn, may result in significant future disability.

The results of knee trauma illustrate how these differences between the pediatric and adult skeletal system predispose the patient to different types of injury. In the knee, as elsewhere in a child's body, the ligaments are stronger than the bones, which in turn are stronger than the growth plates. There-

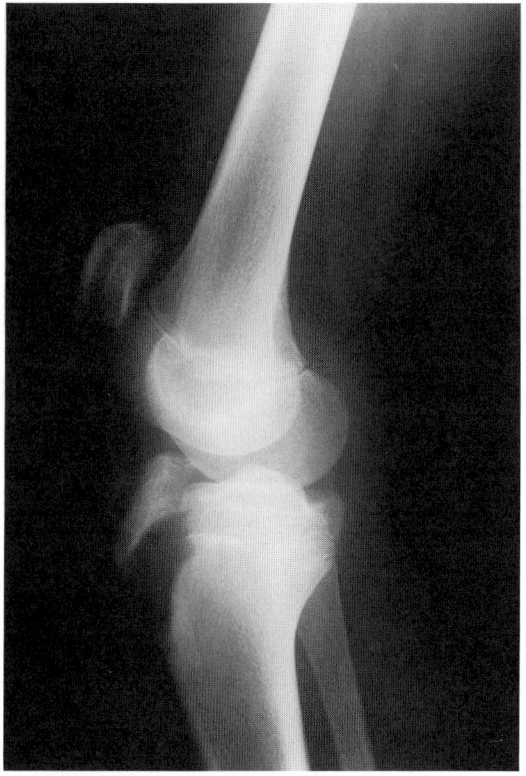

Figure 5–13 Salter IV fracture of the proximal tibia in a 13-year-old boy as the result of excessive force by the patella tendon. The fracture fragment is displaced anteriorly and superiorly resulting in superior dislocation of the patella.

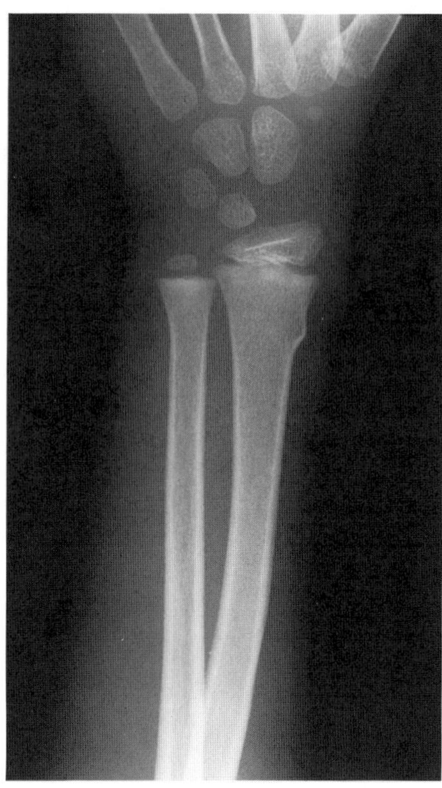

Figure 5–14 Torus or buckle fracture of the distal radius in a 5-year-old boy.

fore a sprain or injury to a ligament without a fracture is exceedingly rare in pediatric trauma. A mechanism that causes a ligament to rupture in an adult causes an avulsion or epiphyseal fracture in a child or adolescent.

In a child's knee, the medial and collateral ligaments originate from the distal femoral epiphysis and insert distal to the proximal tibial epiphysis. Consequently, the tibial physis is protected from varus or valgus forces, whereas the femoral epiphysis is at greater risk of injury from these same forces. Fracture through the distal femoral physis is, therefore, relatively common in childhood up until the time that the growth plates close. Forces that cause a cruciate ligament tear in the adult cause fracture of the tibial spine in children. Although the tibial epiphysis is protected from lateral stresses, it remains at risk for injury from stress on the patellar tendon. Both avulsion of the tibial tubercle and fracture through the proximal growth plate of the tibia occur in adolescent athletes as the result of excessive contraction of the quadriceps against force (Fig. 5-13).

Patellar injury is rare in children. Avulsion fracture of the patella occurs with sufficient tension from the quadriceps. A bipartite patella, which is a normal variant often seen in children less than 10 years of age, is easily confused with a fracture. A bipartite patella is usually bilateral and can often be ruled out by a comparison x-ray of the opposite knee.

The examination of an injured knee is more difficult in a child than in an adult. A child has a lower threshold for the pain caused by manipulation and a poorer ability to localize the pain. The physician should assume that a fracture exists when evaluating a traumatic injury to the knee of a child or adolescent until evidence proves otherwise. Although an x-ray of the knee may yield normal findings, an effusion or instability in the joint indicates the need for stress views or arthroscopy to rule out a self-reduced epiphyseal fracture.

The rapid growth of the periosteum in young children adds width to the bone. The periosteum is thicker in children than in adults, and the cortex has a higher concentration of Haversian canals, resulting in more porous bone. This anatomy, however, does not protect the child from significant

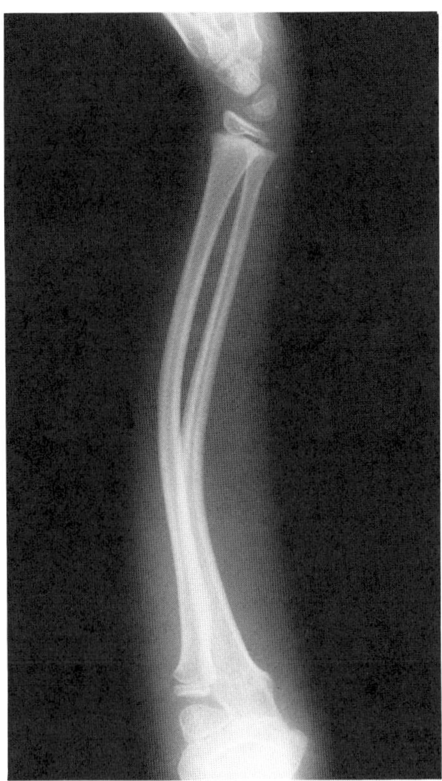

Figure 5–15 Bowing fractures of the radius and ulna in a 3-year-old child.

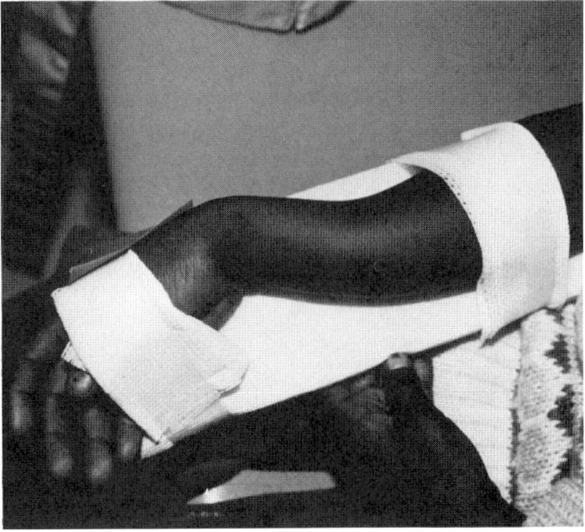

Figure 5–16 Forearm of a young girl with bowing fractures as the result of a shopping cart injury.

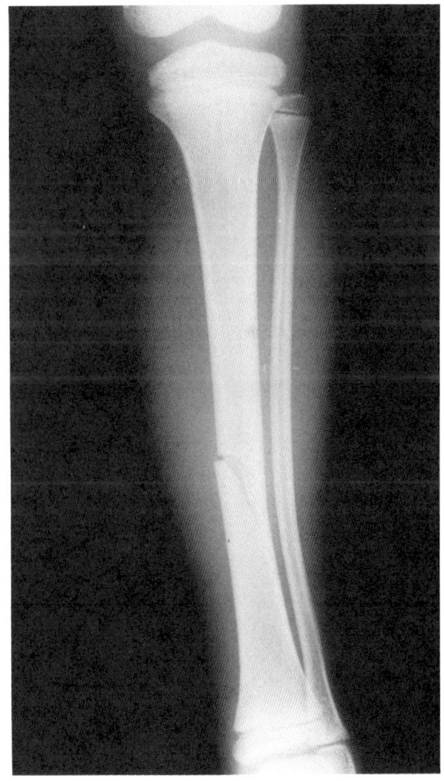

Figure 5–17 Greenstick fracture of the tibia with an associated bowing fracture of the fibula.

blood loss associated with fractures of the shaft of the femur. Blood loss from injured vessels within the bone, torn arteries, or muscles occasionally exceeds 500 ml. The porosity and the lack of ossified material results in the increased compliance of pediatric bones and an ability to tolerate greater deformation than adult bones. This resiliency provides less protection to internal structures. Significant viscous injury can occur in the infant or young child that may not be appreciated by x-ray. Chest contusion and laceration of the liver and spleen can occur in children without evidence of overlying rib fracture.

Certain fractures are found exclusively in children. The torus or buckle fracture is a folding or compression of the cortex without actual evidence of a break (Fig. 5-14). A bending or bowing fracture is also a distortion of the bone without evidence of cortical disruption (Figs. 5-15 and 5-16). Greater force produces a greenstick fracture, which consists of a bending fracture with a break in the cortex of the convex side (Fig. 5-17). These fractures are most common in toddlers and early school-aged children, but can be seen up to the early teenage years.

Rapid periosteal growth accounts for the remarkable ability of pediatric bone to remodel following injury. The younger the child and the closer the fracture to the physis, the greater the potential

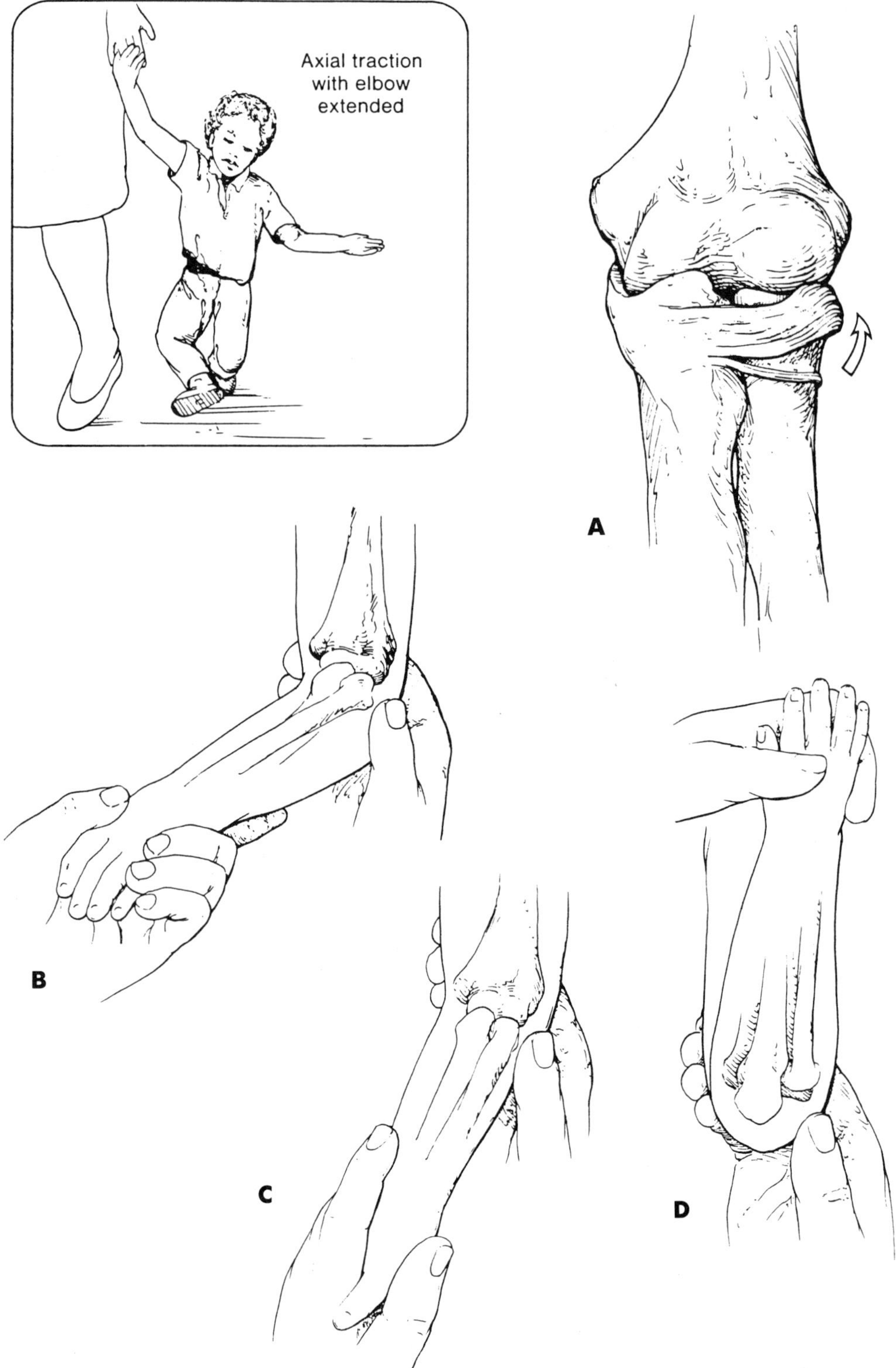

Figure 5–18 Nursemaid's elbow. Excessive traction *(upper left)* resulting in interposition of torn annular ligament between capitellum and radial head (**A**). Reduction involves grasping the wrist and elbow with thumb over the annular ligament (**B**) followed by supination (**C**) and flexion (**D**). (From Fleisher G, Ludwig S, editors: *Textbook of pediatric emergency medicine*, ed 2, Baltimore, 1988, Williams & Wilkins, p 1322.)

of the bone to remold malunions. In some instances, up to 30 degrees of angulation can be corrected through remodeling. The ability of bone to remodel diminishes as a child grows. A femur fracture requires only 2 weeks to heal in a newborn, 4 weeks in a young child, and up to 8 to 10 weeks in an adolescent.

Subluxation of the radial head, or "nursemaid's elbow," is another uniquely pediatric injury resulting from sudden longitudinal traction on the wrist of a child under age 5 (Fig. 5-18). This mechanism results in a tear of the annular ligament which, because of its laxity in this age group, becomes caught between the capitellum and the radial head. The initial presentation is often confusing as the child refuses to move the arm and has difficulty localizing the pain; x-ray examination is unrevealing. The subluxation is easily reduced through supination and flexion at the elbow once a fracture has been ruled out. The injury does not occur in children over 5 years of age because annular ligaments in older children are thicker and stronger and will not tear.

Abdomen

Injury to a child's abdomen results more frequently from blunt, rather than penetrating, trauma. The pediatric abdomen affords less protection from this type of injury than the adult abdomen. The abdominal wall is thinner, with less muscle and subcutaneous tissue. The liver and spleen are the most commonly injured abdominal viscera. They are proportionately larger in children than in adults, and are thus more exposed below the rib cage. Furthermore, the absence of rib fractures does not rule out significant splenic or liver injury in pediatric trauma victims, because of the increased compliance of the bones in this age group.

Other organs are also more predisposed to injury in a child than in an adult. The kidney is located more anteriorly and contains less perinephric fat as protection; more of the bladder is exposed in the abdomen of a child. Duodenal hematoma, disproportionately more common in children than in adults, may be a result of the increased lordosis, the decreased anterior-to-posterior abdominal diameter, and the lack of rib cage protection.

In infants, gastric distension, as a result of aerophagia, can result in a tense abdomen mimicking an acute process and impinging upon the diaphragm. Gastric decompression with a nasogastric tube may calm the infant, allow improved chest expansion, and improve the sensitivity of the abdominal examination.

Because menarche occurs at an average age of 13, pregnancy should not be a concern solely in adult trauma victims. Vaginal bleeding in the adolescent female is always an indication to test for pregnancy.

Straddle injuries are the most common cause of genital trauma in young girls. Such injuries are most likely to cause bruising and bleeding that are visible in an external examination. Sexual abuse must be considered in the young female with vaginal injury, and an examination under general anesthesia is often indicated for evaluation and treatment of persistent vaginal bleeding.

Circulatory system

The heart of a 5-year-old child is anatomically and physiologically equivalent to the heart of a small, healthy adult. There are, however, pronounced differences between the heart of a newborn and that of an adult that diminish during the course of normal development. The left ventricle and right ventricle are the same size at birth. In early development, the left ventricle, left atrium, and aorta all increase linearly with age. The right ventricle grows less rapidly, and by 2 months of age the left ventricle is twice the size of the right ventricle. This differential growth is a response to the increased volume of blood flow and afterload to which the left ventricle is subjected after birth.

The young heart has a relatively limited functional capacity when compared with the adult heart. This is partially the result of differences in microstructure. Myofibrils are arranged in a disorganized manner, and contractile proteins make up only 30% of cell volume in the infant heart, as compared with 60% in adult heart cells. This limits the extent of fibril shortening and ultimately the ventricular compliance of the immature heart.

Anatomic differences are reflected in the functional capacity of the infant and the adult hearts. The young heart is less compliant. Stroke volume reaches a plateau at low filling pressures in the immature heart, which shifts the Starling curve to the left. The young heart is more sensitive to volume or pressure overload than the healthy adult heart and is at greater risk of failure from either cause. Cardiac output is almost completely dependent on the heart rate until the heart has reached adult proportions. Although the immature heart is capable of maintaining higher rates than the adult heart, functional capacity remains lower and progressively increases with age.

The heart of a newborn or infant has a higher tolerance from hypoxemia than the adult heart as a result of the increased capacity of ventricular muscle mitochondria for anaerobic glycolysis. This tolerance, however, is limited to a certain extent by the higher myocardial oxygen consumption in the infant heart and the decreased ability of the peripheral vessels to compensate for hypoxia. The

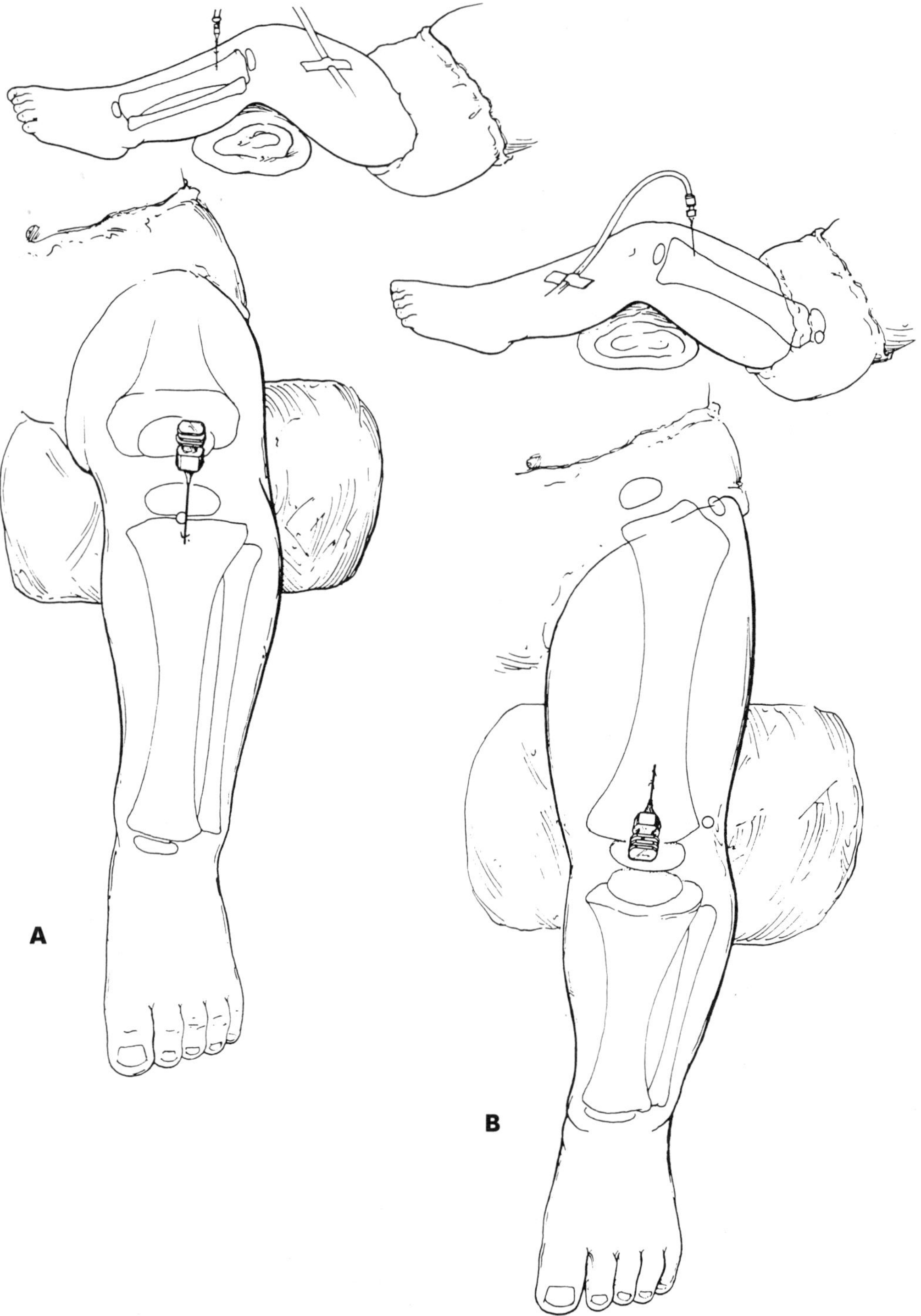

Figure 5–19 Intraosseous line placement in the proximal tibia **(A)** and distal femur **(B)**. (From Fleisher G, Ludwig S, editors: *Textbook of pediatric emergency medicine*, ed 2, Baltimore, 1988, Williams & Wilkins, p 1268.)

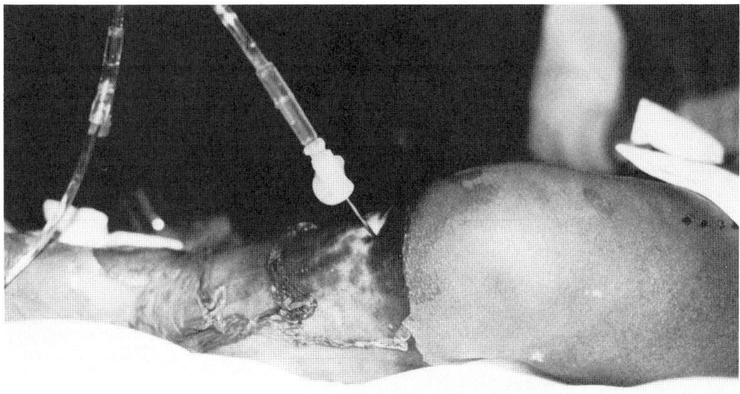

Figure 5–20 Intraosseous line infusing fluids into the proximal tibia of a young burn victim.

immature heart and peripheral vessels have a diminished number of sympathetic fibers and, consequently, are less responsive to sympathetic nerve stimulation. The parasympathetic system, however, is more fully developed in the infant. Clinically, this accounts for the relative increase in vagal tone, the differential response to certain pharmacologic agents, and the immature response of the circulatory system to stress in the infant.

The most obvious differences between the adult and pediatric circulatory systems are in vessel size and blood volume. What would be considered relatively small blood losses in an adult may lead to critical hypovolemia in a child. Although it may be crucial to obtain intravenous access in a critically ill infant or child, such access may be exceedingly difficult to achieve and is frequently the time-limiting step in pediatric resuscitation. Vessel size limits the gauge of intravenous catheters, often to 24 peripherally and 22 centrally in the infant. Flow rate is subsequently restricted, and maintenance of the line is more difficult. Subcutaneous tissue further interferes with visualization of peripheral sites. Access to the jugular veins is compromised by the short, stubby neck of the infant and must await stabilization of the airway, leaving the femoral veins as the first choice for cannulation once peripheral attempts have failed. Children also have a greater risk of complications from central line placement than adults. For instance, their smaller size predisposes them to pneumothorax with jugular or subclavian line placement.

There are alternative sites for venous access in the infant. A frequently overlooked site is the umbilical vein in the infant under 2 weeks of age. Scalp veins, although not the first choice, are often more visible and are a common site of peripheral access.

Intraosseous lines have recently been revived as a rapid means of obtaining access in the critically ill child (Fig. 5-19). Initially recommended only in children under 3 years of age, the use of intraosseous lines is now accepted in older children as well. Placement in children under 3 years of age is generally in the anterior tibial plateau (Fig. 5-20), and in children over 3 years in the medial malleolus. The distal femur and the iliac crest are acceptable alternative sites. Care is necesssary to avoid injury to the physis during placement, as this could lead to future growth abnormalities. Besides specially made intraosseous needles, bone marrow needles, spinal needles, and even butterfly needles can be used to pass through the porous bone of the child. The intraosseous line has proven effective in infusing drugs as well as fluids with flow rates of over 100 ml/hr.[10] Advantages over central lines include speed of access and a minimal rate of complications. The low fat content of marrow in children may account for the lack of fat emboli complicating the procedure. Blood obtained on initial aspiration is useful for determining electrolyte values, hematocrit levels, blood type, as well as for cross matching blood and blood culture.

Intravenous access remains a difficult problem in young children. Because of anatomical differences, however, alternative means of access are available in children that are not available in adults.

NEUROCOGNITIVE GROWTH AND DEVELOPMENT

As the child progresses through stages of physical growth and anatomic change, there are concomitant changes in neurologic, cognitive, and personality development. It is important to understand how these differences play a part in the etiology of injury and the management of the child who has sustained trauma injury (Table 5-4).

A brief review of the Denver Developmental Screening Test (Fig. 5-21) gives an overview of neurologic development during the first 4 years of

Table 5–4 Effects of growth and development on etiology and management of injury

Age (yr)	Period	Trauma type	Communication pattern	Management concepts
Birth–1	Dependency	Abuse Neglect MVA-passenger	Tactile Preverbal	Meet needs
1–2	Individuation	Exploration injury Abuse	Receptive language good Expressive language poor	Use parental contact
2–4	Imitative	MVA-pedestrian Fires Falls	Expressive language excellent Fantasy life rich	Use fantasy and make-believe
5–9	Competence	MVA-pedestrian Sports injury	Mature language Understanding of concepts, including death	Describe mechanics Project outcome
10–14	Peer oriented	MVA-pedestrian, passenger Inflicted trauma Suicide	Mature language "Slang"	Use adult communication Childlike reassurance
15–19	Young adult	MVA-driver, passenger Inflicted trauma Suicide	"Adult" interaction	Use informed consent Decision making

life. Although this test is constructed to screen for developmental delay, it provides an easy listing of neurologic milestones in the areas of gross motor development, fine motor development, and higher cognitive functions such as social interaction and language development.

Through the first year of life the newborn (first 28 days) and infant (first 12 months) can best be described as "dependent." Even at the moment of birth the newborn is equipped with some competency; however, overall the period is marked by dependence on the surrounding environment for survival. Neurologic skills are not complete but progress rapidly. Infants require help with most body functions including eating, temperature regulation, protection, and communication. For the most part, these dependency needs are met, but in some cases they are not and the dependency of the infant makes him or her highly vulnerable.

The major mechanisms of trauma during this period are those resulting from injuries at the hands of abusive parents or those that result from neglect or inadequate supervision, such as in falls, fires, bathtub drownings, or accidents to unrestrained motor vehicle occupants.

In caring for an injured infant, one must recall all the dependency needs of the patient. Because infants are unable to speak for themselves, the health care team must anticipate their needs. When feasible, it is important to involve parents at the earliest possible point in the process.

By the second year of life, basic neurologic competency is in place; a child has the ability to walk, use of the hands for exploration, and a sense of autonomy. This period may be called the period of "individuation." Indeed, some of the trauma that occurs in this period is caused by the child's need to express his or her individuality. Thus, trauma results from exploratory behavior, for example, touching or biting electrical wires, ingesting pills or other toxins, and a period of individual defiance that is commonly called "the terrible twos." This period begins in the second year of life and may continue for the next year or two and accounts for a certain amount of caregiver-inflicted trauma.

Although *individuation* is the watchword of the period when the child is under stress or injured, parental presence is required to decrease fears and anxiety. Illness or injury leads to psychological regression. During this period dependency behaviors may again predominate. At times a vestige of the past, such as a special toy, blanket, or pacifier, will be of comfort. As to language development, receptive abilities are far more developed than are expressive abilities. Talking to the child victim is important and helpful even though there may not be any interactive verbal response.

Through years 2 to 5, the developmental period may be characterized by the term *imitative*. During this time neurologic development has proceeded to the point where children can imitate adult behaviors. They do not yet have the appropriate judgment to go with their new-found motor skills. Initiative behavior and the fantasy life of the toddler may lead to a variety of different mechanisms of injury, for example, falls, cooking fires, unintentional

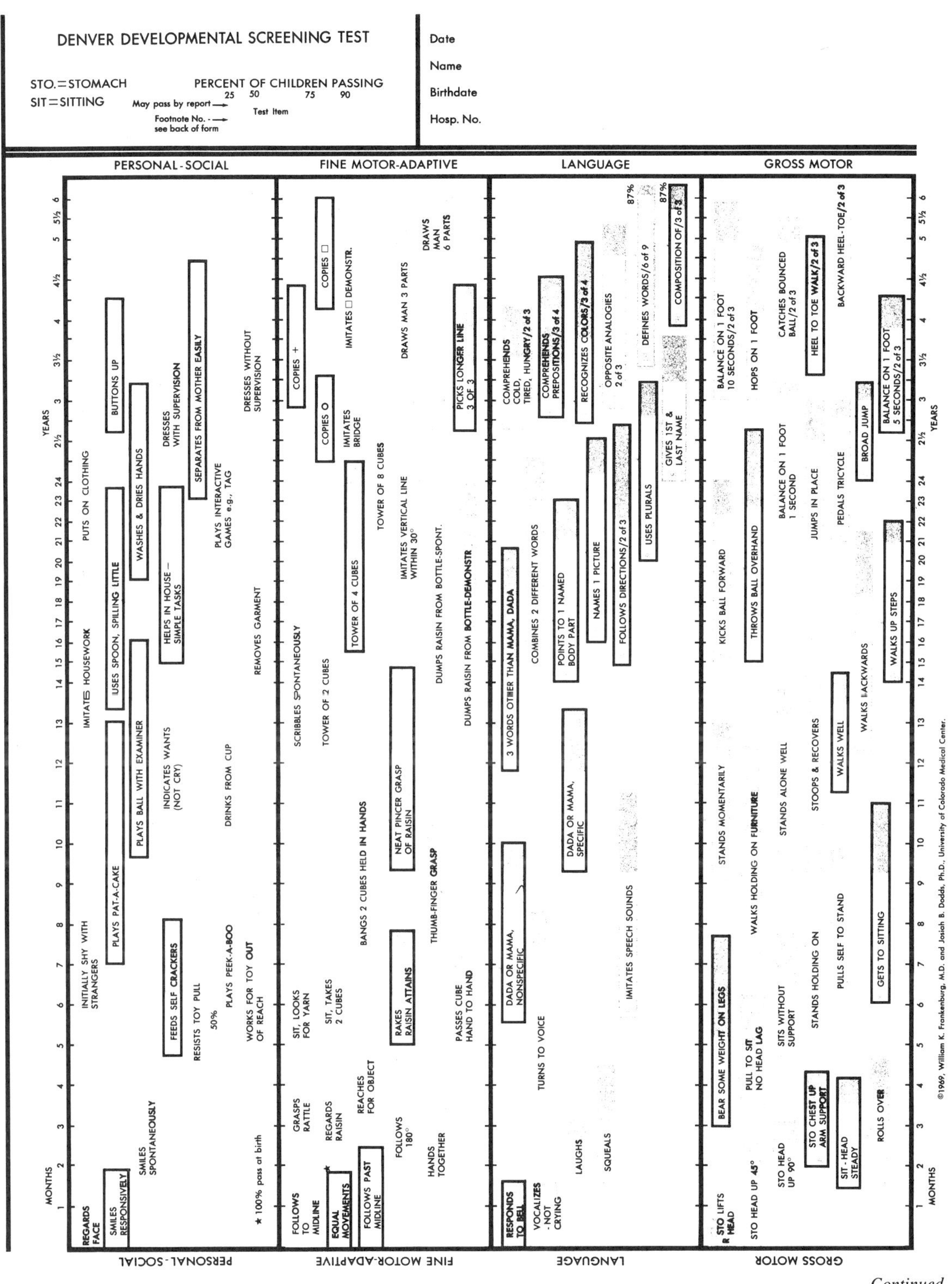

Continued.

Figure 5–21 Denver Developmental Screening Test. (© 1969, William K. Frankenburg and Josiah B. Dodds, University of Colorado Medical Center.)

<pre>
                                    DATE
                                    NAME
              DIRECTIONS   BIRTHDATE
                                    HOSP. NO.
</pre>

1. Try to get child to smile by smiling, talking or waving to him. Do not touch him.
2. When child is playing with toy, pull it away from him. Pass if he resists.
3. Child does not have to be able to tie shoes or button in the back.
4. Move yarn slowly in an arc from one side to the other, about 6" above child's face.
   Pass if eyes follow 90° to midline. (Past midline; 180°)
5. Pass if child grasps rattle when it is touched to the backs or tips of fingers.
6. Pass if child continues to look where yarn disappeared or tries to see where it went. Yarn
   should be dropped quickly from sight from tester's hand without arm movement.
7. Pass if child picks up raisin with any part of thumb and a finger.
8. Pass if child picks up raisin with the ends of thumb and index finger using an over hand
   approach.

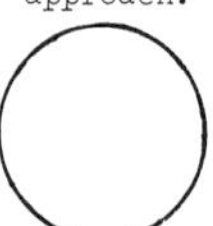 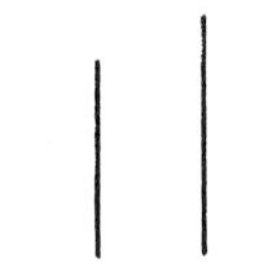 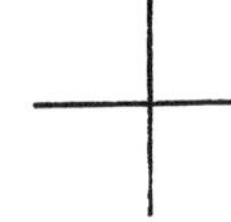 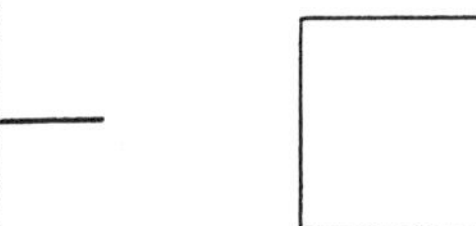

9. Pass any en-   10. Which line is longer?   11. Pass any   12. Have child copy
   closed form.   (Not bigger.) Turn   crossing   first. If failed,
   Fail continuous   paper upside down and   lines.   demonstrate
   round motions.   repeat. (3/3 or 5/6)

   When giving items 9, 11 and 12, do not name the forms. Do not demonstrate 9 and 11.

13. When scoring, each pair (2 arms, 2 legs, etc.) counts as one part.
14. Point to picture and have child name it. (No credit is given for sounds only.)

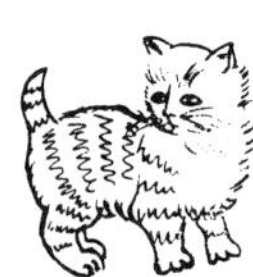 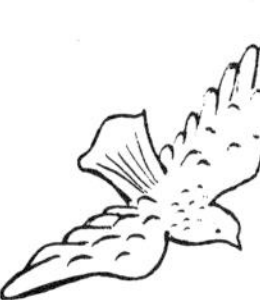 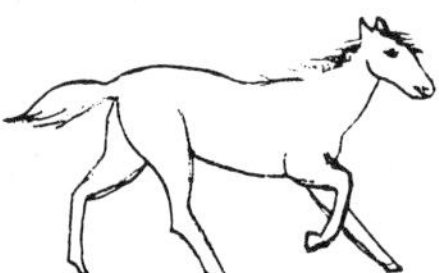 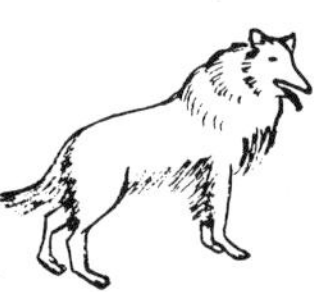 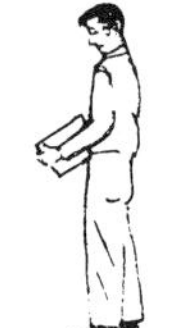

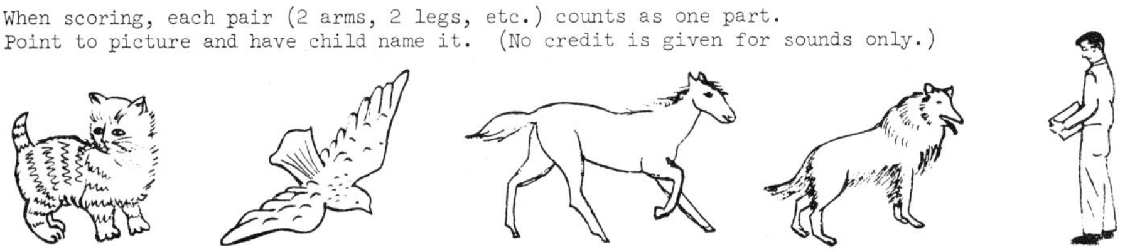

15. Tell child to: Give block to Mommie; put block on table; put block on floor. Pass 2 of 3.
    (Do not help child by pointing, moving head or eyes.)
16. Ask child: What do you do when you are cold? ..hungry? ..tired? Pass 2 of 3.
17. Tell child to: Put block <u>on</u> table; <u>under</u> table; <u>in front</u> of chair, <u>behind</u> chair.
    Pass 3 of 4. (Do not help child by pointing, moving head or eyes.)
18. Ask child: If fire is hot, ice is ?; Mother is a woman, Dad is a ?; a horse is big, a
    mouse is ?. Pass 2 of 3.
19. Ask child: What is a ball? ..lake? ..desk? ..house? ..banana? ..curtain? ..ceiling?
    ..hedge? ..pavement? Pass if defined in terms of use, shape, what it is made of or general
    category (such as banana is fruit, not just yellow). Pass 6 of 9.
20. Ask child: What is a spoon made of? ..a shoe made of? ..a door made of? (No other objects
    may be substituted.) Pass 3 of 3.
21. When placed on stomach, child lifts chest off table with support of forearms and/or hands.
22. When child is on back, grasp his hands and pull him to sitting. Pass if head does not hang back.
23. Child may use wall or rail only, not person. May not crawl.
24. Child must throw ball overhand 3 feet to within arm's reach of tester.
25. Child must perform standing broad jump over width of test sheet. (8-1/2 inches)
26. Tell child to walk forward, 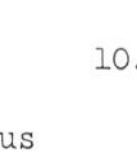 heel within 1 inch of toe.
    Tester may demonstrate. Child must walk 4 consecutive steps, 2 out of 3 trials.
27. Bounce ball to child who should stand 3 feet away from tester. Child must catch ball with
    hands, not arms, 2 out of 3 trials.
28. Tell child to walk backward, 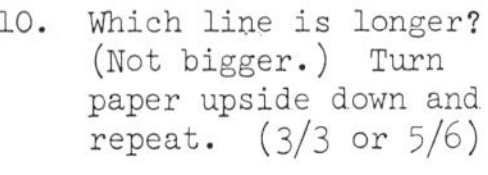 toe within 1 inch of heel.
    Tester may demonstrate. Child must walk 4 consecutive steps, 2 out of 3 trials.

<u>DATE AND BEHAVIORAL OBSERVATIONS</u> (how child feels at time of test, relation to tester, attention
span, verbal behavior, self-confidence, etc,):

157. 10-70

Figure 5–21, cont'd For legend see p 55.

gunshot injuries, tool-related injuries, and drownings.

Imitative interaction may be used in a positive way by the medical care team to gain the cooperation and compliance of the child. For example, it is possible for a child to allow a face mask of oxygen to be held to the face because that is what the astronauts do. Communication with a toddler is much easier than with a younger child because the toddler both understands and gives some feedback. Thus, expressions of anxiety and fear may be elicited and addressed more individually and more directly.

The period between the ages of 6 to 10 may be characterized by the term *competence*. It is at this time that school-aged children gain competence and control over their own functions. Neurologically, they can perform quite complex functions, and in language development they are virtually mature. They are now interacting with the written word as well as the spoken word.

Trauma during the competency period is relatively infrequent and often results from the school-aged child's incomplete competence and, certainly, lack of adequate judgment. Trauma rates at this age fall because children are more careful, realizing that they are vulnerable. Trauma during this age occurs in the form of motor vehicle pedestrian injury, bicycle and sledding injury, sports injury, and others. Adult-inflicted injuries occur in the form of overvigorous attempts at discipline, often for poor school performance or behavior.

In working with the injured school-aged child, it is important to explain how the body functions and to stress the child's competence and ability to handle physical pain and psychological stress. The school-aged child is usually able to communicate fully if allowed the opportunity. It is important to clarify and correct any misconceptions the child harbors. Gender identification is strongly in place during this time, and modesty an important issue.

Between ages 11 and 14 (the early adolescent age range) the term *peer person* best describes the age. Living for peer group interaction, peer contact, and peer acceptance is the norm. Neurologically, children at this stage are quite capable. Psychologically, they have a sense of invincibility that results in risk-taking behavior. Traumatic injury occurs with more frequency in this period. It is the beginning time for both significant nonintentional (accidental) and intentional injury. The early adolescent is typically the passenger in the automobile unskillfully driven by a slightly older peer. During early adolescence, teens begin experimentation with drugs and alcohol. They may also behave in ways described as rebellious as they try to make their own statements of independence. Reports indicate that in some urban environments young adolescents have an increased incidence of penetrating trauma because of their employment as messengers and delivery agents in illegal drug trafficking.

In working with adolescents of this stage, it is important to communicate with them as if they were adults while reassuring them as if they were children. The adolescent's right to confidentiality and capacity for decision making must be safeguarded. The physician must, furthermore, protect the teen's sense of physical modesty. Reassuring a young adolescent about his or her peer group acceptability is important and helpful in forging an easy working relationship.

The period of late adolescence or "young adulthood" comes between ages 15 and 19 years. Late adolescents have often assumed adult roles and responsibilities. Periodic emotional vulnerability and weak coping mechanisms, however, may lead them into challenging and dangerous situations. Trauma at this age comes primarily from three sources: motor vehicle driver and passenger injury, self-inflicted injury (that is, suicide), and homicide. It may be difficult to differentiate these forms of trauma. With individuals of this age, communication and interaction should be conducted on an adult level. Older adolescent patients should be permitted to give informed consent and allowed independent decision making.

SUMMARY

The child's anatomy, as well as his or her stage of growth and development has an important impact on the form of trauma the child sustains and the techniques for trauma management. Caring for a 6-month-old victim of child abuse is very different from caring for the 16-year-old victim of a motor vehicle injury. How the child became injured, the patterns of injury, the treatment techniques, the method of interaction with the child and family, the means of preventing similar injuries—all these vary with the individual patient. Treatment protocols and techniques should never become so mechanized that these important differences are overlooked.

REFERENCES

1. Catell HS, Filtzer DL: Pseudosubluxation and other normal variations in the cervical spine in children, *J Bone Joint Surg* 47-A:1295-1309, Oct 1965.
2. Committee on Trauma, American College of Surgeons: *Advanced trauma life support course*, Chicago, Ill, 1989, The Committee.
3. Eckenhoff JE: Some anatomic considerations of the infant larynx influencing endotracheal anesthesia, *J Am Soc Anesthesiol* 12(4):401-410, July 1951.
4. Fleisher G, Ludwig S, editors: *Textbook of pediatric emergency medicine*, ed 2, Baltimore, Md: 1988, Williams & Wilkins.

5. Hasue M, Hashino R, Omata S et al: Cervical spine injuries in children, Fukushima *J Med Sci* 20:115-123, June 1974.
6. Herzenberg JE, Hensinger RN, Dedrick DK et al: Emergency transport and positioning of young children who have an injury of the cervical spine, *J Bone Joint Surg* 71-A:15-22, Jan 1989.
7. Kissoon N, Dreyer J, Walia M: Pediatric trauma: differences in pathophysiology, injury patterns and treatment compared with adult trauma, *Can Med Assoc J* 142(1):27-34, 1990.
8. Lubitz DS, Seidel JS, Chameides L et al: A rapid method for estimating weight and resuscitation drug dosages from length in the pediatric age group, *Ann Emerg Med* 17(6):576-581, June 1988.
9. Swischuk LE: *The spine and spinal cord: emergency radiology of the acutely ill or injured child*, ed 2, Baltimore, Md: Williams & Wilkins, 1986.
10. Tocantins LM, O'Neill JF: Infusions of blood and other fluids into the general circulation via the bone marrow, *Surg Gynecol Obstet* 73:281-287, July 1941.

6 Pathophysiology of Injury

David K. Magnuson and *Ronald V. Maier*

The physiology of trauma in childhood, that is, the collection of functional derangements and adaptations that accrue from an abrupt alteration of internal homeostasis, is a subject about which more information is rapidly becoming available. The physiologic "uniqueness" of the acutely injured child, as compared with the adult, is frequently debated. Although trauma is the leading cause of death in children, the absolute incidence of severe injury in children fortunately remains relatively small. Because of this, as well as ethical restraints on the use of children as study subjects, clinical research has been conducted mainly in adults. Basic research is usually conducted in mature animal models and compared with adult human subjects. Furthermore, the wide spectrum and continuously changing parameters of normal physiology in the growing child make it difficult or impossible to define pediatric trauma patients as a single group. This chapter delineates some of the more common pathophysiologic changes in organ system function that underlie the clinical manifestations of mechanical trauma in the child. It also reviews some of the adaptive responses that occur and discusses the physiologic ramifications that transpire when the immunoinflammatory response becomes generalized and unregulated. Whenever possible, differences between children and adults, with respect to their responses to injury, are delineated.

ACUTE ORGAN-SYSTEM PATHOPHYSIOLOGY

Several factors contribute to the differing effects of mechanical trauma on the various organ systems of children and adults. Among these factors are differences in size and proportion, differences in tissue elasticity and compliance, and a relative absence in children of the preexisting diseases that tend to limit physiologic reserve in the adult. The cumulative influences of these differences result in discrepancies, both subtle and overt, in injury patterns and manifestations between children and adults. Recognition of these differences must be tempered with a realization that the same resuscitation principles apply to children as to adults, and that failure to adopt the same urgency and com-pulsive management in children will result in catastrophic and unnecessary morbidity, mortality, and long-term disability.

Nervous system

Because of its lack of resiliency and the limited potential for reparative therapies, injuries to the central nervous system (CNS) are the most common cause of mortality and long-term disability in children. Intracranial injuries are often more difficult to diagnose in children because of their inability to cooperate with the examination and respond appropriately to commands and inquiries. The widespread early use of computed tomography, however, has made feasible the rapid diagnosis of serious head injuries. Children suffer from focal intracranial lesions, such as subdural hematoma and intraparenchymal hemorrhage and contusion, less frequently than adults. They do, however, seem to have a higher incidence of epidural hematoma, perhaps because the thinner, less rigid skull is more apt to fracture and lacerate meningeal arteries. Although progressive neurologic decompensation can be dramatic with epidural hematoma, the long-term neurologic outcome is better than for subdural hematoma because associated cerebral contusion is less severe. In general, the outcome for children older than 3 years of age is better than for adults with comparable injuries and Glasgow Coma Scale (GCS) scores.[2,3] Young children less than 3 years of age, however, do not enjoy this same advantage.

Although children develop fewer intracranial hematomas than adults, they have a significant propensity for diffuse axonal injury (DAI). This entity is defined clinically as prolonged, severe neurologic dysfunction unassociated with an intracranial mass lesion and usually presents as coma immediately following injury without a "lucid interval." DAI is histologically characterized by disruption of ascending and descending axonal tracts, particularly in the corpus callosum and internal capsule, and is caused by shear forces generated by rapid angular and rotational acceleration. The proportionately larger size of the cranium in children, along with a less muscular and more flexible ligamentous cervical spine, may account for this finding.

In addition to axonal disruption, these injuries are frequently associated with markedly elevated intracranial pressures which cause secondary brain injury by impairing microvascular perfusion and oxygen delivery. It is widely recognized that intracranial hypertension (ICH) in the absence of an intracranial mass lesion is more common in pediatric than adult trauma victims.[4,5] In infants, such pressure elevations may be decompressed by open fontanelles until rapid decompensation occurs. Children frequently display a more severe form of "malignant ICH," which may be due to alterations in microvascular permeability and resistance. Seizures are also more common in children, but tend to be self-limited and do not necessarily portend a worse prognosis.

Because the head is highly vascularized and relatively larger in small children, strict attention should be paid to all head lacerations and cephalohematomas. A relatively larger blood loss may be experienced by children with soft-tissue head injuries, therefore having a greater impact on resuscitative needs. As hypotension and hypovolemia cause significant secondary morbidity in the setting of associated intracranial injuries, prompt recognition and treatment of bleeding lacerations and expanding hematomas is imperative.

Injury to the thoracic and lumbar spine is less common in children, probably because of the lower incidence of high-velocity injury mechanisms and the relatively resilient vertebral column. Spinal cord injuries are frequently not associated with any bony abnormality of the spine as defined by radiologic survey; therefore careful examination and clinical follow-up are essential to exclude potentially serious cord trauma. The relatively large head, however, may generate considerable momentum and cause significant cervical spine injury, particularly in car-versus-pedestrian vehicular trauma. Because of the momentum generated by the child's large head, dislocations of the occiput on the cervical spine are more common. Such atlantooccipital dissociations may cause devastating injuries to the spinal cord at the foramen magnum and are a cause of nonresuscitability in the bluntly injured child. Appropriate radiographic evaluation of the cervical spine should be performed in the unresponsive, agonal child who has not exsanguinated before embarking on more aggressive interventions.

Cardiovascular system

The considerable cardiopulmonary reserve possessed by most injured children is well recognized by most practitioners. The absence of the usual medical comorbidity that often complicates adult trauma in advanced age accounts for the frequent ability of children to survive significant torso trauma with surprisingly little physiologic derangement. It must be borne in mind, however, that because of this reserve children seldom manifest hemodynamic evidence of hypovolemia, hypoxia, or hypercarbia until relatively late in their physiologic decline. When cardiovascular decompensation does occur, it is frequently marked by progressive bradycardia rather than the tachycardia exhibited in the preterminal adult. To avoid the precipitous and often catastrophic decompensation that inevitably accompanies unrecognized injuries, a low threshold of suspicion based on the mechanism of injury and a careful scrutiny of physiologic parameters and clinical signs must be applied at all times.

The upper limits of normal heart rates decline in children from approximately 160 beats per minute at birth to 120 beats per minute during the preadolescent stage. In adolescence, hemodynamic parameters correspond roughly to adult values. Furthermore, children are more likely to develop tachycardia after trivial injuries as the result of an exuberant catecholamine response to the anxiety induced by the traumatic incident and the emergency room environment. Similarly, systolic pressures are commonly under 100 torr in the preschool child, making interpretation difficult. More helpful is the recognition that peripheral signs of tissue perfusion, such as skin temperature, color, and capillary refill, are not confused by atherosclerotic peripheral vascular disease in the child. These are consistently reliable, albeit imprecise, indicators of the adequacy of cardiac output. An injured child with a normal blood pressure and a heart rate of 120 beats per minute who has cool, clammy extremities and delayed refill mandates aggressive evaluation and intervention. Once a child has unexpectedly decompensated to cardiac arrest from ongoing hemorrhage, the potential for successful intervention is miniscule and long-term salvage anecdotal.

Pulmonary system

The thoracic cage of a child is extremely compliant, and the mediastinum more mobile than that of an adult. This presents a particular pattern of thoracic injuries seen in children. In blunt trauma, more kinetic energy is transmitted to the pulmonary parenchyma and less is absorbed by the bony thorax. Therefore, there can be severe pulmonary contusions in the absence of rib fractures, and unexplained hypoxemia without clinical or radiographic signs of major chest wall injury should suggest this diagnosis. The presence of air and/or blood in the pleural space may have early and profound consequences, as the mediastinal structures of the child are highly mobile. Accordingly, tension hemopneumothorax is common and causes mediastinal shift and cardiac preload compromise at lower displacement pressures in children than in adults. Major injuries of the tracheobronchial tree are rare in children and carry an extremely high mortality rate. It has been suggested that the mobility of the tracheobronchial tree accounts for its susceptibility to "sheer force" injuries, including parenchymal lacerations and tracheobronchial disruptions.[18]

The airways are obviously smaller in children, making obstruction by foreign bodies with concomitant lobar or segmental collapse more frequent. In addition, because of the small size of the trachea, emergent intubation in the field may be traumatic and performed without standard pediatric uncuffed endotracheal tubes. Care of the airway and reevaluation of the appropriateness of the endotracheal appliance is mandatory as soon as exigent issues have been resolved. Inability to secure the airway with an endotracheal tube is an absolute indication for surgical airway control via the cricothyroid membrane. As the cricoid cartilage is the only circumferential support for the trachea, needle cricothyroidotomy is preferrable to open cricothyroidotomy in the child under 12 years of age who has a small, easily injured tracheal apparatus. This maneuver allows time for a controlled tracheostomy to be performed, rather than a cricothyroidotomy as is commonly performed for surgical control of the airway in adults.

Other systems

The differences between child and adult with regard to other organ system trauma are less obvious. In small children with proportionately larger stomachs, acute gastric dilatation resulting from aerophagia and paralytic ileus is a common occurrence. This condition may have a number of consequences, including an increased risk of aspiration on anesthetic induction, significant impairment of ventilation secondary to increased intraabdominal pressure, and vagally mediated alterations in heart rate. The liver and spleen are the most commonly injured intraperitoneal organs in blunt trauma. These injuries are usually isolated in children and, hence, are frequently appropriate for observational management. In adults, the higher incidence of associated hollow viscus injuries makes exploration more common.[10] Renal function is somewhat different in small children, who have less tubular concentrating ability. This accounts for the fact that children will continue to produce urine in spite of hypovolemia as long as compensatory mechanisms support an adequate cardiac output. Thus, in chil-

dren, a minimum urine output of 1 to 2 ml/kg/hr is considered adequate, compared with 0.5 ml/kg/hr for adults.

NEUROENDOCRINE RESPONSE TO INJURY

At the time of injury, and in the reparative period that follows, a number of noxious stimuli are recognized by the neuroendocrine, immune, and reticuloendothelial-hematologic systems. These systems respond in turn by elaborating humoral substances that act to counter traumatic events and protect the organism from further injury. Some of the stimuli include pain, hypotension, hypovolemia, hypoxemia, degradation products of direct and indirect tissue injury, and bacterial toxins such as gram-negative bacterial lipopolysaccharides (LPS, endotoxin). Neuroendocrine mediators generally have systemic effects on metabolism, intravascular volume, and cardiovascular performance.

Neuroendocrine stimulation and response

Specialized receptors in the peripheral nerves, vascular tree, and central nervous system transduce specific stimuli associated with trauma into afferent impulses, which are integrated and interpreted at higher centers such as the hypothalamus, and which elicit a variety of efferent neural and endocrine responses. The cumulative effect of these neuroendocrine reflexes is to conserve intravascular volume, raise blood pressure, improve oxygen delivery, and mobilize energy substrates and amino acids from peripheral muscle and fat to support the metabolism and synthesis of glucose and acute-phase proteins by the liver. There is a great deal of redundancy in this system, with various combinations of different afferent inputs having additive or synergistic effects on the magnitude of a largely stereotypical response.

Pain. Pain is perceived by specific nociceptors in the periphery, which respond to mechanical stimulation as well as to a variety of chemical substances. Resultant neural impulses are transmitted via A-delta (mechanical) and C (polymodal) fibers to the spinal cord, where they ascend in the anterolateral quadrant (for example, the spinothalamic tract) to the thalamus and hypothalamus. In transit, they synapse at multiple levels with competing somatosensory input in the modulation, or "gating," of nociceptive awareness. The CNS, in turn, responds by elaborating a variety of endocrine substances, including adrenocorticotropic hormone (ACTH), antidiuretic hormone (ADH), and endorphins, and stimulates via sympathetic output the secretion of catacholamines and renin from the adrenal medulla and kidney, respectively. Fear and anger, emotional states associated with injury and mediated by the limbic system, project directly to the hypothalamus and potentiate the effects of pain on neuroendocrine outflow.

Hypovolemia and hypotension. Hypovolemia and hypotension, produced by hemorrhage, isotonic fluid sequestration ("third-spacing"), or profound vasodilatation, are also potent stimuli of the neuroendocrine axis. Low-pressure stretch receptors in the atria and high-pressure baroreceptors in the aorta, carotid sinus, and renal arteries monitor intravascular pressure and volume and their rate of change. When negative changes occur, tonic inhibition of CNS outflow is released, allowing the increased secretion of ACTH, ADH, growth hormone (GH), endorphins, catecholamines, and renin. Direct stimulation of the adrenal medulla resulting in the secretion of circulating catecholamines appears to require both baroreceptor and stretch-receptor discharge, as hypotension is a potent stimulus for adrenomedullary catecholamine output, but repeated nonhypotensive hemorrhages resulting in hypovolemia alone do not elicit enhanced catecholamine secretion. Renin is also elab-elaborated directly by the renal juxtaglomerular apparatus, which can function autonomously as a stretch receptor.

A recently isolated counterregulatory hormone, termed atrial natriuretic factor (ANF) or atriopeptin, appears to act in direct opposition to the agents mentioned above. This family of small peptides with a common 17-amino-acid sequence is synthesized in the atrial myocytes and is released in response to atrial stretch. Actions of ANF include inhibition of ADH and aldosterone, direct stimulation of renal natriuresis by tubular epithelium, and direct peripheral vasodilatation. Hypovolemia resulting in a reduction of atrial stretch causes a reduction in ANF production.

Oxygen, carbon dioxide, and pH. Other receptors in the carotid bifurcation and aortic arch serve as chemoreceptors, which respond to alterations in P_{O_2}, P_{CO_2}, and pH. These highly specialized neuroreceptors transduce alterations in oxygen, carbon dioxide, or hydrogen ion concentration into autonomic afferent activity, which brings about an increase in ventilatory rate. The mechanism by which these receptors function is still undefined, but one theory implicates receptor tissue pH as the final common pathway by which the receptors are stimulated. The response by the CNS is an increased respiratory rate, increased parasympathetic tone, and decreased sympathetic tone, leading to an increase in minute ventilation (V_{min}) and a decrease in myocardial and peripheral oxygen consumption (V_{O_2}). The afferent response to pH and P_{CO_2} appears to be linear, but that to P_{O_2} tends to be sigmoidal, mimicking the oxyhemoglobin dissocia-tion curve and linking autonomic compensatory activity to hemoglobin saturation rather than P_{O_2}.[7]

Temperature. Core temperature is monitored directly by the CNS in the preoptic hypothalamus. A reduction in temperature may be the result of direct exposure with conductive and convective losses, hemorrhage, crystalloid resuscitation, or destruction of insulating barriers as seen in thermal injury. Such temperature alterations directly augment the secretion of ACTH, ADH, GH, and thyroid-stimulating hormone. They also stimulate sympathetic outflow to produce increased levels of circulating epinephrine, which redistributes blood flow to central core organs.

Neuroendocrine environment

Hormones are defined as chemical substances that are synthesized by specialized tissues, circulate in the vascular system, and produce functional changes at distant target sites via receptor-mediated alterations of cellular function. Many of the functional changes induced by the hormonal milieu that characterizes the postinjury state are metabolic, that is, changes in the mobilization, balance, and utilization of energy substrates. Others involve fluid balance, cardiac performance, and vascular tone. The result is a highly redundant and complex system of functional adaptations evolved to promote survival in the acute posttraumatic period, but which may have disadvantageous effects when prolonged for long periods of time after injury (Table 6-1).

Cortisol. All steroid hormones are derived from cholesterol, which is obtained largely by receptor-mediated internalization of plasma (LDL) by the stimulated adrenal and, to a lesser extent, by *de novo* synthesis. Cholesterol is converted to pregnenolone, in a rate-limiting step mediated by ACTH, angiotension II, and potassium, and then enters one of a variety of pathways in which hydroxylation and other modifications determine the final product. The specific biosynthetic pathway that pregnenolone enters is dependent on the particular enzymes expressed in a specific adrenal cell type. The glucocorticoid hormones, of which cortisol is by far the most physiologically significant, are steroid compounds synthesized in the adrenal cortex, predominantly in the zona fasciculata.

Cortisol production is regulated by ACTH, which is derived by hydrolytic cleavage of pro-opiomelanocortin in the pituitary, and is secreted in response to afferent input to the hypothalamus. ACTH circulates in the plasma as an unbound peptide with a half-life of 10 minutes and stimulates increased cortisol secretion from the adrenal cortex by accelerating the conversion of cholesterol to pregnenolone via a cAMP-dependent mechanism.

Table 6–1 Characteristics of neuroendocrine mediators

Agent	Structure	Source	Stimuli	Mechanism	Effects
Cortisol	Steroid	Adrenal cortex	ACTH	Cytoplasmic receptor DNA binding	↑ Proteolysis, lipolysis, gluconeogenesis, glycogenolysis, hepatic acute phase protein synthesis; Potentiates catecholamines and glucagon; Insulin antagonism; Inhibits phospholipase cleavage of arachidonic acid
Aldosterone	Steroid	Adrenal cortex	ACTH, K^+ Angiotensin II	Cytoplasmic receptor DNA binding	↑ Na and H_2O resorption in renal tubule and intestinal mucosa
Angiotensin II	Peptide	Pulmonary microvasculature	↓ GFR	Membrane receptor	↑ Cardiac contractility and rate, vasoconstriction; ↑ Aldosterone, ADH, gluconeogenesis; Potentiates epinephrine
Epinephrine	Catecholamine	Adrenal medulla	Sympathetic outflow	Membrane receptor	↑ Cardiac contractility and rate, CO, MAP, AV conduction; Vasodilatation, bronchodilatation; ↑ Lipolysis, ketogenesis, insulin antagonism
Norepinephrine	Catecholamine	Sympathetic neurons	Sympathetic outflow	Membrane receptor	↑ Cardiac contractility and rate, MAP, arrhythmias; ± CO; Vasoconstriction, bronchoconstriction
Dopamine	Catacholamine	Sympathetic neurons	Sympathetic outflow	Membrane receptor	Low dose: ↑ renal and splanchnic blood flow; Medium dose: beta-adrenergic effects; High dose: alpha-adrenergic effects
Vasopressin	Polypeptide	Posterior pituitary	↑ OSM, ↓ BP, ↓ volume	Membrane receptor	↑ Renal H_2O resorption; Vasoconstriction; ↑ Gluconeogenesis, glycogenolysis
Glucagon	Polypeptide	Pancreatic alpha cells	Hypoglycemia Adrenergic stim	Membrane receptor	↑ Gluconeogenesis, glycogenolysis, ketogenesis
Insulin	Polypeptide	Pancreatic beta cells	Hyperglycemia ↑ Amino acids ↑ Fatty acids	Membrane receptor	Glucose and amino acid uptake, glycogen synthesis; ↓ Gluconeogenesis, glycogenolysis, proteolysis, lipolysis
β-Endorphin	Polypeptide	CNS	Fear, pain, shock	Opiate receptor	↓ Pain, anxiety, catecholamine activity; ↑ Cardiac contractility, vasodilatation

Normally, negative feedback inhibition exists between glucocorticoids and ACTH. There is considerable evidence, however, that in the acute response to trauma ACTH secretion stimulated by multiple sequential stimuli is not inhibited by cortisol, but may in fact be potentiated.

Cortisol circulates primarily in the bound state, mostly to corticosteroid-binding globulin (CBG, transcortin), and a smaller fraction to albumin. The role that CBG plays in uncertain, as cortisol is soluble itself, and the free form of cortisol accounts for its effects. Cortisol, being hydrophobic, readily crosses cellular lipid bilayers and binds to specific cytoplasmic receptors. As a result of cortisol binding, a DNA-binding domain on the receptor changes conformation, thus allowing the receptor-hormone complex to migrate into the nucleus and bind to specific DNA regulatory regions termed glucocorticoid regulatory elements. Cortisol therefore acts to increase the transcription of a specific set of genes.

The effects of glucocorticoids on intermediary metabolism are legion and serve to increase available substrates for energy production in the posttraumatic period. In peripheral tissues such as skeletal muscle, cortisol inhibits insulin-dependent glucose uptake and metabolism. It also promotes catabolism of skeletal muscle proteins with the release of free amino acids into the circulation. In adipocytes, it increases lipolysis and inhibits lipogenesis. These actions tend to increase blood levels of glucose, fatty acids, glycerol, and amino acids. In the liver these substrates are taken up and enter various biosynthetic pathways. Gluconeogenesis and glycogen deposition are increased; acute-phase protein synthesis is stimulated. Furthermore, cortisol appears to potentiate the similar effects of epinephrine and glucagon on both peripheral and core tissues. The brain, myocardium, and erythrocytes are insensitive to the glucose-inhibitory effects of cortisol, allowing these critical tissues to utilize glucose for energy substrate during stress.

Aldosterone. Aldosterone, like cortisol, is a steroid hormone derived from cholesterol by a series of hydroxylation and oxidation steps. It is produced in the zona glomerulosa, where the predominant intermediate enzymes favor mineralocorticoid synthesis, the end product of which is aldosterone. Stimulation of aldosterone synthesis and secretion is governed by three factors: ACTH, angiotensin II, and potassium. ACTH acts through a cAMP-dependent, Ca^{2+}-dependent process, whereas angiotensin II and potassium act via cAMP-independent, Ca^{2+}-dependent processes. All three stimuli accelerate the rate-limiting proximal conversion of cholesterol to pregnenolone. During acute stress states, ACTH-mediated processes predominate,

with angiotensin II playing a lesser role. In more chronic postinjury states, angiotensin II may predominate. It is unlikely that potassium plays a significant role in the hyperaldosteronemic state following injury.

The effects of mineralocorticoids on target cells are mediated through cytoplasmic receptor mechanisms similar to the glucocorticoids. The principle target cells for aldosterone are in the distal convoluted tubule and proximal collecting duct of the renal nephron. Here, aldosterone-sensitive gene products enhance Na^+/K^+-ATPase-dependent sodium and water resorption. Potassium and hydrogen are excreted in exchange for sodium, either by direct enzyme-linked exchange, or passively by moving down the electrochemical gradient created in the tubular lumen by the egress of sodium. Similar effects are seen in the mucosal cells of the small and large intestines. The overall result is an augmentation of intravascular volume to offset that lost by hemorrhage or sequestration due to "third spacing."

Angiotensin II. Angiotensin II is an octapeptide produced by a complex set of processes that begins with the production of renin in the nephron. The synthesis, secretion, and regulation of renin occurs in the juxtaglomerular apparatus (JGA), a highly specialized cellular network that bridges the afferent and efferent arterioles. The JGA comprises the juxtaglomerular cell (a myoepithelial cell associated with afferent arteriolar endothelium), the macula densa (a specialized group of epithelial cells in the distal tubule closely approximated to the afferent arteriole), and the juxtaglomerular neurogenic receptor. As renal perfusion falls, chloride presentation to the macula densa falls. This information is translated from the macula densa to the adjacent juxtaglomerular cell, which responds by cleaving intracellular prorenin into renin, a 274-amino-acid glycoprotein that is secreted into the lumen of the afferent arteriole. Renin secretion can also be stimulated by direct beta-adrenergic stimulation of the juxtaglomerular neurogenic receptor via norepinephrine and by decreased tension on renal baroreceptors (possibly the juxtaglomerular cell itself).

In the circulation, renin catalyzes the conversion of angiotensinogen, a protein containing more than 400 amino acids, to the decapeptide angiotensin I. Angiotensinogen is an acute-phase protein produced by the liver that is manufactured after hepatic stimulation by cortisol and other stress-response hormones. Angiotensin I is hydrolyzed by angiotensin-converting enzyme (ACE) in pulmonary microvascular endothelial cells to the octapeptide angiotensin II.

Angiotensin II has a half-life of approximately

90 seconds, and its effects are of rapid onset and short duration. Angiotensin II is one of the most potent direct arteriolar vasoconstrictors yet identified. As previously described, angiotensin II is an important inducer of aldosterone production by the adrenal, especially in more chronic states. Chronic aldosterone hypersecretion is also mediated by the trophic effects of angiotensin II on the zona glomerulosa. Other important effects of angiotensin II in the traumatized patient include an increase in the inotropic and chronotropic state of the myocardium, potentiation of adrenal epinephrine secretion, stimulation of vasopressin (ADH) release, and up-regulation of hepatic glycogenolysis and gluconeogenesis. Angiotensin II appears to exert its effects at the cellular level via classic receptor-mediated increases in intracellular Ca^{2+} levels and accelerated membrane phospholipid turnover.

Catecholamines. The neurotransmitters dopamine and norepinephrine and the amine hormone epinephrine are all catecholamines; that is, they all have aromatic 6-carbon (catechol) rings substituted at one position with an amine group. Dopamine is the common precursor and is synthesized from tyrosine prior to storage in neurosecretory granules. In sympathetic postganglionic neurons, dopamine is hydroxylated to norepinephrine, which functions at the synapse. In the adrenal medulla, norepinephrine is further methylated to epinephrine, the principle circulating catecholamine.

Catecholamines bind to specific adrenergic cell surface receptors that are linked to adenylate cyclase via stimulatory or inhibitory guanine-nucleotide–binding regulatory proteins (G-proteins). Adenylate cyclase catalyzes the degradation of ATP to cAMP, which activates cytoplasmic serine-threonine protein kinases by binding to regulatory subunits on the kinases. Depending on whether the receptor is linked to a stimulatory or inhibitory G-protein, occupation of that receptor will result in greater or lesser intracellular protein phosphorylation, which in turn will alter the balance of metabolic events inside the cell.

Adrenergic receptors are ubiquitous, and the effects of sympathetic autonomic activity and adrenal medullary secretion on hemodynamic and metabolic events are therefore widespread. Receptors are classified as $alpha_1$, $alpha_2$, $beta_1$, and $beta_2$, and the catecholamines have differing effects determined by their relative affinities for the various receptor subclasses. $Alpha_1$ receptors mediate arterial and venous vasoconstriction, as well as hepatic glycogenolysis and gluconeogenesis, and pancreatic islet cell inhibition. $Alpha_2$-receptor stimulation results in platelet aggregation and mediates presynaptic feedback mechanisms. $Beta_1$ receptors are found in the myocardium and govern both the positive inotropic and chronotropic effects of catecholamines, as well as increased atrioventricular conduction velocities. Other important $beta_1$-mediated effects are lipolysis and ketogenesis in adipose and hepatic tissue. $Beta_2$ receptors, found on smooth muscles cells of the arterial and bronchial trees, mediate relaxation and dilatation. They also exert a stimulatory effect on pancreatic islet cell endocrine secretion, an inhibitory effect on peripheral insulin-dependent glucose utilization, and augment glycogenolysis in muscle. Since beta receptors predominate in the alpha islet cells whereas alpha receptors predominate in the beta islet cells, adrenergic influences following trauma favor the secretion of glucagon and the inhibition of insulin release.

The three physiologically relevant catecholamines, epinephrine, norepinephrine, and dopamine, have receptor-specific effects that appear to be dose-dependent. Epinephrine tends to exert beta-mediated effects at lower doses, whereas alpha effects predominate at higher concentrations. Norepinephrine appears to exert primarily alpha effects through the entire concentration range, although significant beta activity is present. Because of these differences, epinephrine tends to increase myocardial contractility and heart rate and cause peripheral vasodilatation, resulting in increased cardiac output, mean systemic pressure, and systolic pressure, while lowering diastolic pressure. Norepinephrine, on the other hand, augments systolic, mean, and diastolic arterial pressures, but may result in an unchanged or even lowered cardiac output due to increased afterload. Both agents cause an increase in myocardial oxygen consumption and arrythmogenicity. Dopamine principally stimulates dopaminergic receptors in the renal and mesenteric vasculature at low doses, but causes beta and alpha receptor stimulation at intermediate and high concentrations, respectively. The effects of increased sympathetic and adrenomedullary outflow following injury therefore include enhancement of cardiac output, elevation in systemic pressures, mobilization of fatty acids, and maintenance of the hyperglycemia required by certain glucose-dependent tissues.

Vasopressin. Vasopressin (antidiuretic hormone, ADH) is an octapeptide that is synthesized in the hypothalamus and transported to nerve terminals in the posterior pituitary, where its release is dependent on several factors. Afferent stimuli that promote the secretion of ADH originate in the cerebral osmoreceptors, carotid baroreceptors, and atrial stretch receptors. Increased serum osmolarity, hypotension, and hypovolemia can therefore cause elaboration of vasopressin. The threshold for osmolarity-dependent vasopressin secretion appears to be about 280 mosm/L, and vasopressin concentrations rise linearly with increases in serum osmolarity. Hypovolemia-dependent vasopressin secretion requires at least a 7% isotonic intravascular volume depletion before stimulation occurs, beyond which vasopressin concentrations rise exponentially with further reductions in total blood volume. Vasopressin release is potentiated by trauma, pain, and hypoxia and is inhibited by alcohol.

The actions of vasopressin are multiple. Serum osmolarity and volume are restored by cAMP-mediated increases in the permeability of renal collecting ducts to free water resorption. Blood pressure is augmented by systemic arteriolar vasoconstriction, particularly in the splanchnic bed. This mechanism may contribute to the development of nonocclusive mesenteric ischemia observed in low-flow states. Other effects of vasopressin include enhancement of hepatic glycogenolysis and gluconeogenesis.

Glucagon and insulin. The balance between these two counterregulatory hormones, glucagon and insulin, contributes significantly to the overall metabolic milieu in the postinjury state. The cumulative effects of their actions determine the flow and utilization of energy substrates. They are both under the control of substrate concentrations as well as the autonomic nervous system, and changes in one hormone are usually countered by reciprocal changes in the other.

Glucagon is a 3000-dalton polypeptide hormone synthesized in the alpha cells of the pancreatic islets. Synthesis and secretion are promoted by hypoglycemia, increased levels of circulating gluconeogenic amino acids, and increased adrenergic tone. The principal effects of glucagon are mediated through the liver: glucagon causes a cAMP-dependent increase in glycogenolysis, gluconeogenesis, and ketogenesis. Lipolysis and peripheral glucose metabolism are largely unaltered.

Insulin is a 6000-dalton polypeptide synthesized in the beta cells of the islet and is released in response to hyperglycemia and increased levels of free amino and fatty acids. Its release is inhibited by glucagon, somatostatin, and endorphins. Its functions are essentially anabolic: hepatic glycogenolysis and gluconeogenesis are inhibited, peripheral tissue uptake of glucose and processing via glycogen synthesis and glycolysis are enhanced (except in hematopoietic, cerebral, and inflammatory tissues), and amino acid oxidation and lipolysis are inhibited. The effects of insulin on peripheral tissues are largely negated by the actions of corticosteroids on target cell responses to insulin. Since the neuroendocrine environment in the postinjury state favors a shift toward glucagon-me-

diated metabolism, a state of hyperglycemia and increased substrate availability exists for a highly variable but prolonged time period.

Endorphins. A family of endogenous neuropeptides, endorphins comprise a large number of substances that share a common pentapeptide sequence at their amino terminus. Although they appear to act principally within the central nervous system as neurotransmitters or modulators, certain peptides such as beta-endorphin have been observed in elevated concentrations in circulating blood following stress events such as shock and sepsis. The effects of endorphins on the physiologic response to injury are varied. On one hand, they occupy opiate receptors on neural tissue and moderate the perception of noxious stimuli, thus producing a sense of well-being and hypothetically allowing the individual to function in spite of the pain associated with trauma. On the other hand, endorphins have been demonstrated to elicit a number of physiologic changes that might be considered counterproductive in the posttraumatic state. These include a depression of myocardial contractility, inhibition of sympathetic activity, and peripheral arteriolar and venous dilatation. Studies in primates on the ability of naloxone, an opiate antagonist and competitive inhibitor of endorphins, to alter the response to shock have documented that in the absence of acidosis and hypothermia naloxone can increase myocardial contractility and mean arterial pressure during hypovolemic and endotoxemic shock.[13] Randomized, prospective trials of naloxone infusion during septic shock in humans have not convincingly shown an improvement in outcome. Routine use of opiate antagonists for the treatment of either hypovolemic or septic shock cannot be recommended.

METABOLIC RESPONSE TO INJURY

The cumulative effect of the various neuroendocrine responses outlined above is the production of a hemodynamic state that augments oxygen delivery to core structures by optimizing myocardial performance, vascular tone, and fluid retention, and the creation of a metabolic milieu that maximizes the availability of energy substrates to match obligatory requirements that occur during the period of acute stress. As opposed to starvation, the postinjury state is one of increased metabolic rate and energy requirements to support the reparative process. These increases are mediated, in large part, by the sustained increase in catecholamine activity. As children already exhibit an elevated basal metabolic rate to provide for normal growth, further increases to satisfy the needs of the posttraumatic reparative process may not be easily sustained. The metabolic parameters that characterize this state are somewhat stereotypical, regardless of the type of injury, and are prolonged beyond the acute event even in well-resuscitated trauma victims. An understanding of this environment is requisite for the apropriate management of the critically injured child and for the anticipation of potential posttraumatic complications.

In their classic studies, Moore and Cuthbertson divided the metabolic response to injury into three phases. A brief "ebb" phase occurs immediately following injury and is characterized by hyperglycemia resulting from a variety of factors. After tissue perfusion is restored, either by endogenous adaptive mechanisms or resuscitative intervention, the "flow" phase begins. This phase is also marked by hyperglycemia, although the mechanisms are different. The distinguishing features of this phase are hypermetabolism and protein catabolism, resulting in a negative nitrogen balance. The flow phase persists until euvolemia is restored, tissue oxygenation normalized, wounds closed, and infection controlled. At this point, metabolism reflects a definite anabolic trend and positive nitrogen balance ensues. Energy production, metabolic rate, and serum glucose levels return to normal, and the lypolytic state is reversed. These three phases are the cumulative result of distinct variations in the metabolism of carbohydrate, fat, and protein as energy substrates, which in turn are the result of the dynamic hormonal environment previously described.

Carbohydrate metabolism

Although simple starvation is associated with reduced serum glucose concentrations, hyperglycemia characterizes much of the posttraumatic period. The degree of hyperglycemia observed appears to correlate roughly with the severity of injury and, presumably, with the intensity of the neuroendocrine response. The survival advantage afforded by hyperglycemia is twofold. Carbohydrate-dependent tissues, such as erythrocytes, leukocytes, neurons (including brain), renal medulla, and the wound itself, are ensured of an adequate supply of energy substrate. Furthermore, the hyperosmolarity associated with elevated glucose levels contributes to an osmotic gradient favoring passive movement of free water from the intracellular space to the intravascular space and the restoration of circulating volume. The hyperglycemia of stress is produced by three separate events: increased glycogenolysis, enhanced gluconeogenesis, and diffuse insulin resistance.

Glycogenolysis occurs principally in the liver (because peripheral muscle lacks a necessary phosphatase to release glycogen into the circulation) and is the primary source of glucose during the acute

ebb phase. Elevated catecholamine and cortisol levels as well as decreased insulin levels promote the induction of glycogenolytic enzymes and the release of glucose. Hepatic glycogen stores, however, are modest and supply only about 1 g of glucose per kg of body weight.

During the flow phase, new glucose production occurs through gluconeogenesis, a process by which 3-carbon fragments are rechanneled into the glycolytic pathway, where substrate concentrations and several unique enzymatic steps favor the regeneration of glucose (Fig. 6-1). The carbon fragments are derived from several sources. Glycerol produced from triglyceride breakdown can enter the gluconeogenic pathway directly. Furthermore, most amino acids can participate via deamination to their respective alpha-keto acid, followed by entry into the tricarboxylic acid (TCA) cycle and conversion to pyruvate. The most important amino acid in this regard is alanine, which is deaminated directly to pyruvate. Finally, the wound is an important source of lactate, which is transported to the liver for conversion to glucose and redistribution back to the wound and other glucose-dependent tissues (Cori cycle).

Glucose uptake and glycolysis are increased in the wound from the outset, resulting in significantly increased production of lactate. This process has been previously attributed to the relatively anaerobic environment of the wound. Recent evidence, however, suggests that the process is an aerobic one, as both oxygen consumption and CO_2 production are simultaneously enhanced. Aerobic glycolysis and lactate production is a characteristic of inflammatory cell metabolism, hence this aspect of wound substrate utilization may be a consequence of the intense inflammatory infiltrate that occurs almost immediately in mechanically disrupted tissue.

Like glycogenolysis, gluconeogenesis is driven by cortisol and catacholamines, although glucagon also plays an important role. The process of gluconeogenesis is endothermic, that is, it requires a net input of energy to drive. It therefore does not alleviate the energy requirements of the injured child, but instead increases them, and can be viewed as an energy investment in supplying certain tissues with a requisite energy source. The energy required for gluconeogenesis comes largely from the beta-oxidation of fatty acids in the liver. If the starvation state continues longer than 3 to 7 days, neural tissue undergoes a process of ketoadaptation, in which membrane transport mechanisms and metabolic pathways designed to utilize ketones (end products of fatty acid oxidation) appear, thereby reducing the requirements for gluconeogenesis and protein catabolism. In the setting

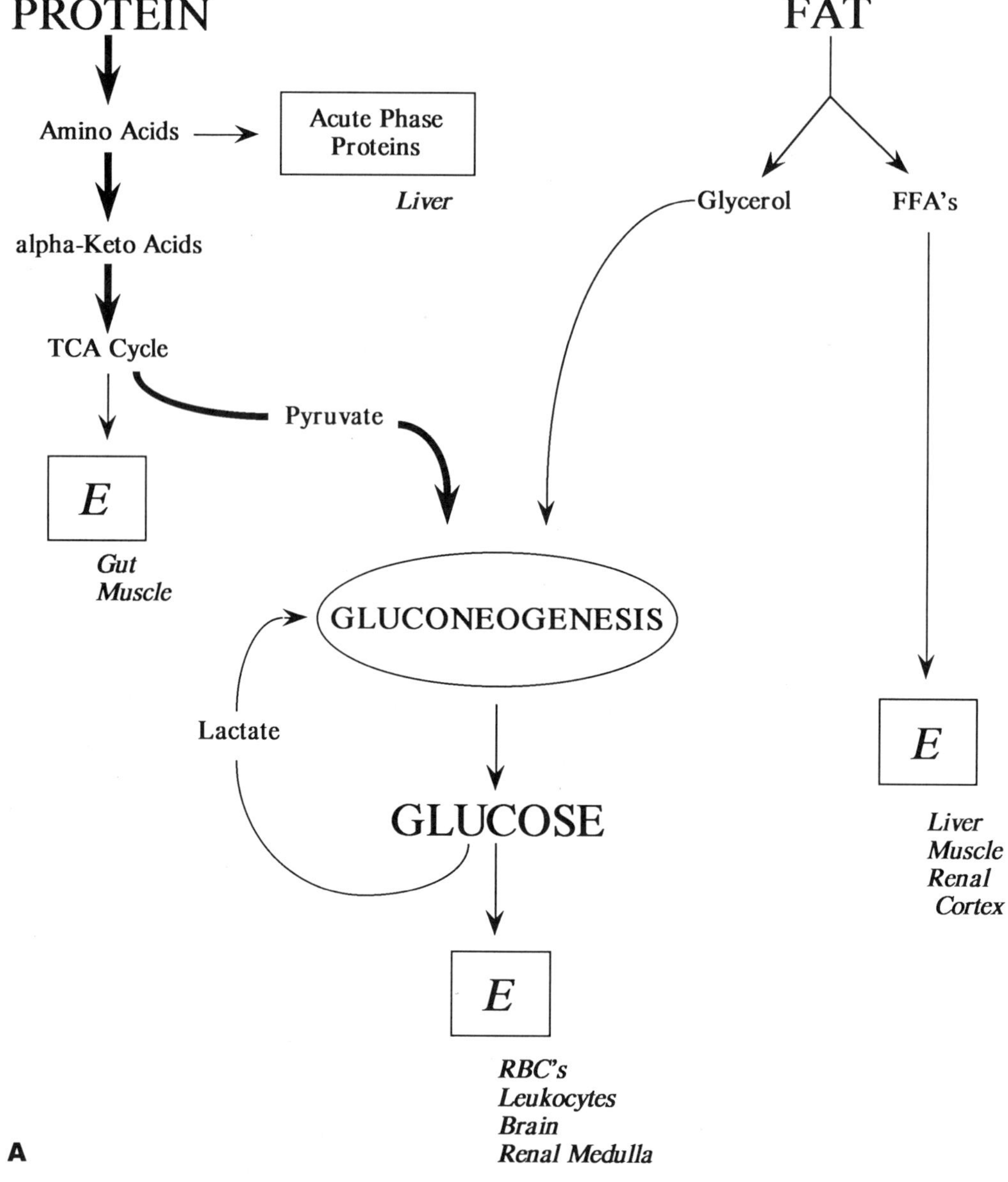

Figure 6–1 A, Metabolic fates of protein, fat, and glucose for energy production *(E)* during the stress response to trauma. Gluconeogenesis is required by crucial glucose-obligate tissues and is a central process that drives the persistent protein catabolism that characterizes this period. Keto-adaptation of neural tissue and enhanced ketogenesis from fatty acid oxidation, which combine to reduce markedly the gluconeogenesis requirements and protein catabolism during simple starvation, are both significantly inhibited after injury.

of severe trauma, however, the ketoadaptive process may not occur, and protein catabolism may continue unabated, as discussed below.

Although glycogenolysis and gluconeogenesis serve to increase glucose availability, insulin resistance resulting from the hormonal environment (the "diabetes of injury") serves to maintain high serum glucose levels and directs glucose to tissues that require it. Initially, circulating insulin levels are low secondary to an adrenergic-mediated decrease in beta-islet sensitivity. During the flow phase, however, insulin synthesis and levels are actually increased, but peripheral tissues under the influence of catecholamines and cortisol become resistant. That lipolysis and gluconeogenesis continue in the face of elevated insulin levels reflects the insulin-resistant state. Glucose levels rise until the gradient for transmembrane glucose transport

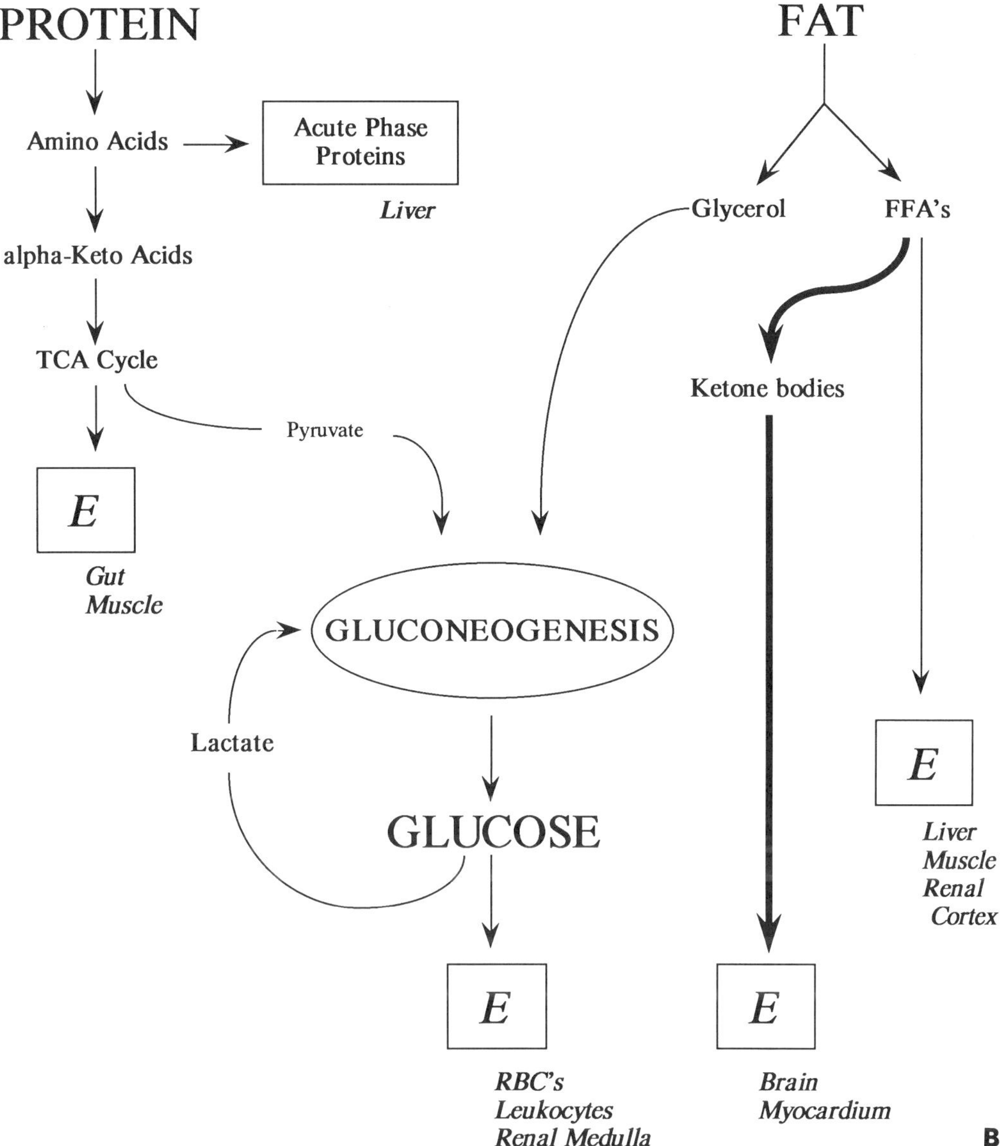

Figure 6–1, cont'd B, Metabolic adaptation to simple starvation. Keto-adaptation by brain tissue and increased ketogenesis during free fatty acid oxidation result in reduced requirements for amino acid gluconeogenic precursors.

exceeds the inhibitory effects of the hormonal environment, and glucose uptake and utilization commences. In spite of the insulin-resistant state, glucose consumption during the flow phase is actually increased relative to baseline.

Fat metabolism

Requirements for energy metabolism are increased during all phases of the posttraumatic state. Most of the energy produced in this setting is derived from the beta-oxidation of fatty acids, as suggested by respiratory quotient (RQ) of 0.7 to 0.8 in trauma victims. The increased levels of catecholamines, glucagon, and cortisol favor lipolysis and discourage further fatty acid synthesis. Fatty acids cleaved from triglycerides are sequentially oxidized to acetyl-CoA on hepatocyte mitochondrial membranes, and acetyl-CoA is shuttled into the mitochondrial core for further metabolism to CO_2 and H_2O in the TCA cycle. Alternatively, acetyl-CoA can be converted into ketone bodies, which are released from the liver and are usable fuel sources in cardiac and skeletal muscle, and in the brain if ketoadaptation occurs. Ketogenesis, however, is suppressed initially after major trauma and shock and may contribute little to the early postinjury state.

Protein metabolism

The catabolism of proteins after major injury is associated with dramatic clinical sequelae and has therefore undergone a great deal of investigation. Marked muscle wasting and increased urinary nitrogen losses following long bone fractures were first noted by Cuthbertson and were later documented in patients with burns, head injury, mechanical trauma, and sepsis. This net negative nitrogen balance peaks within 2 to 3 days following trauma and, if healing and restoration of function ensue, gradually normalizes over several weeks as oxygen consumption and metabolic rate return to baseline. Nitrogen balance is the cumulative result of protein synthesis and catabolism. After minor trauma, as after starvation, protein catabolism is unchanged but synthesis is decreased. After major trauma or burns, or in the setting of uncontrolled sepsis, synthesis may actually be increased, but is offset by a much larger increase in protein degradation.

Proteolysis of skeletal muscle liberates free amino acids which can be deaminated to their respective alpha-keto acids and used by the TCA cycle to drive the oxidative phosphorylation of ADP to ATP. Only about 20% of the hydrolyzed protein, however, is used in this manner as energy substrate. Another small amount is used for the synthesis of structural proteins by the wound and acute-phase proteins by the liver. Most of the amino acids, however, are utilized in the liver as precursors for gluconeogenesis. As previously described, gluconeogenesis is absolutely necessary for continued energy metabolism in a variety of essential tissues including the wound, inflammatory cells, erythrocytes, and brain. Severe trauma is not followed by the ketoadaptation observed in simple starvation, and requirements for glucose therefore do not significantly diminish over time. The mechanism behind this inhibition of ketoadaptation is unknown, but has been postulated to involve either interleukin-1 (IL-1) or a novel proteolysis-inducing factor (PIF).[9]

Although peripheral proteins appear to be broken down in a somewhat nonselective fashion, more than 50% of the released amino acid pool is composed of alanine and glutamine. This suggests that other amino acids are converted to alanine and glutamine, and that these amino acids are the predominant nitrogen carriers from peripheral muscle to protein-synthetic and gluconeogenic tissues. Alanine is the major gluconeogenic precursor, whereas glutamine is a major source of nitrogen for renal ammonia synthesis and now appears to be the preferred fuel for enteric mucosal epithelium and for some inflammatory cells as well. In addition, glutamine may be utilized to maintain adequate intracellular levels of glutathione, an endogenous antioxidant thought to be involved in cellular repair and in host protection against the inflammatory response. For these reasons, glutamine-supplemented diets are advocated, as glutamine appears to become a relatively essential amino acid during stress. Branched-chain amino acids, aspartate, and aspargine are principally used by peripheral muscle as TCA-cycle precursors in energy generation. Unless exogenous glucose and protein sources are aggressively and appropriately administered after severe trauma, protein catabolism will continue unchecked. Persistent catabolism is associated with increased mortality in direct relation to the loss of lean body mass.

Thermoregulation

Core temperature is consistently elevated following trauma, even in the absence of infection. This phenomenon appears to be due to a change in the central hypothalamic thermoregulatory center, induced by interleukin-1 and other inflammatory cytokines and resulting in a higher equilibrium temperature "set point." Depressed temperature levels are usually associated with overwhelming sepsis and critically diminished physiologic reserve and should be regarded as an ominous sign of impending demise.

The regulation of core body temperature depends on manipulating the two determinants of temperature, that is, heat production and heat loss. Heat production is a direct result of metabolic rate and oxygen consumption and is elevated in the posttrauma setting. The increase in metabolic rate is a consequence of increased energy requirements (not an attempt to raise core temperature primarily), but has been shown to contribute to the host defense against bacterial and viral pathogens. Shivering, which begins at approximately 32° to 33° C, is a reflex response to hypothermia designed to increase oxygen consumption and generate heat.

Heat loss is effected via evaporation, radiation, conduction, and convection and therefore may be significantly altered by the intensive care setting. Unnecessary exposure, failure to change blood or fluid-soaked sheets and dressings, the use of air beds, and the administration of unwarmed fluids in large volumes all cause increases in heat loss and may result in the deleterious effects of hypothermia. Toddlers and young children who are rapidly growing have increased surface area/volume ratios, less insulating fat, and less muscle mass for shivering and are therefore more susceptible to inappropriate heat loss. Infants may have lower surface area/volume ratios, but have far less muscle mass and reduced abilities to generate heat and are therefore also at high risk for hypothermia in the ICU environment.

Consequences of hypothermia are manifold. The myocardium is particularly sensitive to temperature changes, and hypothermia is accompanied by increased ventricular irritability to potassium and calcium concentrations. Premature ventricular contractions are seen at approximately 30° to 32° C, with a threshold for ventricular fibrillation at about 28° to 30° C. Cold also shifts the oxyhemoglobin dissociation curve to the left, impairing peripheral oxygen delivery. Other effects of hypothermia include central nervous system depression, respiratory depression, coagulopathy, and loss of peripheral vasomotor tone. All of these effects may initiate or exacerbate metabolic acidosis, hemodynamic instability, and organ dysfunction.

IMMUNOINFLAMMATORY RESPONSE TO INJURY

Much of the altered physiology and organ dysfunction that occurs after trauma results from the large number of immunoinflammatory mediators elaborated in response to stimuli associated with the wound. These mediators include various protein products of enzymatic cascades, eicosanoid products of membrane lipid metabolism, cytokines produced by cells of the inflammatory response, and toxic oxidants, proteases, and cationic proteins released by activated neutrophils and macrophages. Under normal circumstances this response serves to activate, modulate, and effect localized inflammatory events in a contained and well-coordinated fashion. In situations in which the inflammatory stimulus is overwhelming, however, the distribution of these mediators is systemic and unfocused. The generalized proinflammatory state that results may cause "bystander injury" to parenchymal cells in distant organ sites, leading to dysfunction and failure. There is a significant degree of overlap in the effects of the various mediators, which makes the discrete assignment of certain clinical phenomena to a specific agent impossible. This multiplicity has also frustrated attempts to alter pharmacologically the pathophysiologic course of organ dysfunction and the onset of multiple organ failure syndrome (MOFS) following major trauma.

Humoral inflammatory response

Complement. The complement system consists of several serine esterases and their substrates, which play a prominent role in localized and systemic inflammatory responses. Following activation by a variety of stimuli, the enzymatic cascade generates several peptides that participate in the host response against invading organisms. The mechanisms by which complement components act include opsonization, cell lysis, and the recruitment and activation of inflammatory cells such as neutrophils (PMNs).

The activation of the complement cascade occurs via two pathways. The classical pathway involves the binding of the Fc domain on antigen-complexed IgG or IgM immunoglobulins to C1, a macromolecular complex of C1q, C1r, and C1s. Activated C1 cleaves C2 and C4, allowing the formation of C4b2b, which is a C3-convertase. The other, or "alternative" pathway of C3-convertase formation involves the binding of preexisting C3b, normally present in small concentrations as a product of spontaneous hydrolysis, with factor B. This event requires a "protective" surface or environment such as lipopolysaccharides (bacterial endotoxins), polysaccharides (for example, zymosan), or other cell surface constituents of invading microorganisms. Once bound to C3b, factor B is split by factor D, leaving a C3bBb complex, the other major C3-convertase. This complex requires stabilization by properdin for prolonged activity.

The central event in the complement cascade involves the enzymatic conversion by either C3-convertase of C3 to C3b, an activated enzyme which in turn converts C5 to C5b. C5b then assembles C6 and C7 and inserts into membrane lipid bilayers. Once anchored, this complex binds C8 and C9 and polymerizes to form a transmembrane pore that allows unimpeded flow of water and solute into the cell, culminating in osmotic lysis. C3b also functions as an opsin, binding to particulate surfaces and promoting phagocytosis by leukocytes via C3b membrane receptors.

The other cleavage products of C3 and C5, C3a and C5a, are termed *anaphylatoxins* and play prominent roles in initiating and amplifying the inflammatory response. Both peptides are highly cationic, provoke histamine release from basophils and mast cells, and cause smooth muscle contraction and increased microvascular permeability. In addition, C5a promotes activation, receptor-mediated chemotaxis, and adherence of PMNs. This activation includes respiratory burst activity with production of toxic oxygen radicals, degranulation of lysosomal proteases, IL-1 secretion, and release of prostaglandins and leukotrienes.

All of these mechanisms participate heavily in localized defense against injury and infection, but may also lead to diffuse organ dysfunction and parenchymal damage if generalized and indiscriminant after excessive activation by devitalized tissue or systemic bacterial infection. Both in vivo animal models and actual clinical settings, such as renal dialysis, have demonstrated that systemic complement activation may result in diffuse tissue injury. Observed pathologic changes in the lung include pulmonary microvascular leukoaggregation, membrane lipid peroxidation secondary to PMN-derived toxic oxygen radicals, and histologic evidence of endothelial cell injury with increased permeability culminating in hypoxemia and respiratory failure.[20] Furthermore, reductions in hepatic, renal, and mesenteric perfusion have been noted, again associated with microcirculatory leukocyte aggregation and microthrombosis. Such observations suggest a prominent role for complement cascade by-products in the pathophysiology of posttraumatic organ dysfunction.

Eicosanoids. The eicosanoids comprise a large number of biologically active derivatives of arachidonic acid, a ubiquitous 20-carbon polyunsaturated fatty acid found in the lipid bilayer of cell surface membranes. These substances have protean effects on the modulation of host responses to shock and sepsis that are mediated via autocrine, paracrine, and endocrine mechanisms. Although all cells share the capacity to mobilize arachidonic acid and generate eicosanoids, the specific metabolite produced is both cell-type and stimulus dependent.

Arachidonic acid is cleaved from membrane phospholipids by phospholipase A or C in response to cell-specific stimuli. This initial step is potently inhibited by glucocorticoids through the induction of an intermediate inhibitory substance (lipocortin), accounting for the antiinflammatory properties of steroid hormones. Once liberated, arachidonic acid is degraded by one of two membrane-associated enzymes: cyclooxygenase or lipoxygenase. Products of the cyclooxygenase pathway include the prostaglandins (PGD, PGE, PGF series), prostacyclin (PGI_2), and thromboxane (TxA_2).[14] This pathway involves oxidation to unstable intermediates, which then decompose spontaneously to form the cyclic end products, and is inhibited by nonsteroidal antiinflammatory drugs (NSAIDs) such as indomethacin, ibuprofen, and aspirin. The lipoxygenase pathway results in production of the leukotrienes LTB_4, LTC_4, and LTD_4, and 5- and 12-HETEs.

TxA_2 is produced primarily by platelets and macrophages, and elevated plasma levels have been documented during endotoxemia and posttraumatic shock. Platelets aggregated in response to epinephrine, ADP, or platelet activating factor release TxA_2, which is also a potent platelet aggregator and causes a "second wave" of aggregation. TxA_2 is likewise a potent constrictor of pulmonary and systemic vascular smooth muscle, as well as bronchial smooth muscle. Among the principal biologic consequences of TxA_2 activity are, therefore, va-

soconstriction, stasis, and microvascular thrombosis. These properties contribute significantly to the development of the early pulmonary hypertension commonly observed secondary to endotoxemia.

In contrast to TxA_2, PGI_2 inhibits platelet aggregation and causes relaxation of bronchial and both pulmonary and systemic vascular smooth muscle. PGI_2, one of the principal eicosanoids produced by endothelial cells in response to endotoxins and hemorrhagic shock, serves a homeostatic function by counteracting the effects of TxA_2 in intact vascular beds where thrombosis would be inappropriate. Although PGI_2 has no direct effects on microvascular permeability, its vasodilatory properties augment fluid efflux in vascular beds where barrier function has already been altered by other inflammatory mediators.

Perhaps the most diverse set of activities among eicosanoids belongs to PGE_2, the favored arachidonate product in the renal medulla, gastric submucosa, and endothelium. PGE_2 release is observed during endotoxemic and hemorrhagic shock and after experimental splanchnic ischemia-reperfusion injury. In addition to causing bronchial and microvascular dilatation, nonvascular smooth muscle contraction, and inhibiting platelet aggregation, PGE_2 also modulates lymphocyte and macrophage function, renal tubular sodium absorption, and neurotransmission. It is a primary regulator of renal and gastric microperfusion and therefore has protective as well as functional effects on both organs. PGE_2 also appears to function in a paracrine/autocrine capacity as a negative feedback down-regulator of tumor necrosis factor and interferon-gamma inflammatory activities. However, overproduction and/or prolonged release of PGE_2 are associated with impaired humoral and cell-mediated immunity and lead to an increased incidence of infectious complications.

Leukotrienes are produced from arachidonic acid by the action of lipoxygenase. LTA_4 can be further metabolized to LTC_4 and D_4, or to LTB_4. LTC_4 and D_4, previously known as slow-reacting substances of anaphylaxis, are potent bronchoconstrictors and vasoconstrictors. They also dilate some microvessels, increase capillary permeability, and stimulate mucous production. LTB_4, on the other hand, has a different repertoire of effects, directed exclusively at augmenting PMN function through enhanced PMN adherence, diapedesis, lysosomal enzyme release, and toxic oxygen radical generation. LTB_4 is the most potent chemoattractant for neutrophils in the human lung, and elevated lung levels of both LTB_4 and neutrophils have been observed in the adult respiratory distress syndrome (ARDS). Clearly, the leukotrienes possess the potential for important participation in the systemic inflammatory response that characterizes the posttraumatic state.

Platelet activating factor. Platelet activating factor (PAF) is an endogenous phosphoglyceride with many potential roles in the posttraumatic response. PAF is synthesized primarily by PMNs, macrophages, platelets, and endothelial cells in response to a wide variety of stimuli, including LPS, tumor necrosis factor (TNF), calcium, bradykinin, and thrombin. The first step in PAF synthesis is the cleavage of arachidonic acid from the phosphoglyceride backbone, thus eicosanoid and PAF production are intimately linked. This compound is generated from membrane phospholipids and is either secreted or displayed on the cell-surface membrane to participate in cell-cell interactions. The effects of PAF are widespread and mediated by specific membrane receptors.

One principal effect of PAF during endotoxemia is systemic hypotension. It is postulated that leukocyte-derived PAF causes profound pulmonary vasoconstriction, bronchoconstriction, and capillary leak. This results in acute elevations in pulmonary vascular resistance, followed by right ventricular decompensation, left ventricular preload reduction, and systemic hypotension. Hypoxemia secondary to pulmonary interstitial and alveolar edema also ensues. PAF appears to produce these effects in part by stimulating local production of multiple eicosanoids. TxA_2 is a potent pulmonary vasoconstrictor and platelet aggregator, and TxA_2 levels correspond to the pulmonary pressure changes. Indomethacin pretreatment blocks TxA_2 production and abolishes the pulmonary hypertensive response.

Recently, PAF has also been implicated in acute bowel mucosal injury. When infused into the mesenteric circulation, PAF appears to act synergistically with both LPS and TNF to produce necrotic lesions in intestinal mucosa. Although studies have implicated PAF in the pathogenesis of necrotizing enterocolitis, there are also direct implications for posttraumatic intestinal barrier dysfunction and bacterial translocation. The mechanism for this is unclear, but may involve the chemoattraction by PAF of activated PMNs and their cytotoxic products to the epithelial barrier. A similar role for PAF in the etiology of hepatic and myocardial dysfunction following shock has been postulated.

Cytokine response

A great deal of attention is currently focused on a class of inflammatory mediators collectively referred to as cytokines.[12] These polypeptides, synthesized and secreted from stimulated immunocompetent cells in the blood and various tissues, function in the regulation of the immune and inflammatory responses. Unlike the classic stress hormones, it is likely that most cytokines exert physiologic effects while acting both as paracrine agents in local environments and as systemic mediators via the general circulation. Localized and appropriately directed cytokine activity in response to microbial invasion or local trauma clearly has beneficial effects for the host. When the inflammatory response becomes unfocused and generalized, however, and excessive cytokine dissemination occurs, a broad spectrum of pathologic events ensues that may have profoundly deleterious effects.[7] This occurs through a complex process of cytokine networking in which a cascade of inflammatory mediators is generated, resulting in diffuse activation of multiple molecular and cellular cytotoxic mechanisms. A complete description of the complex events associated with these agents is beyond the scope of this chapter, but several important participants are discussed (Table 6-2).

Tumor necrosis factor. Cachectin/tumor necrosis factor-alpha (TNF) is a 17 kD polypeptide of approximately 160 amino acids that is produced primarily by cells of the macrophage line (circulating monocytes, alveolar and peritoneal macrophages, Kupffer cells, etc.) in response to bacterial endotoxins, exotoxins, and other microbial products. Other cell types, notably microvascular endothelium and lymphocytes, also produce TNF. TNF production in response to LPS involves transcription and new protein synthesis. The secreted product is short-lived, having a half-life of about 15 minutes in humans.

The effects of TNF on immune and inflammatory function, metabolic activity, and hemodynamic parameters are widespread. TNF infusions mimic closely the known effects of acute endotoxemia, that is, hypotension, tachycardia, fever, acidosis, disseminated intravascular coagulation, and increased capillary permeability. These effects are manifested by diffuse organ damage involving the kidneys, adrenals, lungs, and gut.

Because the lethal effects of LPS infusions in animals can be blocked experimentally by passive immunization or by pretreatment with monoclonal antibodies to TNF, this agent is thought to be a central mediator in the pathophysiology of septic shock. Peak TNF levels occur approximately 90 minutes after endotoxemic challenge, then decline rapidly. This pulse is thought to be perhaps the initial signal governing the hemodynamic response to sepsis. Further evidence is provided by studies that have demonstrated a close correlation between peak and sustained TNF levels and mortality in meningococcal septicemia, particularly in children.

Other effects of TNF include PMN and mono-

Table 6–2 Characteristics of cytokine mediators

Cytokine	Structure	Sources	Stimuli	Effects
TNFα	17kD polypeptide	Monocyte/macrophages, lymphocytes, endothelium	LPS, exotoxins, fungi, viruses	Hypotension, shock; PMN release, activation, adherence; Macrophage proliferation, activation; Endothelial activation, leak; ↑ Lymphokine production; ↑ Acute phase protein synthesis, proteolysis, lipolysis
IL-1β	17kD polypeptide (soluble)	Monocyte/macrophages, lymphocytes, PMNs, endothelium	LPS, TNF	PMN release, adherence; Macrophage release, activation; Endothelial activation; T-cell proliferation, activation, lymphokine production; ↑ Acute phase protein synthesis, proteolysis, lipolysis; Fever
IL-2	15kD polypeptide	T-lymphocytes	IL-1	T-cell proliferation, activation, lymphokine production; Hypotension, capillary leak
IL-6	Phosphoglyco-proteins	Monocyte/macrophages, endothelium	LPS	T-cell proliferation and cytotoxicity; ↑ B-cell antibody production; ↑ Acute phase protein synthesis
IL-8	Polypeptide	Monocyte/macrophages	LPS	PMN chemotaxis, activation
IFNγ	Glycoprotein	T-lymphocytes	Bacteria, viruses, IL-2	Macrophage activation; Antigen presentation; ↑ B-cell antibody production; PMN activation

cyte/macrophage activation, increased lymphokine production, enhanced PMN-endothelial adherence by both endothelial and neutrophil-dependent mechanisms, increased endothelial procoagulant activity, and increased hepatic acute-phase protein synthesis accompanied by peripheral proteolysis and lipolysis. That TNF production in response to LPS has been documented in fetal and neonatal macrophages, and that elevated TNF levels have been observed in a variety of pediatric groups with severe infections, suggest that TNF plays a central role in the pathophysiology of organ dysfunction that follows shock and sepsis in post-traumatic patients of all ages.

The interleukins. Interleukin I (IL-1) comprises two distinct 17 kD species, one (IL-1α) that is predominantly membrane-associated and another (IL-1β) that is soluble and capable of being converted to a bioactive form by many nonspecific proteases present in inflamed tissues. Both species interact with the same specific cell-surface receptors on target cells. Following receptor binding, the peptide is internalized and translocated to the nucleus where it interacts directly with chromosomes.

IL-1 is synthesized primarily by macrophages in response to LPS, but also by neutrophils, lymphocytes, and endothelial cells in response to other stimuli. IL-1 increases circulating numbers of PMNs and monocytes through direct effects on bone marrow maturation and release, and also activates macrophages. It is a potent stimulus for T-lymphocyte proliferation, activation, and lymphokine production. The effects of IL-1 on hepatic metabolism are similar to those of TNF-increased acute-phase protein synthesis at the expense of peripheral proteolysis. IL-1 is also the original "endogenous pyrogen," responsible for resetting the hypothalamic thermoregulatory center via intracellular eicosanoid production and producing the febrile response to infection.

IL-1 has important effects on vascular endothelium, which may participate in many processes underlying organ injury during sepsis. Procoagulant activity on endothelial cell surfaces is up-regulated by IL-1, which causes enhanced tissue factor expression and inhibition of thrombomodulin (an endogenous anticoagulant). Several inflammatory mediators, including PAF and IL-1 itself, are produced by endothelial cells in response to IL-1 exposure, and these in turn are known to strongly activate PMNs. IL-1 also stimulates endothelial cells to synthesize and express several classes of cell-surface adhesion molecules that promote the adherence of PMNs, monocytes, and lymphocytes. Such functions serve to promote the tight adherence of activated PMNs and other cellular elements to microvascular endothelium, resulting in endothelial barrier injury, increased permeability, and transendothelial migration.

The role played by IL-1 in the hemodynamic response to sepsis is less clear. IL-1 alone has not reproducibly caused hypotension during experimental systemic infusion, but may act synergistically with TNF to produce hypotension. Because elevated serum levels of IL-1 have not been observed consistently during infection and endotoxemia, its role in the acute systemic response to trauma has not been established. It is more likely that the membrane-associated form plays an important role in the modulation of localized cellular responses to inflammatory stimuli in the wound and elsewhere.

Several other interleukins may also participate, to a lesser extent, in the posttraumatic state. IL-2 is elaborated by T cells in response to IL-1 and serves an amplification feedback function by activating T cells, promoting T-cell proliferation, and further stimulating lymphokine production. Although exogenous administration of IL-2 causes profound hypotension and capillary leak, it is not thought to be an important participant in shock following trauma and sepsis.

IL-6 represents a family of several related phosphoglycoproteins produced by macrophages and endothelial cells in response to LPS and other cytokines. This cytokine family stimulates both B- and T-lymphocytes and enhances their antibody production and cytotoxic potential, respectively. Like IL-1 and TNF, they also augment hepatic acute-phase protein synthesis and inhibit the production of albumin and other structural proteins. Elevated levels of these peptides are found circulating in response to trauma, endotoxemia, and thermal injury. Like TNF, they can be detected early in the course of injury and have a short half-life.

IL-8 is a recently described product of LPS-stimulated macrophages that acts as a potent chemoattractant and activator of PMNs. It has recently been established that IL-8 is identical to two other mediators, neutrophil activation protein (NAP-1) and macrophage inflammatory protein (MAP-2). Its role in the posttraumatic state is still undefined, but has recently been detected in bronchoalveolar lavage fluid from patients with ARDS, suggesting a role in the etiology of posttraumatic lung injury.

The interferons. In addition to its antiviral and lymphocyte-stimulatory properties, interferon-gamma (IFN-gamma) has been shown to be a potent stimulator of macrophage/monocyte cytotoxicity by enhancement of respiratory burst activity. It also enhances antigen presentation by up-regulating membrane HLA-Dr expression. The observations that these events are both inhibited by PGE_2, and that IFN-gamma levels are reduced in the posttraumatic period, have suggested that PGE_2-inhibition of IFN-gamma may be one mechanism by which immunosuppression associated with severe injury is brought about. The efficacy of enhancing immune function and preventing infectious complications in multiply injured trauma patients by administering exogenous IFN-γ is currently undergoing randomized, double-blind multicenter trials.

Others. The roles of other cytokines in the response to trauma are currently the subject of much investigation. Some of these include the colony-stimulating factors (GM-CSF, G-CSF), and the various growth factors (EGF, TGF, PDGF). All play major roles in the host response to injury and in the processes governing wound healing. As these agents undergo investigation, however, stringent criteria should be applied to conclusions regarding their clinical relevance and any potential therapeutic implications.

Cellular inflammatory responses

Monocytes and macrophages. As the above sections have described, the interplay between the many inflammatory mediators and various effector cells of the immune system is complex and extensive. The monocyte/macrophage appears to be the most proximal signal processor in many components of this response to trauma. Although circulating monocytes can be recruited to areas of inflammation, it is the resident macrophage populations in various tissues (for example, hepatic Kupffer cells, lung alveolar macrophages, and intestinal submucosal macrophages) that are responsible for early cytokine generation and the initiation and augmentation of the systemic inflammatory cascades.

In response to LPS, macrophages secrete TNF, IL-1, and various other cytokines. In addition, they have cell-surface receptors for C3b, C5a, the immunoglobulin Fc site, and a formyl-peptide receptor that recognizes formylated microbial proteins. Occupation of these receptors by opsonized bacteria or their products leads to the elaboration of various cytokines, cytotoxic products, and PMN chemotactic agents (for example, C5a, LTB4, IL-8). Macrophage procoagulant activity, which appears to be linked to tissue factor synthesis, is also stimulated by LPS and bacterial products, thus involving the coagulation cascade in the inflammatory response.[7]

It is attractive to envision a central role for alveolar and hepatic macrophages in the generation of systemic inflammatory response in the trauma victim. These cells are strategically located at two important portals of entry for bacteria in the critically ill trauma patient: the lungs and the enterohepatic axis. Exposure of macrophages to bacteria and their endotoxins that have transgressed the usual biologic barriers causes an immediate localized and systemic inflammatory response effected by cytokines and other mediators. In addition, local cytotoxic activity by these resident macrophages may produce considerable direct parenchymal damage.

Neutrophils. The neutrophil (PMN) is a primary effector cell of the posttraumatic response. It is rapidly recruited to sites of tissue injury by a host of chemoattractants and by specific adherence mechanisms that allow it to attach preferentially to appropriately stimulated endothelium. Its many phagocytic and cytotoxic functions allow it to engulf and dispose of both bacteria and necrotic debris.

The PMN contains several mechanisms for causing microbial death: membrane-generated toxic oxygen metabolites, and granule-based proteolytic enzymes and cationic proteins. Following cell activation, membrane-bound NADPH-oxidase generates superoxide anion ($O_2 \cdot {}^-$) from oxygen. Superoxide anions can combine spontaneously in a dismutase reaction to form hydrogen peroxide (H_2O_2) or can react with H_2O_2 itself in the presence of certain transition metals to form the hydroxyl radical ($OH \cdot$). All three compounds are strong oxidants and have been shown to be destructive to a wide variety of cellular components in vitro. In vivo, however, the principal oxidizing agent may be hypochlorous acid (HOCl), formed by H_2O_2 in the presence of myeloperoxidase, an enzyme that is abundant in PMN granules. In addition to being a potent oxidizing agent, hypochlorous acid causes oxidative inactivation of alpha-1-antiprotease, a ubiquitous enzyme that protects host tissues against PMN-derived proteases such as elastase and cathepsin-G. Observations in vivo suggest that nearly all H_2O_2 generated from superoxide may be preferentially channelled into the production of hypochlorous acid.

The other major limb of PMN-mediated tissue injury is the disgorgement of granular proteolytic enzymes, primarily elastase, collagenase, and cathepsin G. When a microbe is successfully engulfed during phagocytosis, extracellular release of granular enzymes is limited. If a PMN inappropriately attacks a nonmicrobial surface too large for ingestion, however, frustrated phagocytosis occurs in which an abortive phagocytic vacuole releases its toxic products into the immediate environment. These enzymes may disrupt the extracellular matrix and cause alterations in barrier function, parenchymal support, and cellular growth, migration, and differentiation.

With increasing frequency, the PMN is being implicated as a primary effector of tissue injury and organ dysfunction during the generalized inflammatory state that exists following trauma and shock. The role of PMN-mediated endothelial injury in the pathogenesis of this process is now well established.[14] Evidence of PMN infiltration into dysfunctional organs following shock and endotoxemia has long been available, but a causative role has not been proven. Neutrophil depletion studies have suggested that injury to the lung and other tissues by endotoxemia can be mitigated or entirely prevented by prior removal of circulating PMNs. More recently, monoclonal antibodies directed against PMN-membrane adherence molecules have been used to block PMN-endothelial adherence in vivo. Pretreatment with such antibodies protects against diffuse organ injury and death after hemorrhagic shock and resuscitation in rabbits and primates.[17,19] Histologic examination reveals that blocking PMN-endothelial adherence attenuates injury to the stomach, intestine, and liver, but surprisingly confers little protection to the lung. Inhibition of PMN-endothelial adherence has also been effective in ameliorating the microvascular injury observed in experimental ischemia-reperfusion injury and frostbite.

Endothelium. The endothelium has traditionally been thought of as a passive component of vascular conduits. More recently, however, an active role has been proposed for the endothelial cell in the pathogenesis of multiple organ dysfunction during shock and sepsis. It is now recognized that the endothelial cell displays a capacity for activation to a proinflammatory state characterized by cell-surface procoagulant activity, cytokine production, generation of toxic oxygen metabolites, and MHC-antigen presentation.

Perhaps its most significant proinflammatory property, however, is the synthesis and cell-surface expression of various intercellular adhesion molecules that serve to promote the tight adherence of PMNs and other immune cells to the endothelial surface. These adhesion molecules, termed endothelial-leukocyte adhesion molecules (ELAM-1

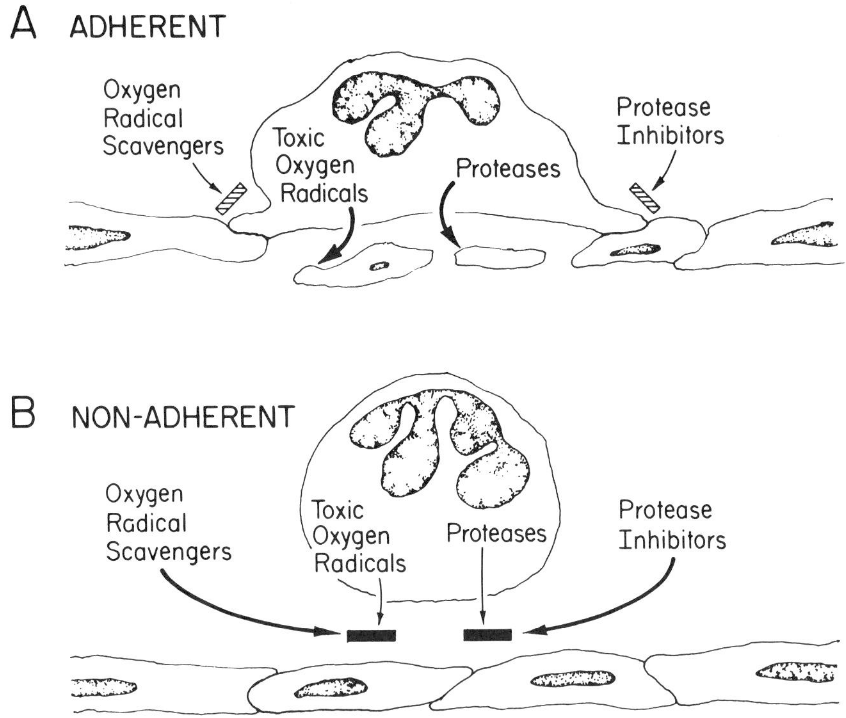

Figure 6–2 A, Adherent PMN has protected microenvironment for release of toxic products. **B,** PMN-derived toxic products are inactivated by circulating oxygen scavengers and protease inhibitors.

and 2) and intercellular adhesion molecules (ICAM-1 and 2), combine with specific ligands on PMNs, monocytes, and lymphocytes to promote their margination and emigration into tissues. Endothelial cells express these properties only after specific activation by LPS, TNF, or IL-1. Increased expression of these adhesion molecules by activated endothelial cells, as well as enhanced cell-surface procoagulant activity, results in leukocyte adherence, capillary plugging, and thrombosis of the microcirculation.

One important aspect of this relationship between endothelial cells and immune effector cells is the requirement for tight adherence in neutrophil-mediated endothelial injury. In vitro studies have established that the blocking of PMN-endothelial adherence completely protects against neutrophil-mediated destruction of endothelial monolayers. A similar requirement for adherence is likely to exist in vivo. Endogenous antioxidants and antiproteases are ubiquitous and highly effective in limiting the destruction of host tissues by toxic PMN-derived products. The tight adherence of PMNs to activated endothelial surfaces, however, provides an interface into which PMNs may release their toxic products. This protected microenvironment is inaccessible to circulating inhibitors, thus permitting the unopposed destruction of the underlying endothe-

lial barrier (Fig. 6–2). Loss of barrier function with increased permeability and cellular transmigration ensues, culminating in edema formation and direct injury to parenchymal tissues.

Ischemia-reperfusion injury

One of the primary mechanisms by which inflammatory cascades and effector cells become activated after injury and shock is through the functional derangements that occur in ischemic tissues when they are reperfused. Although restoration of oxygen delivery to ischemic tissues is requisite to cellular recovery and survival, much recent evidence illustrates that delivery of oxygen to ischemia-altered cells frequently causes more damage than the original ischemic insult alone. This paradox is explained by the fact that enzymatic pathways exist in ischemic cells which convert molecular oxygen to a variety of toxic oxygen metabolites. These metabolites, in turn, can cause direct biochemical injury or initiate proinflammatory and chemotactic signals that recruit activated PMNs.[6] Ischemia-reperfusion injury is a common consequence of trauma, whether confined to an injured limb or experienced diffusely by the gut and other organs as a consequence of hemorrhagic shock followed by resuscitation. Recent studies have documented an association between experimental ischemia-reperfusion injury of the gut and diffuse lung injury that is mediated by PMNs and has histologic and clinical similarities to ARDS.[8]

Purine components of nucleic acids are recycled by sequential degradation to hypoxanthine, xanthine, and uric acid. In normal cells, xanthine dehydrogenase catalyzes the conversion of hypoxanthine to xanthine and xanthine to uric acid, using NAD^+ as the electron acceptor during this oxidation. During cellular ischemia, however, xanthine dehydrogenase is converted to xanthine oxidase, which can perform the same degradation reactions, but requires oxygen as the electron acceptor. Upon reperfusion, large quantities of hypoxanthine that have accumulated from the breakdown of ATP to adenosine are converted to xanthine and uric acid. This reaction occurs in the presence of available oxygen and generates superoxide radical ($O_2 \cdot ^-$) and (H_2O_2). As in the PMN, this results in generation of highly reactive hydroxyl radicals.

Toxic oxygen metabolites produce cellular damage in a variety of ways. They oxidize nucleic acids and cause DNA "nicking." They cause membrane lipid peroxidation, which alters membrane fluidity and results in leakage. They also cross-link and degrade proteins, rendering them nonfunctional. The premise that such processes are clinically important is supported by many investigations that have documented protection against ischemia-reperfusion injuries by pretreatment with a variety of reactive oxygen scavengers and inhibitors such as allopurinol, superoxide dismutase, and catalase. Microvascular endothelial and intestinal mucosal epithelial cells contain particularly high concentrations of xanthine oxidase. It is self-evident that diffuse injury to these barriers by reactive oxygen metabolites would have profound and far-reaching consequences.

MULTIPLE ORGAN FAILURE SYNDROME

In the late 1960s and 1970s critical care technology became sufficiently advanced to support patients with posttraumatic organ dysfunction caused by a variety of causes. Patients who previously would have died in the early postinjury phase now survived weeks or months after the initial insult, and a few were able to leave the hospital and return to productive lives. Unfortunately, this prolongation of survival also led to the recognition of a new pattern of sequential, progressive multiple organ failure that was marked by an exceedingly high mortality rate.[1]

It was initially thought that this multiple organ failure syndrome (MOFS) was caused solely by uncontrolled infection. Accordingly, there was temporary enthusiasm in several centers for considering the onset of MOFS an indication for exploratory laparotomy in the absence of other identifiable infections. It soon became recognized, however, that MOFS was frequently, but not uniformly, associated with ongoing bacterial invasion. It is now understood that MOFS represents a state of altered physiology that accompanies the generalized activation of inflammatory cascades, one cause of which is concurrent, untreated sepsis. Frequently, however, the proinflammatory state is self-sustaining and persists long after invasive infections have been eradicated. In this syndrome, the delicate balance between controlled, local inflammatory activity and generalized protection of the host from the effects of inflammation is upset, leading to "malignant systemic inflammation."

The mechanisms by which ongoing systemic inflammation causes progressive organ dysfunction and failure at sites distant from the initiating stimuli are not fully understood. Although direct injury to tissues by the products of inflammatory cascades is possible, it is more likely that chemical mediators activate cells of the immunoinflammatory response in a nonspecific fashion, and that these cells are the common pathway by which most tissue injury is produced. Recent investigations have implicated PMN-mediated injury to endothelial barriers and other tissues as a primary causative event in MOFS.[7]

The patterns of organ dysfunction and failure that occur after trauma are relatively characteristic, implying that each system has a somewhat stereotypical response to a variety of injurious stimuli. The most frequent and consequential organs to fail are the lungs, liver, heart, kidneys, and gastrointestinal tract. The bone marrow, central nervous system, and endocrine systems also exhibit characteristic changes, but these are usually not the ultimate cause of patient demise. Whatever the combination of involved systems is, it is clear that mortality rate rises steeply with the number of systems failing, reaching nearly 100% when three or four systems are involved for more than 3 to 4 days.

Although not well quantified, the incidence of MOFS in pediatric trauma victims is perceived to be lower than that in the adult population. Two frequently stated explanations for this impression are that children have less preexisting medical comorbidity than adults, and that they may have better regulated immunoinflammatory responses. Given the widespread availability of handguns and the increasing exposure of children to violent crime associated with drug use, it is becoming clear that children and adolescents are becoming more frequent victims of serious injury. Pediatric surgeons therefore can expect to treat serious blunt and penetrating injuries more frequently than in the past;

they can also expect to encounter more patients with progressive organ dysfunction who require long-term physiologic support.

Respiratory failure

The adult respiratory distress syndrome (ARDS) is a frequent component of MOFS, usually occurring within 48 to 72 hours of the initial injury. The list of conditions thought to be etiologically related to ARDS is extensive: it includes pneumonia, aspiration, pulmonary contusion, toxic inhalation, sepsis, shock, massive transfusion, and pancreatitis. In spite of the wide variety of initiating insults, the pulmonary response is extremely constant and is manifested clinically by progressive hypoxemia resistant to supplemental oxygen, reduced lung compliance, and diffuse bilateral pulmonary infilrates on chest radiographs in the absence of cardiac failure.

The pathophysiology of ARDS can be thought of as noncardiogenic (or nonhydrostatic) pulmonary edema, caused by pulmonary microvascular endothelial injury and increased permeability. As the endothelial barrier is disrupted, the interstitial space is flooded with protein-rich fluid and cells, resulting in reduced compliance and increased work of breathing. When the interstitial space is exceeded, alveolar flooding occurs, leading to several events. As gas-exhange spaces fill, areas of low V/Q increase, as does the shunt fraction (Q_s/Q_t). This results in hypoxemia resistant to supplemental oxygen administration. Sensitive type I pneumocytes that line alveolar walls slough and leave a denuded basement membrane that accumulates cell debris and fibrin, forming a hyaline membrane. Surfactant is also inactivated, contributing to premature airway closure, loss of alveolar units, and decreased compliance. These changes are all similar to those seen in infant respiratory failure (IRF).

After this exudative phase, a proliferative phase is entered, in which thick, cuboidal type II pneumocytes divide to replace the alveolar membrane and fibroblasts migrate into both the interstitium and airways, laying down collagen in a process of progressive fibrosis. This gross distortion of pulmonary architecture has several consequences. The pulmonary capillary bed is progressively destroyed, leading to increased resistance and contributing to pulmonary hypertension. Fibrosis progressively disconnects the alveoli from the remaining capillaries, increasing both dead space and shunt. Cavities that form by coalescence of alveoli damaged by barotrauma also add to dead space ventilation and are more susceptible to rupture, leading to pneumothorax.

As activated PMNs have been found sequestered in the pulmonary microcirculation and interstitium, and have been retrieved from bronchoalveolar lavage fluid in patients with ARDS, a primary causitive role for PMNs has been hypothesized. This concept is supported by animal studies in which lung injury secondary to endotoxemia and other stimuli is attenuated by neutrophil depletion. In addition to causing endothelial injury as previously described, PMNs elaborate both PAF and TxA_2. These mediators lead to microthrombosis and pulmonary vasoconstriction, respectively, and contribute significantly to the production of pulmonary hypertension. Such conclusions must bc tcmpcrcd, however, by the realization that ARDS has been documented in severely neutropenic patients, implying a multifactorial etiology for this stereotypical response to injury.

The principal treatment strategies in ARDS are directed at two goals: recognition and treatment of the underlying inflammatory stimulus, and supportive measures to allow time for resolution and healing of the pulmonary injury to occur. Supportive measures usually include mechanical ventilation with positive end-expiratory pressure (PEEP), which is designed to recruit and maintain functional alveolar units and to reduce V/Q mismatch and shunt. Although recognition and monitoring of those patients who are at highest risk to develop ARDS is important, no benefit is derived from the prophylactic use of PEEP. In spite of many important advances in the understanding and treatment of this disorder, mortality rates of 40% to 60% are still commonly reported for this syndrome.

Cardiovascular failure

Altered myocardial performance is a frequent contributor to MOFS following trauma. Quantifiable reductions in myocardial contractility (for example, stroke-work index) in the absence of cardiac contusion have been documented in sepsis and following hemorrhagic shock. A variety of substances collectively referred to as "myocardial depressant factors" (MDFs) have been isolated from experimental animals subjected to a wide variety of injuries. It is postulated that these factors are released from the wound or from poorly perfused tissues, such as the splanchnic bed, and circulate to the heart where they exert negative effects on contractility. In addition to MDFs, certain well-characterized stress-response mediators such as beta-endorphin are known to depress the inotropic state. Myocardial edema and functional membrane abnormalities that accompany the widespread effects of sepsis also have negative effects on caridac performance.

The clinical manifestations of left-ventricular dysfunction range from systemic hypotension to more subtle indicators of inadequate tissue perfusion, such as increased peripheral oxygen extraction and decreased oxygen consumption. Careful monitoring of peripheral oxygen delivery and consumption, and enhancement of these parameters when necessary by increasing blood oxygen content and cardiac output, represent important therapeutic interventions in MOFS.

An emerging concept in the hemodynamic management of the posttraumatic patient is an appreciation for right ventricular performance.[11] Even in the absence of obvious left ventricular dysfunction, right ventricular function may be seriously compromised. With relatively little muscle mass and a highly compliant chamber, the right ventricle has evolved as an efficient "volume pump," but a poor "pressure pump." Changes in circulating volume and preload are well tolerated, but increases in afterload frequently lead to decompensation.

As previously noted, endotoxemia and posttraumatic pulmonary dysfunction are characterized by an acute increase in pulmonary vascular resistance. If this increased afterload exceeds the narrow margin within which the right ventricle can operate, the right heart will distend and fail. The increase in end-diastolic volume and pressure will elevate myocardial oxygen demand and simultaneously reduce subendocardial coronary flow, thereby exacerbating myocardial ischemia. Finally, right-sided output will fall, resulting in a reduction in left ventricular preload, decreased stroke volume, increased heart rate, and, ultimately, in hypotension and shock. Judicious use of inotropes and pulmonary vasodilators improves right ventricular function. PGE_1 is a direct pulmonary vasodilator that is metabolized during first passage through the lung and, therefore, has few systemic effects. This agent may become the drug of choice in treating isolated right ventricular failure in the posttraumatic period.

Renal failure

Posttraumatic renal dysfunction has been well recognized since World War II. The advent of hemodialysis, providing an effective means of supporting fluid and electrolyte clearance until renal function recovers, has allowed the study of the natural history of acute renal failure following trauma. Although virtually all renal dysfunction in this setting is referred to as acute tubular necrosis (ATN), there is widespread agreement that ATN is not simply one entity. Before a diagnosis of ATN can be made, renal failure due to inadequate renal perfusion (prerenal failure) and obstruction (postrenal failure) must be excluded.

Acute renal failure in the posttraumatic setting may be related to one or more of several factors. Classically, ATN referred to direct tubular epithelial damage either from ischemia (the medullary tubular loops are the most ischemia-sensitive elements in the kidney), or from direct toxins (for example, aminoglycosides and myoglobin). As tubular epithelial cells become swollen from membrane dysfunction, the tubular lumen becomes obstructed. This condition is exacerbated by cellular desquamation and cast formation. Tubular obstruction leads to increased intraluminal pressure, culminating in diminished glomerular filtration. Another related cause of oliguria and azotemia is the passive backflow of tubular luminal contents through the damaged epithelial barrier, and into the renal interstitium and capillary bed.

A separate mechanism of acute renal failure relates to the maldistribution of renal parenchymal blood flow. In ATN, renal cortical blood flow appears to be disproportionately reduced, reflecting a diffuse afferent arteriolar vasoconstriction. Increased afferent resistance directly decreases glomerular flow and, therefore, filtration. The stimulus for this vasoconstriction is unclear, although a primary role for prostaglandins has been postulated. Prostaglandin inhibition, however, does not appear to alter and may worsen the course of ATN associated with MOFS.

Treatment of progressive renal dysfunction in the posttraumatic state is mainly supportive. Of paramount importance is aggressive hemodynamic monitoring and management to ensure that blood volume and renal perfusion are normalized. Beyond this, the use of diuretics and low-dose dopamine infusion (1-3 $\mu g/kg/min$) may stimulate water and sodium excretion but do not appear to alter outcome. It is well accepted that nonoliguric renal failure carries a much better prognosis for full recovery than does oliguric failure. Consequently, clinicians frequently attempt to "convert" oliguric renal failure to nonoliguric azotemia by the use of forced diuresis and dopamine. These measures may, in fact, only identify those patients with enough renal reserve to respond to aggressive treatment and may not represent a real improvement in outcome.

Gastrointestinal failure and bacterial translocation

Progressive dysfunction of the gastrointestinal tract is a well-recognized problem in the management of the multiply injured patient. Patients with no significant injuries to the GI tract itself nevertheless display several types of enteric failure. For many years, attention centered primarily on two of these entities: paralytic ileus and stress-induced gastritis with hemorrhage. With the advent of parenteral nutrition in the late 1960s, routine decompression of the nonfunctional GI tract and provision of adequate energy and protein substrate by the intravenous route became standard supportive measures in the ICU. Subsequently, neutralization of gastric acidity accompanied by careful monitoring of gastric pH dramatically reduced the incidence of stress gastritis and bleeding and the associated high morbidity and mortality.

These therapeutic maneuvers brought to light several other manifestations of GI compromise. Long-term total parenteral nutrition is associated with multiple potential complications, including catheter-related sepsis, acalculous cholecystitis, cholestatic jaundice, fatty infiltration of the liver with inflammation, and a variety of metabolic and electrolyte abnormalities. Gastric alkalinization promoted bacterial overgrowth of the normally sterile stomach, leading to microaspiration in the ventilator-dependent patient and an increased incidence of serious gram-negative pneumonias. Prevention of stress gastritis by cytoprotective agents while maintaining the normal inhospitable acidic environment has been shown to decrease the incidence of serious nosocomial pneumonias, one of the principal contributors to the morbidity of long-term respiratory support. These developments highlight the risks that attend prolonged intestinal disuse and alterations in normal gut flora.

Perhaps the most physiologically devastating consequence of enteric dysfunction is the loss of mucosal barrier function and the subsequent translocation of bacteria and endotoxin from the gut lumen to the lymphatic and portal venous systems. The gut normally relies on three basic mechanisms to protect against invasion from commensal bacterial flora: physical, microbiologic, and immunologic. Physical aspects of host protection include an intact epithelial barrier that undergoes continuous renewal and desquamation, intact aboral peristalsis, and mucous production. Second, a delicate microbiologic balance exists between inhabitant flora, preventing colonization and overgrowth of pathogens. The anaerobic species are proposed to play a major role in this process. Finally, there exists an active immunologic barrier composed of secreted immunoglobulins and a complex system of resident immunocompetent cells, referred to as gastrointestinal-associated lymphoid tissue (GALT). Alterations in any or all of these components will place the host at risk for translocation of bacteria and endotoxin. Once internalized, these inflammatory stimulants may escape filtration and neutralization by macrophages in the intestinal wall, regional mesenteric lymph nodes, or hepatic reticuloendothelial system (Kupffer cells) and may gain entry into the systemic circulation. Furthermore, stimulated Kupffer cells may elaborate

TNF and other mediators of systemic inflammation, in addition to altering normal adjacent hepatocyte function.

Impairment of these defenses is common in the critically ill patient. Intestinal mucosa atrophies when not fed enterally, probably as a result of diminished perfusion, the lack of luminal glutamine, and the absence of normal trophic substances that are stimulated by feeding. Ischemia associated with hypotension and sepsis, as well as reperfusion injury during resuscitation, add to the disruption of the epithelial barrier. Alterations in gut microflora are also common, owing not only to gastric alkalinization, but also to systemic antibiotics used for other indications and to the abnormal environment of the ICU. Much recent investigation has documented that multiply injured patients are immunocompromised, and it is no surprise that this should affect defenses against invasion from gastrointestinal bacteria.

Although translocation of bacteria and endotoxins from the gut is an attractive hypothesis for the pathogenesis of MOFS in patients with no other identifiable infection, evidence to support this theory is incomplete. Multiple studies in animals have correlated various physiologic insults (endotoxemia and shock, for example) with translocation of intestinal bacteria to the mesenteric lymph nodes, liver RES, and spleen. Whether this represents a causative relationship or an epiphenomenon is unclear. Several trials of selective decontamination of the gut ("selective" in that the anaerobic population is preserved) by the prophylactic enteral administration of nonabsorbable antibiotics have been undertaken in a variety of patients, including trauma victims. Although infectious complications such as bacteremia, pneumonia, and urinary tract infection were reduced, no reduction in overall mortality was observed.[16] Infection may merely identify yet another organ system failure: the immune system. Such patients may be dying, not from infection, but with infection. Whether or not such regimens will be efficacious in preventing MOFS in the postinjury state awaits further clinical investigation.

Therapeutic approaches

In spite of steady progress in the physiologic support of multiply injured patients, MOFS continues to be a common complication of trauma and carries an extremely high mortality rate. It has become abundantly clear that simply substituting technology for failing organs may prolong survival without improving it. For this reason, attempts to alter clinically the ultimate course of MOFS have focused on interrupting or modifying the cycle of autoinflammation that defines the syndrome.

Several trials of selective bacterial decontamination of the gastrointestinal tract have documented a reduction in nosocomial infections but have failed to improve rates of survival. This may be because other impaired mechanisms of maintaining intestinal barrier function are not addressed, namely, underlying immunocompromise and the damaged epithelial interface itself. With new modalities of immunologic support and emphasis on early enteric feeding with glutamine-supplemented diets, selective decontamination may contribute to an improvement in outcome.

Several attempts to alter the course of MOFS by inhibiting the activation and perpetuation of the inflammatory cascade have been reported. The contribution to ARDS and MOFS by eicosanoid products has been extensively studied in animals, suggesting an important pathogenic role. Cyclooxygenase inhibitors (NSAIDs) have been shown to improve hemodynamic and respiratory parameters, as well as survival, in animal models of septic shock. Similar benefits have not yet been reproduced in human trials.

Another recent approach has relied on the proximal inhibition of the systemic inflammatory response by administering monoclonal antibodies directed against constant determinants on the lipid A moiety of LPS to patients with gram-negative endotoxemia and sepsis. Lipid A is the component of LPS that confers biologic toxicity to this molecule. Early results have indicated that survival is improved in "septic" patients who have documented episodes of gram-negative bacteremia, but not to the majority of patients who have physiologically defined "sepsis" without identifiable bacteremia.[22] Although these results may suggest a specific role for anti-LPS in documented gram-negative sepsis, they also emphasize the frequent nonbacteremic nature of sepsis syndrome. Inhibition of TNF by monoclonal antibody infusion has demonstrated marked attenuation of the hemodynamic consequences of endotoxemia and might also be expected to have a beneficial effect in nonbacteremic, autoinflammatory pathologic states as well. Given the extremely short circulating time and transient activity of TNF, however, the utility of anti-TNF therapy in the clinical setting is likely to be limited, and pretreatment of animals prior to abdominal sepsis has actually decreased survival rates.

Another potential adjunctive modality in the treatment of MOFS may be the selective inhibition of PMNs, which are thought to be common effector cells in many aspects of diffuse organ injury following trauma and sepsis. As previously discussed, monoclonal antibodies directed against PMN-membrane adhesion complexes have been used to block PMN-endothelial adherence in vivo and to protect against organ injury and death after hemorrhagic shock and resuscitation in several animal models. Although the safety and efficacy of anti-PMN therapy in humans suffering from MOFS have not been established, such findings support a central role for diffuse endothelial injury mediated by activated PMNs in the pathogenesis of multiple organ dysfunction following shock and trauma, and they suggest exciting new therapeutic modalities in the treatment of the multiply injured patient.

REFERENCES

1. Baue AE: Multiple, progressive, or sequential systems failure: a syndrome of the 1970s. *Arch Surg* 110:779, 1975.
2. Becker DP, Miller JD, Ward JD et al: The outcome from severe head injury with early diagnosis and intensive management, *J Neurosurg* 47(4):491, 1977.
3. Berger MS, Pitts LH, Lovely M, et al: Outcome from severe head injury in children and adolescents, *J Neurosurg* 62(2):194, 1985.
4. Bruce DA, Raphaely RC, Goldberg AI et al: Pathophysiology, treatment, and outcome following severe head injury in children, *Child's Brain* 5(3):174, 1979.
5. Bruce DA, Schut L, Bruno LA, et al: Outcome following severe head injuries in children, *J Neurosurg* 48(5):679, 1978.
6. Carden DL, Smith JK, Zimmerman BJ et al: Reperfusion injury following circulatory collapse: the role of reactive oxygen metabolites, *J Crit Care* 4(4):294, 1989.
7. Carrico CJ, Meakins JL, Maier RV et al: Multiple-organ failure syndrome, *Arch Surg* 121:196-208, 1986.
8. Caty MG, Guice KS, Oldham KT et al: Evidence for tumor necrosis factor-induced pulmonary microvascular injury after intestinal ischemia-reperfusion injury, *Ann Surg* 212(6):694, 1990.
9. Clowes GHA, George BC, Viller CA et al: Muscle proteolysis induced by a circulating peptide in patients with sepsis or trauma, *N Engl J Med* 308:545, 1983.
10. Coran AG: *Pediatrics: perioperative care.* vol 8(1):23. In D.A. Willmore et al, editors: *Care of the surgical patient,* New York, 1991, Scientific American.
10a. Cuthbertson DP: Observations on the disturbances of metabolism by injury to the limbs, *Q J Med* 1:233, 1932.
11. Eddy AC, Rice CL: The right ventricle: and emerging concern in the multiply injured patient, *J Crit Care* 4(1):58, 1989.
12. Fong Y, Moldawer LL, Shires GT et al: The biological characteristics of cytokines and their implications in surgical injury, *Surg Gynecol Obst* 170:363, 1990.
13. Gurll NJ, Reynolds DG, Holaday JW: Evidence for a role of endorphins in the cardiovascular pathophysiology of primate shock, *Crit Care Med* 16(5):521, 1988.
14. Jaffe BM, LaRosa CA, Kimura K: Prostaglandins and surgical disease, II, *Curr Prob Surg* 25(11):715, 1988.
15. Kronenberg R, Hamilton FN, Gabel R et al: Comparison of three methods for quantitating respiratory response to hypoxia in man, *Respir Physiol* 16:109, 1972.
16. Ledingham IM, Alcock SR, Eastaway AT et al: Triple regimen of selective decontamination of the digestive tract, systemic cefotaxime, and microbiological surveillance for prevention of acquired infection in intensive care, *Lancet* i:785, 1988.
17. Mileski W, Winn RK, Vedder NB et al: Inhibition of CD18-dependent neutrophil adherence reduces organ injury after hemorrhagic shock in primates, *Surgery* 108:206, 1990.

18. Nakayama DK, Romenofsky ML, Rowe MI: Chest injuries in childhood, *Ann Surg* 210(6):770, 1989.
19. Vedder NB, Winn RK, Rice CL et al: A monoclonal antibody to the adherence-promoting leukocyte glycoprotein, CD18< reduces organ injury and improves survival from hemorrhagic shock and resuscitation in rabbits, *J Clin Invest* 87(3):939, 1988.
20. Ward PA,Till GO, Heatherill JR et al: Systemic complement activation, lung injury, and products of lipid peroxidation, *J Clin Invest* 76:517, 1985.
21. Weiss SJ: Tissue destruction by neutrophils, *N Engl J Med* 320(6):365, 1989.
22. Ziegler EJ, Fisher CJ Jr, Sprung CL et al: Treatment of gram-negative bacteremia and septic shock with HA-1A human monoclonal antibody against endotoxin, *N Engl J Med* 324(7):429, 1991.

7 Psychosocial Aspects of Care

Thomas Walsh

Among the multitude of medical and surgical factors in the area of pediatric trauma, the psychosocial aspects of trauma care may seem the least urgent and can at times be relegated to secondary status. In reality, however, the emotional aspects of trauma care should be viewed as being equal in importance to the various medical interventions. Probably no other type of emergency creates a situation in which the potential for anxiety and emotional impact is as great and as wide-ranging. One must consider the psychological implications not only for the child but also for parents, siblings, and all caregivers. Although important for all trauma victims, the dependence of the child on others, the special relationship to the family, and the emotional response that childhood injury evokes in all adults make these considerations more pressing for the injured child.

To care for the injured child adequately, therefore, it is important for professionals to understand the specific areas of trauma care that take on special importance for the child, the basic concepts of child development, and the complexities of parental emotional interactions.

THE CHILD

Pediatric trauma care is different from adult trauma care in a multitude of ways. Because of the vulnerability of the child, emergency care itself can become a second emotional trauma, adding to the stress caused by physical injury. Unlike the adult patient, the child does not have the cognitive ability to process and understand the complexities of medical care. The child has less well-developed defense mechanisms and thus does not have the same emotional ability to cope with stress. Because of inability to communicate, especially with medical personnel, a child may have problems in understanding what is taking place and in making known his or her needs and concerns. Even innocent comments are often misinterpreted by children and become significant sources of anxiety and fear. In addition, even more than adults, a child needs to have family available at a time of stress. In this setting parents may be emotionally unavailable or physically not present.

To understand how children at different ages are affected and the specific reactions typical of each age group, it is necessary to understand the basic concepts of child development. Each developmental stage has its own predictable hallmarks and issues. These are generally seen in all children, but may have subtle differences based on the individual child and family.

Age 0 to 3 years

For the infant, the emergence of a strong attachment to the mother is the central focus of development. Through much of the first year there is little appreciation of strangers, and the need for comforting, soothing, and nurturing is paramount. At about 9 months the child can appreciate strangers and begins to experience distress when separated from the comfort of the nurturing figures in his or her life. Thus, in the first 6 months the central issue to attend to is comfort and the provision of appropriate pain management. The need for parents to be close by for this age group is more for the parent's sake than for the child's.

By the end of the first year, children become more aware of the world around them, and the central emotional issue becomes separation from those with whom they have developed strong attachment for a sense of security. Children in this age group have little appreciation of space and time and possess little ability to delay gratification or to tolerate frustration. Language skills are poorly developed; thus the ability to communicate with strangers is difficult. These children are in the early stages of cognitive development and so have a limited sense of reality, routinely demonstrating illogical and "magical" thinking. The toddler is more sensitive to the disruption in trauma care than the infant. For a child of this age, even a brief separation can be overwhelming when he or she is in pain or when the surrounding world is strange and chaotic. The issue of separation is important when transportation is necessary, as well as when a child must be cared for in the hospital. The presence of one of the child's parents, a familiar person, or at least a calm, comforting adult, and the availability of a special object such as a blanket or a teddy bear can help to alleviate the stress of separation.

Age 3 to 6 years

For the preschool child (aged 3 to 6) the ability to tolerate separation is greater even though the availability of parents is still important. Children of this age can tolerate longer separations and understand that they will be reunited with parents. When under stress, however, the preschool child may well regress and demonstrate the same sensitivity to separation as the toddler. In preschool children the ability to think more rationally is noticeable, although their thinking continues to be more concrete and their view of what happens in the world around them egocentric. In this age group there is also an extreme sensitivity to body integrity and intactness; there can be confusion and anxiety about painful medical and surgical procedures, which may be perceived as punishment or an intentional attack on the child, especially if in the genital or anal areas. It is possible to explain medical procedures to the preschool child, to reassure, to respond to questions, and to allow the child to express feelings either verbally or through play.

Age 7 to 12 years

By age 7 there is a noticeable change in the way a child thinks, the ability to think abstractly becoming gradually more pronounced and refined, a process that continues through adolescence. With this increased ability to process information the child is more logical and rational and so can make use of explanations to understand illness, injury, and treatment. Thus the child will be more amenable to accepting unavoidable procedures and to cooperate with caregivers. This is a situation in which a child needs to feel somewhat in control of self and, at the same time, needs control from the environment—a balance that is difficult to achieve in the emergency setting.

In addition to enabling the child to process information more effectively, increased abstract cognitive ability after age 7 allows the child to perceive death as a real and irreversible entity, and this becomes an acute and an unavoidable concern. In caring for the child in this age group, therefore, it is necessary to appreciate the presence of the fear of death accompanying any injury and to provide reassurance when necessary.

Adolescence

Adolescence is a period of continued cognitive development and increased psychological difficulty. The struggle for autonomy (independence from parents), the need to develop a future orientation, the sense of invulnerability to danger, illness, and death, and extreme sensitivity to the issues of body image and appearance all provide challenges to medical caregivers, especially in a time of emergency. Although adolescents have the cognitive ability to understand information about medical care, their emotional preoccupation with independence can produce noncompliance and lack of cooperation. Adolescents need firm limits, but with an understanding, empathic presence, to allow them to voice concerns about disfigurement, handicap, and death. Given the potential of emotional difficulty in adolescence with resultant depression, caregivers in a trauma situation must always question the nature of an injury and be alert to the possibility that an injury has been self-induced and to the obvious implications for appropriate consultation and treatment planning.

Other variables

Even though there is a significant predictability of emotional reaction for each age group, the manner in which any individual child responds to a particular stress is determined by other factors in addition to developmental stage. Thus there can be a noticeable variability of response among children of the same age. Constitutional factors, commonly referred to as temperament, account for a broad range of responses in any given developmental phase. Some children are intrinsically more adaptive and less reactive; therefore they are able to negotiate a stressful event more smoothly than others. Environmental and cultural factors also influence emotional reaction to stress. Prior experience with hospitals can at times provide some familiarity with care and thus facilitate adjustment. On the other hand, if past experience has been unpleasant or if there have been negative experiences, either directly or indirectly (for example, a serious injury or death of a friend or family member), adjustment and coping skills may be impaired. Because the child is sensitive to surroundings, the presence of extreme circumstances or the witnessing of tragic events can make adjustment more complex. In addition, because of the child's being so dependent on others, absence of parental support, anxiety, disorganization, or insensitivity to his or her needs by medical caregivers will make the child more vulnerable and impede the ability to cope.

Although symptoms such as agitation, withdrawal, or other disruptive behaviors can be seen as a function of an emotional response to a stressful situation, some children demonstrate abnormal or bizarre behavior that goes beyond the scope of adjustment phenomena. Symptoms such as disorders in thought process, hallucinations, delusions, agitation, panic, and disorientation are possibly a function of an encephalopathic process or delirium. These symptoms require not only behavior management but also an active evaluation of underlying physiologic causes. For the injured child the most common causes of delirium are head injury, drug toxicity, hypoxia, fluid and electrolyte disturbance, and abnormal metabolic states. The treatment of delirium is multidimensional, including correction of the underlying cause and environmental intervention, such as a decrease in extraneous stimuli, increased contact with staff and family, reassurance, and reorientation. Sedation is occasionally required. Fortunately, most acute confusional states are relatively short-lived.

THE FAMILY

The reactions of parents to the child, his or her injury, and the necessary care are critical factors in the child's ability to cope. Children who respond best to the stress of medical care are those whose parents demonstrate the least anxiety at each step of care from initial injury to the return home. As one might expect, the child from a disturbed environment in which parental support is poor will do less well under the stress of emergency medical care.

An injury to a child always precipitates a crisis for the family. The stress of an injury to their child subjects parents to a variety of emotions. Initially, they are shocked and numbed by the sudden, overwhelming threat to their child's well-being. At this time, parents' responses may be dulled and questions may be few while they try to comprehend what has happened. This reaction then gives way to a search for meaning and fear of the possible outcome. Parents begin to question everything, both of themselves and others, as they try to make sense of the situation and achieve some measure of control. The information they begin to receive about the injury and the child's condition may be so overwhelming that they need to deny the seriousness of the threat to their child's well being. This denial may be frustrating to the caregivers who wish to help the family; it is necessary to understand that the process of emotional stabilization and acceptance must move at its own rate. Not only are these reactions variable from case to case, but they may also vary between the two parents of one child. Unfortunately, this difference can become the source of marital conflict and discord.

Parents may also develop a sense of guilt that they did not protect their child or, in a search for some degree of control, may feel that they are somehow responsible and that the incident is punishment for a past transgression. Although a sense of guilt may help to move parents to effective problem solving, feelings of excessive guilt may have the opposite effect, paralyzing them and impairing their ability to cope. Anger or depression may follow, resulting in attacks on medical staff and emotional unavailability to the child.

Because parents are the most important source of comfort to the child and because psychological fallout from this experience may affect the family for years to come, the parents' ability to cope with the episode is important. Each family requires support and guidance in its efforts to cope, and proper communication with the parents is essential. This communication is the foundation for the relationship with the child's physician, providing a stabilizing force for the family and demonstrating that the child's care is important to others. To be most effective, communication should be the responsibility of one physician.

Mental health staff must be available to assist the child and family as soon as possible, when indicated. For parents to function adequately, emergency staff must also be supportive. It is important for all staff to avoid being drawn into a conflict with an angry parent, but rather to remain objective and empathic in an attempt to assist parents in moving forward in the adjustment process. Withdrawn, depressed parents often need to be gently pursued and drawn into the care of the child if only minimally, such as in discussing progress. Staff must be careful to avoid reinforcing nonproductive anger or withdrawal.

Siblings are also stressed at a time of medical emergency. They are often confused because little or no information is shared with them in an attempt to spare them the pain that parents are experiencing. Brothers and sisters are, in fact, quite aware of the tension and changes in the family; without concrete information they are left to imagine the worst. They may begin to think that the injured sibling has died, that they are somehow responsible, and that they too will soon experience the same tragedy. As care progresses, siblings may also feel resentment that the injured child is receiving special attention or that parents seem interested only in the sick child. All of these concerns require special consideration. Efforts to support and help parents to cope will ultimately benefit siblings, but in the acute phase parents may need specific guidance to help their other children. Direct intervention by medical staff, providing information and support, may be necessary for siblings in a time of crisis.

THE CAREGIVER

Professionals engaged in care of injured children also are subject to emotional stress, especially in the care of the child with major injury. While health care staff are making life-saving judgments and interventions almost daily, they are constantly exposed to suffering, disfigurement, and loss—persistent reminders of their own vulnerability. In response to intense stress and anxiety, staff may react with emotional detachment, denial of feelings, depression, stress-related physical disorders, and even impaired clinical judgment. Frustration may produce or increase anger at parents for not protecting the child or for allowing injury to the child, even when the parents did nothing to cause the trauma. This, unfortunately, can begin a vicious circle that affects the emotional outcome for all involved. Staff often become so overwhelmed that they shut themselves off from the useful support of the group and become isolated and alone. In many cases, intervention, including supportive debriefing, can help to sustain trauma staff and avoid pathologic defenses and burnout.

DEATH

Unfortunately, death is a common part of trauma care. The death of a child and its impact on the family (and sometimes the death of a family member in the same traumatic event) presents special challenges to patients and caregivers alike.

Confronting the death of a child is possibly the most difficult task a parent can face. The parent's response can vary dramatically, depending on the circumstances of the injury or death, past experiences with death, family support, and preexisting personality factors. Some parents are so overwhelmed that they are unable to be available to the dying child, spouse, and other children. Initial reactions, which may be predominant in the case of accidental death, include disbelief and shock followed by denial and avoidance. At times, when death is sudden, a parent may be seemingly unaffected and appear calm and in control; in these cases those involved in trauma care may never see the true emotional reactions. The guilt, anxiety, and depression felt upon a child's death can produce withdrawal, intrusive behavior, criticism of care provided, and anger, which may gradually give way to regret and acceptance of the inevitable. Some parents react with extreme panic or total withdrawal and depression. Because grief is a gradual process, emergency medical staff are not usually part of more than the initial phase. The role of emergency staff is to provide initial support and remain nonjudgmental. It is important to ensure some monitoring of the grieving process, and a follow-up protocol can be of great value in aiding parents' long-term adjustment.

An often-forgotten part of a grieving family is the dead child's sibling. A sibling typically experiences confusion about the child's hospitalization and death and has to cope with this without the emotional support of parents. The sibling may feel a sense of guilt and can become depressed. There is a strange ambivalence between resentment of the attention the injured child has received and sadness over the child's death. Because siblings often fear that a similar fate will befall them soon, they can become fearful and clinging.

Another difficult situation is that in which an injured child survives but a family member dies. This presents special challenges regarding decisions about how much information the child should be given, when, and by whom. It is important to assess the point at which a child is able to process such news, and it is wise to convey bad news when a supportive family member can be with the child.

EMOTIONAL SEQUELAE

There is often a delayed emotional reaction to a traumatic event, both in the acute phase or over the long-term adjustment period. Immediately following a critical period, a child may become overcautious and fearful, exhibiting a variety of behaviors and emotions not seen earlier. Anxiety and confusion become more noticeable as time passes. It is in the period after the acute phase that the child is more amenable to emotional support, which may enable him or her to master the emotional trauma. In some cases, if the stress of a traumatic event is ignored, a posttraumatic stress disorder (PTSD) emerges with symptoms such as a preoccupation with safety and injury, recurrent nightmares, anxiety, hypervigilance, irritability, and extemes of emotion. The stressful event causing PTSD may be the accident, injury, or the emergency medical care itself. Parents should be warned about long-term sequelae and helped to understand the need for intervention.

It is important to be aware that long-term emotional sequelae in a child with a head injury are often difficult to differentiate from the relatively frequent neuropsychiatric symptoms of postconcussion syndrome. Symptoms resulting from traumatic brain injury, which are mild but can persist for a year or more, include difficulty with memory and attention, confusion and disorganization, anxiety, mood lability and depression, and vague sensory and somatic symptoms. Although these symptoms are more frequent than those associated with circumscribed cortical lesions, they tend to go unrecognized or, when evident, to be interpreted as psychosocial in nature. Once the link to neurologic injury is appreciated, the potential for appropriate intervention, both pharmacologic and behavioral, helps to ameliorate the symptoms or at least to prevent the development of secondary emotional complications.

Long-term adjustment is a problem for the family as a whole and may continue through a rehabilitation period beyond the recovery phase before the return of physical health. In fact, in many cases the emotional aftermath is the only true long-lasting complication of a traumatic injury for both the child and the family. The unrecognized emotional trauma to the child and siblings, the stress on a marriage, the reactions of each parent, and the change in the parent-child relationship can all have irreversible effects. The potential for a maladaptive overprotection of a child who has in fact returned to a state of good health (the vulnerable child syndrome) needs to be anticipated.

Given the clear risk of adjustment problems in the child, family, and staff, it is crucial that professionals involved in trauma care be prepared to anticipate and respond to the emotional needs of all the victims. Provision of a mechanism for the detection of maladaptive patterns and anticipation of the need for appropriate mental health intervention are essential components of truly comprehensive trauma care for the child.

REFERENCES

1. Green M, Solnit AJ: Reactions to the threatened loss of a child: a vulnerable child syndrome, *Pediatrics* 34:58, 1964.
2. Gualtieri CT: Pharmacotherapy and the neurobehavioral sequelae of closed head injury, *Brain Injury* 2:101-129, 1988.
3. Harris BH, Schwaitzberg SD, Seman TM: The hidden morbidity of pediatric trauma, *J Pediatr Surg* 24(1):103-6, Jan 1989.
4. Jellinik MS, Herzog D: *Psychiatric aspects of general hospital pediatrics*, Chicago, 1990, Year Book Medical Publishers.
5. Jost E, Haase JE: At the time of death: help for the child's parents, *Child Health Care*, 18(6):146-152, Summer, 1989.
6. Livingston MG, McCale RJ: Psychosocial consequences of head injury in children and adolescents: implications for rehabilitation, *Pediatrician* 17(4):255-61, 1990.
7. Martini DR, Regan C, Nakagama D: Psychiatric sequelae after traumatic injury, *J Am Acad Child Adolesc Psychiatry*, 29(1):70-5, Jan 1990.
8. Perrin EC, Gerrity PS: There's a demon in your belly: children's understanding of illness, *Pediatrics*, 67(6):841-849, 1981.
9. Rutter M, Hersov L: Child and adolescent psychiatry, Oxford, 1987, Blackwell Scientific Publications.
10. Schlump-Urquart ST: Families experiencing a traumatic accident: implications and management, *Crit Care Nurs*, 1(3):522-34, Nov 1990.
11. Tichy AM, Braam CM, Meyer TA et al: Stressors in pediatric intensive care units, *Pediatr Nurs* 14:40-42, 1988.

PART THREE

Components of Pediatric Trauma Care

8 Continuum of Care: General Philosophy

Geraldine S. Pratsch and Martin R. Eichelberger

It took nearly 10 years for treatment of injured children to be accepted as part of the Emergency Medical Services (EMS) system in this country. Much persistence on the part of pediatric professionals who recognized a need, formed committees, passed resolutions, and educated legislators was necessary to develop an Emergency Medical Services for Children (EMSC) system, which complements the EMS system for adults.

With the recognition that children do have physiologic and psychological differences separate from adults, the development of pediatric guidelines, designation criteria, and standards of care was accomplished.[2] It was not intended that children have their own EMS system, but that health care professionals and prehospital providers of the existing EMS system be knowledgeable about the necessarily unique treatment and emotional needs of injured children and their families. However, because injured children do require specialized equipment and highly trained pediatric professionals to achieve optimal outcome, every EMS system needs a designated pediatric trauma center to provide the best care for severely injured children.

REGIONAL PEDIATRIC TRAUMA CENTER

A regional pediatric trauma center provides the mechanism to maximize resource utilization without duplication within a particular state or community. The designation of a pediatric trauma center is a politically based process representing the consensus of the community, which defines the standards of care for injured children. A regional pediatric trauma center provides the *immediate* availability of highly trained pediatric specialists and the application of hospital resources in a timely, coordinated, and efficient manner.

CONTINUUM OF CARE PHILOSOPHY

Care for the injured child and family requires a global commitment by the pediatric trauma center. Because injury is the leading cause of death of children in this country, care goes far beyond the walls of the center. There is a commitment of service to the child and family that involves prevention efforts in the community and the willingness to share pediatric knowledge with the physician, nurse, and prehospital provider who provide care to injured children.

The "continuum of care" philosophy requires a commitment to the injured child that includes prevention, acute care, and rehabilitation.[6] The conceptual framework (Fig. 8-1) defines the need for an interdisciplinary approach to care and focuses on the essential components of the EMSC, a federally funded program.[4] The components are prevention, prehospital, acute, restorative, and posthospital care. The horizontal axis indicates the passage of time, and the vertical axis indicates resource utilization. Research, education, and quality assurance are continuous throughout the model.

MODEL FOR CONTINUUM OF CARE

There are a multitude of services to assist the injured child and family who enter the EMSC system (Table 8-1).

Prevention

Prevention is the first line of defense to save lives, reduce disability, and avoid the high cost of trauma care. Prevention programs require incorporation into the overall EMSC system in averting pediatric injury and its consequences. The resources of the pediatric trauma center are of no avail if a child dies before reaching the center or within the first hour of care. There must be a balance between injury control programs and treatment services. Prevention requires a massive education effort aimed at parents, teachers, and day-care center staff. Education should include not only information on how to prevent injury, but also what to do until the EMS team arrives. Manufacturers of toys and of sports and recreational equipment also need education about how to "childproof" their products in anticipation of any potential hazard to the child. Children's National Medical Center (CNMC) channels its prevention efforts through the National SAFE KIDS Campaign. This program focuses parents and the lay public on specific initiatives to reduce the mortality and morbidity related to childhood injury. Creation of a safe environment for the

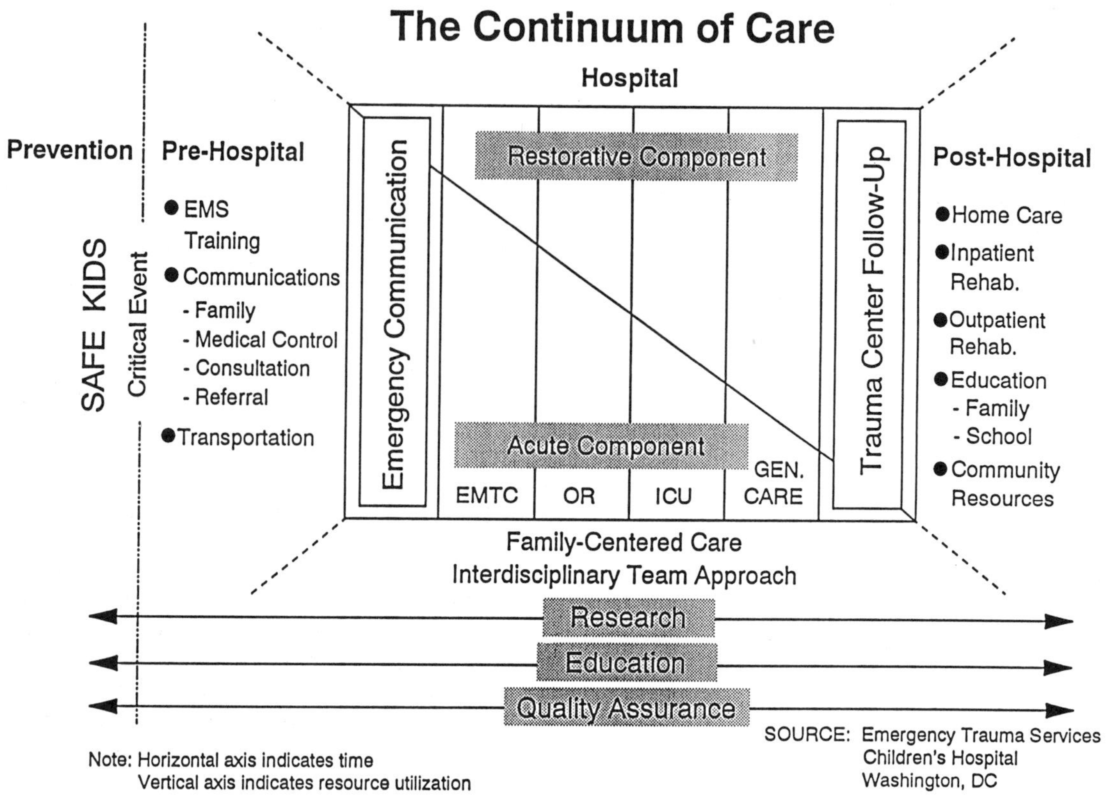

Figure 8–1 Conceptual framework for continuum of care.

growing child is imperative and can be achieved through knowledge about injury prevention (see Chapter 2).

Prehospital care

The prehospital phase of the continuum of care encompasses a wide range of activities. The most critical component of this phase is the prehospital provider who begins the definitive care of injured children and whose knowledge and skill in managing childhood injuries will effectively improve outcome. The skill of the prehospital provider, however, depends on several factors: (1) the amount of pediatric emergency training incorporated into the basic curricula and into EMS continuing education programs, (2) the type of drugs and equipment specifically designed for children that are carried on the ambulance for resuscitation and immobilization before and during transport, and (3) the involvement of pediatric health care professionals in the development of standardized prehospital pediatric treatment protocols and their communication by medical control to the prehospital provider.

Prehospital care also includes the Emergency Communication and Information Center (ECIC), which provides systematic triage of incoming communication from the field provider during transport, and from the local emergency department physician preparing a child for transfer to the pediatric trauma center. The ECIC, also the agency to arrange for air or ground transport of a child, is the pivotal link to the pediatric trauma care system for the region.

Acute care

A child entering the CNMC pediatric trauma center is given resuscitative care in the emergency department by a trauma team, which maximizes the utility of acute care resources.[3] Following resuscitation, stabilization, and radiologic assessment, the child moves on to surgery in the operating room for definitive treatment and subsequent transfer to the intensive care unit; continuous communication with the child's family is imperative. Optimal care of the child is achieved in the pediatric trauma center because of the highly skilled and dedicated professionals of the trauma team. This team functions according to a predetermined pediatric trauma protocol, in which the role and responsibility of each team member is clear.

In the emergency department the inner-core team consists of surgeons, pediatricians, anesthesiologist, and nurses, who function at the bedside in the

Table 8–1 The continuum of care

Accident prevention and injury control
Parent education
Public information
Accident prevention
Community programs
School and day-care education

Prehospital care
Seminars and workshops for prehospital providers, physicians, and nurses
Medical control for advanced life-support paramedics
Consultation with community hospitals
Transfer and transport arrangements

Acute care
Level I pediatric trauma center designation
Trauma resuscitation area, emergency department
Pediatric intensive care unit
Burn intensive care unit
Pediatric medical-surgical general care units
Restorative care services

Posthospital care
Interdisciplinary follow-up trauma clinic
Coordinated patient placement in appropriate rehabilitation facilities
Transition to home, school, and community
Long-term pediatric rehabilitative services

Research
Consistent, reliable data collection on all trauma patients throughout the continuum of care
Data analysis to determine improved care
Research abstracts and papers
Clinical research

Education
Continuing education for physicians, nurses, and prehospital providers
Standardized training programs sponsored and supported by professional organizations and agencies
Prevention programs offered to the community

Quality assurance
Data collection
Data analysis
Identification of areas for improvement
Improved patient care services

resuscitation area. The support team members of the department of social work, radiology, blood bank, central supply, and security are in liaison with the operating room and administrative staff. These support services are immediately accessible at any time during the resuscitation process. A group pager sounding the "Trauma Stat" activates the team in 1 to 2 minutes. Such organization of a trauma response team facilitates a standard of care that permits simultaneous diagnosis and treatment of life-threatening injuries of children. The trauma team is not exclusive to the emergency department. All hospital personnel who care for injured children within the hospital, including the general care units, are considered part of the trauma team.

Restorative care

Rehabilitation of a child with a disability resulting from acute injury and restorative care services begins at the moment of the critical incident and increases throughout the child's care and return to community living. The goal of rehabilitation is to achieve an optimum level of function by restoring or enhancing impaired or residual biologic function, by enhancing compensatory systems unaffected by the injury, and by adapting biotechnical equipment to enhance an individual's performance.[5] Disability can be minimized through attention to rehabilitation needs during the early phases of care. This information is used to develop short- and long-term goals directed at attaining an optimum level of functioning for the child and family.

Posthospital care

Long-term treatment of multiple-system injury in a child requires a mechanism to make available the many specialty physicians and restorative services. An interdisciplinary follow-up trauma clinic maintains continuity for children and families within a variety of services after discharge, without the inconvenience of multiple postdischarge hospital visits. If a long-term pediatric facility is necessary for a child's rehabilitation, continued services and consultation by team members of the follow-up trauma clinic are an important component of ongoing care.

Research

It is through the research process of data collection and analysis that discoveries are made that will ultimately reduce mortality and morbidity in childhood injury. Through their observations, a trauma team garners a wealth of information throughout the continuum of care. The trauma registry reflects clinical practice and EMSC systems services and adds dimension to the preventive aspects of caring for injured children. Such data collected ultimately provide descriptive information about the population using the services, as well as scientifically valid data for clinical research. Data are also collected to monitor the delivery of care and to identify deficiencies within the pediatric trauma center system in order to effect change through the quality improvement process.

Education

Education is a major component of a successful pediatric trauma system. This means not only education of health care professionals pertaining to acute care, but also community prevention education for parents, teachers, and day-care staff members.

Education of the trauma team is essential to provide rapid, efficient, and effective care to the seriously injured child and family. The continuing education and updating of trauma team members has become a standard of practice.

The emphasis in a pediatric trauma education program for the health care professional is the identification of areas in which the child differs from the adult, both anatomically and physiologically. Pediatric trauma centers working with community organizations can facilitate the introduction of pediatric injury prevention programs to the general lay public (see Chapter 2).

Quality care improvement

The most important part of quality improvement (QI) is proof of improvement as a result of the QI effort—the improvement being better patient care services. The objective of QI is not only to identify and resolve problems that affect quality of care, but also to identify and address opportunities for improvement.[1] Components of the quality-related process are (1) *quality control activities,* such as emergency department policies, prehospital provider treatment protocols, and trauma registry data collection, (2) *quality improvement activities,* such as revising policies and procedures, conducting inservice and continuing education programs, and analyzing data collected. These tasks are performed to foster continuous improvement within the system. *Quality improvement* means review and continuous assessment of all activities to assure a reliable program for children and their families.

Quality care for injured children depends on standards that are consistent within the pediatric trauma center and standards that are implemented throughout the regional EMS system served by the pediatric trauma center.[7]

SUMMARY

To improve outcome for injured children throughout the continuum of care, administrators and pediatric professionals must commit financial and human resources to integrate prevention, acute care, and rehabilitation. In addition, the pediatric trauma center needs the cooperation of state and local resources and decision makers to achieve delivery of optimum pediatric trauma care. Commitment to the continuum of care enhances the ability to provide the best care to injured children and their families.

REFERENCES

1. Benson, DS: Quality assurance in emergency services. In van de Leuv JH, editor: *Management of emergency services,* Rockville, Md, 1987, Aspen Publishing.
2. Committee on Trauma of the American College of Surgeons: *Resources for optimal care of the injured patient,* 1990, The Committee.
3. Eichelberger MR, et al: 1988. Pediatric trauma protocol: a team approach. In Eichelberger MR, Pratsch GS, editors: *Pediatric trauma care,* Rockville, Md, 1988, Aspen Publishing.
4. *Public Health Services Act,* Law of the 99th Congress, section 1910, 1985. Washington DC Sept 30, 1985, US Government Printing Office.
5. Rodriguez JG, Brown ST: Childhood injuries, *Am J Dis Child* 144:627-646, 1990.
6. Seidel JS, Henderson DP, editors: Emergency medical services for children: a report to the nation. Washington, DC, 1991. National Center for Education in Maternal and Child Health.
7. Standard guide for development and operation of Level I pediatric trauma facilities (F 1286-90), *Annual Book of ASTM Standards* 13.01:616-622, 1990.

Emergency Medical Services for Children: General Considerations

J. Alex Haller Jr.

Comprehensive pediatric emergency care should be integrated into an overall emergency care system and organized regionally to address the special needs of children. Some pediatric specialists have suggested that emergency care for children should be organized separately in a system parallel to adult emergency systems, but this plan would put children in competition with adults for national and regional funding. Equally pertinent is the natural overlap of many pediatric emergency services with obstetric, perinatal, adolescent, and young adult programs; all of these will be strengthened by integration and weakened by separation. The one nonnegotiable principle must be that any emergency medical system that includes children must use the best and most experienced pediatric specialists available in the area. The location of a regional pediatric emergency care facility (that is, a self-standing children's hospital versus a children's component of a general hospital) is not as important as the total commitment of that institution and its medical personnel to the optimal care of acutely ill and severely injured children.

ROLE OF TRAUMA SPECIALISTS AND PEDIATRIC SURGEONS IN ORGANIZING EMSC

How can trauma specialists and pediatric surgeons offer leadership in the organization of such Emergency Medical Services for Children (EMSC)? How can they use their experience in trauma care of children as a model to include children with life-threatening illness as well as multiple organ injuries?[2] Basically, the answers lie in reviewing what has been learned from the study and management of trauma in children and addressing objectively the challenges that lie ahead.

First, pediatric specialists must face the sobering fact that 50% of children who die between the ages of 1 and 18 die of injuries, and then ask why and what can be done about it. Second, they should focus on what has been learned about the diagnosis and management of serious trauma in children. Finally, they must ask how treatment of life-threatening illnesses can be integrated into a comprehensive EMSC that was originally designed to address life-threatening injuries.

CHANGES IN CURRICULA

Traditionally, pediatricians and internists have been excluded from the treatment of trauma victims during their residency training. This omission of experience in trauma management should be corrected in medical school and residency curricula. Indeed, several medical centers have begun introducing principles of trauma care, such as the didactic and skill materials of the Advanced Trauma Life Support (ATLS) course, into the undergraduate and postdoctoral curricula. Few pediatricians and emergency physicians have any operative experience or instruction in surgical skills as part of their formal training programs. Until surgical experience can be more widely disseminated and then implemented in a true surgical-pediatric partnership, the simple act of taking and passing an ATLS course, however laudable, cannot produce instant trauma experts. It is hoped that because of these ongoing curricular changes, pediatric surgeons and emergency pediatricians will work even more closely in a team approach to the management of one of the most complex of pediatric diseases, life-threatening trauma.

From pediatric surgeons within the ranks of general surgery came the new component of the ATLS course, management of trauma in children. Whenever and wherever the ATLS course is given regionally, to surgeons and emergency physicians, pediatric surgeons are asked to supervise the special pediatric skill stations and to lecture on resuscitation of severely injured children.

STANDARDS OF CARE

From the accumulated experiences in regional trauma systems came the endorsement by the American College of Surgeons for standards of care for critically injured pediatric patients.[1] This body of knowledge was developed by the Committee on Trauma of the American Pediatric Surgical Asso-

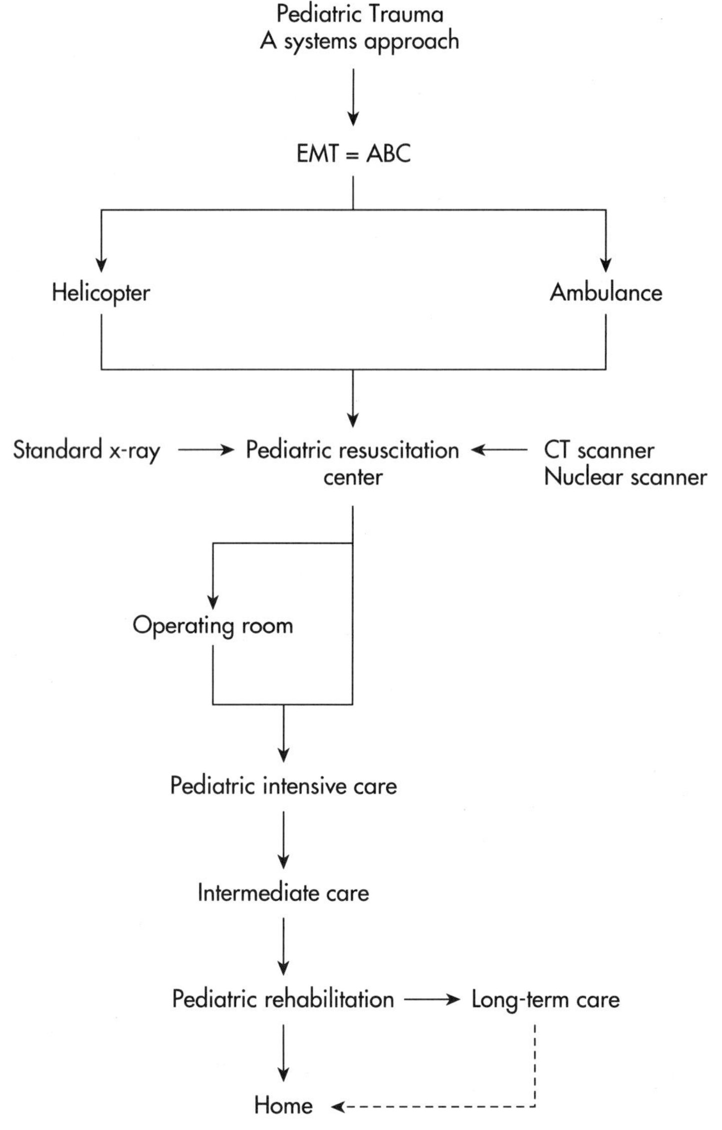

Figure 9–1 Components of regional trauma system for children emphasizing sequential use of integrated facilities and personnel. (From Touloukian RJ: *Pediatric trauma,* ed 2, St Louis, 1990, Mosby–Year Book.)

ciation.[7] These pediatric surgeons received much valuable input from emergency pediatricians in several regional emergency systems, notably those of Mobile-Birmingham, Alabama; Jacksonville, Florida; Boston; Salt Lake City; Philadelphia; and Baltimore.

SYSTEMS OF REGIONAL TRAUMA CARE

Extensive experience in the management of multiple systems injuries in children led to the establishment of systems of regional trauma care such as that at the Johns Hopkins Children's Center, which opened in 1973 in Baltimore.[4] The components of this system are illustrated in Fig. 9-1, which is a prototype of a regional pediatric trauma program.

In providing this initial leadership in the care of childhood trauma victims, pediatric surgeons with trauma experience have actively sought the cooperation and input of their emergency pediatrician colleagues. This close interaction is best illustrated by the role of pediatric surgeons in the development of the Advanced Pediatric Life Support course (APLS) of the American Academy of Pediatrics (AAP), whose effort was orchestrated through the Section on Emergency Medicine of the AAP. As a result of this cooperative venture in which pediatricians asked pediatric surgeons to provide ex-

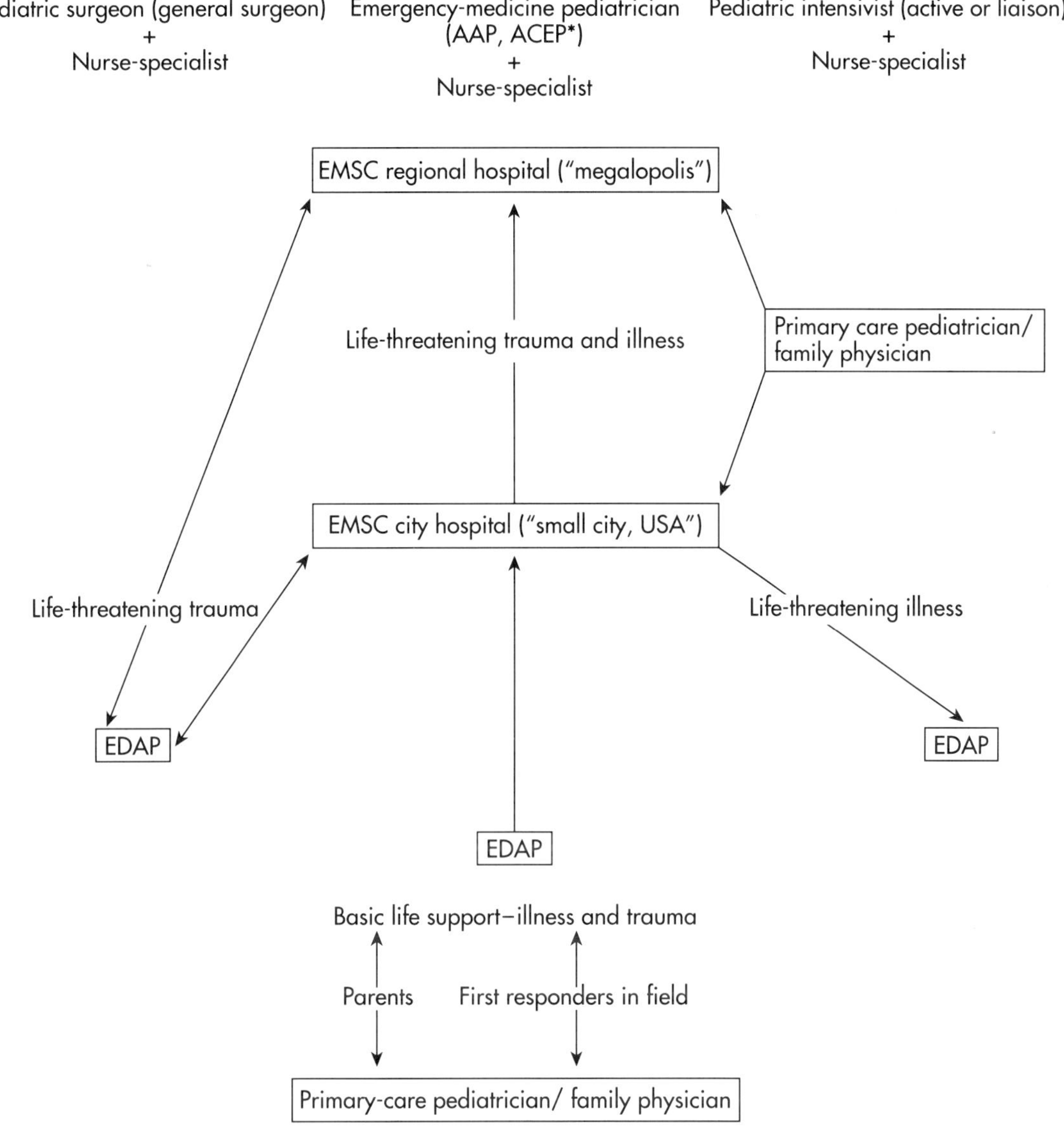

Figure 9–2 Chart of a proposed integrated and comprehensive system of emergency medical care for children. In this chart, *emergency medicine pediatricians* includes emergency medicine physicians with special skills and experience in the management of life-threatening illnesses and injuries in children as well as pediatricians with additional training in emergency care. EMSC = emergency medical services for children; EDAP = emergency department appropriate for pediatric care; AAP = American Academy of Pediatrics; ACEP = American College of Emergency Physicians. (From Haller JA: *Emergency medical services for children.* Report of the 97th Ross Conference on Pediatric Research, Columbus, 1989, Ross Laboratories.)

pertise in treatment of trauma, the APLS course is now available to all—pediatricians, emergency physicians, and surgeons—who care for children with life-threatening trauma.

This concept of echelons of trauma care based on the severity of a child's injuries can be extended to include life-threatening illness. A model for such a comprehensive EMSC was first proposed by a Ross Conference in 1989.[5] This prototype of an integrated program like the EMSC is shown in Fig. 9-2.

Experience in trauma care for children can and must be extended to include management of life-threatening illness. Access to EMSC systems is variable, however, and a strong educational effort by pediatric health care providers is needed to facilitate entry into the EMSC system. Entry into the systems of emergency care may occur directly from the field via paramedics (for example, in trauma care), by parents (for example, for a child with a high temperature or seizures), or by primary care pediatricians and family physicians from their offices to a regional center directly or, more commonly, to emergency departments appropriate for pediatric care. Emergency rooms that have organized components and staffing for treatment of life-threatening conditions in children have been called EDAP (Emergency Departments Appropriate for Pediatrics).[8,9] This whole system is then integrated by central EMSC communication and alarm, and transport is controlled on-line by dedicated, experienced, pediatric emergency physicians (see Fig. 9-2).

EARLY DETECTION OF LIFE-THREATENING CHILDHOOD ILLNESS

A major challenge remains: How can criteria be developed *for early detection of childhood illness* that may rapidly become life-threatening, so that affected children can be appropriately entered into the system *before death is impending?* Such a proposed Illness Severity Score, similar to an Injury Severity Score,[6] is obviously needed to provide a basis for the surveillance of the EMSC system and quality assessment of the delivery of emergency care. With further integration of emergency systems and close cooperation between pediatric emergency physicians and pediatric surgeons, such systems management offers an important opportunity to extend modern pediatric critical care to children in the home, in the field, and during transport to designated centers for emergency medical care.[3]

Working side by side in the emergency room and in the pediatric intensive care unit, pediatric surgeons and pediatric critical care intensivists can deliver state-of-the-art management to children with life-threatening trauma or illness. This is the urgent challenge for the 1990s.

REFERENCES

1. American College of Surgeons Committee on Trauma: Field categorization of trauma patients and hospital trauma index, *Bull Am Cell Surg* 65:28, 1980.
2. Haller JA: Emergency medical services for children: what is the pediatric surgeon's role? *Pediatrics* 79:576, 1987.
3. Haller JA: Toward a comprehensive emergency medical system for children, *Pediatrics* 86:120, 1990.
4. Haller JA, Beaver B: A model: systems management of life threatening injuries in children for the state of Maryland, USA, *Intensive Care Med* 15:S53-S56, 1989.
5. Haller JA, editor: *Emergency medical services for children: report of the 97th Ross Conference on Pediatric Research,* Columbus, Ohio, 1989, Ross Laboratories.
6. Mayer T et al: The modified injury severity scale in pediatric multiple trauma patients, *J Pediatr Surg* 15:719, 1980.
7. Ramenofsky ML, Morse TS: Standards of care for the critically injured pediatric patient, *J Trauma* 22:921-933, 1982.
8. Seidel JS: EMS-C in urban and rural areas: the California experience. In Haller JA, editor: *Emergency medical services for children: report of the 97th Ross Conference on Pediatric Research,* Columbus, Ohio, 1989, Ross Laboratories, pp 22-30.
9. Seidel JS, Hornbein M, Yoshiyama K et al: Emergency medical services and the pediatric patient: are the needs being met? *Pediatrics* 73:769-772, 1984.

10 Prehospital Care of the Injured Child

Joan M. Burg and *Gary R. Fleisher*

Injuries are the most common cause of death in children ages 1 to 14 years. To decrease the frequency of these injuries and the resultant morbidity and mortality, a systemwide approach must be applied that incorporates prevention, access to care, prehospital personnel, in-hospital personnel, and rehabilitative services. Prehospital care providers have a critical role in the initial stabilization and transport of the injured child.

The initial development of organized Emergency Medical Services (EMS) systems was brought about in an attempt to decrease the morbidity and mortality resulting from acute illness. Early legislation to achieve this goal included the Highway Safety Act of 1966, which authorized the Department of Transportation to improve the quality of emergency medical services, and the Emergency Medical Services Act of 1973. These acts and their subsequent amendments, served as catalysts to the development of the EMS systems and personnel structure as we know them today. The systems were modeled on the premise that early intervention and rapid transport would result in increased patient survival. Significant overall progress has occurred in this arena, but the pediatric component of prehospital care has been slow to evolve.

Unfortunately, the unique needs of children within the emergency medical system have not been a priority. There is a relative underutilization of basic and advanced life support vehicles for the transport of critically ill pediatric patients or those with urgent needs. Children, although representing 30% to 35% of the population, account for only about 10% of ambulance runs. The outcome of those children who have required advanced life support (ALS) intervention in the field has been disappointing. Children who suffer out-of-hospital cardiac arrests have a poor outcome compared with their adult counterparts. Whereas adult cardiac arrest is often the result of a readily treatable ventricular dysrhythmia, pediatric arrest usually is the end stage of a serious medical illness such as respiratory failure or sepsis. Recent reports have indicated that attempts at ALS intervention in the prehospital setting have a higher failure rate among children than in the adult population. Unlike adult patients, in whom prehospital endotracheal intubation has a high success rate (86% to 97%), the success rate in children, particularly those under 1 year, is as low as 50%. In addition, IV placement and intubation prolong field time and have not yet demonstrated an increased rate of survival to hospital discharge.

The curriculum used to train emergency medical technicians and paramedics in most states follows that developed by the National Highway Traffic Safety Administration of the Department of Transportation. The training of prehospital providers in pediatrics includes a limited number of lecture hours and little hands-on clinical experience. The mean number of hours of didactic pediatric training is 8 hours for Emergency Medical Technicians (EMTs) and 15 hours for paramedics, of the total 100+ hours required for EMT and the 1000+ hours for paramedic training.

Despite the limited impact of prehospital care on survival of the pediatric cardiac arrest victim, appropriate management may decrease the morbidity resulting from medical illness. Additionally, prehospital care personnel play an integral role in the initial evaluation and stabilization of the child trauma victim. They provide the first medical contact the child has following injury and can serve to relieve some of the anxiety related to the incident. The initial field evaluation is essential in the diagnosis and management of potentially life-threatening emergencies, such as cervical spine fracture or upper airway obstruction. Early recognition and treatment of these emergencies can improve chances for survival. Prehospital care personnel can relay to physicians a clear description of the type and location of the accident, an estimate of the amount of force involved, and a description of damage at the scene. In addition, they can provide information on the child's condition at the time of their arrival at the scene of the accident and any changes in status prior to hospital arrival. This information provides essential clues to the type and severity of expected injuries.

Childhood trauma presents both an intellectual and an emotional challenge to all health care professionals. Despite the prevalence of trauma in

Table 10–1 Suggested Pediatric Equipment and Medications

Medication	Standard supply	Minimum quantity
Albuterol sulfate 0.5%	20 ml bottle	1
Atropine sulfate	0.1 mg/ml in 10 ml prefilled syringe	2
Dextrose 25%	12.5 gm in 10 ml prefilled syringe	2
Dextrose 50%	25 gm in 50 ml prefilled syringe	2
Diazepam	5.0 mg/ml in 2.0 ml vial	1
Diphenhydramine HCL	50 mg/ml in 1.0 ml vial	1
Epinephrine 1:1,000	1.0 mg/ml in 1.0 ml ampule	2
Epinephrine 1:10,000	0.1 mg/ml in 10 ml prefilled syringe	3
Glucagon	1.0 mg in vials (mixing required)	1
Lidocaine HCL	10 mg/ml in 10 ml prefilled syringe	2
Metapreterenol sulfate 5%	10 ml or 30 ml bottle	1
Naloxone HCL	1.0 mg/ml in 2.0 ml ampule	2
Normal saline	500 or 1000 ml bag	3
Sodium bicarbonate 4.2%	1.0 mEq/ml in 10 ml prefilled syringe	2
Sodium bicarbonate 8.4%	1.0 mEq/ml in 50 ml prefilled syringe	1
Sodium chloride injection 0.9%	10 ml vial	4
Airway		
Laryngoscope handle	Penlite size	1
Miller blades	#0, #1, #2, #3	1 each
Macintosh blades	#2, #3	1 each
Stylet	6F and 14F	1 each
Oropharyngeal airways	00-5	1 each
Nasopharyngeal airways	5.5, 6.0, 7.0, 8.0	1 each
Endotracheal tubes (uncuffed)	2.5, 3.0, 3.5, 4.0, 4.5, 5.0, 5.5	2 each
Endotracheal tubes (cuffed)	6.0, 7.0, 8.0	2 each
Nasogastric tubes	5F, 8F, 10F, and 14F	1 each
Suction catheters	6F, 7F, 10F, 12F, and 14F	1 each
Magill forceps	Pediatric size	1
Magill forceps	Adult size	1
Oxygen supply tubing		1
High concentration mask	Pediatric size	1
Nebulizer		1
Bag-valve-mask resuscitator	Child and infant size	1 each
Transparent ventilation masks	Premature, newborn, infant, child, and small adult sizes	1 each
Bulb syringe		1
Syringes		
1 cc		3
3 cc		3
5 cc		5
10 cc		5

children, only about 5% of all prehospital calls involve a child who has sustained traumatic injury. Some of these children die at the scene, and others succumb in the hospital emergency department, in surgery, or during hospitalization. The injury-related death rate in children is two times that in adult patients, and investigators have estimated that 15% to 20% of in-hospital deaths could have been prevented.[7] The limited number of children requiring EMS intervention results in a rapid degradation of caregiver skills. Ongoing training is essential, as is a well-organized, systematic approach to the care of the childhood trauma victim.

Injury prevention

The cost of injury to society is enormous, estimated at over 8 billion dollars annually. Health care providers, including emergency care personnel, can play an important role in raising the awareness of community members, and information on injury prevention should be incorporated into routine medical practice.

Table 10–1 Suggested Pediatric Equipment and Medications—cont'd

Medication	Minimum quantity
Needles—straight metal	
23 gauge	5
21 gauge	5
19 gauge	5
Needles—butterfly	
25 gauge	2
23 gauge	2
Intraosseous needle	
Jamshidi/Kormed disposable bone marrow needle (sternal/ileac aspiration needle), 15 gauge	2
Intravenous catheters	
24 guage	2
22 gauge	2
20 gauge	2
18 gauge	2
16 guage	2
14 gauge	2
Miscellaneous	
Pediatric defibrillator paddles	1 set
Child size sphygmomanometer	1
Baby No Neck, pediatric, and short Stifneck extrication collars	1 each
Stockinette cap	1
Pediatric monitoring electrodes	6
Minidrip administration set	2
Maxidrip administration set	2
Intravenous extension set	2
Alcohol prep pads	
Band Aids	
Tape, 1 in and ½ in	
Arm boards	
Topical antiseptic ointment (single use)	
Isolation masks	
Venous constricting bands (Penrose drain, elastic band)	
Spare AA batteries	
Spare laryngoscope bulb	

Consensus Document of Pediatric Task Force: Joan Burg, M.D., FACEP, FAAP, Attending Physician, Emergency Services, Children's Hospital; Patricia O'Malley, M.D., FAAP, Director, Pediatric Emergency Services, Massachusetts General Hospital; Robert Vinci, M.D., FAAP, Director, Pediatric Emergency Services, Boston City Hospital; William J. Schneiderman, Assistant Director, Metropolitan Boston Hospital Council, MEDIC IV/EMS Project; Charlotte Yeh, M.D., FACEP, Medical Director, MEDIC IV Emergency Medical Services Project.
© 1990 by Medic IV Emergency Medical Services Project, Metropolitan Boston Hospital Council, Burlington, Mass.

Ambulance equipment recommendations

If proper care is to be provided to the ill or injured child, emergency vehicles must be properly equipped to handle pediatric emergencies. Equipment adequate to care for the adult patient is often inadequate for the child, and all vehicles should be stocked with items necessary to care for children of all ages. A sample equipment list used in the Boston metropolitan area is shown in Table 10-1. Essential components include airway equipment for children of all sizes: infant and child bag-valve-mask (BVM) devices; premature, newborn, infant, and child ventilation masks; and an assortment of laryngoscope blades and endotracheal tubes. Pediatric defibrillator paddles, blood pressure cuffs, and cervical collars should be available as well.

Access to care

Emergency medical care must be available to any child who needs it, irrespective of background or socioeconomic status. Unfortunately, there are a number of barriers to accessing emergency medical services, including language, lack of telephone or transportation, and lack of awareness of when to seek medical assistance. These problems are most common in lower-income communities, the same groups that have a higher incidence of medical emergency, violent injury, and death. In addition, an estimated 12% of all children have chronic illness or a disabling condition, almost half of whom have conditions that require specialized health services. Many of these children are more prone to sustaining traumatic injury and are, in many instances, being cared for by their families at home, which requires the availability and adequate training of EMS personnel to serve their needs.

Arrival on the scene

It is essential for health care providers to protect themselves from unsafe environments at all times. Upon arrival at the scene, the ambulance must be positioned in a location where it is near the victim, yet not in danger from traffic or other hazards. Once the victim is reached, immediate removal from an unsafe environment should occur following proper immobilization. On-scene witnesses may provide important information about the mechanism of injury that can give clues to the presence of potentially life-threatening injuries. For a motor vehicle accident, the scene itself can provide further evidence of the type and extent of injuries; the use of helmets or safety belts, the presence of steering wheel or car damage, and the distance of the patient from the car should be noted. Caregivers can help to explain what is happening, and familiar items used to calm the child. Emergency personnel should take any significant medical history and look for Medic Alert identification.

PRIMARY SURVEY

During the initial phase of assessment a search for any immediately life-threatening conditions is made, and resuscitation proceeds simultaneously. The primary survey follows the guidelines published by the American College of Surgeons. Ideally, it should be accomplished within the first 5 to 10 minutes after the arrival on the scene by the prehospital care provider. On-scene time should be determined not only by the severity of injuries, but also by transport time to the receiving facility. For example, a child with airway compromise who is within 5 minutes of the hospital may be better served by immediate transport than by attempted field intubation. If the same child faced 50-minute transport time, intubation before transport would be advantageous. Components (ABCs) of the primary survey include:

A: *A*irway and cervical spine control
B: *B*reathing
C: *C*irculation and hemorrhage control
D: *D*isability
E: *E*xposure

Airway and cervical spine control

Cervical spine immobilization. The number one priority in managing the trauma patient is to assure airway patency. In any child who has sustained significant trauma, assume the presence of a cervical spine injury; immobilization of the head and neck is mandatory. Cervical spine injuries are less common in children than in adults, but when they occur they often involve the upper cervical spine. Movement of the head and neck can convert an injury without neurologic deficit into one with an irreversible neurologic injury.

Some of the indications for cervical spine immobilization are listed in Table 10-2. If the provider is uncertain as to whether immobilization is indicated, immobilizing unnecessarily is preferable to failing to immobilize a child who has a potential neck injury. Prehospital providers should assume a cervical spine injury in any child who has significant trauma above the level of the clavicles, including children with head trauma. In addition, any child who has a significant mechanism of injury needs immobilization, as does any child with altered mental status or complaints of neck pain.

A variety of equipment is available to assist in cervical spine immobilization, including rigid collars, KED and long boards, sandbags and tape. A papoose or a KED board may be used to immobilize an infant, along with sandbags or a blanket roll and tape to provide immobilization to the cervical region. A toddler can be immobilized in a similar manner; if available, a properly fitting rigid cervical collar is preferred over sandbags or a blanket roll. The older child is most appropriately immo-

Table 10–2 Indications for cervical spine immobilization

High-speed motor vehicle accident
Fall from a significant height
Significant trauma above the level of the clavicles
Complaints of neck pain
Altered mental status
Diving injury
Neurologic deficit or paresthesias
History of a loss of consciousness

bilized like an adult, using a rigid collar and a long board.

Airway management. In managing the pediatric airway, simple airway maneuvers such as repositioning, airway-opening techniques, and bag-valve-mask ventilation will most often allow for adequate ventilation to initiate transport. Only when these measures are unsuccessful, or if transport time is excessive, may endotracheal intubation be necessary. In both medical and traumatic emergencies, orotracheal intubation is the preferred method of establishing an airway. Nasotracheal intubation, a useful procedure for adult trauma victims, is not indicated for children. Blind nasotracheal intubation is often unsuccessful in children because of anatomic differences; nasotracheal intubation using Magill forceps is an even more difficult and time-consuming procedure. If attempts at intubation are unsuccessful and an airway cannot be managed through bag-valve-mask ventilation, needle cricothyroidotomy may be indicated (see "Cricothyroidotomy").

Opening the airway. Assessing for airway patency in the older child is as simple as asking, "What happened?" or "How are you?" The child who is able to answer appropriately with normal phonation has a patent airway. Similarly, the younger child with normal phonation or a strong, normally pitched cry is not likely to immediately obstruct the airway. The common causes of airway obstruction after an injury are an altered level of consciousness, foreign body (blood or vomitus), trauma (maxillofacial fractures), and inflammation (burns). Signs of upper airway compromise include stridor, hoarseness or high-pitched voice, drooling, retractions of the respiratory muscles, and noisy or labored respirations. If any of these signs are present, transport should be initiated immediately while the child receives blow-by oxygen.

Simple maneuvers to open the airway need to be performed without manipulation of the cervical spine. Particularly in the unconscious child, the tongue may displace posteriorly, causing partial airway obstruction. Placement of one or both hands at the angle of the mandible while applying gentle forward traction (jaw thrust) allows the tongue to move anteriorly without movement of the cervical spine. Often the cause of airway obstruction is foreign material such as blood or vomitus in the oropharynx. A suction machine should be available and ready for use. Suctioning the mouth with a large tonsil or Yankauer device can remove foreign particles and will often relieve a partially obstructed airway. Keep in mind that infants are obligate nasal breathers; suctioning of the nares can assist in providing an adequate airway.

The optimal technique for opening the airway *once the presence of a cervical injury has been eliminated* is to place the child in the "sniffing position," in which the neck is slightly flexed on the chest and the head slightly extended on the neck. This can be accomplished by placing a folded towel under the occiput to raise it slightly above the level of the shoulders. Unfortunately, field personnel can rarely rule out cervical spine injury.

Oral and nasal airways. Oropharyngeal airways are useful in bringing the tongue forward to allow for adequate ventilation in the unconscious child. These airways should be used only in a comatose child, as they may cause a conscious child to gag and thus increase the risk of vomiting and aspiration. To determine the proper size, hold the airway against the child's face; it should extend from the corner of the mouth to the angle of the mandible. In the adult patient the airway can be inserted backward and rotated 180°, but this may cause significant trauma to the teeth and oropharynx in children. The best way to insert an oral airway is by pulling the tongue forward with a tongue blade or gloved hand.

Nasopharyngeal airways are a helpful and underutilized alternative for opening the airway in a conscious child. They extend from the nares to the posterior pharynx and prevent the tongue from falling backward and completely occluding the airway. After lubrication, insert the airway parallel to the palate. A nasopharyngeal airway of proper length will extend from the corner of the child's mouth to the tragus of the ear. This airway is tolerated better than the oral airway in a semiconscious patient or a child who has an intact gag reflex.

Esophageal obturator airways. Esophageal obturator airways *are not* indicated in chldren under 16 years of age.

Pediatric airway anatomy. Prior to intubation of the pediatric patient, it is important to review the anatomic differences of the pediatric airway. The occiput of the infant is relatively large and in the supine position will cause some flexion of the neck. Infants are obligate nose breathers, and their nasal passages are narrower and more easily occluded by secretions. The tongue is larger in relation to the mandible, and the tonsils and adenoids are more prominent. The larynx is more cephalad and anterior, making it easier to visualize the vocal cords using a straight, rather than a curved, laryngoscope blade in the child under 2 or 3 years of age.

Endotracheal intubation. A child who cannot be adequately ventilated with a bag and mask device, or who is unable to protect his or her airway during a prolonged transport, should be intubated if ALS staff are at the scene. Some of the indications for endotracheal intubation are listed in

Table 10-3. Oral intubation is difficult under the most controlled circumstances, and, if the child has an adequate airway, field time should not be prolonged by attempted intubation.

The key to successful intubation is adequate preparation. It is essential to have all equipment ready to use, including the appropriate size endotracheal tube (as well as one size larger and one smaller), laryngoscope handle with the appropriate blade, a Yankauer or tonsil suction device, and a nasogastric tube. To determine appropriate endotracheal tube size, one can use the formula

$$\frac{Age\ +\ 16}{4}$$

or find a tube the size of the child's little finger or nostril. In children under 8 years of age, uncuffed tubes should be used; the cricoid cartilage is the narrowest part of the airway and provides an adequate seal. Cuffed tubes should be used in older children. Endotracheal tube guidelines are listed in Table 10-4.

Prior to intubation, if time allows, hyperoxygenate the child with 100% oxygen or with bag-valve-mask ventilation. An assistant should maintain the cervical spine in a neutral position by holding in-line stabilization during intubation. Placement of a stylet in the endotracheal tube lumen may make the procedure easier. Clear the oropharynx well, using a Yankauer suction device. The application of gentle pressure to the cricoid cartilage, known as the Sellick maneuver, may allow for better visualiza-

tion of the glottis and help to prevent aspiration of gastric contents. If attempts at intubation are unsuccessful after 30 seconds, or if the heart rate begins to drop, resume bag and mask ventilation for several minutes prior to repeated attempts. Passing a nasogastric or orogastric tube after intubation will decompress the stomach and may assist ventilatory efforts.

Once the endotracheal tube has been placed correctly, an air column should be seen with ventilations, and condensation may be seen in the tube lumen. Look for symmetric chest wall movements and auscultate the lung fields to determine equal breath sounds bilaterally. Also listen over the stomach because breath sounds can be transmitted to the lung fields with esophageal intubation. If breath sounds are louder on the right, most likely the tube has slipped into the right mainstem bronchus and needs to be pulled back slightly. Secure the tube well before transporting the patient.

Gastric tube. Placement of an orogastric tube is reasonable after intubation, particularly if transport time is long. Artificial ventilation inevitably causes gastric distension, which can result in vomiting and aspiration. In addition, a distended stomach may interfere with diaphragmatic excursion and significantly impair ventilation. Nasogastric tube placement is contraindicated in cribriform plate fractures. If there is significant facial trauma, particularly with blood or clear fluid draining from the nose, an orogastric rather than a nasogastric tube should be placed to avoid accidental entry into the cranial vault.

Cricothyroidotomy. Traumatic upper airway obstruction in children is uncommon but can occur in cases of severe maxillofacial injuries or direct trauma to the neck or larynx. In rare instances, when bag and mask ventilations are unsuccessful and endotracheal intubation cannot be achieved, cricothyroidotomy may be necessary. An assistant should hold the patient's head in the neutral position with the neck exposed. Palpate the cricothyroid membrane in the midline; it is the space located below the laryngeal prominence or Adam's apple (thyroid cartilage) and above the cricoid cartilage. Use sterile gloves and prepare the area with betadine solution. A 12- or 14-gauge angiocatheter (or other over-the-needle catheter) with an attached 5- to 10-cc syringe is used to puncture the skin midline, with the needle directed 45° caudally. Advance the unit until air is rapidly aspirated into the syringe, then advance the catheter into the lumen of the trachea. The syringe should be reattached and the position rechecked by aspirating on the syringe.

The adapter from a 3.0- or 3.5-mm endotracheal tube is attached to the catheter, and manual ven-

Table 10–3 Indications for endotracheal intubation

Cardiopulmonary arrest
Respiratory failure (unable to ventilate with
  BVM or prolonged transport)
Absent gag reflex (vomiting child or prolonged
  transport)
Complete airway obstruction

Table 10–4 Endotracheal tube guidelines

Age	Tube size	Blade size
Premature	2.5–3.0	0
6 months	3.5	1
18 months	4.0	1–2
3 years	4.5	2
5 years	5.0	2
8 years	6.0	2
12 years	6.5	2–3
16 years	7.0–8.0	3

tilation with an Ambu bag attached to the connecter may be attempted. This will allow for oxygen delivery but not ventilation. An alternative is to attach the endotracheal tube adapter to a Y connector. A pressurized oxygen source (25 to 50 psi) with tubing is attached, and ventilation is provided by intermittent occlusion of the open port of the Y with the thumb. Remember that needle cricothyroidotomy is a temporizing measure only. It can provide a maximum of only 30 to 40 minutes of oxygenation, during which a significant buildup of CO_2 occurs.

Breathing

It is essential to provide adequate cellular oxygenation for the injured child. Airway and pulmonary injuries may be subtle and high-flow oxygen via face mask should be provided to all children, even if there is no evidence of respiratory distress. Potential injuries can often be recognized if one remembers to "look, listen, and feel" for them. Inspect the chest, looking for any evidence of external trauma and asymmetry of chest wall movement with respirations or flail segments. Evidence of respiratory difficulty, including muscular retractions, nasal flaring, or grunting, should be noted. Listen to both sides of the chest for breath sounds, which should be equal and clear.

Circulation

Signs of shock in children may be subtle; they are often unapparent until approximately 25% of blood volume has been lost. The rate, quality, and regularity of the pulse should be noted. In a child with hypovolemia, an increase in heart rate is the first adjustment made by the cardiovascular system and may be seen long before a drop in blood pressure. Keep in mind that a child's heart rate will also increase in response to fear, pain, temperature, hypoxemia, and a multitude of other factors. An increase in capillary refill time is further evidence of hypovolemia. The thenar eminence, or nail bed, is pressed for 5 seconds; when released, normal skin color should return within 2 seconds. A delay in refill, particularly if greater than 4 seconds, is indicative of volume loss. In a hypothermic child the capillary refill time may be prolonged in the absence of hypovolemia.

Other useful signs in assessing the injured child are those that evaluate end-organ perfusion. An alteration in mental status may be due to a decrease in cerebral blood flow, although it can also result from numerous other causes. In the absence of renal disease, urine output is an indication of renal blood flow and will be decreased if shock is present. A urine output of greater than 1 cc/kg/hour in general indicates adequate renal blood flow. Un-

fortunately, this value has limited use in the prehospital stabilization of the injured child, except during prolonged transport. Table 10-5 lists normal pediatric vital signs.

Vascular access. Vascular access should be considered as part of the circulatory assessment and resuscitation of children who have sustained significant trauma. Ideally, a large-bore intravenous catheter should be inserted into a large peripheral vein, such as that in the antecubital fossa. Obtaining vascular access may be useful in the field, but transport should not be delayed for IV attempts. Particularly if internal bleeding is suspected, rapid transport to the hospital and operating room may have much greater positive impact than the intravenous fluids administered during the same time period. If transport time is less than 15 to 20 minutes, consider making IV attempts only en route to the hospital. In longer transports, one or two attempts at IV access should be made in the ambulance, but rapid transport should not be delayed. If the child is in full cardiopulmonary arrest and percutaneous venous access cannot be established after one attempt, intraosseous placement can be attempted during transport.

For a child who has evidence of shock, fluid resuscitation should be instituted immediately in accordance with the guidelines given above. An initial fluid bolus of 20 cc/kg of an isotonic crystalloid solution (lactated Ringer's solution or normal saline) should be infused as rapidly as possible by having the tubing clamps wide open and elevating the solution. All fluids should be administered via large-bore IV tubing; use of microdrips should be avoided. Glucose-containing solutions may lead to hyperglycemia and an osmotic diuresis and should not be used as the initial solution.

Keep in mind that the child's total blood volume is 80 cc/kg. If vital signs fail to improve after the initial infusion, another 20 cc/kg bolus should be administered. When conditions allow, vital signs and clinical parameters should be followed en route to the hospital to determine changes in circulatory status. If the child still fails to respond after the second bolus, there is likely to be significant internal blood loss and the need for surgical inter-

Table 10–5 Normal pediatric vital signs

Age	Heart rate	Blood pressure	Respiratory rate
1 Month	110–170	>70	<50
1 Year	100–160	>80	<40
5 Years	80–130	>90	<30
Adolescent	<90	>90	<20

vention. In this case, rapid transport to the hospital is crucial.

External hemorrhage. Bulky pressure dressings and direct pressure should be applied to any evident bleeding site. Blood loss from scalp lacerations may be excessive but can almost always be controlled with direct pressure. Pressure dressing plus elevation of an extremity will decrease ongoing blood loss. The use of tourniquets should be avoided. Immobilization is helpful in preventing further bleeding or ongoing trauma.

Internal hemorrhage. Internal bleeding is not nearly so obvious as external blood loss, and subtle historical or physical examination findings must serve as clues to occult injury. Significant injury to any of these areas should raise the suspicion of internal bleeding. Immobilization with traction splinting for femur fractures or with a pneumatic antishock garment (PASG) for suspected pelvic injuries may help diminish ongoing blood loss. Rapid transport to a facility with surgical capability or, preferably, pediatric trauma expertise, is imperative.

Pneumatic antishock garment. The PASG has been used as an adjunct to the treatment of shock in both pediatric and adult trauma victims. Its effectiveness, previously thought to be largely a result of "autotransfusion" by increasing the total peripheral resistance, is probably limited to only 5% to 10% of the blood volume. There are limited data on the effectiveness of the PASG in children, although there is speculation that it can be useful in the stabilization of lower extremity and pelvic fractures and in tamponading blood loss. Disadvantages to its use in children include the frequent unavailability of the proper size; the time required for proper application; and the difficulty in subsequent exposure of lower extremity veins for venous access.

Transport time must be taken into consideration when deciding whether PASG placement is indicated. If significant pelvic or femur fractures are suspected and transport time is long, the garment may be placed on the long spinal board after neck immobilization and before general immobilization is completed. The garment need not be inflated prior to transport, but if it is so placed will then be available should hemodynamic instability ensue en route to the hospital. As in adults, the garment is contraindicated if there is pulmonary edema or diaphragmatic disruption and must be used with caution in children with cardiac disease. Once inflated, the PASG should be deflated gradually only after intravenous fluid administration; deflation should be stopped if a 10 mm Hg drop in blood pressure occurs. If a child develops respiratory distress after trouser inflation, the garment should be rapidly deflated to avoid further respiratory compromise.

Disability

A rapid assessment of mental status should be included in the field evaluation of a trauma patient. Appropriate answers to questions such as, "What happened?" or "What is your name?" indicate that the child is alert and adequately responsive. The mnemonic AVPU can be used to assess mental status rapidly:

A: *A*lert
V: Responds to *V*erbal stimuli
P: Responds to *P*ainful stimuli
U: *U*nresponsive

Pupillary response may be assessed and movement of all extremities should be observed to identify any gross motor deficit. Transport should not be delayed in order to do a more thorough neurologic evaluation.

Exposure

Remember that because of a larger body surface area and less subcutaneous tissue than that of adults, children may readily become hypothermic. Blankets and hats should be used to help maintain a normal core temperature.

Traumatic arrest. Rarely will the prehospital provider confront a pediatric traumatic arrest victim; therefore this situation, when it occurs, may cause significant anxiety on the part of the health care provider. Cardiopulmonary resuscitation should be initiated according to the standard BLS protocols, and oral intubation may be necessary if field personnel are unable to provide ventilation to the child with BVM ventilation or if transport time is prolonged. If IV access can be established en route to the hospital, fluids should be administered as rapidly as possible, but under no circumstances should transport be delayed to establish access. The only hope of resuscitating a child with traumatic arrest is through aggressive in-hospital management, through appropriate chest tube placement, pericardiocentesis, or open thoracotomy. The more prolonged the transport to the medical facility, the less likely the child is to be successfully resuscitated. In general, the only medications that should be administered to such a patient are oxygen and IV fluids. A sample algorithm for traumatic arrest is shown in Table 10-6.

RESUSCITATION

As mentioned previously, one should interrupt the primary survey in order to initiate patient resuscitation. The following measures should be accomplished prior to further evaluation. All children should receive high-flow supplemental oxygen.

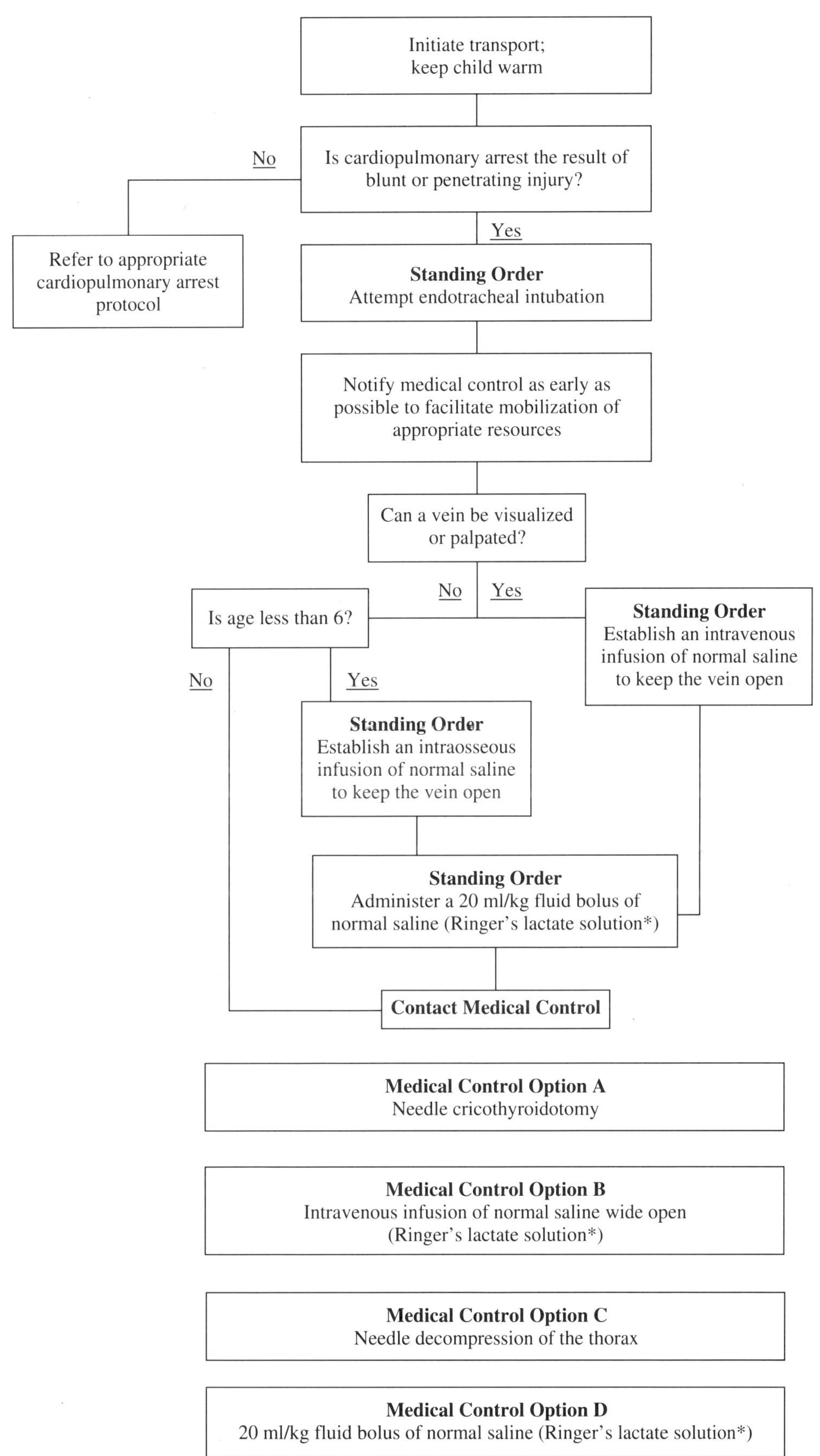

Modified from Medic IV Emergency Medical Services Project Treatment Protocol, Metropolitan Boston Hospital Council, Burlington, Mass, 1990.
*Editor's modification.

This is optimally administered using a rebreather mask to provide a concentration approaching 100% oxygen; a nasal cannula is not as effective. If at any time the child develops evidence of airway compromise, the airway and ventilation must be reevaluated.

Monitoring

All injured children should have ongoing cardiac monitoring. Cardiac arrhythmia may be a warning sign of hypoxemia, hypoperfusion, or cardiac contusion. Blood pressure readings should be obtained during the initial survey and repeatedly at regular intervals during long transports. Some EMS systems may have pulse oximetry, which may be useful during long transport as a clue to respiratory embarrassment.

SECONDARY SURVEY

The secondary survey in prehospital care of an injured child is a rapid head-to-toe assessment that may, if time allows, be performed after any immediately life-threatening injuries have been managed. The survey may require interruption if there is any change in the patient's status, in order to reassess cardiorespiratory status. A sequential, head-to-toe evaluation is best accomplished en route to the hospital.

Head

Head injuries are a leading cause of morbidity and mortality in childhood and occur in approximately 75% of children sustaining multiple trauma. Specific head injuries and their management are described elsewhere in this text. Examination of mental status is an integral part of the neurologic assessment. The AVPU assessment should have already been performed as part of the primary survey. The Glasgow Coma Scale (Table 10-7) serves as a guide for assessing mental status, and a modified form is available to help assess the infant or young child (Table 10-8).

In a child who fails to have spontaneous movement or activity, it is necessary to determine whether there is a response to verbal command. If there is no reaction to shouting, assess for response to noxious stimuli. This can be determined by application of digital pressure to the nail beds of the fingers or toes. Ability to follow commands indicates intact cortical and brainstem function. Asymmetric movements of the extremities may result from focal lesions of the cerebral cortex. Decorticate posturing (abnormal flexion response of the upper extremities) indicates diffuse cerebral dysfunction but an intact brainstem. Decerebrate or abnormal extensor posturing usually indicates diffuse damage to the upper midbrain, although it can

Table 10–7 Glasgow Coma Scale

Eye opening response	
Spontaneous	4
Verbal stimuli	3
Painful stimuli	2
None	1
Verbal response	
Oriented	5
Confused conversation	4
Inappropriate words	3
Incomprehensible sounds	2
None	1
Motor response	
Follows commands	6
Localizes	5
Withdraws	4
Abnormal flexor response (decorticate)	3
Abnormal extensor response (decerebrate)	2
None	1

Table 10–8 Modified Glasgow Coma Scale (young children)

Eye opening response	
See Table 10–7	
Verbal response	
Appropriate words, social smile, or fixes and follows	5
Cries but consolable	4
Irritable or inconsolable	3
Restless, agitated	2
None	1
Motor response	
Spontaneous intentional movement	6
Localized withdrawal to pain	5
Generalized withdrawal	4
Decorticate	3
Decerebrate	2
None	1

occur in severe anoxic encephalopathy. The child who fails to exhibit any motor response and has areflexia has sustained a severe brainstem injury; the prognosis is relatively poor.

Pupillary response and eye movements also provide clues to the level of brain injury. Equal, briskly reactive pupils indicate an intact midbrain as well as second and third cranial nerves. Pinpoint pupils suggest narcotic overdose or pontine hemorrhage. Small pupils that react are also seen in the early stage of herniation as well as in metabolic disorders. A unilateral fixed and dilated pupil indicates herniation of the temporal lobe through the tentorial notch, resulting in damage to the ipsilateral third cranial nerve; this finding warrants immediate intervention. If both pupils are fixed and dilated, there is likely to be severe ischemic brain damage or ingestion of a catecholamine. Midposition fixed pupils indicate severe midbrain injury. Subconjunctival hemorrhages are seen in the "shaken baby" syndrome and may serve as a clue to child abuse.

The respiratory rate and pattern should be noted as part of the neurologic evaluation. An abnormal respiratory pattern may indicate the etiology of underlying cerebral dysfunction. Apnea is a nonspecific finding that may occur in a multitude of neurologic, respiratory, toxic/metabolic, or other conditions. Cheyne-Stokes respirations, a crescendo-decrescendo pattern with intermittent periods of apnea, may indicate diffuse bilateral cerebral damage. Hyperventilation may result from anxiety, hypoxemia, respiratory embarrassment, or acidosis.

The scalp should be examined for lacerations and the skull palpated for deformities. Significant blood loss can occur through scalp lacerations, and these should be controlled immediately by pressure dressings. If there is blood or fluid draining from the nose or ears, be suspicious of a basilar skull fracture with cerebrospinal fluid rhinorrhea or otorrhea. Other clues to this diagnosis include a Battle's sign (ecchymosis behind the ears) or raccoon eyes (ecchymosis around the eyes).

Neck

Cervical spine injuries are less common in children than in adults, but they do occur. Unlike older patients whose spinal injuries are usually in the lower cervical vertebrae, children more commonly fracture the upper cervical spine. This is probably due to the increased laxity of the ligaments, a more horizontal alignment of the facets, and a proportionately larger head size in the child. Any child who has sustained multiple trauma should be assumed to have a cervical spine injury and requires adequate immobilization. One EMT or paramedic should hold in-line stabilization while the other inspects the neck for evidence of penetrating trauma, subcutaneous emphysema, tracheal deviation, or jugular venous distension. In-line stabilization should be maintained until a cervical collar or other appropriate device is applied.

Blunt or penetrating injuries to the neck can cause airway compromise either by direct injury (a stab wound with laryngeal or tracheal disruption, for example) or by indirect injury (soft tissue swelling or hematoma resulting in airway compromise). These injuries must be managed aggressively by establishment of an airway through intubation if possible or by needle cricothyroidotomy if complete airway obstruction occurs.

Chest

Chest injuries in children under 14 years of age are usually the result of blunt trauma. Because of the compliancy of the pediatric chest wall, severe intrathoracic injury can be present without any external evidence of trauma. Inspect the thorax for symmetric movement, adequate motion with respirations, abrasions or flail segments. Palpate the chest wall for evidence of musculoskeletal injury, crepitus, or rib deformities. The lungs should be auscultated for bilateral breath sounds, the absence or asymmetry of which suggest a hemothorax or pneumothorax, requiring early treatment. Some of the more common chest injuries and treatment modalities are discussed below.

Pneumothorax and hemopneumothorax. These injuries can result from either blunt or penetrating injury. A large pneumothorax often results in respiratory distress and cyanosis. On chest auscultation, breath sounds are decreased or absent on one side. The extreme, a tension pneumothorax, is poorly tolerated by a child and is an immediate threat to life. Following the development of a pneumothorax, the mobility of the mediastinum may allow structures to shift, resulting in compression of the large vessels and the opposite lung. Tension pneumothorax is a clinical diagnosis based on the findings of neck vein distension and tracheal deviation in the presence of muffled heart and breath sounds.

Open pneumothorax. This is usually the result of penetrating trauma, although occasionally it can result from a rib fragment's puncturing the skin. Physical examination reveals a chest wound with blood or air bubbling from the injury on expiration. Treatment is by application of an occlusive dressing that is taped on three sides, which prevents air from entering the thoracic cavity during inspiration but allows it to escape through the opening during expiration. This is only a temporizing measure; definitive care involves chest tube insertion and surgical repair. Application of a dressing taped on all sides may result in a tension pneumothorax and should be avoided.

Flail chest. Owing to the flexibility of the child's chest wall, a flail segment may result when several ribs are fractured, even if at only one site. This segment becomes detached from the rest of the thoracic cage and moves paradoxically with respirations, resulting in respiratory insufficiency. This is an uncommon injury in children because of the pliability of their ribs. Physical findings include respiratory distress, rib tenderness or deformity, subcutaneous emphysema, and a rib segment that moves in during expiration and out on inspiration.

Pericardial tamponade. Cardiac tamponade may result from penetrating trauma or severe blunt injury. Even a small amount of blood accumulating in the pericardial sac will restrict myocardial contractions and decrease cardiac output. On physical examination, Beck's triad may be present: shock, jugular venous distension, and muffled heart sounds. Many children with cardiac tamponade, however, will have no physical signs other than hypotension; thus sophisticated modalities, such as ultrasound, are often required for diagnosis in the emergency department.

Abdomen

The abdominal musculature in children is meager, and as a result the child is less protected than an adult from injuries to the viscera. The organs most commonly injured in abdominal trauma are the spleen, liver, bowel mesentery, and kidney. The onset of symptoms may be rapid or quite gradual, and the clinician must maintain a high level of suspicion for intraabdominal injury. Serial physical examinations of the trauma patient are essential in helping determine the need for operative intervention. Any child who is hemodynamically unstable without another obvious source of blood loss, or who has an expanding abdomen, is likely to need surgical exploration. Physical examination should include evaluation for ecchymosis, abdominal distension, rigidity, tenderness, and evidence of peritoneal irritation. The bony pelvis should be firmly palpated for evidence of discontinuity.

Urinary tract

In children the kidney is proportionally larger, has less rib and muscle protection, and has a more anterior location than in adults, making it more vulnerable to blunt injury. In addition, the bladder has a more abdominal location and is less protected by the bony pelvis, also making it more susceptible to disruption. Pediatric patients with congenital renal anomalies are particularly prone to renal injury following even only minor trauma. Children should be evaluated for abdominal, lower chest, and flank abrasions, ecchymosis, and tenderness.

Extremity injuries

Extremity fractures are relatively more common in children than in adults, as a result of their bones being less well developed. The bones in adults have ceased to grow and ligamentous injuries commonly occur. The cartilaginous growth plate in the child is weaker than the ligaments, making growth plate (epiphyseal plate) injuries common. Fractures through the epiphysis have been described by the Salter-Harris classification, which divides these injuries into five types.

Initial assessment of the extremities includes inspection for deformity, swelling, and ecchymosis. As previously described, any sites of active bleeding must be controlled by elevation and pressure dressings, and pulses distal to the injury evaluated. Movement may cause further injury and blood loss, so any obviously deformed extremity should be splinted to minimize further damage. Ice packs may be applied to decrease soft tissue swelling. An open fracture should be covered by a sterile, moist dressing, and a splint applied prior to transport. Amputated parts should be wrapped in moist saline-soaked gauze, placed in a plastic bag, and transported on ice. They should not be placed directly in ice water or packed on dry ice. As described previously, a PASG may be useful in splinting suspected pelvic or lower-extremity fractures.

FIELD TREATMENT PROTOCOLS

Many geographic locations now have field treatment protocols for both basic and ALS personnel. The development and implementation of these protocols allow for physician-directed standardized care that corresponds to both the needs of the community and the level of personnel training. Unfortunately, although there are protocols for the care of adult patients in many communities, pediatric protocols are lacking in many locations. Standardized protocols serve as an extension of physician-directed medical care, not a replacement for direct communication with a physician, and medical control contact prior to or during transport is often advantageous. Table 10-6 illustrates a sample pediatric protocol.

FIELD TRIAGE GUIDELINES

Field triage guidelines aim to accomplish two objectives. First, they raise prehospital caregiver's awareness about certain anatomic, historical, and physiologic conditions that increase the risk of death and disability. Second, through attempts to match the severity of an illness or injury with the capability of an institution, the guidelines should result in a reduction of the associated morbidity and mortality. Once these guidelines are adopted by an EMS system, hospitals are categorized according to their capability, and field personnel are authorized to bypass one institution for another of greater capability when necessary. Experience nationwide suggests that prior to development of field triage criteria for injured children, an alarming number of children were transported to institutions that lacked the ability to provide them with necessary care. Through the development of such guidelines and their implementation, optimal care can be provided for all children.

PREPARATION FOR TRANSPORT

All injured children require appropriate immobilization and stabilization prior to and during transport. Adequate cervical spine immobilization through the use of a rigid cervical collar and long backboard or other devices has been previously discussed. Any child who has had a significant mechanism of injury, who has head or upper chest injuries, or who complains of neck pain, requires immobilization (see Table 10-1). Any potentially constricting clothing or jewelry should be removed, particularly those distal to injuries in an extremity. For example, rings should be taken off if there is an upper extremity injury; the subsequent development of edema may interfere with their removal at a later time. As previously described, areas that are suspected of having sustained injuries should be immobilized prior to moving the child in order to decrease subsequent pain and tissue damage. Injured extremities may be elevated and ice packs applied when time allows.

The hemodynamic or neurologic status of the patient may change rapidly, and it is important to monitor injured children as carefully as possible during transport. Cardiac and respiratory monitoring should be continuous throughout transport, and blood pressure may serve as a useful indicator of hemodynamic status. Pulse oximetry, if available, may be useful as an early clue to respiratory embarrassment. A change in mental status during initial stabilization or transport is important to document and report to the receiving facility as early as possible. Finally, young children, particularly infants, readily become hypothermic and need to be wrapped appropriately prior to and during transport. Because infants have a disproportionatly large head circumference, the head should be covered with a hat or blanket to help preserve body temperature.

MEDICAL CONTROL

Medical care provided by EMS personnel by law requires the active involvement of a physician. Medical control serves as the link between prehospital personnel and the medical director or a physician representative. These individuals serve as a resource for medical direction in the management of critically ill or injured patients, or whenever field personnel feel the need for physician assistance. Medical control contact should be established when the administration of optional drugs or deviation from standard protocols is warranted, when a patient who requires intervention refuses transport, or when on-scene individuals interfere with patient care. Contacting medical control or the receiving facility whenever possible not only allows for physician direction but appraises the receiving facility of the situation and allows staff to prepare for the patient. This is particularly advantageous in the case of a critically injured child who will require immediate intervention upon arrival. Notification allows the facility to have essential equipment and medical staff available at the time of the child's arrival in the emergency department.

DOCUMENTATION

The need for careful documentation has been largely overlooked by many EMS systems. Similar to any other medical record, a trip report is a measure of accountability and should document the provision of quality care.

CHILD ABUSE

The incidence of child abuse, unfortunately, has increased significantly, and prehospital personnel may be called to assist injured children who have sustained intentionally inflicted trauma. The incidence of physical, emotional, and sexual abuse is 9.2 in 1000 children, or close to 1% of the population. Evidence of abuse, such as multiple fractures, bruises of different ages, or suspicious burns, should be recognized. A history should be obtained in a nonthreatening way; if a parent or caregiver senses blame, he or she may resist transport to the hospital. If a violent individual is present at the scene, prehospital personnel must use caution to protect themselves and the patient from further injury. Police should be notified immediately, and efforts to remove the child forcibly from a guardian should be avoided. Careful documentation of both the history and physical findings is essential, and it is the responsibility of prehospital care providers to notify and provide written documentation for the local child protection agency.

ROLE OF EMS PERSONNEL UPON ARRIVAL IN THE EMERGENCY DEPARTMENT

The EMS provider's role does not end immediately upon arrival in the emergency department. It is the responsibility of the prehospital care provider to care for the child until treatment can be turned over to medical personnel with an equal or higher level of training. Prehospital personnel are responsible for presenting the history and pertinent physical findings to the receiving facility, in addition to noting any change in status from their time on-scene to arrival at the emergency department. It is important to convey information from the scene of the injury, such as the height from which a child has fallen or the condition of a vehicle involved in an accident. Prehospital personnel should remain to assist hospital staff until the necessary hospital personnel are available to handle the situation adequately.

QUALITY ASSURANCE

No discussion of EMS can be complete without mentioning quality assurance. Every system must have a method to review system performance in order to assess the quality of patient care and its impact. Regular review, with input from both medical control and prehospital personnel, should include all aspects of patient care from notification of EMS (dispatch) to completion of duties in the emergency department. Any system changes that result should be incorporated into prehospital care training programs. A carefully built working relationship between EMS providers and medical personnel is essential if optimal patient care is to be provided.

SUMMARY

Prehospital care providers serve as an extension of physician caregivers before arrival in the emergency department and are an essential part of the medical team that cares for the injured child. Their general approach to pediatric trauma victims should be similar to the ABC approach recommended by the American College of Surgeons. A knowledge of the anatomic and physiologic differences between child and adult will facilitate the recognition and treatment of potentially life-threatening injuries. An ongoing review of field interventions, particularly ALS runs, will help to ensure provision of high quality care for all injured children.

REFERENCES

1. Aijan P, Tsai A, Knopp R et al: Endotracheal intubation of pediatric patients by paramedics, *Ann Emerg Med* 18:489-494, May 1989.
2. Eichelberger MR, Ball JW, Pratsch GS et al: *Pediatric emergencies: a manual for prehospital care providers*, Englewood Cliffs, NJ, 1992, Brady, Prentice-Hall.
3. Eichelberger MR, Ball JW, Pratsch GS et al: Pediatric emergencies: instructors manual, Englewood Cliffs, NJ, 1992, Brady, Prentice-Hall.
4. Eichelberger MR, Ball J, Runion E et al: *Pediatric Emergency Medical Services Training Program: a national program for the instructors of emergency medical technicians.* Sponsored by the US Department of Health and Human Services and the US Department of Transportation, 1987.
5. Eisenberg M, Bergner L, Hallstrom A: Epidemiology of cardiac arrest and resuscitation in children, *Ann Emerg Med* 12:672-674, Nov 1983.
6. Burg JM, O'Malley P, Vinci R et al: Medic IV emergency medical services project: paramedic treatment protocols for pediatric patients and suggested pediatric equipment and medications, Metropolitan Boston Hospital Council, 1990, Burlington Mass.
7. Ramenofsky ML, Luterman A, Quindlen E et al: Maximum survival in pediatric trauma: the ideal system, *J Trauma* 24:818-823, 1984.
8. Rockwood CA, Mann CM, Farrington JD et al: History of emergency medical services in the United States, *J Trauma* 16:299-307, 1976.
9. Seidel JS, Hornbein M, Yoshiyam K et al: Emergency medical services and the pediatric patient: are the needs being met? *Pediatrics* 73:769-772, 1984.
10. Seidel JS: Emergency medical services and the pediatric patient: are the needs being met? II. Training and equipping emergency medical services providers for pediatric emergencies, *Pediatrics* 78:808-812, 1986.
11. Smith P, Bodai BI, Hill AS et al: Prehospital stabilization of critically injured patients: a failed concept, *J Trauma* 25:65-70, 1985.
12. Tsai A, Kalisen G: Epidemiology of pediatric prehospital care, *Ann Emerg Med* 16:284-292, March 1987.

11 Pediatric Trauma Center: Essential Criteria and Organization

Dennis W. Vane

Although there have been many recent advances in trauma care, trauma remains the leading cause of death in North American children over the age of 1 year.[3] Studies have demonstrated that children have special needs and problems as compared with adults and that when treated in centers specializing in the care of children, outcomes appear to be improved.[6,8] For this reason, numerous organizations have begun to derive standards, or concepts, for centers specializing in the care of injured children. Since pediatric trauma represents only approximately 25% of cases seen in large trauma centers, centers specializing specifically in pediatric care are most likely to be regionalized to conserve limited resources.

The concept and design of centers treating injured children might seem to be self-evident: those hospitals with the most resources will treat children and those without adequate resources will not. Unfortunately, given the present medical climate, any system that attempts to exclude existing facilities is bound to fail.

The best model for creation of a pediatric trauma center is regionally based. In addition, it is historically evident that any sort of trauma treatment system for children must be inclusive of regionally available facilities, rather than exclusive. No functional hospital wishes to be excluded from the care of children and, when impartially analyzed, *any* facility can contribute *something* to a well-functioning pediatric trauma system. The task is to define exactly what the contribution of each facility will be. Experience has taught that the best way to determine this is to allow each unit to define carefully its resources, capabilities, and, subsequently, the role in the system it wishes to assume. These determinations will be different for any given geographic or population base. Rural hospitals or care centers with minimal capabilities and facilities will have a larger role in such a system than similarly equipped urban centers. They may be called upon, because of their remote location, to see all patients initially and resuscitate severely ill children before transport. A similar urban hospital might be by-passed entirely by a severely traumatized child, injured just blocks away, for transport to a larger definitive care facility in juxtaposition. That same urban hospital, however, may receive all single-system orthopedic injuries in order to free beds in the definitive care facility for more needy patients.

The critical point is that in attempting to organize an effective trauma care system for children, the entire medical community must have input. Each aspect of care (prehospital, hospital, rehabilitation unit, physician's office) has a place in the system and should be allowed to determine what general form the system should take. Organizers will find that using this approach, although cumbersome, will allow for more effective regionalized treatment systems with better chance for success.

ESTABLISHING THE CENTER

The first step in the development of a pediatric trauma system is the determination of the region of care. Participants must identify the patient population or geographic area to be served. This determination should be based on one facility's acting as the "flagship" institution, which can be classified as the optimal care center for injured children in the area, or the Level I pediatric trauma center. It is best to allow natural referral patterns to determine this region if possible. This permits a free flow of children to the center without creating unnecessary political upheaval. In some cases, political patterns must be redrawn when optimal care for the child is not presently best served or is unnecessarily duplicated. Essentially, timely transport of the most critically ill children to the institution best able to serve the needs of those children should determine the regionalization of the system. Once the service region is defined, the pediatric trauma optimal care center must be identified. Four sets of established criteria are presently popular.[1,2,5,7] One set comes from the American College of Surgeons *Resource Document for Optimal Care of the Injured Patient* and essentially identifies a Level I pediatric trauma center as a Level I adult trauma center with special facilities and personnel.[1]

A second document from the American Pediatric Surgical Association remains as yet unpublished, but essentially briefly reiterates the American College of Surgeons document and another criteria list from the American Society for Testing and Materials.[5] The third document comes from the Pennsylvania Trauma Systems Foundation and is quite extensive, but very specific to the special needs of Pennsylvania.[7] The fourth document deals with all aspects of an optimal care center for injured children and is a consensus standard from the American Society for Testing and Materials.[2] Any attempt to establish a local standard should certainly include a review of these documents, as they all have important points to be taken into consideration. Of critical importance is that each region modify its own criteria as to what will work for that particular area, assuring that as a minimum standard the optimal care of the most severely injured child will be established.

Organizers should keep in mind that it is often more prudent to accept compromise in the system design at its inception than to become bogged down in emotional details. As the system begins to function and hospitals realize their optimal roles, variations in treatment plans and referral agreements can be modified with much less dispute.

DEFINITION

The second step in the development of a trauma care system is to identify the participants. Any institution that desires to become an optimal or Level I pediatric trauma center must have an institutional commitment to provide care to the most severely injured child. This does not mean the most cost-effective care or simply better care than is available at an alternative institution. All participating institutions must be willing to commit themselves to developing the facilities and personnel that provide the most advanced treatment for the most severely ill child. These resources include, but are not limited to, personnel, diagnostic equipment, intensive care, operating suites, transport capabilities, laboratory facilities, and a program of continuing education for the facility itself, referring hospitals, and the community.[1,5,7]

INTEGRATION OF THE SYSTEM

The third step provides for the integration of the participating facilities into a referral and treatment system. Clearly, any Level I pediatric trauma center must be compatible with criteria established by the local, state, and federal governing bodies that claim jurisdiction for this designation. In addition, the center must commit itself to being available at all times to receive children from its referral area. If not available for reception of children, the center must have in force an organized system for their transfer to another institution, given that transfer will not unfavorably affect the outcomes for those children. This mandates participation in regional and statewide systems of prehospital and hospital care. Established and formalized transfer agreements between referral institutions must be in place, clearly describing the priorities of interhospital transfer both in and out of the Level I center. These agreements must be available to the local prehospital care and transport authorities. In addition, participating institutions must identify which children should be preferentially transported to the Level I center and which should be taken to other institutions. This reduces inappropriate delivery of children and possible delay of optimal care. Clearly, this identification of children will take into consideration the individual capabilities of participating institutions and their willingness to treat children.

Relatively few states have legislation evaluating the capabilities of local institutions and the types of patients they are best able to care for. Experience teaches that the determination of which children are to be transferred and which are to be kept should initially be left to the participating hospitals. If attempts are made to impose criteria on these institutions, significant resistance can be expected. Generally, facilities define their capabilities, equipment, and personnel fairly and accurately and, subsequently, can reasonably determine which children they are capable of managing in a definitive fashion. Participating hospitals can best accomplish this determination by listing their equipment, personnel, and facilities on paper and then, working from that document, defining their patient capabilities. Questionable areas usually resolve over time, as participants realize that to treat certain types of injuries requires a dedication of personnel and finances they are not willing to commit.

SERVICES

The fourth is the determination of what services will be available at which institution. The obligation of an institution in identifying itself as a Level I pediatric trauma center implies that it will provide optimal care for the most severely injured child. In addition to medical care, centers must provide appropriate support services for injured patients: social services, psychological counseling for the patient and family, spiritual counseling when appropriate, and family support contacts to assist with parental responsibilities during the hospitalization of a child. Specific guidelines for such services are beyond the scope of this chapter but are available in the referenced criteria.[1,2,5,7] All support services must be available 24 hours a day, 365 days a year.

Early intervention in these areas has dramatically affected family dynamics, as guilt associated with the injured child often plays a significant role.

Requirements for medical services in a Level I pediatric trauma center are extensive. It is understood that the hospital designated to be a Level I center must have immediately available all subspecialists necessary to provide acute care and definitive treatment for an injured child. An expanded definition of exactly what this entails, again, can be obtained from the referenced criteria.[1,2,5,7] In addition, the term *immediately available* is necessarily ill defined and is very much regionally determined. In rural areas where only one subspecialist may be available, *immediately* has an entirely different definition than it might in an urban center where 15 subspecialists may practice.

Any hospital with an active trauma population must establish a separate trauma service, and this requirement is similarly necessary for a Level I pediatric trauma facility. Presently all published, nationally accepted criteria for pediatric centers define the director of a trauma service optimally as a pediatric surgeon. This point has undergone considerable debate with widespread input from the medical and lay communities. This conclusion was reached because pediatric surgeons are trained in the surgical physiology of children and their illnesses. In addition, their training *requires* formal education in the definitive and contemporary treatment of pediatric trauma. In instances where a pediatric surgeon is not available, effort must be made to obtain one as director of the unit so that it can be a maximally functioning Level I facility. When this is impossible, the role may be assumed by a trained adult trauma surgeon with significant education, interest, and experience in the care of injured children.

Other hospital personnel must also be educated in and familiar with not only the care of children, but the care of injured children as well. Nursing, radiology, respiratory therapy, and laboratory personnel, as well as participating physicians, must participate in programs familiarizing them with injured children. Courses such as those designed by the Advanced Trauma Life Support Course of the American College of Surgeons and the Pediatric Advanced Life Support Course of the American Academy of Pediatrics are recommended. In addition, the hospital must define the roles of these health care providers to delegate their responsibility, authority, and accountability in the immediate treatment of the injured child.

Perhaps the most important appointment to the trauma team, for the organization and continuing success of the unit, is the trauma nurse coordinator. This individual is charged with the overall balance of the service, as well as its integration into the general hospital functions. It is critical that this person be committed to the goals and organization of the trauma team. Historically, the trauma nurse coordinator has been responsible for maintaining the patient documentation of the unit and for functioning as the public relations contact for the community. In these roles, the nurse coordinator can greatly facilitate the day-to-day workings of the center as well as inspire community support. Another critical aspect of the nurse coordinator's job is the maintenance of communications with referring hospitals, physicians, and prehospital units. This permits identification of potential or minor problems before they become significant and allows them to be addressed in a timely fashion. The nurse coordinator also follows up on the care and rehabilitation of the child. This person functions often as a sounding board and essentially runs the administrative function of the trauma center.

A Level I pediatric trauma center must be staffed appropriately to tend to the needs of any injured child. This requires physicians with specific training and interest not only in the care of children, but specifically in the care of injured children. The list of subspecialists required is quite long and may be obtained from the references standards.[2] Of essential importance is that the institution provide the optimal care available in the region for these patients.

PHYSICAL RESOURCES

The fifth step establishes the hospital resources available to the center. One of the most difficult areas in which to obtain consensus regarding a pediatric trauma center is the hospital resources that must be available. It is clear to anyone caring for severely injured children that maximum care resources *should* be available 24 hours a day, 365 days a year. Unfortunately, most hospitals find that staffing emergency room and operating rooms on this schedule is somewhat inefficient, given the relatively low incidence of pediatric trauma late at night.[4] However, this is no argument. If a center is to call itself a Level I pediatric trauma center, then it must commit itself to optimal patient care, not just cost-effective patient care. Patients are frequently transferred between institutions at any hour of the day or night. In addition, the currently widely accepted practice of observation for certain cases of traumatic intraabdominal bleeding makes operating room availability essential at all times. This means staffing an operating room 24 hours a day with an anesthesiologist, comfortable with the care of children, and a fully functioning emergency room. Lesser models, after somewhat heated and extensive discussion, were considered inadequate.

Some arguments considered abrogating certain duties of a physician to a nurse clinician, particularly a nurse anesthetist. Subsequent discussion determined that a nurse anesthetist could not function independently of a physician. If, on the other hand, such a shift were possible, and the duties of an anesthesiologist could be replaced by the nurse clinician, then the responsibilities and duties of the surgeon could, likewise, be replaced by a nurse clinician. This was deemed unacceptable and it was felt that essential criteria should mandate the presence of physicians to fulfill physician roles.

In addition to specific facilities available at a Level I pediatric trauma center, certain equipment is also necessary. The list is extensive and includes, essentially, that equipment felt to be mandatory for the proper monitoring, medical care, and special needs of children. The range of equipment comprises that necessary in emergency rooms, operating rooms, and all other patient care areas. The specifics are available in the essential criteria previously referenced.[1,2,5,7]

OTHER PROGRAMS

After the center is established, with systems and staff in place, other programs must be integrated. After an injury, many children require some sort of rehabilitative intervention. It is imperative that a Level I pediatric trauma center be capable of providing such rehabilitative care. Because the number of children who suffer severe trauma is small and the rehabilitative process is often long and not acute in nature, present standards do not mandate that a rehabilitative unit be immediately available or on site. What is necessary is that the institution demonstrate that the needs of any child requiring rehabilitation are met. This may be accomplished through a self-contained unit or through a referral agreement with an off-site center. In addition, some minimal rehabilitative services, such as occupational therapy and physical therapy for children, must be provided at the acute-care center until children are stable and may be transferred to another institution. If the unit is off-site, a mechanism must be in effect to provide follow-up to the Level I center regarding children's outcome and progress. These reports must be included in the children's records for adequate follow-up and for quality assurance.

A similar requirement is standard for pediatric burn centers. It is recognized that not all Level I pediatric trauma centers necessarily require an on-site burn unit for the definitive treatment of burned children. These children may best be served at large burn referral centers, particularly when the patient population of a given region will not support a self-contained unit. Again, the Level I center must be equipped for the immediate care and resuscitation of the acutely burned child and, then, if appropriate transfer agreements are in effect, undertake later transport of the child, when stable, for definitive treatment.

COMMUNITY RELATIONS

Relationship with the community is essential for the successful function of any trauma center, particularly a pediatric center. The community must see itself as part of the center, and, subsequently, the center must take a leadership role in childhood trauma-related issues. Specifically, the Level I center must form the nucleus of community education programs for the prevention of trauma and its early treatment. It should provide programs for referral hospitals, community physicians, prehospital care providers, and the lay community. Each must be targeted to the population being served. It is helpful for the trauma center, through the nurse coordinator, to develop programs for the local physicians and hospitals to enhance their roles and participation in the regionalized care system. If the concept of community-based participation is developed when the trauma center starts, the success rate of the unit will be increased. Community members will feel that they have a stake in the center and assure its viability.

Clearly, any Level I trauma center must make preparations for potential mass casualty disasters. The pediatric trauma center must create and test disaster plans that incorporate the referral patterns of the community. The inclusion of local hospitals in the planning and protocols for any such plan will ensure their feeling of participation and the realistic provision of optimal care for the greatest number of children, should a significant disaster occur. In any multiple-patient tragedy, the vast number of children are only slightly injured. These patients can and should be triaged to outlying hospitals with relatively minimal pediatric capabilities. This prevents the more comprehensive centers from becoming incumbered with traffic problems resulting from an influx of patients with relatively minor injuries. It also allows the more timely treatment of a larger number of children, who might otherwise be forced to wait significant periods of time while the diagnostic equipment of the Level I center is occupied with the most seriously ill patients.

Centers must also develop transport protocols both within the unit and between hospitals. These protocols allow the free flow of children and prevent the possibility of disasters that may result when a child is inappropriately moved from one area to another.

RESEARCH AND SELF-ASSESSMENT

Finally, in addition to providing leadership in educational programs for the community, the Level I pediatric trauma center must actively participate in pediatric trauma research. Research activities should not be confined to accumulation of bench data, but should be part of the ongoing process of self-evaluation of the institution. Treatment protocols should be evaluated for their effectiveness, and clinical trials to improve care should be undertaken. Given the relatively rare incidence of severe trauma to children, it is essential that patient data be collected and, when appropriate, pooled with other data banks to evaluate treatment effectively at each institution. Moreover, common trends in the care of injured children that might improve results nationwide may be identified when large groups of data are analyzed. To this end, national registries such as the National Pediatric Trauma Registry have become useful.

In addition to the obligation of collecting regionalized data and participating in national protocols, each institution has a mandate to perform an exercise of self-evaluation. Each Level I center should also provide leadership in self-evaluation for the entire network of the system. This is a critical requirement for any institution dealing in patient care, not just the pediatric trauma center. All deaths must be reviewed and determination made, with currently obtainable standards, whether each death was preventable or not. Critical evaluation of outcome statistics for varying levels of injury is also essential. Failures of the system must be analyzed methodically to assure that flaws are worked out. It is very helpful to include participants from all prehospital care systems as well as representatives from referring hospitals. Not only are these people interested in ascertaining the outcomes for their referred or transportable children, they are also generally interested in trying to improve care if possible. Their suggestions often provide a different perception than can be obtained from workers at the Level I center and can be very helpful in identifying solutions to problems. Members of the trauma team and the nursing staff, as well as all paramedical personnel, should be included in these sessions. They can provide valuable insight into the workings of the trauma service and can often make extremely helpful recommendations on improving protocols and operations within the unit.

CONCLUSIONS

The creation of a Level I pediatric trauma center is not an easy feat. In addition to understanding the very specialized medical care that children require, organizers must realize that obtaining the equipment and personnel for the center is the easiest part of their task of organization. Hospitals must be committed to the concept because, at least at the outset, significant resources and funds are necessary for start-up costs. Community approval is also critical. Without support from the medical and lay community, the center will be destined to fail. Regional referral hospitals cannot assume a competitive role within the system. Expenditure of funds for competitive publicity means withdrawing those funds from improvement in facilities or patient care in an already financially strapped medical community. Organizers must assume an inclusive approach with both the lay and medical community in initial proposals if success is to be assured. In each instance when this approach has been utilized, centers have grown and patient care has benefitted. Conversely, when exclusive methodology was attempted to try to "corner the market" in pediatric trauma care, those centers spent significant amounts of money, only to become underutilized and occasionally face bankruptcy over the long run.

REFERENCES

1. Committee on Trauma American College of Surgeons, *Resource document for optimal care of the injured patient*, Chicago, Il, 1990, American College of Surgeons. pp 51-54.
2. F 1286-90 Standard guide for development and operation of Level I pediatric trauma facilities. In: *Annual book of ASTM standards* 13:01, Philadelphia, Pa, 1990, American Society for Testing and Materials.
3. Greensher J: Recent advances in injury prevention, *Pediatr Rev* 10:171-177, 1988.
4. Haller JA, Beaver B: A model: systems management of life threatening injuries in children for the State of Maryland, USA, *Intensive Care Med,* 15:S53-S56, 1989.
5. Harris BH, Barlow BA, Ballantine TV et al: American Pediatric Surgical Association: principles of pediatric trauma care, *J Pediatr Surg* 274(4):1-3, 1992.
6. McKoy C, Bell MJ: Preventable traumatic deaths in children, *J Pediatr Surg* 18:505-508, 1983.
7. Pennsylvania Trauma Systems Foundation: *1990–1991 pediatric* standards for trauma center accreditation, Pennsylvania Trauma, Harrisburg, Pa, 1990, The Foundation.
8. Ramenofsky ML, Luterman A, Quindlen E, et al: Maximum survival in pediatric trauma: the ideal system, *J Trauma* 24:818-823, 1984.

12 Nursing Roles in the Continuum of Care

Cynthia J. Wright and Leslie M. O'Brien

Traumatic injury affects the physical, cognitive, psychosocial, and emotional components in the lives of the injured child and family. Trauma nursing care occurs throughout all phases of the continuum of care (see Table 8-1, p. 93) and involves the injured child, parents or guardians, siblings, extended family, and the community. Hospitalization after a traumatic injury is a sudden, unanticipated situational crisis for the child and family. Throughout the course of treatment, nurses provide direct clinical care, education and anticipatory guidance, emotional and tangible support, and assistance in understanding and interfacing with the interdisciplinary trauma team and health care system. The nursing team establishes the foundation for reuniting child and family and facilitating reestablishment of the parental role in advocacy for the child.

Nursing practice has been described as both an art and a science. The specialty of pediatric trauma nursing requires the expertise and skill to create an environment that promotes the well-being of the injured child and family within the highly technical care system throughout the continuum of care. Nurses have practiced in the home, hospital, school, community, and prehospital arenas, advocating injury prevention, rapid and appropriate specialized care, as well as reintegration into the home and activities of daily living. Scientific advances in trauma nursing have grown from the MASH units and resuscitation bays in the field and in hospitals through computerized or mechanized mobility, respiratory, communication, and environmental control systems established in rehabilitation centers. During the past 3 decades of ever-increasing technology, nurses and their colleagues throughout the world of health care have retained the "human touch" in caring for the injured family unit. The pediatric nurse is well known for his or her strong advocacy and surrogate parenting of the injured child. In today's "high-tech" and fast-paced environment, these efforts can be valuable assets for the child, family, and health care team in maintaining a family-centered care practice. The injured child and family need a strong advocate to keep them from becoming lost among multiple services. At the Children's National Medical Center (CNMC) in Washington, D.C., the trauma coordinator (TC) and the trauma rehabilitation coordinator (TRC) function as liaison personnel for the interdisciplinary team. In the absence of these roles, responsibility reasonably shifts to the staff nurse. *The continuity link afforded by the nursing staff is of additional importance when resident teaching programs provide a significant portion of medical care. Residents can benefit from instruction regarding this link and the advantages of drawing from the knowledge and experience of pediatric nurses.*

The child who sustains a traumatic injury has a unique set of physical and psychological needs and priorities. The highly specialized care begins in the prehospital area with stabilization and initial resuscitation and continues into the emergency and critical care areas. As the child's condition is stabilized, the restorative and rehabilitative needs emerge, and a care plan initiated based on the child's developmental and physiologic status. Nurses in all areas of health care focus on the stages of development of both the child and the family.

CONTINUUM OF CARE: TRAUMA COORDINATORS

Using the continuum of care as a philosophical framework and a daily practice model, nurses in all phases of care promote a holistic approach to care of the injured child and family. Through a coordinated system of services and programs, the TC and TRC ensure that appropriate resources are effectively and efficiently marshalled for the injured child and family. The coordinators interface with the entire health care team in both the hospital and the community to facilitate an interdisciplinary plan of care. This plan of care involves many disciplines and departments, each evaluating the child within a specific area of expertise and developing a plan of care based on input from all disciplines to promote the highest level of health and functioning. *The interdisciplinary model does not presuppose that all team members think alike, but*

118

rather that they act, plan, intervene, and evaluate care together. Through interdisciplinary interactions, opportunities for education and research are frequently identified.

The roles of the TC and TRC intertwine to ensure that the injured child and family benefit from all resources available throughout the continuum of care. The role of the TC at CNMC is diverse and dynamic and includes responsibility for ensuring that the entire system of care for the acutely injured child is functioning as intended. This includes coordinating the plan of care provided by prehospital, medical, nursing, and ancillary personnel at the scene, through the emergency department, operating room, intensive care and intermediate care units. The child and family need an advocate to help them navigate an often confusing system. The TC meets with the child and family daily to answer questions, provide education, offer support, coordinate patient care conferences, and ensure that information is clear, concise, and consistent.

In addition to family support, responsibility for quality assurance for all services involved in the care of the acutely injured child lies with the TC. This includes preparation for monthly interdisciplinary mortality and morbidity meetings and reviewing code room, operating room, and intensive care unit documentation, trauma debriefing forms, and videotapes. Feedback to care providers on a regular basis creates an opportunity for staff education, problem solving, and increased communication between departments.

The TRC facilitates clinical, educational, and research programs during the restorative phases of care for the injured child and family. On a day-to-day basis the TRC coordinates the plan of care with all team members, working closely with the primary nurse and attending physician. The key to successful interdisciplinary care delivery is two-fold. The first essential ingredient is effective oral and written communication between disciplines. The second is a consistent core group of professionals who establish rapport with the child and family. In a complex hospital and university system, the coordinators provide both consistency and ongoing communication. The TRC initiates contact with rehabilitation programs for outpatient, home care, or inpatient needs. Serving as a liaison to community education and health care professionals, the TRC assists the family in accessing new resources for either temporary or permanent disabilities. Reintegrating the child and family into their home, school, and community requires specific planning among all disciplines, as well as a central referral source.

In the outpatient setting, the interdisciplinary trauma follow-up clinic provides the mechanism and staff to link specialized acute trauma and rehabilitation care experts with primary care providers. Commonly known as the "trauma clinic," the outpatient follow-up program requires a commitment from each discipline, ensuring that the resources of the hospital will be centralized for the child and family. Availability and accessibility for evaluations, diagnostic tests, therapy, and counseling are keys to the success of any follow-up program. This program provides a central contact point for interdisciplinary evaluation and recommendations for school and community programs and an essential link to primary care providers. Additionally, the trauma clinic serves as an excellent resource for the educational and research components of a tertiary Level I trauma center and university-affiliated hospital program. *Perhaps the most important function of an interdisciplinary trauma follow-up program is to promote the supportive networks built between families and children who have had similar experiences and now face unique challenges together.*

NURSING ALONG THE CONTINUUM

In every phase of the injured child's care, the nurse is the common denominator. From admission to discharge, nurses facilitate communication between members of the trauma team, additional specialists and departments involved in the child's care, and personnel in other areas of the hospital. A key factor in determining the child's progression through the "golden hour" is the expertise of the nursing members of the trauma response team. A centralized trauma team that draws its nursing support from the emergency department staff has distinct advantages in ensuring an expert, smooth resuscitation. Increased experience and the opportunity to function routinely as a team improves the level of care provided to each child. A decentralized nursing team, however, can provide other advantages. Response by nurses from other areas in the hospital interjects expertise of different backgrounds and may open lines of communication between nursing units. Staffing patterns, commitment to the care of injured children, and levels of nursing knowledge and experience will assist in determining which concept is appropriate for each institution.

Nurses play a vital role in the trauma response team at CNMC. The team is centralized and, therefore, nurses are drawn from the Emergency Medical Trauma Center (EMTC), also known as the Emergency Room, unless multiple emergencies arrive simultaneously. In this situation, nursing staff respond from the pediatric intensive care unit, the burn unit, or the intensive care nursery. A brief description of each nursing role follows.

Nurse in charge

The nurse in charge ensures that all care is clearly documented in the child's record. This minute-by-minute chronology benefits all members of the team. During resuscitation, the chronology provides ready access to the progression of vital signs, medications and fluid boluses administered, and changes in Glasgow Coma Scale (GCS) scores. The nurse in charge assists the team by providing frequent summarized updates and ensuring that newer team members are familiar with the center's trauma protocols. The step-by-step nursing documentation in the code room also provides a clear record of the resuscitation and provides individuals who were not involved in the initial events with the ability to determine the child's prognosis and plan of care.

Nurse Left

The nurse on the child's left maintains a strong link with the child throughout resuscitation by providing a calm, reassuring influence. Nurse Left's primary role is to talk to the child and explain the perceived confusion in a manner most appropriate for the child's developmental age. Nurse Left also assists in obtaining vital signs, in monitoring left-sided infusions and medications, and in other left-sided procedures. If the child is in cadiac arrest, Nurse Left initiates CPR.

Nurse Right

The nurse on the child's right removes the child's clothing, places ECG leads, monitors right-sided infusions, and assists the surgeon with all procedures. If the child is a burn victim, this role is performed by a nurse from the burn unit.

Medication nurse

The medication nurse draws up all medications, flushes, and blood-drawing equipment as they are needed. All medication dosages and concentrations are communicated to the team as they are used.

Nursing administrator liaison

The nursing administrator liaison functions as the communication link between the trauma response team and all other departments involved in a child's care. These include the laboratory and blood bank, consulting physicians, radiology, public affairs, the social worker caring for the child's family, and the admitting department, among others. This role is filled by a nursing supervisor and is critical in ensuring that resuscitation proceeds smoothly and efficiently.

Operating room nurse

The operating room (OR) charge nurse responds to the trauma bay and assesses the potential for surgical intervention, both in the EMTC and in the operating room. If an immediate thoracotomy is necessary, the OR nurse is available to assist in the EMTC. If the child requires surgery, the OR nurse triages current OR cases and prepares the operating room.

Emergency department paramedics

Paramedics are successfully utilized in the emergency department at CNMC as an adjunct to nursing care. A paramedic well trained in prehospital management is a natural asset for the trauma response team and fills the Nurse Left or Nurse Right role effectively. In addition, the presence of paramedics in the emergency department augments nursing staff capabilities.

Intensive care

When a critically ill child is stabilized and ready for transport to radiology or to the intensive care unit (ICU), an ICU nurse responds, receives a report from the emergency department nurse, and assumes responsibility for the child's care. This system maintains continuity of care and decreases the child's fear and confusion that may occur if numerous caregivers are involved.

Specialized general care

The injured child who is transferred from the critical care unit to a specialized general care unit faces yet another new and unknown environment. Both the child and family will experience mixed feelings. *Although the transition to a less intensive level of care is one step closer to returning home, there is also a change in frequency of many aspects of care, which can produce additional stress for the family.* The primary nursing staff on each specialty care unit works with the social workers and coordinators to assist the child and family to understand and adapt to changes. The nursing staff is actively involved in coordinating new routines and daily schedules, as well as facilitating greater parental involvement in care. Each family unit has unique responses and individual coping patterns, but all require empathy and support during this and future changes in environments.

Discharge planning and restorative care components are integrated into the nursing care plan from the day of admission. Specialists in home care, school, public health, and rehabilitation programs are available to work with the nursing and social services staff to evaluate needs and available resources. The current health care financing climate poses an additional challenge when ensuring that the child and family receive appropriate and timely clinical care and equipment in rehabilitation and at home. The TRC and the social worker are available to work with the family, nursing and physician staff, and the reimbursement source or case management services.

The unique requirements of the injured child and family necessitate a unique system of care. A variety of expanded roles have been created out of the necessity to bridge gaps in a system that did not meet these special needs. Nurses trained in children's psychiatric needs assist the child and family in resolving stressful aspects of hospitalization, such as nightmares, behavioral difficulties, pain management, and coping with loss. The challenge of managing children at different developmental levels is met by the child life workers who use play therapy to prepare children for various procedures, explore their reactions, and assist their siblings with coping mechanisms. Social workers nurture the child and family through all phases of the continuum of care and ensure the provision of

adequate support systems during and after hospitalization.

Quality assurance

The quality assurance and improvement (QA/QI) program of the trauma service is the responsibility of the TC and the TRC in collaboration with the trauma director. Just as in the clinical program, the QA/QI program represents interdisciplinary input from all services. Concurrent chart and care audits are combined with medical records, flow sheets, and audit filters to form the basis for case and systems review. The trauma morbidity and mortality conference, which can occur weekly or monthly, requires input from all departments in peer review of individual clinical cases. The trauma management committee meets monthly, serving as a forum for discussion of hospitalwide systems and

Table 12–1 Resources for trauma nursing

American Trauma Society Trauma Coordinators Subcommittee 8903 Presidential Parkway Suite 512 Upper Marlboro, MD 20772-2656 (800)556-7890	Annual meeting: May in Washington, DC National Database of Trauma Coordinators Regional networks for consultation/collaboration Focus on injury control and EMS systems
Society of Trauma Nursing 888 17th Street N.W. Suite 1000 Washington, DC 20006	National meetings: March in Baltimore December in California Written standards for trauma nursing and trauma education
Society of Pediatric Nurses P.O. Box 626 Danville, CA 94526-0626 (510)820-9652	
Emergency Nurses Association 230 East Ohio Street Suite 600 Chicago, IL 60611-9900 (312)649-0297	
American Association of Critical-Care Nurses 101 Columbia Aliso Viejo, CA 92656 1-800-899-AACN	
American Association of Neuroscience Nurses 224 N. Des Plaines Suite 601 Chicago, IL 60661 (312)993-0043	
Association of Rehabilitation Nurses 5799 Old Orchard Road First Floor Skokie, IL 60077-1024 (708)966-3433	

programs and acting as a focal point for initiation of change and improvement of the systems of care.

Education and research

Education and research are a prime focus in all phases of the continuum of care. To ensure that physicians, nurses, families, prehospital personnel, and ancillary departments are cognizant of and following trauma protocols requires frequent interaction and constant monitoring. Education occurs within many forums: on a daily basis at the bedside and on clinical rounds, through weekly trauma lecture series for residents and fellows, and as part of an annual schedule of continuing education lectures for each nursing unit. The coordinators and clinical nurse experts from specialty units participate in local, regional, and national conferences for professionals in the prehospital, emergency department, critical care, and specialty care areas, and in rehabilitation programs (Table 12-1). The trauma center has also established an International Pediatric Trauma Conference, held every 2 years, which focuses on current advances in the nursing practice of pediatric trauma care through the entire continuum. Through clinical research grants and interdepartmental projects, staff are able to assess the current protocols and develop more effective means of caring for injured children and families.

Injury prevention

At CNMC, nurses are involved in every phase of the care of the injured child and family, including injury prevention. Through the National Safe Kids Campaign and other unit-based programs, nurses teach in the community to help prevent childhood injuries. They speak to students, parents, school nurses, and community service groups, using a core lecture and slide presentation developed in collaboration with the trauma service and the Safe Kids Campaign. The ultimate goal of these activities is, in essence, to "put ourselves out of business."

CONCLUSION: ADVOCACY

The pediatric nurse possesses numerous exceptional qualifications, of which expertise in advocating for the child and family is perhaps the most important. In light of the challenges of health care in the 1990s, the child can easily be engulfed by an ever-changing, fast-paced environment. When the child is also a trauma victim, the likelihood of becoming lost in the system increases unless there is appropriate advocacy through each phase of care.

The interdisciplinary trauma team faces a major challenge in reintegrating a physically and psychologically healthy child and family into their home, school, and community. The pediatric nurse can be the strongest link in this integration and negotiation of the health care delivery system.

CASE STUDY

On a crisp, clear Sunday morning, Johnny is riding with his big sister, Linda, on their way to church along a quiet country road. As Linda's compact car rounds a sharp curve, it is met head-on by an out-of-control, full-sized auto driven by an elderly woman. Fortunately, both Linda and Johnny are in three-point restraints. Linda is found alert and well-oriented by the prehospital flight team, but is pinned under the steering wheel, her head against the gearshift. Five-year-old Johnny is unresponsive and has extensive injuries. A difficult and prolonged extrication delivers Linda and Johnny into the care of the flight nurse and paramedic.

Pediatric resuscitation often begins with a nurse/ paramedic team. Therefore, a commitment to comprehensive training in the care of injured children is critical. The PALS certified prehospital team knows that Johnny has special care requirements. He is at greater risk for hypovolemia and hypothermia. In addition, his patterns of injury differ from those typical of the adult population.

On arrival in the emergency department, Johnny is moaning and minimally responsive to pain. The nurse in charge documents his GCS score of 5 and trauma score of 12. The nurse on his left speaks calmly to Johnny, despite his unresponsiveness, and obtains vital signs. The nurse on his right assists with physical assessment, drawing blood, and IV access while calling

out information for documentation. The flight nurse advises the team that Johnny's respiratory pattern has changed dramatically. The medication nurse anticipates intubation and draws up the necessary medications. The anesthesiologist then proceeds with intubation, assisted by respiratory therapy and Nurse Right. Meanwhile, the nursing supervisor calls radiology, requesting a CT scan of the head and abdomen, and pages the neurosurgeon to consult in the emergency department (ED) for a possible spinal cord injury.

The ICU nurse receives the radiology report and assumes Johnny's care, thereby linking the ED and ICU nursing staff and easing the transition for the child and family. When an L2 spinal column injury is detected, the ICU nurse provides emotional support and clinical explanations throughout the acute phase of care. The assignment of primary nurses in the ICU promotes further continuity and trust in the injured child and family. Primary nursing also aids in early recognition of subtle, physiologic changes, such as the cardiac contusion diagnosed on day 2 in Johnny's case. The list of Johnny's injuries includes:

Concussion with loss of consciousness
Multiple abrasions and contusion to face and left eye
CN VI nerve palsy on right
Orbital floor fracture on left

Bilateral pulmonary contusions
Myocardial contusion
Deep lacerations to abdomen
L2 and L3 spinal column fracture
L2-4 incomplete spinal cord injury
Neurogenic bladder and bowel

As Johnny's cardiorespiratory status stabilizes, initial consults were communicated to physical and occupational therapy with a request to begin splinting, positioning, and passive range of motion therapy. Over the next week, a daily care routine is established by the nurses and therapists for daily care and exercises along with the numerous continuing radiographic and cardiac tests. Daily care includes not only typical AM and PM care, meals, and a new bladder and bowel regimen, but also most important activities in a 5-year-old boy's day, Teenage Mutant Ninja Turtle cartoons and Matchbox car races with another child and Dad.

A general surgery, neurosurgery, plastic surgery, physiatry, ophthalmology, and cardiology team make rounds each day, evaluating Johnny's progress and planning for appropriate changes in care. At each visit a nurse is present to help Johnny talk about how he feels and to provide current information to the physicians of all disciplines. Twice a week, representatives from each service meet on the nursing unit with the TC, the TRC, primary nurses, social worker, child life worker, physical and occupational therapist, and a representative from utilization review. From the day of admission, contact has been made with insurance providers and Medicaid to begin the process of applying for Social Security Insurance (SSI) and planning for referrals to a pediatric inpatient rehabilitation facility. Meetings with the family occur at all major decision and transfer points, as well as spontaneous conferences as opportunities for education and support emerge at the child's bedside and in the parents' lounge.

Before discharge, Johnny, his sister, and his parents spend 2 weeks learning about cardiac monitors, spinal cord anatomy, the CT scanner, and the schedule of medications for his bladder and bowel care. The primary nurses teach the family as they demonstrate care and individualized written material about each skill and routine. When the day comes for transfer to the rehabilitation program, a discharge conference is held with the family and the interdisciplinary trauma team. The primary nurse helps Johnny and his mother to write out a list of clothes and toys to pack, and staff from each service writes a summary of care and a plan for long-term follow-up. On the day of transfer, one 5-year-old, two parents, four Ninja Turtles, 10 summaries, and 20 x-ray copies leave the hospital, headed for 3 months of continued learning, practice, and therapy at the rehabilitation facility. Johnny and his family will visit the nursing and medical teams on the first of many visits to the trauma clinic after discharge from rehabilitation.

REFERENCES

1. Cardona VC, editor: *Trauma nursing from resuscitation through rehabilitation*, Philadelphia, 1988, WB Saunders Company.
2. Donahue MP: *Nursing: the finest art*, St Louis, 1985, Mosby–Year Book.
3. Eichelberger MR, Pratsch GL: *Pediatric trauma care*. Rockville, Md, 1988, Aspen.
4. Joy C, editor: *Pediatric trauma nursing*, Rockville, Md, 1989, Aspen.
5. Seidel JS, Henderson DP, editors: *Emergency medical services for children: a report to the nation*, Washington, DC, 1990, National Center for Education in Maternal and Child Health.

13 Disability from Injury and Rehabilitation

Michael A. Alexander, Jane A. Crowley, Lynn E. Patten, and Barbara A. McHugh

The comprehensive rehabilitation of children requires an interdisciplinary team approach throughout the continuum of care. This approach begins with the trauma team and continues in the transition of the child and family from the acute care setting to the comprehensive pediatric rehabilitation center and, ultimately, to home, outpatient follow-up, school reintegration, and independence.

Rehabilitation, of necessity, constantly works at multiple levels with each child and family system. The first level is that of working in the present with the existing abilities, strengths, and weaknesses to maximize the child's function. The second level requires remedial work on current deficits and problem areas in the hope of returning the child to normal capability and function. The third and most difficult part of pediatric rehabilitation is dealing with developmental aspects and effecting the transition of the child from childhood-onset disability to adult competence.

The World Health Organization (WHO) definitions of *disease, impairment, disability,* and *handicap* provide a template for conceptualizing intervention levels.[13] *Disease* is defined as the actual insult to the human being, such as a traumatic brain, spinal cord, or multisystem injury. *Impairment* is a diminution in the physiologic capability of an organ system as the result of disease or trauma, whereas *disability* is the resultant impact of that diminished capability on function and activities of daily living. Disability, however, is a condition that can be compensated for with assistive devices, medications, and/or support systems. *Handicap* reflects those situations in which disability cannot be compensated for, owing to existing behavioral or attitudinal considerations, environmental or architectural obstacles, or legal impediments in society.

REHABILITATION PROCESS

The interdisciplinary team model for rehabilitation includes physical medicine and rehabilitation specialists (physiatrists), nursing and allied health professionals, working in coordination to maximize the outcome of the child. The child is viewed as an intact being who has unique problems or disabilities that are the result of the impairments sustained through trauma. The team addresses rehabilitation issues as problem areas and develops integrated and coordinated treatment goals. A master problem list serves as the template for team conferences, treatment planning, and documentation (Table 13-1).

The rehabilitation process is often based on a compromise between teaching the patient skills that can minimize existing impairments and attempting remedial measures toward a prospective outcome. For instance, when a child is not ambulating, the team may recommend a wheelchair for increased mobility. The family, however, may feel that this is giving up on the child's ability to relearn walking. The point is that it is important to give the child some measure of autonomy and increased potential for mobility and activity early in the rehabilitative process. In fact, it has never been shown that teaching wheelchair mobility while waiting for physical recovery and ambulation has impeded the final outcome. Families have to be supported in understanding that the decision to provide the wheelchair is not, in fact, giving up on the child but simply allowing the child to have maximal success now. Rehabilitation progresses in a series of compromises that allow the child to function optimally while working toward future goals.

Rehabilitation has two underlying philosophies, in addition to that of dedication to the maximal restoration of function. First, discharge planning begins on admission, with program structure based on the development of long-term and short-term goals. Goal achievement determines length of stay.

Second, process is justified through evaluation of outcome measures. Rehabilitation clinicians are obliged to continual evaluation of treatment programs in terms of functional effectiveness and efficiency, as measured against resource expenditure. Many families whose child sustains traumatic onset disability have but a limited resource of available funds. A major portion of these funds is, of necessity, expended in stabilizing the child's life; what remains must be used judiciously. In recognition of this reality, the Commission on Accred-

Table 13–1 Master problem list

1. *Cognitive/language/perception.* Includes alertness, reality orientation, intellectual function, memory, attention span, judgment, perceptual deficits; receptive and expressive language; school and prevocational skills.
   a. Rancho Level of Cognitive Function
   b. Cognitive Assistance Scale (CAS)
   c. Patient/family teaching
2. *Neuromuscular/skeletal.* Includes abnormal tone, reflexes, strength, balance, coordination, range of motion, and oral motor control.
   a. Physical Assistance Scale (PAS)
   b. Frankel Classification for SCI patient, including sensory/motor level and motor index score
   c. Patient/family teaching
3. *Nutrition.* Includes nutritional parameters, weight, oral feeding, tube feedings, special diets, and adequate hydration.
   a. Patient/family teaching
4. *Mobility.* Includes transfer, ambulation, wheelchair mobility, bed mobility, and level of assistance needed.
   a. Patient/family teaching
5. *Sensory.* Includes hearing, tactile, temperature, visual, olfactory, and vestibular acuity, proprioception, and sense of taste.
   a. Patient/family teaching
6. *Activities of daily living.* Includes self-care, daily hygiene and dressing skills, sleep patterns; home, leisure, and community skills; driving and therapeutic community visits.
   a. Patient/family teaching
7. *Preexisting medical problems.* Includes any medical problem that existed prior to current hospitalization.
   a. Patient/family teaching
8. *Emergent medical problems.* Includes any medical problem that develops during current hospitalization.
   a. Patient/family teaching
9. *Respiratory system.* Includes tracheostomy, mechanical ventilation, and/or reactive airway disease.
   a. Patient/family teaching
10. *Cardiovascular system.* Includes blood pressure, pulse rate, arrhythmia, hypertension, pacemaker, cardiac arrest, cardiac surgery and/or injury.
    a. Patient/family teaching
11. *Gastrointestinal system.* Includes gastroenteritis, gastroesophageal reflux, vomiting, bowel incontinence, diarrhea, constipation, neurogenic bowel.
    a. Patient/family teaching
12. *Genitourinary system.* Includes urinary incontinence, catheterization problems, vaginitis, neurogenic bladder.
    a. Patient/family teaching
13. *Skin.* Includes rashes, wounds, pressure areas, turgor, and edema.
    a. Patient/family teaching
14. *Pain.* Includes acute, chronic, and headache.
    a. Patient/family teaching
15. *Safety.* Includes physical, medical, and cognitive factors related to chronologic age-appropriate expectations.
    a. Patient/family teaching
16. *Sexuality.* Includes medical factors that alter sexual functioning and communication of these factors to patient and family.
    a. Patient/family teaching
17. *Social/emotional status of patient.* Includes inappropriate behavior; self-related, task-related, environment-related, and interpersonal behaviors; mental disorders; insight; and adjustment to disability.
    a. Patient/family teaching
18. *Social/emotional status of family/significant other.* Includes emotional and physical health of family members; family composition, expectations, and resources; and all items listed in 17, above.
    a. Patient/family teaching
19. *Adaptive equipment/supplies.* Includes augmentative communication devices, environmental control units, home modifications, durable medical equipment, adaptive equipment, respiratory equipment, and other home care supplies.
    a. Patient/family teaching
20. *Discharge planning.* Includes therapeutic leaves of absence, home evaluation, receptivity to discharge, community reintegration (including appropriate postdischarge services), and written plan of follow-up care.
    a. Patient/family teaching

itation of Rehabilitation Facilities (CARF)[4] requires systematic program evaluation. The rehabilitation facility has to assign functional classification scores to patients at admission, ascertain improvement at discharge, and, at subsequent follow-up, determine whether those functional gains have been maintained.

Commitment includes the orchestrated transition of control from team members to the family, and then to the child. Families are recognized as integral to the team process as they, on behalf of their child, join in setting goals, for the family lives with the ramification of the decisions made. Ultimately, this responsibility must be transferred from the parents to the child or adolescent as that individual becomes capable of developing and helping to coordinate a long-term care strategy.

OVERVIEW OF PROBLEM AREAS
Cognitive deficits

In traumatic brain injury (TBI), cognitive deficits are the most common even in those injuries judged to be mild by the Glasgow Coma Scale. A body of literature is emerging, documenting previously undetected neuropsychological deficits concurrent with spinal cord injury[5], presumably resulting from trauma or hypoxia to the brain. There is a well-known progression that marks emergence from coma, including passage through a stage of agitation and confusion. Only with the return of a patient's orientation can definitive statements be made about cognitive deficits.

Generally speaking, typical cognitive deficits vary between open and closed head injuries. Closed head injuries are more likely to show the effects of global disruption of the cortex. In general, those cognitive skills performed most automatically are those that return strongest. Cognitive tasks requiring active analysis, such as reading comprehension and mathematic calculation will be impaired in predictable ways within general age categories. New learning is impaired because of posttrauma difficulty in memory formation, as well as metacognitive difficulties (speed of processing, task approach, concentration, etc.). Classic syndrome appearance can occur, but is less common. When there are discrete symptoms, these are sometimes correlated with evidence of intracranial hematoma, as seen on structural imaging studies. Generally speaking, imaging studies have not been found to be predictive of the cognitive deficit pattern, despite the age of the child.

Open head injuries, although sometimes demonstrating more global disruption, typically demonstrate a more syndrome appearance, given a certain level of maturity of the brain. This syndrome appearance is due to the focal disruption of specific areas. Considerably less often is there a period of protracted sensorium disturbance. Most individuals with open head injuries may have genuine memory of the injury acquisition itself (usually a penetrating wound), whereas this is most uncommon, if not totally absent, in those with closed head injuries.

Full neuropsychological evaluation by psychologists with specialized training in this area is required on a serial basis to plan for educational needs of injured children, as well as to render opinions about the level of community safety, and other concerns. The influence of premorbid status is currently recognized as a predictive factor in the ultimate recovery of not only cognitive, but also behavioral, competence. Some cognitive deficits can lead to behavioral problems, particularly when they exist in the context of heightened irritability or loss of capacity for initiation. The effect of any injury on the long postnatal developmental course of the brain is a serious consideration. There are few guidelines, as the severity of injuries that are currently survived is much more serious and our awareness of cognitive functions much greater than in the past. The extant literature should be examined carefully if prognostication is sought in legal cases.

Somatic problems

Autonomic dysfunction. Autonomic hyperreflexia is seen in patients with spinal cord injuries above the level of T6, but may occur with injuries at any level over L1. Although uncommon in prepubertal children, it may develop after puberty. It is characterized by pounding headache and elevated blood pressure and may be accompanied by sweating, flushing of face and neck, blurred vision, nasal congestion, piloerection, and bradycardia. Autonomic hyperreflexia may be caused by any stimulus that creates excessive sympathetic nervous system activity below the level of the lesion. Most commonly, it is caused by a stimulus to the bladder, bowel, or skin, such as urinary retention, bladder calculi, urinary tract infection, fecal impaction, rectal stimulation, pressure sores, sunburn, ingrown toenails, or constricting clothing.

Intervention consists of placing the child in the sitting position and removing the offending stimuli, if possible. The bladder is checked for distention, and the child is catheterized to empty the bladder. The bowel is carefully checked for stool, using a numbing gel, and any impaction removed when symptoms lessen. The child's position is changed to reduce pressure. Tight clothing is loosened. If blood pressure remains elevated, vasodilators may be indicated, as autonomic hyperreflexia is potentially life threatening. Prevention consists of strict adherence to bladder, bowel, and skin regimen.

Neurosweats. It is common to see a type of autonomic dysfunction referred to as "neurosweats" in the severely brain-injured child or adolescent. This is characterized by diaphoresis of the face and upper trunk, elevated blood pressure, tachycardia, and generalized increased tone. These symptoms tend to occur early in the recovery process and are associated with discomfort caused by wet or soiled diapers or undergarments, casts or splints, positioning, or illness. They may last several minutes or hours. Severe neurosweats may result in significant fluid loss, as well as interfere with the therapy regimen.

With the onset of a neurosweat the child's diaper or undergarment is checked and changed if needed, and the child is repositioned. If symptoms are unrelieved, it may be necessary to remove any inhibitive cast. A general examination and workup for infection and neurologic pathology are indicated if symptoms persist. Recurrent neurosweats are treated with beta-blockers, commonly Inderal. The child is given a low dose that is gradually increased as the frequency of neurosweats is monitored. Treatment is continued if there is significant improvement.

Temperature regulation. In the child or adolescent with a spinal cord injury, the ability to regulate body temperature below the level of the lesion may be lost. As a result, the child will be greatly affected by exposure to extreme temperatures. Family and child education is important to prevent the occurrence of hypothermia, hyperthermia, sunburn, and frostbite. Preventive measures include dressing appropriately, limiting time spent outdoors in hot or cold weather, and, with frequent monitoring, gradually increasing time spent in areas of extreme temperature.

Central fever may occur in the severely brain-injured child. This diagnosis is made when there is persistent fever with no identifiable cause. Fever is managed by maintaining a cool environment and avoiding the use of heavy clothing and covers. Acetaminophen may be administered if other measures are unsuccessful.

Sleep cycle and arousal. A disturbance in the level of arousal and the normal sleep-awake cycle is common after a traumatic brain injury. A decreased level of daytime arousal can lead to a decreased responsiveness to the therapeutic interventions of the rehabilitation team. Conversely, in an agitated child, lack of sleep may well produce heightened irritability, similar to that seen in neonates. To achieve an increased level of arousal during the day, several different measures are taken. All members of the team attempt to maintain an appropriate degree of arousal in the child during the therapeutic day, using varied stimulation techniques. Rest periods are provided, with a gradual increase in the duration and intensity of treatment sessions. A short-acting sedative may be used temporarily at night to adjust the child's sleep schedule. Methylphenidate may be used to increase the level of arousal and alertness. In our experience, it is usually given twice a day, 1 hour prior to the start of therapy sessions. Medications having a sedative effect are not used during the day.

Sleep apnea. Central sleep apnea resulting from an insufficient central respiratory drive is occasionally seen in children with severe brain injury. Ventilatory response to hypercapnia and hypoxia is inadequate or absent with periods of apnea occurring during sleep. The problem is identified by the use of end-tidal carbon dioxide and oxygen saturation monitoring. A sleep study is done to monitor the number and duration of apneic episodes.

Apnea monitoring may be sufficient intervention if the apneic episodes do not occur frequently or result in a significant drop in oxygen saturation. In response to the apnea alarm, a caregiver stimulates the child by gentle shaking, which generally results in initiation of spontaneous breathing. With frequent and significant periods of apnea, intervention may involve the use of mechanical ventilation or continuous positive airway pressure during sleep.

Obstructive sleep apnea may result from the collapse of the pharyngeal airway during inspiration in patients who have sustained tracheal insult. Loud snoring and breathing difficulties may be associated with obstructive apnea. In addition to a sleep study, fluoroscopy of the airway is performed to ascertain the presence of obstruction and identify its site. Apnea monitoring and continuous positive airway pressure are provided during sleep.

Bowel and bladder dysfunction

The goal of bowel and bladder management is the development of predictable patterns of elimination. A basic bowel program consists of a high-fiber diet with adequate fluid, a stimulative laxative such as Senokot, and a Biscodyl rectal suppository. The medication schedule is determined by the desired time for defecation and may be given daily or every other day. The suppository is inserted before mealtime, and the child is toileted immediately after the meal is completed in order to utilize the gastrocolic reflex. If stools become hard or impaction occurs, the child (adolescent) is treated with mineral oil, administered either orally or by feeding tube, and daily Fleet or Biscodyl enemas.

Neurogenic bladder dysfunction is treated with an intermittent catheterization program. Indwelling catheters are not used, owing to the risk of infection. Initially, the child is catheterized every 4 hours, and the frequency then decreased to four times a day if residuals remain low for several days. In general, catheterization is done in early morning, at lunch, at dinner, and before the child retires. The frequency of catheterization must be increased if fluid intake is significantly increased. Antibiotics such as Bactrim, Macrodantin, and Mandelamine may be used to prevent urinary tract infections.

The brain-injured child or adolescent with severe memory dysfunction may have a lack of awareness of the need to urinate or make frequent requests to urinate. The child is toileted upon awakening, and then every 2 to 3 hours throughout the day and at bedtime. Fluids are limited after 6:00 to 8:00 PM. If incontinence persists, disposable diapers are used. If memory function is disturbed, notes are kept as a guide for toileting and to increase patient awareness of the frequency of requests. External catheter devices are not used with brain-injured male children because of the risks of skin irritation or breakdown and those associated with forceful removal.

Nutrition

Impairment of oral motor functioning is common after traumatic brain injury and includes disorders such as delayed or absent swallowing, failure of airway protection valves to close, uncoordinated or weak pharyngealperistalsis, and the presence of pathologic reflexes. Nutrition is vital because often significant weight loss has occurred during coma. An evaluation is done by the speech pathologist to determine whether the child is an appropriate candidate for an oral feeding program. When appropriate, the child's feeding begins with pureed substances and progresses to thickened liquids and, finally, to thin liquids if there is no evidence of aspiration. During this process, nutritional needs are met through an enteral or nasogastric feeding tube and the child is closely monitored by the clinical dietician.

Consideration of the child's daily therapeutic regimen determines the feeding schedule. Whenever possible bolus feedings will be used during the day, and continuous feedings at night if needed for additional calories. As oral intake increases, tube feedings are decreased and discontinued when the total caloric and fluid needs of the child are being met through feedings by mouth. Weight is monitored weekly, and nutritional parameters monthly, while the child is receiving enteral feedings.

An evaluation for the placement of a gastrostomy tube is initiated when a lack of progress with oral feeding persists over 2 months. A complete barium swallow is done to identify aspiration, gastroesophageal reflux (GER), and delayed emptying. This is followed by a 24-hour PH probe to identify the presence and frequency of gastroesophageal reflux. In the absence of significant GER, a percutaneous endoscopic gastrostomy is performed. An antireflux procedure is indicated if significant reflux is present despite GER precautions, such as thickening the formula, raising the head of bed during and for 1 hour following tube feeding, and the use of medication such as metoclopramide. A jejunostomy tube is not usually recommended because of the consequent inability to administer bolus feedings.

It is common, once real feeding is accomplished, for some TBI survivors to engage in overeating because of disturbed memory or disruption of the satiation mechanism. This behavior often passes as mental status improves, but occasionally persists so that supervised limitation of intake is required to prevent obesity.

Respiratory problems

Children who have sustained traumatic injuries that affect their respiratory centers will undergo tracheostomy after a reasonable period of time. In our experience,[1] 86% of children with traumatic brain injury required tracheostomy for ventilation during the acute phase of their care. The duration of tracheostomy from time of injury to weaning in our series averaged 49 days. Early complications of pneumonia with subsequent complications include tracheal granulomas, tracheal stenosis, and persistent tracheocutaneous fistula. The decision regarding whether to decannulate is facilitated by lateral films of the neck, CT scans, and bronchoscopy at the beginning of the weaning process and prior to removal. In children or adolescents in whom there is associated or suspected brainstem injury, we recommend 24-hour monitoring respiratory functions for a period of time to determine whether there is evidence of sleep or obstructive apnea. After decannulation children need to be followed for evidence of tracheostenosis.

Posttraumatic seizures

Factors predisposing a child to posttraumatic epilepsy include depressed skull fracture, intracranial hematoma, seizures occurring within 1 week of injury, and prolonged disturbance of consciousness.[8] Children under 2 years of age at the time of injury are more likely to develop posttraumatic seizures than are older children.[10] Posttraumatic epilepsy can evolve months or even years after an injury.

Types of posttraumatic seizure activity include generalized, simple partial, and complex partial seizures. A seizure may be manifested as an altered level of consciousness, change in behavior, or motor activity. The latter, being quite similar to tremors, often makes clinical diagnosis difficult. A routine awake and asleep electroencephalogram or a 24-hour EEG is performed to aid in diagnosis.

The decision to treat a child with anticonvulsants is based on the occurrence of seizure activity more than 1 week after injury, EEG findings, and the type of brain injury. Our experience has indicated that prophylactic anticonvulsants are not indicated unless the child (adolescent) has had seizure activity more than 1 week after injury or the EEG is positive for epileptiform activity. For the child receiving anticonvulsant therapy in the acute-care phase, who does not require continued therapy, a slow weaning process is initiated in our program. For the child who requires continued anticonvulsant prophylaxis, carbamazepine and valproic acid are the medications of choice, owing to the effects on cognitive functioning seen with use of phenytoin and phenobarbital. If the child remains seizure free for 1 year and has a negative EEG, weaning from anticonvulsants is initiated.

Sensory disturbances

Sensation. Trauma to the brain or spinal cord can produce disturbances in the perception of touch, pain, temperature, and position. Depending on the level and extent of a spinal cord injury, there may be a loss of one or more of these senses below the level of the lesion. A child with a loss of sensation will no longer sense discomfort from prolonged pressure to a particular area of the body and is at risk for the development of pressure sores. Early implementation of a timed pressure-release program is essential.

The brain-injured child may experience sensory changes ranging from sensory loss to hypersensitivity of a particular area of the body, as well as impairment of the senses of hearing, vision, taste, and smell.

Hearing. Hearing loss may be conductive or sensorineural and can result from fracture of the petrous portion of the temporal bone or from a basilar skull fracture. Hearing is evaluated by observation of the child's responses to auditory stimulation as evidenced by startle, search, and localization, as well as brainstem auditory-evoked responses and formal audiologic testing. A conductive hearing loss caused by disruption of the ossicular chain may be corrected with surgical intervention. Sensorineural loss caused by transverse fracture of the temporal bone, however, is not amenable to surgery.[3] Hearing loss may improve spontaneously over time. Amplification may be indicated if the loss is below the critical speech range, but in our experience is seldom required.

Vision. Visual disturbances may result from injury to the various structures of the visual system and range from diplopia to complete blindness. Common disturbances seen after a traumatic brain injury include diplopia, visual field deficit, impaired accommodation, and refractive errors. Accommodation may be absent or limited in range, resulting in an inability to focus on near objects and altering focus from near to distant objects or vice versa. A loss or decrease in accommodation will affect visual acuity at different distances.[7] An ophthalmologic consultation is generally arranged to evaluate visual structures and function, in deference to their place as the primary sensory channel in humans and one used in all rehabilitation therapies with mental status improvement. Reexamination is performed to confirm the initial findings.

Diplopia is caused by injury to the extraocular muscles or to the third, fourth, or sixth cranial nerve and is the most common visual sequela in our population. Clinically, the child may exhibit limitations in one or more of the extraocular movements, compensatory head postures, and closure of one eye. Diplopia may increase the brain-injured child's level of confusion and interfere with his or her ability to perform the tasks of rehabilitation therapies. It may also have a further impact on academic functioning and community safety.

Patching is indicated when diplopia is interfering with the child's level of functioning and comfort. For the younger child, the patch is alternated between eyes to prevent amblyopia. This is not necessary for the older child. The sound eye may be patched to encourage movement of the involved eye, or the involved eye may be patched to allow optimal performance. Patching is no longer necessary when the child is able to suppress the second image or when nerve irritation subsides. Spontaneous recovery of ocular muscle function may occur within 1 year of injury. If recovery has not occurred, surgical correction may be indicated after 12 months.

Loss of vision resulting from injury to the optic nerve or its pathway to the occipital lobe is less common. Formal visual acuity and field testing is not possible until the child is able to respond consistently and accurately. Visual function is assessed by observing the child for the presence of visual focus and tracking, convergence, and accommodation and noting whether the child orients more to stimuli approaching from one side or the other. Visually evoked responses may aid in evaluating the integrity of the optic disc and its pathway to the cortex. Cortical blindness results from injury to the occipital lobes and may improve over time as the brain recovers, but is an uncommon occurrence owing to mechanisms of injury and the convexity of the occiput. A referral to the appropriate state agency for the visually impaired is indicated for any child who has a permanent or protracted visual loss. Such referral and involvement should be initiated during the inpatient stay to incorporate this input into the therapeutic approach.

Olfactory system. Damage to the olfactory system occurs with injury to deep structures or to the orbital frontal area. Both anosmia and paranosmia can occur. Odor sensitivity testing can aid in the diagnosis of olfactory impairment, as can family observation of a dramatic change in the child's food preferences. Spontaneous recovery may occur.

Motor impairments

Spasticity. In instances of motor impairments, rehabilitation basically addresses the management of spasticity that develops as a result of injury to motor control mechanisms. The management of spasticity in the traumatically brain-injured child consists of pharmacologic and physical interventions. Therapy is initially aimed at maintaining alignment of the joints while keeping soft tissue and muscles stretched appropriately. Serial casting can be used to facilitate stretching. Orthoplast splints and turnbuckle elbow orthosis may be of help for the upper extremities. Diazepam and Baclofen can be used to decrease spasticity; however, in traumatic brain injury they may contribute to an increase in lethargy. Because the two drugs act pharmacologically at different sites on the anterior horn cell synapses, they can be used together. Sodium dantrolene, which works on the calcium pump at the sarcoplasmic reticulum in the muscles, seems to have a greater effect in weakening the force of contraction of spastic muscles than of nonspastic muscles. A side effect of Dantralene sodium, however, is its association with severe fulminant hepatotoxicity. In our experience, many traumatically brain-injured children arrive at rehabilitation with elevated liver functions and, consequently, cannot receive Dantrolene until liver functions have returned to normal levels.

The injection of peripheral nerves to reduce spasticity in traumatically brain-injured children has great appeal, as such procedures are time limited. A solution of 45% ethanol or 6% phenol can be injected into peripheral nerves to decrease the tone in the groups innervated. There is a significant drawback to this procedure, however, in that it will also create some degree of anesthesia in the extremity. The literature reports production of persistent painful neuromas in adults; however, we do not find that result in the pediatric literature. In our own experience, particularly in traumatically brain-injured children, this is not a significant concern.

Phenol can be injected into the muscle at the area of the motor point innervation, and this will lead to decreased power in that muscle contraction at that particular time. The effect of these injections lasts 2 to 3 months. The injections, when done correctly and the degree of phenol kept at a minimum, can be effective. Use of phenol in deep muscle compartments is theoretically associated with an increased risk of the development of compartment syndrome. For this reason, our use of phenol is reserved for the more superficial muscles. Some children, in spite of aggressive therapy, stretching, casting, and nerve blocks, will rapidly develop contractures of the tendons, particularly of the Achilles tendon and the tibialis posticus. Surgery to lengthen these tendons, placing the feet in proper weight-bearing position, is indicated for severe contractures as early as 3 months posttrauma when other measures have been ineffective.

The disuse syndrome that occurs as a result of severe illness and incapacitation requires that children be placed on a strengthening program. The injury to motor control decreases their ability to voluntarily recruit muscles to a degree that will facilitate progressive resistive exercises. Young children do not ordinarily respond well to resistive exercise programs, and therapists must intersperse diversional and functional activities that enhance the strengthening of muscle groups. A coupling of exercise with games and, at times, biofeedback devices is quite effective in the management of decreased strength in these children.

Children with spinal cord injuries present the same problems of spasticity as do brain-injured children and may have an associated loss of anterior horn cells at the level of the cord injury as well. Young children who sustain muscle imbalance, particularly with a combination of lower motor neuron and upper motor neuron in the same extremity are at high risk of developing deformities. Children who sustain injury to muscle tone of the spine are also at high risk of developing scoliosis and hip dislocation. Young children with cervical or upper thoracic cord injuries will develop scoliosis, which in most cases will ultimately require surgical correction.

Heterotopic ossification. Sudden swelling and pain in an extremity signals heterotopic ossification (HO) in the traumatically injured child or adolescent. Abnormal bone forms in the periarticular soft tissue in both the lower and upper extremities. HO can start at sites distant to trauma and, in our experience, does not require didronol to prevent bone formation. Persistent range-of-motion exercises and nonsteroidals such as Indomethacin usually suffice. In the rare case when persistent bone formation interferes with function, surgery should be delayed until the bone is mature and no longer shows new formation.

SOCIAL CONSEQUENCES

The essence of pediatric rehabilitation mirrors the essence of pediatrics itself, namely the developmental nature of childhood. In classic medical terms, this refers to the progression toward physical maturity. In the social and emotional realms, this development relates to progression toward the psychological product of child development, the concept of self. Self-concept incorporates body image and the individual's perceptions of self-competencies in a vast array of realms: social, intellectual, behavioral, athletic, and so forth. The interposition of trauma, however, presents a dramatic, singular event that demands extraordinary coping efforts of the child and family, as well as an alteration in self-concept. There is little in the standard environment that offers preparation for this eventuality. The coping required relates to an altered physical being, and to the demands of the rehabilitation process itself.

Coping

In an inpatient acute rehabilitation unit, the coping efforts demanded of the child and the family are enormous. First is the issue of survival, which at this point may mean significant temporary or permanent alterations in a child's former competencies. This dramatic change, in addition to any remaining physical discomfort, is a source of fear and anxiety for the entire family. In the initial stages of rehabilitation, we focus on support for the child (adolescent) and the family. An important element is respect for the family, reflected in our policy of encouraging the parent, or parental substitute, to participate in the unit. For the preschool child, the experience of trauma seems to be primarily influenced by the absence of the parent. Separation from a parent can be a primary source of developmentally appropriate anxiety for young children. For the older child, parental support and the intimate knowledge of the child that the parent or family member can provide create the rationale for our policy. Time is spent in interviewing parents or other family members about the nature and coping style of the child. The conversation includes a delineation of likes and dislikes, premorbid sources of fear or anxiety, and unique competencies that can become priorities for the child. For example, when a child is proficient in a certain sport, attempts to make that sport safely accessible can be important in augmenting the child's personal coping. However, weaning from parents of the

school-aged and older child is important, as this mirrors a real-life developmental and functional requirement.

Stress on the child. There are unique demands beyond separation inherent in the inpatient rehabilitation process. Much therapeutic work is done on a one-to-one basis. Although this is important for the quality and intensity of the therapy, it can be intimidating to children. Typically, younger children find this degree of adult attention enjoyable, whereas the older child or adolescent may find it stressful. Consider the normal environment of these older children. When Johnny has an "off day in school," he can hide behind the student in front of him to avoid being called on. In rehabilitation, that sort of hiding is much more difficult in the one-to-one interactions of therapy. It is important to communicate to staff the reality of those "off days" as children face the often time-pressured achievement of certain rehabilitation goals.[6] Inherent in such a process is the team's recognition of the need to build a child's sense of success to form the foundation of the working relationship that will be required for therapy to be maximally successful.

Rehabilitation presents a radical departure from acute care. Essentially, rehabilitation is not recuperation but, rather, remobilization. Further, the demands on the patient escalate during rehabilitation. An integral part of goal achievement is the reality that as soon as one goal has been achieved, another goal is set. For example, a child who is struggling to regain the ability to walk finds that as soon as this is achieved, the ability to run or jump is addressed. These are basic human competencies that evolved in a natural developmental sequence, and so a child has no conscious memory of the previous mastery. Despite the intensive interposition of skilled therapists, the resumption of walking or the use of a prothesis becomes an idiosyncratic challenge to each child or adolescent. Successful completion requires a new level of awareness of one's body that has never been required before.

Stress on the family. For families, the fear and the frustration in their child or adolescent present a situation for which no parenting experience has prepared them. They are unsure about how hard to push, often agonizing over the circumstances that precipitated the trauma. In this state of acute disruption of their own sense of parenting and of the normal family life, and with deep concerns about the future of their child, they feel compelled to be superparents. Often removed geographically from sources of family or community support, parents may feel quite alone. An integral part of our rehabilitation philosophy is support of parents and family members. This is offered not only informally by the individual treatment team members, but quite uniquely by rehabilitation nurses, as well as by parent groups. Parent groups specifically address coping strategies, stress management, and the individual facts about the physiologic and psychological nature of traumatic injuries, within the context of supporting each other as parents in the same situation. The aim is to dissipate some measure of guilt and anxiety and to provide parents with active means of remaining integral to their child's or adolescent's life.

Denial. Only recently has a long-standing "dragon" of rehabilitation been addressed. It has served as perhaps the most enduring barrier between the child and family and the professionals. This dragon is the concept of denial. For several types of trauma (amputation or spinal cord injury, for example), the prognosis for return to prior levels of physical health and competence is known. For traumatic brain injury, prognosis is less certain. Often under pressure from the child and family, the professional staff seek to offer prognostic information. Previously, when the prognosis was not accepted by family members or the child, it was labeled as denial. Through the work of Treischman,[12] we now recognize the vital distinction between hope and denial. What had become apparent in long-term follow-up of such children is that the maintenance of any type of coping strategy is greatly augmented by the prospects offered by hope. This may well be as dramatic a hope as total recovery from a complete spinal cord injury. Unrealistic as it may be, children and their families have now informed professionals that this hope is necessary for their psychological survival.[11]

The passage of time serves to make expectations more realistic. Our interdisciplinary team is aware that it is a matter of profound disrespect to deny the individual survivor and the family the necessary hope. What must be recalled is that many families were told at the time of acute care that their child might die. The welcome survival of the child or adolescent, in the face of this earlier prognosis, engenders a sense of "beating the odds" that is to be nurtured. Ongoing staff education in mental health and the integration of mental health professionals in all aspects of rehabilitation are necessities when the importance of this issue is taken into consideration.

Participation of the child and family. The most essential aspect of coping to be supported in children is mutuality, their sense of ability to offer input, to have their own effect on what is happening to them. As such, in our program it is common for the mental health professional to orchestrate meetings between the child and the treatment team. Mutually agreed-upon goals are negotiated, as are certain therapeutic activities that may cause pain but are essential to the rehabilitation process. The most dramatic example of such an activity is stretching. Although this activity must be performed to maintain muscle integrity, it is often resisted by the child because of the pain or discomfort involved. A variety of techniques are used by our therapists. Sometimes the child is allowed to perform the stretching activities on the therapist first, or allowed to select the time when the activity occurs. Sometimes the child is also permitted to give input about how long the activity must be endured. Mastery of situations, rather than passivity, is nurtured in our model.

The typically passive role of families in the acute-care phase must be significantly altered to an active role during the rehabilitation process. This is fostered through scheduled weekend visits home, where therapeutic goals to assess the child's competence and independence in the home environment are set. Difficulty in handling the physical environment of home and the alterations in expected independence are encountered while the rehabilitation team is readily available for discussion and problem solving. These visits act as a systematic desensitization process in preparation for discharge to home. Difficulties are encountered in carefully mediated "chunks," as opposed to the overwhelming experience that may be encountered upon discharge without such carefully calibrated steps. In addition, these experiences provide the team with a sense of the consistency of competence demonstrated in the real world versus the hospital environment. Motivation is often stronger, or the reality more compelling, when a situation is faced in a child's natural environment as opposed to in the hospital. The interposition of the real world with the hospital environment is vital. On a direct coping basis, it allows the child or adolescent to experience peer and family reaction at a time when it is possible to return to the rehabilitation setting where this experience can be examined.

SELF-CONCEPT

For revision of self-concept, the obvious mandate is to preserve the developmental process. Through this process a child's or adolescent's self-concept is formed and graduated levels of independence are achieved in preparation for adulthood. Preschoolers are approached differently from latency-aged children, who are approached differently from adolescents in this work. It is this constantly changing nature of childhood that differentiates pediatric rehabilitation from its adult counterpart. Consequently, different techniques are needed for the two primary components of our work in this regard: education and direct skills training.

Preschool children

Education of verbal, preschool children is provided through individual contacts. This kind of education is approached in broad terms that concern the nature of the child's injury and how it was acquired. Attention to this latter aspect is important to prevent the development of an egocentric attribution for the cause of the injury. Children of this age tend to view their world primarily as the result of their own direct actions. They can, therefore, easily become convinced that the injury was their fault, often seeing it as a punishment. This promotes an avoidance of grappling with resultant disability. The second portion of education has to do with a simplified but realistic notion of the altered way in which the body may operate. These dual purposes are served primarily in the individual context with the construction of a "lifebook." A lifebook contains drawings by the child and actual photographs that chronicle the details of the injury acquisition and the child's travel through the rehabilitation process. The child's involvement through the drawings becomes important, as they provide the mental health professional and other treatment team members with a first hand view of the child's own construction of the new body image, as well as his or her place in family and comfort in the rehabilitation unit.

Most children of this age are drawn to books, and these become objects and subjects of play. As such, the lifebook functions as a concrete object that the child can review repetitively during the rehabilitation process and upon returning to home. Use of the lifebook also serves to augment the outpatient process, since rehabilitation therapies often continue beyond the inpatient program.

Conceptions found in the popular media about the progression of injuries or about people with disabilities are explicitly covered in the educational process. The most available example for those with traumatic brain injury is the popular conception of coma terminating rapidly, followed by an immediate and complete recovery of all functions. For those who may require mobility devices or who have an apparent physical disability, the common perception of such individuals as always having significant cognitive disabilities is also covered. With such training, the knowledge of the basis on which some misconceptions and consequent prejudices about people with disabilities are formed is provided. A distinction is drawn between understanding the perceptions of some able-bodied people about a person with disability, and the rejection of these perceptions on a personal level.

School-aged children and adolescents

Direct skills training for the pediatric-adolescent population consists of providing role models with disabilities directly and overtly in the educational process. Because of prejudice and lack of access to the environment, children have seldom experienced peers or role models with disabilities. Yet the exposure to realistic role models is broadly acknowledged as an important experience for all children. In our setting, professional staff members with disabilities are discussed with the patient. Age-appropriate storybooks including children with disabilities as a natural part of a story line are read and discussed. Unrealistic or maudlin presentations, including those that characterize children with disabilities as being "brave," are avoided because they deny the natural range of talents and strengths in children with disabilities that are found in the same distribution in their able-bodied peers.

Group education and training

For the adolescent or school-aged child, these two major goals (educational and skills training) are served primarily in a group context. This environment is seen as vital, as it is that in which children and adolescents function and which the developmental mandate presents as an important arena for the formation of self-concept. Groups are used as an initial peer context in which these young people explore their evolving capabilities. It is likely that such a group will be the largest group of children and adolescents with similar disabilities that these young people will ever encounter. Essential to an esprit de corps, which is actively fostered and promoted in the group, is the notion of each child or adolescent as a survivor, not a victim. The pride inherent in the notion of survivor-versus-victim is essential, infusing both the educational and direct-skills training process.

There are a variety of approaches used to foster the dual purpose of these groups. Because of the greater demands of independent functioning for adolescents, as well as increased peer pressure for "sameness," two separate groups are offered, delineated by age.

Educational approaches

An ongoing videotaped recording is made of each older child and adolescent as a vital, concrete record of the rehabilitation course. This is especially important to traumatically brain-injured children and adolescents, since confusional states or memory problems tend to rob them of recall or awareness of the early stages of recovery. Whether these tapes are reviewed in the group, or in an individual session, for all children and adolescents suffering the psychological challenge of rehabilitation, the videotaping is vital. The tapes remove the aspect of interpersonal confrontation relative to altered capacities. For TBI survivors, they provide the insight and awareness that a cognitive function is often lost as a result of global disruption of the brain. When used in the group context, the tapes provide other group members with an opportunity to do the inevitable comparison that is part of self-concept formulation in a more concrete and objective manner.

Within the group context, education takes place in a somewhat structured format, with periodic written and oral "tests" to ensure that acquisition of key concepts is proceeding. Education covers the broad aspects of injury and includes details essential to a child's understanding of the idiosyncratic aspects of his or her own injury. Further, important lifestyle modifications, such as diet alterations for a child or adolescent with spinal cord injury, the use of safety equipment such as helmets in bike riding, or avoidance of alcohol for the brain-injured survivor, are also addressed. These are presented not so much as rigid prohibitions, but as information to enable young persons to make their own informed choices. Obviously, learning is somewhat affected by the age level of the child, but it can include a sense of responsibility for respecting the body's new needs, important because children and adolescents are expected developmentally to function for hours at a time apart from direct parental supervision. In a more overt approach, games are used, carefully engineered and designed according to individual group characteristics. Young survivors are led to appreciate their new "talents" and "untalents" in a setting where they can see that others with similar disabilities also possess individual and unique ranges of ability.

Direct discussions of the wide range of lifestyles that can be enjoyed by people with disabilities are also provided. Guest speakers, either alumni of our rehabilitation program or adults with disabilities, are part of the educational process.

As direct skills are taught in occupational, physical, and communication therapies, so direct social skills are taught in the group context. Despite the professed egalitarian concepts of our culture, it is a reality that people with disabilities require extraordinary social skills to achieve integration. It is with this extraordinary demand in mind that social skills training is offered in a specific context. Extensive role play is done within the group, mirroring situations likely to be encountered in the real-world environment beyond the hospital. This is done to model the essential fact that physical condition, and information about it, is each person's individual property. The matter of decision as to where, when, and how much is shared is expressed as a personal prerogative. These discriminations can be subtle and yet are taught with a reminder that such information is sometimes requested in an intrusive and obnoxious fashion. Particularly for the survivors of traumatic brain injuries, the ability to engage in repartee is often reduced. For those with cognitive deficits, the capacity to respond quickly when nervous, or in an unstructured situation is often particularly impaired. Therefore these survivors are drilled in responses (almost of a "wiseguy" quality) so that they can engage competently within their peer groups and survive with esteem intact.

On a completely different level of social skills training, advocacy skills are offered. The perceptions and misperceptions of able-bodied individuals are specifically discussed. Prejudices are explicitly expressed to the survivors as wrong—sometimes understandable, but always wrong. The young people are taught to view issues of access, both architectural and social, from a civil rights' perspective rather than from that of a victim to whom access is granted out of sympathy. The ability to engage with professionals in the assertion of individual goals and desires is also specifically practiced. The survivors' capacity to call their own "team meetings" within the inpatient setting becomes their initial foray in this endeavor. The group is used both to role-play these encounters and to provide members with peer-generated strategies for approaching the adult professionals who will be part of their lives for a significant period of time to come.

Further practice in direct skills is offered through group-planned outings in the community. Survivor groups are afforded an opportunity to experience, within a supportive peer group, what may be their first attempts in the community. As in any group, some members may be more assertive than others. These persons provide modeling by their responses to such commonly encountered affronts as staring and whispered comments. This vital aspect of our group program is felt to extend beyond the typical professional-laden therapeutic community visits offered in a more traditional plan.

Our approach to the issues of self-concept revision derives primarily from our own experiences in canvassing adults with disabilities in both the available rehabilitation literature and disability rights' movement writings. We feel that this perspective offers children and adolescents the appropriate underpinnings of pride in themselves and an optimistic, but realistic, perception of the possibilities that lie ahead. Without these personal resources, it is our conviction that the rigors of rehabilitation and the energies and heartaches of the families who support them will not have provided these young persons with the engine of the developmental process, that is, hope for a fulfulling and meaningful life.

TECHNOLOGY

Children are amazingly adept at using electronic devices and new computer technologies. Many preschool-age children have mastered the use of the VCR and the computer at home and are often quite skillful at using joysticks for computer games. The provision of a computer to serve as a stimulus and enhancement of cognitive attention while providing opportunity for success, when physical impairment diminishes ability to play and be competitive, is incorporated early and frequently in our rehabilitation program. For a severely motor-injured child, we often endeavor to find an extremity or digit that is capable of turning a switch on and off consistently in order to effect an interaction with the environment. As a child's cognitive function improves, a computer's unflagging ability for repetition and infinite patience provides consistent and intrinsically interesting stimuli. The efficacy of cognitive retraining (as opposed to stimulation or drill), however, has not been substantiated in the literature.

Children who have impairment of communication skills but are cognitively capable of handling symbols and language production may benefit from augmentative communication devices that begin with low-technology items such as two cue cards (one saying "yes" and one saying "no"), progressing to laptop computers that are capable of synthetic speech production.[2]

Power mobility for these children is an option that is often considered. When a high degree of energy is required to propel a manual wheelchair or a one-hand-drive wheelchair, and the length of time it takes to get from one point to another is great, the use of powered mobility as an interim or permanent assist to the child is often quite important. Allowing children to have greater control over their environment and their ability to impact on situations becomes a vital issue. Children as young as 18 months have successfully interacted with power mobility systems.

Children with high cervical cord lesions or with severely impaired motor control can benefit from the ability to control their environment by using environmental control systems. Infrared sensors and transmitters can be built into the same controls that power a wheelchair, allowing a child (adolescent) to enter a room, turn on and off various devices, and use the telephone and other alerting and alarming systems.

Future research will include issues relevant to the application of robotics in the rehabilitation of children. Robot workstations have been developed and used in certain restricted work settings by individuals with severe motor impairments. Obviously, the areas of needed research that will make these resources universally available will be in developing robotic systems that are safe to use around human beings. Inherent sensing abilities, will be required, as well as self-correcting programs, to allow a robot to accomplish many tasks without step-by-step direction from the operator of the system.

Technology, whether used as a stepping stone by children and adolescents with disabilities as they improve their neurofunction or as a lifelong option for enjoying increased control over their environment, provides necessary and important adjuncts to rehabilitation. Regional pediatric rehabilitation centers should have a rehabilitation engineering department that offers expertise in providing children with technologic options.

REFERENCES

1. Alexander MA, Citta-Pietrolungo TJ, Steg NL et al: Complications of tracheostomy and decannulation in pediatric patients with traumatic brain injury, *Arch Phys Med Rehab* 70:21, 1989.
2. Alexander MA, Demasco PW, Gilbert M, et al: Rehabilitation technology for disabled children, *Arch Phys Med Rehab: State of the Art Reviews* 15(2), 1991.
3. Berrol S, Horn LJ, Cope DN: *Cranial nerve dysfunction in traumatic brain injury,* Philadelphia, 1989, Hanley & Belfus.
4. Commission on Accreditation of Rehabilitation Facilities: *Standards manual for organizations serving people with disabilities,* Tucson, 1991, The Commission.
5. Davidoff G, Thomas P, Johnson M, et al: Head injury in acute traumatic spinal cord injury: incidence and risk factors, *Arch Phys Med Rehab* 69:869-872, 1988.
6. Gans JS: Hate in the rehabilitation setting, *Arch Phys Med Rehab* 64:176-179, 1983.
7. Gianutsos R, Perlin R, Mazerolle K, et al: Rehabilitation optometric services for persons emerging from a coma, *J Head Trauma Rehab* 4(2):17-25, 1989.
8. Jennett B, Teasdale G: *Management of head injuries,* Philadelphia, 1981, FA Davis.
9. Kifoyle RM, Foley JJ, Norton PL: Spine and pelvic deformity in childhood adolescent paraplegia: a study of 104 cases, *J Bone Joint Surg* 47A:659-682, 1965.
10. Levin H, Benton A, Grosman R: *Neurobehavioral consequences of closed head injury,* New York, 1982, Oxford University Press.
11. Novack T, Richards J Scott: Coping with denial among family members, *Arch Phys Med Rehab* 72:521, 1991.
12. Treischmann RB: *Spinal cord injury: psychological, social and vocational adjustment,* New York, 1980, Pergamon.
13. World Health Organization (Geneva, Switzerland 1980), Chang R: *International classification of impairments, disabilities, and handicaps: report of the panel on physical, medical, and rehabilitation research,* Washington DC, 1989, The Organization.

14 Education of the Trauma Team

Jane W. Ball and Geraldine S. Pratsch

A major component of a successful pediatric trauma system is the education of the trauma team. In addition to the coordination of available state, local, and hospital resources and the delivery of comprehensive health care and community services, the pediatric trauma system should provide education and training to health professionals and the general public in order to provide optimal pediatric trauma care. The trauma team must be highly skilled to provide rapid, efficient, and effective care to the seriously injured child and family.

EDUCATION FOR AN EMERGENCY MEDICAL SERVICES SYSTEM

Historically, the military services of the United States made a significant number of advances in the care of seriously injured persons before the 1960s. The pressing demands of field surgery, advances in medical care, and education of health professionals to treat war injuries aggressively contributed, in part, to the high level of performance realized during the Vietnam War. Improvements in field resuscitation and transportation efficiency were other major factors contributing to life-saving endeavors.[16] This success was demonstrated by the reduction of deaths among injured soldiers reaching designated facilities from 8% in World War I to less than 2% in the Vietnam War.[7]

The initiation of modern civilian emergency medical services (EMS) systems began in 1966 with the publication of *Accidental Death and Disability: The Neglected Disease of Modern Society* by the National Academy of Sciences, National Research Council.[1] This landmark document reflected a farsighted approach to the need for development of an effective national EMS system to reduce deaths and disabilities from injury among the civilian population. In addition, it reported that *unskilled health care personnel*, working with inadequate transportation and communication system policies and guidelines, were taking the injured to facilities that were not sufficiently prepared to treat them.[16] The federal government passed the Emergency Medical Services Systems Act (EMSS) in 1973, which supported a nationally coordinated and comprehensive system of emergency health care accessible to all citizens.[15] The education of prehospital care providers was addressed in this legislation.

Education of health professionals has always been the responsibility of colleges and universities, both for initial professional training and for continuing medical education. Professional organizations additionally play a significant role in defining the educational criteria for specialty practice, as well as specifying continuing medical education requirements to maintain specialty certification.

In 1976 the Committee on Trauma of the American College of Surgeons (ACS) called for hospitals to commit personnel and facility resources for the care of seriously injured patients in its report "Optimal Resources for the Care of the Seriously Injured."[9] The ACS Committee on Trauma also recognized the extremely delicate relationship between surgical education and provision of optimal care to the trauma patient.

A formal educational program for physicians in the management of critically injured patients was developed and sponsored by the ACS. The Advanced Trauma Life Support (ATLS) Program is an intense, comprehensive program for physicians who do *not* manage major trauma daily, but who must often evaluate and resuscitate seriously injured patients. The ATLS program uses the ABC (*A*irway, *B*reathing, and *C*irculation) approach to set management priorities for the most life-threatening injuries. The course emphasizes that care during the first hour after injury must include the following components: initial assessment and treatment of the trauma patient, life-saving interventions, reevaluation, stabilization, and guidelines for transfer to another health care facility when appropriate.[2] The ATLS program has become a nationally recognized education standard.

The ACS also developed the currently recognized guidelines for the organization and categorization of hospitals providing trauma services by level of service. Hospital facilities can be designated as a Level I, II, or III trauma center by criteria based on resources, personnel, and commitment. The ACS guidelines expect Level I and Level II trauma centers to provide *formal training programs in continuing education for staff physicians, nurses, allied health personnel, and community physicians.*[10]

Trauma service directors (surgeons) are required to participate as instructors in an ATLS program. They are additionally expected to actively participate in other continuing medical education courses and to teach other health care personnel at Level I and Level II centers. Surgeons and emergency physicians practicing in trauma centers are often required by their hospitals to complete successfully the ATLS program. In many cases, specially modified ATLS programs for nurses and paramedics have been developed so that appropriate content is also integrated into their clinical practice.

Trauma centers are required to provide continuing medical education and academic training for health professionals because well trained and educated health professionals are best prepared to provide optimal care to the patients transported to them. These trauma centers generally provide education in three ways: (1) Education is often provided as a community service of the trauma center, targeted to hospital-based professionals and prehospital care providers in the region served. Seriously injured patients transported to local hospitals and subsequently transferred to the trauma center are thus cared for by professionals who understand priorities of injury care. (2) Inservice education is provided to assure that trauma center professionals (for example, emergency physicians, surgeons, nurses) are optimally prepared to diagnose and treat acute injuries. This education is especially important for quality improvement. (3) Most major trauma centers are affiliated with a university medical school, and faculty have an academic obligation to fulfill their roles as educators, preparing future leaders and health professionals in trauma care. Special residency and fellowship programs are often sponsored by the centers.

As a result of these educational programs and improvements in trauma system development, research has documented improved outcomes for injured adults over the past 15 years. Adults sustaining major trauma have a greater chance for survival if they receive optimal care—including immediate field resuscitation and transport to a definitive care facility—during the "golden hour," the first hour after injury.[14] Unfortunately, children were not separately acknowledged in the early EMS system development as having their own unique physiologic and psychological differences. As a result, they were treated as "small adults" and comparable improved outcomes cannot be documented for injured children.

In 1982 a study by Seidel and colleagues demonstrated that approximately 10% of paramedic calls were on behalf of children.[12] Trauma death rates were significantly higher for children than for adults, the highest rates being found among infants and young children. Head trauma was more frequently seen in children than in adults. Study findings suggested that *education of paramedics and emergency department personnel may not have been adequate to provide proper management of the special emergency needs of children.* Lack of timely transport to pediatric centers where definitive care was available also played a role in prehospital and emergency department mortality of the seriously ill or injured child.

Pediatric emergency care and pediatric trauma care are new specialty fields, developing over the past decade. Knowledgeable leaders and scholars in pediatric trauma have organized specialized trauma systems for children that are responsive to their special care needs. Part of their mission includes advocacy for more specialized education of health professionals in pediatric trauma and emergency care. Traditional education for prehospital providers, nurses, and physicians has not yet incorporated the newly evolving knowledge from these specialty fields. For this integration to occur, a *defined body* of essential knowledge, well-prepared instructors, educational resources, and models of programs or methods for teaching the essential content must be widely available. There must also be a strong advocacy for inclusion of pediatric emergency topics as part of established curricula.

In 1985, under the Public Health Service Act, Section 1910, the Emergency Medical Services for Children (EMSC) Demonstration Program was authorized by Congress. This program, administered by the Maternal and Child Health Bureau of the Department of Health and Human Services (MCHB/DHHS), was created to reduce childhood mortality and morbidity in emergency, out-of-hospital, critical illness, and injury. This legislation was an effort to ensure that the successes and benefits of the EMS system for adults were provided for infants and children.[8]

OVERVIEW OF PROFESSIONAL TRAINING IN PEDIATRIC TRAUMA

Virtually no educational program for health professionals provides adequate preparation for practice in pediatric trauma management at a basic or entry level. The defined body of knowledge, skills, and technology is still evolving, as the practice of pediatric emergency and trauma specialties is new. Students may have exposure to injured children during their professional education, but this experience usually occurs after the emergent phase of care. For this reason, the current methods of education of health professionals in the care of injured children are continuing education programs, fellowship programs, graduate education, and on-the-job training.

Physicians

Physicians receive little pediatric trauma education during medical school and residency programs. Pediatric emergency medicine and pediatric trauma surgery are very new disciplines, and there are still limited numbers of medical centers having the resources to train professionals. Only those physicians who chose a pediatric emergency medicine fellowship program or surgeons obtaining a pediatric surgery/trauma fellowship obtain extensive education in pediatric emergency and trauma management. Other physicians receive on-the-job training and participate in continuing education programs to supplement their professional education.

Of the total number of patients seen in the 5000 emergency departments in this country, only 25% to 35% are children, of whom only 3% are critically ill or injured. The relatively small number of these children makes it difficult for emergency medicine physicians to maintain the skills needed to resuscitate the very ill or injured child.[13] Two pediatric emergency continuing education programs have been developed by professional organizations to address this problem.

The Pediatric Advanced Life Support Program (PALS), a program jointly developed and sponsored by the American Heart Association and the American Academy of Pediatrics, was initiated in 1988. The purposes of this advanced life support continuing education program are the following:

1. To review the fundamentals of pediatric cardiopulmonary resuscitation
2. To provide health professionals already familiar with pediatric resuscitation a conceptual framework for application of their knowledge and skills
3. To teach a uniform approach to the resuscitation of the critically ill child with respiratory distress, or respiratory or cardiopulmonary failure.

An optional trauma resuscitation scenario has recently been added to the program.

This program has become a national standard for the education of advanced life support personnel, including physicians, nurses, and paramedics in pediatric emergency care.[11]

Initiated in 1989, the Advanced Pediatric Life Support (APLS) course is a program developed and supported by the American College of Emergency Physicians and the American Academy of Pediatrics. It is aimed at physicians who care for children in emergency settings. It specifically addresses pediatric conditions not covered in the PALS program, such as trauma, poisonings, and child abuse. APLS also reviews the management of pediatric cardiorespiratory failure and provides physicians with the information needed to assess and manage critically ill or injured children during the first hour of emergency department care.

Nurses

Trauma nursing is a specialty area of nursing practice that encompasses all aspects of nursing care for injured persons or those at risk for injury. The practice of trauma nursing is holistic, encompassing the continuum of care for patients, beginning with prevention and including prehospital care, resuscitation, stabilization, supportive care, rehabilitation, and reintegration into society.[15] Virtually no undergraduate nursing programs provide emergency nursing experience or education. Of 13 graduate nursing programs with emergency nursing or trauma-related tracks, only six programs indicate a focus on pediatric trauma care.[3]

To meet the need for continuing education in pediatric emergency nursing, the Emergency Medical Services for Children (EMSC) Demonstration Projects and the Emergency Nurses Association developed a self-guided curriculum that uses case studies to teach practical application of pediatric emergency concepts to nursing practice. Several modules have a pediatric trauma management focus.[11]

The Children's National Medical Center, Washington, D.C., was awarded funding in 1990 for development and implementation of a pediatric emergency nursing program by the Division of Nursing, Bureau of Health Professions, DHHS. The 3-day continuing education program is geared to nurses working in community hospital emergency departments. Nursing management of the acutely injured child and family is heavily emphasized. The program provides lectures, skill practice, and case study scenarios for integration and application of content to practice.

Prehospital providers

Emergency Medical Technicians (EMTs) receive minimal training in the management of adult trauma during their 110-hour basic training according to the Department of Transportation Curriculum for EMT-Ambulance (EMT-A) personnel. Only noninvasive basic life support skills are taught, such as bleeding control, use of pneumatic antishock garments, and spinal immobilization. Only 3 hours of the entire curriculum are devoted to pediatrics with emphasis on neonatal and pediatric assessment, cardiopulmonary resuscitation, and management of respiratory and medical emergencies.[11] Curriculum guidelines are being revised, and the new guidelines may focus more extensively on pediatric emergencies.

Paramedics (EMT-Ps) are taught more extensive adult trauma management in their entry-level training. Guidelines in the Department of Transportation Curriculum for EMT-P require 400 hours of training, but many programs have expanded the training time. Paramedics learn such invasive skills as intravenous access and intubation. However, course content regarding the assessment and management of ill and injured children is limited, offering an average of 12 program hours in pediatrics.[11]

Two continuing education programs in trauma management for prehospital providers have been developed to address weaknesses in their basic training. Basic Trauma Life Support (BTLS) is a program sponsored by the American College of Emergency Physicians (ACEP). Prehospital Trauma Life Support (PHTLS) is a program developed and sponsored by the National Association of Emergency Medical Technicians (NAEMT). Neither of these programs has an extensive focus on pediatric trauma management.

In 1982 the Children's National Medical Center, Washington, D.C., recognized the weaknesses in the training of prehospital personnel for treatment of pediatric emergencies. With private funding from the Devore Trust Foundation, a basic life support training program for EMTs in the Washington metropolitan area was developed. An increase in knowledge and skills for managing pediatric emergencies was demonstrated by the 200 prehospital care providers attending the program.[4] The success of this training effort led to the development of a "train the trainer" model program targeting instructors of prehospital care providers, the Pediatric Emergency Medical Services Training Program (PEMSTP). The National Highway Traffic Safety Administration of the Department of Transportation (NHTSA/DOT) and the MCHB/DHHS provided funding to design, develop, and implement this pediatric emergency training program for national dissemination. More than 250 instructors of prehospital care providers, representing all 50 states, have attended the program.

The PEMSTP curriculum used the ATLS model of the ABC approach to set management priorities in life-threatening events. It further included D and E, *Disability* and *Exposure*, in the model which, in care of the injured child, are of equal concern. This comprehensive program covers both trauma and medical emergencies, and it also emphasizes the emotional response of the child and the family's reaction to the emergency, the unique physiologic responses of the child to the illness or injury, and the prehospital care provider's psychological response when caring for a seriously ill or injured child. Advanced life support was added to the program's content in 1988. This program was the foundation for many of the pediatric prehospital continuing education programs now taught in the United States. *Pediatric Emergencies: A Manual for the Prehospital Care Providers* and *Pediatric Emergencies: Instructor Manual* are products of this program.[5,6]

DEVELOPMENT OF EDUCATIONAL PROGRAMS

The goal of professionals who develop educational programs is to provide adequate information and opportunities for practical application to improve patient care. When programs are developed for employees of an EMS system, the goal includes a risk management focus to ensure that all team members, both prehospital and hospital-based, provide appropriate care to the injured child. The goal of health professionals seeking educational programs is usually to correct a perceived deficiency in knowledge or skills, or a desire to provide high quality care to the injured child in an effective and harmonious manner with other team members.

There is currently no general agreement about the extent and range of education needed (the defined body of essential knowledge) by health professionals of various levels to provide high quality pediatric trauma care. Therefore, educational offerings are used to upgrade the education of health professionals, particularly as new technology is developed for assessment and management of injured children.

Educational methodology

To manage injured children effectively, professionals need high-level skills in rapid assessment and intervention. Education must be directed toward assisting professionals and other students to attain such skills and to work as a team member when providing care. Educational methods must incorporate strategies to promote learning of essential content, skill practice, and competence in performance of patient management. Various considerations, such as time, cost, and instructors available, are also important factors in determining the design of the educational offering.

The designers of continuing education programs must select those methods proven effective in educating the adult learner and practicing professional. Adults have individual learning and teaching style preferences. Because these programs are generally offered to groups of professionals, many learning and teaching style preferences will be represented; it is important to employ as many learning styles as possible within each program. The styles used, however, must be appropriate to the setting (classroom, laboratory, or clinical) in which the program is offered. In addition, learning can be enhanced and retention increased if content is reinforced through a combination of teaching methods.

When education is geared toward health professionals, rather than toward entry-level staff, it should build on their past education and experience. This provides an opportunity for learners to apply new concepts to previously learned information. For example, when teaching pediatric trauma care to professionals who are experienced in adult trauma management, the details of basic trauma management do not have to be addressed. Instead, similarities between child and adult trauma management principles should be illustrated while important differences in management of the two populations are being emphasized. Not only does the instructor demonstrate respect for the professional's current knowledge and learning time, but through this approach focuses the professional on important new concepts for application to practice. Some content repetition is necessary, but it should be planned to enhance application of pediatric trauma management principles.

Designing educational programs

There are several important steps in designing education programs:

1. Establish the need or purpose of the program.
2. Identify the audience (professional level, skill level, for example).
3. Define the standard of care expected at the conclusion of the program.
4. Identify available teaching resources.
5. Determine the program design (formal or informal, instruction methodology).
6. Determine the budget available.

Need or purpose of program. In planning the educational offering, determine the need for it or its purpose. A needs assessment survey is often conducted by professional organizations to determine what new topics should be covered in future conferences or programs. Trauma centers and EMS agencies often have a clear idea of the purpose of educational activities. Examples of reasons for educational programs include the following: new employees need orientation and training to perform their jobs skillfully, quality assurance criteria screens indicate a problem in patient management that can be addressed by educational sessions, and implementation of a new management guideline or protocol requires all staff to be informed about their adjusted responsibilities.

Knowledge of audience. When designing educational offerings, it is important to know the au-

dience and its expectations so that efforts can be made to tailor the program level and content to them. Answering the following questions can help in describing the audience targeted for an educational program.

1. Why are participants attending the program? Is it required or do they have a choice in selecting the program?
2. What is the participants' professional level of practice? Public, prehospital provider (BLS or ALS), nurse (practice specialty), physician (practice specialty)?
3. What is their skill level or practical experience with the program content?
4. What is known about preferred learning experiences?
5. Are there any barriers to the learning process? Do students work the night before a program? Are they on call? Will they have adequate time for class preparation?

One of the more complex issues to address when learning about the audience is their motivation for seeking or attending an educational program. Individuals who voluntarily elect to attend an educational program are more highly motivated to learn. They have self-selected themselves for this program because they perceive that the content is meaningful to their practice or that it meets their individual goals. These participants will generally be more receptive to the material taught. Individuals who attend because of extrinsic motivators, such as threats, salary or award incentives, or recertification or relicensing requirements, are often less motivated to learn and apply the information. In this case, the program design must incorporate some creative teaching strategies to stimulate and motivate students to learn.

Programs should also be geared to the professional level of experience and responsibility of students. To have the most effective program, present specific knowledge and skills to a particular professional group so that the information is most applicable to their practice. This decreases the potential for dilution of content to meet the capabilities of the lowest-level professional. For example, even though all ALS providers (paramedics, nurses, and physicians) need similar content addressing stabilization of an injured child, application of the content to field practice may not occur as readily if management guidelines primarily cover hospital care, or vice versa. In this case, the individuals must take the initiative to apply the content learned to their particular practices, unless opportunities for small group discussions of professional responsibility are provided. Some programs do benefit from a mixed audience, however, particularly when professionals need to learn and understand their patient management responsibilities as members of a trauma team.

Standard of care. Before planning any educational program, review the accepted practice standards, such as an institutional protocol or a professional organization's statement on standard of care. Because continuing education programs should promote this standard of care, make sure that faculty understand the practice standard, even if they are not speaking about its content in detail. If a faculty member does not reflect an understanding of this practice standard, credibility with students is decreased and content taught by this professional may be devalued. Paramedics and other field providers may become confused or frustrated if presented content reflects management strategies not authorized by their protocols.

Teaching resources. Review of available teaching resources for the program is essential during early planning of the educational design. Teaching resources include the program coordinator, faculty, audiovisual resources, textbooks, clinical sites and preceptors, classroom space, training equipment, and funding. A dedicated program coordinator is the most important resource for effective and successful educational offerings. This person should have experience in planning the preferred type of educational offering, including faculty liaison, preparation of the program brochure and materials, scheduling, and so forth.

Other educational resources, such as standardized programs (Advanced Trauma Life Support, for example) or program models (pediatric prehospital programs), lecture outlines, textbooks, videotapes, and slides, may be available free or for a nominal fee from other programs or agencies. Purchase of previously prepared materials may be most cost-effective because development of new teaching resources is expensive and very labor intensive.

Faculty should be selected who can effectively communicate the course concepts to the target audience. Each faculty member should be willing to teach the requested content at the level of this audience. The program coordinator should discuss the knowledge base and skill level of the participants with each faculty member. Try to recruit approved faculty of standardized programs who will need minimal preparation time to teach in the program. If such faculty are not available, provide adequate time for new faculty to research and prepare their presentations.

Program design. When planning an educational program, integrate various methods and teaching resources to present the content, keeping in mind the methods that will enhance retention of content.

In addition, choose methods that fit the size of the group being taught. For example, large groups reduce the amount of interaction possible between faculty and students. Combine lectures with slides or videos to provide stimulation. When possible, break the larger group into small work groups for demonstrations, skill practice, discussions, or case simulations. For small groups, it is possible to be more creative and to blend a variety of teaching methods. Keep in mind that clinical experience is one of the best methods for teaching, so whenever possible provide opportunities for supervised clinical experiences in appropriate settings.

Often it is important to consider methods for evaluation of the participants of the program. Although written tests are frequently used, they generally test recall of content taught. Skill stations can be used to test competence in performance of specific skills. Case scenarios can be used to test the integration of information taught and its application to the practice of the participants.

In many cases, programs designed for health professionals should provide continuing education credit. Criteria for review of continuing education offerings are available from credentialing agencies for specific health professionals:

1. For physicians, seek AMA Category I or II credits through a university medical school or the American Medical Association.
2. For nurses, seek continuing education contact hours from a state nurses' association or specialty nursing organization.
3. For prehospital providers, seek continuing medical education credits from a state EMS agency or the National Registry of EMTs.

It is especially important to obtain approval by the appropriate credentialing agency for a continuing education program when relicensing or recertification of health professionals is dependent upon continuing education attendance. Students will preferentially attend programs that demonstrate approval by a credentialing agency, recognizing that efforts have been made to meet established standards for continuing education credits.

Financing educational offerings. Many educational offerings can be provided without substantial funding if faculty donate their time and no fee is charged for classroom space. Some funding commitment is necessary, however, if refreshments are served and educational materials are provided. There are various options for educational program funding. These include program sponsorship by institutions or vendors, tuition fees or contracts, and private donations or foundation grants. The education coordinator must often be resourceful in finding means to assure adequate funding for programs.

Pediatric trauma educational programs. When planning a pediatric trauma program for health professionals, several elements of content are currently considered essential. The depth and range of content must be tailored to the professional audience targeted by the program. The major content and emphasis of programs should minimally include:

1. An overview of the unique anatomic and physiologic differences between children and adults.
2. The primary trauma survey, with a focus on anticipating specific physiologic deterioration, ABCDEs, and management of life-threatening injuries.
3. The child's and family's response to injury.
4. The management of specific injuries, especially life-threatening injuries (with guidelines specific to providers, that is, nurses, prehospital providers, physicians).
5. Special skills or management techniques and procedures for treating children (for example, intraosseous infusion, fluid boluses, immobilization principles, pneumatic antishock garment, airway management and ventilation, use of oxygen, temperature control).

To provide optimal care for injured children, health professionals involved at each step along the continuum of care should have appropriate educational opportunities, including those professionals who provide care following resuscitation and stabilization. Care must be coordinated to reduce the occurrence of secondary injury and to assure the child's return to the family and community with minimal disability.

Injury prevention has a profound effect on the reduction of trauma death and disability in the pediatric age group. For this reason, it is recommended that injury prevention be a component of all standardized national curricula for health professionals within EMSC systems.[13] A special effort should be made to inform all health professionals about current efforts in pediatric injury prevention, so that they become effective advocates for the ultimate reduction of mortality and morbidity resulting from injury.

REFERENCES

1. National Academy of Sciences–National Research Council: *Accidental death and disability: the neglected disease of modern society,* PHS pub no. 1071-A-13, Washington, DC, 1952, US Government Printing Office.
2. American College of Surgeons, Committee on Trauma: Advanced Trauma Life Support Program, Chicago, Ill, 1990.
3. Annual listing of graduate programs offering emergency nursing or trauma-related nursing tracks, *J Emerg Nurs* 17(4):38A-43A, 1991.
4. Eichelberger MR, Stossel-Pratsch G, Mangubat EA: A pediatric emergencies program for emergency medical services, *Ped Emerg Care* 1:177-179, 1985.
5. Eichelberger MR, Ball JW, Pratsch GS et al: *Pediatric emergencies: a manual for prehospital care providers,* Englewood Cliffs, NJ, 1992, Brady Publishing.
6. Eichelberger MR, Ball JW, Pratsch GS et al: *Pediatric emergencies: instructor manual,* Englewood Cliffs, NJ, 1992, Brady Publishing.
7. Heaton, LD: Army medical service activities in Vietnam, *Milit Med* 131:646, 1966.
8. Law of the 99th Congress, Public Health Services Act, Section 1910, Washington, DC, Sept 30, 1985.
9. American College of Surgeons, Committee on Trauma: Optimal hospital resources for care of the severely injured, *Bull Am Coll Surg* 61:15-22, 1976.
10. American College of Surgeons, Committee on Trauma: Resources for optimal care of the injured patient, *Bull Am Coll Surg* 68:11-21, 1983.
11. Seidel JS, Hendersen DP, editors: *Emergency medical services for children: a report to the nation,* Washington, DC, 1991, National Center for Education in Maternal and Child Health.
12. Seidel JS, Hoenbein M, Yoshiyma K et al: Emergency medical services and the pediatric patient: are the needs being met? *Pediatrics* 73:769-772, 1984.
13. Silverman BJ, editor: *Advanced pediatric life support manual,* Dallas, 1989, American College of Emergency Physicians.
14. Trunkey DD: Trauma, *Scientific American* 249:29-36, 1983.
15. US Congress: *Emergency Medical Services Systems Act* (Public Law 93-154). Ninety-third Congress, SB2 410, Washington, DC, 1973, US Government Printing Office.
16. Veise-Berry SW: Evolution of the trauma cycle. In Cordoba VD, editor: *Trauma nursing,* Philadelphia, 1988, WB Saunders, pp 4-5.

PART FOUR

Initial Evaluation, Resuscitation, and Critical Care

15 Algorithm for Pediatric Trauma

James M. Chamberlain

The pediatric victim of multiple trauma presents a unique opportunity for the emergency physician. Children rarely sustain lethal injury. However, failure to recognize subtle signs of physiologic derangement may result in significant morbidity or preventable mortality. The injured child may appear deceptively well, yet subsequently decompensate. Therefore, an organized and thorough approach by the emergency team is necessary for each child.

Two points bear emphasis. First, frequent reassessment is essential. The stable child may worsen because of progression of the injury, because of initial failure to recognize a problem, or because of difficulties related to transport or to the administration of medications. Transport to the radiology suite or to another hospital may result in loss of an airway or displacement of an intravenous line. Even modest doses of sedative medication can cause hypotension or loss of airway reflexes. Therefore, any deterioration should prompt an immediate step back to the "ABCs" (airway, breathing, circulation) to reassess the child. The astute physician repeatedly examines the child throughout the stay in the emergency department, reaffirming the patency of the airway, effectiveness of breathing, and the adequacy of circulation. Reassessment is also the best means to evaluate the effects of therapy. If a particular intervention does not achieve the desired effect, a more direct, aggressive approach is necessary.

The second point of emphasis is the need for an organized team of physicians, nurses, and ancillary personnel to treat the patient with multiple trauma rapidly and effectively (see Appendix 15-1). Optimal medical care is ensured when each member of the team assumes his or her role without redundancy and without confusion. Regionalization of trauma care is desirable for economic reasons, but every hospital that cares for children should prepare a team to stabilize and treat the injured child. Although the algorithm for pediatric trauma care (Fig. 15-1) is presented sequentially in order of urgency, the trauma team performs several steps simultaneously, thus improving the efficiency of care.

ABCs: LIFE SUPPORT PHASE OF RESUSCITATION

The ultimate common pathway to death in the injured child is inadequate delivery of oxygen to the tissues. Therefore, the purpose of the initial phase of resuscitation is the rapid evaluation and treatment of immediately life-threatening injuries that compromise oxygenation or circulation.

Airway with cervical spine immobilization

The child with multiple trauma or a serious mechanism of injury is presumed to have a cervical spine injury until it is proven otherwise. Movement of the neck can convert a bony or ligamentous injury into a permanent neurologic deficit. The following guidelines are vital: At the scene of the injury, immobilize the cervical spine with the head in a neutral position, using a stiff cervical collar or sandbags and tape (Fig. 15-2). After the child arrives at the hospital, provide gentle manual in-line immobilization to further stabilize the neck. Children or infants involved in motor vehicle accidents in their car seats are best immobilized and transported without removing them from the car seat until arrival in the trauma unit (Fig. 15-3).

There are several anatomic features that predispose the child to airway obstruction. A child's relatively large head causes flexion of the neck in the supine position. The large tongue occludes the airway proximally, and the narrow trachea is more susceptible to occlusion with vomitus or blood. Loose teeth in the preschool child are easily dislodged and may obstruct the airway. These anatomic problems are compounded by loss of pharyngeal tone and the gag reflex in the obtunded or comatose child.

The child with airway obstruction appears agitated or, more commonly, obtunded. Breath sounds are diminished and there is often stridor, which suggests upper airway obstruction. Retractions and nasal flaring indicate resistance to air movement. Cyanosis is a late sign; pulse oximetry is useful for the early detection of hypoxia (<95% saturation).

If the child has any sign of airway obstruction, perform the jaw thrust maneuver and administer

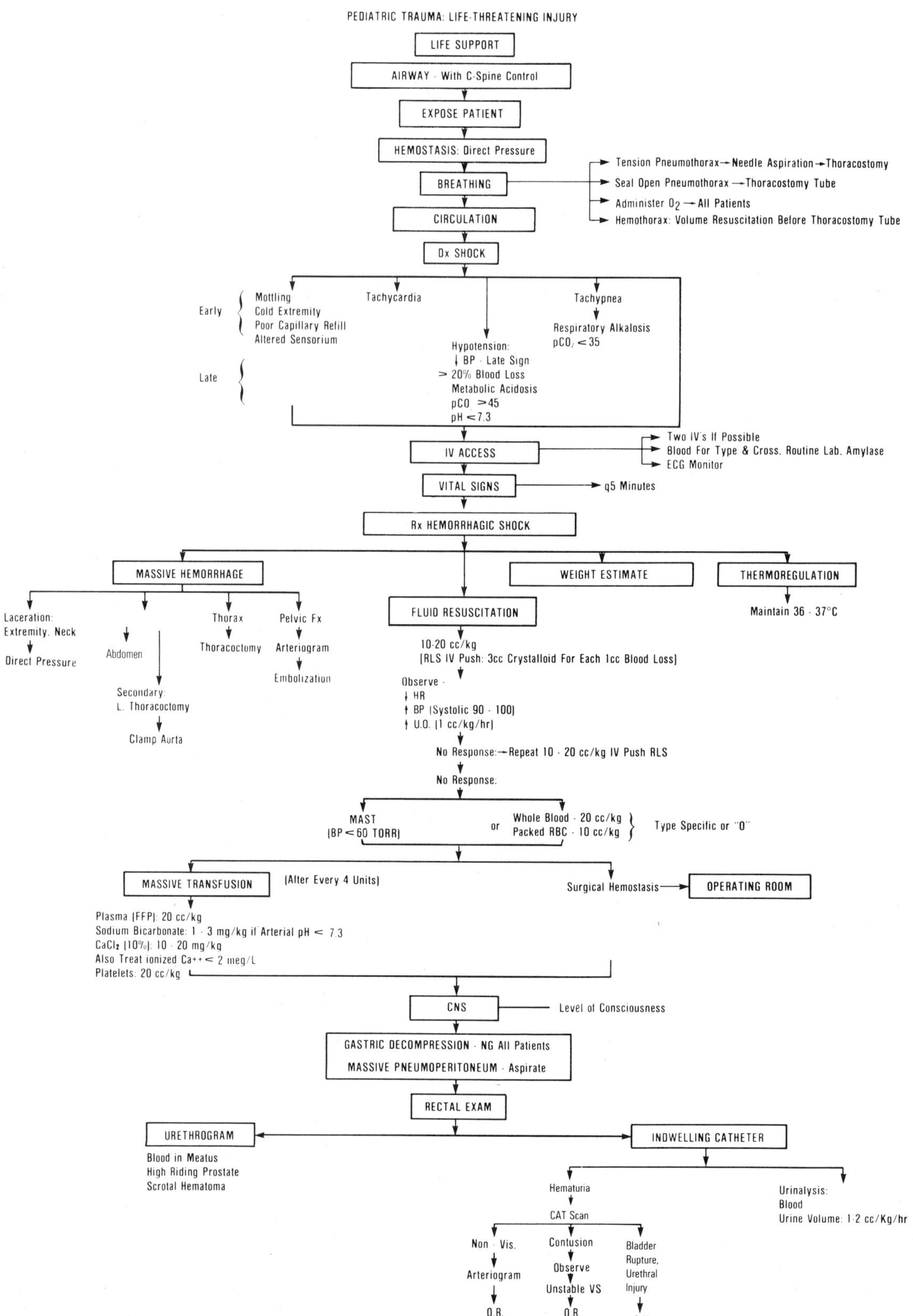

Figure 15–1 An algorithm for treatment of the pediatric trauma victim.

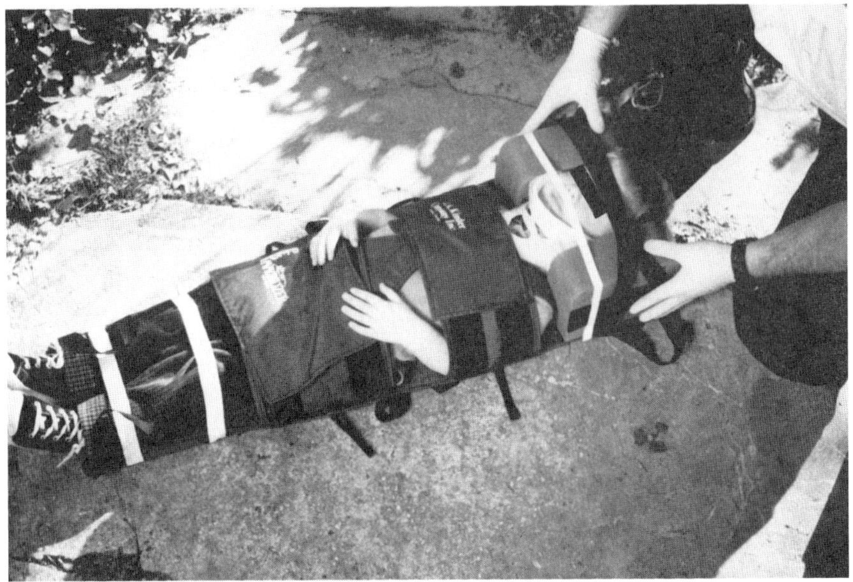

Figure 15–2 Cervical spine immobilization in the young child.

100% oxygen. This simple approach results in marked improvement in most children. If the child does not improve with the jaw thrust, proceed in the following order of increasingly aggressive airway management:

1. Suction the oropharynx.
2. Assist ventilation with bag and mask.
3. Intubate the trachea and assist ventilation.

Intubation of a child is difficult because of an anterior and cephalad glottis, but is indicated for any child requiring prolonged assisted ventilation. Use of the bag and mask without intubation results in gastric distention and emesis, which further compromises the airway and ventilation. Do not use an oral airway, because the device causes emesis in the semicomatose child and is not necessary in the comatose child. A child in coma requires an airway secured by endotracheal intubation, which facilitates hyperventilation for treatment of increased intracranial pressure.

Occasionally, a child sustains severe maxillofacial or laryngeal trauma that impedes intubation. In this case, surgical cricothyroidotomy is necessary. Needle cricothyroidotomy can provide the child with a route for oxygenation, but adequate ventilation is not possible with this technique without jet ventilation. Optimal management involves conversion to a surgical airway as soon as possible.

Breathing

Once the airway is secured, attention should be focused on the chest and abdomen for mechanical

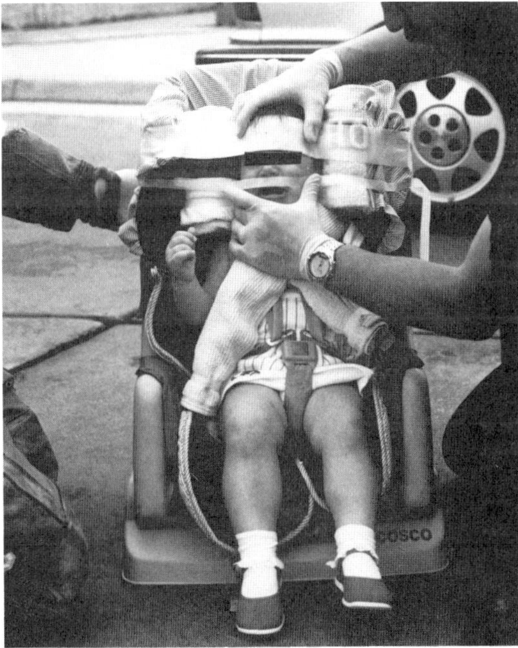

Figure 15–3 Immobilization using the infant car seat.

problems that interfere with adequate ventilation and oxygenation. There are physiologic and anatomic reasons that a child may be more prone to tissue hypoxia following traumatic insult. Oxygen needs are proportionately higher for a child than an adult. A child has limited ability to increase cardiac output because stroke volume is relatively fixed; therefore, there is less reserve for the child. Anatomically, airways in the child are smaller and have higher resistance, and dead space is proportionately greater than in the adult. One frequently overlooked cause of ventilatory compromise is gastric distention, which is common in the frightened child prone to crying and aerophagia. Finally, flexible ribs and a relatively mobile mediastinum provide less protection for the lung parenchyma and the mediastinal structures following blunt trauma.

The child with compromise of oxygenation appears agitated or obtunded and exhibits retractions or flaring of the nostrils. Pulse oximetry is useful to detect hypoxia before the appearance of cyanosis. Hypoxia is suspected when oxygen saturation is less than 95%. Treatment depends on reassessment of the airway, since occurrence of right mainstem bronchus intubation is common in children. Reposition the endotracheal tube if there are diminished breath sounds on the left. Occasionally the left bronchus is intubated, so repositioning is indicated for diminished breath sounds on the right as well. If the child does not improve after proper placement of the endotracheal tube, suspect a tension pneumothorax. Bilaterally diminished breath sounds require suctioning of the endotracheal tube to remove mucous plugs and laryngoscopic examination to ensure correct placement of the tube in the trachea. If the child does not respond to these maneuvers, remove the endotracheal tube, assist ventilation with bag and mask, and reintubate the trachea.

Failure to improve after reintubation requires needle thoracentesis of the affected side(s). This is a useful procedure both diagnostically, to confirm the presence of pneumothorax or hemothorax, and therapeutically, to relieve pneumothorax temporarily. Insert a plastic over-the-needle catheter or a small butterfly needle into the pleural space in the second intercostal space in the midclavicular line. Use a large syringe (30 or 60 cc) to temporarily decompress a pneumothorax. A stopcock between the catheter and the syringe is useful for repeated decompression, but definitive treatment of pneumothorax or hemothorax is tube thoracostomy. Attend to volume replacement carefully in the event of hemothorax, since tube thoracostomy results in acute decompression of the thorax and loss of tamponade. Poor oxygenation even with a patent and properly placed endotracheal tube and bilateral chest tubes usually indicates severe chest trauma with pulmonary contusions. Since lung compliance is poor, PEEP (positive end-expiratory pressure) and high inspiratory pressure are indicated.

Because of their flexible ribs, flail chest is uncommon in children. Flail chest is treated with positive pressure ventilation. Open pneumothorax is usually caused by penetrating trauma and is treated with an occlusive dressing followed by tube thoracostomy.

Circulation

After provision of adequate ventilation and oxygenation, delivery of oxygen to the tissues is the priority. Shock is a pathologic state of inadequate tissue perfusion that results in tissue hypoxia. Shock is *not* defined by a specific blood pressure.

As a general rule, most children have a normal systolic blood pressure of at least 80 torr (the neonate is an exception and may have a normal systolic blood pressure of 60 torr). However, children maintain blood pressure until late in the course of shock. Treatment must therefore begin before blood pressure decreases. Early signs of shock include tachycardia and peripheral vasoconstriction. Diastolic pressure may increase because of vasoconstriction.

Children have a deceptively small blood volume of 80 cc/kg, or 8% of body weight. For example, a 10/kg child has a blood volume of only 800 cc. Loss of 400 cc, well tolerated in an adult, in a child results in severe shock and probable death unless fluid resuscitation begins.

Treat shock with mechanical pressure on any active bleeding site and fluid resuscitation. Bleeding from the scalp is often overlooked or regarded as minor when, in fact, significant blood loss is occurring. Treat scalp bleeding with direct pressure followed by large hemostatic sutures, if necessary. Pneumatic antishock trousers are seldom used in treating children, because inflation of the abdominal compartment interferes with ventilation and may cause pulmonary edema. The trousers are a useful adjunct for refractory shock caused by pelvic fracture. If a child arrives with pneumatic antishock trousers inflated, deflate them slowly, with fluids ready to infuse, to prevent shock resulting from sudden loss of circulating blood volume into the lower extremities.

Intraabdominal bleeding is the most common cause of reversible shock. Intracranial hemorrhage can lead to blood loss sufficient to cause shock in the young child or infant, but this is rare. Intrathoracic bleeding that interferes with ventilation and cardiac output must be decompressed; however, careful evacuation is prudent since rapid decompression of the tamponade may cause refractory hypotension.

Intravenous catheter access to the circulation is often the rate-limiting step in resuscitation of the critically ill child. The antecubital fossa and saphenous veins at the ankle are preferred sites for percutaneous cannulation. If intravenous access is delayed, perform a cutdown on the saphenous vein at the ankle or the groin, or percutaneous catheterization of the femoral vein using the Seldinger technique. Access with two large-bone intravenous catheters is ideal, but proceed with resuscitation as rapidly as possible; often only a single access site is available.

In the critically ill child intravenous access is essential within 2 to 3 minutes; insert an intraosseous needle if access is delayed. A bone marrow needle or spinal needle is introduced with a twisting motion into the flat (medial) surface of the tibia, 1 to 3 cm below the tibial tuberosity. Other sites include the distal femur and the medial malleolus. A distinct "pop" is evident upon entry into the medullary cavity. Unfortunately, extravasation is common, because the needle penetrates through the marrow into the lateral cortex. Confirm proper placement by aspiration of marrow or by the ability to infuse saline without causing edema of the surrounding tissue. Infuse fluids or medications into the marrow. Fluid administration usually requires mechanical infusion with a pump or syringe, because gravity is ineffective.

If a child exhibits signs of shock, infuse a rapid fluid bolus of 20 cc/kg Ringer's lactate. Reassess the circulation. If improvement is evident, administer a maintenance fluid infusion and continue evaluation. If improvement is transient, administer a second bolus infusion of 20 cc/kg. If there are continued or recurrent signs of inadequate perfusion after administration of two challenges with crystalloid solution, transfuse 10 cc/kg of packed red blood cells. The need for repeated transfusions of blood of more than 40 cc/kg indicates ongoing bleeding, which requires surgical hemostasis.

Exploratory laparotomy to identify the bleeding site is indicated if more than 50% of the child's blood volume must be replaced. Penetrating trauma causing hemothorax in a hemodynamically unstable patient is an indication for open thoracotomy in the trauma unit.

The child in cardiopulmonary arrest following blunt trauma may respond to attempts at correcting the airway and circulation. Often the cause of arrest is massive head injury with apnea and resultant hypoxia. The patient improves with endotracheal intubation, but brain death frequently occurs within 24 to 48 hours. If the child does not improve after establishment of a secure airway and administration of fluids, insert chest tubes bilaterally. Proceed with pericardiocentesis if cardiac arrest persists. These maneuvers treat mechanical causes of cardiopulmonary arrest. The child's failure to respond frequently indicates a lethal head injury or, uncommonly, disruption of a great vessel. The resuscitation should be stopped after two complete sequences of drugs to stimulate return of spontaneous circulation. Thoracotomy is ineffective to reverse cardiopulmonary arrest caused by blunt trauma but should be considered in cases of penetrating trauma to the thorax. Figure 15-4 depicts the sequence for treating the child with hemorrhagic shock.

Disability (neurologic)

A child's head is proportionately very large. This affects the outcome of trauma in several ways. First, head injury is a leading cause of death. Second, blood loss can be significant from either scalp bleeding or intracranial hemorrhage; this will worsen injury to the brain by exacerbating shock. Finally, cervical spine injuries are more likely to be high injuries (above C3) in children younger than 8 years of age. Consequently, respiratory arrest occurs frequently, causing hypoxia and further damage to the spinal cord and brain. Head injury and cervical spine injury often occur concomitantly.

The most common type of severe injury sustained by the central nervous system of children is diffuse cerebral edema. Initial treatment consists of endotracheal intubation, administration of 100% oxygen, hyperventilation to maintain P_{CO_2} at 28 to 30 torr, and positioning of the head in the midline and elevated 30°. Delay in treatment of head injury makes elevated intracranial pressure more difficult to control, and prognosis is poor in many cases. Subarachnoid hemorrhage occurs when the subarachnoid vessels are subjected to shearing forces, as in the shaken baby syndrome or in whiplash injury. Subdural and epidural hemorrhage are less common.

Initial assessment of the central nervous system is made by using the AVPU mnemonic. Describe the child as *A*lert, responsive to *V*erbal stimuli, responsive to *P*ainful stimuli, or *U*nresponsive. Children with withdrawal response to pain or higher brain functioning can be further stabilized and reassessed during the secondary phase of evaluation. Children who are unresponsive or have abnormal posture responses to painful stimuli require intubation and hyperventilation to decrease intracranial pressure. Lidocaine (1 mg/kg IV) is useful to blunt the rise in intracranial pressure associated with the intubation procedure.

Primary injury to the brain occurs at the time of trauma and includes contusion, laceration, and local edema. The goals of treatment are to minimize secondary injury caused by anoxia or ischemia. Loss of autoregulation of cerebral blood flow occurs with head injury so that cerebral perfusion pressure becomes directly dependent on arterial blood pressure. Pay careful attention to the ABCs in order to perfuse the injured brain or spinal cord with well-oxygenated blood. Do not withhold fluids because of concern for cerebral edema if the

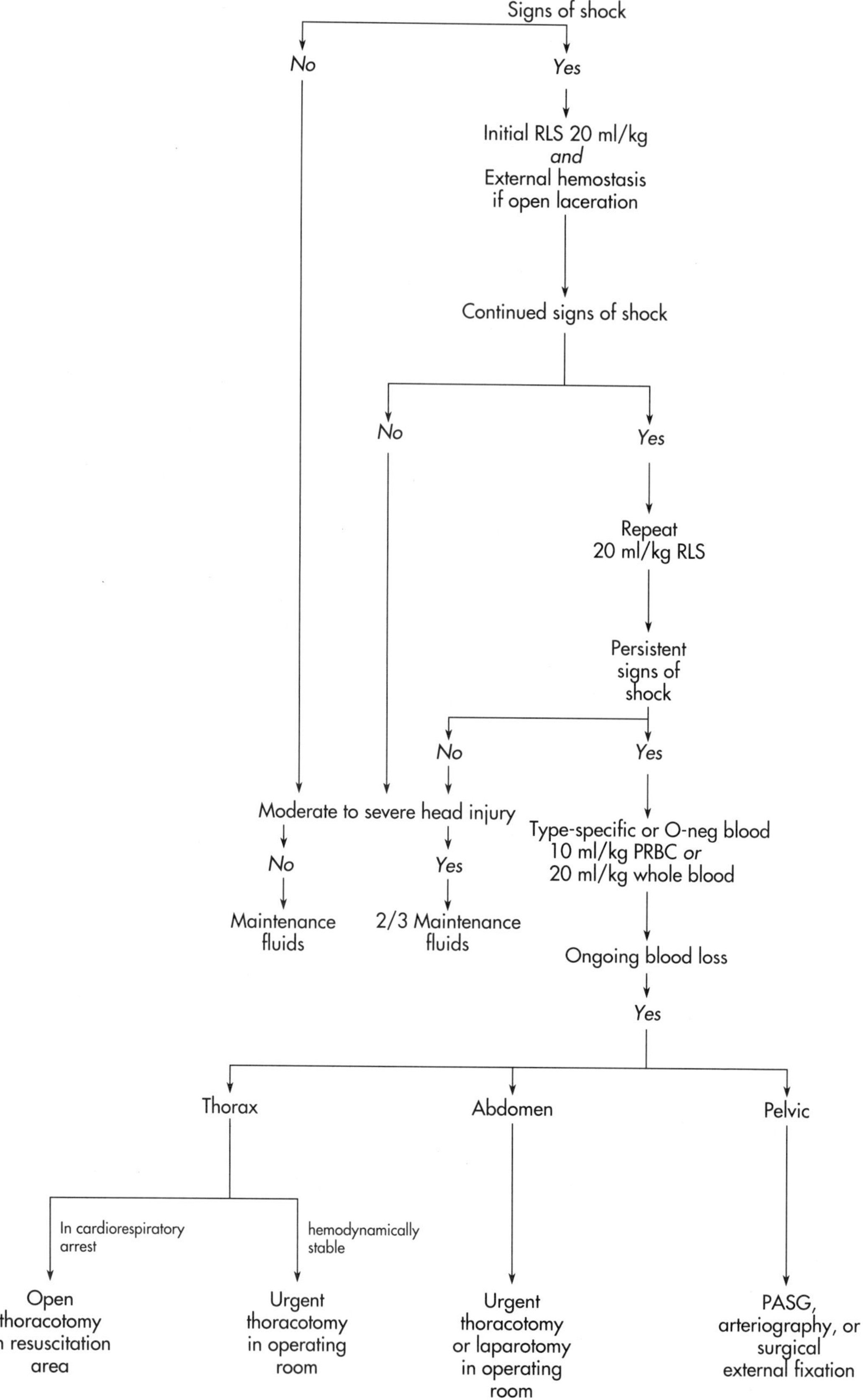

Figure 15–4 An algorithm for treating hypovolemic shock. (From Young G, Eichelberger MR: *Initial resuscitation of the child with multiple injuries.* In Grossman M, Dieckmann RA, editors: *Pediatric emergency medicine,* Philadelphia, 1991, JB Lippincott, p 233.)

child manifests hypovolemic shock. In the euvolemic child with good tissue perfusion, however, fluid restriction and even diuresis are desirable. Furosemide or osmotic diuresis by administration of mannitol is acceptable. Treatment also includes maintenance of correct head position. Analgesia and sedation help to blunt the reactive increase in intracranial pressure associated with painful procedures. Corticosteroid administration, hypothermia, and barbiturate-induced coma are not indicated for severe head injury. Early use of corticosteroids may have a role in preventing some of the neurologic sequelae of spinal cord injury.

Exposure and examination

Once the child is stable, remove all of his or her clothing to permit a thorough head-to-toe examination. Reassess the ABCs before proceeding to the secondary survey and definitive therapy. Careful attention to thermoregulation is mandatory in treatment of young children. Use heat lamps and warmed intravenous fluids to maintain body temperature at 36° to 37° C.

SECONDARY SURVEY AND DEFINITIVE THERAPY

A complete set of vital signs should be obtained while the physician completes the physical examination. The Glasgow Coma Scale provides a standardized and repeatable method of describing cerebral function and should be used to chart the patient's progress over time. In assessing infants, use a modification of the scale (Table 15-1) or simply describe the mental status of the child. Words such as *lethargic* and *unconscious* are vague; use descriptive phrases, such as "Sleeping comfortably at rest, cries vigorously and fights attempts at venipuncture," that describe the child's awareness of his or her environment. Apply monitors for heart rate, respiratory rate, oxygen saturation, and blood pressure. Place an indwelling urinary catheter after rectal examination; ongoing urine output is a sensitive measure of tissue perfusion. Place a nasogastric tube to decompress the stomach unless there is concern about possible basilar skull fracture; use an orogastric tube in that case.

The rest of the examination focuses on the presence of bleeding or fractures that will need therapy. Pay particular attention to the abdomen and pelvis since massive blood loss may occur at these sites. Abdominal distention and tenderness with guarding usually accompany intraabdominal injury but may be absent if there is head injury.

Examination of the abdomen may be very difficult in the infant and toddler. Young children have naturally protuberant abdomens that appear somewhat distended. Aerophagia with subsequent gas-

Table 15–1 The Glasgow Coma Scale score modified for young children

Glasgow Coma Scale		Pediatric scale	
Eye opening			
Spontaneous	4		
To speech	3	*Same as*	
To pain	2	*adult scale*	
None	1		
Best verbal response			
Oriented	5	Oriented	5
Confused	4	Words	4
Inappropriate words	3	Vocal sounds	3
Incomprehensible		Cries	2
sounds	2	None	1
None	1		
Best motor response			
Obeys commands	6		
Localizes pain	5		
Withdraws	4	*Same as*	
Flexion posturing	3	*adult scale*	
Extensor posturing	2		
None	1		

Normal aggregate score	
Birth-6 mo	10
6-12 mo	12
1-2 yr	13
2-5 yr	14
>5 yr	15

Adapted from Simpson D, Reilly P: Paediatric coma scale, *Lancet* 2:450, 1982.

tric dilatation is common. In addition, infants tense the abdominal muscles upon palpation (simulating guarding), and toddlers may scream uncontrollably during the entire examination. A physiologically stable child can be reassessed over time, whereas the child with evidence of blood loss or altered mental status needs CT scan of the head, chest, abdomen, and pelvis because of the nonspecific nature of the physical examination.

Obtain arterial blood gas levels and hemoglobin/hematocrit results and send samples to the blood bank for type and cross matching. Send coagulation profiles to the blood bank if the child requires massive blood transfusion, and blood and urine samples for toxicology screening if there is altered mental status. Elevated liver enzymes are a helpful indicator of hepatic injury.

Obtain roentgenograms of the cervical spine, chest, and pelvis. An alert child whose physical examination reveals a normal cervical spine requires a portable lateral roentgenogram that visualizes all seven cervical vertebrae to rule out injury. For a patient with neck pain or tenderness, perform a full cervical spine series if the portable lateral roentgenogram is normal. Occasionally, CT scan or MRI (magnetic resonance imaging) of the neck is necessary. The cervical spine is discussed in detail in Chapter 22.

The child with suspected head injury or abdominal trauma requires CT scan of the suspected area(s). Abdominal CT scan is the best technique for assessment of blunt trauma and has replaced the diagnostic peritoneal lavage for two reasons. First, and most important, management of most intraabdominal bleeding in children does not require surgery. CT scan can define the site of bleeding, most commonly the liver or spleen, and the type of injury (hematoma or laceration). The child's physiologic status and response to fluid resuscitation, combined with information obtained by CT scan, determines whether the child will need laparotomy. Peritoneal lavage subjects many children to unnecessary laparotomy. Second, the retroperitoneum can be better explained by CT scan than by lavage. Assessment of renal function through the use of intravenous contrast enhances evaluation. Lavage is a useful adjunct to CT scan to detect perforation of the hollow viscera (as in lap belt injury) or injury to the pancreas.

The mechanism of injury assists the physician in differential diagnosis. An infant restrained in a rear-facing car seat is virtually immune from serious injury unless the car seat itself has been dislodged or impacted in a high-speed crash with collapse of the passenger compartment. The forward-facing toddler in a car seat does nearly as well, except for occasional whiplash injury to the head and neck with cervical spine fracture. Children restrained with lap belts may sustain injury to the lumbar spine and the hollow viscera; duodenal or jejunal hematoma or perforation are classic injuries with this mechanism. Pedestrians or bicyclists struck by motor vehicles may have lethal head or thoracic injury. Falls from a bed or couch rarely result in anything more than a superficial bruise. Similarly, a fall downstairs is generally benign because of the tumbling nature of the fall. Occasionally, an infant in a walker may fall down the stairs and suffer significant head injury. Falls from heights greater than 10 feet are associated with injury to the head and spine (usually cervical or thoracic). Finally, the possibility of subarachnoid hemorrhage should be considered in any infant or toddler with possible shearing injury (for example, whiplash) or with unexplained irritability (the shaken baby syndrome).

SUMMARY

The pediatric victim of trauma requires quick assessment and treatment to prevent morbidity and mortality. Frequent reassessment and a smoothly functioning team are indispensable. The child has unique anatomic and physiologic factors that are important in the treatment of trauma. Initial management focuses on the ABCs to identify and treat immediately life-threatening injuries and to ensure delivery of well-oxygenated blood to the tissues. After stabilization of the ABCs, the secondary survey identifies injuries that are not immediately life-threatening but that will require definitive therapy. Consideration of the mechanism of trauma is useful in predicting likely injuries.

APPENDIX 15-1
Pediatric Trauma Team*

SURGICAL COORDINATOR (SURGICAL ATTENDING OR SENIOR SURGICAL FELLOW)

I. General responsibilities
  A. Assumes primary responsibility for patients and directs all involved personnel
  B. Ensures priority of diagnosis (primary survey)
  C. Defines order of therapy
  D. If absent, EMTC attending or surgical fellow assumes coordinator's position
II. Life support (ensures order of priority)
  A. Airway
    1. Assume cervical spine injury in all patients while performing airway maneuvers in priority order
      a. Protect neck: in-line immobilization or rigid neck collar (ensured by respiratory therapist)
      b. Administer O_2 (5 to 10 L/min)
      c. Suction secretions; remove any foreign body
      d. Perform chin-lift or jaw thrust
      e. Insert oral airway if patient is lethargic (*caution:* can stimulate vomiting)
      f. Ventilate (bag-valve-mask)
      g. Intubate (orotracheal)
      h. Assess for upper-airway obstruction
        • cricothyroidotomy [needle (16 gauge) or surgical]
      i. Esophageal obturator airway (EOA contraindicated in children)

---

*From Eichelberger MR, Zwick HA, Pratsch GL, et al: Pediatric trauma protocol: a team approach. In Eichelberger MR, Pratsch GL, editors: *Pediatric trauma care*, Rockville, Md, 1988, Aspen, pp 11-31.

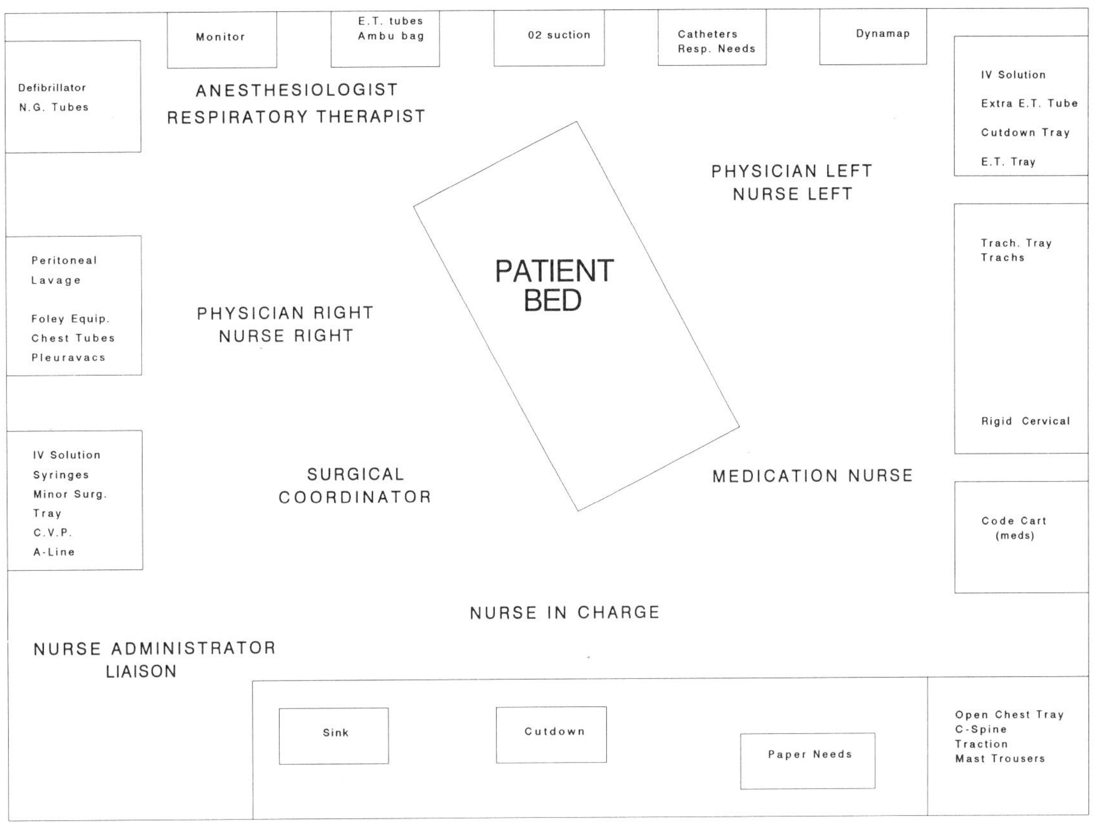

2. If suspected neck injury, no stridor but apparent upper-airway obstruction
   a. Perform a through f as above
   b. Two attempts at endotracheal intubation
   c. If unsuccessful, needle cricothyroidotomy (16 gauge)
3. If anterior neck injury, stridor, and upper-airway obstruction
   a. Suspect laryngeal crush injury, laryngotracheal separation
   b. Proceed to cricothyroidotomy or tracheostomy without prior attempt at endotracheal intubation

B. Breathing
   1. If pneumothorax
      a. Needle thoracentesis: midclavicular line into the second intercostal space (20-gauge)
      b. Thoracostomy tube: directed to lung apex
         • small infant, 12 Fr
         • children, 20-24 Fr
   2. If tension pneumothorax
      a. Needle thoracentesis
      b. Tube thoracostomy

3. If hemothorax
   a. Fluid resuscitation before insertion of thoracostomy tube
   b. Thoracostomy tube directed posterior and inferior (use larger tube if possible: e.g., 28 Fr in adolescents)
4. If open pneumothorax
   a. Cover defect: petroleum jelly–impregnated gauze and sterile dressing
   b. Thoracostomy tube

C. Circulation
   1. If external bleeding
      a. Provide hemostasis with direct pressure to external bleeding sites
      b. Determine source of bleeding
   2. If cardiac arrest (asystole)
      a. Evaluate and treat mechanical reasons for arrest; i.e., tension pneumothorax, pericardial tamponade
      b. Physician Left assumes simultaneous cardiac medical resuscitation
      c. Check carotid and/or femoral pulse; brachial pulse in small child or infant
   3. If shock
      a. Administer crystalloid, 20 ml/kg

Ringer's lactate solution (RLS) IV push

- repeat if vital signs not improved, followed by
- type-specific/O negative packed red blood cells, 10 ml/kg IV push
- maintain patient with RLS 10 ml/kg/hr for 2 hours, then maintenance fluids (See D—for isolated head injury treatment)

b. If head injury, imperative to treat shock with fluid resuscitation; maintain blood pressure at 80 mm Hg systolic (minimum)

c. If blood pressure less than 60 mm Hg and unresponsive to fluid resuscitation (unabated shock), use pneumatic antishock trousers (PAST) and inflate leg compartment only; inflate abdominal compartment with severe pelvic fracture (*caution:* injudicious inflation of abdominal compartment may lead to respiratory embarrassment

4. Cardiac tamponade
   a. Shock unresponsive to volume with decreased pulse pressure
   b. Neck vein distention
   c. Pulsus paradoxus
   d. Treat with pericardiocentesis

5. Indications for open thoracotomy
   a. Immediate
      - penetrating wound of heart
      - massive or continuous intrapleural hemorrhage
      - massive intraabdominal hemorrhage (for aortic cross-clamping)
      - open pneumothorax with major defect of chest
   b. Urgent (OR)
      - cardiac tamponade following pericardiocentesis
      - widened mediastinum with left hemothorax or aortogram confirming aortic transection
      - ruptured esophagus
      - massive pleural air leak suggestive of ruptured bronchus
      - traumatic diaphragmatic hernia

D. Disability (central nervous system)
   1. Treat shock: maintain blood pressure at 80 mm Hg systolic (minimum)
   2. Ventilate (Po_2, 80 to 100 torr; Pco_2, 25 to 30 torr)
   3. Immobilize cervical spine
   4. Treatment
      a. Restrict fluids (⅔ maintenance 5% dextrose in ½ normal saline if vital signs are stable)
      b. Elevate head of bed 30° in absence of neck flexion or spinal injury
      c. If severe injury (Glasgow Coma Scale score less than 8)
         - orotracheal intubation with hyperventilation
         - see anesthesiologist role for drug sequences

5. Neurosurgery consultation to assess nature and extent of brain or spinal cord injury

6. Computed axial tomography (CAT) scan (preferred diagnostic tool if clinically indicated)

E. Coordinate radiologic examination (transition to poststabilization phase)
   1. Lateral cervical spine (visualize levels C1 to C7)
   2. Anterior-posterior (AP) chest
   3. AP pelvis

F. Abdomen
   1. Quick assessment: tenderness, rigidity, distention
   2. Insert nasogastric tube (orogastric tube for severe facial fracture or basilar skull fractures)
   3. CAT scan
   4. Indications for lavage (rarely used)
      a. Central nervous system trauma (lethargic to unresponsive with hemodynamic instability)
      b. Unexplained shock, unresponsive to fluid resuscitation
      c. Penetrating chest wounds below nipples
      d. Operation for other major system repair
   5. Abdominal hemorrhage or severe pelvic fracture
      a. Fluid resuscitation essential
      b. Proceed to OR for unabated shock requiring transfusion equal to or greater than 50% blood volume
      c. PAST for severe pelvic fracture (rarely used)
         - apply only if blood pressure less than 60 mm Hg and unresponsive fluid resuscitation
         - decompression sequence directed by surgical coordinator with close monitoring of vital signs and blood pressure (maintain blood pressure at or above 80 mm Hg)
      d. Left thoracotomy: clamp aorta (last resort; infrequently required)

6. Proceed to OR for penetrating injury of abdomen
G. Genitourinary (GU)
1. Rectal exam: precedes insertion of indwelling bladder catheter
2. Insert indwelling bladder catheter
   a. Allow patient to void if awake and alert with no clinical indication of potential GU injury
   b. Obtain urologic consultation and do not insert indwelling bladder catheter if
      • blood at urethra meatus or gross hematuria
      • high-riding prostate
      • perineal hematoma or injury
      • alert and responsive patient is unable to void for significant period of time
      • pelvic fracture (severe)
   c. If urethral injury excluded, urethral catheter may be placed and CAT scan performed with indwelling bladder catheter clamped
   d. Usual catheter sizes: infant, 8 Fr; child, 10 Fr; adolescent, 14 Fr
3. Patient should be evaluated with abdominal CAT scan (preferred) or intravenous pyelogram (IVP) and voiding films
4. IVP (infrequent; intravenous injection of contrast medium, 1 ml/16, maximum 100 ml)
5. Cystogram, performed if bladder injury is remotely possible (pelvic fracture, abdominal trauma); if patient arrives with catheter in place after pelvic fracture or if urethral injury is suspected, CAT scan should be performed first, then cystogram without removal of catheter
H. Fracture stabilization
1. Reduce fracture dislocation and splint
2. Fractured femur: splint stabilization before operative procedure
3. Evaluate for vascular or neurologic compromise
4. Orthopedic consultation
III. Poststabilization
A. Surgical coordinator receives EMTC (Emergency Medical Trauma Center) attending physician's briefing on family status, medical history, and so forth
B. Triage
1. Determine sequence: radiology, OR, intensive care unit (ICU)
2. Determine specialty service needs: neurosurgery, orthopedics, urology, ENT (ear, nose, throat), plastic surgery, ophthalmology, cardiovascular surgery, dental surgery
3. Coordinate triage with attending surgeon, anesthesia
C. OR transition: communicate with OR trauma nurse
D. Coordinate with nurse administrator liaison (NAL) (the nursing supervisor)
E. Establish contact with family if this is possible
F. Direct further radiologic sequence as needed
G. Determine need for tetanus toxoid and antibiotic prophylaxis

SURGICAL TEAM: PHYSICIAN RIGHT AND NURSE RIGHT
Physician right (surgical resident)

I. General responsibilities
A. Know sequence for diagnosis and treatment in surgical coordinator's absence
B. Know right-side procedures and all other surgical procedures
C. Work in cooperation with Physician Left
1. If cardiac arrest, evaluate and treat mechanical reasons for arrest (tension pneumothorax, pericardial (tamponade, inadequate volume infusion)
2. Physician Left responsible for drug sequence
D. Radiologic sequence
1. Cervical spine, chest x-ray, AP pelvis
2. Special studies (in radiology department as required)
   a. CAT scan
   b. IVP, cystogram, urethrogram
   c. Arteriogram
E. Documentation
F. Accompany patient to OR, radiology, ICU, or other destinations throughout transport phase and until admitted to receiving unit
II. Life support
A. Protect neck: in-line immobilization (by respiratory therapist) or rigid neck collar
B. Assist cricothyroidotomy if necessary
C. Chest tube (chest trauma)
1. Fourth to fifth interspace, midaxillary line
2. Catheter without trocar
   a. Infant, 12 Fr
   b. Young child (less than 30 kg), 20 to 24 Fr
   c. Older child (greater than 30 kg), 28 Fr

  d. If hemothorax
- use largest bore possible for patient's size
- fluid resuscitation before insertion of thoracostomy
- clamp chest tube if excessive blood present

  3. Pleurevac suction:
  a. Infant, 10 cm H_2O
  b. Older child, 20 cm H_2O
  4. If bleeding rate is 1 to 2 ml/kg/hr, proceed to thoracotomy
D. Hemostasis: right side; direct pressure of external bleeding; do not clamp vessels
E. IV access
  1. General
  a. Percutaneous attempt (twice), then proceed to cutdown
  b. Shock-saphenous vein cutdown (first choice)
  c. Chest injury (saphenous vein cutdown)
  d. Abdominal injury: upper extremity if possible; if not use lower extremity
  e. Proximal femoral vein cutdown
  f. Femoral vein, percutaneous (quickest)
  g. Intraosseous
  2. Priority
  a. Saphenous (distal) cutdown (best access for pediatric patient in shock)
  b. Upper extremity, right
  c. Right femoral, percutaneous
  d. Femoral cutdown, 18- or 20-gauge
  e. Subclavian venous catheter (last resort, dangerous resuscitative maneuver; high incidence of iatrogenic injury)
  3. Catheter sizes
  a. Small infants, 22 gauge
  b. Older children, 18 to 20 gauge
  c. Cannulas preferable
F. Resuscitate from shock: administer 20 ml/kg RLS IV push; if shock persists administer second bolus
G. Check femoral pulses during cardiac arrest
III. Poststabilization
A. Assist with patient movement during radiologic evaluation
B. PAST (decompression sequence)
C. Pelvis (evaluate for fracture)
D. Rectal exam: before insertion of indwelling catheter, obtain stool sample for hemetest
E. Indwelling bladder catheter
  1. Head, neck, chest, pelvis

  2. Extremities (splint and check pulses)
  3. Femur fracture (splint)
F. Nasogastric tube
  1. Maintain in-line cervical spine immobilization during insertion
  2. Check aspirant for content and blood
  3. Guarantee patency of tube
  4. Contraindications: cribriform plate fracture, major facial fractures, basilar skill fracture (assume if rhinorrhea or drainage from the ear present); use oral route as alternate
G. Peritoneal lavage ("mini-laparotomy" technique, rarely used; see indications under "Surgical Coordinator" section)
  1. "Mini-laparotomy" technique:
  a. Insert urinary catheter to decompress bladder
  b. Insert nasogastric tube
  c. Infiltrate with 1% xylocaine with epinephrine (to minimize subcutaneous bleeding)
  d. Perform midline, vertical infraumbilical incision, 3 to 4 cm in length (use supraumbilical approach for pelvic fractures or previous lower quadrant incisions, e.g., appendectomy)
  e. Open linea alba and peritoneum under direct vision
  f. Insert pediatric peritoneal lavage catheter:
- direct toward left pelvis
- remove trocar before insertion into abdomen

  g. Aspirate catheter (if greater than 10 ml blood present, tap is positive)
  h. Infuse 15 ml/kg RLS, recover by gravity
  i. Obtain red and white blood cell counts (RBC and WBC), amylase in fluid (do not spin down); positive results include more than 100,000/mm RBC, bile, bacteria, stool, greater than 175 mg/dl amylase level, greater than 500/mm WBC
  2. Perform all in OR if other major operative procedure is undertaken
H. Accompany patient to OR, radiology, ICU, continuously monitoring for respiratory, circulatory, and neurologic instability
I. Documentation
  1. Trauma score: immediately and 1 hour after injury
  2. Trauma form: physical
  3. Standard orders: check off

4. Admission office: call as soon as possible
5. Guarantee that all forms from trauma stat resuscitation sheets are present and signed
6. Obtain parental signatures on necessary permits

Nurse right (emergency department/nursery nurse)

Note: If patient has burn injuries, this position will be filled instead by a burn unit nurse. Notification for this change will be accomplished by the group page: Trauma Stat—Burn

  I. Assist Physician Right

  II. Expose patient, except for PAST

  III. Turn on monitor and place electrocardiogram (ECG) leads

  IV. Assist with IV percutaneous stick of cutdown and secure all right-side lines (stopcock and extension tubing added to IVs of all potential OR patients)

  V. Monitor and control all right-side infusions, blood products, lavages and all right-side outputs (blood, urine, drainage, vomitus, etc), and announce to nurse in charge

  VI. Operate trauma table

  VII. Assist with insertion of chest tubes, nasogastric tube, and Foley catheter and set up pleurevacs

  VIII. Apply dressings to all open wounds

  IX. Operate warming lamps as needed for patient exposure

  X. Apply identification bracelet and guarantee patient identification before transport to other areas

  XI. May accompany patient to radiology, OR, ICU, burn ICU, or other destinations as directed by nurse administrator liaison

**MEDICAL TEAM: RESIDENT LEFT
AND NURSE LEFT**
Physician left (ICU fellow)

I. General responsibilities
  A. Work in cooperation with Physician Right
  B. Perform all left-side procedures
  C. Manage medical resuscitation during cardiac arrest at discretion of surgical coordinator
  D. Guarantee that all blood specimens are drawn and given to medication nurse
    1. Venous specimen (12 ml) for complete blood count, platelets, electrolytes, creatinine, blood urea nitrogen, glucose, amylase, bilirubin, prothrombin time/partial thrombin time (PT/PTT)
    2. Arterial gases (all patients)

  E. Monitor ECG
  F. Push all medications during medical sequence

II. Life support (circulatory priority)
  A. Assess pulse: femoral or carotid; if none, Nurse Left begins chest compression
  B. If cardiac arrest
    1. May assume medical leadership at discretion of surgical coordinator
    2. Call medications (e.g., epinephrine, $NaHCO_3$, $CaCl_2$)
    3. Coordinate defibrillator
  C. Hemostasis (left side; direct pressure for external bleeding)
  D. IV access (left side)
    1. Insert percutaneous vein catheter (femoral stick if necessary)
    2. Use 22- to 18-gauge cannulas
    3. Draw venous blood (12 ml, all patients)
    4. Alternate IV site (see IV access sequence in "Physician Right" section)
  E. Arterial blood gas specimen (all patients)

III. Poststabilization
  A. Evaluate respiratory and circulatory status in conjunction with anesthesiologist/respiratory therapist
  B. Insert arterial line as needed

Nurse left (EMTC nurse)

  I. Compress chest during cardiac arrest until relieved by other personnel

  II. Expose patient except for PAST

  III. Communicate to patient, giving reassurance and explanations

  IV. Observe cervical spine precautions

  V. Obtain vital signs (temperature, pulse, respiration, blood pressure, neurologic signs) every 5 minutes (four times) until the following criteria are met (Rule of 5)
    A. Temperature: taken once; repeat every 5 minutes if below or above normal (36° to 38° C)
    B. Pulse: stable within 5 beats of each reading (rate less than 30 beats/Min)
    C. Respiration: stable within 5 respirations (rate, 20 to 30 per minute)
    D. Blood pressure: stable within 5 mm Hg (pressure, greater than or equal to 80 mm Hg systolic)
    E. Neurologic signs: until not deteriorating
    F. When vital signs are stable to the above criteria, obtain every 15 minutes

  VI. Assist with left-side procedures

  VII. Assist with IV access and blood drawing, secure all left-side lines (stopcock and extension tubing added to IVs of all potential OR patients)

VIII. Monitor and control all left-side infusions, blood products, lavages and all left-side outputs (blood, urine, drainage, vomitus, and so forth) and announce to nurse in charge

IX. Coordinate PAST inflation/deflation with Physician Right

X. May accompany patient to radiology, OR, ICU, burn ICU, or other destinations as directed by nurse administrator liaison

Anesthesiologist

I. Protect cervical spine throughout airway maneuvers and team procedures

II. Airway management (in order of priority)
   A. Suction of secretions, blood, debris, foreign body
   B. Chin lift or jaw thrust
   C. Oral airway (cation: can stimulate vomiting)
   D. Mask ventilation
   E. Orotracheal intubation
      1. Drug sequence:
         a. Flaccid, unresponsive patient: no drugs
         b. Reactive patient, cardiovascular (CV) stable, rapid airway control not mandatory: Surital, 5 mg/kg; Pancuronium, 0.1-0.15 mg/kg; ventilate with bag-mask O_2 for 3 minutes; use cricoid pressure (omit if patient is retching); intubate
         c. Reactive patient, CV stable, rapid airway control not mandatory: Surital, 5 mg/kg; succinylcholine, 2 mg/kg; ventilate for 60 seconds; use cricoid pressure (omit if patient is retching); intubate
         d. Reactive patient, CV unstable and increased intracranial pressure not of concern: omit Surital
      2. Oral route preferred unless severe maxillofacial injuries present
      3. Tube size: $16 + age \div 4$, or estimate by matching diameter of tube to child's small finger or external nares
   F. Cricothyroidotomy/tracheostomy by surgical team
   G. EOA contraindicated in children

III. Ventilation
   A. O_2, 5 to 10 L/min to all injured patients
   B. Observe and auscultate the chest for:
      1. Symmetric breath sounds
      2. Symmetric chest expansion
      3. Absence of cyanosis
      4. Absence of gastric distention
      5. Subcutaneous emphysema
      6. AP chest x-ray (tube position above carina)

   C. Ventilate via hand resuscitator

IV. Circulation:
   A. Cardiac (assess heart sounds)
   B. Capillary refill

V. Monitor central nervous system status:
   A. Level of consciousness
   B. Pupil size and symmetry
   C. Pupil reaction to light

VI. When patient is stable, respiratory therapist may assume airway management

Respiratory therapist

I. Support anesthesiologist; assume airway management when patient is stable

II. Ensure O_2 at 5 to 10 L/min

III. Provide suctioning, bagging, monitoring of endotracheal tube placement

IV. Guarantee in-line immobilization of cervical spine

V. Accompany patient during transport and assure ventilation and oxygenation (O_2: must have 1500 lb in tank before transport)

Medication nurse (emergency department nurse)

I. Before patient arrives:
   A. Take succinylcholine and Pavulon from ICU medication refrigerator to resuscitation room (backup supply available in EMTC medication refrigerator)
   B. Draw up and label four 6-ml normal saline flushes
   C. Draw up and label 5-ml normal saline flushes for Foley catheter (3 ml for #8 catheter)
   D. Assemble all blood-drawing equipment

II. After patient arrives:
   A. Prepare all medications and infusions as requested
   B. Know and verbalize all drug actions, incompatibilities, and dilutions
   C. Communicate to Physician Left exact dosage in milligrams of drugs
   D. Place correct amounts of blood in proper tubes to send to laboratory
   E. Assemble pressure lines and transducers as needed
   F. Draw up medications for transport as needed
   G. Assume other duties and responsibilities as directed by nurse in charge (e.g., assisting to expose or restrain patient)
   H. May accompany patient to ICU, burn ICU, OR, radiology, or other destinations as directed by nurse administrator liaison

III. If cardiac or respiratory arrest occurs:
   A. Draw up and label the following in this order (19- or 21-gauge needles):

1. $NaHCO_3$, 50 ml (one; Bristoject without cardiac needle)
2. Epinephrine, 1:10,000 × 10 ml (one; Bristoject without cardiac needle)
3. Atropine, 1:10,000 × 10 ml (one; Bristoject without cardiac needle)
4. $CaCl_2$, 500 mg in 5 ml syringe (one)
5. Glucose 50%, 20 ml (one)

B. Draw up and label all the above drugs again and keep at least one dose ahead on all medications and flushes (arrange in alphabetical order on cart)
C. Prepare other medications according to standard resuscitation chart unless otherwise instructed
D. Set up pressure lines, transducers, and pumps for dopamine or epinephrine drips

Nurse in charge (EMTC nurse)

I. Record entire trauma stat event; acquire data from all team members (e.g., all input and output, vital signs every 5 minutes, sizes of inserted tubes and catheters, and so forth)
II. Communicate to surgical coordinator and other team members status of vital signs, pending medication times, trends from data, and the like on frequent basis; give periodic summary reports of fluid infusion
III. Monitor all nursing activities and patient needs; anticipate and communicate priorities to nurse administrator liaison
IV. Label all specimens and note time sent to laboratory
V. Cosign blood slips as necessary
VI. Guarantee that appropriate paperwork is completed before transfer and that all necessary forms are completed
VII. Coordinate release of team members with surgical coordinator and nurse administrator liaison when appropriate
VIII. Ensure that necessary equipment, supplies, medications, and personnel are ready to transport
IX. Telephone report to receiving unit (patient condition, treatments, and so forth)
X. May accompany patient to radiology, OR, ICU, burn ICU, or other destinations as directed by nurse-administrator liaison

OUTER CORE TEAM
Nurse administrator liaison (Monday to Friday, 0800 to 1500 hours: Director of EMTC nursing services; all other times, assistant director of nursing)

I. Serve as communication link between trauma room and rest of hospital system
II. Maintain team to established number and roles

III. Trouble shoot with consulting departments as needed
IV. Receive laboratory results and report them to surgical coordinator
V. Initiate and expedite triage process to facilitate patient disposition
VI. Communicate with admissions office, OR, nurse staffing office, ICU, or receiving unit regarding status of patient, approximate time of transfer, required equipment, supplies, and so forth
VII. Adjust nurse staffing to ensure nursing care of trauma patient during and after stabilization and disposition
VIII. Communicate with administration, public relations, and police as needed
IX. Designate nurses to accompany patient during transport for special procedures (CAT scan, x-ray) or to receiving unit
X. Communicate status of receiving unit to team members
XI. Stamp additional slips, labels and forms as needed
XII. Decide who is dismissed from code room after discussion with nurse in charge and surgical coordinator
XIII. Double-check chart components before patient is transported

EMTC attending or surgical fellow

I. Act as trauma team coordinator if surgical coordinator not present
II. Debrief personnel, family, police
III. Determine and report to surgical coordinator:
A. Mechanism of injury
B. Essential medical history
C. Allergy
D. Weight of patient
IV. Provide medical liaison to family while team is involved with resuscitation
V. Provide medical back-up for Physician Left if not functioning as team coordinator

OR trauma nurse

I. Respond to trauma room to assist with emergency surgical procedure if indicated
II. Call in additional OR personnel if they are needed
III. Prepare OR suites
IV. See OR protocol

Laboratory technician

I. Stat blood and urinalysis studies; review laboratory slips and samples for accuracy; communicate any problems to nurse administrator liaison
II. Deliver samples to all appropriate laboratories and expedite processing

III. Ensure that laboratory results are reported to nurse administrator liaison promptly by phone

X-ray technician

I. Obtain lateral cervical spine, AP chest, AP pelvis, respectively, in trauma resuscitation area

II. Responsible for processing, developing, and expediting return of x-rays to resuscitation area

III. Positioned outside resuscitation area and receives direction from surgical coordinator or nuse administrator liaison

Security

I. Secure helicopter pad for landings and take-offs

II. Control traffic flow in resuscitation area

III. Obtain elevator for transport

Transport technician

I. Obtain ice for laboratory specimens and take to resuscitation bay

II. Obtain supplies and equipment and transport specimens (particularly blood gas specimens) to laboratory

III. Positioned outside resuscitation area and receives direction from nurse administrator liaison

Social worker (see Department of Social Work, Trauma Protocol)
Surgical specialties immediately on call

I. Neurosurgery
II. Orthopedics
III. Urology
IV. Cardiovascular surgery
V. Plastic surgery
VI. ENT
VII. Ophthalmology
VIII. Dentistry

APPENDIX 15-2
Trauma Protocol: Operating Room

GENERAL

I. Room: there is no specific trauma room; however, a trauma room is designated by charge nurse at 1500 hours each day

II. Room readiness check (or trauma team will ensure that designated trauma room contains the following basic supplies and that all equipment is in working order)

A. Standard equipment: IV poles (two); operating room table; Mayo stand; back table, prep table; overhead lights; suction (two); Bovie machine

B. Stand-by case carts for all specialities

C. Drugs and solutions such as paint, prep, water, saline, thrombin, surgical, antibiotics

D. Equipment for insertion of Foley catheter, central/arterial lines

E. Power equipment for opening chest, skull

NURSING ROLES: TRAUMA STAT OR
OR trauma nurse (0900 to 1500 hours)

I. Carry group page beeper

II. Respond to communications when code beepers are tested

III. Check availability of emergency stand-by carts and emergency drugs at beginning of each shift

IV. Respond to trauma bay in person unless impossible; then respond by telephone

A. Remain outside code room unless otherwise instructed by surgical coordinator; if instructed to enter, assist surgical coordinator and Physician Right with emergency surgical procedures in resuscitation area

B. Communicate with operating room/anesthesia staff as to age, injury, condition of patient, immediate plan of care (i.e., destination of patient)

C. If no surgical intervention in trauma area, return to OR

D. Communicate with anesthesia staff, prepare OR suite to receive patient

E. Function as primary circulator and complete all documentation on patient care records

OR trauma nurse (1500 to 2300 hours)

I. Evening nurse (only nurse on duty from 1800 to 2300 hours); carry group page beeper and respond to trauma area as described above

II. Call on-call personnel if multiple trauma patient needs surgical intervention

III. Check room and case carts as described above

OR trauma nurse (2300 to 0700 hours)

I. Check room and case carts as described on arrival

II. Carry group page beeper and respond to trauma area as described above

III. Respond to OR for nontrauma surgical emergencies

DUTIES OF OR TRAUMA NURSE WHEN PATIENT IS TRANSPORTED TO SURGERY

* Alert trauma technician and back-up team if necessary
* Prepare OR with technician and anesthesia team
* If patient is too unstable to place adequate monitoring lines in trauma area, be prepared to assist with insertion of these lines on arrival in OR
* On patient's arrival, quickly assess condition and status of resuscitation
* Assist with transfer to OR table and positioning
* Attend to needs of anesthesia and surgical teams
* Monitor aseptic technique as defined in event of life-threatening injuries
* Control traffic flow in OR
* Document surgical event on patient's record
* Attend to needs of scrub technician
* Monitor blood loss (through suction and discarded sponges)
* Do sponge and needle counts if possible, arrange for x-ray examination
* During closing, report to ICU nurse
* Assist with patient transfer to ICU bed
* Assist technician with care of instruments and room
* Alert central supply to replace stand-by cart
* Return unused blood products to blood bank

TRAUMA COVERAGE: OPERATING ROOM

From 0700 to 1500 hours

The OR is open and working the elective schedule. Trauma cases are given first priority and assigned to the first available room and staff. The charge nurse carries the group page beeper and responds to the trauma room. The charge nurse is the primary circulator on the case.

From 1500 to 2300 hours

The OR is open to finish the elective schedule and for urgent and emergency cases. Room 3 is designated the trauma room unless otherwise specified. The evening nurse carries the group page beeper and responds to the trauma room. The evening nurse is the primary circulator for the trauma case. The operating room on-call team may be called to assist if deemed necessary by the trauma nurse.

From 2300 to 0700 hours

The OR is closed but with on-call coverage for all surgical emergencies. The trauma nurse is in-house and carries the group page beeper. The trauma technician is on-call at home Monday to Friday from 2300 to 0700 hours. There is only one call team available for all surgical emergencies.

WEEKEND AND HOLIDAY TRAUMA COVERAGE

The OR staff provide in-house coverage 24 hours a day on weekends and holidays. The trauma nurse is in-house and carries the group page beeper. The trauma technician is on-call at home. A separate call team is designated to cover other surgical emergencies. The back-up call team may be called to assist the trauma team as deemed necessary by the trauma nurse.

REFERENCES

1. Cooney DR: Splenic and hepatic trauma in children, *Surg Clin North Am* 61:1165-1180, 1981.
2. Eichelberger MR, Randolph JG: Thoracic trauma in children, *Surg Clin North Am* 61:1181-1197, 1981.
3. Eichelberger MR, Randolph JG: Pediatric trauma: an algorithm for diagnosis and therapy, *J Trauma* 23:91-97, 1983.
4. Eichelberger MR, Zwick HA, Pratsch GL et al: *Pediatric trauma protocol: a team approach.* In Eichelberger MR, Pratsch GL, *Pediatric trauma care*, Rockville, Md, 1988, Aspen, pp 11-31.
5. Fuchs S, Barthel MJ, Flannery AM et al: Cervical spine fractures sustained by young children in forward-facing car seats. *Pediatrics* 84:348-354, 1989.
6. Hennes HM, Smith DS, Schneider K et al: Elevated liver transaminase levels in children with blunt abdominal trauma: a predictor of liver injury, *Pediatrics* 86:87-90, 1990.
7. Hill SA, Miller CA, Kosnik EJ et al: Pediatric neck injuries: a clinical study, *J Neurosurg* 60:700-706, 1984.
8. Joffe M, Ludwig S: Stairway injuries in children, *Pediatrics* 82(3 Pt 2):457-461, 1988.
9. Newman KD, Bowman LM, Eichelberger MR et al: The lap belt complex in children, *J Trauma* 30:1133-1138, 1990.
10. Orenstein JB, Klein BL, Ochsenschlager DW et al: Pediatric cervical spine injury: results of an 11-year review (submitted for publication).
11. Ramenofsky ML: Pediatric abdominal trauma, *Pediatr Ann* 16:319-326, 1987.
12. Ruge JR, Sinson GP, McLone DG et al: Pediatric spine injury: the very young, *J Neurosurg* 68:25-30, 1988.
13. Selbst SM, Baker MD, Shames M: Bunk bed injuries, *Am J Dis Child* 144:721-723, 1990.
14. Simpson D, Reilly P: Paediatric coma scale, *Lancet* 2:450, 1982.
15. Yager JY, Johnston B, Seshia SS: Coma scales in pediatric practice, *Am J Dis Child* 144:1088-1091, 1990.
16. Young GM, Eichelberger MR: *Initial resuscitation of the child with multiple injuries.* In Grossman M, Dieckmann RA, editors: *Pediatric emergency medicine: a clinician's reference*, Philadelphia, 1991, JB Lippincott.
17. Young GM, Klein BL, Ochsenschlager DW et al: The child with multiple injuries: resuscitation priorities, *Indian J Pediatr* 55:705-713, 1988.

16 Airway Management

Linda Jo Rice and *John T. Britton*

Children are not just small adults. Most health care providers learn airway management skills using adult models and patients. Their clinical experience usually involves adult patients as well. Just as in every other aspect of care, children require special consideration in airway management. The smaller the child, the less anatomic features resemble those of adults, and the more critical are those special considerations.

ANATOMY

To put it simply, infants have smaller airways than adults. There are five important differences between the infant airway and that of older patients (Fig. 16-1).

1. The infant larynx is higher in the neck, located between C3 and C4, whereas in the older patient it is between C4 and C5. The angle for insertion of a laryngoscope blade is therefore slightly different. Upon laryngoscopy, this more superior location makes the vocal cords appear to be more anterior. A stylet is often useful to help direct the endotracheal tube through the cords.

2. The infant tongue is large in relation to the rest of the oropharynx. Thus more rapid upper airway obstruction is possible because of the large tongue and the shorter distance between the tongue and the hard palate. Even a small amount of pressure on the soft tissues under the mandible by the hand holding the mask may be enough to cause airway obstruction. In addition, the position of an infant's tongue is more difficult to control with a laryngoscope blade.

3. The infant epiglottis is short, stubby, and angled away from the axis of the trachea. The adult epiglottis is broad, floppy, and has an axis parallel to the axis of the trachea. The infant epiglottis may therefore be difficult to control with a laryngoscope blade.

4. The infant vocal cords are more cartilaginous, distensible, and easily damaged. They have a lower attachment anteriorly than posteriorly, as compared with adult vocal cords, which are perpendicular to the axis of the trachea.

5. In the child, the narrowest diameter of the airway is at the cricoid ring, whereas in the adult it is at the glottis. Thus an endotracheal tube may readily pass through the vocal cords of a child but become "tight" in the subglottic region.

The pediatric trachea is also shorter than the adult trachea. Failure to appreciate this difference may result in endobronchial intubation, hypoxia, or perforation.

MANAGEMENT

The goals of airway management in the injured child are (1) optimal oxygenation and ventilation, (2) cervical spine protection, and (3) minimal increases in intracranial pressure. Any child who sustains trauma is presumed to have a cervical spine injury until normal anatomy is evident by radiographic examination. All injured children must have the cervical spine managed by in-line immobilization with the head in a neutral position, or by application of a rigid cervical collar. Uncontrolled manipulation of the cervical spine may lead to spinal cord injury. A lateral x-ray of the cervical spine (C1 to C7) is necessary to evaluate vertebral skeletal alignment.

Airway management in a spontaneously breath-

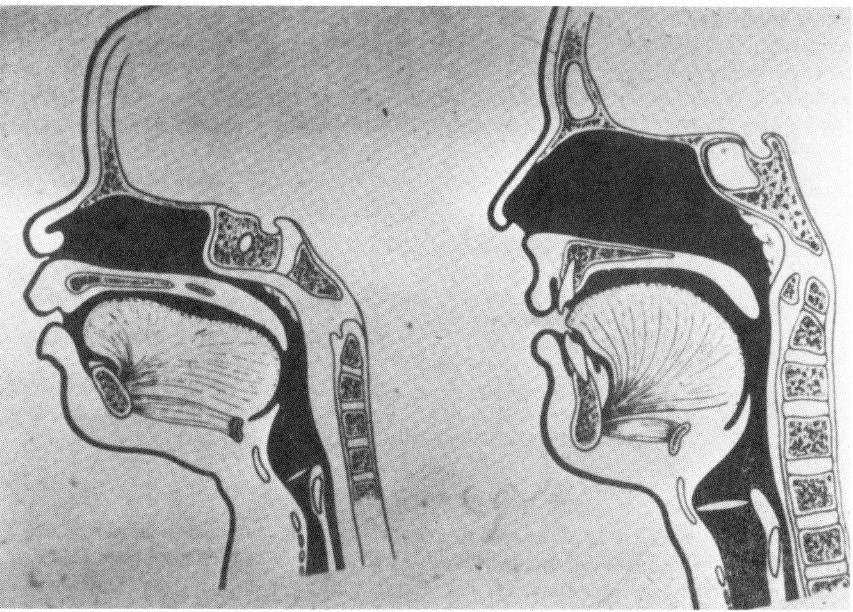

Figure 16–1 Comparison of adult and child airways. (From McGill WA: Airway management. In Eichelberger MR, Pratsch GL, editors: *Pediatric airway management,* Rockville, Md, 1988, Aspen Publications. Reprinted with permission from Aspen Publications, Inc.)

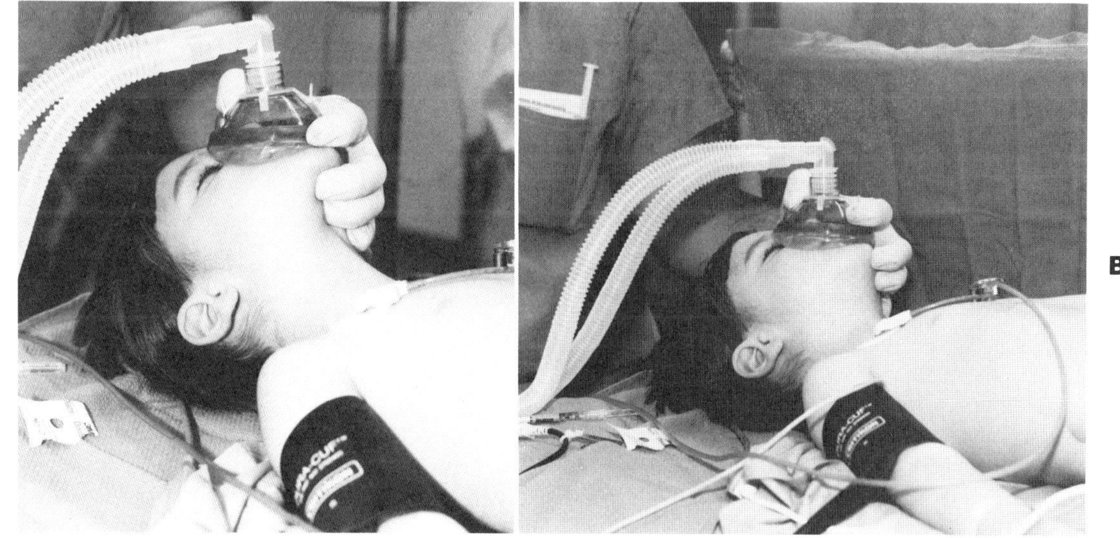

Figure 16–2 A, Incorrect finger placement. **B,** Correct finger placement.

ing child requires the following maneuvers: open the airway by means of a jaw thrust; suction the mouth and oropharyngeal areas clear of secretions and debris, while simultaneously administering supplemental oxygen (5 to 10 L/min). Excessive extension of the neck to open the airway must be prevented until the cervical spines are confirmed to be intact.

During assisted or controlled ventilation, the airway manager must prevent the application of undue submental pressure while achieving an effective mask seal around the mouth and nose. This maneuver, usually successful in adults, can result in complete airway obstruction in a small child as the tongue is pushed upward and backward into the relatively small oropharyngeal space (Fig. 16-2).

Table 16–1 Oral and nasopharyngeal airways: complications

Complication	Treatment
Induction of retching and vomiting	Suction: Turn patient on side, head down if conditions permit; remove airway; intubate trachea
Pushing tongue or foreign materials posteriorly, causing obstruction	Remove airway and/or foreign substance; intubate trachea
High airway resistance owing to inadequate lumen of nasopharyngeal airway	Remove airway; intubate
Epistaxis from nasopharyngeal airway placement	Remove airway; apply suction; intubate

From McGill WA: Airway management. In Eichelberger MR, Pratsch GL, editors: *Pediatric airway management*, Rockville, Md, 1988, Aspen Publications. Reprinted with permission from Aspen Publications, Inc.

ORAL AND NASAL AIRWAYS

Oral and nasal airways do not protect the lungs from aspiration of vomitus, blood, or foreign material and cannot reliably ensure a patent airway. These devices are meant to displace the tongue so that adequate air movement is ensured. Table 16-1 lists some of the common problems encountered when these airway adjuncts are used. They are useful only as temporizing measures to enhance gentle positive-pressure mask ventilation during preparation for tracheal intubation or cricothyrotomy. Strong suction is essential for proper management of an injured child, as it may be required to keep the airway clear. Adequate oral suction and oxygen administration are all that is necessary to treat respiratory insufficiency in a large number of injured children.

TRACHEAL INTUBATION

Endotracheal intubation is necessary in any child who cannot control his own airway or maintain oxygenation or ventilation (Table 16-2). Oral endotracheal intubation is the "gold standard"; nasotracheal intubation has no place in a newly injured child. Nasotracheal intubation is specifically contraindicated if a basilar skull fracture is present. This approach to intubation is also slower, more difficult to perform, and much more stimulating to the child than a swift, facile orotracheal intubation. Moreover, the larger amount of tonsil and adenoid

Table 16–2 Situations in which tracheal intubation is indicated

For cardiopulmonary resuscitation
In an unconscious patient
    To overcome soft-tissue obstruction
    To prevent aspiration of vomitus and foreign matter
    To ensure proper O_2/CO_2 exchange and thus prevent secondary brain injury
To bypass direct airway obstruction from airway or facial trauma
For prophylaxis in a child whose facial or airway burn or trauma will probably lead to a subsequent obstruction from edema
Under any circumstance in which inadequate gas exchange is life threatening, e.g.,
    Apnea
    Cyanosis
    Trauma to lung or bellows mechanism

From McGill WA: Airway management. In Eichelberger MR, Pratsch GL, editors: *Pediatric airway management*, Rockville, Md, 1988, Aspen Publications. Reprinted with permission from Aspen Publications, Inc.

Table 16–3 Recommended tracheal tube sizes in relation to age

Age	Internal diameter (ID) (mm)
Premature (2.5 kg)	2.5
Term newborn	3.0
6 months	3.5
12 months	4.5
18-24 months	4.5
4 years	5.0-5.5
6 years	5.5-6.0
8 years	6.0-6.5
10 years	6.5
12 years	7.0
14 years	7.5
Adults	8.0-9.5

Note: Children of the same age vary in size; occasionally a tube 0.5 mm smaller or larger in ID may be required. General formula for children older than 2 years of age:

$$\text{Tube ID (mm)} = \frac{\text{age (years)}}{4} + 4.5$$

From McGill WA: Airway management. In Eichelberger MR, Pratsch GL, editors: *Pediatric airway management*, Rockville, Md, 1988, Aspen Publications. Reprinted with permission from Aspen Publications, Inc.

tissue present in school-aged children is subject to injury during nasotracheal intubation.

Uncuffed tubes of proper sizes are recommended for children less than 6 to 8 years of age to minimize vocal cord trauma, subglottic edema, and ulceration. Although there are a number of formulas for calculating correct endotracheal tube size, a quick and available index for tube size selection is to choose a diameter equal to that of the distal phalanx of the child's little finger (Table 16-3). A range of endotracheal tube sizes should always be available. Stylets may be very useful; they should be lubricated before insertion into the endotracheal tube. Lubrication with surgical jelly, or even the patient's own saliva, reduces friction so that the stylet can be removed from the endotracheal tube following proper placement into the trachea.

It is important to remember to maintain neutral alignment of the cervical spine during all airway manipulations.

Always check the endotracheal tube position by listening to breath sounds over both lung apices and by observing the symmetry of the thoracic excursion. If chest wall excursion or breath sounds are unequal, the endotracheal tube should be withdrawn slowly until breath sounds are equal at both apices. Although breath sounds and evidence of CO_2 on a capnogram or detection device indicate that the endotracheal tube is positioned in the trachea, it must be noted that endotracheal tubes frequently move during the turbulence of a resuscitation. This is a particular problem in small children, in whom a 1-cm movement of an endotracheal tube can cause endobronchial intubation or unrecognized extubation. Constant vigilance regarding proper endotracheal tube position is essential.

If the endotracheal tube position is proper, but breath sounds are absent in one lung, it is reasonable to suspect a pneumothorax. Auscultation of the epigastric area to detect esophageal intubation is also important. Inflation of the stomach or gurgling sounds heard with the stethoscope indicate esophageal intubation. In this event, withdraw the endotracheal tube, reestablish mask ventilation, and replace the endotracheal tube into the trachea.

After the primary survey, a chest x-ray examination is essential in checking for proper endotracheal tube placement. It is also essential to secure the endotracheal tube prior to transporting the child, in order to prevent extubation and esophageal or endobronchial migration. Markings on the tube are used to verify the position of the endotracheal tube; 12 cm at the gums in a 1-year-old, with an additional centimeter of depth for each year of age, is a reasonable depth. These markings permit surveillance of endotracheal tube position at all times. Bilateral breath sounds must be assessed after every move of the patient. It is possible for an unrecognized extubation to occur, wherein the endotracheal tube is out of the trachea while still in the oropharynx.

Uncertainty regarding cervical spine stability makes it desirable to wait for cervical spine films prior to laryngoscopy. However, emergency intu-

Table 16–4 Controlled intubation sequence

1. Clear and support airway (suction)
2. Ventilate with 100% O_2 by bag and mask
3. Administer cricoid pressure
4. Administer pentothal (4 mg/kg, only if cardiovascular system is stable) and vecuronium (0.1 mg/kg)
5. Intubate 3 minutes after administering vecuronium
6. If suspected or existing cervical spine fracture, perform laryngoscopy and intubation while assistant provides in-line traction on neck

From McGill WA: Airway management. In Eichelberger MR, Pratsch GL, editors: *Pediatric airway management*, Rockville, Md, 1988, Aspen Publications. Reprinted with permission from Aspen Publications, Inc.

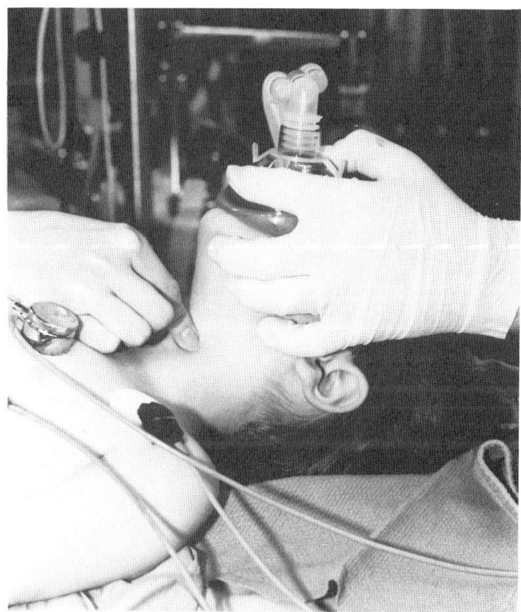

Figure 16–3 Cricoid pressure.

bation is frequently necessary (Table 16-4). Prior to laryngoscopy, gentle mask ventilation with cricoid pressure permits maximum oxygenation prior to the apneic period during laryngoscopy (Fig. 16-3). Cricoid pressure is used only to prevent regurgitation, not to prevent active vomiting. In-line cervical immobilization to keep the cervical spine in the neutral position requires an additional assistant during laryngoscopy (Fig. 16-4). If a hard collar is in place, remove the anterior piece of the collar during laryngoscopy in order to displace the mandible and tongue forward.

Increased intracranial pressure is likely in an unconscious child with a head injury. Attempts to

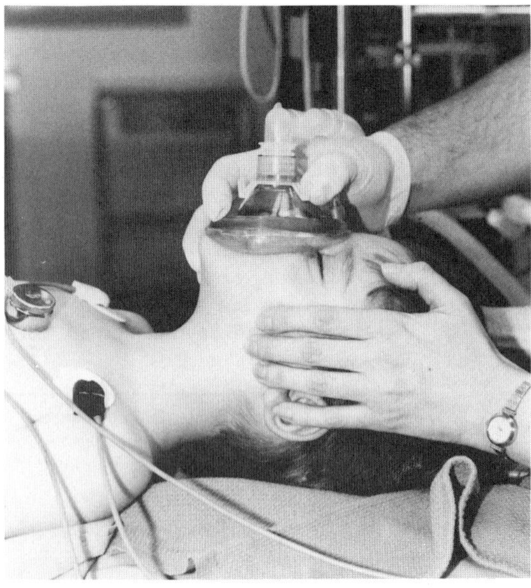

Figure 16–4 In-line cervical traction.

intubate a partially responsive, coughing, gagging, combative child will cause further elevation of intracranial pressure. Optimal conditions for intubation are possible with administration of a short-acting barbiturate (pentothal or surital 2-4 mg/kg) and a muscle relaxant such as vecuronium (0.1 mg/ kg). Optimal relaxation will be present in 2 to 3 minutes, during which time maintenance of oxygenation and ventilation with a bag and mask are essential. A shorter-acting muscle relaxant (succinylcholine 2 mg/kg IV) and a benzodiazepine are reasonable alternatives. These drugs, however, are less protective against the intracranial pressure response resulting from laryngoscopy. Atropine (0.02 mg/kg) or glycopyrrolate (0.01 mg/kg) prevents bradycardia associated with succinylcholine. These anticholinergics may also be administered to children less than 10 years of age to prevent bradycardia secondary to the vagal stimulation of laryngoscopy.

It is important to differentiate between children who require amnesia and muscle relaxation from those who are undergoing resuscitation. All amnestic agents are myocardial depressants, which contraindicates administration of a sedative to a child who is hypovolemic or hypotensive. In addition, administration of a muscle relaxant requires certainty on the part of the clinician that he or she can maintain the child's airway and ventilate him or her. These potent drugs *should not be administered* unless the clinician possesses the skills to control the child's airway. Finally, it should be kept in mind that any sedative or muscle relaxant can im-

Table 16–5 Situations in which intubation may be impossible

Massive maxillofacial trauma
Inability to visualize larynx or need for blind intubation because cervical fracture precludes proper tube position
Unusual patient anatomy (Goldenhar's syndrome, Pierre Robin syndrome, and the like)
Absence of personnel skilled in procedure
Foreign body and upper airway obstruction

From McGill WA: Airway management. In Eichelberger MR, Pratsch GL, editors: *Pediatric airway management,* Rockville, Md, 1988, Aspen Publications. Reprinted with permission from Aspen Publications, Inc.

Table 16–6 Considerations for airway management in burned children

Indications for careful airway evaluation
Patients burned in confined space
Patients with soot on nares, face, or mouth

Evidence of upper airway burn (indications for tracheal tube placement)
Facial burns from fire in closed space
Singed nasal hairs
Carbonaceous sputum
Edema, erythema, or searing of any part of airway from lips to larynx

From McGill WA: Airway management. In Eichelberger MR, Pratsch GL, editors: *Pediatric airway management,* Rockville, Md, 1988, Aspen Publications. Reprinted with permission from Aspen Publications, Inc.

pair a child's neurologic status. Shorter-acting agents are more appropriate if the child's level of consciousness is a clinical concern.

CRICOTHYROTOMY

Occasionally, maintenance of the airway by endotracheal intubation is impossible (Table 16-5). Needle cricothyrotomy (14-gauge needle) is preferable to surgical cricothyrotomy. Insertion of a needle requires less technical skill and can save a child's life. Surgical cricothyrotomy is technically much more difficult in a small child than in an adult, because the neck structures are closer to each other in a small child. Although cricothyrotomy provides a means of emergency oxygenation, ventilation (maintaining normocarbia) is much more difficult. In addition, the patient can still aspirate stomach contents during this procedure.

More definitive airway management methods, such as retrograde intubation or tracheostomy, facilitate ventilation and provide definitive airway control. Needle tracheostomy is preferable in children.

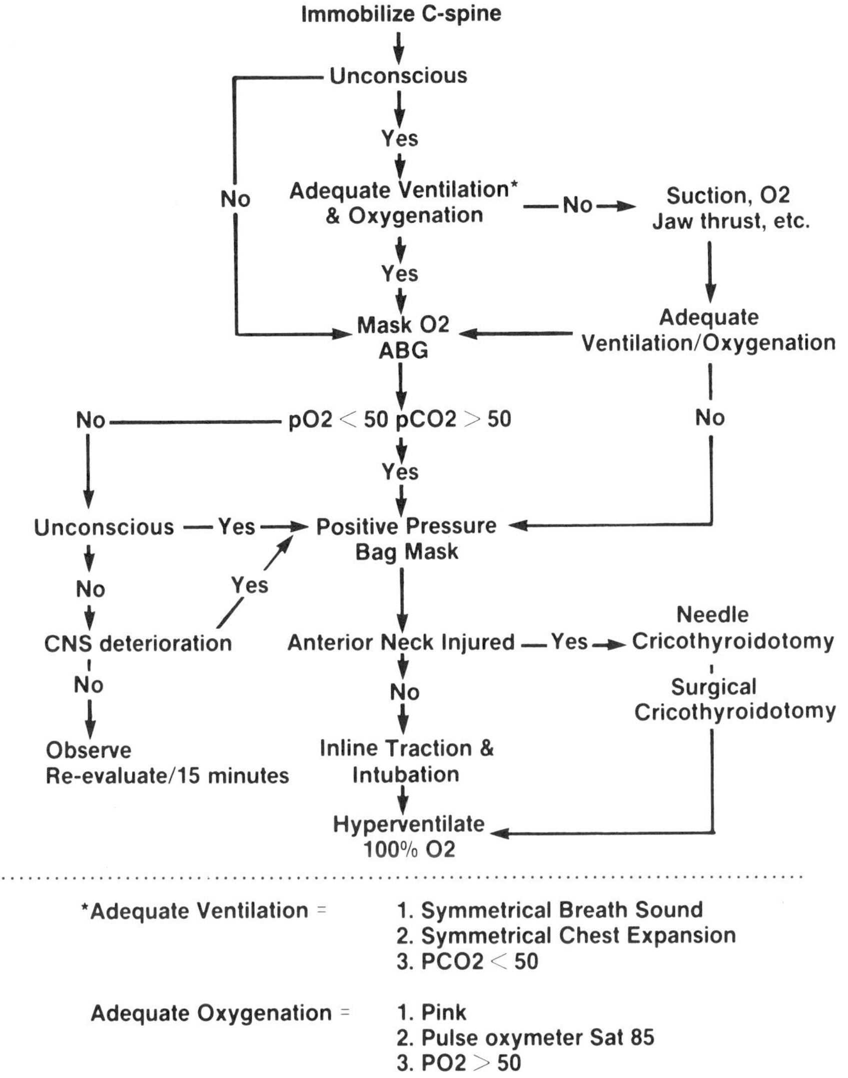

Figure 16–5 Airway management in children with head injury. (From McGill WA: Airway management. In Eichelberger MR, Pratsch GL, editors: *Pediatric airway management*, Rockville, Md, 1988, Aspen Publications. Reprinted with permission from Aspen Publications, Inc.)

AIRWAY MANAGEMENT FOR BURNED CHILDREN

Children with burn injuries require early airway evaluation. Heat injury to the upper airway leads to rapid development of edema of the tongue, pharynx, and larynx (Table 16-6). The upper airway becomes obstructed, and mask ventilation increasingly difficult; as tissues become swollen and distorted, endotracheal intubation is likewise progressively more difficult. Prophylactic intubation is useful if heat injury to the upper airway is suspected. Removal of an endotracheal tube is easier than placement of the critically necessary one.

Inhaled toxic fumes and carbonaceous particles produce chemical injury at all levels of the airway and lung, leading to bronchospasm, pulmonary edema, and hypoxia. When cyanosis or respiratory distress persists in spite of 100% oxygen administration by mask, tracheal intubation ensures efficient delivery of high concentrations of inspired oxygen and permits application of positive end-expiratory pressure in the treatment of pulmonary edema and hypoxia.

Carbon monoxide poisoning produces hypoxia, because carbon monoxide binds the hemoglobin molecule more tightly than does oxygen. High carboxyhemoglobin levels produce tissue hypoxia, which affects the central nervous system. Because pulse oximetry and arterial blood oxygen may be normal, blood carboxyhemoglobin levels are necessary for diagnosis. The half-life of carboxyhemoglobin in a child breathing room air is 4 hours, but only 30 minutes with administration of 100% oxygen.

SUMMARY

Situations requiring intervention with mask ventilation and endotracheal intubation include

1. Unconscious child who is not breathing
2. Any child who is not moving enough air to maintain oxygenation or who is cyanotic
3. ABGs with pO_2 <50 and/or respiratory acidosis or SpO_2 <90

The ABCs of resuscitation of the injured child (airway, breathing, and circulation) stress *airway:* support the airway, secure the airway, and protect the cervical spine in any injured child (Fig. 16-5). Of course, techniques necessary to provide an airway vary with the age of the child.

REFERENCES

1. Latto IP, Rosen M: *Difficulties in tracheal intubation,* London, 1986, Balliere Tindall.
2. McGill WA: Airway management. In Eichelberger MR, Pratsch GL, editors: *Pediatric airway management,* Rockville, Md, 1988, Aspen Publications.
3. Roberts JT: *Fundamentals of tracheal intubation,* New York, 1983, Grune & Stratton.
4. Whitten CE: Anyone can intubate, San Diego, Calif, 1989, Medical Arts Press.

17 Ventilation Essentials

Mary E. Fallat

Ventilation is the cyclic process of air exchange. Ventilation disturbances in injured children may be caused by a number of anatomic or physiologic derangements that are not necessarily related to a direct chest injury. Ventilation abnormalities are detected through a combination of clinical skills and laboratory investigations, and their treatment ranges from the simple administration of oxygen to complex surgical procedures. The effect of a ventilation disorder is functional and potentially life-threatening, which is why it is important for every clinician to develop the skills necessary to recognize respiratory insufficiency. Regardless of the cause of the disturbance, every injured child is approached with a high level of suspicion for injury until normal ventilation is established.

Blunt trauma accounts for the majority of life-threatening injuries causing respiratory compromise in children. Specific injuries to the chest or upper airway are often associated with trauma to other anatomic sites, as a result of the force required to cause an injury to the chest or neck in a child. Approximately 5% of injured children less than 14 years of age who receive treatment at a trauma center have a chest injury, and mortality in this group is 25%.[11]

NORMAL PHYSIOLOGY AND ANATOMY OF VENTILATION

Normal ventilation provides for maintenance of arterial oxygen, carbon dioxide, and pH at the least level of work.[2,3,10] The alveolar-capillary membrane is thin, and normally there is no difference in oxygen tension between the alveolar gas and pulmonary venous blood, or in arterial and alveolar carbon dioxide tensions. Ventilation involves movement of air in and out of the lungs. The diaphragm is the most important muscle for normal inspiration, although intercostal and accessory respiratory muscles aid in maximal inspiratory effort. Quiet expiration results from elastic recoil of the lungs and chest wall and relaxation of the diaphragm. The mechanical factors in lung expansion include flow-resistive or dynamic properties and elastic or static properties, known as compliance. The dynamic properties of lung expansion are air-way resistance and tissue viscous resistance, which combine to make up total pulmonary resistance. The work of breathing requires energy to overcome inertia, surface active forces, airflow and elastic resistance, and tissue viscous resistance. Rate and depth of breathing are adjusted so that alveolar ventilation is maintained at a minimum of respiratory work. Approximately 1% of total basal metabolism is normally expended on the work of breathing.

The mechanism that regulates and maintains pulmonary gas exchange is normally remarkably efficient. In healthy children, the level of arterial P_{CO_2} is maintained within a very narrow range in spite of varying demands for oxygen and CO_2 production during exercise and rest. A precise match of the level of ventilation to the output of CO_2 is achieved by a combination of neural and chemical controls.

In the normal situation, pulmonary ventilation is maintained with rhythmic contraction and relaxation of respiratory muscles. The central neural control of respiration is in the medulla, where tonic activity in the inspiratory center is periodically inhibited by the excitement of neurons in the adjacent expiratory center (Fig. 17-1). In addition, medullary chemoreceptors regulate alveolar ventilation and maintenance of normal arterial P_{CO_2} and P_{O_2}. The central chemoreceptors are located in the medulla but are anatomically separate from the respiratory center. They respond to changes in hydrogen ion concentration in the adjacent cerebral spinal fluid, rather than to changes in arterial P_{CO_2} or pH. Peripheral chemoreceptors react rapidly to changes in Pa_{CO_2} and pH and contribute to the respiratory drive. The primary role of peripheral chemoreceptors is their response to changes in arterial P_{O_2}. Moderate to severe hypoxemia (Pa_{O_2} less than or equal to 64) results in a significant increase in ventilation in children of all ages with the exception of newborns.

A child has an increased metabolic rate with oxygen demands that are two to three times greater than an adult's. Oxygenation is dependent on the adequacy of pulmonary circulation or pulmonary perfusion. Maintenance of the ventilation-perfu-

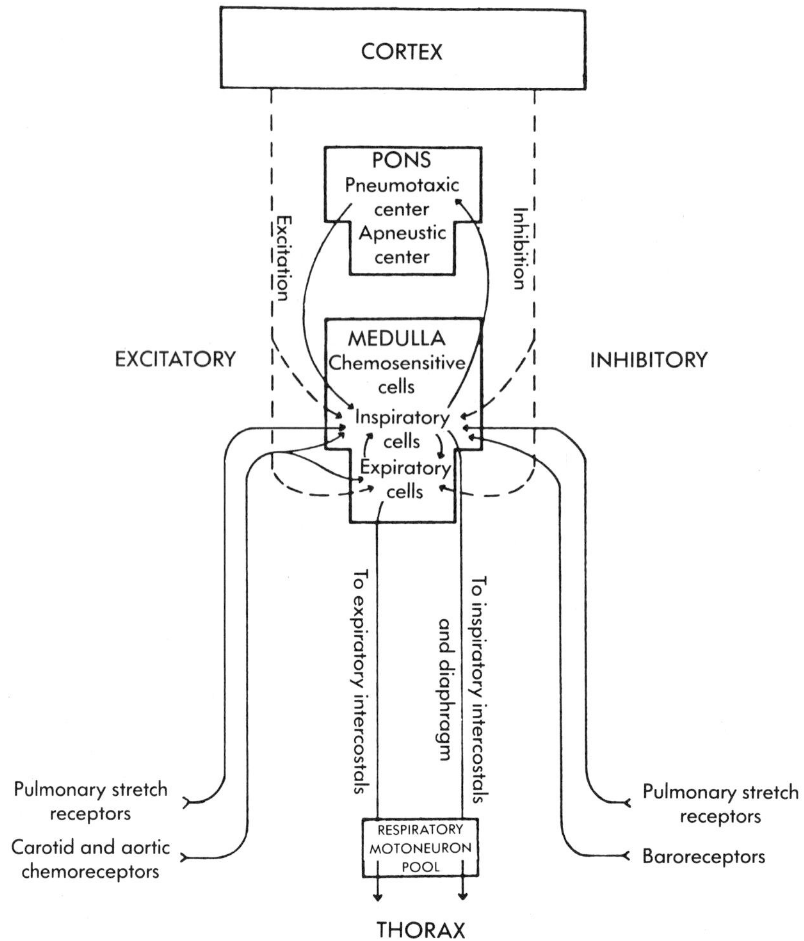

Figure 17–1 Schematic representation of the respiratory centers and their important connections. (From Mountcastle VB, editor: *Medical physiology,* ed 13, St Louis, 1974, Mosby–Year Book.)

sion relationship is instrumental to adequate pulmonary function. With disease, the mechanism providing for ventilation-perfusion adjustment may be sufficiently damaged to result in regional imbalances, leading to a decrease in arterial oxygen tension. Minimal overall alveolar hyperventilation can maintain carbon dioxide tension at normal or low levels until much later in an injury process, because of the greater ease of diffusion of carbon dioxide across the alveolus.

The pediatric airway differs from that of the adult in several important ways.[5,7] Anatomic differences of the upper airway include a larynx that is relatively cephalad in position and an epiglottis that is U-shaped and protrudes into the pharynx. The vocal cords are short and concave, and in children less than 8 years of age the narrowest portion of the airway is at the cricoid cartilage rather than at the level of the vocal cords. The larynx and lower airways are smaller, and the supporting cartilage is less developed in the infant and small child than

in the adult. This predisposes these structures to a higher rate of obstruction by secretions, swelling, spasm, or foreign material. It is relatively difficult to visualize a clear plane from the mouth through the pharynx to the glottis for endotracheal intubation in the small child. The selection of endotracheal tube size must be based on the size of the cricoid ring rather than the glottic opening. A child has a relatively large tongue, compared with the surface area of the oral cavity, which may drop back when the child is in the supine position and cause an upper airway obstruction. Laxity of the arytenoid muscle attachment of the tongue, however, permits mobility during visualization of the larynx.

The ribs and sternum normally support the lung and help it to remain expanded. The intercostal muscles and diaphragm alter intrathoracic pressure and volume leading to movement of air. In young children, the ribs often fail to support the lung since the chest cage is so pliable, thereby leading to paradoxic sternal and intercostal retractions during active inspiration, rather than lung expansion. Tidal volume in the child is much more dependent on function and movement of the diaphragm. When intrathoracic processes or increased intraperitoneal pressure interferes with diaphragmatic movement, effective respiration is compromised since the chest wall is unable to compensate.

The child has a compliant chest wall that ordinarily resists fracture, but a force is more easily transmitted to the underlying lung parenchyma, resulting in pulmonary contusion or hemopneumothorax. The mediastinum of the child is more mobile than that of an adult, accounting for a low incidence of major vessel or airway injury. In addition, the child lacks calcifications in the great vessels, which allows them to shift with the mediastinum rather than shear against it, producing less susceptibility to transection. The more mobile mediastinum of the child, however, may result in rapid cardiovascular and ventilatory compromise owing to dislocation of the heart, angulation of the great vessels, compression of the lung, and angulation of the trachea.

ALTERATIONS IN PHYSIOLOGY CAUSED BY SPECIFIC INJURY

Partial or complete upper airway obstruction is probably the most common indication for airway support in the injured child. There are many factors that influence the duration of total airway obstruction that a child will tolerate before becoming profoundly hypoxic. These factors include the inspired oxygen concentration prior to obstruction, lung capacity, ongoing rates of oxygen consumption and carbon dioxide production, intravascular blood volume and hemoglobin concentration. When airway obstruction occurs, the increase in intrathoracic pressure also causes an elevation of intracranial pressure, owing to a decrease in return of cerebral venous blood to the heart. This situation is particularly detrimental in the child with a head injury.[1]

In a child who sustains a head injury, the most common cause of airway obstruction is posterior displacement of the tongue. The muscles of the upper airway are activated synchronously with the inspiratory effort to ensure a patent oropharynx. If the negative pharyngeal pressure created during inspiration overcomes the distending pressure exerted by the upper-airway muscles, airway obstruction occurs. A loss of protective airway reflexes, including cough, gag, and swallowing, also commonly occurs in the child with acute brain injury. This loss of protective reflexes occurs with or without lower cranial nerve dysfunction and imposes the threat of regurgitation and aspiration resulting from an inability to protect the airway. Absence of cough results in inability to mobilize mucus and debris in the trachea and peripheral pulmonary tree, thus causing predisposition to atelectasis and pneumonia.

Pneumothorax

Pneumothorax is a collection of air within the pleural space resulting from a disruption of lung parenchyma, a tear in the tracheobronchial tree, penetration of the chest wall, or an esophageal perforation. If a child suffers a blow to the chest when the glottis is closed, the direct force is applied to the alveoli, resulting in localized rupture. With blows sufficient to cause rib fractures, the sharp bone fragments can cause parenchymal lacerations. The presence of blood in the pleural space or hemothorax is also associated with lacerations and penetrating injuries.[4]

The child with a pneumothorax may be asymptomatic or have severe respiratory distress. Physical findings include decreased breath sounds on the ipsilateral side, hyperresonance to percussion, external abrasions on the chest, or subcutaneous emphysema of the chest wall. Subcutaneous emphysema results from air escape into the subcutaneous tissues through a tear in the parietal pleura. Tension pneumothorax occurs with the progressive entry of air into the pleural space, which cannot escape. Intrapleural pressure rises with ensuing collapse of the ipsilateral lung, shift of the mediastinum to the opposite side, and compression of the contralateral lung. As air fills the ipsilateral pleural space, the diaphragm may be significantly depressed, further embarrassing respiratory function.

In open pneumothorax, there is a traumatic communication between the pleural space and the environment. An immediate equilibration of intrathoracic and atmospheric pressure occurs with collapse of the lung and shift of the mediastinum. A large opening allows air to pass freely in and out of the chest. A small opening allows air entry during inspiration, but may obstruct air exit during expiration, producing a further shift of the mediastinum and a tension phenomenon. There may also be a to-and-fro movement of the mediastinum, resulting in a decrease in venous return to the right heart. The mediastinal shift causes angulation of the vena cava, which interferes with blood return to the right atrium, decreases cardiac output, and leads to cardiovascular collapse.

Traumatic asphyxia

Traumatic asphyxia occurs with direct compression of the chest wall caused by a blow or severe crush injury to the chest. If the child takes a deep inspiration with the glottis closed, it results in transient venous hypertension in the upper part of the body.

There is an absence of valves in the venous system of the inferior and superior vena cava, resulting in transmission of the hypertension to the brain. Patients usually exhibit disorientation and evidence of respiratory compromise. Signs of traumatic asphyxia include cyanosis of the face and neck; petechiae of the head, neck, and chest; subconjunctival hemorrhages; and retinal hemorrhages. Associated intrathoracic and upper abdominal injuries are common.

Flail chest

A flail chest is an injury associated with multiple rib fractures, usually resulting from high-velocity trauma. The flail segment is characterized by paradoxic movement resulting from loss of continuity with the rest of the chest wall. The free segment of the chest wall moves inward with inspiration and outward with expiration. This paradoxic movement is pathognomonic of a flail chest, and it greatly interferes with normal ventilatory physiology. The lung parenchyma underlying the flail segment frequently sustains a contusion. This decreases the volume of pulmonary parenchyma available for respiratory efforts and results in a diffusion abnormality caused by blood within the alveoli. Hypoxemia results from a ventilation-perfusion defect through the poorly ventilated and contused pulmonary parenchyma.

Pulmonary contusion

Pulmonary contusion resulting from blunt injury to the chest is common and frequently associated with both localized pulmonary edema and atelectasis. A pulmonary contusion disrupts the effectiveness of the alveolar-capillary interface, causing a diminution in PaO_2 and an increase in intrapulmonary shunt, and results in swelling of endothelial cells. Plasma moves into the basement membrane and alveolar spaces, causing edema of the alveolar epithelium; this results in progressive hypoxia. The extravasation of fluid and blood into the alveolar and interstitial spaces provides an excellent culture medium for bacteria, and extensive involvement by contusion may effect a predisposition to adult respiratory distress syndrome (ARDS).

Adult respiratory distress syndrome

Common synonyms for ARDS include shock lung, posttraumatic pulmonary insufficiency, and pulmonary insufficiency syndrome. The common etiology for ARDS is injury at the alveolar-capillary interface with leakage of proteinaceous fluid from the intravascular space into the interstitium and alveolar spaces. Common denominators in the injuries leading to ARDS are systemic hypotension and extensive tissue damage. Unfortunately, many of the therapeutic maneuvers used to treat specific traumatic injuries may contribute to or aggravate the respiratory failure that ensues.

The pathophysiology of ARDS is a loss of functional residual capacity (FRC) or of gas volume left in the lung at the end of a normal tidal volume. The FRC is a buffer against hypoxia, and its decrease in ARDS is due to alveolar collapse, atelectasis, hemorrhage, edema, exudate, and hyaline membrane formation. The loss of FRC results in ventilation-perfusion mismatch or a shunt. In other words, the alveoli no longer oxygenate the blood that perfuses the parenchyma, making treatment by increases in inspired oxygen futile. A marked increase in dead space ventilation results, further resulting in hypercarbia and the need for hyperventilation. Cardiovascular dysfunction is also common in ARDS.

The pathologic appearance of ARDS is well documented. The acute phase is characterized by interstitial edema and fibrin thrombi in the microvasculature, resulting in focal destruction of the blood-gas barrier and endothelial cell damage. Progression of the disease leads to alveolar epithelialization and interstitial fibrosis. Oxygen toxicity is the proposed mechanism responsible for these findings.[6]

The symptoms of ARDS include tachypnea, dyspnea, and hypoxemia, which develop over time, associated with radiographic evidence of diffuse fluffy infiltrates, loss of lung volume, and development of extra parenchymal lung water. Although the symptoms of pulmonary contusion are similar, they appear almost immediately following injury. Radiographic evidence of pulmonary contusion is usually apparent on initial chest x-ray, is focal in nature, and tends to resolve over 2 to 6 days. The clinical evolution of ARDS occurs some time after the injury, symptoms usually becoming apparent 12 to 24 hours after injury.

Adult respiratory distress syndrome is often seen in children who exhibit profound shock, or for whom treatment of profound shock is delayed. The infusion of lactated Ringers', plasma, and blood products to restore effective circulating volume may enhance fluid leakage into the alveoli. Additional iatrogenic insults that may contribute to ARDS include the use of high oxygen concentrations, which may predispose to oxygen toxicity, and high ventilating pressures that result in barotrauma and secondary air leak, which may further exacerbate the disease process.

Inhalation injuries

Inhalation injuries usually result from fires within closed spaces. The injury to the respiratory tract is the result of irritation and inflammation caused by noxious gases and smoke in combination with asphyxia resulting from carbon monoxide poisoning. Carbon monoxide enters the circulatory system, causing a shift of the carboxyhemoglobin curve to the left and inability of the tissues to extract oxygen, thereby resulting in hypoxia. The products of combustion cause a chemical tracheobronchitis that leads to mucosal slough, injury to mucus-producing cells, and injury to respiratory cilia that clean the airway. This loss of normal airway maintenance can permit entry of bacteria into the lung parenchyma and atelectasis. Atelectasis that is not cleared promptly predisposes to bacterial colonization and pneumonia.[8]

There are three temporal stages of pulmonary injury: (1) respiratory insufficiency with bronchospasm occurring at 1 to 12 hours following injury, (2) pulmonary edema at 6 to 72 hours, and (3) bronchopneumonia after 60 hours.[12] Herndon and colleagues[9] found that inhalation injuries are associated with an increase in extravascular lung water (EVLW) during the first 24 hours after injury; lung edema is attributed to the toxic effects of smoke inhalation. This increase in lung microvascular permeability is attenuated by increasing cardiac output to normal levels with appropriate fluid resuscitation. Fluid resuscitation is increased on the order of 2 ml/kg/percent body surface area burned above calculated resuscitation volumes. Fluid restriction may lead to excessive pulmonary fluid formation and hypoxia. Inhalation injury renders a child at risk for recurrent chest infections for several weeks following injury, owing to lack of the normal protection of mucous and ciliary action. The complication of pneumonia in respiratory injury poses a significant threat and increases risk of mortality.

GENERAL MANAGEMENT SCHEME

The initial symptoms of a ventilatory disturbance may appear soon after the injury occurs or up to several hours later. Signs of respiratory compromise are hoarseness or stridor, subcutaneous emphysema in the head or neck area, cyanosis, dyspnea, or frank respiratory distress with or without apnea.

Initial radiologic evaluation that may help to establish a diagnosis of injuries contributing to ventilation disturbance include a lateral cervical spine film to document fractures or impingement on the airway, and a chest x-ray to evaluate the pulmonary parenchyma, mediastinum, and cardiac silhouette. An arteriogram is essential if one suspects an injury to the great vessels in the chest or neck. Laryngoscopy, bronchoscopy, and esophagoscopy help define injuries not readily apparent in examination or in radiologic studies. The electrocardiogram and echocardiogram are useful to define further a suspected injury to the heart.

Resuscitation of any injured child begins with *A*irway, *B*reathing and *C*irculation, the ABCs of basic and advanced life support. A high level of suspicion should be maintained for an injury to the airway throughout resuscitation. Possible airway adjuncts may be required, including oxygen, the jaw thrust maneuver, suction, an oral airway, a bag-valve-mask device, or an endotracheal tube.[5]

Upper-airway obstruction

Upper-airway obstruction poses a threat in almost all traumatic injury, particularly if there is a loss of consciousness. Rarely does an injured child have an empty stomach. The risk of vomiting and of aspiration is considerable in the unconscious child who has a loss of normal reflexes. Upper-airway obstruction in small infants and children occurs as a consequence of posterior displacement of the relatively large tongue in comparison with a small oropharynx. Obstruction by the tongue is common in a child in the supine position; a simple manual jaw thrust can displace the tongue forward to relieve the obstruction.

Foreign body

The presence of a foreign body in the airway is a true emergency because of the potential for total airway obstruction. The clinical presentation reflects the location of the obstruction. Laryngotracheal foreign bodies are evidenced by stridor, cough, and dyspnea. A foreign body lodged in the more distal tracheobronchial tree produces a ball-valve effect, which causes hyperaeration on the side of aspiration and compensatory atelectasis in the opposite lung. The most common symptoms and signs of lower-airway foreign bodies are wheezing, dyspnea, decreased air entry, and cough. Differential breath sounds upon auscultation are a helpful diagnostic finding. If coughing and phonation are present, encouragement of the cough is helpful. The Heimlich maneuver is indicated for victims of aspiration who are choking and cyanotic.

Injury precluding endotracheal or nasotracheal intubation

Alternative maneuvers are indicated if the child has a facial or neck injury and respiratory embarrassment that preclude endotracheal or nasotracheal intubation. It is imperative to ascertain whether the injured child has an oxygenation or ventilatory disturbance, in order to guide the establishment of an emergency airway. If the child is able to maintain an airway, as was the case of the boy in Fig. 17-2, resuscitation, diagnostic tests, and tracheostomy

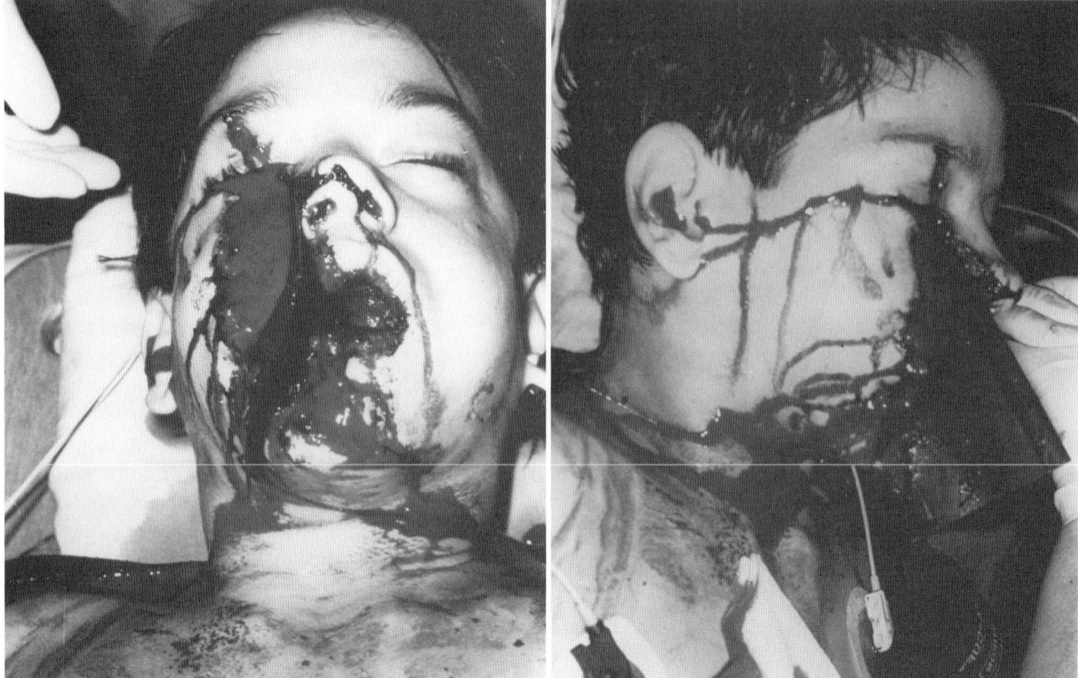

Figure 17–2 A, B, Adolescent who suffered the impact of a fan belt on his face while he was working under a vehicle. The patient was able to maintain his own airway during emergency evaluation, and a semiurgent tracheostomy was performed in the operating room.

are best performed under controlled conditions in the operating room. Further injury to the airway or loss of airway is possible if attempts are made to intubate a child under adverse circumstances, especially if the child is breathing without difficulty. The exception to this rule is the child with severe head, neck, or facial injury who requires transportation over a long distance to another facility.

Laryngeal trauma

Laryngeal trauma is rare in children and adolescents, but can occur with penetrating injuries, with suicide attempts by hanging, or with a car or motorcycle crash in which the victim collides with a horizontal fixed object, such as a dashboard or a fence that is at neck level. The presenting signs and symptoms of laryngeal trauma include stridor, subcutaneous emphysema of the neck area, and hoarseness if the child is able to vocalize. The most common anatomic sites of laryngeal fracture are the hyoid bone, thyroid cartilage, or cricoid cartilage. Cricotracheal separation may occur, a situation that warrants urgent cricothyrotomy or tracheostomy.

Pneumothorax

An open or tension pneumothorax or hemopneumothorax may pose a life-threatening problem in children owing to the mobility of the mediastinum and consequent cardiorespiratory compromise. In the presence of an open wound, it is important to place a sterile occlusive dressing over the area to stop the inflow of air into the chest. Subsequently, evacuation of intrapleural air is essential. Both types of pneumothorax may be initially managed with a needle thoracostomy placed in the second intercostal space at the midclavicular line. This maneuver is simple and will result in almost immediate relief of the tension. Upon stabilization of the child, insertion of a closed-tube thoracostomy permits continuous evacuation of air from the thorax.

Open or tension pneumothorax may be associated with more significant injuries to the tracheobronchial tree. This would be indicated by a continuous air leak from the chest tube following placement, or continued clinical respiratory distress. Bronchoscopy and bronchography are useful adjuncts in evaluating a potential tracheobronchial tear. Management of a distal injury to the tracheobronchial tree is possible by the infusion of fibrin-thrombin clot into the injured airway via a catheter through a bronchoscope. A major tracheobronchial injury requires thoracotomy or sternotomy for repair. Blood loss from the tube should be carefully monitored to avoid hypotension and assess the need for thoracotomy.

Flail chest

A flail chest, rare in children, is frequently associated with an underlying pulmonary contusion or penetrating injury to the lung parenchyma. Signs and symptoms of contusion, or associated pneumothorax or tracheobronchial injury, include hemoptysis, subcutaneous emphysema in the base of the neck, and persistent air leak after chest tube placement. A significant pulmonary contusion will result in hypoxemia from a ventilation-perfusion mismatch. In addition, the child may have a decrease in circulating blood volume secondary to the traumatic event, or a decrease in venous return secondary to the mediastinal shift compressing the vena cava. Occasionally a child is able to maintain normal blood gas levels by receiving mask or nasal oxygen, which permits management with intermittent rib blocks, pain medication, and aggressive pulmonary toilet consisting of nasotracheal suction, incentive spirometry, chest percussion and postural drainage, and ultrasonic nebulizer treatments.

In the presence of paradoxic motion and hypercarbia, most children require stabilization of the flail segment by endotracheal intubation and positive pressure ventilation. Positive pressure ventilation minimizes atelectasis and helps reapproximate the rib ends for healing, and endotracheal intubation allows for an improvement in pulmonary toilet. Unfortunately, the endotracheal tube also acts as a potential route for the introduction of bacteria and secondary iatrogenic infection. Appropriate management requires gradual removal of ventilator support. Infusion of crystalloid fluids during resuscitation is limited, if possible, to decrease pulmonary edema in the injured segment. Severe fluid restriction for an extended time, however, results in thickened secretions which make respiratory toilet difficult and iatrogenic infection more likely. Controlled ventilation with positive end-expiratory pressure (PEEP) is usually required for 2 to 3 days until the chest wall becomes stable enough to permit spontaneous respiration. Therapy related to the parenchymal injury is the major determinant for recovery; use of a servoventilator improves the ability to wean a child from mechanical respiratory support.

Cardiac injury

Although pericardial effusion and injury to the heart are rare in children, a pericardiocentesis is an important, and possibly lifesaving, technique. Beck's triad—muffled heart sounds, increased jugular venous distention, and decreased pulse pressure—suggests pericardial tamponade. If the condition of the child deteriorates, a pericardiocentesis helps to establish the diagnosis and provide immediate treatment. A positive pericardiocentesis for blood indicates the need for an urgent thoracotomy or median sternotomy to identify the cardiac injury in need of repair.

Myocardial contusion is also quite rare in children. It occurs more commonly in adolescents who drive cars and during a crash strike the steering wheel column at the sternum. The resulting chest pain and myocardial dysfunction may result in respiratory embarrassment. Diagnosis of myocardial contusion requires evaluation of cardiac isoenzymes, review of serial electrocardiograms, and performance of echocardiography to define the anatomy of the injury. Management is similar to that for a victim who has incurred a myocardial infarction.

Aerophagia

Aerophagia is a much greater problem in small children who are injured than in injured adults. The subsequent increase in intraabdominal girth and pressure can cause respiratory compromise, vomiting, and aspiration, particularly in a child with a head injury. Nasogastric tube decompression of the stomach reduces the potential of these complications. If a nasogastric tube fails to decrease abdominal distention, suspect intraabdominal hemorrhage or an intestinal perforation with free intraabdominal air. Abdominal distention limits ventilatory efforts owing to impingement upon the diaphragm; occasionally, endotracheal intubation is necessary when distention persists.

Diaphragmatic laceration

Diaphragmatic laceration can result from a fall from an excessive height or from a crush injury to the chest. The combination of chest wall pain and loss of diaphragm function makes ventilation extremely inefficient. When an injury to the diaphragm results in herniation of the intraabdominal contents into the chest, respiratory efforts are further compromised. The negative phase of the respiratory cycle draws the abdominal viscera into the chest, compromising lung expansion. Treatment consists of positive pressure ventilation, decompression of the stomach and upper intestinal tract with a nasogastric tube to prevent further gaseous distension of viscera in the thorax, and laparotomy to reduce the intraabdominal contents and repair the diaphragm.

Esophageal rupture

Esophageal rupture is rare and usually the result of forceful vomiting or ingestion of irregular foreign bodies, rather than blunt trauma; esophageal injury may occur with penetrating trauma. The child exhibits dysphagia, tachypnea, tachycardia, and fever. A chest roentgenogram may show a foreign body, mediastinal air, or a mediastinal air-fluid level indicative of an abscess. Esophagoscopy can remove a foreign body or document the injury; a contrast esophagram aids in diagnosis.

Inhalation injury

Inhalation injury results in considerable disturbances in both ventilation and oxygenation. Between 3% and 15% of children admitted to a burn unit have associated inhalation injury. Ventilation injury has been found to be the most important determinant of mortality in burn patients. An inhalation injury produces singed nasal hair, perioral and intraoral soot, and severe facial burns. The normal mechanism of injury is a fire occurring in a closed space. Clinical signs include carbonatious sputum and hoarseness. The child who appears symptom-free a few hours after injury may develop significant respiratory distress within a few more hours owing to respiratory irritation caused by the products of combustion. Arterial blood gas analysis and a carboxyhemoglobin blood level are laboraory studies that aid in the diagnosis of a respiratory injury. Diagnostic bronchoscopy and/or laryngoscopy help confirm the diagnosis. Treatment of severe injury of the tracheobronchial tree is best managed by endotracheal intubation in anticipation of airway edema and asphyxia. The primary goals of endotracheal intubation and ventilatory therapy are (1) to provide an adequate airway while edema subsides and (2) to maintain adequate oxygenation and ventilation. Vigorous suction, saline lavage, positive end-expiratory pressure, humidification of inspired gases, chest percussion, and postural drainage can optimize respiratory care. Laryngoscopy and bronchoscopy help to determine the appropriate time to remove the endotracheal tube. Children with severe chest injury or ventilatory disturbance require placement in a pediatric intensive care unit. This allows for continuous observation and provides an opportunity for more frequent pulmonary toilet.

Fluid management

Initial fluid management of the child with a ventilation disturbance depends on the nature of the injury. The child in shock or with a cutaneous burn requires fluid infusion until hemodynamic stability occurs; maintenance of a urine output of 1 to 2 cc/kL is appropriate. Alternatively, children with pulmonary contusion require fluid restriction, if possible, to minimize fluid egress into the injured parenchyma.

Antibiotics

Administration of a systemic antibiotic is indicated only after establishment of a culture-proven infection. Prophylactic antibiotic use to prevent infec-

tions tends to allow the airway to colonize with resistant bacteria. Systemic steroid use prior to extubation in children with anatomic airway injuries is controversial.

Adult respiratory distress syndrome

The identification and treatment of ARDS is instrumental to eventual outcome. This disorder may be due to blunt or penetrating trauma, head or spinal cord injury, direct injury from thermal or chemical burns, near drowning, or aspiration pneumonia. Clinical signs and symptoms begin approximately 12 to 24 hours following injury. The usual initial sign is hypoxemia unresponsive to increased FiO_2, decrease in pulmonary compliance, loss of lung volume, and decrease in FRC. An increase in EVLW results in a radiographic appearance of bilateral diffuse, fluffy infiltrates. The child manifests an increase in minute ventilation, tachypnea, dyspnea, hypoxemia, and respiratory alkalosis.

Management of posttraumatic respiratory failure consists of endotracheal intubation, controlled ventilation, and restoration of functional residual capacity using PEEP. The goal is to match ventilation and perfusion, using the lowest inspired oxygen concentration possible to minimize further pulmonary damage resulting from oxygen toxicity.

To monitor the physiologic progress of the child with a ventilation disturbance, several techniques are possible. An arterial catheter allows frequent blood gas determination and continuous blood pressure assessment. A central venous catheter permits measurement of central venous pressure on the right side of the heart. A Swan-Ganz catheter is best for assessment of pulmonary capillary wedge pressure, mixed venous oxygen levels, cardiac output, and systemic resistance. Physiologic surveillance of the child permits appropriate therapy to decrease extraparenchymal lung water and to reduce the need for excessive PEEP. As the child improves, reduction of FiO_2 precedes reduction of PEEP. Mixed venous oxygen determinations from the pulmonary artery catheter help guide removal of FiO_2, to minimize oxygen toxicity.

Injured children with posttraumatic respiratory failure may require protracted assisted ventilation. Many will manifest complications, including massive air leaks with a need for bilateral closed-tube thoracostomy. Airleak problems often persist until removal of the child from the respirator. The mortality rate associated with respiratory failure is high; autopsy specimens usually demonstrate alveolar duct fibrosis consistent with oxygen toxicity. Pulmonary function tests in survivors often show mild restrictive or obstructive changes long after recovery from the acute illness.[6]

SUMMARY

This chapter reviews the normal respiratory anatomy and physiology of the child and how they relate to the mechanics of breathing. A disruption of normal ventilation results in physiologic changes that have implications for treatment and recovery of the injured child. The identification of injuries that affect ventilation is imperative, and adequate understanding of the pathophysiology of these disturbances is critical to allow timely diagnosis and treatment.

REFERENCES

1. Anas NG: *Airway management and ventilation.* In *Brain insults in infants and children,* 1985, Orlando, Fla, Grune & Stratton.
2. Ayres SM: *Ventilation.* In Shoemaker WC, Thompson WL, Holbrook PR et al, editors: *Textbook of critical care,* Philadelphia, 1980, WB Saunders.
3. Backofen JE, Rogers MC: *Upper airway disease.* In Rogers MC, editor: *Textbook of pediatric intensive care,* vol 1, Baltimore, 1987, Williams & Wilkins.
4. Burrington JD: Chest injuries in children, *Can J Surg* 27(5):466-469, 1984.
5. Chameides L, editor: *Textbook of pediatric advanced life support,* Dallas, 1988, American Heart Association.
6. Effmann EL, Merten DF, Kirks DR et al: Adult respiratory distress syndrome in children, *Radiology* 157:69-74, 1985.
7. Eichelberger MR, Randolph JG: Thoracic trauma in children, *Surg Clin North Am* 61(5):1181-1197, 1981.
8. Fallat ME, Longmire-Cook SJ: Successful early management of adolescent inhalation injuries, *Pediatr Surg Int* 5:322-326, 1990.
9. Herndon DN, Barrow RE, Traber DL et al: Extravascular lung water changes following smoke inhalation and massive burn injury, *Surgery* 102(2):341-349, 1987.
10. Motoyama EK, Cook CD: *Respiratory physiology.* In Smith RM, editor: *Anesthesia for infants and children,* ed 4, St Louis, 1980, Mosby–Year Book.
11. Peclet MH, Newman KD, Eichelberger MR et al: Thoracic trauma in children: an indicator of increased mortality, *J Pediatr Surg* 25(9):961-965, 1990.
12. Stone HH: Pulmonary burns in children, *J Pediatr Surg* 14:48-52, 1979.

18 Hypovolemic Shock

Yeheskel Waisman and Martin R. Eichelberger

Hypovolemic shock is a clinical state of inadequate tissue and organ perfusion resulting from the escape of blood or plasma from the intravascular compartment.[3,7] The most common cause of shock in children is acute blood loss as a result of trauma. In the United States, it is estimated that more than 23,000 children die[13] annually, and even more remain disabled owing to complications of traumatic injuries, among them hypovolemic shock.

Successful management of hemorrhagic shock remains a challenge to the clinician, and understanding the concept of shock is important in instituting appropriate therapy. The current concept of hypovolemic shock is that it results from insufficient tissue perfusion resulting in inadequate delivery of oxygen and nutrients to the cells, and accumulation of metabolic wastes, creating a substrate-depleted and toxic cellular environment.[3,9] Prompt restoration of the intravascular volume may reverse this cellular damage; however, prolonged tissue hypoperfusion beyond a critical period results in irreversible shock that leads to cell and organ death.[1,8] The treatment of shock requires rapid restoration of cellular and organ perfusion with adequately oxygenated blood.

Although end-stage shock is easy to recognize, identification of early shock remains a challenge. There is no single clinical or laboratory test that can immediately establish the diagnosis of early shock. Therefore, diagnosis relies on the appreciation of a *complex* of signs including tachycardia, decreased pulse pressure, cold extremities, increased capillary refill time, disorientation, pallor, and hypotension. However, each one of these signs alone is not specific. Despite clinical uncertainty about the diagnosis of early shock, it is critical to begin treatment promptly rather than delay it until a more clear clinical picture is evident.

The diagnosis of shock depends on a comprehensive understanding of physiology, which leads to appropriate management of children.

PATHOPHYSIOLOGY
Physiologic response to hypovolemia

Hemorrhage is a model of hypovolemic shock[7] that results in a decrease of circulating blood volume, reduction of mean circulatory filling pressure, and a fall in cardiac output. As a result, mean arterial pressure (MAP) falls and reduces regional perfusion, which affects delivery of oxygen and nutrients to the tissues. Severe hemorrhage not only creates an anaerobic environment in which the cells must function, it also results in a toxic environment by disabling the mechanism for clearance of cellular waste products.[3]

The intrinsic physiologic response to shock adjusts the cardiovascular and respiratory systems to improve blood flow and to deliver essential nutrients to the cells. This physiologic response correlates with clinical signs that enable the clinician to assess shock (Table 18-1).

Hypotension caused by blood volume loss stimulates baroreceptors in the aortic arch and the carotid sinus; these increase the sympathetic discharge and transmit information to the cardiovascular centers within the central nervous system. Tachycardia and increased myocardial contractility

Table 18–1 Clinical physiologic correlates

Clinical response	Physiology
Delayed capillary refill	↑ PVR
	↓ Capillary flow
Pale, mottled, cool skin	↑ PVR
	↓ Capillary flow
	↓ Hct
Poor skin turgor	Interstitial dehydration
Tachycardia	↑ Sympathetic tone
	↑ Release of catecholamines
	↓ Parasympathetic tone
Thread pulse	↓ Pulse pressure
	↑ PVR
	↓ Mean circulatory filling pressure
	↓ Cardiac output (MAP may be normal)
Tachypnea and ↑ Respiratory effort	↑ pco₂
	↓ po₂
↓ Level of consciousness	↓ Cerebral flow
	↑ pco₂
	↓ po₂

ensue, improving stroke volume and cardiac output (cardiac output = stroke volume × heart rate). Arterial vasoconstriction also occurs, causing an increase in systemic vascular resistance (SVR). This physiologic response allows an increased MAP (pressure = flow × resistance) and diversion of blood flow from less critical organs, such as the skin and the gastrointestinal tract, to those of vital importance such as the brain, heart, and kidneys. Active venoconstriction owing to the increased vascular tone (sympathetic activity) enables shift of blood from the capacitance veins to the circulation, increasing the mean circulatory filling pressure.

Cellular hypoxia and acidosis, which result from tissue hypoperfusion, stimulate chemoreceptors that initiate a compensatory increase in respiratory rate and force. Hyperventilation is an attempt to reverse tissue hypoxia and local acidosis by increasing oxygen delivery to the cell and carbon dioxide removal from the tissue, respectively. The effectiveness of this compensation, however, is related to the adequacy of blood flow through the capillary bed. The chemoreceptor stimulation also increases sympathetic discharge that affects both the cardiovascular and endocrine systems. The endocrine system responds with an outpouring of cortisol and epinephrine to the circulation, resulting in an increased blood glucose concentration to deliver more nutrients to energy-depleted cells and bronchodilatation to improve oxygen delivery and carbon dioxide removal.

At the tissue level, the fall in MAP reduces pre-capillary hydrostatic pressure and capillary blood flow, altering the fluid dynamics of the microcirculation and causing redistribution of extracellular fluid in accordance with Starling's law of capillary exchange.[9] The distribution of fluids between intravascular and extravascular spaces is governed by two balanced but opposing forces: (1) capillary hydrostatic pressure, which forces fluids across the capillary endothelium out of the vascular space into the interstitium; and (2) colloid osmotic pressure, which retains fluid within the vascular space. In early shock, hydrostatic pressure falls, disturbing the balance with colloid osmotic pressure and allowing a shift of fluid into the vascular space, which increases circulating blood volume and interstitial dehydration. A schematic summary of physiologic changes and responses to hemorrhage is shown in Fig. 18-1.

Thus the cardiovascular and metabolic responses are powerful compensatory mechanisms activated in an attempt to improve delivery of oxygen and nutrients to hypoxic cells. Appreciation of the presence of these compensatory mechanisms enables the clinician to recognize shock and assess the response to treatment.

Clinical-physiologic correlates

The circulatory responses to blood loss are manifest by clinical signs that reflect the degree of activation of the compensatory mechanisms. A summary of these correlates is tabulated in Table 18-1. Tachycardia is the primary response to hypovolemia in children; however, it is a nonspecific sign. Tachy-

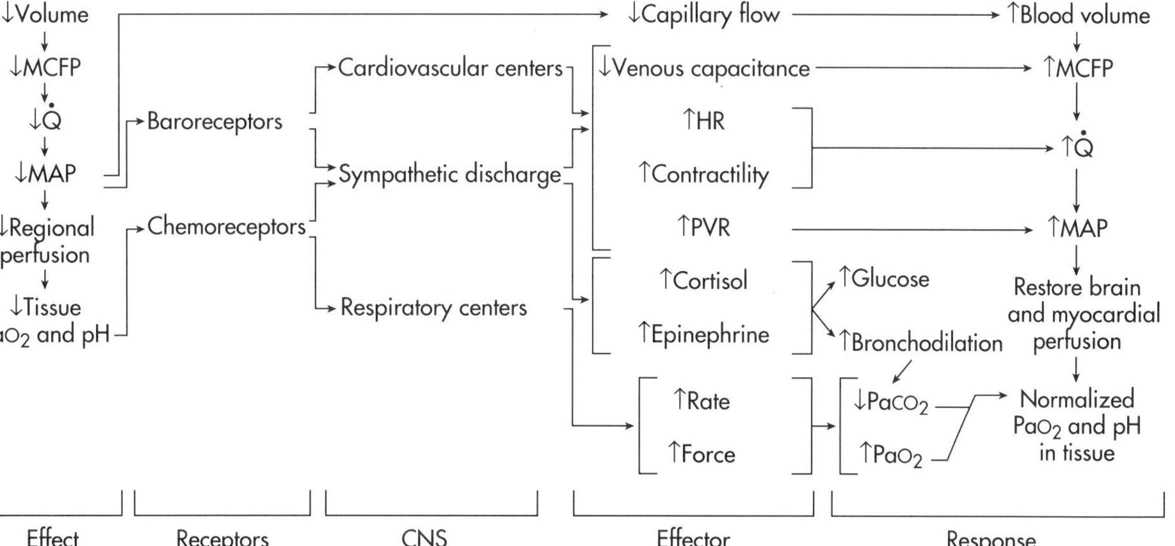

Figure 18–1 Physiologic response to hemorrhage. (From Mangubat EA, Eichelberger MR: Hypovolemic shock in the pediatric patient: a physiologic approach to diagnosis and treatment, *Trauma: Clinical Update for Surgeons* 2:2-8, 1984, Nassau Publications.)

cardia may occur in children as the result of various stimuli such as fear, pain, or even the psychological stress that occurs when children are separated from their parents. Thus the diagnosis of hypovolemia cannot rely on a single measurement but, rather, on the complex of signs. As blood volume loss increases, more signs become evident. A thready pulse reflects a narrow pulse pressure caused by a decrease in systolic blood pressure secondary to decreased cardiac output, and an increase in the diastolic blood pressure secondary to increased vascular tone. Progressive cutaneous vasoconstriction is indicated by cool and mottled skin, particularly over the extremities. A delayed capillary refill time (greater than 2 seconds) reflects increased SVR and decreased capillary flow. This sign is a sensitive and reliable indicator of shock in children.[9] Because of the activation of compensatory mechanisms, especially catecholamine release, changes in blood pressure appear rather late in hypovolemic shock. MAP remains stable until a 20% to 30% loss of blood volume occurs (a liter of blood in an adult [70 Kg] patient). A slight and transient increase in diastolic pressure and a decrease in systolic pressure precede changes in MAP. Changes in these measurements in a canine model of graded hemorrhage (Fig. 18-2) demonstrate the physiologic response in cardiac output, blood pressure, and peripheral resistance from baseline up to a 50% loss of intravascular blood volume. Similar physiologic changes occur in children.[12] Thus, because 95% of all children older than 1 year of age have a systolic pressure greater than 80 mm Hg, a systolic pressure less than 80 mm Hg indicates a blood volume loss of at least 20%. Remember that children with normal blood pressure can manifest clinical shock.

Tachypnea and increase in respiratory effort occur when compensatory mechanisms are activated in response to cellular hypoxia and hypercarbia, which result from decreased microcirculatory perfusion. The hyperventilation that occurs in early shock is evident in an arterial blood gas analysis that commonly reveals a normal PaO_2 and respiratory alkalosis. In late shock, decompensation occurs, respirations become shallow and less effective, and blood gas analysis reveals increasing metabolic followed by combined metabolic and respiratory acidosis.

In summary, early diagnosis of shock is accomplished by recognition of the clinical signs of increased PVR and decreased capillary perfusion (for example, skin mottling, cold extremities, increased capillary refill time), and signs of compensation for decreased cardiac output reflected by tachycardia and decreased pulse pressure. Early recognition of the shock complex is important to prevent circulatory decompensation, hypotension, hypoxemia, or metabolic acidosis. Optimal treatment depends on early clinical recognition and rapid initiation of therapy.

PHYSIOLOGIC CHARACTERISTICS OF CHILDREN

The general physiologic concepts of hemorrhagic shock apply to both adults and children. Children, however, are unique in several aspects of anatomy and physiology that necessitate special consideration in the assessment and management of hemorrhagic shock.

Physical size is the most notable difference between children and adults. Variability in size and weight poses a problem in ensuring the availability of appropriate equipment and medications for the resuscitation of the child.

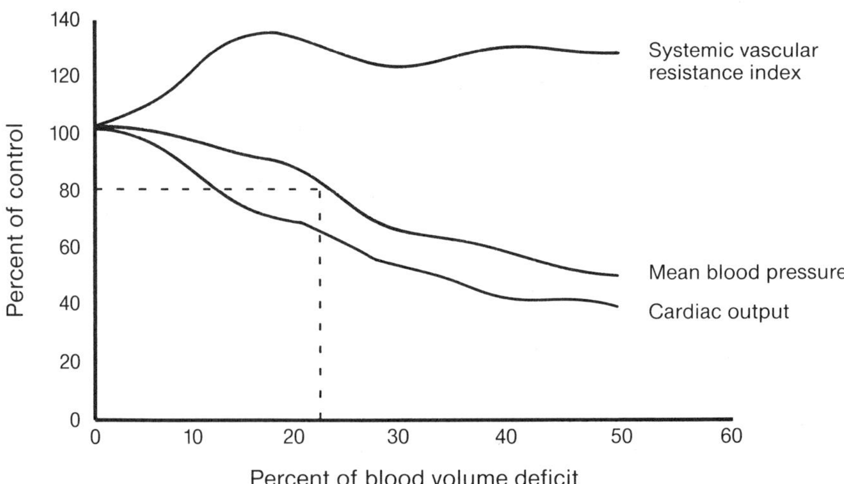

Figure 18-2 Physiologic response to blood loss in a canine model of graded hemorrhage.

The normal blood volume in children varies from 7% to 8% of body weight (80 ml/kg body weight). In relative terms, this corresponds to a 20% to 25% larger volume than in adults (normal = 5% to 6%). What may appear to be a small amount of blood loss in an adult, however, is significant in a young child. For example, a 10-kg child with a blood volume of 800 ml who loses 160 ml of blood depletes his blood volume by 20%. Furthermore, children tend to have lower hemoglobin and hematocrit levels than adults, even up to the teenage years (Table 18-2).[2]

Children have a high body-surface area:mass ratio that is highest at birth and diminishes through infancy and childhood. The relatively large surface area is important for two reasons: (1) increased conductive and convective heat losses can result in hypothermia, which in turn adds the additional stress of pulmonary hypertension and metabolic acidosis to the hypovolemic child and (2) a greater insensible water loss by evaporation makes children more susceptible to dehydration and hypovolemia.

In young children, regulation of body temperature is a major problem encountered in resuscitation. Particularly vulnerable are infants less than 6 months of age, who lack the insulation of subcutaneous fat and an involuntary shivering mechanism. Hypothermia is devastating in these children, causing pulmonary hypertension, hypoxia, and progressive metabolic acidosis. If hypothermia persists, a marked increase in oxygen consumption and severe vasoconstriction depletes metabolic energy stores and exacerbates metabolic acidosis resulting from shock.

The compliant mediastinum in children decreases tolerance to pneumothorax. Wide swings in mediastinal structures seen in tension pneumothorax in young children not only angulate the vena cava, decreasing venous return and cardiac output, but also compress the contralateral lung, impairing ventilatory capacity.

Because vital signs are age-related in the pediatric population, it is crucial for the clinician who is assessing shock in a child to be familiar with the normal vital signs of the patient. For example, a heart rate of 150 beats per minute is normal for an infant but means tachycardia for an adolescent. Similarly, a systolic blood pressure of 80 mm Hg is normal for an infant, whereas it reflects hypotension in an adolescent. Values for normal vital signs for children of different ages are presented in Table 18-3. A good approximation of blood pressure is possible by using the following formulas: *80 + (2 × age in years)* and *70 + (2 × age in years)* for estimation of the fiftieth percentile and the lower limit of systolic blood pressure, respectively, in children over the age of 2 years.

TREATMENT OF SHOCK

Once a patent airway and adequate ventilation exist, treatment of shock becomes the priority. Successful management of shock in children requires simultaneous diagnosis and treatment. Direct pressure controls active sites of bleeding effectively. Avoid attempts to clamp bleeding vessels in acute situations because of the risk of injury to adjacent structures, especially nerves.

Recognition and assessment

The first step in the management of hypovolemic shock is appreciation of its presence. Although signs of late hypovolemic shock may be easy to recognize, the clinical presentation of early or evolving shock is subtle and requires a high level of suspicion. There are no laboratory tests that can immediately make a diagnosis of shock. Therefore

Table 18–2 Lower limits of normal hemoglobin and hematocrit at sea level, by age

Age	Hemoglobin (g/100 ml)	Hematocrit (percent)
7 months-4 years	11.0	33.0
5-9 years	11.5	34.5
10-14 years	12.0	36.0
Adult male	14.0	42.0
Adult female	12.0	36.0
Pregnant woman	11.0	33.0

From Committee on Iron Deficiency, AMA: Iron deficiency in the United States, *JAMA* 203:407, 1968.

Table 18–3 Normal vital signs

	Heart rate (beats/minute)	Minimum systolic BP (mm Hg)	Respiratory rate (respirations/minute)
Infant	100-160	60	30-40
Preschool	80-140	70	20-30
Adolescent	60-110	90	16-20

Table 18–4 Systemic responses to hemorrhage in the pediatric patient

	Early < 25% **blood volume loss**	**Prehypotensive 25%** **blood volume loss**	**Hypotensive 40%** **blood volume loss**
Cardiac	Increased heart rate; weak, thready pulse	Increased heart rate, thready pulse, positive Tilt test	Frank hypotension, tachycardia to bradycardia
CNS	Normal, anxious, irritable, combative	Confused, lethargic, dulled response to pain	Comatose
Skin	Cool, clammy	Cyanotic, decreased capillary refill, cold extremities	Pale, cold
Kidneys	Decreased urinary output, increased specific gravity	Increased BUN, decreased urinary output	No urinary output

the clinician must rely on the assessment gained from the physical examination. By evaluating the *heart rate, peripheral pulses* (present or absent, volume), *skin perfusion* (capillary refill time, temperature, color, mottling), *blood pressure* and *CNS perfusion* (recognition of parents, reaction to pain, lethargy, coma), the clinician is able to recognize the presence of hypovolemic shock and estimate the amount of blood volume loss. Tachycardia, weak thready pulse, capillary refill time greater than 2 seconds, and mottled and cool extremities are clinical signs of early shock, whereas hypotension and changes in level of consciousness are late signs indicating a loss of at least 20% to 25% of the blood volume. Table 18-4 provides some clinical correlates of systemic responses to different degrees of blood volume loss that assist evaluation of the child's blood volume status and requirement of fluid replacement.

Laboratory evaluation

There is no useful and rapid method to estimate blood volume deficit or to establish immediately a diagnosis of shock. In a canine model of slow hemorrhage, however, of 36 variables studied (physiologic, metabolic, and hematologic measurements), arterial base deficit was found to be the most sensitive indicator of volume loss. Arterial base deficit increased with additional hemorrhage of the dogs, remained unchanged over time when hemorrhage ceased, and did not overestimate blood volume loss. These responses suggest that arterial base deficit is a useful measure for accurate and rapid assessment of actual or ongoing blood volume loss in injured children.[11] Validation in the hypovolemic child is necessary before this laboratory study can be adopted.

Fluid resuscitation

Venous access. The establishment of venous access for infusion of fluid is critical in the care of children with life-threatening injuries. The insertion of an intravenous (IV) catheter requires experience and patience, especially in hypovolemic children whose vessels are maximally constricted. Because flow is directly related to the diameter and inversely related to the length of the catheter, a large-bore short IV catheter facilitates rapid infusion of fluids. At least two functioning IV catheters are inserted during resuscitation of an injured child; placement of the catheters in veins above and below the diaphragm is optimal. After the intravenous lines are established, blood samples are drawn for laboratory analyses, including type and cross match. Arterial blood gas analysis is also helpful.

Access to the peripheral vascular system must be prompt; central venous access is unnecessary in children during initial resuscitation. The most desirable sites for peripheral IV lines are (in order of priority) (1) percutaneous access via antecubital or distal forearm veins, (2) percutaneous access to distal saphenous vein, and (3) cutdown on the distal saphenous vein. Plastic catheters, 22-gauge for infants, 22- to 20-gauge for children, and 18- to 16-gauge for adolescents, are recommended. Small T-connectors in the IV line should not be used because they only decrease flow. Two or three attempts at percutaneous catheterization are reasonable before proceeding to a cutdown technique. The jugular veins are difficult to cannulate during resuscitation, and catheterization of the subclavian vein risks the potential complications of pneumothorax or hemothorax even in experienced hands.

If peripheral cutdown is unsuccessful, intraosseous infusion is possible. The intraosseous route is safe, efficacious, and requires less time than a venous cutdown. Complications in this procedure include cellulitis and osteomyelitis, but are very rare (0.7% and 0.6%, respectively).[4] A 16- to 18-gauge bone marrow aspiration needle is used to cannulate the bone marrow compartment of the anterior superior tibia, 2 to 3 cm below the tibial tuberosity. Entry of the needle is perpendicular to the bone or 60 degrees inferiorly with the bevel

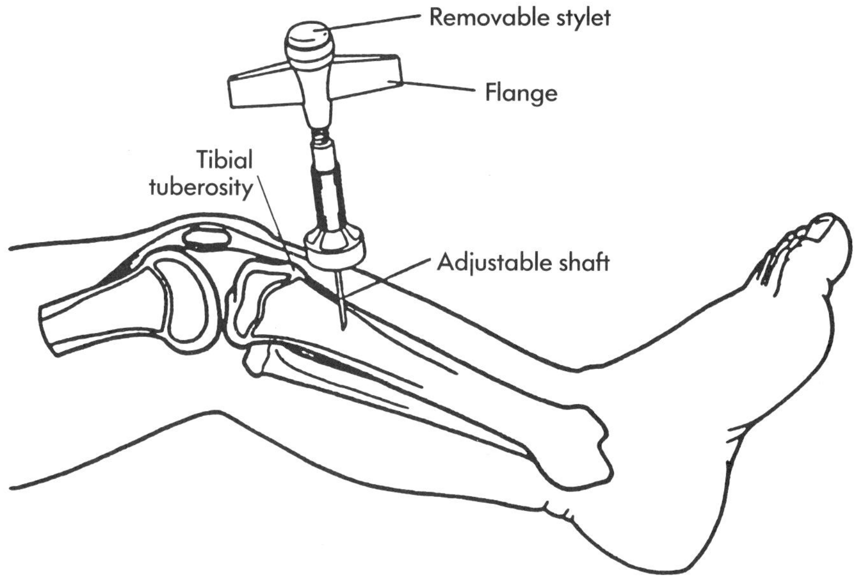

Figure 18–3 Placement of bone-marrow aspiration needle in the proximal tibial location. (From Fiser DH: Intraosseous infusion, *N Engl J Med* 322:1579-1581, 1990. Reprinted with permission from *The New England Journal of Medicine*.)

directed upward; aspiration of bone marrow indicates adequate needle position (Fig. 18-3). Administration of crystalloid, blood products, and medications is possible via the intraosseous route at a reasonable rate. If the tibia is fractured, a bone marrow needle can be inserted into the femur, 3 cm above the external condyle, anterior to the midline.

Fluids: volume, rate, type. Once shock is identified, administer fluids by bolus infusion. Infusion of 20 cc per kilogram (25% of blood volume) of a crystalloid (Ringer's lactate solution [RLS]) is appropriate for an initial rapid bolus. The physiologic responses to this treatment are a slowing of the heart rate, increase in the pulse pressure, decrease in skin mottling, increase in the warmth of extremities, faster capillary refill, clearing of sensorium, and increase of urinary output. Repeat the 20 cc/kg bolus if reassessment of the child shows inadequate tissue perfusion. Following the rule of "three-for one,"[1] three aliquots of crystalloid for each aliquot of blood loss, estimate the volume of crystalloid required to replace blood volume deficit. A third 20-cc per kilogram bolus (60 cc/kg total) is appropriate if necessary; however, if shock persists after two bolus infusions of crystalloid solution, administer 10 ml per kilogram of packed red blood cells (type specific or O negative). If blood is unavailable, use a colloid such as albumin (20 ml/kg of albumin 5% or 4 ml/kg of albumin 25%) for infusion (Fig. 18-4).

The use of *vasopressors* is *contraindicated* in hypovolemic shock.

Acid-base balance

Children in hypovolemic shock may initially develop respiratory alkalosis in the body's attempt to compensate for cellular hypoxemia and carbon dioxide retention. If shock persists, a combined respiratory and metabolic acidosis may ensue. If acidosis (pH <7.2) persists despite correction of the respiratory component, administer a dose of bicarbonate (1 mEq/kg IV), and repeat every 10 minutes if indicated by reassessment. Recent studies regarding the use of bicarbonate in canine hemorrhagic shock, however, did not show any improvement in outcome.[6]

Thermoregulation

Because hypothermia complicates shock, a small hypothermic child may be refractory to the therapy for shock. Therefore, while the child is exposed during the resuscitation phase, overhead heaters or thermal blankets are necessary to maintain body temperature at 36° to 37° C.

Pneumatic antishock trousers

Use of pneumatic antishock trousers (PAST) is not indicated in children because (1) inflation of the abdominal compartment may impair diaphragmatic excursion, causing respiratory arrest, (2) the frequent use of saphenous vein for IV access is thereby precluded, (3) pulmonary edema results when preload (fluid infusion) accompanies an acute increase in afterload (application of PAST), and (4) current evidence suggests that outcome is worse following application of the device.[10] The authors' current

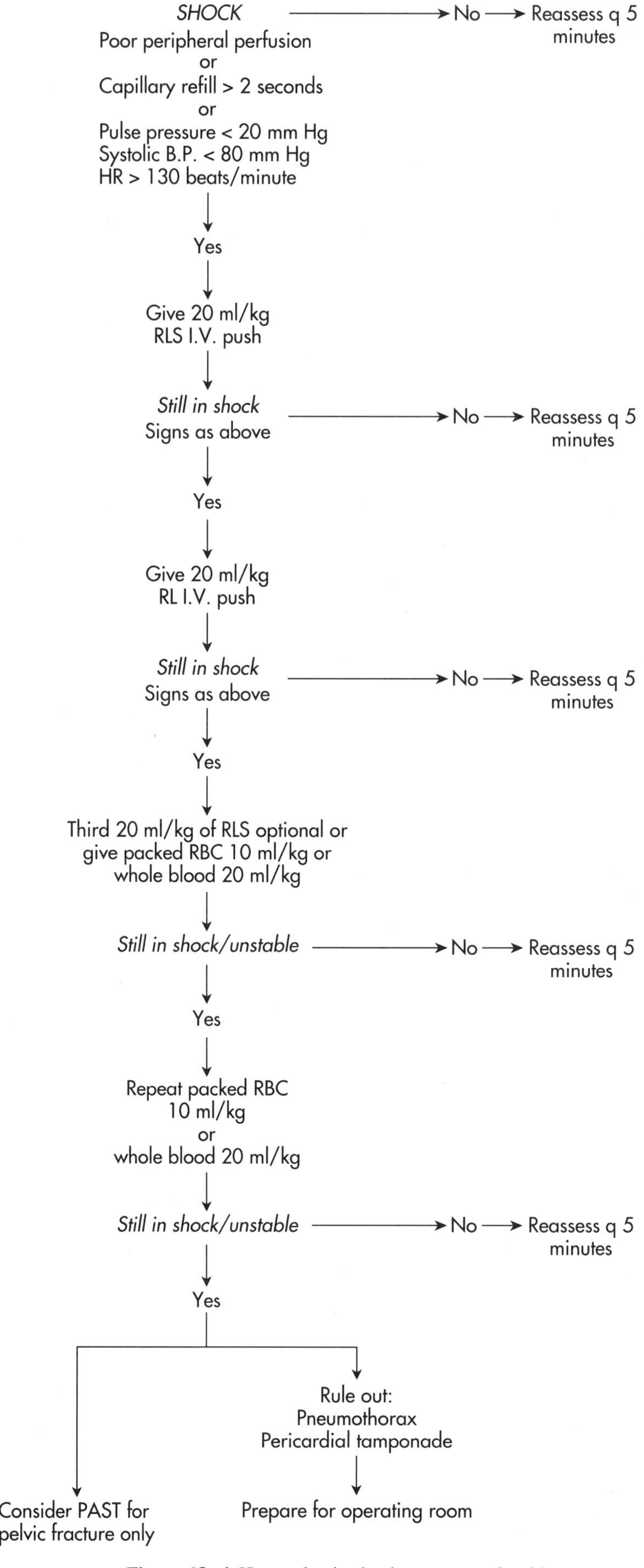

Figure 18–4 Hypovolemic shock treatment algorithm.

recommendation is application of pneumatic antishock trousers in ongoing hemorrhage resulting from pelvic fracture.[5] Children needing inflation of the abdominal compartment usually require endotracheal intubation and positive pressure ventilation.

Other etiologies of shock

If shock persists, other treatable etiologies require exclusion. The unilateral absence of breath sounds and asymmetric movement of the chest are indicative of a newly developed *tension pneumothorax,* which requires immediate treatment by insertion of an 18-gauge plastic catheter into the fourth costal space in the midaxillary line, followed by chest tube placement. Muffled heart sounds with a pulse paradox may indicate the presence of *pericardial tamponade* requiring pericardiocentesis.

After these maneuvers, the treatment of shock is successful in most children. If these measures are not effective, the child usually requires immediate operative intervention to provide surgical hemostasis.

OUTCOME

Data on the prognosis of children with posttrauma hypovolemic shock are currently limited, and available data are difficult to interpret because of the lack of a universal scoring system for all trauma centers. In addition, outcome in hemorrhagic shock is affected by the nature and extent of associated injuries. Of 90 children who had a measurable systolic blood pressure of 80 mm Hg or less (hypotensive hypovolemia) upon arrival at the pediatric trauma center at the Children's National Medical Center in Washington D.C., 79 (87.8%) survived to be discharged from the hospital. Mean ($\pm$ standard error) systolic blood pressure of survivors was 73.4 ($\pm$ 1.3) and of nonsurvivors 37.4 ($\pm$ 10) mm Hg, respectively ($p < 0.004$). Mechanisms of

injury for nonsurvivors included motor vehicle accidents, burns with or without associated smoke inhalation, and gunshot wounds. Organs involved were primarily head, abdomen, and chest. The authors' experience as well as most studies indicate that early and effective treatment of hypovolemic shock improves outcome.

REFERENCES

1. American College of Surgeons Committee on Trauma: *Advanced Trauma Life Support Instructor Manual,* Chicago, Ill, 1988, The Committee.
2. Committee on Iron Deficiency, AMA: Iron deficiency in the United States, *JAMA* 203:407, 1968.
3. Crone RK: Acute circulatory failure in children, *Pediatr Clin N Am* 27:525-538, 1980.
4. Fiser HD: Intraosseous infusion, *New Engl J Med* 322:1579-1581, 1990.
5. Garcia V, Eichelberger M, Ziegler M et al: Use of military antishock trouser in a child, *J Pediatr Surg* 16:544-546, 1981.
6. Iberti TJ, Kelly KM, Gentili DR et al: Effect of sodium bicarbonate in canine hemorrhagic shock, *Crit Care Med* 16:779-782, 1988.
7. Kallen RJ, Lonergan JM: Fluid resuscitation of acute hypovolemic hypoperfusion states in pediatrics, *Pediatr Clin N Am* 37:287-294, 1990.
8. Lillehei RC, Longerbeam JK, Bloch JH et al: The nature of irreversible shock: experimental and clinical observations, *Ann Surg* 160:682-710, 1964.
9. Manguhat EA, Eichelberger MR: Hypovolemic shock in the pediatric patient: a physiologic approach to diagnosis and treatment, *Trauma: Clinical Update for Surgeons* 2(13):2-8 1984. (Nassau Publications).
10. Mattox KL, Bichell WH, Pete PE et al: Prospective MAST study in 911 patients, *J Trauma* 29:1104, 1989.
11. Waisman Y, Eichacker PQ, Richmond S et al: Arterial base deficit predicts volume loss in canine hemorrhage, *Pediatr Res* 29:35A, 1991.
12. Wilson RF, editor: *Critical care manual: principles and techniques of critical care,* Kalamazoo, Mich, 1976, Upjohn.
13. Ziegler MM: Major trauma. In Fleisher G and Ludwig S: Textbook of pediatric emergency medicine, ed 2, Baltimore, 1988, Williams & Wilkins.

19 Resuscitation Pharmacology

Arno L. Zaritsky

Clearly, resuscitation of the traumatized child is a complex process requiring an integrated team approach. Advanced planning and preparation are key to achieving a successful outcome. This chapter reviews the epidemiology of pediatric cardiac arrest, resuscitation drug therapy, practical elements of advanced pharmacologic life support, and decisions on when to discontinue therapy.

Resuscitation of the injured child is challenging because of the technical demands of vascular access and airway control. A knowledge of pediatric equipment and drug dosages based on patient size is essential. Unfortunately, selection of equipment is often based on estimation of the child's weight. Age-related variables affecting implementation are rarely a problem in adult resuscitation. However, because of the tremendous size variation in children (from a 3-kg newborn infant to the 100-kg adolescent), therapeutic modalities that are size-dependent require some adjustment (as does resuscitation time expended) for the individual child. Consequently, precious seconds or minutes can be lost at a most critical time.

Correct drug dosage for children requires four steps: knowledge of the drug dose, estimation of the child's weight, calculation of the dose, and, finally, error-free delivery of the drug to the child. Equipment selection is equally size-dependent and requires accurate estimation of age or weight, as well as knowledge of the corresponding equipment sizes appropriate for different children. There are 10 different endotracheal tube sizes, ranging from a 2.5-mm endotracheal tube for use in the premature infant to a 7.0-mm endotracheal tube for the adolescent, as compared with only three common sizes used in adults. These differences in patient size, and therefore in drug dosage and equipment, can cause error and delay in the pediatric resuscitation process.

The need to calculate drug doses and to select equipment led to the development of the various resuscitation aids in current use. Early attempts consisted of posting a list of drug doses and equipment sizes in accessible areas where they might be needed for resuscitation. The problem with this method was that the child's size had to be estimated

and calculations performed within the stressful situation of pediatric resuscitation. Later efforts employed the use of precalculated drug doses for all pediatric weight ranges, thus precluding the necessity of calculating drug doses in a situation of crisis. This method, however, still required an accurate estimate of the child's weight. Unfortunately, whether the situation is one of crisis or not, accurate weight estimation does not always occur.[5] This is especially likely when the clinician in charge of a resuscitation is one who treats critically ill children infrequently.

Recently, a system permitting accurate drug dosage and equipment selection for pediatric patients has been developed. This system is based on direct measurement of a given child's length. The Broselow Pediatric Emergency Tape is based on the relationship between body length (which can be measured directly in an emergency) and body weight. The reliability of the tape in estimating weight correctly has been established[5] (other length-based systems to estimate body weight for selection of pediatric resuscitation drugs and equipment have also been developed). One side of the Broselow tape indicates drug dosage, as well as drug and fluid volumes precalculated for each kilogram of body weight. On the reverse side of the tape are length-based, color-coded equipment zones that indicate appropriate emergency and resuscitation equipment in relation to length. Recent evidence suggests that child length correlates better than conventionally used measurements for endotracheal tube selection.[6] Other equipment, as well as appropriate basic life-support techniques in relation to length, are also displayed on the reverse side of the tape.

The outcome following cardiac arrest in children is poor. As seen in Table 19-1, the mortality following out-of-hospital cardiac arrest is 90% to 95%.[10] The outcome following resuscitation of hospitalized children is also poor, with 85% to 90% mortality. There are limited data on outcome after traumatic cardiac arrests; adult data report high mortality. Thus, the resuscitation of the pulseless, nonbreathing pediatric victim is often frustrating.

Cardiac arrest refers to the clinical state char-

Table 19–1 Outcome following pediatric resuscitation*

Study author	Patient source	Number of patients by type of arrest			Survival to discharge (%)	
		Resp	CRA	NR	Overall	CRA
DeBard	Hospital	—	—	44	55	NR
Ehrlich	Hospital	—	—	219	47	NR
Ludwig	Hospital	—	—	130	55	NR
Nichols	Out-of-hospital	—	—	13	23	NR
Nichols	Hospital	—	—	34	44	NR
Eisenberg	Out-of-hospital	—	119	—	—	7
Friesen	In-hospital and out-of-hospital		66	—	—	9
Gillis	Hospital	9	33	—	17	9
Lewis	Hospital	16	58	—	28	15.5
O'Rourke	Out-of-hospital	—	34	—	—	21
Rosenberg	Emergency department	—	26	—	—	15
Wark	Hospital	—	—	41	42	NR
Zaritsky	Hospital	40	53	—	34	9.4
Torphy	Emergency department	—	91	—	—	5.5
Losek	Emergency department	—	114	—	—	8

*Patient outcome is stratified by the type of arrest and location, as reported in this study. Overall outcome is the total survival-to-discharge rate reported in the study for all types of arrest. Abbreviations: Resp = respiratory arrest; CRA = cardiorespiratory arrest (absence of pulse and respiratory effort); NR = not reported.

acterized by the absence of *detectable* cardiac activity, recognizing that some children with clinical cardiac arrest may have measurable aortic pressure if an arterial line is inserted. Cardiac arrest usually results from profound hypoxemia, hypercarbia, and/or ischemia. Respiratory arrest is the absence of respiratory effort with ongoing cardiac activity. Outcome following respiratory arrest is much better than that following cardiac arrest, as seen in Table 19-1.

ADVANCED LIFE SUPPORT TECHNIQUES

The initial priorities of securing the airway and providing adequate ventilation in cardiac arrest remain the same in the child with trauma-induced arrest. These aspects of care are covered in other chapters. Securing vascular access is a high priority, since traumatic arrest is often complicated by profound hypovolemia that may be clinically represented by electromechanical dissociation. Providing adequate fluid resuscitation is therefore essential. Tension pneumothorax and pericardial tamponade are the other two common reversible causes of electromechanical dissociation in the injured child.

Vascular access

Rapid vascular access is often difficult to achieve in the pulseless child, but is vital since intravenous epinephrine administration is often essential to restart the heart. Rapid delivery of the drug to the central circulation, combined with effective chest compression–induced blood flow, is necessary to deliver epinephrine to its site of action in the arterial vascular bed. Therefore, central venous drug administration is ideal, but is difficult to achieve in cases of arrest. Peripheral venous administration is used with the recognition that different peripheral venous sites may not be equivalent. Animal and adult studies suggest that a peripheral vein that drains into the superior vena cava is a superior injection site to those that drain into the inferior vena cava.[9] This presumably occurs secondary to the to-and-fro flow of blood in the inferior vena cava, which is not as effectively collapsed as the superior vena cava during chest compression. Limited pediatric animal studies have not shown the route of drug administration to have an important effect on drug delivery. Thus, whichever venous route is available should be used. When using peripheral venous routes, it is essential to flush the catheter with at least 2 to 5 ml of saline to help deliver the drug to the central circulation.

Besides intravenous routes of drug administration, the intraosseous route is effective for rapid drug delivery.[3] The bone marrow space of long bones in children is very vascular and provides a ready means of both drug and fluid administration. The bone marrow space functions as a noncollapsible venous plexus. Intraosseous injections are usually given in the proximal tibia, but the distal femur and anterior superior iliac spine have also been used. Intraosseous needles should not be placed in fractured long bones, since the administered fluids and drugs will leak from the fracture site. Similarly, do not place a needle into a long bone where a needle was placed previously and was subsequently displaced. Drugs may leak out of the previous insertion site.

Resuscitation drugs, vasoactive infusions, and rapid fluid boluses have been given by the intraosseous route; any drug or fluid that can be given intravenously can be given by the intraosseous route. Indeed, some studies suggest that the intraosseous route is superior to the intravenous route, inasmuch as it can effect higher central venous and arterial drug concentrations. Newer intraosseous needles make it possible to give resuscitation drugs and fluids by this route in children up through the age of 6.

Fluid therapy in pediatric resuscitation can be simplified as follows:

1. If the child is in full arrest, IV access and fluids are used only to provide a vehicle for drug delivery. In general, intravenous lines should be maintained at a KVO rate. If the patient is thought to have traumatic blood loss, fluid boluses of 10 to 20 ml/kg may be given while monitoring for pulmonary edema.

2. If the child has an organized rhythm and detectable pulse, but is hypotensive, a fluid bolus of 10 to 20 ml/kg may be given. If hypotension persists after two to three boluses of fluids, or if the child develops pulmonary edema, vasoactive drugs are started. Complicated fluid calculations based on maintenance and deficit therapy are reserved for the postresuscitation phase.

Isotonic non–glucose-carrying fluid should be used for fluid boluses in resuscitation; a glucose-containing solution running at a maintenance rate is appropriate for maintenance fluids. A micro drip or infusion pump should be standard equipment for pediatric resuscitation preparedness in order to avoid inadvertent fluid overload.

Endotracheal drug administration

The intravenous or intraosseous routes are the preferred sites for drug administration during cardiopulmonary arrest. In children older than 6 years of age and in infants and children in whom intraosseous access is delayed, certain drugs may be given by the endotracheal route.[4] These include *l*idocaine, *e*pinephrine, *a*tropine, and *n*aloxone (remember as *lean*). Although the endotracheal route has the theoretic advantage of allowing more rapid delivery of drugs to the arterial circulation by absorption from the pulmonary capillaries, the kinetics of drug absorption do not favor this route.

About 10 times the amount of drug given intravenously must be given by the endotracheal route to achieve equal plasma concentrations and peak drug action.[4,7] The administration of these large doses is limited, however, by the lung's action as a drug depot.[4,7] Thus, if restoration of spontaneous circulation occurs, the child may have prolonged and profound hypertension secondary to slow epinephrine absorption from the lung. Profound hypertension following restoration of circulation may be harmful to cerebral recovery, and excessive afterload may further compromise cardiac function when it is already diminished by arrest-induced myocardial ischemia.

The optimal dose and method of drug delivery by the endotracheal route have not been determined. Current recommendations are based on anecdotal reports and limited experimental data.[9] More recent data show that a larger dose of resuscitation medications than normally given intravenously should be given by the endotracheal route.[7] Therefore, at least two to three times the currently recommended dose (that is, 0.02 to 0.03 mg/kg) of epinephrine 1:10,000 should be used initially. If this dose is ineffective, use 10 times the current dose if IV access is still not available.

The most efficient drug absorption occurs in the alveoli and small airways; thus, effective delivery of the drug to these absorptive surfaces is important. This is achieved by injecting the drug through a catheter positioned into the lower airway, but this procedure is cumbersome because of delays in finding the right catheter. A better alternative is to follow the drug injection with 1 to 2 ml of saline. The latter carries the drug into the lower airway and washes it from the endotracheal tube where it may be adherent owing to capillary action. With any technique, it is important to follow drug administration with several deep positive pressure breaths to help distribute the drug into the lower airways.

The priorities for the site of drug administration are seen in Fig. 19-1. Drug injection into an intravascular location (intravenous or intraosseous) is always preferred over the endotracheal route. Central venous injection is always preferred over peripheral venous injection. When the intraosseous and intravenous routes are not immediately available, the first dose of epinephrine should be given by the endotracheal route.

RESUSCITATION PHARMACOLOGY

The following section reviews the action, indications, doses, routes, and toxicity of resuscitation drugs. Note that recommendations for some of the drugs have changed since the initial American Heart Association guidelines were published in 1986.[1]

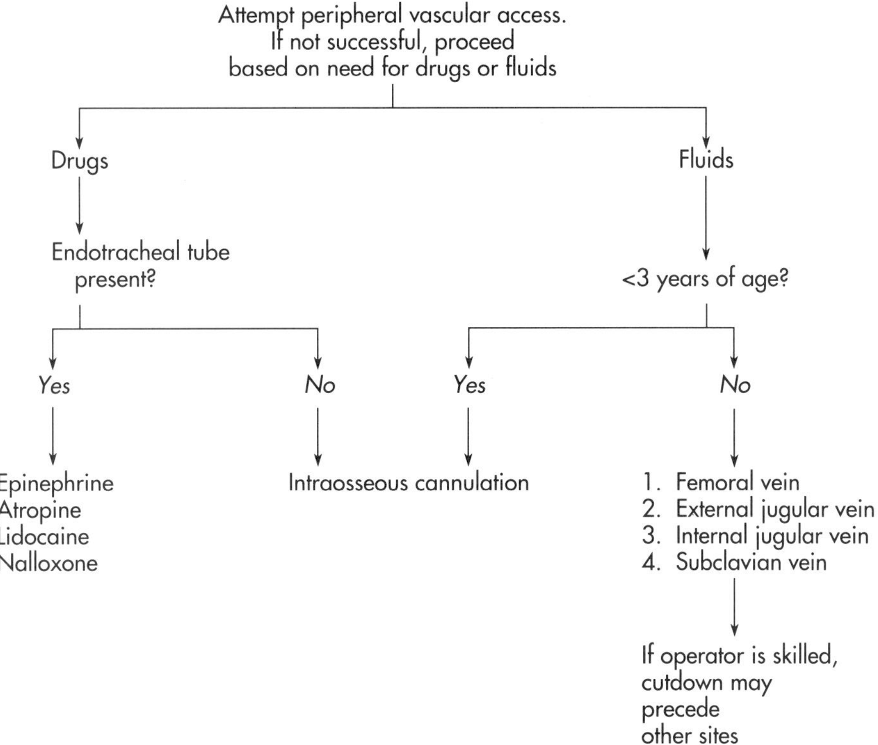

Figure 19–1 Approach to vascular access in the child with cardiac arrest or decompensated shock.

Epinephrine

Epinephrine has both α-adrenergic and β-adrenergic actions, but the large doses used in cardiac arrest produce predominant α-adrenergic effects. This action increases coronary perfusion pressure and myocardial and cerebral blood flow by preventing arterial collapse of intrathoracic arteries and selectively increasing vascular resistance in the skin, muscle, and splanchnic vascular beds. Based on experimental studies, epinephrine's positive inotropic and chronotropic actions are not deemed important in resuscitation from cardiac arrest,[1] but these actions can be useful to reverse bradycardia.

Epinephrine is indicated in all cardiac arrest settings (that is, asystole, electromechanical dissociation, and ventricular fibrillation). The recommended dose is 0.01 mg/kg (0.1 cc/kg of 1: 10,000 solution) IV, or 0.02 to 0.03 mg/kg by the endotracheal route (Table 19-2). If after 2 to 5 minutes this dose is not effective, give *ten times* the initial dose. This latter recommendation is based on experimental data showing that the currently recommended dose is suboptimal and that larger doses (10 to 20 times the currently recommended dose) are more effective.[1] Recent anecdotal data support the use of higher doses of epinephrine in children. The urgency to restart the heart with an effective dose of epinephrine is emphasized by clinical data showing that children who do not have restoration of organized spontaneous cardiac activity with two rounds of epinephrine do not survive to leave the hospital.[11] Thus, giving a larger second dose of epinephrine to help restart the heart outweighs any potential risk from the use of larger drug doses. Note that there is nothing magical about waiting 5 minutes to repeat the dose. If the child remains asystolic 2 minutes after the epinephrine is given, give another, larger dose.

Acidosis in cardiac arrest

A combination of low blood flow and poor ventilation during a cardiac arrest leads to a mixed respiratory and metabolic acidosis. Traumatic hypovolemic shock adds an additional insult by depleting oxygen-carrying capacity and, thus, tissue-oxygen delivery. Severe acidosis depresses myocardial contractility, blunts myocardial and peripheral vascular responses to exogenous catecholamines, increases pulmonary vascular resistance, dilates systemic vascular beds, and decreases glycolytic pathway activity, thus impairing adenosine triphosphate synthesis. Correction of acidosis during an arrest is therefore an appropriate concern, but the optimal treatment method is controversial.

Table 19–2 Pediatric resuscitation drugs

Drug	Dose	How supplied*	Remarks
Epinephrine	0.01 mg/kg (0.1 ml/kg)	1:10,000 (0.1 mg/ml)	Most useful drug in cardiac arrest; IV or ET. Give 2-10× dose if >1 dose needed
Atropine	0.02 mg/kg (0.2 ml/kg)	0.1 mg/ml	Minimum dose of 0.1 mg (1 ml) IV or ET
Sodium bicarbonate	1 mEq/kg (1.0 ml/kg)	1 mEq/ml (8.4% soln)	Infuse slowly *only* when ventilation is adequate; IV only
Calcium chloride	20 mg/kg (0.2 ml/kg)	100 mg/ml (10% soln)	Use for hypocalcemia, hyperkalemia, hypermagnesemia, and calcium entry blocker toxicity; IV only
Glucose	0.5-1.0 g/kg 2-4 ml/kg $D_{25}W$	0.5 gm/ml $D_{50}W$	Dilute 1:1 with sterile water to make $D_{25}W$; very hyperosmolar; IV only
Lidocaine hydrochloride	1 mg/kg volume depends on form used	10 mg/ml (1%) 20 mg/ml (2%)	IV or ET; if needed, repeat dose in 15 min and begin infusion
Bretylium tosylate	5 mg/ml (0.1 ml/kg)	50 mg/ml	IV only; use when lidocaine is not effective. If second dose needed, use 10 mg/kg

*Prefilled syringe form used in resuscitation.
IV = intravenous; ET = endotracheal.

Recent data show that the acidosis noted during a cardiac arrest is poorly reflected by an arterial blood gas. With intubation, ventilation, and chest compression, the blood passing through the lungs may be well oxygenated and have a low P_{CO_2}. The total blood flow through the lungs, however, is often low. Thus, even though arterial blood gases may show a normal or high pH with a respiratory alkalosis, simultaneous mixed venous blood gases show a profound acidosis which is secondary to a severe respiratory acidosis combined with a metabolic acidosis.

The cause of mixed venous hypercarbia is explained by the fact that the difference between arterial and venous CO_2 contents will increase when cardiac output falls or when CO_2 production increases. Ventilation can influence the venous CO_2 content only by changes in arterial CO_2 content; this effect is minor when cardiac output is low. The combination of low blood flow and increased tissue CO_2 production generates venous hypercarbia.

The key to therapy of acidosis, therefore, is to restore tissue perfusion. This often requires administration of packed red blood cells in the injured child to restore circulating blood volume and tissue oxygen delivery.

Sodium bicarbonate

Sodium bicarbonate buffers the accumulated metabolic acids through the following reaction:

$$NaHCO_3 + H^+ \leftrightarrow Na^+ + H_2CO_3 \leftrightarrow H_2O + CO_2$$

Unless ventilation is adequate, the reaction cannot proceed to the right by the elimination of formed CO_2. Unfortunately, ventilation is not usually the limiting factor; instead, inadequate blood flow results in poor CO_2 elimination. Administration of sodium bicarbonate will increase CO_2 production, which may worsen intracellular acidosis even when the measured arterial pH improves. An unfavorable change in intracellular pH results from the increased permeability of the cell membrane to CO_2 compared with bicarbonate. A negative inotropic effect and other adverse effects from an acute worsening of respiratory acidosis may therefore result from the administration of sodium bicarbonate.

Based on concerns about the adverse effects of sodium bicarbonate and the limited data showing its beneficial effect in cardiac arrest models, the most recent American Heart Association guidelines deemphasize its use.[9] Sodium bicarbonate in a dose of 1 mEq/kg may be infused intravenously or intraosseously only *after* the airway has been secured, the victim has been hyperventilated, effective chest compressions are being delivered, and epinephrine administration has been ineffective (see Table 19-2). Subsequent doses (0.5 mEq/kg; 0.5 ml/kg) may be given every 10 minutes of continued arrest. Administration of sodium bicarbonate in the postarrest setting to correct acidosis is controversial, but may be helpful as long as the previous caveats regarding effective perfusion and ventilation are remembered.

Besides adverse effects on intracellular pH, sodium bicarbonate may produce a metabolic alkalosis that shifts the oxyhemoglobin dissociation curve to the left, impairing oxygen delivery to the tissues and depressing ionized calcium concentration. Sodium and water overload may result from excessive administration; sodium bicarbonate is hyperosmolar (2000 mOsm/L) and therefore causes sclerosis to the veins. Catecholamines are inactivated and calcium salts will precipitate in bicarbonate solutions, so careful flushing of the intravenous line is necessary following bicarbonate administration.

Glucose

Glucose is the major energy substrate of the brain and the neonate's myocardium; vigorous myocardial contractility may not be possible when hypoglycemia occurs. Infants and small children are predisposed to hypoglycemia since they have limited glycogen stores. Severe hypoglycemia can mimic hypoxemia (that is, poor perfusion, diaphoresis, tachycardia, and hypotension). Therefore, a rapid bedside test of blood glucose concentration should be performed in all pediatric resuscitation patients.

If hypoglycemia is present, the dose of glucose is 0.5 to 1.0 g/kg given intravenously (see Table 19-2). This is most conveniently administered by using $D_{50}W$, making sure to dilute this solution since it is very hyperosmolar. A 1:1 dilution with sterile water results in $D_{25}W$; the recommended dose is then 2 to 4 ml/kg of this solution given intravenously. Repeated administration is usually not required and may result in a hyperosmolar state. In addition, note that giving a fluid bolus of a glucose-containing solution will also correct hyperglycemia. For example, 20 ml/kg of D_5NS will deliver 1 g/kg of glucose. Repeated doses of this solution are not recommended, however, since profound hyperglycemia may result.

The major side effect of glucose administration is related to local irritation from infusion of this hypertonic solution. Of theoretic concern is the adverse effects of hyperglycemia on the central nervous system during low flow states. Both experimental and clinical data suggest that hyperglycemia predisposes the brain to a more severe ischemic insult by providing increased substrate for lactate formation during anaerobic glycolysis. The increased production of lactate produces a severe intracellular acidosis, which injures the cell. Therefore, the goal of treatment is to normalize glucose concentration and avoid hyperglycemia.

Atropine

Atropine is a competitive antagonist at muscarinic receptors and therefore inhibits vagal activity. This action increases sinoatrial node firing rate and atrio-

ventricular conduction. At low doses, atropine has central and peripheral parasympathomimetic actions that may produce paradoxic vagotonic effects. Through its vagolytic actions, atropine may be helpful in the treatment of bradycardia accompanied by poor perfusion and hypotension. It may also be used to inhibit bradycardia during intubation attempts. In the latter case, other methods to monitor oxygen saturation are essential (for example, pulse oximetry) since the inhibition of bradycardia may mask hypoxemia. Similarly, bradycardia in a child is initially treated by assessment of the airway and ventilation rather than administration of atropine or other drugs, since airway problems with secondary hypoxemia are more common than primary cardiac causes of bradycardia.

If bradycardia persists despite adequate ventilation, administration of atropine is appropriate. Atropine may be given by the intravenous, intraosseous, or endotracheal route (see Table 19-2). A minimum dose of 0.1 mg is used to avoid paradoxic bradycardia. A maximum single dose of 1.0 mg may be used and repeated to a total maximum dose of 1.0 mg in a child and 2.0 mg in an adolescent. These maximum doses produce complete vagal inhibition, and additional doses are not helpful.

Tachycardia may follow atropine administration, but is usually well tolerated in children. Mydriasis may obscure the neurologic examination, and atropine administration should be considered when evaluating the ocular examination of a child following an arrest.

Calcium

Calcium is essential in excitation-contraction coupling. Normally, calcium entry into the cardiac myocyte stimulates calcium release from the endoplasmic reticulum; the increase in intracellular calcium concentration stimulates actin-myosin coupling. Infants have greater inhibition of cardiac contractility by calcium channel blockers, which suggests that intracellular calcium release is deficient and cardiac contractility is more dependent on extracellular calcium influx. Thus, hypocalcemia in an infant may be accompanied by poor contractility and a clinical picture of cardiogenic shock.

Acquired ionized hypocalcemia may be more common in the injured child receiving blood product administration than is clinically recognized. Both packed red blood cells and fresh frozen plasma contain citrate which forms complexes with calcium, lowering the ionized concentration without changing the total calcium concentration. Only the ionized fraction is physiologically important, and low ionized calcium concentrations are apparent only by measurement with an ion-selective electrode. Nomograms to calculate the ionized calcium concentration based on pH and albumin are not accurate in critically ill children. Normally, the citrate in blood products is rapidly metabolized by the liver, but in severe shock or cardiac arrest, citrate clearance will be delayed.[8] Furthermore, blood products are cold and may produce profound hypothermia when rapidly infused into the small child. The hypothermic state markedly impairs hepatic clearance of citrate.[8]

Based on adult studies, there is no evidence to support the use of calcium in asystole and its use in electrical-mechanical dissociation (EMD) is questionable. Only limited data are available for children. Hypocalcemia occurs in children with cardiac arrest, but in the majority it was associated with septic shock.[11] More recent data suggest that calcium antagonizes the action of epinephrine and other adrenergic agents and exerts its major action on blood pressure by producing systemic vasoconstriction rather than a positive inotropic effect. For these reasons, calcium is indicated only to correct documented ionized hypocalcemia, to antagonize the adverse cardiovascular actions of hyperkalemia and of hypermagnesemia, and to reverse the hypotension produced by calcium channel blocker toxicity.[9] In addition, empiric calcium administration should be considered for hypotensive children receiving large volumes of blood products.

For its indicated conditions, calcium is given intravenously or intraosseously in a dose of 20 mg/kg of $CaCl_2$ (see Table 19-2). Note that different calcium salts contain widely differing amounts of elemental calcium; calcium chloride has almost three times the amount of elemental calcium contained in an equal volume of calcium gluconate. Repeated doses increase the risk of morbidity, so the initial dose should be repeated only once in 10 minutes, if needed; subsequent doses should be based on measured deficiencies of ionized calcium concentration.

Rapid calcium administration should be avoided since bradycardia or sinus arrest may occur. Calcium chloride solution is hyperosmolar and causes sclerosis; severe chemical burns may occur if the solution extravasates from peripheral injection sites.

Lidocaine

Lidocaine is an antidysrhythmic agent with membrane-stabilizing effects mediated through inhibition of sodium channels. Sodium channel inhibition reduces automaticity and the difference in the effective refractory period between normal and ischemic tissue; these effects inhibit the propagation of reentrant arrhythmias.

Table 19–3 Preparation of infusion medications using the "Rule of 6"

Drug	Calculation basis
Epinephrine	0.6 * (the body weight in
Norepinephrine	kg) is the number of mg
Isoproterenol	to add to make a final
Prostaglandin E_1	volume of 100 ml
Then, 1 ml/hr delivers 0.1 µg/kg/min	

Drug	Calculation basis
Dopamine	6 * (the body weight in kg)
Dobutamine	is the number of mg to
Nitroprusside	add to make a final vol-
Nitroglycerine	ume of 100 ml
Amrinone	
Then, 1 ml/hr delivers 1 µg/kg/min	

Drug	Calculation basis
Lidocaine	60 * (the body weight in
	kg) is the number of mg
	to add to make a final
	volume of 100 ml
Then, 1 ml/hr delivers 10 µg/kg/min	

Lidocaine is indicated for the unusual pediatric arrest rhythms: ventricular tachycardia and fibrillation. Ventricular fibrillation is seen in less than 10% of pediatric cardiac arrest victims.[10] When ventricular fibrillation is seen in a young patient, a search for a metabolic etiology is indicated unless the child is known to have an underlying cardiac disorder such as structural heart disease, myocarditis, or digoxin toxicity. Metabolic causes of ventricular dysrhythmias include hyperkalemia, hypermagnesemia, and hypothermia as well as toxin-induced causes, such as tricyclic antidepressant overdose.

Lidocaine is given in an initial bolus dose of 1 mg/kg and is repeated, if needed, in 10 to 15 minutes (see Table 19-2). If a second dose is required, a lidocaine infusion is started at 20 to 50 µg/kg/min; lower infusion rates are used in children with liver disease or persistent low cardiac output states, since lidocaine clearance is depressed in these conditions. A suggested method of infusion penetration is seen in Table 19-3. Lidocaine is rapidly redistributed from the plasma compartment following bolus injection, and the plasma concentration may transiently fall to subtherapeutic levels if a single bolus is followed by an infusion. Administration of a second bolus of 1 mg/kg 10 to 15 minutes after starting the infusion will maintain therapeutic plasma concentrations.

High lidocaine plasma concentrations can depress myocardial contractility and produce hypotension through peripheral vasodilation. Additional toxicities result from central nervous system effects. These symptoms range from drowsiness and disorientation to muscle twitching and generalized seizures. Discontinuation of the infusion is usually effective treatment of toxicity. If necessary, diazepam, lorazepam, or phenobarbital may be given to control seizure activity.

Bretylium

Bretylium is an antiarrhythmic agent of complex pharmacology. Its antiarrhythmic actions probably result from adrenergic stimulation which shortens the refractory period, combined with direct myocardial effects to lengthen the effective refractory period. Bretylium has a biphasic sympathetic nervous system effect: it initially increases blood pressure and heart rate by stimulating catecholamine release, followed in several minutes after a bolus injection by a fall in blood pressure and heart rate, owing to inhibition of catecholamine reuptake, which depletes catecholamine stores.

There are no pharmacokinetic or pharmacodynamic studies of bretylium use in children; anecdotal reports note its effectiveness in treating ventricular fibrillation in pediatric patients. Its effectiveness in adults led to its recommended second-line use in children.[9] Some data suggest that it may be effective in hypothermia-induced ventricular fibrillation when electrical defibrillation is not effective. The recommended dose is 5 mg/kg, followed by another attempt at defibrillation (see Table 19-2). If a second dose is needed, 10 mg/kg may be given and the countershock repeated. The most common side effect is hypotension, which typically responds to head-down positioning and fluid administration.

DRUG THERAPY BASED ON CARDIAC RHYTHM

Most rhythm disturbances encountered in the resuscitation of infants and children are secondary to hypoxia and acidosis. Usually, correction of these underlying abnormalities through appropriate airway management and adequate fluid resuscitation is adequate therapy.

Figure 19-2 illustrates a clinical classification of rhythms based on the presence or absence of a pulse, and whether the pulse rate is slow or fast. If the patient has a fast heart rate, it is critical to decide whether it is due to a primary rhythm disturbance or is a secondary phenomenon. In most injured children, the latter is true. Only unstable children with cardiac rhythm disturbances require immediate drug and/or electrical treatment. The clinical definition of instability is usually based on evidence of poor perfusion (that is, cyanosis, mental status changes, hypotension, and prolonged capillary refill). In making an objective determination of a symptomatic arrhythmia (that is, measuring blood pressure and pulse), it is important to know the lower limit of normal hemodynamic parameters from adolescents to newborns. *A blood pressure ≤70 mm Hg in infants, or ≤70 + 2* age in years in children, combined with evidence of poor tissue perfusion would be evidence of a patient with an unstable rhythm disturbance.* In newborns and young infants, the blood pressure value is often difficult to obtain; a heart rate less than 80 beats per minute rather than a specific blood pressure value is used as another objective measurement of instability.

Bradycardic rhythms

Bradycardic rhythms are the second most common types of arrest rhythm seen in children. Their management is based on the underlying cause of the bradycardia (Fig. 19-3). In the injured child, bradycardia typically results from hypoxemia and a severe hypoxic-ischemic insult. In the latter case, the resulting rhythm is often a wide-complex and not preceded by identifiable p waves. The therapeutic approach to symptomatic bradycardia always begins with intubation and ventilation before drug therapy.

Epinephrine is the drug of choice in hypoxia-ischemia–induced bradycardia.[1] It is not likely that atropine will be helpful in this setting. If bolus administration of epinephrine is only transiently effective in postarrest bradycardia, a continuous chronotrope infusion is needed. Epinephrine infusion is preferable to isoproterenol for this indication because the latter often compromises coronary perfusion pressure, whereas epinephrine will maintain coronary blood flow.[1]

The administration of sodium bicarbonate may be considered for the child who fails to respond to epinephrine, or for the child whose response is suboptimal because of severe acidosis. The limitations of bicarbonate therapy are detailed in the section on asystole, below, as well as in the previous section, "Resuscitation Pharmacology."

Asystole

Asystole is the most common pediatric arrest rhythm. The approach to asystole is seen in Fig. 19-4. Epinephrine is the drug of choice,[1] as there are no clinical data showing that any other drug is more effective in the treatment of asystole. Basic life support with optimal ventilation, oxygenation,

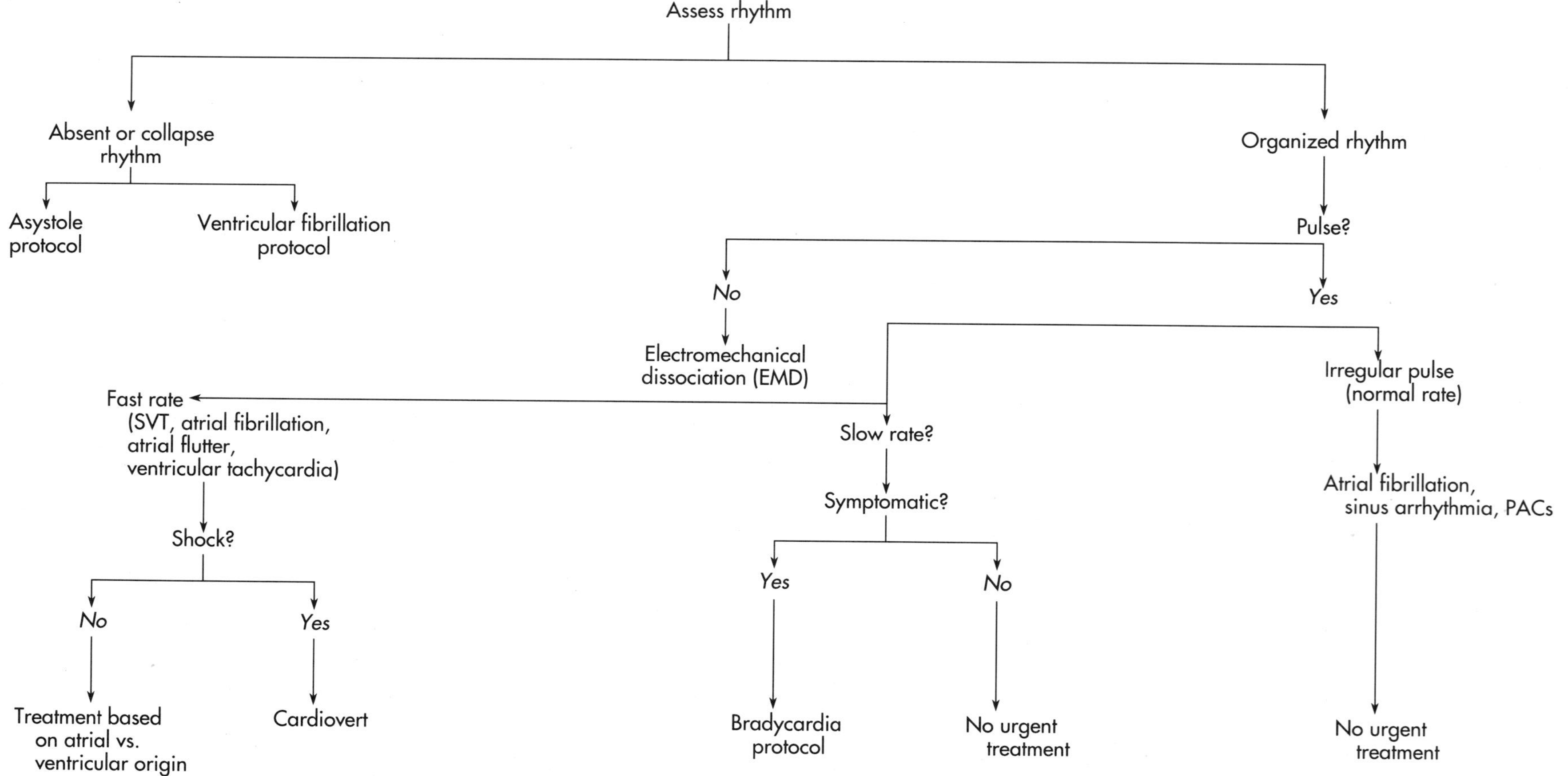

Figure 19–2 Approach to therapy of the child with a rhythm disturbance. Absent or collapse rhythm refers to rhythms without organized activity and lacking detectable perfusion. PAC = premature atrial contraction.

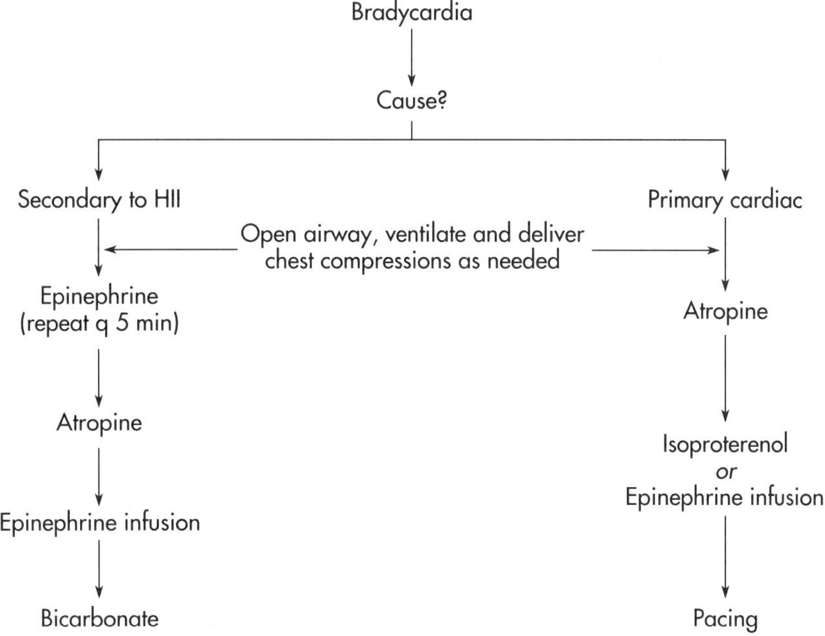

Figure 19–3 Management of symptomatic bradycardia. HII = hypoxic-ischemic insult, such as following severe shock or a cardiac arrest.

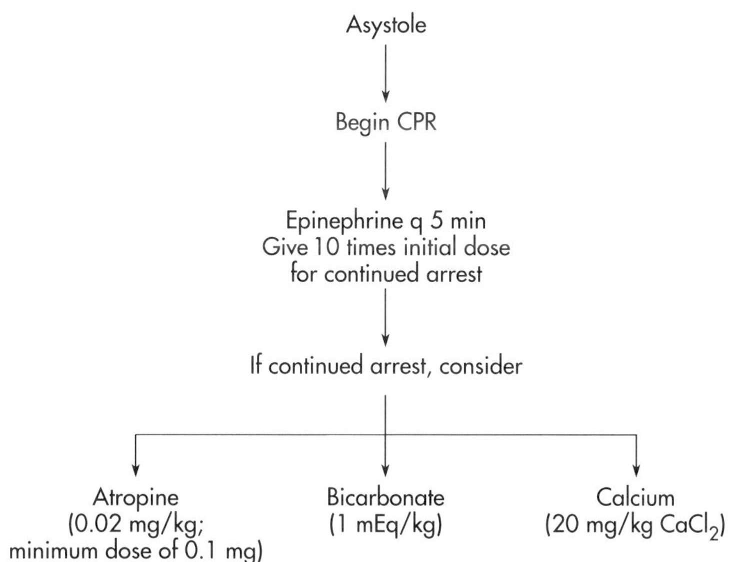

Figure 19–4 Management of asystole.

and circulation (chest compressions) is essential and always precedes drug administration.

Epinephrine is given in a dose of 0.01 mg/kg (0.1 cc/kg of 1:10,000 solution) IV, or 0.02 to 0.03 mg/kg by the endotracheal route. If after 2 to 5 minutes this dose is not effective, give *ten times* the initial dose. This recommendation is based on experimental data showing that the currently recommended dose is suboptimal and that larger doses (10 to 20 times the currently recommended dose) are more effective in experimental models and clinical studies.[2] In addition, clinical data show that patients who do not have restoration of organized spontaneous cardiac activity with two rounds of epinephrine do not survive to leave the hospital.[11] Thus, giving a larger second dose of epinephrine to help restart the heart outweighs any potential risk from the use of larger drug doses.

Although no longer a first-line drug, bicarbonate may be given if the initial dose of epinephrine is not effective. Bicarbonate will *be effective only* if the child undergoes oxygenation, ventilation and blood perfusion. Remember to flush the intravenous line with normal saline following bicarbonate administration.

There is no evidence that either atropine or calcium is useful in asystolic arrest. Therefore, if used, neither should be given in preference to epinephrine. Calcium is given only to treat documented or suspected ionized hypocalcemia (such as resulting from citrate administration) and to reverse the effects of hyperkalemia, hypermagnesemia, and calcium entry blocker toxicity.

Electromechanical dissociation

Electromechanical dissociation (EMD) is a clinical state characterized by organized cardiac activity, but absent pulses. This is most commonly seen as a wide-complex bradycardia in the postarrest setting. Drug therapy is the same as for asystole (that is, epinephrine is the drug of choice), with an important caveat. Always consider the three correctable causes of EMD that are most commonly seen in the injured child: hypovolemia, tension pneumothorax, and pericardial tamponade. When severe hypovolemia causes EMD, a narrow-complex tachycardia or normal heart rate, rather than a wide-complex bradycardia, may be seen. Similarly, tension pneumothorax and pericardial tamponade may produce narrow-complex rhythms, particularly in the early phase of these conditions.

Ventricular fibrillation and pulseless ventricular tachycardia

Ventricular fibrillation and pulseless ventricular tachycardia are uncommon pediatric rhythms. Electrical defibrillation (2 watt-seconds/kg) is the treatment of choice for both rhythms (Fig. 19-5).

If defibrillation is unsuccessful, epinephrine is used in the management of ventricular fibrillation for the same reason that it is helpful in asystole: it increases coronary perfusion pressure and, therefore, myocardial blood flow. Augmenting myocardial blood flow helps restore myocardial cellular function and makes the heart more susceptible to defibrillation. Epinephrine should be repeated every 5 minutes as required, with subsequent doses larger than the first (as described for asystole).

Lidocaine is helpful in preventing the recurrence of ventricular fibrillation, but its administration should *not* delay the only effective treatment: defibrillation. Lidocaine is administered following successful defibrillation, or following three attempts at defibrillation without success. A second dose may be given in 10 to 15 minutes. A continuous infusion should be started if the child has

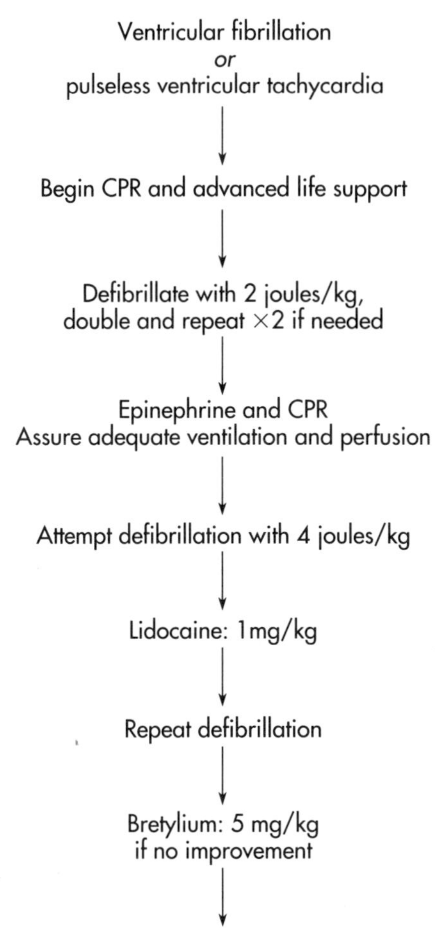

Figure 19–5 Management of ventricular fibrillation.

structural heart disease, recurrent ventricular fibrillation, or runs of premature ventricular contractions. If the child does not respond to defibrillation, epinephrine, or lidocaine, bretylium should be used. The initial bretylium dose is infused rapidly; the dose may be doubled if a second is needed.

In treatment of children, it is important to consider correctable causes of ventricular tachycardia and ventricular fibrillation. These include metabolic abnormalities (for example, hyperkalemia), drug intoxication (for example, tricyclic antidepressant or digoxin overdose), and profound hypothermia (core temperature <33° C).

Defibrillation and cardioversion

Electrical conversion of arrhythmias on an emergent basis is rarely employed in the pediatric population. Tachydysrhythmias are usually seen in relatively stable children, thus allowing for consultation and elective drug therapy or cardioversion.

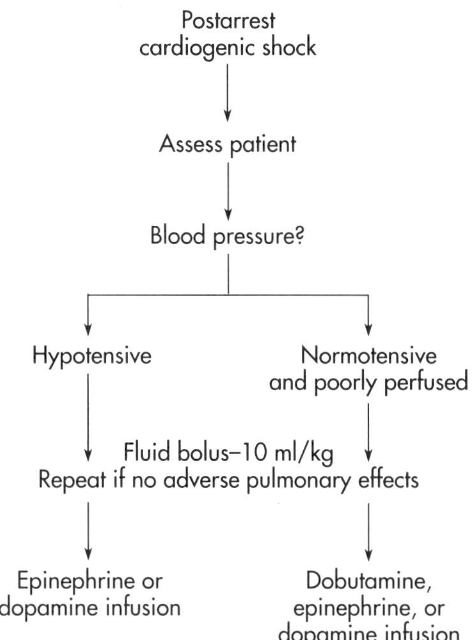

Figure 19–6 Management of postarrest acquired cardiogenic shock. Note that therapy is based on the presence of normal or low blood pressure.

Since children vary in size, there is a range of paddle sizes. The 4.5-cm size is usually adequate for infants, and the 8-cm size for older children. A good principle to remember is that the paddle should contact the chest wall over the entire paddle surface area. In choosing a paddle–chest-wall interface, it is important to avoid allowing the interface substance from one paddle to come in contact with the substance from the other paddle. This is most likely to occur in the treatment of small children and infants, creating a short circuit and precluding energy delivery to the heart.

The defibrillation dose is 2 watt-seconds/kg. If this is unsuccessful, the energy dose should be doubled and attempted twice at the higher energy level. If the second attempt at the higher level is unsuccessful, epinephrine and lidocaine should be given, along with attention to oxygenation and the acid-base status; increasing the energy dose at this point is usually not helpful.

For cardioversion of tachydysrhythmias such as atrial fibrillation or supraventricular tachycardia, small energy doses of 0.25 to 1.0 watt-second/kg can be used. The higher energy dose is used in the treatment of ventricular tachycardia.

POSTRESUSCITATION STABILIZATION

Following successful resuscitation, children often require additional support to maintain a stable rhythm and improve perfusion. The following practical approach to drug selection in the postresus-

citation phase is also applicable to the general management of critically ill infants and children with cardiogenic shock. (The latter may occur as an acquired form of shock following severe hypotension or cardiac arrest.)

When deciding on postresuscitation therapy, it is important to recall the goals of initial drug therapy. These goals include rapid restoration of adequate blood pressure and effective perfusion, and correction of hypoxia and acidosis. These goals are vital to neurologic resuscitation following a hypoxic-ischemic insult. Therefore, I recommend using potent drugs initially to stabilize the child. If the child does well, then less potent agents can be substituted. Figure 19-6 summarizes this approach to postarrest stabilization by outlining the treatment plan for cardiogenic shock.

Following resuscitation, children are often poorly perfused, hypotensive, and very acidotic. After a cardiac arrest, a common reason for persistent poor perfusion is cardiogenic shock, resulting from arrest-associated myocardial ischemia.[1] Thus, a previously healthy child with normal cardiac function may have acquired cardiogenic shock following cardiac arrest or severe decompensated shock secondary to trauma. Some children may also have poor lung compliance following arrest owing to aspiration, cardiogenic pulmonary edema, or lung contusion. Poor respiratory function complicates the ability to achieve adequate oxygenation and ventilation. After an arrest in any child, primary attention is focused on stabilizing the airway and providing adequate oxygenation and ventilation. Application of positive end-expiratory pressure may help improve oxygenation and ventilation.

Pharmacologic treatment of poor tissue perfusion is based on the child's hemodynamic state as reflected by the physical examination. In all children postarrest, administration of a 10 to 20 cc/kg fluid bolus over several minutes, with careful observation for signs of fluid overload, is reasonable. In addition to replacing blood volume lost secondary to trauma, acidosis and severe shock can cause vasodilation and, thus, relative hypovolemia, increasing the amount of fluid resuscitation required to restore an adequate circulating blood volume.

Epinephrine infusion

There are three vasoactive agents commonly used in the postarrest setting for the treatment of hypotension or very poor perfusion: dopamine, dobutamine, and epinephrine. Although dopamine is often the drug of choice for adults with postarrest shock, epinephrine by infusion is the initial treatment of choice for children.[1] Epinephrine is a more potent vasoactive agent and more effectively increases myocardial perfusion pressure. Since coronary artery disease is rare in children, there is less concern about epinephrine's dysrhythmogenic effects and the risk of myocardial ischemia resulting from an increase in myocardial oxygen demand in excess of coronary artery delivery. The required infusion rate of epinephrine varies between 0.05 and 1.0 μg/kg/min; 0.2 to 0.3 μg/kg/min is typically adequate. A method for preparation of the drip is given in Table 19-3. Remember that a higher starting infusion dose may be required in the hypotensive child.

Dobutamine infusion

Dobutamine may be an effective agent following arrest in the *normotensive* child who remains poorly perfused secondary to diminished cardiac function. Dobutamine tends to decrease systemic vascular resistance, which is not helpful in the hypotensive child. In children with cardiogenic shock, dobutamine increases cardiac output and decreases pulmonary wedge pressure, central venous pressure, and systemic and pulmonary vascular resistances. The usual infusion dose is 5 to 20 μg/kg/min (see Table 19-3). Dobutamine may produce hypotension and tachycardia. The former may require the use of epinephrine or its combined administration with dopamine to increase systemic vascular resistance.

Dopamine infusion

Dopamine has positive inotropic and chronotropic effects and tends to increase systemic and pulmonary vascular resistance, especially at the high infusion rates often required following arrest in children. The advantage of this drug, when used at low infusion rates (2 to 5 μg/kg/min), is its selective effect to enhance renal and splanchnic perfusion. Usual infusion rates are 5 to 20 μg/kg/min (see Table 19-3). Dopamine is indicated for children with persistently poor perfusion and low normal blood pressure. The decision to use dopamine instead of dobutamine is often arbitrary and based on personal preference.

Caveats of drug infusion therapy

When infusing any of the inotropic and vasoactive agents discussed above, remember that at the recommended infusion rates, the drug may take 20 or more minutes to reach the child depending on where it is connected to the IV line. There are two alternatives to achieve a more rapid onset of action. The first is to run the drip initially at 5 to 10 times the usual initial starting rate while carefully monitoring the heart rate and blood pressure. When the heart rate begins to increase, quickly decrease the drip rate to the desired infusion dose. The rapid clearance of these drugs prevents drug toxicity resulting from higher infusion rates as long as the rate is readjusted when the effect of a drug is first seen.

An alternative approach is to Y-connect the vasoactive infusion with an IV infusion flowing at a faster rate, to carry the vasoactive infusion to the child more rapidly. Although this method is effective, it may be dangerous since an increase in the carrier infusion rate results in the delivery of a sudden bolus of a potent drug.

Use the "Rule of 6" (see Table 19-3) to calculate inotrope infusion rates; recognize that this rule does not work as well for larger ($>$20 kg) children. For epinephrine, norepinephrine, and isoproterenol, the calculation requires a large amount of drug when used in a larger child. This is easily adjusted, however, by making an appropriate dilution. Thus, in a 20-kg child, the formula calls for 12 mg of epinephrine (12 1-ml vials). If a 1:10 dilution is made, then adding 1.2 mg to accomplish a final volume of 100 ml produces a solution by which *10 ml/hr* delivers 0.1 μg/kg/min. The higher infusion rates are not a problem for larger children. Note in Table 19-3 that other vasoactive drug infusions, although not discussed in this chapter, can be calculated using the Rule of 6. Details on the indications and dosages of these agents may be found in standard pediatric critical care texts.

TERMINATION OF RESUSCITATION EFFORTS

It is often much more difficult to make a decision to terminate resuscitation efforts in a child than in an adult because of the emotional stress associated with the death of a child. Unfortunately, the overall outcome of cardiac arrest in children is poor (see Table 19-1). Prolonged, aggressive resuscitative efforts may restart the heart, but do not restore brain function. This is particularly the case if the child suffers an out-of-hospital cardiac arrest.

There are limited outcome data to guide the clinician. Two studies have examined predictors of outcome and found that the number of doses of resuscitation medications was predictive of outcome. In one study,[11] none of 31 patients requiring more than two doses of epinephrine survived to hospital discharge. Similarly, the other study found that none of 21 patients receiving more than two doses of epinephrine and bicarbonate survived to hospital discharge.

I suggest the following practical approach to pediatric cardiac arrest: (1) assure adequate ventilation and oxygenation; (2) provide effective chest compression; (3) obtain vascular access and give epinephrine at least every 5 minutes, if not sooner, with the second dose being ten times larger than the first; (4) rule out reversible causes of trauma-induced cardiac arrest (severe hypovolemia, tension pneumothorax, and pericardial tamponade); (5) obtain electrolytes, glucose, and arterial blood gas values, although no electrolyte or blood gas abnormality is predictive of outcome. Recognition and correction of severe metabolic abnormalities may be helpful. If these procedures are not effective, and no correctable metabolic disorder is found, the rescuer should consider the presence of profound hypothermia or, possibly, drug intoxication. The former is easy to exclude; the latter depends on the history and clinical suspicion. If the child fails to develop a stable rhythm that results in tissue perfusion, it is appropriate to stop. In the child who arrives pulseless and asystolic, this approach typically requires not more than 15 to 20 minutes.

REFERENCES

1. American Heart Association: *Drug therapy in pediatric advanced life support*. In Chameides L, editor: *Textbook of pediatric advanced life support* (suppl), Dallas, 1988, the Association.
2. Brown C, Werman H: Adrenergic agonists during cardiopulmonary resuscitation, *Resuscitation* 19:1-16, 1990.
3. Fiser D: Intraosseous infusion, *N Engl J Med* 322:1579-1581, 1990.
4. Hahnel J, Lindner K, Ahnefeld F: Endobronchial administration of emergency drugs, *Resuscitation* 17:261-272, 1989.
5. Lubitz D, Seidel J, Chameides L et al: A rapid method for estimating weight and resuscitation drug dosages from length in the pediatric age group, *Ann Emerg Med* 17:576-581, 1988.
6. Luten R, Wears J, Broselow J et al: Length-based endotracheal tube sizing for pediatric resuscitation, *Ann Emerg Med* 19:476, 1990.
7. Ralston S, Tacher W, Showen L et al : Endotracheal versus intravenous epinephrine during electromechanical dissociation with CPR in dogs, *Ann Emerg Med* 14:1044-1048, 1985.
8. Rutledge R, Sheldon G, Collins M: Massive transfusion, *Crit Care Clin* 2:791-805, 1986.
9. Standards and guidelines for cardiopulmonary resuscitation and emergency cardiac care, *JAMA* 255:2841-2989, 1986.
10. Zaritsky A: Drug therapy of cardiopulmonary resuscitation in children, *Drugs* 37:356-374, 1989.
11. Zaritsky A, Nadkarni V, Getson P et al: CPR in children, *Ann Emerg Med* 16:1107-1110, 1987.

20 Intracranial Pressure Control

Sharon L. Pilmer, Ann-Christine Duhaime, and Russell C. Raphaely

Morbidity and mortality in head injury relate in part to the nature of the primary injury, that is, the damage sustained by the tissues of the central nervous system (CNS) over the milliseconds of injury as a result of traumatic forces acting on the brain. Other than prevention, little can be done to alter that component of CNS damage which is irreversible at the time of the primary injury. It is clear, however, that additional injuries can occur after the mechanical insult has been completed, and it is toward these phenomena that the efforts of the clinician are directed.

Delayed neuronal loss after head trauma can be divided into two main categories. The first can be considered "primary reversible injury" and refers to pathologic processes occurring at the cellular level that are initiated but not completed at the time of the mechanical insult. The sublethally injured neurons may recover or may go on to die within the first 1 to 2 days after trauma, owing to such mechanisms as excitotoxic degeneration, secondary axotomy, lipid peroxidation, and other cascading correlates of cellular disintegration.[6,9,29] Newer therapy designed to interrupt these biochemical cascades and thus promote neuronal salvage is possible. The second type of delayed brain injury after trauma occurs when otherwise viable tissue is compromised by brain swelling, hypoxia, or ischemia. Control of such "secondary injury" by reducing swelling and improvement of substrate delivery has been the focus of most of the efforts in head injury therapy during the past several decades.

Impairment of oxygen and substrate delivery to nervous tissue occurs through either diffuse or regional brain swelling. If swelling is uniform, cerebral ischemia occurs as intracranial pressure approaches mean arterial pressure and cerebral perfusion pressure falls. Regional brain swelling results in displacement of portions of the brain such that local ischemia occurs and substrate delivery declines.

Fortunately, treatment is available to influence brain swelling caused by head trauma and to prevent damage from intracranial pressure. For individuals who care for children with head injury, it is important to understand the pathophysiology and treatment of brain swelling, which affect the oxygen and substrate supply to the brain. The approach to the child with a head injury with brain swelling is to manipulate oxygen and substrate supply to meet the demands of vital structures.

DEFINITION OF DANGEROUS INTRACRANIAL HYPERTENSION

In normotensive individuals without intracranial pathology, the generally accepted cerebrospinal fluid (CSF) pressure measured in the lumbar space equals 5 to 15 mm Hg. Variations in CSF pressure occur with both respiration and cardiac pulsations. Transient, self-limited elevations of CSF pressure above 15 mm Hg occur in normal individuals with certain activities (coughing, straining, etc.) without ill effect. Marked increases in intracranial pressure with minimal neurologic dysfunction occur in individuals with disorders such as pseudotumor cerebri and chronic hydrocephalus, conditions with essentially normal brain and normal cerebrovascular autoregulation. Brain injury with abnormal cerebrovascular autoregulation appears to alter the vulnerability of the intracranial nervous tissue to even modest elevations in intracranial pressure. Institution of treatment for dangerous increase in intracranial pressure is important to preserve brain function (Table 20-1).

INCIDENCE AND PREVALENCE OF INTRACRANIAL HYPERTENSION ASSOCIATED WITH PEDIATRIC HEAD TRAUMA

Children with severe head injury are at highest risk for the development of intracranial hypertension. Severity is frequently measured by using the Glasgow Coma Scale (GCS) (Table 20-2).[13] A child with a GCS score less than or equal to 8 after resuscitation (or, in some studies, at 6 hours after injury) has suffered severe head injury. Approximately 5% of children who sustain head trauma, excluding those with isolated scalp or facial injury, manifest a severe head injury,[1a,8,16,20] and about half of these children will develop intracranial hypertension.[2,28] Occasionally, a surgical mass lesion, such as an epidural hematoma, will be responsible

200

Table 20–1 Dangerous elevations
of intracranial pressure

ICP > 15 mm Hg for 30 min
ICP > 20 mm Hg for 3 min
CPP (SAP-ICP) < 50 mm Hg for 3 min

Table 20–2 Glasgow Coma Scale

Eye opening (E)	
Spontaneous	4
To speech	3
To pain	2
Nil	1
Best motor response (M)	
Obeys	6
Localizes	5
Withdraws	4
Abnormal flexion	3
Extensor response	2
Nil	1
Verbal response (V)	
Oriented	5
Confused conversation	4
Inappropriate words	3
Incomprehensible sounds	2
Nil	1
Coma score (E + M + V) = 3 to 15	

From Jennett B, Teasdale G. Aspects of coma after severe head injury, *Lancet* 878-881, 1977.

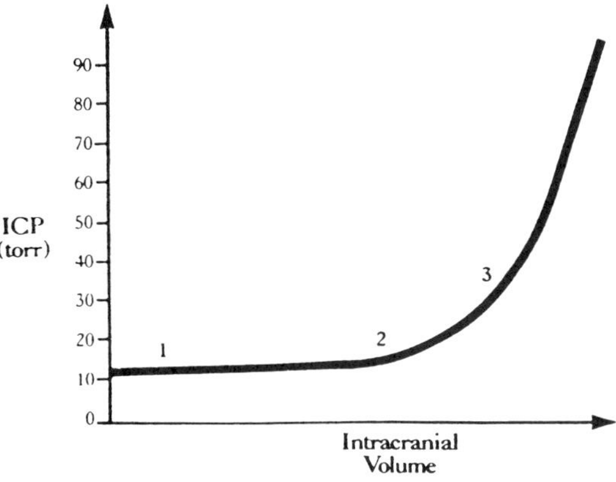

Figure 20–1 Intracranial pressure-volume relationship. The curve describes the compliance characteristics of the intracranial compartment. The flat portion of the curve (1 → 2) illustrates the buffering effect on intracranial pressure of CSF translocation from the intracranial space to the spinal subarachnoid space. As this compensatory mechanism is exhausted, small additional increases in intracranial volume lead to large increases in intracranial pressure (2 → 3).

for the elevation of intracranial pressure; in this case, evacuation leads to prompt resolution of the increased pressure. Treatment of most cases of severe head injury in children, however, is nonsurgical, and resolution of intracranial pressure requires medical management. Conventional thought suggests that dangerous elevations in intracranial pressure in children occurs for 2 to 3 days following injury. Recent experience at the Children's Hospital of Philadelphia indicates that intracranial hypertension in severe injury may become problematic as late as a week after trauma and may persist for several weeks.

PATHOPHYSIOLOGY OF INTRACRANIAL HYPERTENSION

Bony encasement by the skull makes the brain the most protected organ in the body. This becomes a disadvantage when brain injury with swelling occurs. The Monroe-Kellie hypothesis states that the volume of the intracranial compartment is fixed, and is equal to the sum of its contents[13a,22a]:

$$V_{Total} = V_{Brain} + V_{CSF} + V_{Blood}$$

An increase in the volume of one compartment requires an immediate and reciprocal decrease in the volume of another if intracranial pressure is to remain constant. Initially, CSF translocates from the intracranial space to the spinal subarachnoid space. When V_{Brain} or V_{Blood} exceeds the capacity of the space provided by CSF displacement, small additional increments of V_{Brain} or V_{Blood} lead to large increases in intracranial pressure. The relationship between intracranial volume and intracranial pressure is illustrated in Fig. 20-1. As intracranial pressure approaches mean arterial pressure, cerebral perfusion pressure diminishes, capillaries collapse, and tissue ischemia ensues. Intracranial hypertension threatens the viability of nerve cells by global or focal diminution of oxygen and substrate delivery.

Oxygen and substrate demand of the CNS renders it exquisitely susceptible to brief interruptions of blood flow. The brain represents 2% of the body weight, but receives 20% of the cardiac output; the high blood flow to the brain reflects the great demand for oxygen and substrate. Approximately 50% of neuronal energy consumption supports the active transport of ions necessary for the maintenance of transmembrane potentials and transmission of electrical impulses. The remainder consists of biosynthetic work, such as the synthesis of mitochondria and macromolecules. The energy necessary to perform these tasks comes from the degradation of ATP to ADP and orthophosphate. Under normal circumstances the oxidative metabolism of glucose through glycolysis and the citric

Table 20–3 Lesions likely to be associated with brain swelling

---

Large areas of major parenchymal disruption (e.g., gunshot wounds)

Severe impact injuries with multiple contusions

Extreme shear injuries with cortical-subcortical disruption and large intraparenchymal hemorrhage

Subdural hematoma

Superimposed hypoxia or shock

---

acid cycle is the sole source of ATP production in the brain.[24] No reservoir for oxygen or glucose exists in brain cells, hence, they depend on a continuous supply of substrate for normal function. Interruptions in supply of oxygen or glucose lead to cell dysfunction and death.

PATHOGENESIS OF BRAIN SWELLING LEADING TO INCREASED INTRACRANIAL PRESSURE

Secondary brain injury following the primary mechanical injury to nervous tissue has the potential to disrupt the carefully matched substrate supply-demand relationship. Secondary insults relate to disturbances in systemic delivery of oxygen and substrate (hypoxemia, anemia, shock states) or regional factors that interfere with delivery, as is the case in brain swelling and intracranial hypertension. The likelihood of brain swelling in a given child is evident by the history, physical examination, and radiographic findings; this enables the clinician to initiate treatment early (Table 20-3). Brain swelling causes compromise of substrate delivery, which creates a "snowball" effect more difficult to reverse, once established, than to minimize or prevent in its early stages. Common pathophysiologic processes that are associated with brain swelling include cerebral hyperemia, cerebral edema, and the formation of traumatic parenchymal contusion. Conversely, children with pure diffuse axonal injury without superimposed hypoxia or contusion tend to have intracranial pressure that is normal or only modestly elevated.

Cerebral hyperemia, either absolute or relative, frequently contributes to brain swelling in head injury. In health, a number of physiologic variables, including cerebral metabolism, cerebral perfusion pressure, blood viscosity, Pao_2, and $Paco_2$, influence cerebral blood flow (Figs. 20-2 and 20-3). Cerebrovascular autoregulation tightly couples blood flow to metabolic need. Overall cerebral metabolic rate remains remarkably constant during different states of wakefulness and mental activity.

Conditions known to increase metabolic rate include hyperthermia and convulsions. Coma, hypothermia, barbiturates, and general anesthesia all depress cerebral metabolic rate. In individuals with head injuries, cerebral metabolic rate for oxygen ($CMRO_2$) correlates closely with the Glasgow Coma Scale (GCS) score, as shown in Fig. 20-4.[23]

The effect of cranial trauma on cerebral blood flow is less predictable. Some children will exhibit reduced cerebral blood flow, which parallels the reduced metabolic demands of a comatose brain. This situation is seen most commonly with "pure" diffuse axonal injury, without major hemorrhage or superimposed hypoxia. In other children, cerebral flow increases relative to metabolic need; this state of relative cerebral overcirculation, or hyperemia, occurs in both adults and children with posttraumatic intracranial hypertension.[2,18] Vasomotor paresis, with loss of autoregulation such that flow becomes passively dependent on systemic arterial pressure, may be the cause of cerebral hyperemia (Table 20-3). A CT scan reveals small ventricles, obliteration of perimesencephalic cisterns, and increased density of the white matter. This type of transient hyperemia has been hypothesized to be the cause of neurologic decline in some children who appear initially to have sustained clinically less severe injuries. However, the scenario of a mildly injured child who deteriorates to coma from diffuse hyperemia is rare in our experience.

Cerebral edema, defined as an increase in intercellular and/or intracellular fluid, produces deleterious effects on neurologic function through its effect on intracranial pressure and its propensity to cause tissue shifts and resultant focal ischemia. Whether edema is detrimental to brain function itself remains controversial. Both cytotoxic and vasogenic cerebral edema occur with head injury and are likely to be associated with ischemia, hypoxia, or parenchymal disruption. In the setting of ischemia or hypoxia, oxygen deprivation leads to a rapid depletion of high-energy phosphate compounds (ATP). The ATP-dependent Na^+/K^+ pump fails to maintain transmembrane ionic gradients with loss of intracellular potassium to the extracellular space, and leakage of sodium, calcium, and water into the intracellular space. Several mechanisms may contribute to further cellular damage, including calcium-mediated membrane disruption, breakdown of intracellular proteins and lipids, and uncoupling of oxidative phosphorylation. Intracellular acidosis and accumulation of excitatory neurotransmitters may also compromise vital cellular functions.[11] Vasogenic cerebral edema arises from a disruption in the blood-brain barrier, located at the cerebral capillary endothelial junction. Disruption of endothelial cell junctions is pre-

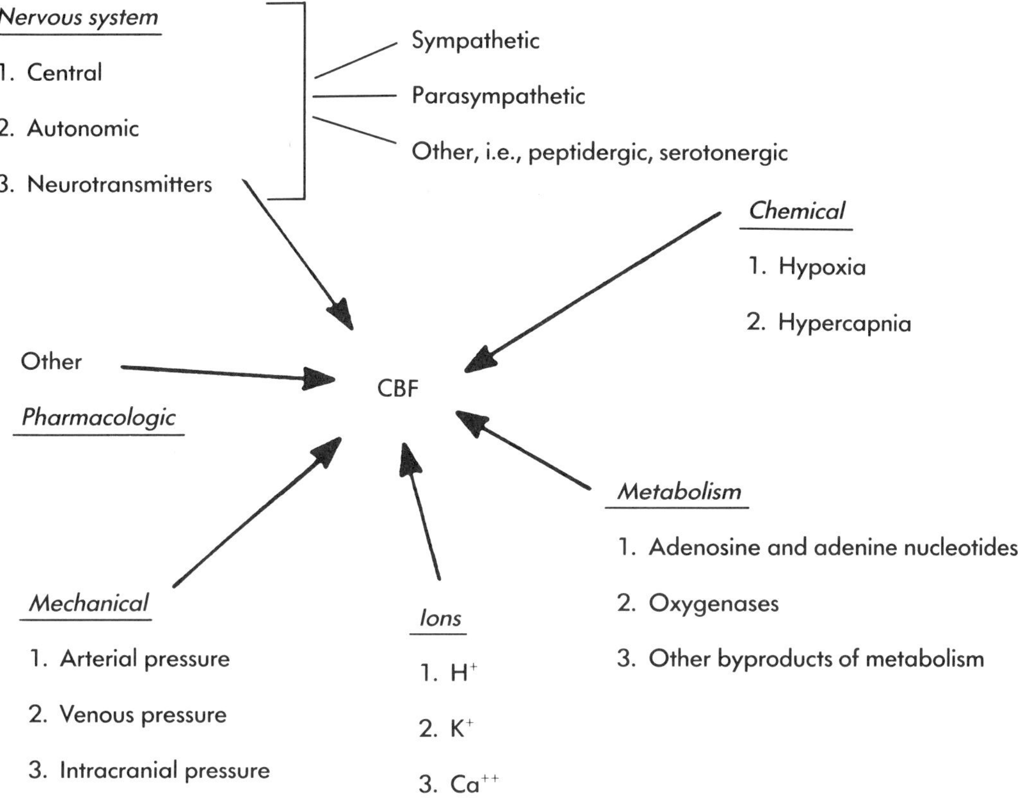

Figure 20–2 Factors controlling cerebral blood flow. (From Traystman RJ: Control of cerebral blood flow. In Vanhoutte PM, Leussen I, editors: *Vasodilatation*, New York, 1981, Raven Press, p 39.)

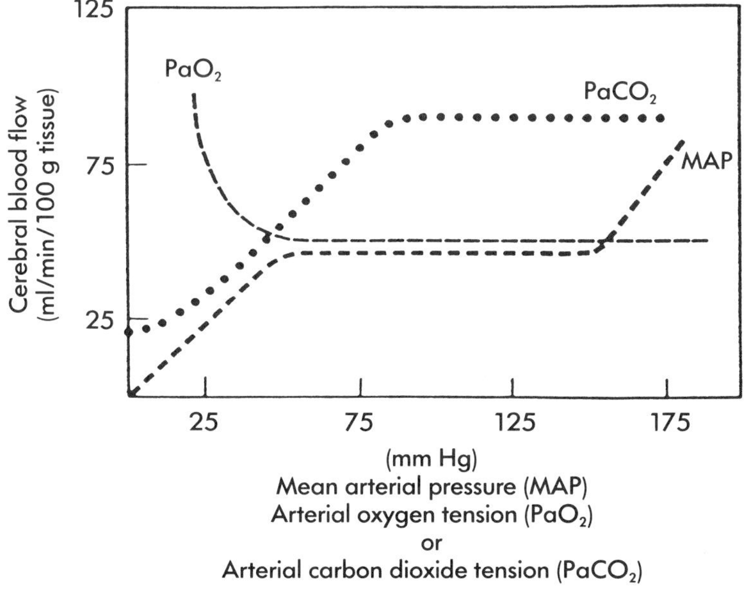

Figure 20–3 The effects of blood pressure and arterial blood gas tensions on cerebral blood flow.

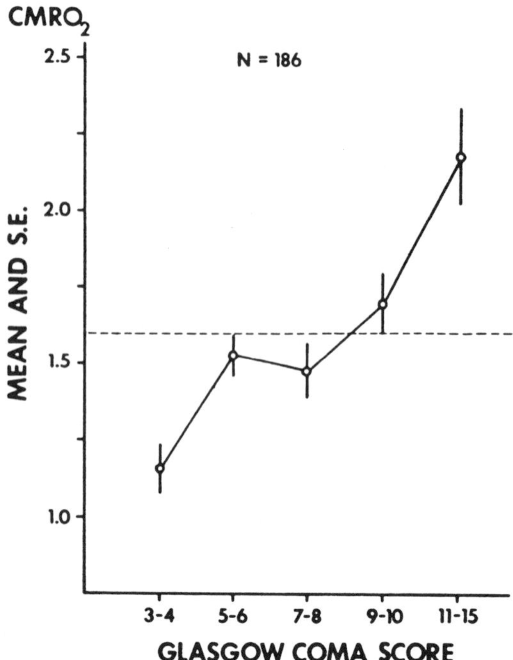

Figure 20–4 Relationship between cerebral metabolic rate and Glasgow Coma Scale score. Mean and standard error of cerebral metabolic rate (CMRO$_2$) plotted against Glasgow Coma Scale score. CMRO$_2$ is expressed in ml/100 gm/min. The findings are based on 186 studies in 65 patients. Patients with a GCS score of 8 or less had a CMRO$_2$ of less than half of the normal mean value of 3.3 ml/100 g/min. (From Muizelaar J, Obrist WD: Cerebral blood flow and brain metabolism with brain injury. In Becker DP, Povlishock JT, editors: *Central nervous system trauma status report, 1985*, Bethesda, Md, 1985, National Institute of Neurological and Communicative Disorders and Stroke, National Institutes of Health.)

sumed to be mechanical, although chemical and neural factors may play a role as well. Edema fluid, rich in plasma proteins and electrolytes, accumulates principally in the extracellular white matter. Hydrostatic pressure gradients shift edema fluid toward the ventricular system, where it is ultimately absorbed. Increases in cerebrospinal fluid pressure may inhibit flow of edema fluid into the ventricular system.

Traumatic intracerebral hematomas (contusions) may be due to direct impact to the brain surface or to movement of the brain within the skull. They often evolve over time, appearing less pronounced or absent on early CT scans. Deterioration in mental status or rising intracranial pressure within the first few days after injury may be due to an enlarging contusion and warrants repeat imaging studies, as surgical evacuation of contused and devitalized brain may be the treatment of choice to maximize salvage of viable tissue compromised by the resultant brain swelling.

DIAGNOSIS OF INTRACRANIAL HYPERTENSION
History and physical examination

As with all other disease, injury, or dysfunctional states, identifying intracranial hypertensions begins with history and physical examination. Many of the physical findings commonly attributed to increased intracranial pressure, such as third-nerve palsy, or signs of tentorial or foramen magnum herniation, are actually due to focal displacement of brain tissue resulting from pressure gradients.[34] Consequently, life-threatening brainstem compromise may occur even when the monitored intracranial pressure is not elevated. Papilledema is a reliable sign of increased intracranial pressure but usually takes several days to occur and may lag behind the child's neurologic deterioration. Hemodynamic responses to intracranial hypertension (systemic hypertension and bradycardia) are not as predictable in the child as in the adult. Decorticate or decerebrate posturing may also appear incompletely; likewise, movements to noxious stimulation occur in forms that are difficult to interpret, such as bicycling or flailing, particularly in infants. In summary, the physical examination may not allow the clinician to make the diagnosis of increased intracranial pressure with precision. It has been found, however, that intracranial hypertension occurs in over half the children with severe head injuries.[2] With moderate to severe head injury, a decline in neurologic function as manifested by a decrease in the Glasgow Coma Scale score represents increased intracranial pressure until proven otherwise.

Imaging studies

The introduction, refinement, and widespread availability of CT scanning have advanced the knowledge of the anatomic response to head injury, and enhanced the ability to care for the child with a serious head injury. CT technology is available in most hospitals and can be employed quickly. With newer CT equipment, an unenhanced CT scan of the head takes approximately 10 minutes. Spiral CT scanning, a relatively new, rapid technique, takes less than 1 minute of actual scan time, and the entire scanning process can be completed in under 5 minutes.

As a general rule, a child with an abnormal neurologic examination following head injury undergoes head and upper cervical spine CT scanning as soon as possible. In the severely injured child with a low Glasgow Coma Scale score at presentation, diffuse axonal injury, multifocal contusions,

Table 20–4 CT scan findings in 262 acutely head-injured children

Anatomical findings	Clinical grade			
	I	**II**	**III**	**IV**
Normal	24	27	21	7
Subarachnoid hemorrhage	1	8	12	25
Depressed fracture	5	12	10	9
Diffuse cerebral swelling	0	8	22	26
Shearing	0	0	0	11
Contusion	3	8	16	15
Focal swelling	0	4	6	6
Intracerebral hematoma	1	1	2	5
Acute subdural hematoma	0	4	8	15
Acute epidural hematoma	2	5	5	6

Grade 1 injury = minimal to no disturbance of consciousness; grade 4 injury = comatose with pain response. (After Zimmerman RA, Bilaniuk LT: Computed tomography in pediatric head trauma, *J Neuroradiol* 8:257-271, 1981.)

and a hemispheric or diffuse hypoxic appearance with small subdural collections (as is often seen in nonaccidental injuries) are the most common injury types seen on CT scan (Table 20-4).[35]

Magnetic resonance imaging (MRI) provides greater resolution of brain parenchymal lesions. Spectroscopy can produce information about regional metabolic activity. Use of MRI in the acute, initial management of the head-injured child is unusual. A satisfactory unenhanced study requires approximately 20 minutes. Human surveillance of the child is limited because of the distance of the child from caregivers when positioned in the magnet. Monitoring of the child with electronic devices while in the MRI scanner has improved in recent years but is still suboptimal when compared with techniques used during CT. Currently, pulse oximetry, digit plethysmography, and noninvasive systemic arterial blood manometry are possible in MRI. Devices that provide electrocardiogram, intracranial pressure measurement, and invasive vascular manometry cannot be used because they interfere with the magnetic field. In some instances, however, MRI and MR angiography are very useful for defining spine injury, vascular lesions, scattered diffuse and brainstem hemorrhages, and other disorders incompletely visualized by CT. In such cases intubated and monitored children in whom intracranial pressure is relatively stable can undergo scanning, with appropriate clinical observation during the study.

Intracranial pressure monitoring devices

Measurement of CSF pressure in the lumbar subarachnoid space has been practiced since the early 1900s. This technique fell from favor in the management of children with severe head injury because of the potential for brainstem compression with herniation, and because pressure in the lumbar subarachnoid space may not accurately reflect intracranial pressure. There are, however, a number of devices for direct placement into the cranial vault.

Ventricular fluid pressure measured through a fluid-filled catheter remains a standard against which all other devices are compared. In patients with normal or increased ventricular size, a ventricular catheter is easily placed through a frontal burr hole into the anterior horn of the lateral ventricle, which offers the advantage of CSF drainage as a means of intracranial pressure control. Placement of the ventriculostomy catheter may be difficult when the ventricles are small, as is often the case when intracranial pressure is increased after trauma, and repeated attempts may injure brain substance or cause hemorrhage. Ventriculitis may occur if the catheter remains in place for more than 72 hours. Finally, because the intraventricular catheter depends on fluid pressure transmission, debris or clot which may clog the tip of the catheter will cause the system to fail, especially as the ventricular system collapses when the maximum translocation of CSF to the spinal subarachnoid space has occurred.

Pressure transducers fluid-coupled to bolts, screws, and catheters have been placed in the epidural, subdural, and subarachnoid spaces. Brain parenchyma, debris, or clot may occlude the orifice or lumen of these devices and interfere with pressure measurement.

At many trauma centers the monitoring device most commonly used currently is a fiberoptic pressure transducer. As shown in Fig. 20-5, changes in intracranial pressure induce changes in the position of the diaphragm located at the tip of the catheter. The changing position of the diaphragm results in alterations of reflected light intensity generated by a fiberoptic bundle reaching the photodetector. The variation in light striking the photodetector results in current change emanating from the photodetector which is amplified, digitized, and displayed after calibration in milliliters of mercury (mm/Hg). This solid-state device does not depend on a continuous column of fluid for pressure measurement. Initial problems with baseline drift have been largely overcome. Crutchfield[4] found an average daily drift of ±0.6 mm Hg with a maximum daily drift of 2.5 mm Hg, as compared with an intraventricular catheter. Over a 5-day period the average drift was 2.1 mm Hg, with a maximum drift of 6 mm Hg. The fiberoptic device may be placed within the ventricle, subdural space, or

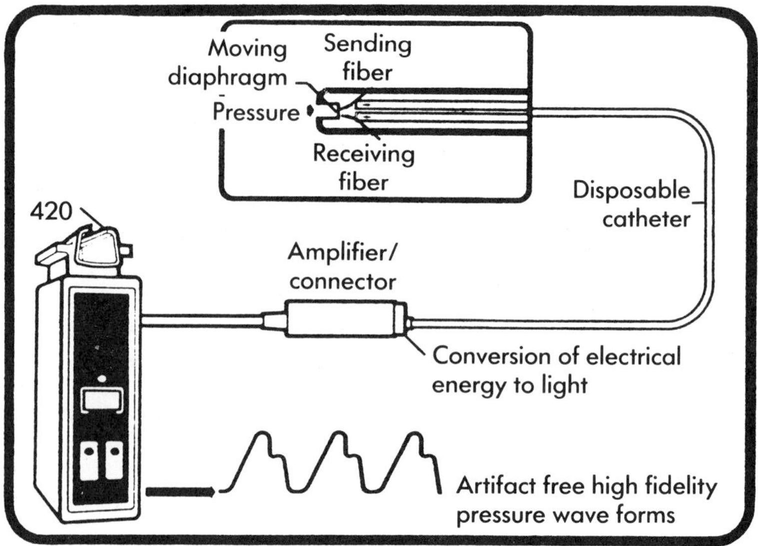

Figure 20–5 Camino Laboratories transducer-tipped fiberoptic catheter for intracranial pressure monitoring. (Courtesy Camino Laboratories, San Diego, Calif.)

brain parenchyma. In our practice, the most common placement of the catheter is within the brain parenchyma. When ventricular size is adequate, we insert a ventricular catheter which permits drainage of CSF along with pressure monitoring. The major disadvantage of the fiberoptic system is its inability to be recalibrated in situ.

Indications for intracranial pressure monitoring

Children with mild to moderate disturbances of consciousness following cranial trauma are unlikely to have dangerous elevations in intracranial pressure. We generally rely on the physical examination to provide us with information about the patient's neurologic functioning in cases of mild to moderate head injury (GCS score >9). Patients with GCS scores ≤8 are considered candidates for invasive intracranial pressure monitoring. Patients with GCS scores of >8 who have traumatic lesions associated with a high likelihood of brain swelling may also be considered for ICP monitoring (see Table 20–3). Less severely injured patients who must receive anesthesia for lengthy diagnostic or therapeutic interventions in the acute posttraumatic period may also be considered candidates for intracranial pressure monitoring because anesthesia interferes with neurologic physical examination.

MANAGEMENT OF INTRACRANIAL HYPERTENSION

Secondary brain injury threatens the seriously head-injured child in the minutes to days following the primary insult. Rapid assessment and treatment of children with potentially elevated intracranial pressure offers them the best chance for recovery from the primary injury. Our approach to such children divides therapeutic interventions into three categories: (1) maintenance of systemic oxygen and substrate delivery, (2) maintenance of cerebral oxygen and substrate delivery, and (3) reduction of cerebral metabolic demand.

Maintenance of systemic oxygen and substrate delivery

The maintenance of systemic oxygen delivery (Do_2) remains a fundamental principle in trauma resuscitation. Inadequate systemic transport will result in a poor outcome, no matter how skillfully intracranial pressure is treated. The Do_2 equals the product of cardiac output (CO), oxygen content of arterial blood (Cao_2) and a factor of 10. Arterial oxygen content is described by the following equation:

$$Cao_2 = Hb \ (gm/dl) \times 1.36$$
$$\times Sao_2 + Pao_2 \times 0.003$$

where 1.36 is the estimate of the mean volume of oxygen in milliliters that can be bound by 1 gm of hemoglobin when fully saturated. The factor 0.003 represents the solubility coefficient of oxygen in plasma. At 1 atmosphere barometric pressure, the amount of oxygen dissolved in plasma is very small and does not make a significant contribution to Cao_2. Cardiac output (CO) is the product of stroke volume and heart rate and by convention is ex-

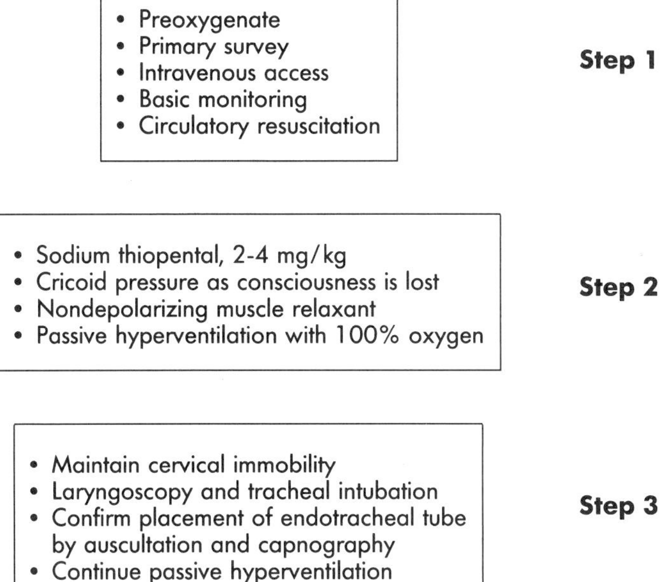

Figure 20–6 Airway management in head injury.

pressed in liters per minute. Oxygen delivery is therefore described by the equation

$$Do_2 \text{ (ml/min)} = Cao_2 \text{ (ml } O_2/dl) \times 10 \text{ dl/L} \times CO) \text{ (L/min)}$$

In a population in which body size may vary 100-fold, it is convenient to express delivery and other variables indexed to a measure of body size, either weight (kilograms) or body surface area (meter^2).

Management of the respiratory and circulatory systems to maintain optimal systemic oxygen delivery improves outcome. Support of these two systems constitutes the first priority in trauma resuscitation and may begin at the scene of injury or in the emergency department.

Respiratory management. Interference with external respiration, the exchange of respiratory gases between inspired atmosphere and pulmonary capillary blood, frequently accompanies head trauma. External respiratory failure results from loss of neurologic control of structures involved in respiration (for example, apnea or loss of airway protective reflexes) or pulmonary edema of neurogenic origin. Extrathoracic gasway obstruction may result from genioglossus hypotonia or obstruction by vomitus, blood, other foreign bodies, or secretions. Swelling or damage to head and neck structures may impede gas flow into the lung. Basic maneuvers such as chin lift, jaw thrust, or artificial airway insertion will help the caregiver to both diagnose and relieve airway obstruction. Cervical movement should be limited until the absence of cervical vertebral or ligamentous injury is confirmed. Once airway pa-

tency is established, administer supplemental oxygen by face piece and reservoir bag while observing respiratory effort. Examine chest wall movement, color, retractions, and use of intercostal and accessory muscle activity, as well as gas flow into and out of the mouth and nose. Imaging studies, pulse oximetry, and arterial blood respiratory gas manometry and acid-base measurement complement the physical assessment.

Perform tracheal intubation in patients who are unconscious and unable to protect or maintain their airway. One should also consider tracheal intubation for agitated or combative patients who may require sedation for diagnostic procedures. A typical sequence for accomplishing tracheal intubation in the head-injured patient is shown in Fig. 20-6. This is usually accomplished by administering thiopental or methohexital and pancuronium intravenously. The ultra-short-acting barbiturate establishes amnesia, blunts increases of intracranial pressure associated with laryngoscopy and intubation, and may lower existing intracranial hypertension. The barbiturates cause venodilation and myocardial depression, which may lead to dangerous reductions in blood flow, especially in hypovolemic individuals. We usually inject sodium thiopental 1 mg/kg and add up to 4 mg/kg, observing the neurologic and hemodynamic responses. Apply cricoid pressure, administer a nondepolarizing muscle relaxant to facilitate laryngoscopy, and begin passive hyperventilation with face piece and reservoir bag immediately upon loss of consciousness. The most accomplished laryngoscopist present exposes the glottis and inserts the tracheal tube when relaxation is adequate. During tracheal intubation, an assistant immobilizes the head in a neutral position to prevent its movement on the cervical spine.

Continue manual hyperventilation and cricoid pressure until acceptable location of the tracheal tube is confirmed. Capnography is employed when possible, along with auscultation of the lung fields with manual inflation to ensure proper position of the tracheal tube within the thoracic trachea. Once an artificial airway has been established and properly located, begin mechanical ventilation. Using a volume preset, time-cycled ventilator, begin with a preset tidal volume of 10 to 15 cc/kg and increase delivered tidal volume if there is insufficient chest motion. Adjust ventilator rate to achieve carbon dioxide tensions in arterial blood of 25 to 35 mm Hg, and add oxygen to inspired air to maintain arterial oxyhemoglobin saturation at 95% or above. Avoid end-exhalatory pressure unless there is decreased lung compliance resulting from reduced lung volumes. Elevated end-exhalatory pressure may worsen delivery of oxygen and substrate to the CNS through two mechanisms. Normal lung compliance permits transmission of raised airway pressure to thoracic veins, impedes cerebral venous return, and may increase intracranial pressure. Impaired systemic venous return will decrease cardiac output and decrease systemic Do_2. When pulmonary edema, pulmonary contusion, or aspiration pneumonitis contributes to decreased functional residual capacity, positive end-expiratory pressure restores gas-containing lung volume and achieves acceptable Pao_2 at a lower concentration of inspired oxygen.

Circulatory management. Suitable hemodynamics allow oxygen and substrate entering the blood to reach the recovering CNS. Of the various influences on cardiac output—preload, afterload, contractility, rate, and rhythm—precise adjustment of preload merits the most attention. In the otherwise healthy child with isolated head injury, preload can be manipulated on the basis of physical findings: pulse quality and rate, capillary refill, extremity temperature, blood pressure, and urine output. In the child with preexisting heart disease, multiple injuries requiring more than 20 ml/kg of fluid resuscitation to achieve acceptable hemodynamics, or myocardial dysfunction from chest trauma, central venous manometry permits more precise intravascular volume adjustment. The femoral route is preferred to either internal jugular or subclavian vein cannulation in patients with head injuries, as positioning necessary to cannulate these veins frequently retards cerebral venous drainage

and may elevate intracranial pressure. Occasionally, in some children, adjustment of preload is insufficient to increase cardiac output to maintain cerebral perfusion. Proper adjustment of contractility and afterload may dictate dilution-based measurements of cardiac output and calculation of systemic and pulmonary vascular resistance indices to determine the contribution of these variables to the low cardiac output state.

The choice of fluid for resuscitation from shock accompanying head trauma remains somewhat controversial. In experimental hemorrhagic shock combined with brain injury, colloid solutions offered no clear advantage over isotonic crystalloid in limiting increased brain water or increased intracranial pressure.[12] Experimental evidence in a similar animal model suggests that hypertonic crystalloid results in lower intracranial pressure, decreased brain water, and improved intracranial compliance when compared with isotonic crystalloid or colloid.[24] We currently favor colloid solutions, such as 5% albumin suspended in 0.9% saline solution, over crystalloid for intravascular volume expansion. It is important to avoid overhydration or the administration of excessive free water, which may contribute to brain swelling.

Maintain hemoglobin concentration between 11 and 12 gm/dl. Evidence in victims of strokes suggests that hemoglobin concentration in this range is optimal for maintaining a balance between improving blood flow from decreased viscosity and preserving oxygen transport as hemoglobin concentration decreases.[12]

Substrate management. The goal of nutritional support in the brain-injured patient is to provide adequate caloric intake in the form of exogenous carbohydrate, fat, and protein to maintain euglycemia and support tissue repair while permitting fluid restriction. Except under conditions of starvation, the CNS depends on an uninterrupted supply of glucose for normal cellular function. Supplying exogenous glucose as a continuous infusion to prevent hypoglycemia is particularly important in young infants, whose glycogen stores are limited. Manipulate the concentration and rate of dextrose infusion to achieve serum glucose levels between 60 and 100 mg/dl and to preserve a state of "euvolemic dehydration" (see "Fluid Restriction").

Recent evidence in studies of animals and humans suggests that hyperglycemia under conditions of tissue ischemia in the CNS predisposes to worse neurologic outcome. Animal studies have shown that preischemic hyperglycemia increases intracerebral lactate concentration and lowers pH. Presumably, the provision of substrate in an oxygen-poor environment fuels anaerobic metabolism, the resulting intracellular acidosis causing greater cellular dysfunction or death.

Severe head injury is accompanied by a dramatic increase in metabolic rate, up to twice the basal metabolic rate. Levels of catecholamines, cortisol, glucagon, and insulin are elevated up to six times the normal in patients with head injuries and are responsible for the increased metabolism. Inflammatory mediators, including Interleukin-1, tumor necrosis factor, prostaglandins, and others may also contribute to tissue catabolism.[15] Caloric requirements parallel motor activity, caloric expenditure increasing by 200% to 300% above baseline in patients with excessive, abnormal motor activity. Endogenous protein and fat serve as the source of calories before full nutritional support can be achieved.

As soon as possible after the injury, we provide 1.5 times the basal energy requirements, including 2 to 2.5 grams of protein per kilogram per day. Nonprotein calories should consist of up to 50% fat, to minimize carbon dioxide production and hyperglycemia, which may complicate excessive carbohydrate administration. Enteral feeding remains the route of choice, using parenteral alimentation only when the gastrointestinal tract is dysfunctional. Select a formula of high caloric density (1 to 2 kcal/ml) that will provide the required calories with a minimum of free water. Gastric emptying is frequently delayed in patients with brain injuries. In spite of this, institute feedings via the orogastric or nasogastric route, monitoring gastric emptying carefully. If gastric stasis is present, insert a transpyloric feeding tube to minimize the risk of regurgitation and soiling of the respiratory tract.

We adjust electrolytes in infused solutions so that patients receive 2 and 3 mEq/kg/24 hr of sodium potassium and sodium chloride, respectively.

Therapies to reduce intracranial pressure

At our institution, all children with head injuries at risk for elevated intracranial pressure are treated presumptively until their clinical examination, imaging studies, and/or intracranial pressure monitoring shows that pressure elevation is not present or likely to occur. Therapies available include those that lower the volume of the intracranial parenchymal, blood, or CSF compartments. All children are treated initially with moderate hyperventilation (Paco$_2$ 30 to 35 mm Hg), and fluids are kept to the minimum necessary to maintain adequate systemic perfusion (usually two thirds calculated normal maintenance requirements). As more information becomes available about the individual

Table 20-5 Physical and laboratory findings in euvolemic dehydration

Daily weight loss of 0.5-0.7% of usual body weight
Serum sodium 145–150 mEq/L
Serum osmolality 295–305 mOsm/L
Urine output 0.75 ml/kg/hr
Urine specific gravity 1.020–1.025
Urine osmolality 800–1000 mOsm/L

child's clinical status, injury type, and intracranial pressure risk, treatment is matched to the child's needs. More aggressive therapies such as barbiturate infusion are reserved for those patients who are refractory to conventional measures. A discussion of the various treatments available for intracranial hypertension follows.

Therapies to reduce V$_{Brain}$

Fluid restriction. "Euvolemic dehydration" is achieved by restricting fluids. This implies maintenance of intravascular volume, with dehydration of extravascular spaces. We consider this condition to exist when the clinical and laboratory features listed in Table 20-5 have been achieved. The combination of colloid solutions plus diuretic therapy facilitates the maintenance of this state.

Osmotic diuresis. Osmotic agents, such as mannitol, decrease brain bulk by creating an osmotic gradient between normal brain with an intact blood-brain barrier and the intravascular space, drawing fluid from brain tissue. Extravascular dehydration occurs principally in areas of normal brain tissue, improving intracranial compliance by providing compensatory volume for injured areas of the brain. In doses of 0.25 to 1.0 g/kg intravenously, it reduces intracranial pressure within 10 to 20 minutes and may last up to 4 hours.[12] It can be administered repeatedly in the acute setting to achieve serum osmolality of 310 to 320 mOsm/L. Serum osmolality in excess of 320 mOsm/L may be associated with renal tubular injury, renal failure, and rebound cerebral edema.[12] Mannitol's effectiveness decreases over 2 to 3 days of repeated use as brain tissue osmolality rises and the gradient between brain substance and blood diminishes.

Mannitol's salutory effect on intracranial pressure may not be exclusively due to its osmotic effects. Recent data in studies of cats suggest that intravenous mannitol, 1 gm/kg of body weight, lowers blood viscosity and increases cerebral blood flow, but decreases cerebral blood volume.[23] The relationship between blood viscosity, blood vessel diameter, and intracranial pressure is shown in Fig.

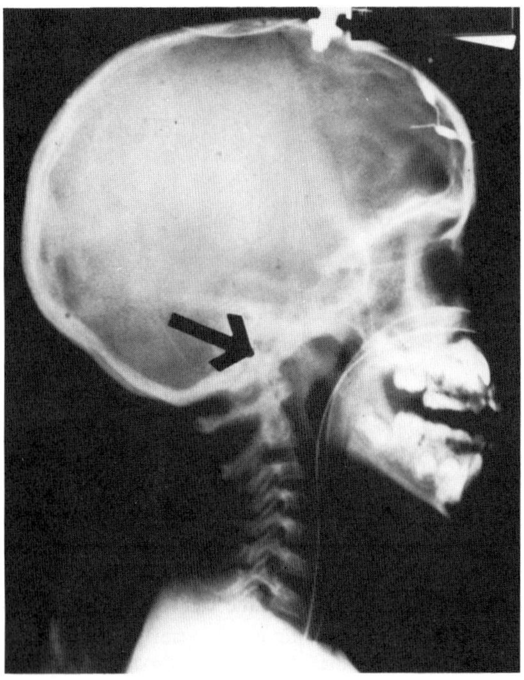

Figure 20–9 Lateral skull roentgenogram showing proper positioning of the tip of the jugular venous bulb catheter just beyond the outer table of the skull *(arrow)*. (From Hayek DA, Veremakis C: Intracranial pathophysiology of brain injury. *Problems in critical care: resuscitation following acute brain injury* 5:135-155, 1991.)

Table 20-6 Interrelationship of CBF, $CMRO_2$, and $AJDO_2$

	CBF	CMRO$_2$	AJDo$_2$
Normal (N)	N	N	N
Compensatory flow-metabolism coupling	↓	↓	N
Compensatory flow-metabolism coupling	↑	↑	N
Ischemia	↓	N	↑
Infarction	↓	↓	↓
Hyperemia	↑/N	↓	↓

From Hayek DA, Veremakis C: Intracranial pathophysiology of brain injury. *Problems in critical care: resuscitation following acute brain injury* 5:135-155, 1991.

centration exist, the clinician may employ the jugular venous bulb oxygen tension alone to judge the match of supply and demand. Studies in normal human volunteers indicate that jugular venous bulb oxygen tensions between 20 and 26 mm Hg are associated with evidence of cerebral anaerobic metabolism.[1,2a] Using this information, the clinician can adjust mechanical hyperventilation to achieve minimal jugular venous bulb oxygen tensions of 28 to 30 mm Hg if intracranial hypertension demands this therapy.

A modification of the Kety-Schmidt technique using nitrous oxide is used to measure CBF.[30] In the 1940s Kety and Schmidt applied the Fick principle to the brain's uptake of nitrous oxide, an inert gas that is taken up by the brain but not metabolized.[14] Cerebral blood flow is computed by using the modified Fick equation:

$$CBF = \frac{100 \cdot \lambda \cdot V(t)}{\int (a - v)dt} cc/100 \ g/min$$

where λ is the brain:blood solubility coefficient, $V(t)$ is the venous N_2O reading at saturation and $\int (a - v)dt$ is the area circumscribed by the arterial and venous curves.[30] The technique as modified by Swedlow and colleagues permits sampling of small aliquots of blood (5 cc total) and can be performed at the bedside with results available within 45 minutes. $CMRo_2$ can be obtained by multiplying $AJDo_2$ times the CBF.

Therapies to reduce cerebral metabolic demand

Ordinary therapies. As a rule, $CMRo_2$ is depressed as a function of depth of coma, as measured by the Glasgow Coma Scale. In the child with severe head injury, pathologic states may exist that increase the cerebral metabolic rate. Hyperpyrexia without an infectious source is frequently present in patients with head injuries. Fever increases cerebral metabolic rate as much as 10% to 15% for every degree centigrade elevation above normal.[25] Increased blood flow, in an attempt to meet increased metabolic demand, may elevate intracranial pressure if compliance is low. Aggressive fever control with antipyretics and surface cooling is indicated in the febrile child with severe head injury.

Convulsions increase cerebral metabolic rate and blood flow, which will in turn increase intracranial pressure if compliance is reduced. Prolonged seizure activity can lead to neuronal ischemia as metabolic demand exceeds delivery of oxygen and substrate. Convulsions should be treated promptly with phenytoin (loading dose 20 mg/kg, intravenously, followed by a maintenance dose of 3 to 8 mg/kg/24 hr in two divided doses). The rate of administration of intravenous phenytoin should not exceed 1 mg/kg/min. In a recent large, randomized prospective study, phenytoin prophylaxis in patients with head injuries significantly reduced the incidence of seizures in the first week following injury.[32]

Extraordinary therapies

High-dose barbiturates. High-dose barbiturates reduce cerebral metabolic demands, produce cerebral vasoconstriction, and diminish CBF. When used as prophylactic therapy in patients with severe head injuries, high-dose barbiturates do not improve neurologic outcome or morbidity.[33] However, they improve intracranial pressure control and decrease morbidity when used in patients with refractory intracranial hypertension that could not be controlled with conventional therapy, as compared with patients who received conventional therapy alone.[5] Thiopental, pentobarbital, and phenobarbital have been used to treat intracranial hypertension.

Maximum suppression of cerebral metabolism and intracranial pressure obtained with pentobarbital correspond to a burst suppression or isoelectric pattern of electroencephalographic activity. Further reduction in energy requirements must come from physical forces such as body cooling. This level of cerebral cortical depression is usually achieved with a serum concentration of pentobarbital of 20 mg/L. This serum concentration of pentobarbital is achieved by administering a loading dose, followed by a constant infusion of pentobarbital. The loading dose of pentobarbital is calculated by using an estimated volume of distribution at steady state (V_{ss}) of 0.9 L/kg, or approximately 20 mg/kg.

Loading dose (mg)
= desired serum concentration (mg/L) $\times$ V_{ss}(L/kg)

Swedlow and co-workers found a large variation in peak serum level of pentobarbital in children when the loading dose was calculated using an estimated volume of distribution of 0.9 L/kg.[31] They found a close association between the cardiac index at the time of the loading dose and the apparent volume of distribution. When cardiac index is known, the apparent volume of distribution of pentobarbital at steady state may be more precisely calculated using the following equation:

$$V_{ss} \ (L/kg) = 0.17 \times CI \ (L/min/m^2) + 0.2$$

This loading dose is infused over 1 to 2 hours, the rate of infusion guided by the response of the intracranial pressure to the barbiturate and systemic hemodynamics. Serum pentobarbital levels rise rapidly and reach peak levels within 4 hours of initiation of therapy. Following the loading dose, continuously infuse pentobarbital, 1 mg/kg/hr. Measure serum pentobarbital level 2 hours after the loading dose has been administered; supplement the initial loading dose and adjust the continuous infusion rate to achieve and maintain desired serum levels. The serum concentrations of pentobarbital can be adjusted to produce a burst suppression pattern on an electroencephalogram.

Hemodynamic depression may occur when high-dose barbiturates are employed as a result of diminished systolic function and systemic vasodilation. Guided by the central venous pressure, infuse albumin in combination with packed red cells to maintain adequate intravascular volume in the presence of increased vascular capacity. When cardiac output is insufficient with adequate preload, contractility is augmented, usually with dopamine. Serum levels of between 20 and 30 mg/L usually result in systemic arterial hypotension or a requirement for inotropic agents in approximately 50% of patients.

Hypothermia. Reducing body temperature to between 30° and 32° C by surface cooling, intravenous infusion of chilled solutions, and gastric lavage with chilled saline decreases neuronal energy requirements. Cerebral metabolic rate for oxygen is reduced 7% to 10% per degree centigrade between 37° and 22°.[22] Cerebral blood flow parallels decreased metabolic requirements. When used in conjunction with chemical suppression of neuronal metabolic activity, hypothermia reduces energy requirements to a lower level than chemical suppression alone, implying a reduction in cellular energy demand for structural maintenance as well as function.

To induce hypothermia, the child is placed on hypothermia blankets and cooled to an esophageal temperature of 33° to 34° C. The blankets are then turned off and the temperature allowed to drift down to 31° C. The patient receives a barbiturate infusion and neuromuscular blockade to prevent shivering. Once 24 hours have passed without dangerous increases in intracranial pressure, the patient is rewarmed at a rate no faster than 0.5 degrees/hour.[26]

Hypothermia has been induced in children with intracranial hypertension caused by trauma and metabolic encephalopathy that has been refractory to other therapies, including barbiturate coma.[26] Although useful in controlling intracranial hypertension, hypothermia induces widespread physiologic perturbations that complicate patient management and preclude its routine use in the child with refractory intracranial hypertension. As body temperature approaches 30° C, cardiac output falls in parallel with systemic oxygen consumption, and dysrhythmias may occur. Plasma volume decreases significantly during hypothermia, and cardiovascular collapse may occur if rewarming is too rapid. Fluid management in the hypothermic patient is further complicated by decreases in renal blood flow, urine output, and renal tubular concentrating and diluting ability. Leukopenia and depression of polymorphonuclear-leukocyte phagocytic activity occur during moderate hypothermia. Finally, confusion in interpreting arterial blood gas tensions and pH arise in managing patients whose body temperature is reduced. For these reasons, extreme hypothermia is rarely employed in cases of head injury.

NEW EXPERIMENTAL THERAPIES

Intense interest has been generated during the past decade in the potential for interventions based on an improved understanding of the basic pathophysiology of neural injury after a variety of insults, including ischemia, hypoxia, hypoglycemia, status epilepticus, and mechanical trauma. Increasing evidence from basic science laboratories suggests that these processes have in common the initiation of a complex, interrelated set of parallel biochemical cascades, which, if unchecked, eventually lead to irreversible cell death. It appears, however, that several steps in these cascades are amenable to therapeutic intervention, resulting in preservation of neurons that would otherwise have succumbed, even when treatment is initiated after the insult.[10,29] Clinical trials of excitatory amino-acid antagonists, calcium channel blockers, lipid peroxidation inhibitors, aminosteroids ("lazaroids"), and other agents designed to thwart delayed neuronal degeneration will be forthcoming during the next several years, replacing the era of supportive care with that of specific brain-injury therapy.

OUTCOME

The obvious measure of success of any therapeutic intervention is a demonstrated decrease in long-term morbidity and mortality. With respect to the latter, the relationship between elevated intracranial pressure and death is clear. The vast majority of patients who survive the initial injury but later succumb in the acute postinjury period do so because of brain swelling resulting in herniation. A smaller number of patients die of systemic complications, usually infection. It is likely that children in whom intracranial pressure is refractory to current aggressive treatment in the acute period have sustained primary brain injuries that are extremely severe and largely irrecoverable. These children typically have major parenchymal disruption or severe superimposed hypoxia or ischemia, a very low Glasgow Coma Scale score (usually 3 or 4), and sustained intracranial pressure in the range of 40 to 50 mm Hg or greater, which becomes increasingly difficult to control. For such children, the likelihood of an outcome better than severe disability is extremely small. As discussed previously, whether newer treatments to interrupt the potentially reversible components of the primary injury will reduce mortality remains to be investigated.

There is little doubt, however, that there is a subset of patients with severe head-injury in whom intracranial pressure can be controlled (that is, intracranial pressure less than 20 mm Hg) with aggressive management, and that these patients would likely die of their head injuries without such intervention.[5] The more difficult question is whether the quality of survival in these patients justifies the level of intervention. Although more studies are needed to answer this question, it is worth noting that a significant percentage of patients in the severely injured category go on to make a good recovery, and that the presence of at least transiently elevated intracranial pressure alone does not preclude a more favorable outcome.[19] It is suggested that the degree of structural disruption or superimposed severe global hypoxia or ischemia are the main determinants of eventual vegetative survival, and that aggressive treatment, especially when it is found to control intracranial pressure successfully, is warranted unless these conditions can be shown unequivocally to exist.

The effect of elevated intracranial pressure on morbidity after head injury is less well studied. Many authors have addressed the complexities of outcome from serious head injury in both adults and children.[3,7,17,21] In brief, all but a few children will eventually regain consciousness, although the duration of coma is sometimes measured in months. Even patients making a good motor recovery are nearly always left with significant deficits in memory, attention, and behavior. Although IQ may approach premorbid levels, there is usually a discrepancy between a relatively preserved verbal IQ and an impaired performance IQ.

Whereas a recent study failed to demonstrate a clear correlation between intracranial pressure elevation in the first 72 hours postinjury and 1-year neurobehavioral measures in adults with severe head injuries, other researchers have found more significant memory impairment in those patients with higher intracranial pressures.[3] As in other aspects of outcome determination, separating various factors such as injury severity, injury type, and premorbid status has confounded efforts to assess treatment efficacy. Intracranial pressure, in particular, lends itself with difficulty to such assessment because it is an ongoing and fluctuating variable that is influenced by treatment effects and the underlying level of responsiveness of the patient. For example, a child who is beginning to recover from fairly severe injury may have a more "normal" pattern of transient elevations in intracranial pressure in response to environmental stimuli. In such a situation, a higher intracranial pressure would not be expected to correlate with an eventual poor outcome. In addition, difficulty with intracranial pressure control may occur later in children and thus be missed in some investigations in which analysis is limited to the first few postinjury days.

Some experimental evidence suggests that certain populations of neurons may be selectively vulnerable to elevation in intracranial pressure; these neurons are likely to subserve subtle functions such as memory and selective attention.[27] For these reasons and the clinical data cited, it is our opinion at present that control of intracranial pressure is likely to improve long-term neuropsychological outcome, although additional work must be done before such an effect can be demonstrated unequivocally.

CONCLUSION

Head injury is the leading cause of accidental death in children. Those that survive severe injuries may suffer cognitive, behavioral, and social impairments that may preclude independent functioning later in life. Brain swelling with intracranial hypertension threatens at least half of those with severe head injuries. Meticulous supportive care, combined with aggressive intracranial pressure control guided by an understanding of the pathophysiology of injury and ongoing assessment of the relationship between oxygen supply and demand in the CNS, offers the child with severe head injuries the best chance for meaningful recovery. The next few decades will, it is hoped, bring improved efforts at prevention of head injury through improved safety devices and public education, as well as therapy directed at primary reversible injury occurring at the cellular level.

REFERENCES

1. Alexander SC, Cohen PJ, Wollman H et al: Cerebral carbohydrate metabolism during hypocarbia in man. *Anesthesiology* 25(5):624-632, 1965.
1a. Brookes M, MacMillan R, Cully S et al: Head injuries in accident and emergency departments: how different are children from adults? *J Epidemiol Community Health* 44(2):147-151, 1990.
2. Bruce DA, Schut L, Bruno LA et al: Outcome following severe head injuries in children, *J Neurosurg* 48:679-688, 1978.
2a. Cohen PJ, Alexander SC, Smith TC et al: Effects of hypoxia and normocarbia on cerebral blood flow and metabolism in conscious man, *J Appl Physiol* 23(2), August 1967, 183-189.
3. Costeff H, Groswasser Z, Goldstein R: Long-term follow-up review of 31 children with severe closed head trauma, *J Neurosurg* 73:684-687, 1990.
4. Crutchfield JS, Narayan RK, Robertson CS et al: Evaluation of a fiberoptic intracranial pressure monitor, *J Neurosurg* 72:482-487, 1990.
5. Eisenberg HM, Frankowski RF, Contant CC et al, and the Comprehensive Central Nervous System Trauma Centers: High-dose barbiturate control of elevated intracranial pressure in patients with severe head injury, *J Neurosurg* 69:15-23, 1988.
6. Faden AI, Demediuk P, Panter SS et al: The role of excitatory amino acids and NMDA receptors in traumatic brain injury, *Science* 244:789-790, 1989.
7. Filley CM, Cranberg LD, Alexander MP et al: Neurobehavioral outcome after closed head injury in childhood and adolescence, *Arch Neurol* 44:194-198, 1987.
8. Gallagher SS, Finison K, Guyer B et al: The incidence of injuries among 87,000 Massachusetts children and adolescents: results of the 1980-81 Statewide Childhood Injury Prevention Program surveillance system, *Am J Public Health* 74:1340-1347, 1987.
9. Gennarelli TA, Adams JH, Graham DI: Diffuse axonal injury—a new conceptual approach to an old problem. In Baethmann A, Go KG, Unterberg A, editors: *Mechanisms of secondary brain damage,* New York, 1986, Plenum Press, pp 15-28.
10. Gill R, Foster AC, Woodruff GN: MK-801 is neuroprotective in gerbils when administered during the postischaemic period, *Neuroscience* 25(3):847-855, 1988.
11. Hayek DA, Veremakis C: Intracranial pathophysiology of brain injury, *Problems in Critical Care: Resuscitation Following Acute Brain Injury* 5:135-155, 1991.
12. Hayek DA, Veremakis C: Therapeutic options in brain resuscitation, *Problems in Critical Care: Resuscitation Following Acute Brain Injury* 5:156-186, 1991.
13. Jennett B, Teasdale G: Aspects of coma after severe head injury, *Lancet* 1:878-881, 1977.
13a. Kellie G: An account of the appearances observed in the dissection of two of three individuals presumed to have perished in the storm of the 3rd, and whose bodies were discovered in the vicinity of Leith on the morning of the 4th November 1821 with some reflections on the pathology of the brain, *Trans Med Chir Soc Edinb* 1:84-169, 1824.
14. Kety SS, Schmidt CF: Determination of cerebral blood flow in man by the use of nitrous oxide in low concentrations, *Am J Physiol* 143:53, 1945.
15. Kirkland LL, Wilson GL: Extracranial effects of acute brain injury, *Problems in Critical Care: Resuscitation Following Acute Brain Injury* 5:292-307, 1991.
16. Kraus JF, Fife D, Cox P et al: Incidence, severity, and external causes of pediatric brain injury, *AJDC* 140:687-693, 1986.
17. Kriel RL, Krach LE, Sheehan M: Pediatric closed head injury: outcome following prolonged unconsciousness, *Arch Phys Med Rehabil* 69:678-681, 1988.
18. Langfitt TW, Obrist WD, Gennarelli TA et al: Correlation of cerebral blood flow with outcome in head injured patients, *Ann Surg* 186:411-414, 1977.
19. Levin HS, Gary HE, Eisenberg HM et al: Neurobehavioral outcome one year after severe head injury: experience of the Traumatic Coma Data Bank, *J Neurosurg* 73:699-709, 1990.
20. Luerssen TG, Klauber MR, Marshall LF: Outcome from head injury related to patient's age: a longitudinal prospective study of adult and pediatric head injury, *J Neurosurg* 68:409-416, 1988.
21. Mahoney WJ, D'Souza BJ, Haller JA et al: Long-term outcome of children with severe head trauma and prolonged coma, *Pediatrics* 71:756-762, 1983.
22. Michenfelder JD, Theye RA: Hypothermia: effect on canine brain and whole body metabolism, *Anesthesiology* 29:1107, 1968.
22a. Monro A: Observations on the structure and function of the nervous system. Edinburgh, Creech and Johnson, 1783.
23. Muizelaar J, Obrist WD: Cerebral blood flow and brain metabolism with brain injury. In Becker DP, Povlishock JT, editors: *Central nervous system trauma status report, 1985,* Bethesda, Md, 1985, National Institute of Neurological and Communicative Disorders and Stroke, National Institutes of Health.
24. Nordstrom CH, Rehncrona S, Siesjo BK: Cerebral metabolism. In Youmans J, editor: *Neurological surgery,* Philadelphia, 1990, WB Saunders, pp 623-651.
25. Olesen WD: Cerebral function, metabolism and blood flow, *Acta Neuro Scand* 57:38, 1974.
26. Raphaely RC, Swedlow DB, Downes JJ et al: Management of severe pediatric head trauma, *Ped Clin North Am* 27:715-727, 1980.

27. Ross DT, Duhaime AC: Degeneration of neurons in the thalamic reticular nucleus following transient ischemia due to raised intracranial pressure: excitotoxic degeneration mediated via non-NMDA receptors? *Brain Res* 501:129-143, 1989.
28. Shapiro K, Marmarou A: Clinical applications of the pressure-volume index in treatment of pediatric head injuries, *J Neurosurg* 56:819-825, 1982.
29. Siejo BK, Wielock T: Brain injury: neurochemical aspects. In Becker DP, Povlishock JT, editors: *Central nervous system trauma status report 1985,* Bethesda, Md, 1985, National Institute of Neurological and Communicative Disorders and Stroke, pp 513-532.
30. Swedlow DB, Lewis LE: Measurement of cerebral blood flow in children, *Anesthesiology* 53:S160, 1980.
31. Swedlow DB, Schreiner MS: Management of Reye's syndrome, *Crit Care Clin: Symposium on Neurologic Intensive Care* 1:285-310, 1985.
32. Temkin NR, Dikmen SS, Wilensky AJ et al: A randomized, double-blind study of phenytoin for the prevention of post-traumatic seizures, *N Engl J Med* 323:497, 1990.
33. Ward JD, Becker DP, Miller JD et al: Failure of prophylactic barbiturate coma in the treatment of severe head injury, *J Neurosurg* 62:383-388, 1985.
34. Wilkinson HA: Intracranial pressure. In Youmans J, editor: *Neurological surgery,* Philadelphia, 1990, WB Saunders, pp 623-651.
35. Zimmerman RA, Bilaniuk LT: Computed tomography in pediatric head trauma, *J Neuroradiol* 8:257-271, 1981.

21 Anesthesia

Willis A. McGill

The quality of care an injured child receives can determine ultimate outcome. A trauma team provides a mechanism to concentrate the resources necessary for quality care beginning when an injured child first enters an institution. Anesthesiologists as team members fill two roles. First, they bring unique skills in airway management and resuscitation—both vital during the first few minutes of assessment and intervention. Second, they initiate the information gathering that will be used in planning anesthetic management should the child ultimately require surgery.

Upon arrival of the child in the trauma unit, the anesthesiologists' primary responsibility (and, indeed, the team's first priority in resuscitating the injured child) is assuring a patent and secure airway, optimal ventilation, and oxygenation. Treatment procedures range from evaluation to providing an enriched O_2 atmosphere by mask or tracheal intubation (see Chapter 16). The objectives of emergency tracheal intubation are as follows:

1. To provide airway protection in an unconscious child.
2. To prevent secondary brain injury resulting from hypoxia/hypercarbia and to facilitate hyperventilation as treatment of elevated intracranial pressure in a child with a closed head injury.
3. To ensure an airway in a child with an actual or threatened compromised airway owing to mechanical or thermal injury. (Although the airway may be initially patent, edema caused by injury such as a burn may make later intervention difficult and risky.)
4. To optimize oxygen delivery in a child in shock.
5. To improve gas exchange in the presence of a thoracic or pulmonary injury.

It is essential that airway intervention and subsequent induction and maintenance of anesthesia be undertaken with consideration for other injuries or precarious physiology. Examples include:

1. *Cervical spine fracture.* In-line immobilization or cervical spine support must be maintained to stabilize the fracture in order to prevent spinal injury.
2. *Increased intracranial pressure.* The drugs and techniques chosen to facilitate intubation should minimize the adverse effects of laryngoscopy or intubation on increased intracranial pressure.
3. *Hypovolemia.* The drugs selected to facilitate intubation must also be selected with consideration of the patient's volume status and cardiovascular stability.
4. All injured children have a full stomach. Thus, airway management must minimize the risk of aspiration of gastric contents.

TRANSPORT AND OPERATING ROOM STABILIZATION

Transport of an injured child is a dangerous maneuver, especially when transport includes a detour to the radiology department. It is essential to minimize risk during this period by (1) maintaining close observation of the child's physiologic compensation (there is a tendency for caregivers to relax following successful resuscitation), (2) continuing to monitor the child at the same level established in the trauma unit, (3) ensuring complete communication of information regarding the child's condition and ongoing resuscitation to team members responsible for the child's care. This is particularly important when the child is transferred to the care of the operating room anesthesia team.

As the child is being prepared for surgery, the anesthesia team performs a rapid reassessment of respiratory, circulatory, and neurological status. If the child was previously intubated, the anesthesiologist establishes that the tracheal tube is properly positioned by observing symmetrical chest expansion, by listening to both lung fields for equal breath sounds, and by measuring CO_2 in the expired atmosphere, while simultaneously assessing adequacy of oxygenation by clinical examination and by pulse oximeter. Mechanical ventilation is instituted soon after arrival in the operating room both to free the anesthesiologist's hands and to ensure uninterrupted ventilation. Insertion of an esophageal stethoscope with thermistor permits continuous auscultation of breath and heart sounds and measurement of core temperature. Adequacy of cir-

"

culation is quickly evaluated by palpating peripheral pulse and by measuring capillary refill time. These assessments are followed by placement of electrocardiogram leads and application of a blood pressure cuff. Insertion of an arterial catheter permits monitoring of the arterial waveform and confirms adequacy of blood pressure. Once the child's condition is stable, analysis of arterial blood reveals acid-base status and reflects pulmonary function.

The anesthesiologist must also ensure adequate and accessible intravenous catheters. The largest gauge catheter that the vein will accommodate guarantees rapid replacement of intraoperative blood lost. Intravenous catheters placed in the emergency room are usually satisfactory, but a final check for function is essential. Unlike an adult's, a child's limbs are inaccessible during surgery. Trying to place an intravenous catheter once surgery has started is difficult and disruptive. Intravenous fluids and tubing should be prepared before the child's arrival in the operating room. These replace those the child arrives with and should include extension set, injection port, and double stopcocks; the first makes sure that the anesthesiologist has access to the fluid line, and the latter two provide alternate injection sites, the ability to change fluid infusion easily, and the option of pumping fluid and blood by the syringe method, which helps to quantify fluids precisely. Blood pumps, fluid warming devices, and blood infusion sets must be ready for use.

MONITORING

The American Society of Anesthesiologists has established minimal standards for intraoperative monitoring. These require that physiologic stability be evaluated continually by ongoing assessment of oxygenation, ventilation, circulation, and temperature. Devices and monitors required to provide the proper information, include, at a minimum, precordial (or esophageal) stethoscope, blood pressure recording device (noninvasive or invasive), electrocardiograph, pulse oximeter, inspired oxygen gas analyzer, thermometer, and a circuit-disconnect alarm and capnogram for any intubated patient. Technology development during the past decade has greatly improved and simplified intraoperative monitoring of children.

More extensive monitoring is required for the severely injured child. Additional monitors that are used frequently are arterial and central venous catheters with displayed arterial and venous waveforms as well as urinary catheters and intracranial pressure measuring devices.

An arterial cannula is essential for proper surveillance of a severely injured child during surgery and throughout postoperative management. Arterial catheter placement is usually performed percutaneously, even in a small infant, by using a 22- or 24-gauge catheter, although cutdown is often necessary. Direct transduction of the arterial waveform is the gold standard for blood pressure measurement; it also provides an immediate beat-to-beat reading of blood pressure and assessment of the adequacy of intravascular volume. The radial artery site is most useful, but the dorsalis pedis, posterior tibial, and femoral arteries provide alternate locations for cannulation. It is best to avoid use of the temporal artery because of the potential for air embolization into the cerebral circulation when the cannula is flushed.

An arterial cannula also allows withdrawal of blood throughout surgery for analysis of hematologic profile, of blood gases for acid-base status, and of electrolytes. This information guides blood component and fluid replacement, as well as ventilatory support during resuscitation.

The availability of noninvasive measures of ventilation and oxygenation has not replaced the need for blood gas analysis. In fact, comparison of blood gas values with pulse oximetry and capnograph readings provides valuable insight into respiratory and cardiovascular physiology in unstable children. For instance, a large alveolar-arterial oxygen difference (A-a DO_2) may be present but missed by pulse oximetry. It will be apparent, however, when arterial oxygen tension is measured. Normally, end-tidal carbon dioxide ($ETCO_2$) reflects arterial CO_2 tensions ($PaCO_2$) within 4 to 6 mm Hg. However, when pulmonary blood flow decreases (as occurs with depressed cardiac output), dead space ventilation increases (there is more ventilation of underperfused alveoli) and there is a decrease in $ETCO_2$, even though $PaCO_2$ remains unchanged or increases. Likewise, a progressively wide gradient between end-tidal and arterial CO_2 (A-a DCO_2) will help to warn of clinically important circulatory problems in trauma, such as hypovolemia, decreased cardiac output, and pulmonary embolism.

Central venous pressures (CVP) and urine output provide the best measurement of the adequacy of volume replacement. The CVP provides immediate information on intravascular volume, and urine output reflects adequacy of tissue perfusion. Although CVP measurement is extremely useful in assessing intravascular volume, it is not the highest priority during the resuscitation of a severely injured child. In contrast, the ability to administer fluids rapidly is of utmost importance, and it may be appropriate to abandon trying to insert a CVP cannula in favor of placement of a large gauge peripheral intravenous catheter.

In contrast to adults, healthy children show little intraventricular disparity in cardiac function. Since measuring only right atrial pressure is not likely to give misleading information about the adequacy of

Table 21-1 Commonly used anesthetic agents

Drug	Dose	Indication and advantages	Drawbacks and side effects
Thiobarbiturates (thiopental/ thiamylal)	4-6 mg/kg IV	Rapid anesthetic induction; Reduces ICP	CV collapse in hypovolemia Poor analgesia Accumulation with repeat dose
Ketamine	2 mg/kg IV	Rapid induction; Good analgesia Sympathetic stimulation; maintains blood pressure	Postanesthetic delerium Elevates ICP Accumulation with repeat dose
Midazolam	0.05-0.3 mg/kg IV	Potent amnesia Rapid onset Rapidly cleared	Hypotension in hypovolemia Anesthetic induction unreliable Poor analgesia
Fentanyl	0.002-0.005 mg/kg IV (incrementally)	Maintenance of anesthesia Excellent analgesia Rapid onset Sole agent in high doses (0.03-0.05 mg/kg)	Rapid infusion causes hypotension in hypovolemia Large doses produce prolonged respiratory depression Poor amnesic agent
Nitrous oxide	30%-70% inhalation	Analgesic Rapid onset Supplements other drugs	Weak anesthetic Hypotension in hypovolemia or with other drugs Limits O_2 concentration Expands closed air spaces
Halothane	0.5%-2% inhalation	Anesthesia maintenance Rapid onset Ease of administration	CV depression and hypotension in hypovolemia Arrhythmogenic Increases CBF
Forane	0.5%-2% inhalation	Anesthesia maintenance Rapid onset/low solubility Maintains peripheral blood flow Nonarrhythmogenic	Hypotension in hypovolemia Increases CBF

venous filling, the need for pulmonary artery catheterization is rare. The most common sites for central venous cannulation are the internal jugular (right preferred), subclavian, or femoral vein. The Seldinger technique has become popular because of the availability of prepackaged catheter placement kits in a wide variety of sizes. Nevertheless, placement of invasive catheters to monitor a child is more difficult in small children and requires expertise (Chapter 58).

Intracranial pressure monitoring is necessary in any child with significant head injury undergoing a nonneurosurgical emergency operation. The Camino monitor is in common use; the goal is to maintain ICP below 20 mm Hg.

ANESTHETIC AGENTS AND TECHNIQUES

The nature of injuries, cardiovascular stability, and neurologic status are all important factors to be considered in choosing the anesthetic; priorities are determined accordingly. For instance, the severely injured child arriving in the trauma unit unconscious and in profound shock does not initially require anesthetic drugs. Ischemic hypoxia will have rendered the child flaccid, unresponsive, and unaware of surgical stimulation. Rapid thoracotomy or laparotomy to control hemorrhage may be an essential part of resuscitation. The anesthesiologist's efforts during this phase will be directed toward airway management, ventilation, oxygenation, and cardiovascular resuscitation. Commonly used anesthetic agents are listed and described in Table 21-1.

Pharmacology of anesthetics in trauma

Virtually all anesthetics depress the myocardium, cause vasodilation, and blunt cardiovascular compensatory mechanisms. This combination of effects can be catastrophic in cases of shock. Patients who are hypovolemic have a reduced need for intravenous anesthetics for the following reasons: (1) total volume of distribution of drug is decreased; (2) dilutional hypoproteinemia occurs during resuscitation, so that drugs are less protein bound and a greater proportion of free drug is available; and (3) during periods of reduced cardiac output, blood flow to the myocardium and brain is maintained at the expense of other organs. Therefore, in the child in shock the myocardium and brain receive an overdose of anesthetic if normal doses are used. Hypovolemia has a similar effect on the kinetics of inhalational anesthetics. Decreasing blood volume causes decreasing cardiac output which, in turn, reduces pulmonary blood flow. As a consequence, alveolar concentrations of anesthetic agents rise more rapidly, resulting in a higher concentration of the agent in arterial blood. Because perfusion to the heart and brain is maintained in shock, a higher concentration of anesthetic agent is delivered to those organs, resulting in excessive depth of anesthesia and myocardial depression unless the inspired concentration of the agent is adjusted.

Within the framework of the dynamic pharmacology, the anesthesiologist plans the rational use of anesthetics for the injured child. If injuries are minor, there will have been little disruption of organ function and minimal loss of blood volume. Therefore, usual techniques of anesthesia administration to children are reasonable.

When multiorgan injury occurs, however, major physiologic disruption is common. Blood loss, hypovolemia, and shock will occur, and the child may also have sustained head injury. Under these circumstances anesthetic management must be modified in order to avoid further physiologic deterioration.

Once resuscitation is successful, induction of anesthesia proceeds by administration of muscle relaxants, narcotics, amnestic drugs, or inhalation agents. Frequent adjustment of dosages is required based on the child's response.

Induction of anesthesia

In most situations a child's blood volume restoration proceeds before induction of anesthesia. The injured child will frequently require immediate intubation; consequently, induction of anesthesia actually occurs in the trauma unit. However, when the child arrives awake in the operating room without endotracheal intubation, induction should occur according to the priorities dictated by the nature of injuries, the child's physiologic stability, and the requirements of the surgical procedure.

Aspiration and hypotension are the two most likely significant complications of anesthetic induction in children. In their study, Bricker and colleagues demonstrated that neither a long ingestion-to-injury period nor an injury-to-surgical time greater than 8 hours resulted in diminution of gastric volumes or an increase of pH into a safe range.[1] Therefore, treatment of an injured child, who invariably has a full stomach, requires a rapid-sequence technique to avoid aspiration.

In the successfully resuscitated child, the following induction sequence is suitable. One hundred percent O_2 by mask is administered for 3 minutes to denitrogenate the lungs fully. During this period curare 0.05 mg/kg (for children less than 5 years old) and atropine 0.01-0.02 mg/kg are given intravenously. While an assistant provides firm but gentle cricoid pressure, thiopental (or thiamylal) 5 mg/kg, followed immediately by succinylcholine 2 mg/kg, is given intravenously. This will produce satisfactory conditions for intubation in 20 to 40 seconds. Following intubation, both lung fields are auscultated for equality of breath sounds, the chest is inspected visually for symmetrical expansion, and vapor is noted in the ET tube during expiration. Cricoid pressure is then released and the tube is taped securely.

If blood loss has been persistent and intravascular replacement inadequate, anesthetic induction sequence could result in cardiovascular collapse. Thiobarbiturates cause myocardial depression, as well as dilation of capacitance vessels, resulting in decreased ventricular filling, decreased stroke volume, and decreased cardiac output; consequently, severe hypotension is predictable. For a child who is hypovolemic it is safer to modify the induction sequence by using ketamine 0.5-1 mg/kg instead of a thiobarbiturate. Ketamine has the theoretical advantage of causing sympathetic stimulation and has produced an improved survival rate in some experimental models.[4] Nevertheless, cardiac arrest can occur in this setting as a consequence of direct myocardial depression when sympathetic stimulation is already at maximum owing to stress. Induction of anesthesia is a high-risk event in the injured child.

Maintenance anesthetic agents

Children who are in shock tolerate anesthesia poorly because of the pharmacokinetic alterations that result in myocardial depression and inhibition of compensatory mechanisms for hypovolemia.

Narcotics have minimal direct cardiac effects and can be titrated against cardiovascular response to surgery. Morphine and meperidine release histamine, which can cause hypotension. For this reason many anesthesiologists prefer fentanyl or its analogues for intraoperative use in the hypovolemic child. Fentanyl provides excellent analgesia and is not associated with histamine release. When used as primary anesthetic agent, small doses (0.002 to 0.005 mg/kg) are titrated incrementally and the hemodynamic response noted. Reduction in sympathetic tone may result in hypotension, which is responsive to further fluid resuscitation. Total doses of 0.025 to 0.05 mg/kg provide adequate analgesia when used alone; however, amnesia is poor and intraoperative recall common.

Benzodiazepines (diazepam 0.1 mg/kg or midazolam 0.05 mg/kg in divided doses) are useful in decreasing recall. In normovolemic children these produce minimal cardiovascular effect. In hypovolemic children, however, depression of the baroreflex response and reduced sympathetic tone increase the incidence of hypotension. Furthermore, this effect is potentiated for children who receive narcotics. Benzodiazepines require titration in small doses when used in the hypovolemic child, particularly in conjunction with other analgesics or anesthetics.

Nitrous oxide is the weakest of the inhalation anesthetics in modern use. It is an excellent analgesic and, when used with narcotics, helps produce amnesia. In healthy normovolemic children it has minimally depressant cardiovascular effects except during hypovolemia. An additional disadvantage of nitrous oxide is that it limits the concentration of oxygen possible in inspired gas.

Both halothane and isoflurane cause dose-dependent hypotension in healthy normovolemic children. Although at equipotent doses the degree of hypotension is similar, there is a subtle but important difference between them.[10] Hypotension produced by halothane is associated with a reduced cardiac output and increased systemic vascular resistance. Isoflurane produces similar levels of hypotension, but cardiac output is preserved and systemic vascular resistance decreases. This suggests that tissue perfusion and oxygen delivery is better in patients receiving isoflurane than those receiving halothane, but there are no outcome data to recommend one agent over the other for hypovolemic children. It is important to remember that in both adults and children, all inhalational anesthetics depress baroreceptor reflexes and interfere with mechanisms compensating for shock in a dose-dependent manner. When these agents are to be used in trauma, slow titration after adequate volume repletion prevents cardiovascular depression. Constant changes in drug doses and levels of anesthesia are likely to be necessary in severely injured children.

Muscle relaxants

Because of the precarious cardiovascular status of severely injured children, muscle relaxants, which have little direct effect on the cardiovascular system, are particularly important in the anesthetic management of trauma patients. Devoid of analgesic and anesthetic effects, they permit maintenance of lighter levels of anesthesia during surgery without the undesirable side effects caused by deep levels of anesthesia. Muscle relaxants used in modern practice include succinylcholine, curare, pancuronium, vecuronium, and atracurium. No one drug possesses all of the desired qualities of the ideal muscle relaxant.

Succinylcholine continues to be unmatched in its ability to provide the rapid onset of paralysis needed for gaining airway control safely during a rapid-sequence induction. Infants are less sensitive to succinylcholine than older children and adults. However, high cardiac output in small children results in rapid onset of action. Intravenous administration of succinylcholine (2 mg/kg) results in profound paralysis in 20 to 30 seconds in infants. Muscle fasciculation is uncommon and is less intense, and intragastric pressure does not rise in children 5 years old. It is therefore possible to omit a nondepolarizing relaxant before rapid-sequence induction in children under 5 years.

Succinylcholine causes vagal stimulation in children, resulting in bradycardia. Injection of atropine (0.02 mg IV) before administration of succinylcholine protects against this response. In normal children intravenous succinylcholine causes slight intracellular potassium release and mild rises (0.5 mg) in serum potassium levels. Following a burn, massive crush injury, upper motor neuron damage, or significant denervation injury, however, succinylcholine causes a rise in serum potassium levels sufficient to produce cardiac arrest. The onset of this sensitivity appears to be from about 48 hours to 6 months following injury. Thus, there is no contraindication to the use of succinylcholine in children immediately following injury.

There is currently a controversy about the propensity of succinylcholine to produce masseter spasm, and whether masseter spasm in this context is a manifestation of malignant hyperthermia (MH). First of all, inadequate jaw relaxation after succinylcholine injection in children appears to be common following induction using potent inhalational agents, but is extremely uncommon following IV anesthetic induction.[9] Second, the incidence of this occurrence (approximately 1%) suggests that factors other than MH susceptibility are at work. Third, the imperative for rapid control of the airway in an injured child who is at high risk for aspiration outweighs the remote possibility of an MH episode.

Nondepolarizing relaxants share a common undesirable feature when compared with succinylcholine: slow onset of action. Although succinylcholine produces satisfactory conditions for intubation in less than 1 minute following IV administration, nondepolarizers typically require 3 to 5 minutes. Several different strategies can be used to shorten time to intubation and may be appropriate when succinylcholine is contraindicated.

Table 21–2 Muscle relaxant dose schedule

	Intubating dose mg/kg	Maintenance dose mg/k	Onset	Duration
Succinylcholine	2		20-60 sec	3-10 min
Curare	0.6	0.2-0.3	2-5 min	45-60 min
Pancuronium	0.1	0.02	2-5 min	45-60 min
Vecuronium	0.1	0.02	2-3 min	20-30 min
Atracurium	0.5	0.125	2-3 min	20-30 min

These include administering a priming dose, giving a very large dose (typically twice the usual intubating dose), and administering the muscle relaxant before the intravenous induction agent. Yet even with these strategies, time to intubation is still a minimum of 90 seconds, and the duration of relaxation is prolonged when a very large dose is used.

Curare is the oldest of clinically available muscle relaxants. It has a slow onset of action, as well as the undesirable side effects of histamine release and hypotension. This is particularly problematic in the injured child with unstable circulatory status. Clinical duration of action following 95% depression of twitch tension with curare is 45 to 60 minutes. In neonates, however, recovery times may be greatly prolonged.

Pancuronium is about 5 to 10 times more potent than curare and has similar characteristics of onset and duration. Its vagolytic action, absence of histamine releasing action, and lack of hypotensive effect make it a suitable choice for use in severely injured children. Occasionally, its accelerating effect on heart rate is excessive.

Vecuronium is chemically related to pancuronium but has a shorter duration of action (except in neonates). At usual doses (Table 21-2) it provides clinical levels of relaxation for 20 to 30 minutes. It is devoid of cardiovascular effects and does not cause histamine release, making it an excellent choice during trauma surgery. Its intermediate duration of action means that one quarter to one third the initial dose must be given every half hour or so.

Atracurium has a chemical structure that results in relatively rapid metabolism by both Hoffman elimination and ester hydrolysis. These elimination mechanisms offer little particular advantage for use in trauma victims under most circumstances. It has a tendency to cause histamine release (although less than curare), which may be a disadvantage. Its onset and duration of action are similar to those of vecuronium.

Unless postoperative mechanical ventilation is planned, children paralyzed with a nondepolarizing muscle relaxant should receive an antagonist for reversal of neuromuscular blockade at the end of surgery. Neostigmine 0.07 mg/kg (preceded by atropine 0.02 mg/kg to counteract the muscarinic effect) is the usual dose to provide full reversal. Intensity of and recovery from neuromuscular blockade should be monitored with a nerve stimulator. Reversal of neuromuscular blockade is unlikely to be effective if the nerve stimulator does not demonstrate some degree of spontaneous recovery. The trachea should be kept intubated and respirations supported until neuromuscular recovery is demonstrated by both testing and clinical measurements.

ANESTHESIA FOR SPECIFIC INJURIES

The nature of injuries suffered and organ system at risk may require modification of anesthetic management to take into account the specific physiologic impairments in progress.

Head injury

Head injury is the most common major injury suffered by children and is associated with a higher rate of mortality.[5] The goal of therapy for significant head injury in the child reaching the trauma center is the prevention of secondary brain injury. This secondary injury results from ischemic brain damage resulting from hypoxia, hypercarbia, systemic hypotension, intracranial hypertension, or a combination of these. Thus, therapy should begin with the initial intervention in the trauma unit and be continued in the operating room. Control of oxygenation and ventilation requires early tracheal intubation and ventilation with 100% oxygen. Cardiac output and blood pressure must be maintained at normal or slightly increased levels. This can usually be achieved with adequate fluid and blood replacement and by maintaining light levels of anesthesia. When necessary, inotropic support should be used.

Elevated intracranial pressure (ICP) leads to secondary injury either by herniation of intracranial contents or by producing cerebral ischemia when cerebral perfusion pressure (CPP) is reduced excessively. Cerebral perfusion pressure is the difference between mean arterial pressure (MAP) and ICP (CPP = MAP − ICP). Although there is little data to define the ideal perfusion pressure in children with head injuries, clinical experience suggests that a CPP of 50 mm Hg is adequate. Common clinical practice is to try to maintain ICP between 15 and 20 mm Hg and to keep the MAP between 65 and 70 mm Hg. This level of ICP can usually be produced by moderate hyperventilation ($PaCO_2$ of 30 to 35 mm Hg), but frequently more aggressive ventilation to a $PaCO_2$ of 25 mm Hg is necessary.

Bruce and colleagues have demonstrated that cerebrovascular congestion and hyperemia, rather than edema (the more common pattern in adults), is the primary pathologic mechanism for intracranial hypertension in children with head injury.[2] Control of this phenomenon is essential to prevent secondary injury and is best achieved with hyperventilation. Mannitol, which can increase cerebral blood flow, is usually unnecessary and is best reserved for those children who develop delayed ICP rises (24 hours to 5 days following injury).[2]

Following head injury in children, mass lesions (epidural or subdural hematomas) are less common than in adults. Thus the child with head injury frequently will arrive at the operating room for nonneurologic surgery. Intraoperative intracranial pressure monitoring is especially important to guide management of ICP while fluid resuscitation and major surgery are under way.

Some anesthetic procedures and agents have deleterious effects on intracranial dynamics. Laryngoscopy is a potent sympathetic stimulator and results in rises in ICP, reducing cerebral perfusion pressure. Thiopental or thiamylal 5 to 6 mg/kg lower intracranial pressure and, when given before laryngoscopy, blunt the intracranial pressure response. Additional measures include IV lidocaine (1 to 1.5 mg/kg) or fentanyl (0.001 to 0.002 mg/kg) 60 to 90 seconds before the induction of anesthesia. Reflex coughing or straining during laryngoscopy and intubation produces surges in ICP as a result of increased superior vena cava pressure. Therefore, it is important to give doses of muscle relaxant at the right interval before laryngoscopy to assure a completely paralyzed child during intubation.

The choice of maintenance anesthetic agents for children with head injuries is controversial. Halothane, enflurane, and isoflurane all cause cerebral vasodilation and, in the presence of reduced intracranial compliance, a rise in levels of ICP. If, however, hypocapnea is established before the administration of inhalation anesthesia, the vasodilating effect is blunted. Among the volatile agents, iso-

flurane causes the smallest ICP elevation with a decrease in $CMRO_2$ and, when used in low concentrations after hypocapnea is established, produces little or no rise in ICP levels.

The most widely accepted neuroanesthetic technique makes use of a combination of nitrous oxide, muscle relaxants, narcotics, and barbiturates. The "balanced" technique has the advantage of maintaining normal systemic circulation and reducing cerebral blood flow and cerebral oxygen consumption. Other intravenous agents such as benzodiazepines are frequently included in the balanced technique. However, ketamine, which increases both cerebral blood flow and oxygen consumption, is best avoided.

Abdominal injury

Most abdominal injuries in children are the result of blunt trauma. Even with bleeding from a ruptured solid viscus, the majority of children are treated nonoperatively if they are hemodynamically stable, have no other abdominal injuries requiring laparotomy, and do not have significant head injury requiring fluid restriction. Penetrating abdominal injuries or hemodynamic instability require surgical exploration.

The anesthesiologist must be prepared to rapidly replace blood lost when the abdomen is decompressed. When abdominal trauma is the primary injury, large-bore intravenous catheters in the upper extremities or jugular or subclavian veins are preferred for rapid replenishment of lost blood volume. Placement of intravenous catheters in the lower extremities in these children may prevent blood, fluids, and drugs from getting to the central circulation if the inferior vena cava is injured.

The stomach is likely to be distended with food, swallowed air, and blood. In the awake child without head injury, a nasogastric tube should be passed to decompress the stomach. This maneuver, however, will not produce an empty stomach, and rapid-sequence induction is still indicated. In the unconscious child with abdominal distension, the trachea is intubated before passing the gastric tube, which can stimulate vomiting and consequent aspiration.

No one particular anesthetic technique has an advantage over another in most cases. Maintenance of anesthesia and selection of agents to be used are guided by the child's response and the pharmacologic principles outlined earlier in this chapter.

Thoracic injury

The compliant chest wall and elastic intrathoracic structures allow for considerable compression during blunt trauma, even with minimal external evidence. Therefore, careful preoperative examination and review of chest x-rays are essential. One of the dangers for the anesthesiologist is that the sequelae of chest injury will not become apparent until a child is in surgery.

The anesthesiologist must maintain a high level of suspicion for pneumothorax in a child with chest injury. Intraoperatively, it may manifest itself with wheezing, increased airway pressure, hypoxia, and hypotension, which can be mistaken for bronchospasm or bronchial intubation. Identifying unilateral breath sounds, tympany to percussion, and subcutaneous emphysema will help to establish the presence of pneumothorax. Although a diagnosis of pneumothorax can be confirmed by examination of the chest x-ray, waiting for a chest film should not delay treatment. Confirmation can be made more quickly and relieved by needle aspiration of the suspected side. Chest tube placement before anesthesia is mandatory for any child with pneumothorax. Positive pressure ventilation will increase intrapleural air in the absence of a chest tube. Nitrous oxide is contraindicated in the presence of pneumothorax, as diffusion of this relatively soluble gas into the pleural space will rapidly expand the pneumothorax.

As in abdominal trauma, massive blood loss may accompany emergency thoracotomy. Large-bore intravenous infusion cannulae must be in place and accessible for massive transfusion of blood and fluids.

In pulmonary contusion, blood fills the alveoli, resulting in increased venous admixture and decreased oxygen saturation. When extensive portions of lungs are involved, hypoxia and decreased pulmonary compliance may require that positive end-expiratory pressure (PEEP) accompany mechanical ventilation with high oxygen concentrations.

Bronchopleura fistula resulting from traumatic bronchial rupture presents a dilemma. When the chest tube is placed, a bronchocutaneous fistula is created. Positive pressure ventilation is then complicated, as a considerable portion of tidal volume may escape through the open bronchus. Developing sufficient airway pressure for ventilation therefore becomes problematic. Strategies for treatment include endobronchial intubation, rapid thoracotomy with control of the air leak, and subsequent repair of the rupture.

Open globe injury

Anesthetic management of an open globe injury in the child has been controversial for years. When this type of injury is present in a child with multiple trauma, the considerations for management of the more life-threatening injuries take precedence. However, when an open globe is the only or primary injury, the priorities of preservation of vision and prevention of aspiration of gastric contents may conflict.

Three possible techniques for management have been suggested. Our practice is to place an intravenous catheter and proceed with a modified rapid-sequence induction. However, in the place of succinylcholine, vecuronium or pancuronium 0.2 mg/kg (twice the usual intubating dose) is administered. Conditions appropriate for intubation will occur in 90 seconds following intravenous injection of the relaxant. To prevent desaturation during this period, cricoid pressure is maintained and ventilation conducted with bag and mask. One concern with this technique is that a child's struggling and crying during attempted venous cannulation will result in a rise in intraocular pressure (IOP), thus risking extrusion of vitreous. The second disadvantage is the somewhat increased likelihood that regurgitation will occur during the rather long interval between induction and tracheal intubation.

Others have recommended that succinylcholine can be used in the induction sequence and that prior administration of a defasciculating dose (one tenth of intubating dose) will prevent a rise in IOP resulting from succinylcholine.[3] Not all authorities agree that IOP is well controlled in this technique.[6]

Some pediatric anesthesiologists advocate inhalation induction to avoid a rise in IOP during IV placement. The risk with this technique is that vomiting or regurgitation will occur during the period in which the airway is unprotected.

SUMMARY

Trauma remains the number one killer of children over the age of 1 year. Thus any practicing anesthesiologist is likely to be called upon to care for an injured child. Safe anesthetic management techniques for children require an understanding of the physiology of shock in children. Modifications in treatment are necessary to take into account the particular psychology, anatomy, physiology, and altered pharmacologic responses of children.

REFERENCES

1. Bricker SRW, McLuckie A, Nightingale DA, : Gastric aspirates after trauma in children, *Anaesthesia* 44:721-724, 1989.
2. Bruce DA, Raphaely RC, Goldberg AI et al: Pathophysiology, treatment and outcome following severe head injury in children, *Child's Brain* 5:174-191, 1979.
3. Libonati MM, Leahy JL, Ellison N: The use of succinylcholine in open eye surgery, *Anesthesiology* 62:637-640, 1985.
4. Longnecker DE, Sturgill BC: Influence of anesthetic agent on survival following hemorrhage, *Anesthesiology* 45:516, 1976.
5. Mayer T, Walker ML, Shasha I et al: Effect of multiple trauma on outcome of pediatric patients with neurological injuries, *Child's Brain* 8:189-197, 1981.

6. Murphy DF: Anesthesia and intraocular pressure, *Anesth Analg* 64:520-530, 1985.
7. Nakayama DK, Davis PJ: Anesthesia for trauma. In Motoyama EK, editor: *Smith's anesthesia for infants and children,* St Louis, 1990, Mosby–Year Book.
8. Pascucci R, Walsh J: Evaluation and management of the injured child. In Capan LM, Miller SF, Turndorf H, editors: Trauma anesthesia and intensive care, New York, 1991, JB Lippincott.
9. VanDerSpek AFL, Fang WB, Ashton-Miller JA et al: The effects of succinylcholine on mouth opening, *Anesthesiology* 67:459-465, 1987.
10. Wolf WJ, Neal MB, Peterson MD: The hemodynamic and cardiovascular effects of isoflurane and halothane in children, *Anesthesiology* 64:328, 1986.

22 Diagnostic Imaging

Carlos J. Sivit and Dorothy I. Bulas

Prompt diagnosis may help save the lives of injured children. To this end, radiographic evaluation provides valuable diagnostic information for detecting skeletal, thoracic, abdominal, and cranial injury. Familiarization with standard radiographic procedures and more complex imaging modalities is critical in delivering early and effective treatment. The radiologist plays a key role in the trauma team, delivering rapid and precise diagnoses and performing interventional procedures when indicated. Although severely injured children whose condition is unstable should be taken directly to the operating room without extensive radiographic evaluation, other children benefit greatly by initial radiographic examination.

IMMEDIATE IMAGING

Prompt, accurate radiographic evaluation of the cervical spine, chest, and pelvis is vital to the treatment of the severely injured child.

Cervical spine

Initial survey of the injured child includes close evaluation of the airway and cervical spine. The typical child may be frightened, uncooperative, and unable to describe and localize neurologic symp-

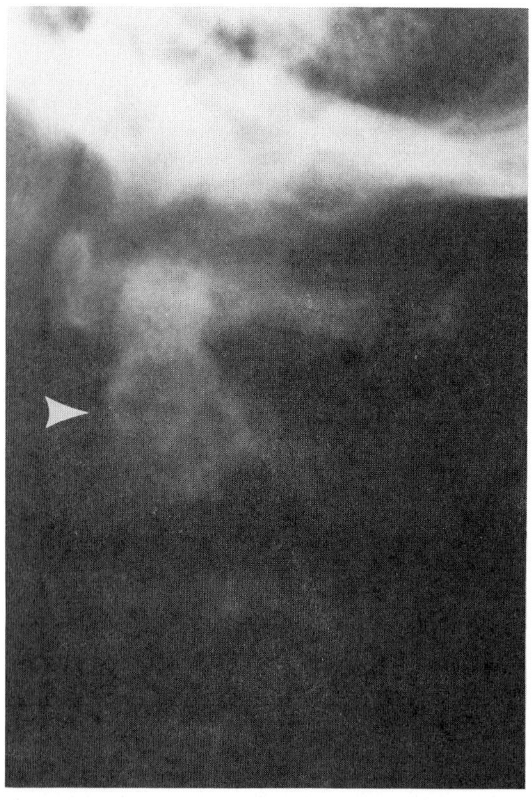

Figure 22–1 Dens body synchondrosis *(arrow)* should not be misinterpreted as a fracture. Fusion usually occurs by adolescence.

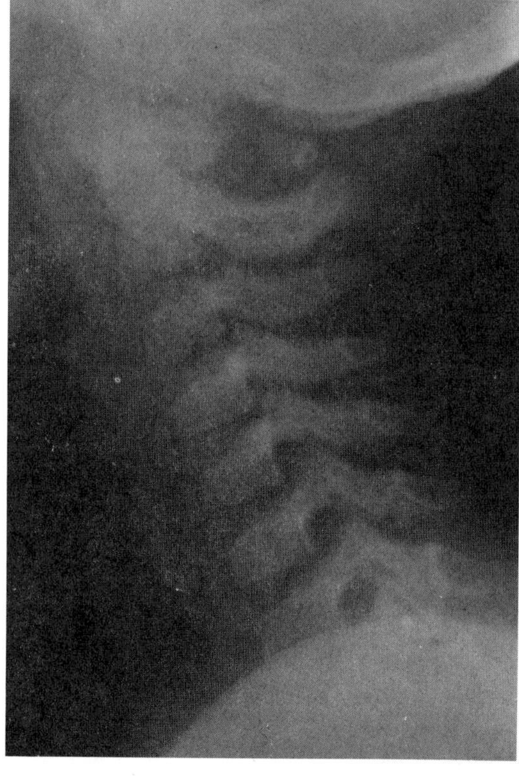

Figure 22–2 Incomplete formation of the posterior arch of C1.

toms. Presumption of cervical spine injury is essential, especially in the comatose child following a high-velocity injury.

A cross-table lateral view of the cervical spine is important in the assessment of cervical spine integrity. If a child arrives at the emergency room with a cervical collar in place, perform a lateral view of the cervical spine with the neck immobilized in the collar.[79]

Normal variants of the developing spine, hypermobility of ligaments and congenital anomalies may make interpretation of the pediatric cervical spine difficult[13,23,41,98] (Figs. 22-1 to 22-4). More important, spinal cord injury without radiographic abnormality (SCIWORA) has been reported frequently in children.[77] A complete neurologic examination is critical in the assessment of cervical spine integrity. Cervical straightening and prevertebral soft tissue swelling provide clues to the presence of a cervical injury, but are not always present.[41,56,115] Overreliance on the initial lateral cervical spine film may lead to errors in treatment.[111]

Cervical spine injuries in children under 8 years of age usually occur in the upper three vertebrae.[4,23,90,98] This is likely a result of the larger size of the head relative to the body, increased laxity of ligaments, horizontally oriented facets, and hypoplastic occipital condyles.[44,97] These injuries are usually characterized by distraction rather than comminution (Fig. 22-5). Synchondroses are vulnerable sites through which fractures are often seen. Dens fractures, usually through the synchondrosis, often result in tilting or displacement of the dens (Fig. 22-6).

The cervical spine attains an adult form by 8 years of age.[4,44,98] The same mechanisms responsible in adult fractures then begin to operate. Familiarity with findings suggesting instability, such as persistent pain and torticollis, is crucial. If a child remains symptomatic despite normal lateral, (AP), and open-mouth cervical spine radiographs, flexion and extension views are necessary, preferably under fluoroscopic observation (Fig. 22-7).[41] These views may need to be delayed until the patient is stable and able to cooperate. If studies

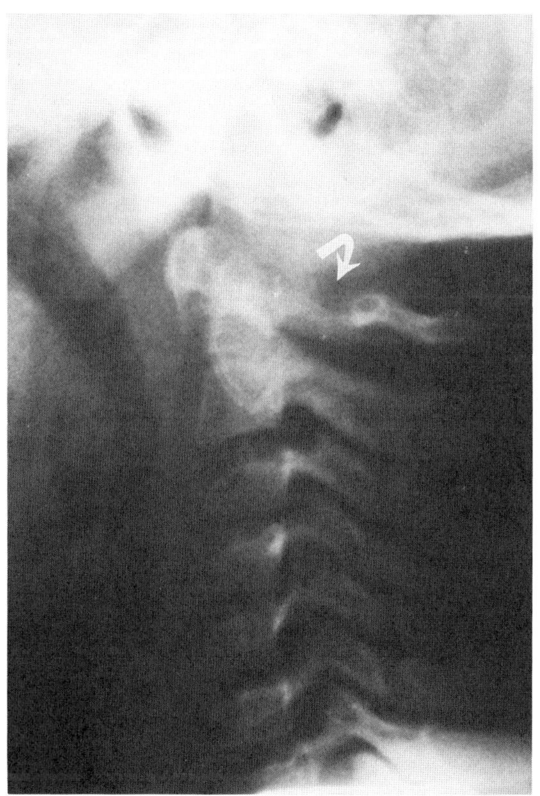

Figure 22–3 Unilateral absence of a portion of the neural arch of C1 *(arrow).*

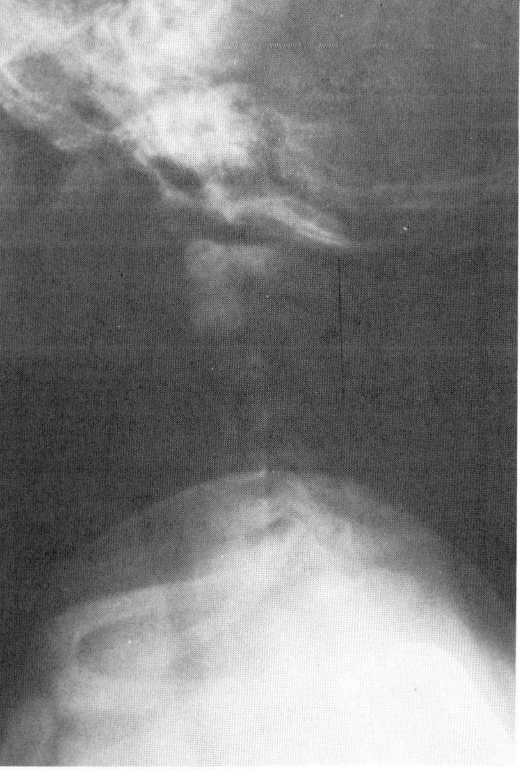

Figure 22–4 C2-3 pseudosubluxation and angulation. Owing to lax spinal ligaments in childhood, excessive motion may erroneously suggest an injury. The posterior cervical line (C1-3) is normal (within 2 mm of the C2 spinous process).

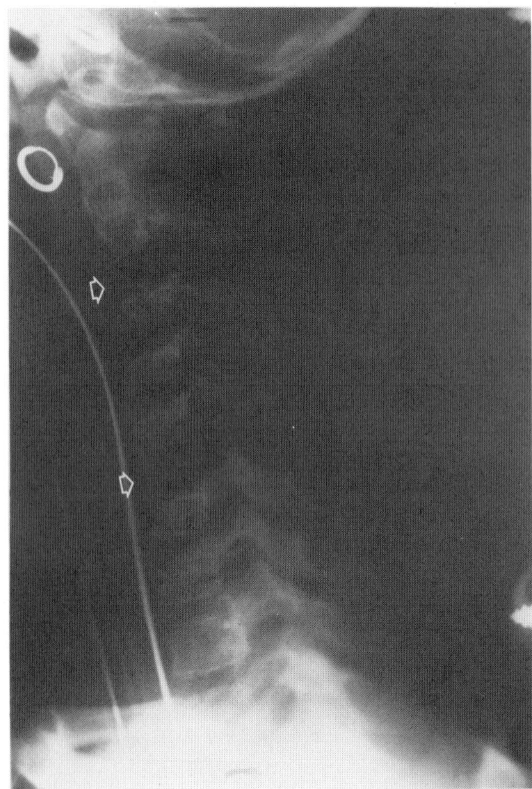

Figure 22–5 Distraction injuries of C2-3 and C5-6 *(arrows)* with tearing of the ligaments of the anterior, middle, and posterior columns.

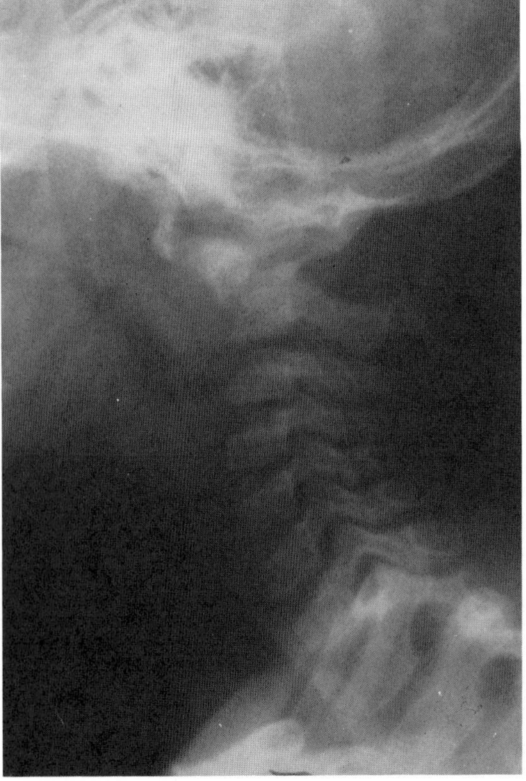

Figure 22–6 Odontoid fracture through the synchondrosis with anterior displacement and angulation.

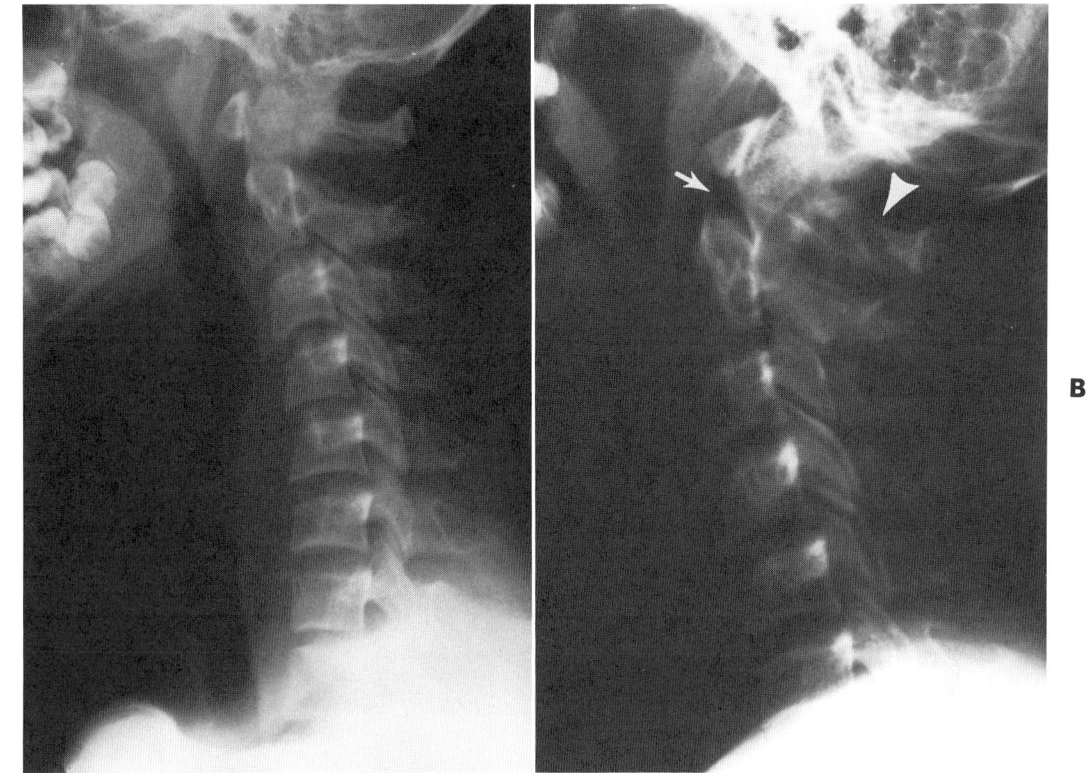

Figure 22–7 Fifteen-year-old adolescent complaining of neck pain following a motor vehicle accident. **A,** Neutral position demonstrates reversal of cervical spine curvature. No fractures are identified. **B,** Extension view demonstrates an oblique fracture through the odontoid *(white arrow)* as well as a fracture of the C1 ring *(white arrowhead)*.

are equivocal or pain persists, immobilization should be continued and repeat studies may be required.

Chest

The portable AP chest radiograph provides immediate information about abnormalities that require immediate intervention but are not clinically obvious. These include pneumothorax, pneumomediastinum, pneumopericardium (Fig. 22-8), hemothorax, mediastinal hemorrhage, diaphragmatic rupture (Fig. 22-9), and major rib fractures. It also provides information on the gas exchange capabilities of the lung, including the presence of pulmonary edema, contusion/laceration (Fig. 22-10), and atelectasis. On the portable AP chest film, apparent mediastinal widening is often the result of magnification or patient rotation. If mediastinal widening is noted on the initial AP chest film, an upright (PA) chest film should be obtained when possible to exclude mediastinal injury. If the mediastinum remains persistently widened, or if clinical suspicion of a vascular injury persists, computed tomography (CT) or arteriography permits further assessment (Fig. 22-11).

Small or moderate pneumothorax and hemothorax may be difficult to detect on supine radiographs. Air may collect medially and anteriorly, with ill-defined lucencies noted adjacent to the cardiac silhouette (Fig. 22-12). If findings are equivocal or the index of suspicion is high, a recumbent AP radiograph or a lateral decubitus film better demonstrates small pleural collections.

Pelvis

The diagnosis of pelvic fractures in multitrauma patients is critical because of the association with internal organ or vascular injury.[8] Early stabilization and realignment of the bony pelvis is often effective in achieving hemostasis. A portable AP examination of the pelvis is included as part of the immediate radiographic evaluation following blunt abdominal trauma. Angled "inlet" and "outlet" views may provide additional information about the sacroiliac joints and sacrum, and demonstrate the spatial relationship of the bones of the pelvic ring

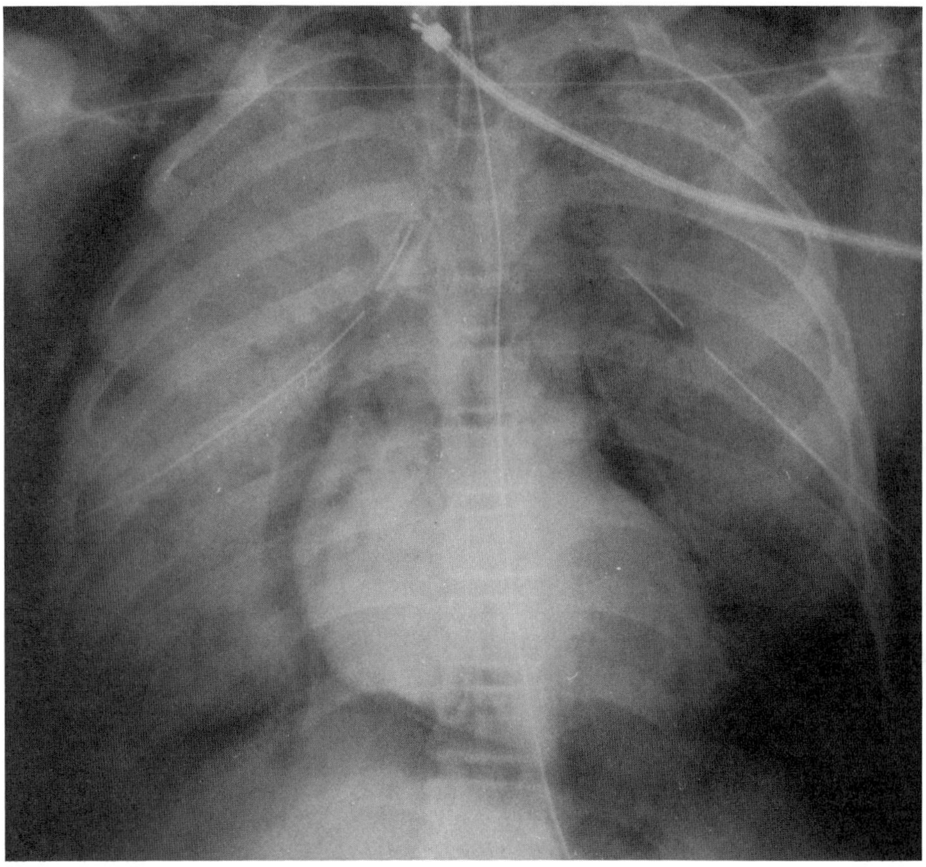

Figure 22–8 Pneumopericardium. AP chest radiograph shows a rim of lucency completely surrounding the cardiac silhouette.

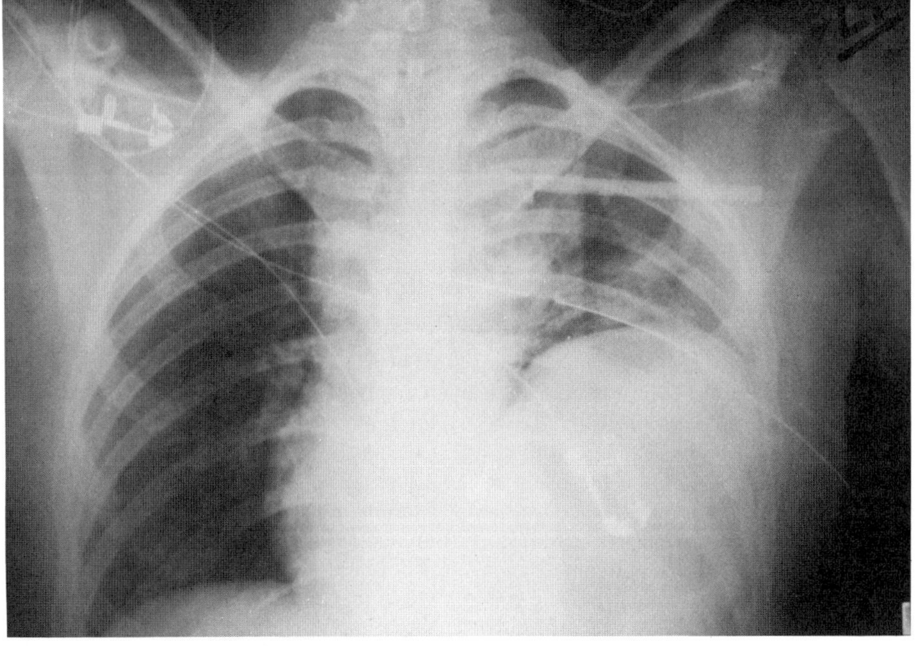

Figure 22–9 Rupture of the left leaf of the diaphragm with herniation of the spleen and stomach into the left pleural cavity.

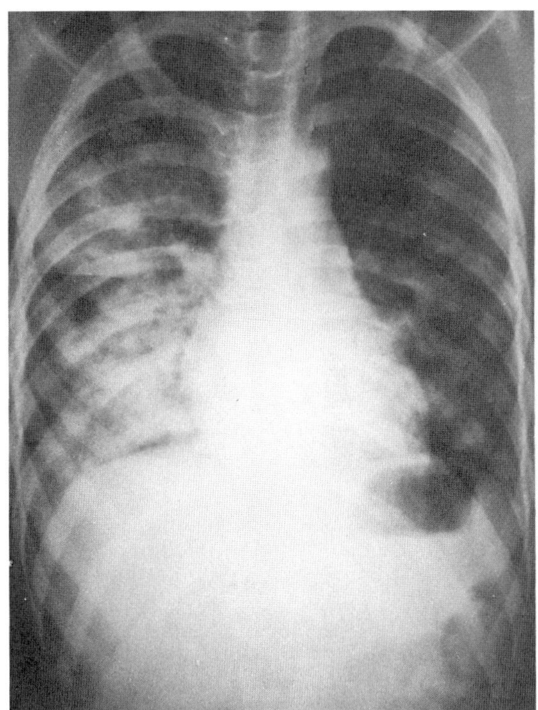

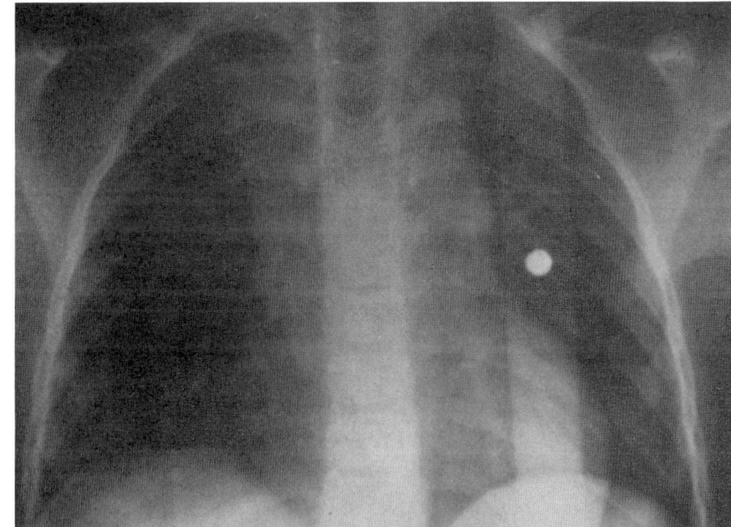

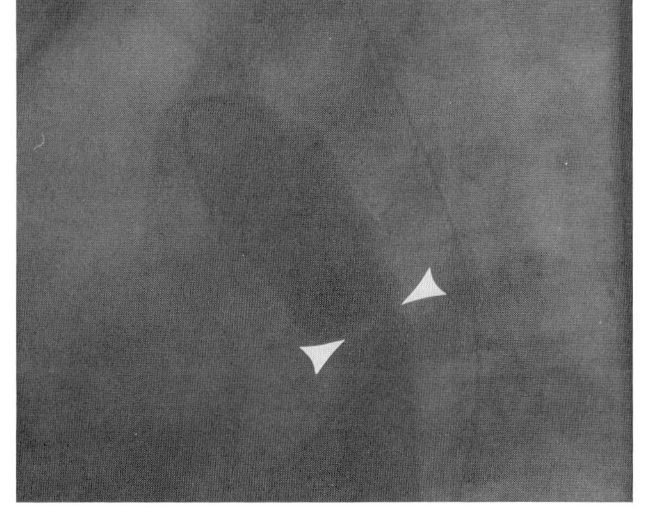

Figure 22–10 Pulmonary contusion. AP chest radiograph shows diffuse opacification of the right lung and left lower lobe.

Figure 22–11 Mediastinal hematoma associated with an aortic tear. **A,** AP chest radiograph shows a widened mediastinum and loss of definition of the aortic arch. **B,** Aortogram demonstrates an aortic laceration *(arrowheads)*.

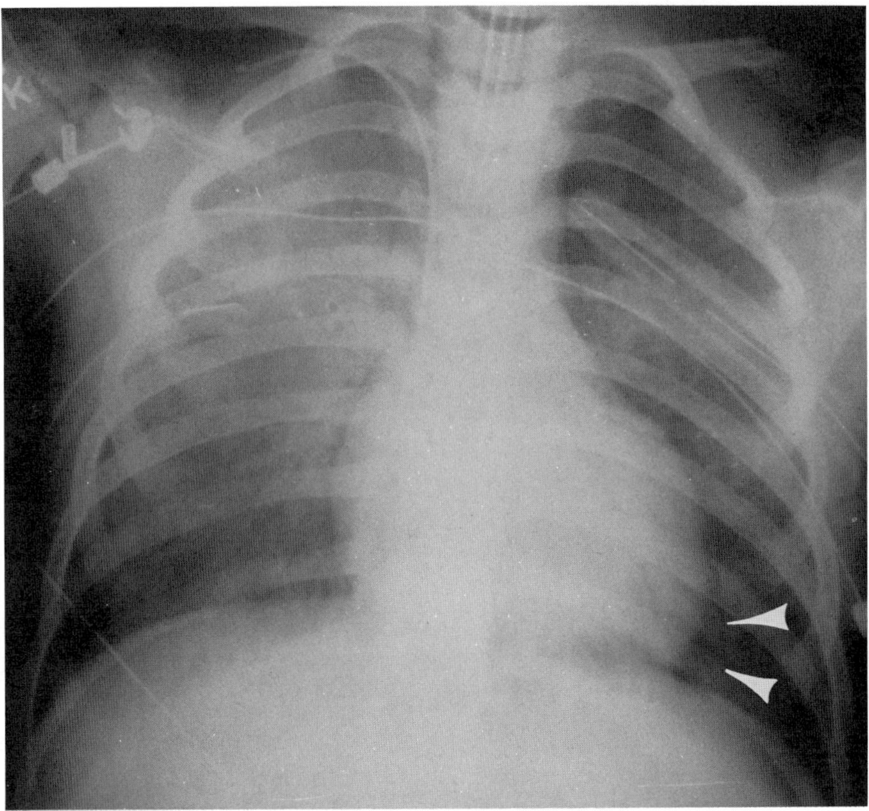

Figure 22–12 Small pneumothorax. AP chest radiograph shows focal area of lucency adjacent to left lower cardiac silhouette *(arrowheads)*.

(Fig. 22-13).[118,119] CT is superior to plain films in the demonstration of diastasis of the sacroiliac joint and pubic symphysis (Fig. 22-14).[65,114,119] In addition, CT provides information concerning the position of fracture fragments, particularly small intraarticular fragments at the level of the acetabulum (Fig. 22-15). CT scanning may be delayed until the patient is stable prior to definitive surgical reconstruction.

Cystography

The bladder, urethra, or both may be injured by blunt trauma to the pelvis. Although most injuries are associated with a fractured pelvis, a direct blow may cause a full bladder to burst against the pubis.[12,116] If gross hematuria is present following blunt pelvic trauma, a retrograde urethrogram or voiding cystourethrogram should be obtained. When a urethral injury is suspected, a retrograde urethrogram should be obtained prior to catheterization. A catheter is inserted in the anterior urethra with contrast-introduced retrograde under fluoroscopic guidance. Contusions and partial or complete ruptures of the bladder become evident with this technique.[12,85]

Bladder examination requires complete filling of the bladder and views obtained in at least two projections. An AP radiograph of the pelvis following voiding is critical in the evaluation of intraperitoneal and extraperitoneal rupture.[84]

THORACOABDOMINAL IMAGING
Computed tomography

CT has become the imaging method of choice in the evaluation of children with suspected thoracoabdominal injury. Its utility in the determination of the presence and extent of injury is well established,[22,48,50,105] and it has largely replaced diagnostic peritoneal lavage in the assessment of hemodynamically stable children.[65] Examination of injured children with CT reduces the need for exploratory laparotomy.[22,48,104] Prompt evaluation with CT will show whether intraperitoneal or retroperitoneal fluid or blood is present and whether the liver, spleen, kidneys, and pancreas are intact. CT may also depict injury to the mesentery or gastrointestinal tract and can usually demonstrate associated fractures or dislocations of ribs, spine, or pelvis.

In this section we present our experience with

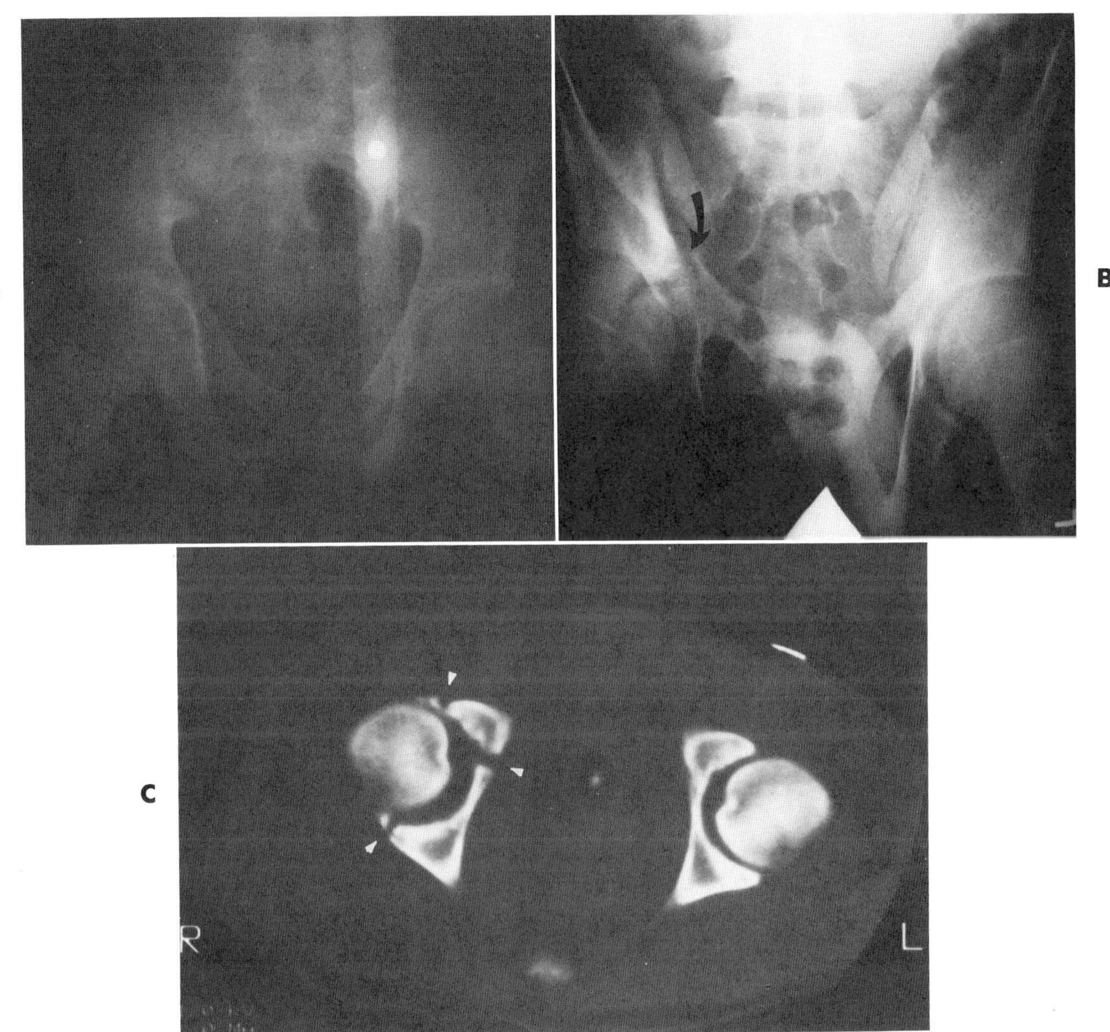

Figure 22–13 A, AP view of the pelvis demonstrates a poorly defined lucency through the right acetabulum. **B,** Inlet view shows an obvious right acetabular fracture *(arrow)*. **C,** CT demonstrates multiple acetabular fractures *(arrowheads)*. No intraarticular fragments were identified.

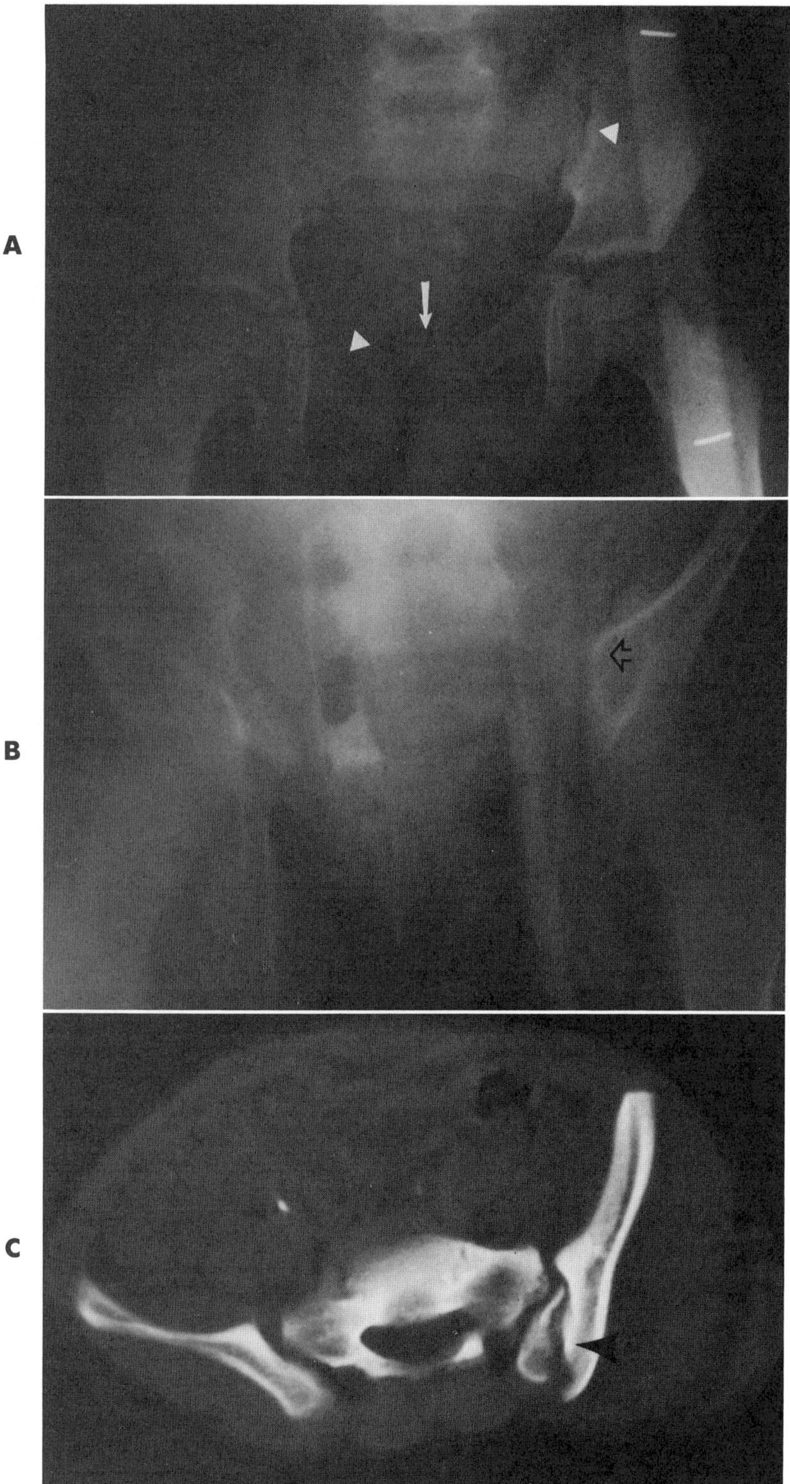

Figure 22–14 A, AP view of the pelvis demonstrates diastasis of the pubic symphysis *(arrow)* and fractures of the right pubic rami and left ilium *(arrowheads).* **B,** Inlet view demonstrates associated widening of the left sacroiliac joint *(arrow).* **C,** CT scan further characterizes the associated fracture through the left ilium *(arrowhead).*

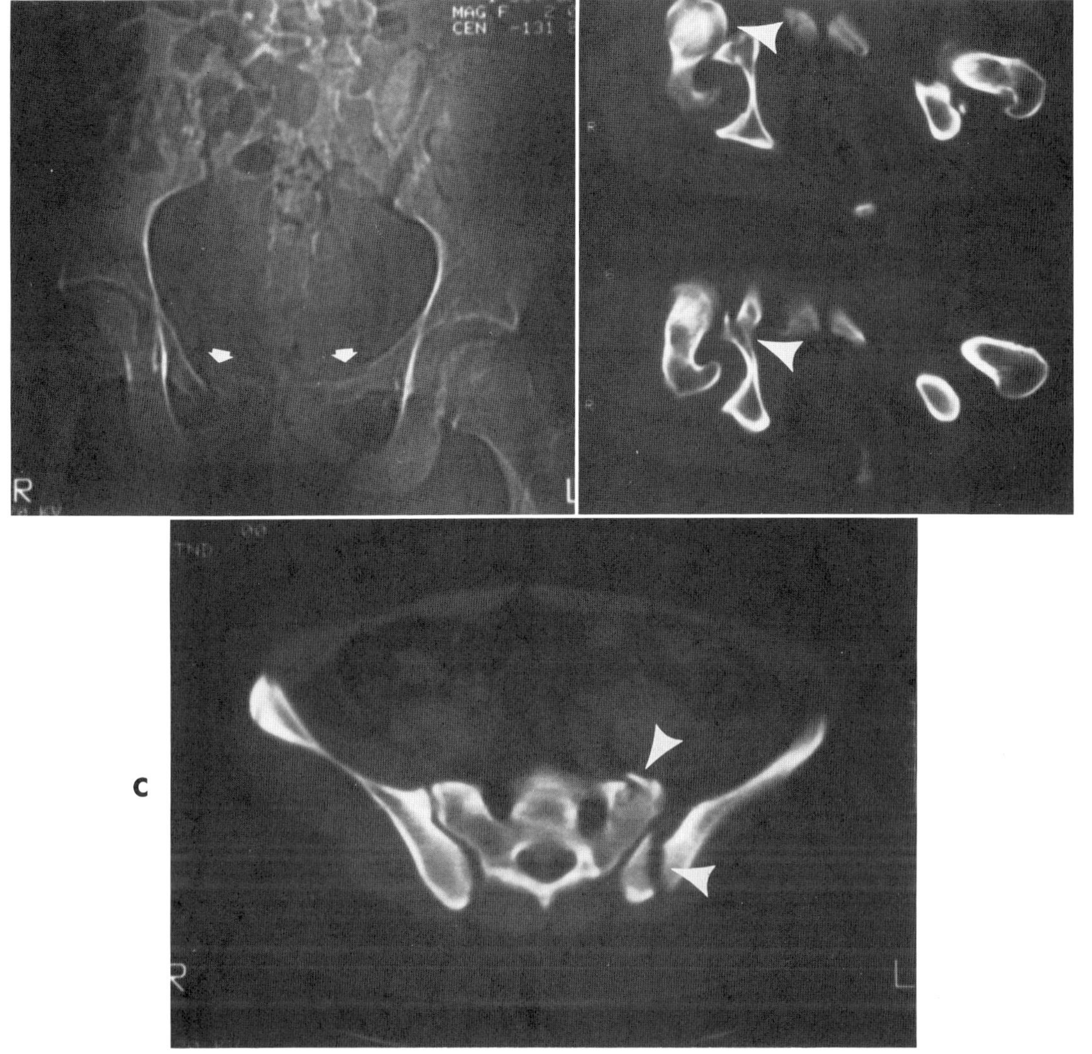

Figure 22–15 A, AP view of the pelvis demonstrates bilateral pubic rami fractures *(arrows)*. CT scan shows associated **(B)** anterior dislocation of the right femoral head *(arrowheads)*, and **(C)** fractures of the sacrum and left ilium with diastasis of the sacroiliac joint *(arrowheads)*.

1000 children, seen consecutively and evaluated with CT for blunt abdominal injury over an 8-year period. Most of these injuries were related to the use of motorized vehicles (Table 22-1).

Technique

The CT technique used is essential to maximize the diagnostic value of the study. Basic principles include patient preparation, proper use of intravenous contrast, location and spacing of CT sections, and image display.

The radius of reconstruction should be sufficiently large to comprise the entire abdomen and pelvis, including soft tissues. The use of low-amperage (70 mA, at 120 kV peak) x-ray technique reduces patient dose and minimizes tube loading.

Table 22–1 Mechanism of injury in children with blunt abdominal trauma

Mechanism	(n = 1000) Patients
Motor vehicle	672 (67%)
Pedestrian	390 (39%)
Occupant	282 (28%)
Falls	142 (14%)
Bicycle	68 (7%)
Assault	55 (5%)
Motorcycle	17 (2%)
Object	15 (2%)
Other blunt	31 (3%)

Table 22–2 CT findings and degree of hematuria

Variable (CT finding)	No hematuria n = 468	Dipstick/microscopic n = 412	Gross n = 90
		(n = 970)*	
Abnormal CT	134 (29%)	118 (29%)	49 (54%)
Renal injury	13 (3%)	28 (7%)	19 (21%)

*Indications available in 970:1000 children.

Image reconstruction with a 256 × 256 matrix speeds processing time. The removal of overlying metallic hardware and withdrawal of nasogastric tubes into the esophagus prior to scanning minimizes streak artifacts. Occlusion of the Foley catheter before the administration of intravenous contrast maximizes bladder opacification.

Vascular enhancement is imperative to identify visceral injury, as a hematoma may be nearly isodense to unenhanced solid viscera. We use a rapid bolus injection of intravenous contrast (3 ml/kg; maximal dose 120 ml) to evaluate the upper abdominal blood supply and parenchymal organs. Approximately two thirds of the total dose is injected before scanning. The remainder is injected continuously throughout the planned scan sequence to maximize vascular and parenchymal opacification. Obtaining scans after an inadequate volume of contrast material may result in an "isodense hematoma." Oral contrast opacification of the gastrointestinal tract is not used routinely in the initial CT study of injured children, but it is used in situations in which an injury to the intestinal tract or pancreas is strongly suspected.

Serial 1-cm–thick slices are obtained at 1-cm intervals from the lower chest to the pelvis. Inclusion of the lower chest is important to identify associated parenchymal or pleural abnormalities. Imaging of the pelvis is necessary to detect intraperitoneal fluid and bony injury. Pause for 2 to 3 minutes before scanning the pelvis to allow for bladder filling with intravenous contrast.

Image display should be at such CT window (W) and level (L) settings as to maximize (1) tissue contrast in the mediastinum and abdominal parenchymal organs (W = 350, L = 100), (2) bone detail (W = 1000, L = 300), and (3) lung parenchymal detail (W = 1500, L = 150).

Indications

Not all children who sustain abdominal trauma are candidates for CT evaluation. The current approach to treatment of children with suspected abdominal injury is as follows. Children with penetrating wounds of the peritoneal cavity are taken directly to the operating room. Children with blunt abdominal trauma who are not hemodynamically stable

Table 22–3 CT findings with asymptomatic hematuria

Variable	Microscopic/dipstick hematuria n = 74	Gross hematuria n = 14
	(n = 88)*	
Renal injury	0	1 (7%)
Nonrenal injury	1 (1%)	0

*Indications available in 970:1000 children. Hematuria was the only sign or symptom in 88 of these children.

Table 22–4 Abdominal injury versus Glasgow Coma Scale

	GCS <8 n = 152	GCS >8 n = 692
	(n = 844)*	
Abdominal injury present	70 (46%)	193 (28%)

p = .0001
*GCS score was known in 844 of 1000 children.

Table 22–5 Solid viscus injury in 1000 children with blunt trauma

Injured organ	Number of children
Solid viscus injury	216 (22%)
Liver	103 (10%)
Spleen	86 (9%)
Kidney	61 (6%)
Adrenal	19 (2%)
Pancreas	16 (2%)

after aggressive attempts at stabilization in the trauma resuscitation unit, or who have suspected peritonitis, are also taken directly to the operating room. Children undergo CT scan evaluation if they fall into one of the following categories (1) children who are hemodynamically stable but in whom se-

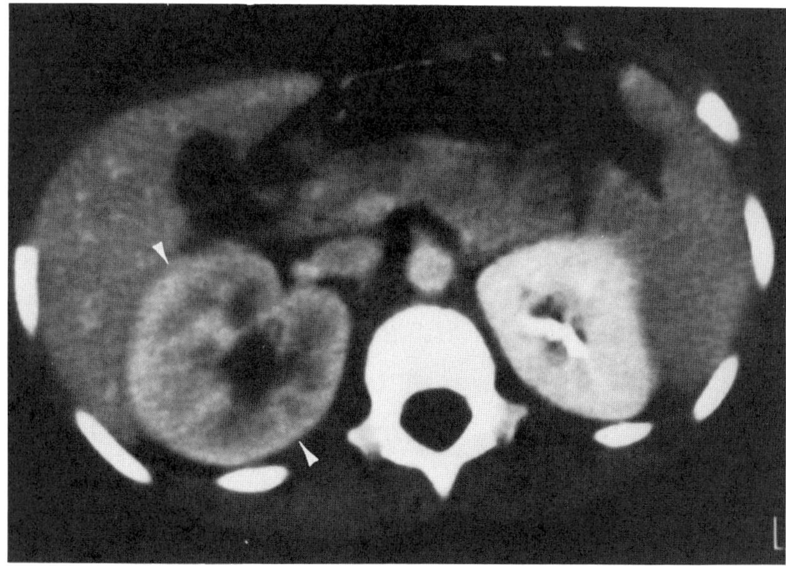

Figure 22–16 Renal contusion. CT shows delayed contrast enhancement of the right kidney *(arrowheads)*.

rious abdominal injury is suspected, (2) those with multisystem injuries (especially head trauma) in whom physical examination suggests injury, and (3) children with gross hematuria.

In the study group, the presence of hematuria was a useful marker of underlying abdominal injury only in association with other suggestive clinical signs and symptoms (Table 22-2).[10] Asymptomatic hematuria is a low-yield indication of injury in children with blunt abdominal trauma (Table 22-3). Significantly, a high proportion of nonurinary injury is associated with hematuria. Splenic and hepatic injury are more common in children with hematuria than are renal or bladder injury. As a result, the use of excretory urography as a screening procedure following blunt trauma is not recommended, because the limited field of view does not permit detection or delineation of injuries to nonrenal organs.

Children with severe neurologic impairment are at higher risk for intraabdominal injury than those without coma (Table 22-4).[100] Neurologic impairment without concurrent abdominal signs, however, is a low-yield indicator of underlying abdominal injury. Only 5 of 65 (8%) neurologically impaired children without abdominal signs had an abdominal injury.

Children who were restrained by safety seats and clinically present linear abdominal or flank ecchymosis caused by the lap belt are at high risk for intraabdominal injury.[74,96] Abdominal or pelvic injury has been present in 63% (39:62) of these children. This compares with a 28% (258:938) rate of

injury in all other children with blunt trauma studied with CT. Additionally, although children with lap-belt ecchymosis represented only 6% (62.1000) of the total examined by CT after blunt trauma, they accounted for 66% (27:41) of all hollow viscus and lumbar spinal injuries seen in this population. Lap-belt ecchymosis is a high-risk indicator of intraabdominal injury and should prompt a careful search for lumbar spine and hollow viscus injury.

Other clinical variables associated with a significantly higher risk of abdominal injury in the study include assault or abuse as a mechanism of injury, abdominal tenderness, a Glasgow Trauma Scale (GCS) score less than or equal to 12, or the presence of more than three clinical indications present at initial evaluation.[103]

Solid organ injury

Blunt abdominal trauma often results in solid organ injury. Twenty-two percent of children studied following blunt trauma had an injury to a solid viscus (Table 22-5). The liver was the most commonly injured organ, followed by the spleen and kidneys, respectively. Adrenal and pancreatic injuries were the least common in the study population. CT has proved to be very accurate in the detection and delineation of hepatic, splenic, and renal injuries.[22,48,50,65,105]

Abnormalities noted on CT include contusion, laceration, fragmentation, subcapsular or intraparenchymal hematoma, or infarction. A contusion is defined as a region of delayed contrast excretion (Fig. 22-16); it may be global or segmental. A

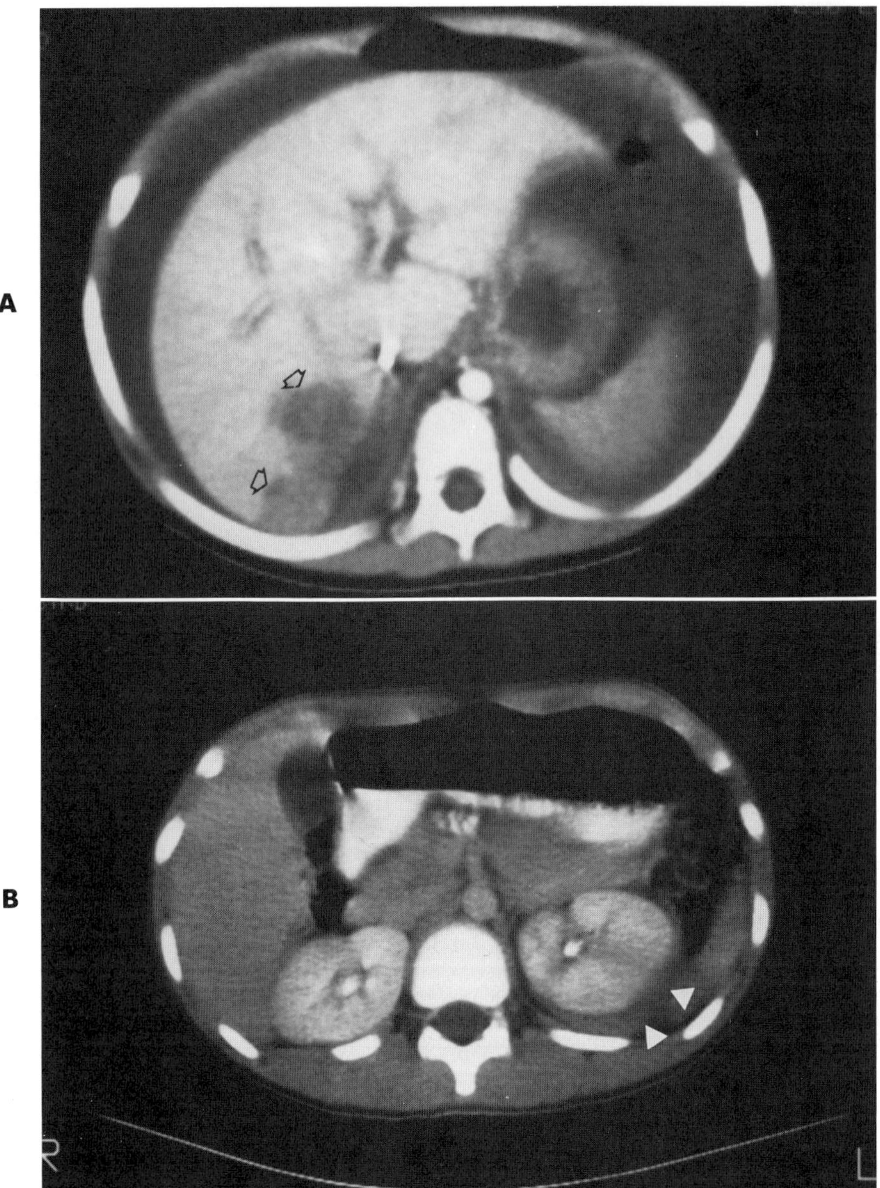

Figure 22–17 CT of the upper abdomen shows **(A)** a right intrahepatic hematoma *(arrows)* and **(B)** a left renal subcapsular hematoma *(arrowheads)*.

hematoma is a focal lesion that does not enhance (Fig. 22-17); it is usually isodense or hyperdense relative to unenhanced solid viscera, but hypodense relative to solid viscera enhanced with intravenous contrast. A laceration is a parenchymal tear (Fig. 22-18), and an infarct is recognized as parenchymal nonenhancement resulting from vascular injury (Fig. 22-19).

A number of classification systems have been proposed for categorizing these injuries through CT, with emphasis placed on the anatomic dimensions of the injury.[68,70,73,110] One system classifies solid organ injury as vascular or nonvascular. Nonvascular injury is further characterized on the basis of the percentage of abnormal parenchyma involved; minor injury (less than 25% of organ volume), moderate (25% to 50% of organ volume), or severe (greater than 50% of organ volume). There are many inherent limitations to any classification system, and a single CT examination cannot precisely determine whether a child is actively bleeding.

Hepatic and splenic injury are frequently, but not always, associated with hemoperitoneum.

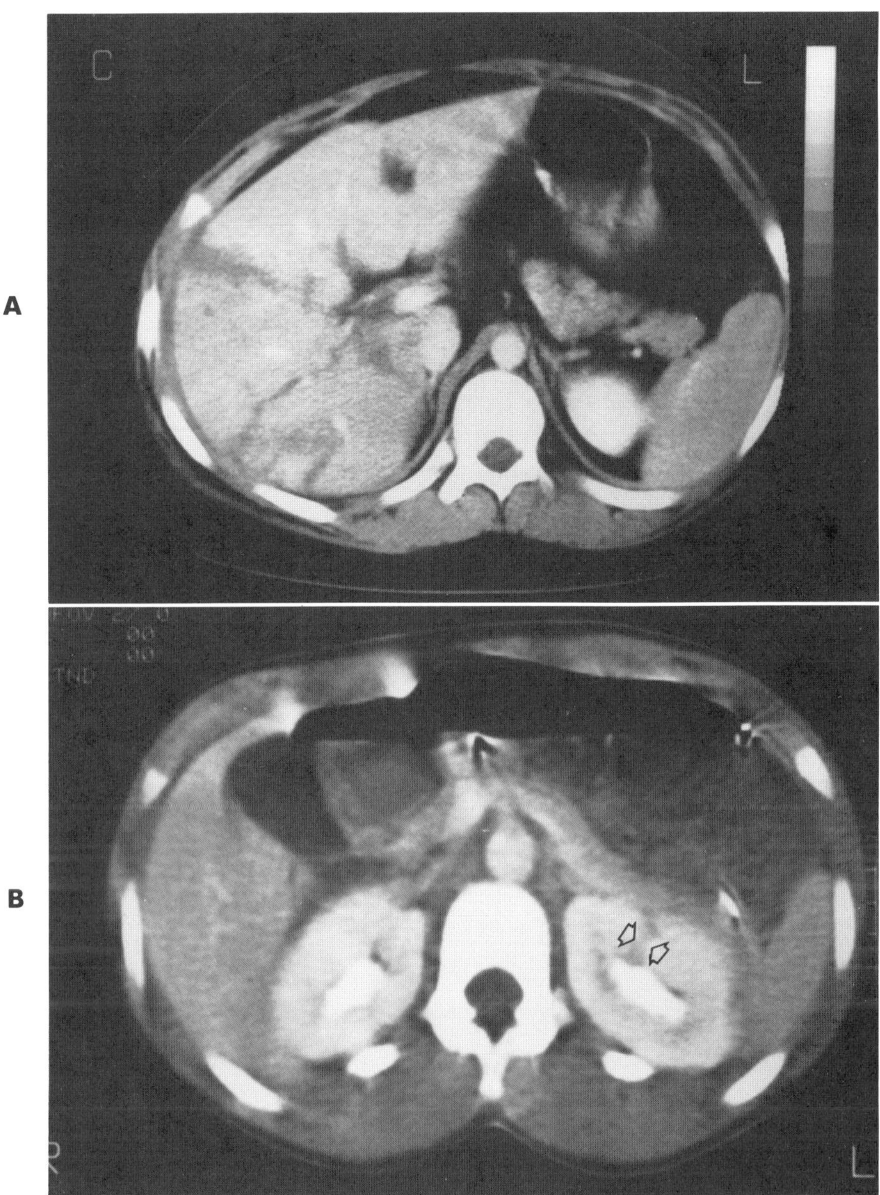

Figure 22–18 Solid organ laceration. CT shows **(A)** a complex hepatic laceration extending to the porta hepatis and **(B)** a laceration of the left kidney *(arrows)*.

Thirty-one percent (56:178) of children in our study population with a hepatic or splenic injury did not have peritoneal fluid at CT. This experience demonstrates a major limitation of diagnostic peritoneal lavage in the diagnosis of solid organ injury. Because peritoneal lavage is sensitive only for identifying the presence of peritoneal fluid, it would have missed nearly one third of these injuries.

Although the information gained by CT is useful in establishing a treatment plan, the decision to manage children with hepatic, splenic, and renal injury operatively or nonoperatively is based on the physiologic status of the child. Regardless of the extent of the injury indicated by CT, hemorrhage stops in the majority of children, and nonoperative management is usually successful.[18,49,75] Of 251 hepatic, splenic, and renal injuries in this population, only 13 (5%) required operative intervention (Table 22-6). Even large parenchymal injuries healed without surgical intervention. Most intraparenchymal lacerations and hematomas undergo spontaneous absorption and healing (Fig. 22-20). The hematoma is replaced by fibrous tissue; if tissue necrosis has occurred, calcific scar may also appear.

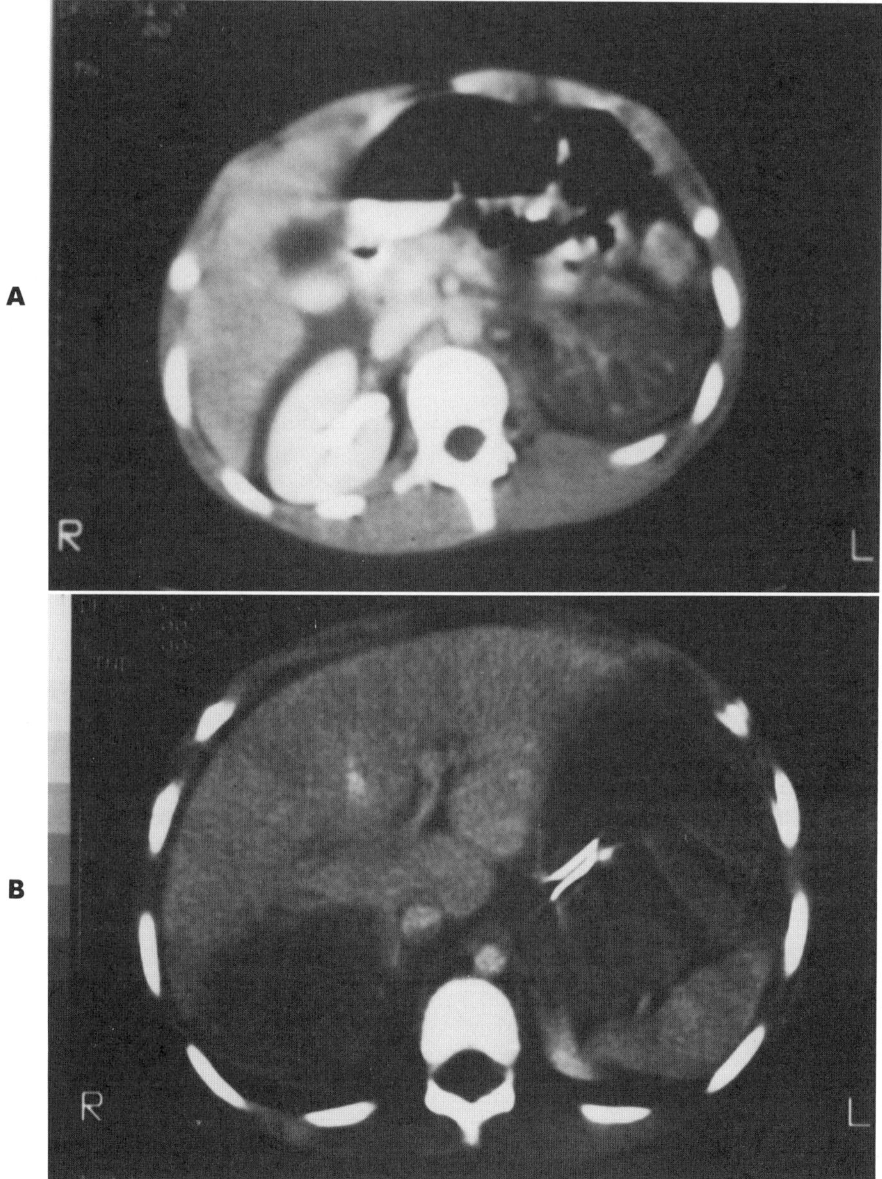

Figure 22–19 Vascular injury. **A,** CT demonstrates absence of contrast enhancement of the left kidney. **B,** Nonenhancement of the posterior segment of the right lobe of the liver is noted.

Table 22–6 Hepatic, splenic and renal injuries requiring laparotomy in 1000 children with blunt trauma

Organ injured	Number requiring laparotomy
Spleen	8:86 (9%)
Splenectomy	6
Splenorrhaphy	2
Renal	4:61 (6%)
Nephrectomy	1
Partial nephrectomy	1
Renal artery graft	1
Infected urinoma drainage	1
Hepatic	1:103 (1%)
Right hepatectomy	1

Pancreatic injury is not easy to identify with CT. Delineation of the margins of the pancreas may be difficult because of the small size of the organ and the relative paucity of surrounding retroperitoneal fat in children. Unlike injury to the liver, spleen, or kidney, laceration or fracture of the pancreas produces little change in density in the acute phase of injury, and such change may be difficult to detect by CT.[16,46,91a] Minimal separation of the lacerated pancreatic fragments may be present. It can also be difficult to distinguish a laceration in the tail of the pancreas from adjacent unopacified bowel loops. In addition, CT cannot directly detect pancreatic duct disruption, which is the major determinant of the clinical significance of pancreatic injury. Adequate bowel opacification with contrast material is useful in the evaluation of the pancreas. Although administration of oral contrast for CT scan following blunt trauma is not routine, instillation of contrast in the upper gastrointestinal tract is useful when there is a high clinical suspicion of pancreatic injury. The presence and location of peripancreatic fluid collections is helpful in establishing a diagnosis of pancreatic injury. The presence of fluid in the lesser sac has been a useful marker for injury to the pancreas (sensitivity, 69%; specificity, 99%) (Fig. 22-21). Fluid in the anterior pararenal space has been less helpful in suggesting injury (sensitivity, 44%; specificity, 98%). On follow-up CT or ultrasound examination, a well-defined pseudocyst may be seen (Fig. 22-22). Serial evaluation with CT or ultrasound is useful in guiding management by characterizing changes in the size of these collections over time. Pseudocysts may resolve spontaneously and not require drainage.

Adrenal hematoma also occurs in severely injured children. The characteristic CT findings are gland enlargement, oval or triangular shape, and decreased attenuation relative to enhanced liver and spleen (Fig. 22-23).[31] Ipsilateral crural thickening is often seen. The right adrenal is more commonly involved than the left, and adjacent solid organ injury is usually present. Posttraumatic adrenal hematoma was noted on CT in 19 children (2%). The hematoma was unilateral in 95% (18:19) and bilateral in 5% (1:19). Adjacent solid organ injury was present in nearly all of these children (95%). Signs of adrenal insufficiency were not observed in any children with adrenal hematoma.

Hollow organ injury

Bowel injury. Gastrointestinal tract injury in children who have sustained blunt abdominal trauma is infrequent. Bowel injury was present in 2% of children (n = 18) examined with CT following blunt trauma. Twelve of these children (67%) were restrained passengers in motor vehicle crashes and manifested linear lap-belt ecchymosis across the lower abdomen or flank. The most common location of injury was the jejunum (50%, n = 9), followed by the duodenum (39%, n = 7), ileum (6%, n = 1), and sigmoid colon (6%, n = 1). Injury types included complete transection (n = 8), partial tear (n = 5), contusion or hematoma (n = 3), and stricture (identified on follow-up upper gastrointestinal series) (n = 2).

CT diagnosis of bowel injury is difficult. Findings of intestinal trauma are subtle and nonspecific; peritoneal lavage or early laparotomy is warranted if the clinical signs and symptoms suggest a bowel injury. The presence of pneumoperitoneum is neither sensitive nor specific for the diagnosis of bowel injury.[11,16,81,89,96] A tear may seal quickly with no chance of air escaping into the peritoneum. Conversely, only fluid contents may extravasate, and the sole sign of injury may be free fluid within the peritoneal cavity.[81,89,96] Pneumoperitoneum occurred in only 39% of bowel injuries in the study (Fig. 22-24) (Table 22-7). "Unexplained" peritoneal fluid is a useful indicator of bowel injury (Fig. 22-25). Peritoneal fluid is rarely seen after blunt trauma as an isolated finding. In the absence of a solid viscus injury, pelvic fracture, or "hypoperfusion" complex, peritoneal fluid occurred in only 17 of the 1000 children (2%) studied by CT following blunt trauma. Nine of these (59%) had a bowel injury, and 1 other child had a perforated appendix. Additional associated CT findings in these children included bowel wall thickening (wall thickness >3 mm in diameter) and localized hematoma (Table 22-7).

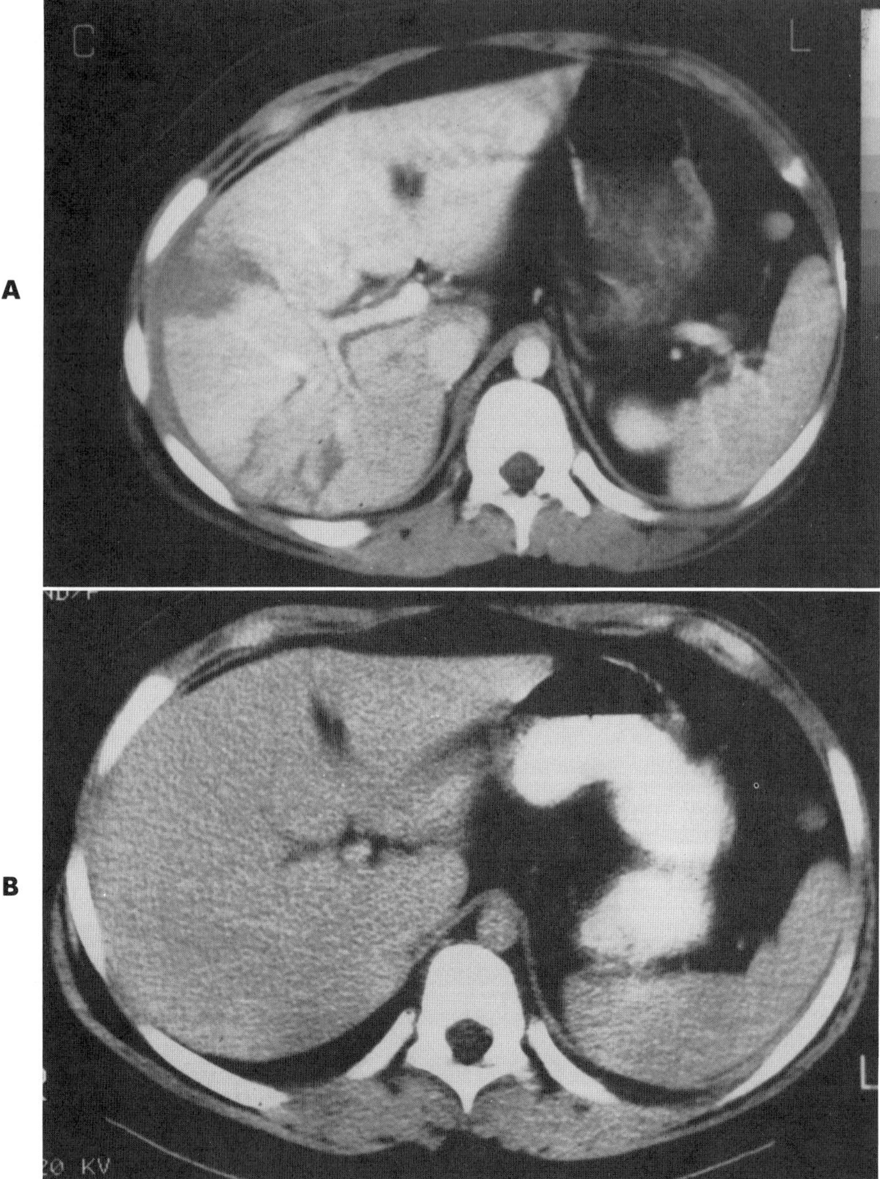

Figure 22–20 Laceration of the liver with healing. **A,** A complex laceration of the right lobe of the liver is noted. The child was managed nonoperatively. **B,** Follow-up CT examination 4 months after the injury shows no residual hepatic abnormality.

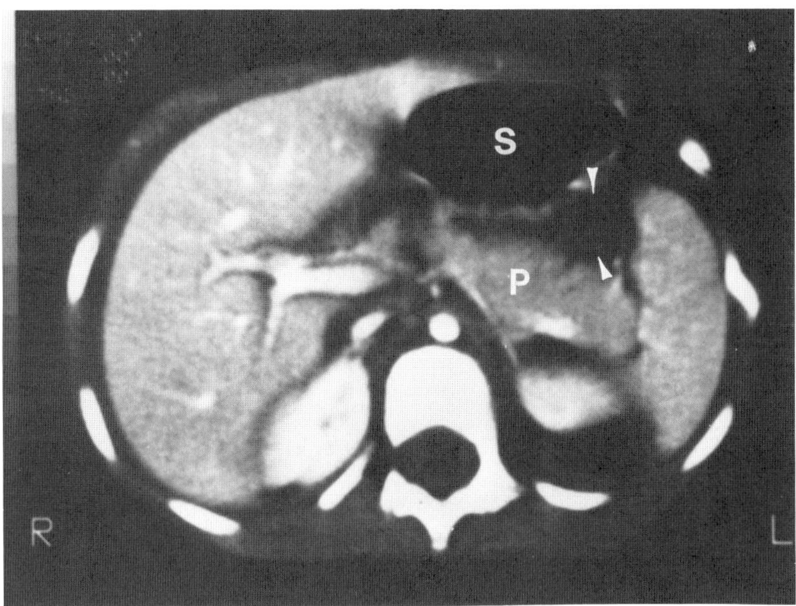

Figure 22–21 CT at level of the pancreas shows fluid in the lesser sac *(arrowheads)*. S = stomach, P = pancreas.

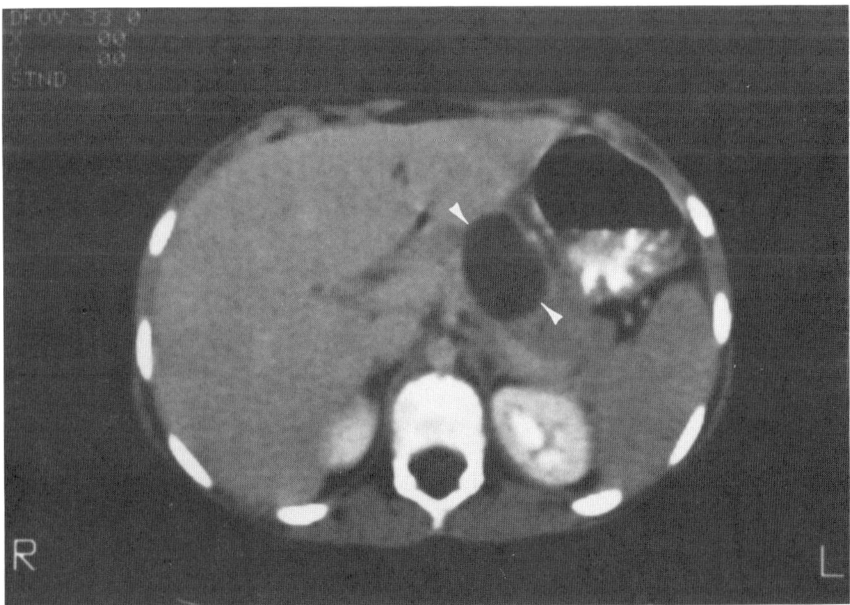

Figure 22–22 Pancreatic pseudocyst. CT shows an intrapancreatic pseudocyst *(arrowheads)*.

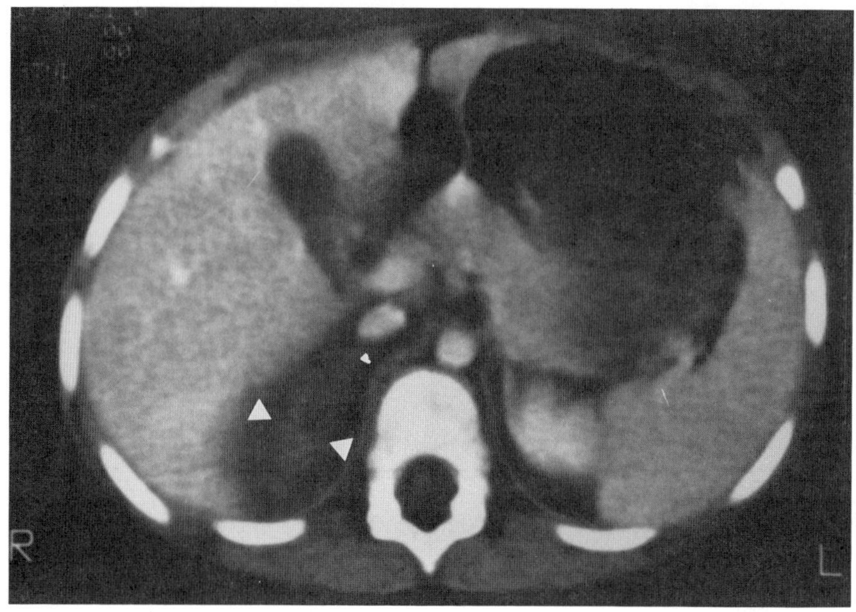

Figure 22–23 Adrenal hematoma. CT demonstrates an oval-shaped adrenal hematoma *(large arrowheads)*. Note ipsilateral thickening of the diaphragmatic crus *(small arrowhead)*.

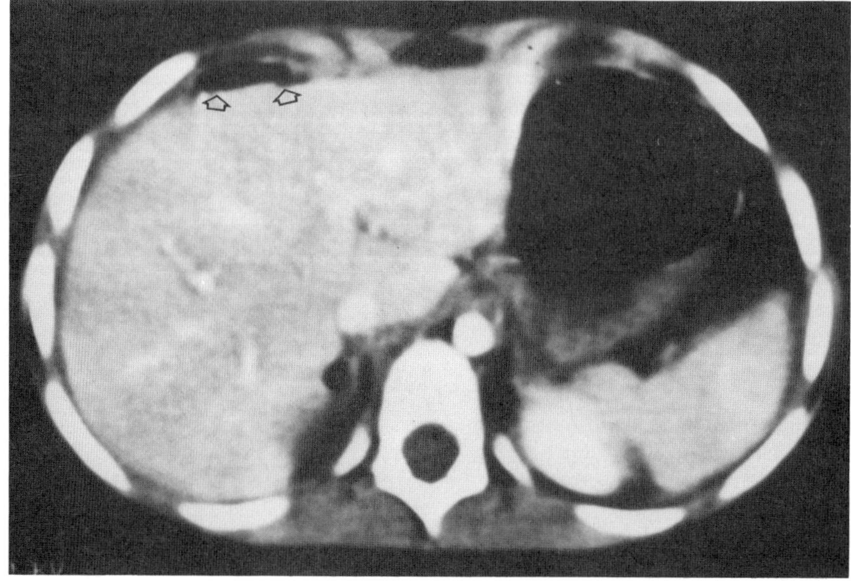

Figure 22–24 Pneumoperitoneum. CT shows free intraperitoneal air anterior to liver *(arrows)*.

Table 22–7 CT findings in children
with bowel injury

CT finding	Present n = 18
Pneumoperitoneum	7 (39%)
Peritoneal fluid	17 (94%)
Associated solid organ or bony pelvis injury	7 (39%)
"Unexplained" fluid	10 (56%)
Bowel wall thickening	8 (44%)
Localized hematoma	1 (6%)
"Unexplained" peritoneal fluid, bowel wall thickening or pneumoperitoneum	15 (83%)

Bladder injury

Injury to the urinary bladder is uncommon in children; there were only five (<1%) cases in the population of the study. Two occurred in children with lap-belt ecchymosis across the lower abdomen, and two were associated with pelvic fractures. Types of bladder injury resulting from blunt trauma include (1) contusion, or tear of the bladder mucosa, (2) intraperitoneal bladder rupture, and (3) extraperitoneal bladder rupture. Treatment of bladder contusion and extraperitoneal bladder tear is usually nonoperative, whereas intraperitoneal bladder rupture requires early surgical repair. The diagnosis of bladder contusion is difficult to determine with imaging techniques[84,86] because CT and cystogram findings may be normal.

Intraperitoneal bladder rupture occurs as a result of blunt force to a distended bladder causing a tear along the peritoneal portion of the bladder wall. Upon CT examination, intraperitoneal extravasation of contrast is noted (Fig. 22-26). In extraperitoneal bladder rupture, there is extravasation first into the paravesical space. With a more extensive tear, extension occurs into the anterior and posterior pararenal spaces, as well as the perinephric space. Diagnosis may be difficult with CT and cystography, as extravasated contrast material may be obscured by a distended bladder. A postdrainage radiographic examination enhances the potential of the cystograph to establish the diagnosis.

Pelvic fracture/dislocation

Six percent of children (n = 56) in the study evaluated with CT following blunt trauma had a pelvic fracture or subluxation. CT is helpful in planning treatment of bony pelvic injury; it can demonstrate the plane of fracture and relationship of bony fragments quite readily. In addition, a CT scan is superior to plain films in providing details of fractures, position of fracture fragments, extent of diastasis or angulation, and presence of intraartic-

ular bone fragments. It is also of value in assessing associated visceral injury and hematoma, as any force powerful enough to fracture a pelvis can result in injury to adjacent body areas. Associated visceral injury was noted in approximately one third of the study population (Table 22-8). Bladder injury rarely occurs with injury to the bony pelvis (4%). Major blood loss associated with pelvic fracture may occur as a result of bleeding from the superior gluteal artery or internal iliac artery. Hemoperitoneum was noted in 22% of children (8:37) with isolated bony pelvic injury. The identification of associated severe hemorrhage is important, as early pelvic immobilization with external or internal fixation reduces the likelihood of further bleeding.

Lumbar spine fracture/dislocation

Injury to the lumbar spine occurred in 2% of children (n = 19) evaluated with CT following blunt trauma. Thirteen of these (68%) shared the same mechanism of injury; they had been passengers in motor vehicle crashes involved in sudden deceleration. All had been secured by an adult lap-style safety belt and, after trauma, manifested linear ecchymosis across the lower abdomen or flank. Spinal injuries in these children occurred because of hyperflexion of the lumbar spine following sudden deceleration, associated with incorrect positioning of the lap belt about the iliac crest.[74,96,99] The injuries occurred primarily in the midlumbar region, some occurred at the thoracolumbar junction. Although CT can depict the cross-sectional anatomy of the spine accurately, it is not a useful screening tool. Lumbar spine injuries are difficult to identify on CT scans of the abdomen because of the limitations of CT in detecting horizontal fractures and facet distractions. Only 32% (6/19) of lumbar spine injuries were noted on abdominal CT scans. All of the injuries were present on lateral radiographs of the spine. Because children with injuries of this type usually present few clinical signs, current practice includes AP and lateral scout radiographs of the lumbar spine as part of the CT evaluation in all children (Fig. 22-27). Scout radiographs are obtained with the child in the CT gantry and serve as a screening devices. Plain radiographs of the lumbar spine are still necessary to visualize the spine in greater detail.

Hypoperfusion complex

Hemodynamic stability is one of the criteria for abdominal CT examination. Occasionally children respond adequately to life-saving measures and undergo CT, albeit with tenuous hemodynamic stability. Normal blood pressure and pulse rate are not always reliable indicators of stable hemodynamic status. Consequently, a new complex of findings on abdominal CT in 26 children became apparent in association with profound shock: the

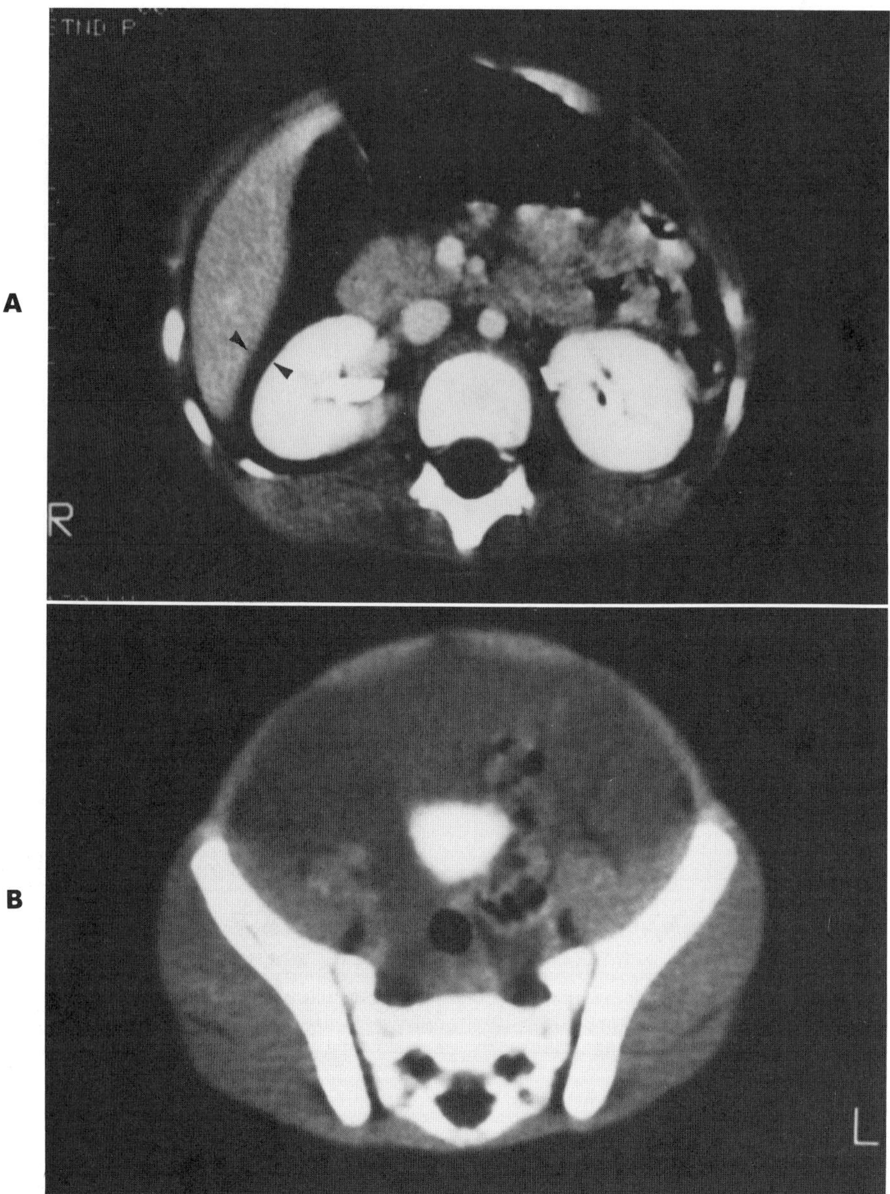

Figure 22–25 Unexplained peritoneal fluid associated with bowel injury. **A,** CT of upper abdomen shows fluid in Morison pouch *(arrowheads)* and **(B)** section through the pelvis demonstrates fluid in the lateral paravesical fossae. No solid organ injury or pelvic fracture was noted.

"hypoperfusion" complex.[102] This constellation of findings has been associated with a poor outcome; 85% of children (22/26) with the complex died.

CT findings in all children with the hypoperfusion complex included diffuse dilatation of the intestine with fluid, intense contrast enhancement of the bowel wall, mesentery, kidneys, abdominal aorta, and inferior vena cava (Fig. 22-28). Variable findings included intense contrast enhancement of the adrenals and pancreas, intense contrast enhancement and diminished caliber of the superior mesenteric artery and vein, persistent dense ureteral filling, decreased splenic and pancreatic enhancement, and bowel wall thickening (Table 22-9). Peritoneal and retroperitoneal fluid collections may be seen in the absence of associated intraabdominal injury.

Familiarity with the CT findings that are part of the complex should help avoid unnecessary laparotomy for suspected abdominal visceral injury. Decreased splenic or pancreatic enhancement may lead to the erroneous inference that a vascular in-

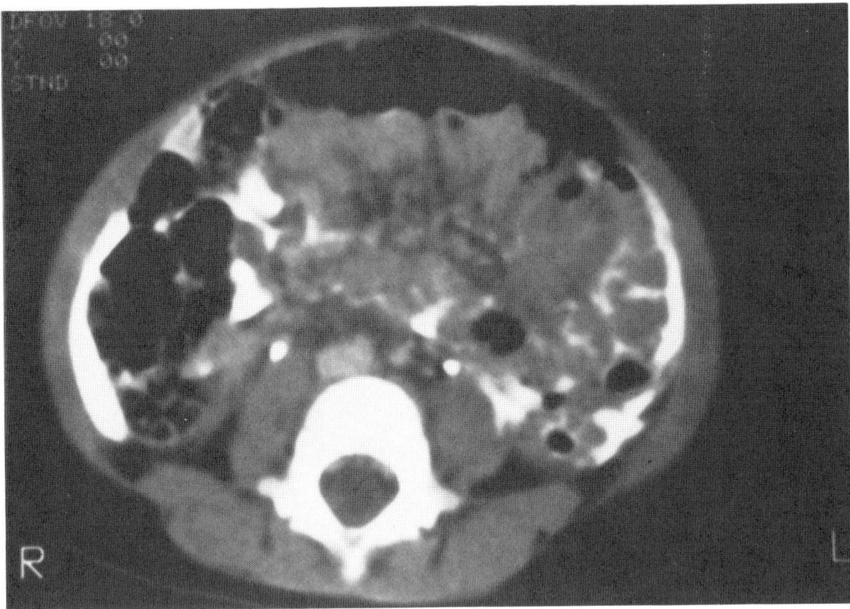

Figure 22–26 Intraperitoneal bladder rupture. CT through the lower abdomen demonstrates diffuse intraperitoneal extravasation of excreted intravenous contrast.

Table 22–8 Children with bony pelvis injury

	(n = 56)
Associated visceral injury	19 (34%)
Solid organ injury	16 (30%)
Bowel injury	3 (6%)
Bladder injury	2 (4%)
No associated injury	37 (66%)

jury, with resultant organ infarction, is present. The finding is probably related to systemic vasoconstriction in response to sympathetic stimulation.[7] Diffuse intestinal dilatation and intense bowel wall and mesenteric enhancement may lead to the conclusion that a bowel or mesenteric injury is present. These findings are likely related to vasoconstriction of the splanchnic vascular bed and "third space" fluid losses into the gastrointestinal tract.[102] Although it is possible that bowel hypoperfusion may lead to ischemia in severe cases, none was observed in the study population, either at surgery or at autopsy. The presence of intraperitoneal or retroperitoneal fluid could suggest the existence of an abdominal visceral injury. This fluid is probably the result of "third space" fluid losses. In summary, the intense multiorgan enhancement pattern seen in the hypoperfusion complex indicates tenuous hemodynamic stability and is associated with a poor outcome.

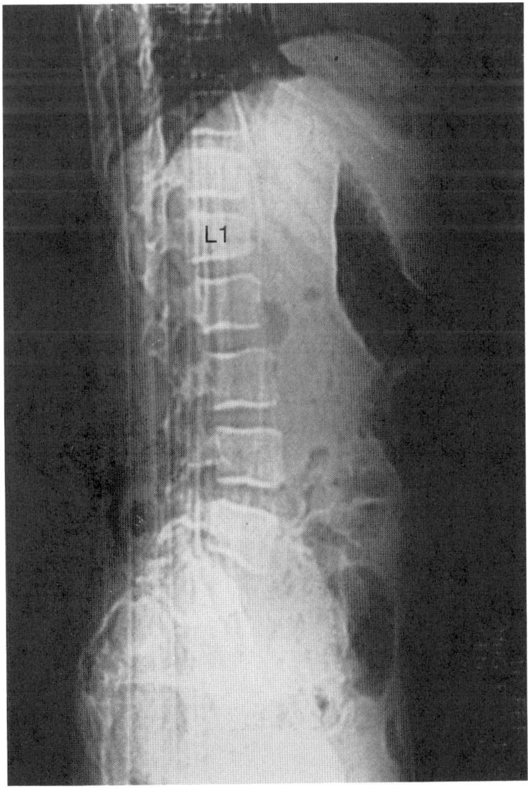

Figure 22–27 Lateral scout radiograph of the lumbar spine demonstrates a compression fracture of the L1 vertebral body.

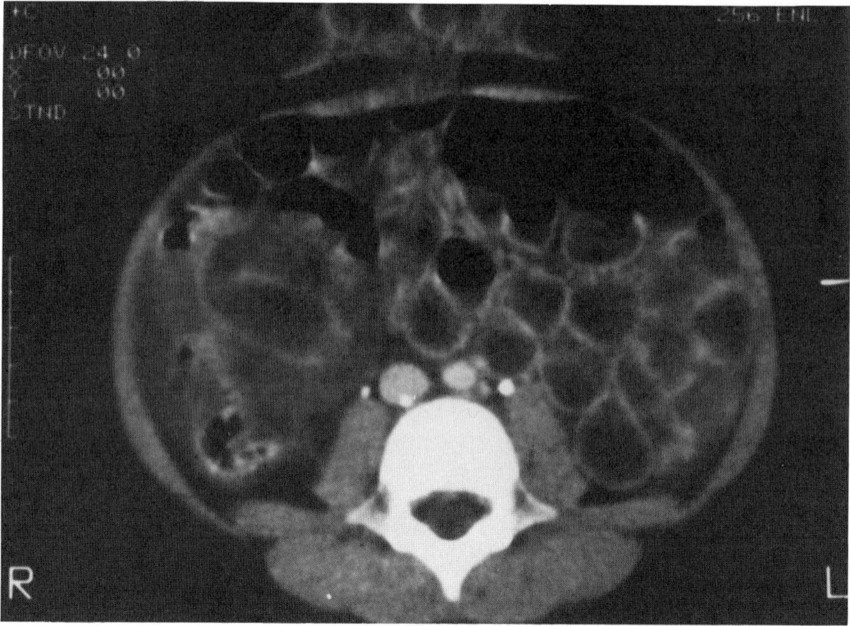

Figure 22–28 Hypoperfusion complex. CT shows diffuse dilatation of the intestine with fluid and intense contrast enhancement of bowel wall, aorta, and IVC.

Table 22–9 Variable CT findings in children with "hypoperfusion" complex

Abnormality	(n = 26) Number of patients
Intense adrenal enhancement	17 (65%)
Intense SMA and SMV enhancement	15 (58%)
Dense ureteral filling	12 (46%)
Intense pancreatic enhancement	3 (12%)
Decreased splenic enhancement	3 (12%)
Bowel wall thickening	2 (8%)
Decreased pancreatic enhancement	1 (4%)

Peritoneal fluid

Following blunt trauma, peritoneal fluid or blood tends to collect in dependent recesses. In the upper abdomen, the most dependent site is in the Morison pouch (Fig. 22-29).[67] The Morison pouch communicates superiorly with the perihepatic space and caudally with the right paracolic gutter, which is wider and deeper than the left gutter (Fig. 22-30). The pelvis is the most dependent part of the peritoneal cavity and is anatomically continuous with both paracolic gutters and the left infracolic space. Fluid collects within the central pouch of Douglas, or laterally in the paravesical fossae (Fig. 22-31).[67] Extensive hemorrhage may result in a large pelvic collection with little blood in the upper abdomen. This is a principal reason that the CT evaluation of children following abdominal trauma must include the pelvis.

The clinical significance of peritoneal fluid or blood observed by CT scan following blunt trauma continues to evolve in this era of nonoperative management of solid organ injury.[95,104] Currently, the decision for operative versus nonoperative management is not based on the extent of peritoneal fluid shown by CT, but on the physiologic condition of the child. Even if all of the fluid represents blood, the amount seen at CT examination reflects the cumulative amount of bleeding that occurred between the time of injury and the time of the CT scan. Although in rare instances extravasation of intravenous material from a bleeding site may be seen, CT cannot usually be used to determine whether active bleeding is present.[46,75,92,95,104] The majority of children with large posttraumatic fluid collections undergo nonoperative management (Table 22-10).

Preferably, fluid collections within the abdomen following trauma are termed *peritoneal fluid* rather than *hemoperitoneum,* because differentiation of blood from other types of fluid is difficult by CT scan. Fluid in children with isolated hollow viscus injury or third-space fluid losses associated with the "hypoperfusion complex" often demonstrates attenuation coefficients equal to those of blood.

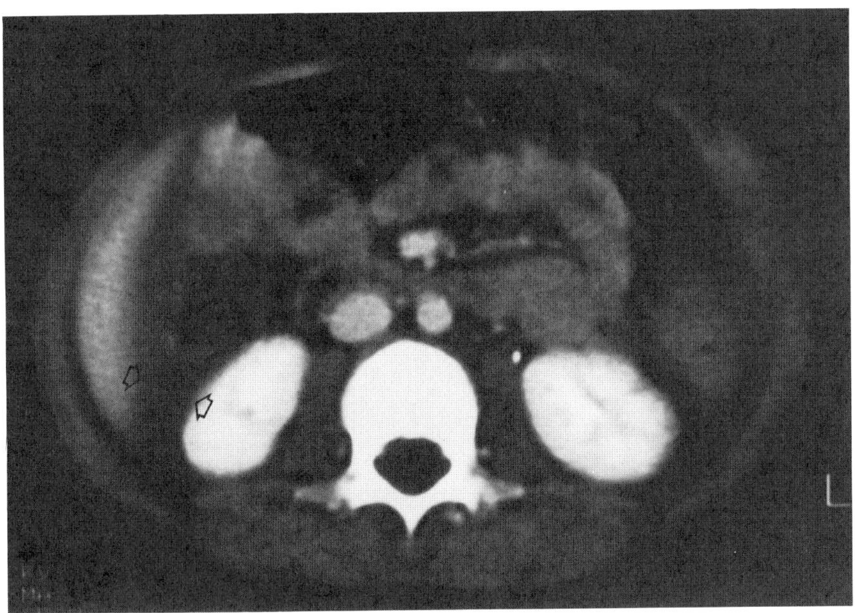

Figure 22–29 CT of upper abdomen shows fluid in Morison pouch *(arrows)*.

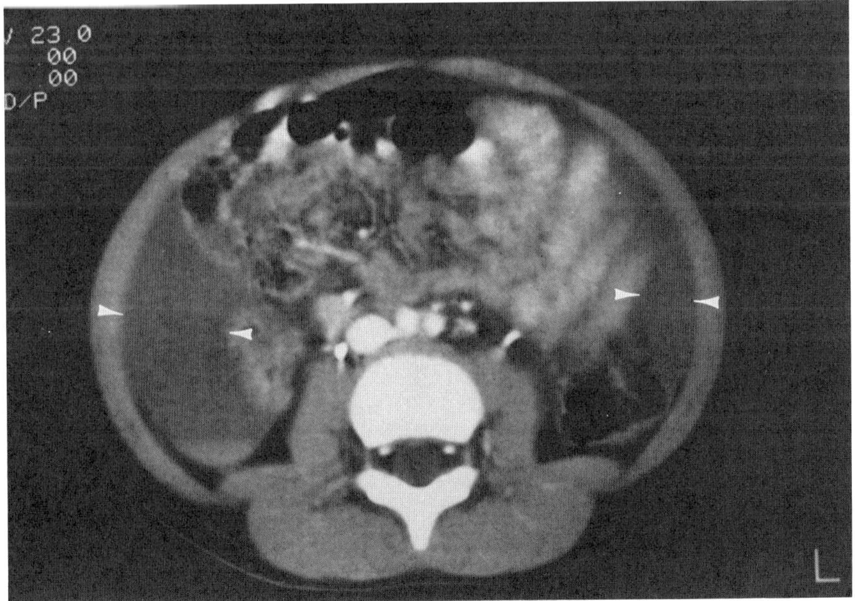

Figure 22–30 CT of mid abdomen demonstrates fluid in the right and left paracolic gutters *(arrowheads)*.

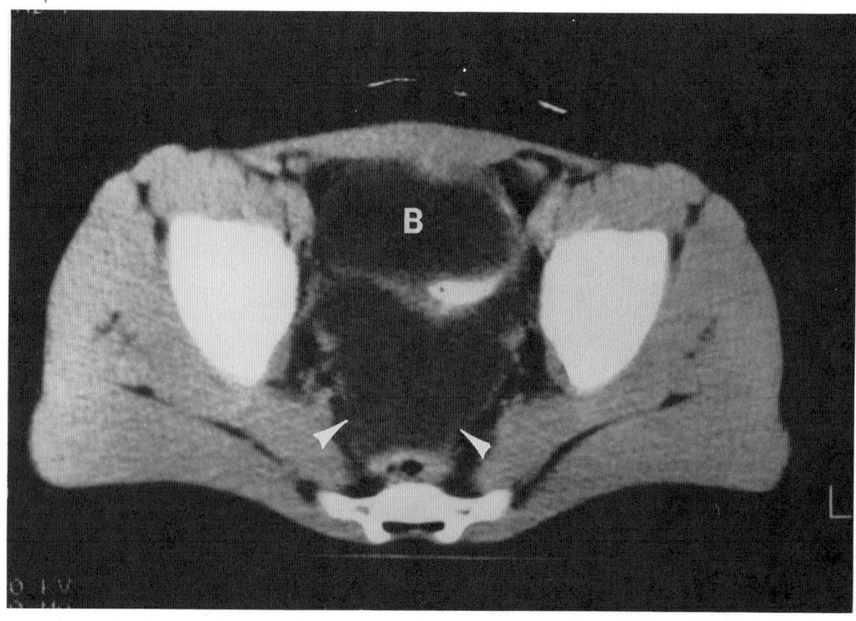

Figure 22–31 CT of the pelvis shows fluid in the central pouch of Douglas *(arrowheads)*. B = bladder.

Table 22–10 Frequency of operative management versus amount of peritoneal fluid in 1000 children with blunt trauma

Amount of peritoneal fluid	(n = 170)* Number of children requiring surgery
None	6/819 (1)
Small	8/67 (12)
Moderate	9/50 (18)
Large	22/53 (42)

p = .0001
*Eleven children had peritoneal lavage prior to CT and are not included.

Table 22–11 Abnormalities associated with peritoneal fluid on CT

Abnormalities	(n = 170) Number of patients
Hepatic/splenic injury	116 (68%)
No intraperitoneal solid organ injury	54 (32%)
Isolated renal, adrenal, or pancreatic injury	10 (6%)
Isolated bowel injury	9 (5%)
Isolated "hypoperfusion" complex	9 (5%)
Isolated pelvic fracture	8 (5%)
Isolated bladder injury	2 (1%)
More than one of the above	8 (5%)
Appendicitis	1 (1%)
No additional abnormality noted	7 (4%)

The presence of peritoneal fluid in the absence of solid organ injury, pelvic fracture, or the hypoperfusion complex should raise a strong suspicion of bowel injury. Fluid in the peritoneal cavity was identified in 17% of children in the study, and more than 50% of all children with peritoneal fluid as an isolated finding had a bowel injury (Table 22-11). Peritoneal fluid following blunt trauma was truly "unexplained" in only 4% of the children. The detection of peritoneal fluid should prompt a careful search for associated injury.

Chest injury

The evaluation and treatment of thoracic trauma is a central feature of the early assessment and management of the injured child because chest injury leads to hypoxia. A reliable clinical diagnosis of chest injury in the acutely injured child is often difficult. Cardiopulmonary symptoms may not be present in the first 24 hours, and there are no consistent relationships between external chest wall injury and underlying abnormalities. This is particularly evident in children in whom increased compliance of the bony thorax allows major inter-

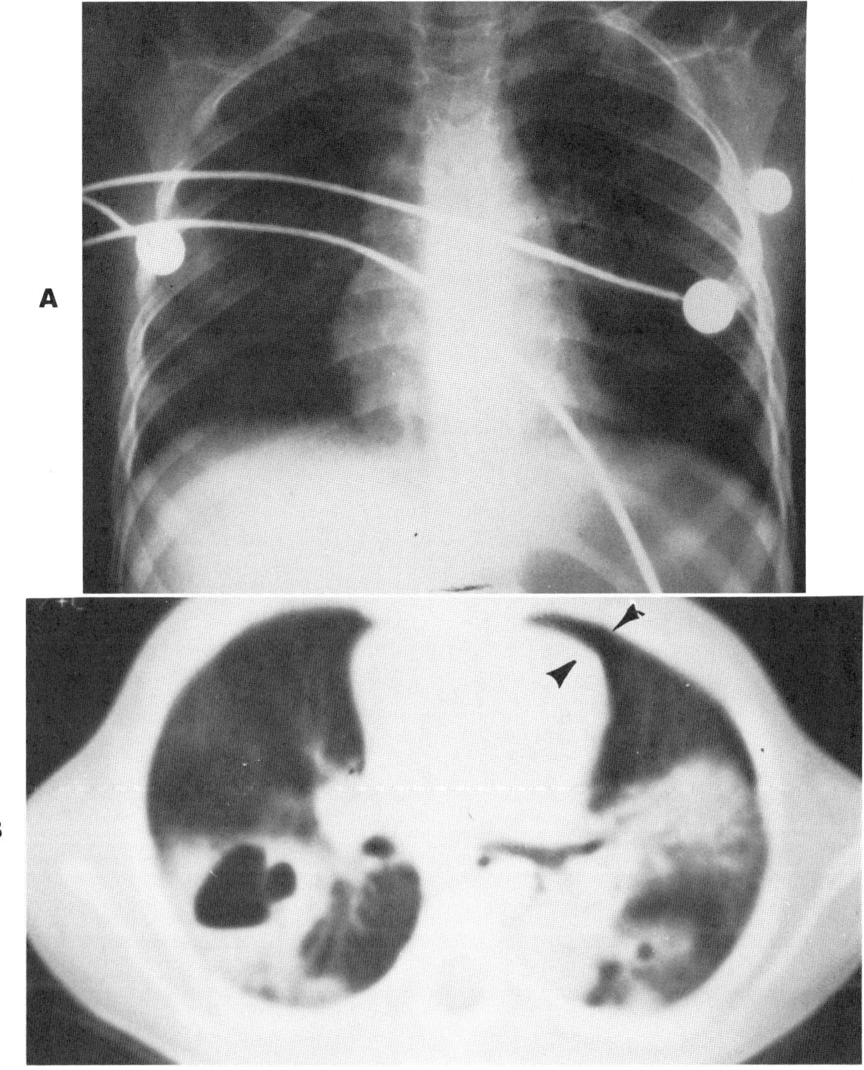

Figure 22–32 A, AP chest radiograph shows no abnormalities. **B,** CT scan of the same patient through the mid chest 1 hour later demonstrates a right pulmonary laceration, left pulmonary contusion, and small left pneumothorax *(arrowheads).*

nal injury to occur without associated skeletal injury.[36]

Chest radiography remains the primary method for evaluation of posttraumatic chest injury. Radiographs are usually obtained with portable equipment, the child supine, and various monitoring devices overlying the areas of interest. As a result, even with optimal technique, the chest radiograph may underestimate or miss significant chest abnormality (Fig. 22-32).[93]

Performance of a lower chest CT scan in conjunction with CT scan of the upper abdomen is helpful in the early recognition of unsuspected chest injury. Often abnormalities in the chest that are far more extensive than suspected on the basis of the plain radiograph become evident. Consequently, three or four CT slices of the lower chest in all children with abdominal trauma enhances diagnostic accuracy; in the study, chest injury was present in 12% of the children. Thirty-eight percent of all abnormalities identified on CT scans had been underestimated or missed on the initial chest radiograph.[93] If a major abnormality is present on these images or suspected on the chest radiograph, obtain additional CT scans on a case-by-case basis. The presence and extent of a chest injury is a marker of the severity of the trauma and a risk factor for a poor outcome.[93]

Battered children

Abdominal CT examination is useful in evaluating battered children with physical signs and symptoms of abdominal trauma. Within the population studied, battered children with abdominal visceral injury represented a select population with severe injury.[95] Battered children with lower thoracic or abdominal injury had greater physiologic derangement and mortality than children without thoracoabdominal injury.[94] The spectrum of abdominal injury in this group of children was similar to that seen in children injured by unintentional trauma. Nonpancreatic solid viscus injury, particularly hepatic and splenic, occurred more frequently than bowel, mesenteric, or pancreatic injury. Although most solid organ injuries do not require operative intervention, the identification of physical abnormalities in these children is important evidence in legal proceedings.

Penetrating injury

Stab and gunshot wounds to the abdomen and back present a serious diagnostic problem because of the high risk of bowel or diaphragmatic injury. The mainstay in the evaluation of children with such injuries continues to be careful local wound exploration and mandatory laparotomy in cases of demonstrated peritoneal penetration. CT can give anatomic information on the presence and depth of injury when it is clinically occult. There is also a role for CT in the postoperative evaluation of children with penetrating trauma who develop sepsis or peritonitis, identifying and localizing intraperitoneal fluid collections and abscesses.

Angiography

Because of the availability of CT, angiography is now rarely used in the evaluation of the child with abdominal trauma. If vascular integrity of a solid organ such as the kidney is evident on CT, emergency surgery rather than arteriography is indicated. As a result of early external fixation of pelvic fractures, hemostasis following iliac and gluteal artery tears is now usually achieved without the use of embolization.

Angiography is essential in the assessment of the thoracic aorta and its major branches in severe chest trauma when the chest radiograph or CT scan indicates a mediastinal hematoma (Fig. 22-11).[62,88] In severe fractures of the extremities in which limb ischemia is noted, angiography may identify an intimal flap, arteriovenous malformation, or traumatic aneurysm.[82,83] Angiography may also be useful in the evaluation of children with posttraumatic renovascular hypertension, as well as those with hematobilia.

CRANIAL AND SPINAL IMAGING

Cranial and spinal injuries are a major cause of mortality and long-term disability in children. The goal during initial assessment of the injured child is to determine rapidly and accurately the extent of injuries that require immediate surgical intervention. Factors that determine which imaging modality is to be used are (1) the speed with which the examination results are needed, (2) the ability of the child to cooperate, and (3) the amount of support equipment and monitoring required.

Skull radiography

Skull radiographs play a minor role in the evaluation of cranial injury. Although skull films are more sensitive than CT in the identification of linear skull fractures, the presence or absence of a linear fracture is a poor predictor of intracranial injury. The time required to obtain a skull film delays the diagnosis and treatment of brain injury.[20,60]

Computed tomography

Since its introduction cranial CT has proved to be invaluable in the assessment of critically injured children, often leading to prompt, lifesaving care.

Technique. Many of the techniques described for abdominal CT scanning are applicable in cranial CT. Removal of overlying metallic hardware and an adequate radius of reconstruction are important considerations. Because of the quick scanning techniques now available with most CT scanners, sedation is rarely required when imaging the brain in the axial plane. Noncontrast, serial 1-cm–thick images are obtained at 1-cm intervals through the brain in the axial plane. Image display includes window (W) and level (L) settings that maximize soft tissue contrast (W = 70, L = 40) and bone detail (W = 1000, L = 300). Radiation exposure is usually less than 2 rads, not significantly more than a skull series.

Acute intracranial hemorrhage appears on CT without the use of intravenous contrast. Contrast media define the extent of a cerebral contusion and prove useful in defining isodense hematoma.[61] Intravenous contrast, however, carries a risk of neurotoxicity that precludes routine use.[40,42,117]

Indications. Many criteria are used in the attempt to identify which children need assessment by cranial CT scan; unfortunately, no clinical findings accurately identify all children whose CT scan findings will be abnormal. Altered mental status, focal neurologic abnormality, and a GCS score of 12 or less have been associated with a higher frequency of abnormal CT findings.[80] However, children with a high GCS score also have unexpected abnormal cranial findings on CT. Criteria for use of CT at our institution include loss of consciousness, palpable depressed skull fracture, persistent vomiting, altered mental status, focal neurologic abnormality, progressive headache, or severe facial fracture. Children with normal CT scan findings

Table 22–12 Cranial CT findings in children with blunt trauma

Type of abnormality	(n = 500) Number of children
Skull fractures	126 (25%)
Linear	96 (19%)
Depressed	30 (6%)
Nonfracture abnormalities	115 (23%)*
Cerebral contusion	59 (12%)
Subarachnoid hemorrhage	40 (8%)
Cerebral edema	40 (8%)
Subdural hematoma	37 (7%)
Intraparenchymal hemorrhage	28 (6%)
Intraventricular hemorrhage	16 (3%)
Epidural hematoma	5 (1%)

*Some children had more than one nonfracture abnormality.

still may have significant intracranial injury.[58] If a child's neurologic status does not correlate with CT findings, an MRI provides additional diagnostic information.[26,122]

Cranial injury. Cranial injuries secondary to trauma may be focal or diffuse (Table 22-12). Focal injury includes epidural hematoma, subdural hematoma, intracranial hematoma, and parenchymal contusion. Diffuse injury can be the result of high-velocity torque which causes axonal shear.[25,26,123]

CT rapidly and reliably demonstrates most subdural, epidural, and intraparenchymal hemorrhage.[21,52,78,120] Acute subdural hematoma appears as a crescent-shaped region of high density, separating the brain from the inner table of the skull and falx (Figs. 22-33 and 22-34). The bleeding results from the rupture of subdural veins that bleed between the arachnoid and pia. Although a large subdural hematoma is readily identified on CT, small subdural collections extending beneath the temporal lobe and convexity and bilateral subdural hematomas are difficult to recognize. Over time, as blood products break down, subdural hemorrhage becomes isodense. Flat sulci and ventricular compression are useful clues in the identification of these collections. Accuracy of diagnosis improves with intravenous contrast enhancement.

Epidural hematoma is most often attributable to arterial bleeding into the epidural space displacing

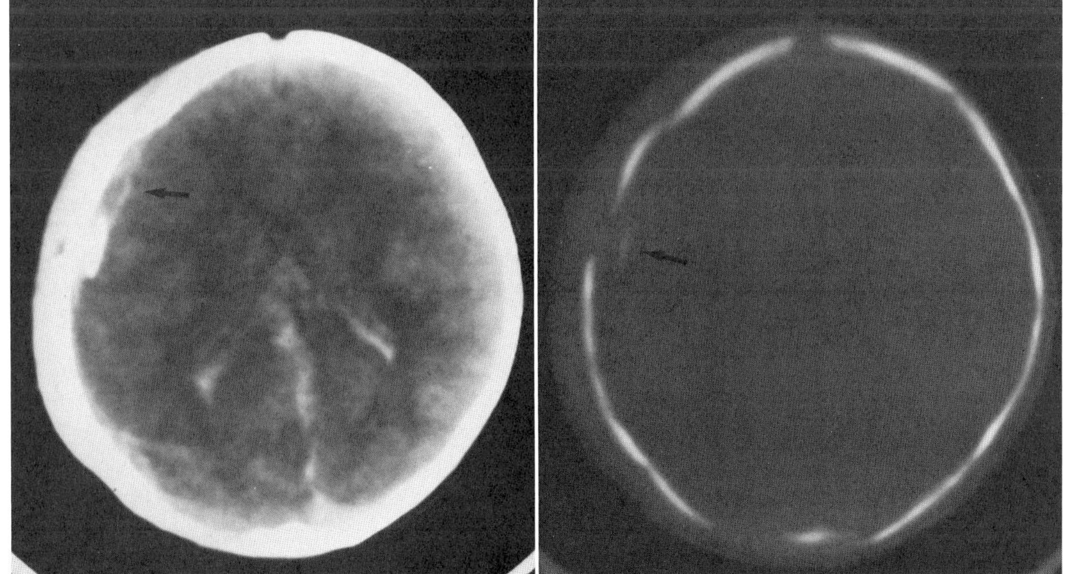

Figure 22–33 A, Six-month-old injured in motor vehicle accident. Soft tissue windows demonstrate subarachnoid hemorrhage, intraventricular hemorrhage, and a right temporal subdural hematoma *(arrow).* **B,** Bone windows demonstrate a depressed fracture fragment at the level of the subdural hematoma *(arrow).*

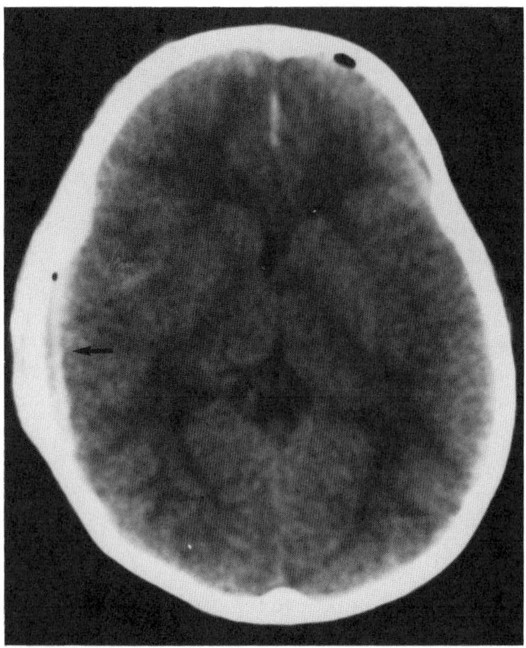

Figure 22–34 CT scan demonstrates a crescent-shaped collection of blood consistent with a subdural hematoma *(arrow)*. Pneumocephalus and subarachnoid hemorrhage within the interhemispheric fissure are present as well.

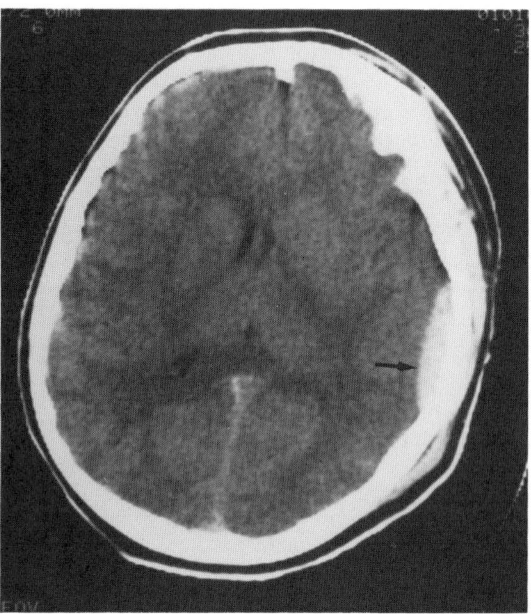

Figure 22–35 Extraaxial convex collection of blood, consistent with an epidural hematoma *(arrow)*.

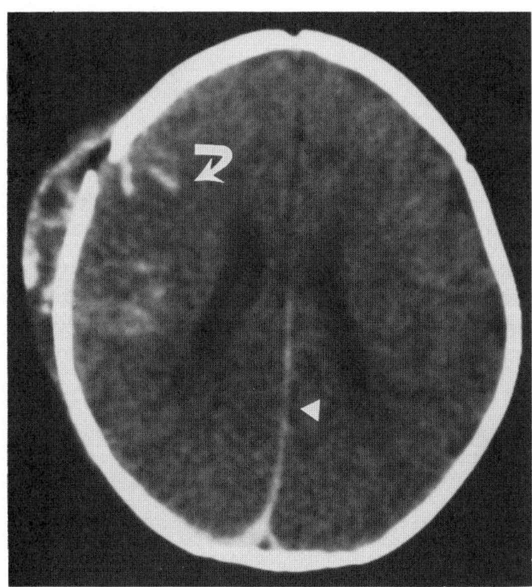

Figure 22–36 Large right intracerebral contusion interspersed with small areas of hemorrhage *(arrow)*. Adjacent fracture through the right frontal suture and scalp hematoma are consistent with a coup injury. Subarachnoid blood is also present along the falx *(arrowhead)*.

the brain parenchyma. Dura, which is bound down at the cranial sutures, defines the margins of the epidural collection, producing an inward convexity (Fig. 22-35). This hemorrhage is often associated with a temporal fracture that disrupts the middle meningeal artery. The epidural hematoma is frequently accompanied by mass effect, which causes transincisural herniation. These findings are well demonstrated by CT and require immediate surgery.[121]

Intracerebral contusion or hematoma results from coup and contracoup injury to small parenchymal vessels. In CT these lesions appear as mottled regions with mass affect. In parenchymal contusions, small areas of hemorrhage intersperse within regions of edema and necrosis, resulting in a "salt and pepper" appearance (Fig. 22-36). Larger collections of clotted blood, termed *hematoma,* appear as regions of high attenuation with adjacent hypodensity secondary to edema (Fig. 22-37). The most frequent site of injury is the frontal lobe; temporal and occipital regions are frequent sites for contracoup injury.[52] Small superficial contusions that lie adjacent to high-density bone are difficult to identify. Wider window settings are effective in separating bone from blood, and coronal images help demonstrate parietal and temporal lobe

contusions. Brainstem injury is especially difficult to visualize owing to the presence of beam-hardening artifacts.[125]

Large subarachnoid hemorrhage appears as a high-density collection conforming to the sub-

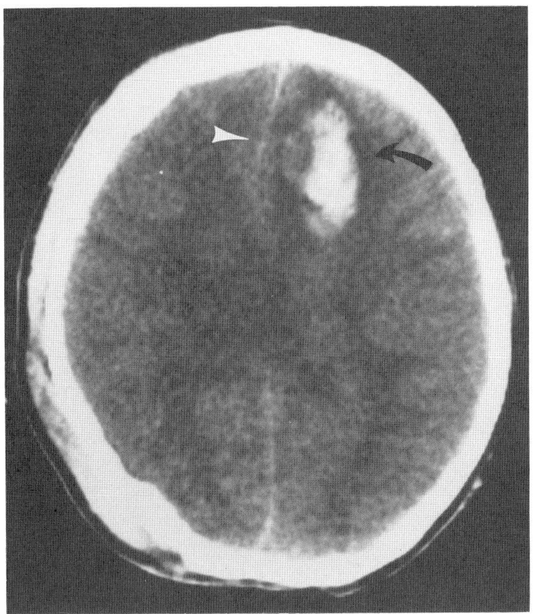

Figure 22–37 Two-year-old injured in a motor vehicle crash. CT scan demonstrates a left frontal lobe parenchymal hematoma with surrounding edema *(black arrow)*. Mass affect is present with shift of the interhemispheric fissure to the right *(arrowhead)*.

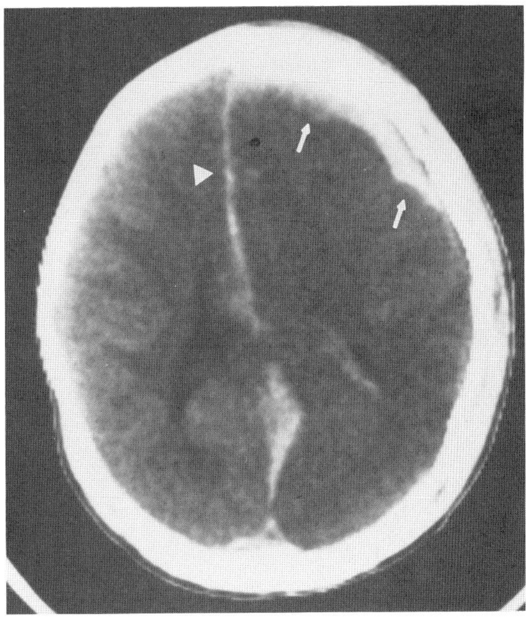

Figure 22–38 A subdural hematoma along the left frontal convexity *(arrows)* with adjacent edema is compressing the left lateral ventricle. The interhemispheric fissure, which is filled with subarachnoid blood *(arrowhead)*, is shifted to the right owing to mass affect.

arachnoid space, a result of leptomeningeal vessel rupture. CT misses up to 10% of subarachnoid hemorrhage as a result of partial volume averaging. Small amounts of subarachnoid blood localize in the interhemispheric region and are difficult to differentiate from normal falx. If there is extension of interhemispheric hyperdensity to the rostrum of the corpus collosum, and hyperdensity is noted to conform to gyri, subarachnoid hemorrhage is present (Fig. 22-38).[76,128]

Diffuse cranial injury is the result of severe rotational force causing axons to tear and shear.[2,123] Axonal injuries occur most commonly at interfaces between grey and white matter, the corpus collosum, basal ganglia, cerebellar peduncles, and the brainstem. Although these injuries may be accompanied by hemorrhage, a large percentage are not well demonstrated by CT because of its low contrast resolution.[123] Unfortunately, these lesions result in severe brain dysfunction, often with a poor neurologic outcome.[58]

Following trauma, hypoxia to the brain occurs for an indeterminant period. Initially, cerebral swelling is a consequence of cerebral hyperemia and increased blood volume[10]; diffuse or focal edema follows. Focal edema often corresponds to a vascular distribution and results in mass affect, compressing ventricles and shifting of midline structures (Fig. 22-39). Regions especially sensi-

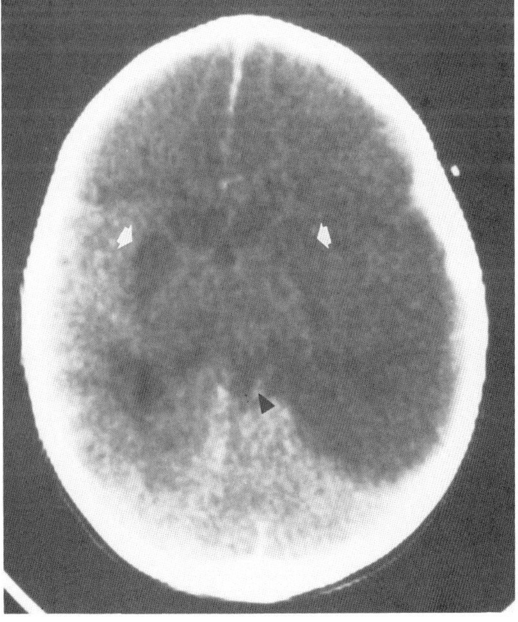

Figure 22–39 One-year-old victim of abuse. CT scan demonstrates edema of the left cerebral hemisphere and right frontal lobe with shift of the interhemispheric fissure to the right. The basal ganglia *(white arrows)* are usually low in attenuation. The cisterns are compressed *(arrowhead)*, consistent with uncal herniation.

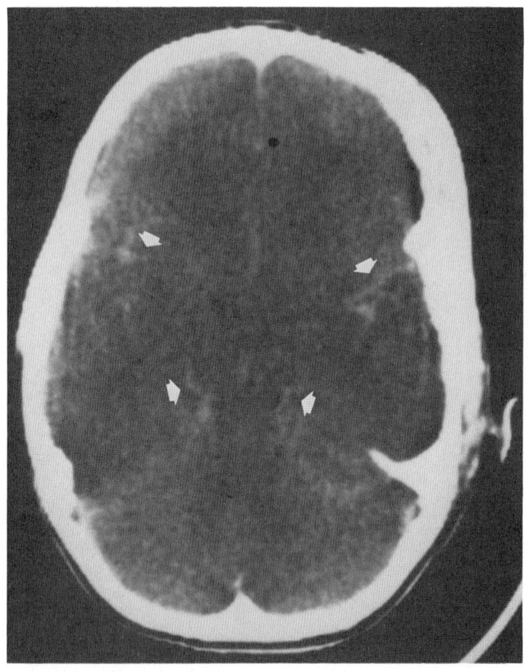

Figure 22–40 Seven-year-old struck by car who was in shock on admission. Cranial CT demonstrates diffuse cerebral edema with compression of ventricles and cisterns. Subarachnoid blood is present within the sylvian fissures and cisterns *(arrowheads)*.

tive to diffuse hypoxia include the basal ganglia and cerebral cortex. Loss of gray-white matter differentiation, effacement of cisterns and sulci, and focal decreased attenuation of the basal ganglia are CT signs of hypoxic injury (Fig. 22-40).[51,108,124] The white matter of the thalamus, brainstem, and cerebellum may be spared with relative high attenuation of these regions as compared with the surrounding brain; this is the "reversal sign" that suggests severe diffuse edema (Fig. 22-41).[39] Although the CT findings of edema are useful in the evaluation of the injured child, a normal CT scan is possible in children with severe neurologic damage and markedly elevated intracranial pressure.[43,106,112]

Spinal injury. CT has an important role in the evaluation of vertebral trauma. Initial plain films miss up to 25% of fractures. Nondisplaced pedicle, and lateral mass fractures are best seen by CT. In addition, CT can reveal the presence of bone fragments and foreign bodies in the spinal canal.[1,9,70]

Scans of the spine with CT require thin sections and the use of a high-resolution algorithm for bone detail. Standard 10-mm sections used for abdominal CT may miss significant fractures or subluxations. Coronal and three-dimensional reconstruction of the radiographic image improves the demonstration of complex fractures. Compression fractures may be missed in the axial plane. Three-

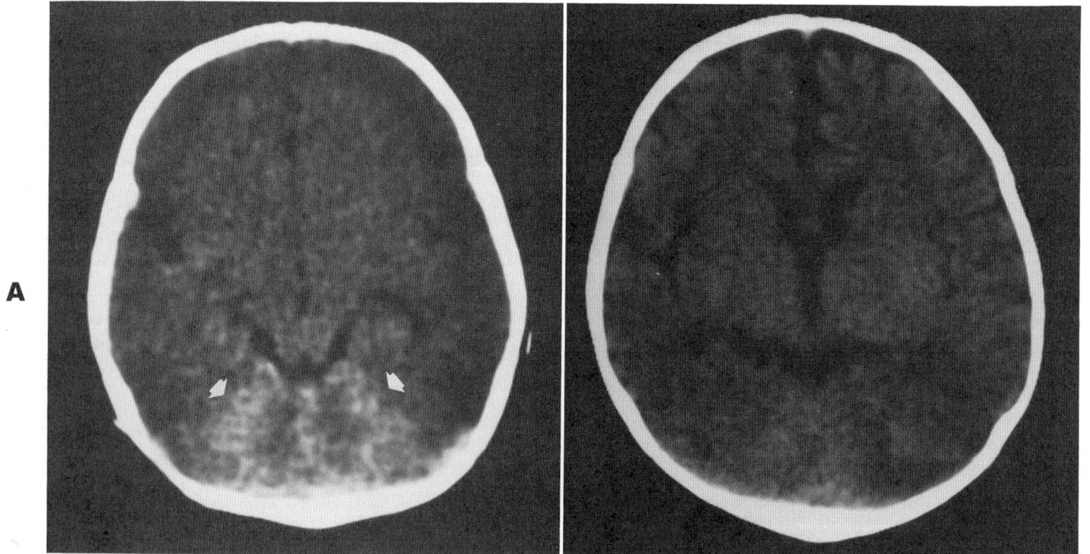

A **B**

Figure 22–41 One-month-old victim of abuse. **A,** CT demonstrates low attenuation of the cerebral cortex with high attenuation of the cerebellum *(white arrows)*. Termed the *reversal sign,* the finding suggests diffuse edema with sparing of the cerebellum. **B,** Follow-up 3 weeks later demonstrates diffuse cerebral atrophy.

dimensional reconstruction identifies up to 30% of spinal fractures missed on two-dimensional displays and is a useful technique in evaluation of children with spinal trauma.[113,129]

Prior to the advent of MRI, CT myelography was used to identify spinal cord trauma. Currently, its use is limited to patients for whom MRI is technically not feasible or unsuccessful (Fig. 22-42). Myelography remains the definitive examination for the diagnosis of a dural tear and the evaluation of bone fragments within the spinal canal (Fig. 22-43).[33,70]

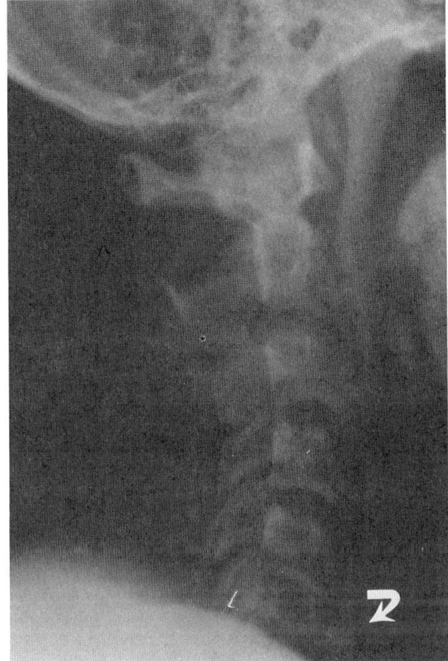
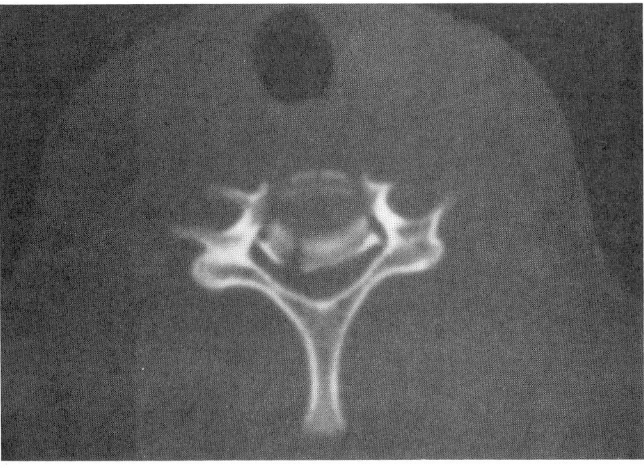

Figure 22–42 Sixteen-year-old paraplegic status following diving accident. **A,** Lateral cervical spine demonstrates compression fracture of C6 *(arrow)*. **B,** CT demonstrates fracture fragments within the spinal canal.

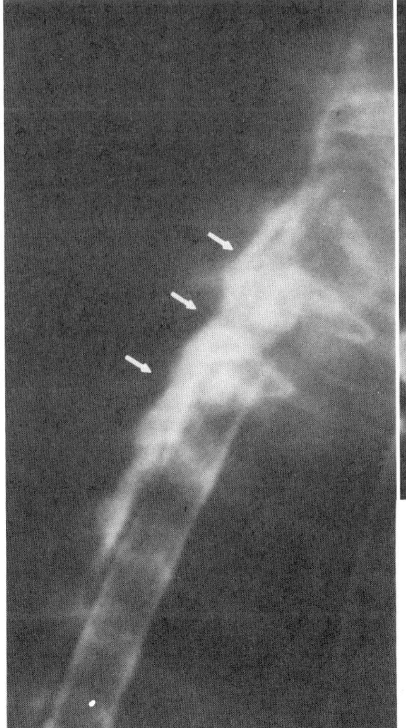
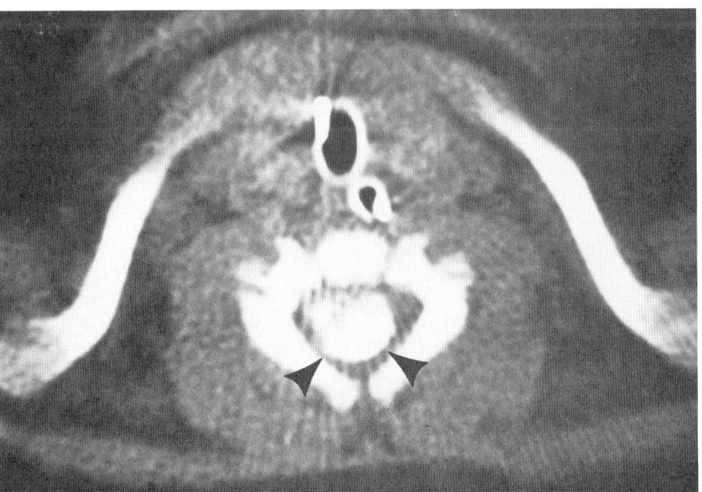

Figure 22–43 One-month-old injured in a motor vehicle crash. **A,** Myelogram demonstrates leakage of contrast, consistent with a dural tear at the T1 level *(arrows)*. **B,** CT following myelogram demonstrates a tear within the upper thoracic spinal cord with contrast filling the spinal canal.

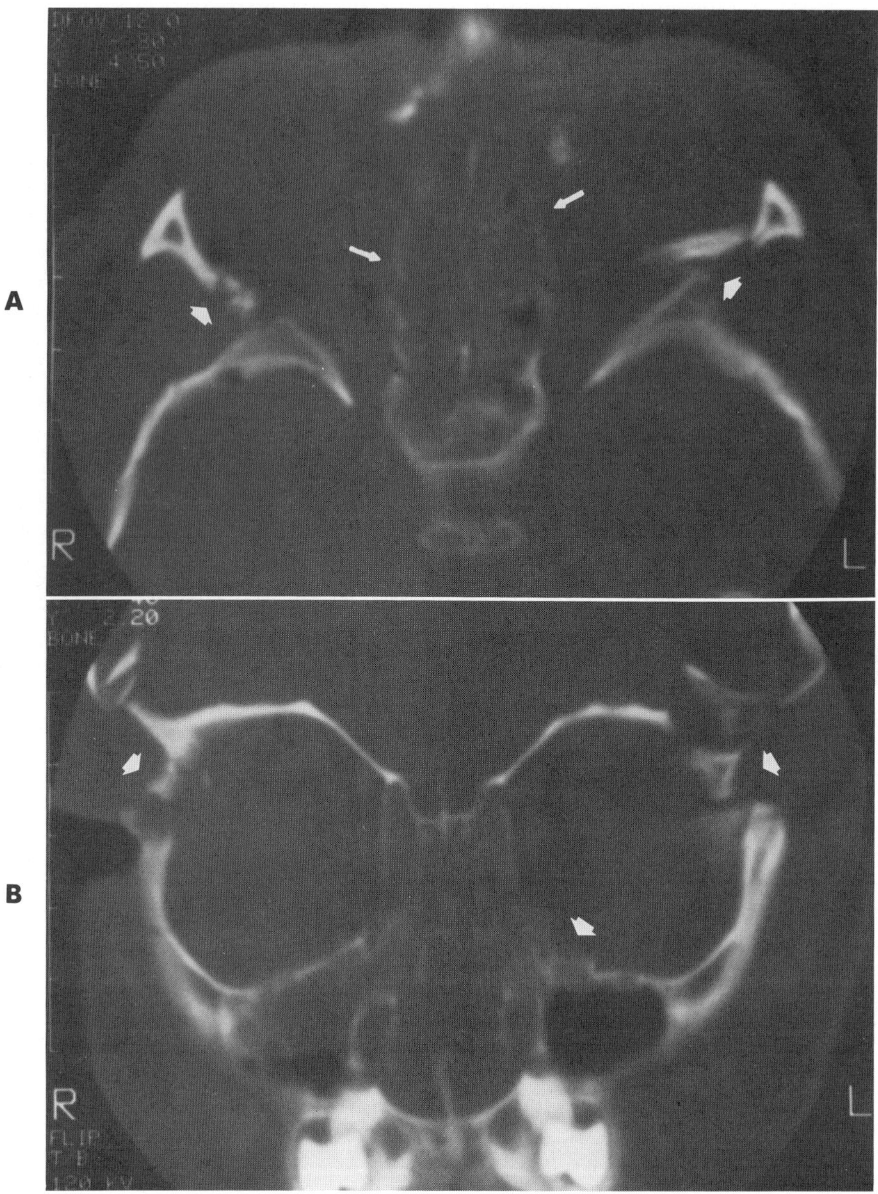

Figure 22–44 Axial **(A)** and coronal **(B)** images of the face demonstrate multiple orbital and ethmoid fractures *(arrows)*. The ethmoid and right maxillary sinuses are filled with blood.

Facial injury. CT is extremely useful in the evaluation of complex facial fractures and associated soft tissue abnormalities.[38] Muscle entrapment, loose bone fragments, and globe damage is evident through CT scan. Complicated facial fractures require coronal images for three-dimensional evaluation (Fig. 22-44).[30] In such cases, the child's head must be placed vertically, often requiring additional time and sedation. If the child's condition is unstable, this additional view must be delayed until it stabilizes.

Magnetic resonance imaging

Magnetic resonance imaging (MRI) is a new modality in the evaluation of acute head and spine trauma. Magnetic resonance images are formed by a strong magnet used in conjunction with a radiofrequency transmitter. Images are formed through the interaction of magnetic fields and radiofrequency pulses with protons of tissue water within the child. Cross-sectional planes can be viewed in almost any orientation without the patient being moved.

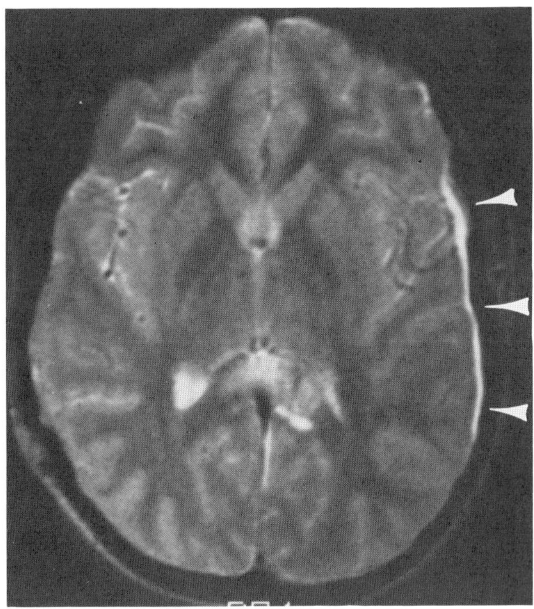

Figure 22–45 Thirteen-year-old child with a left temporal bone fracture. T2 weighted MR image demonstrates a high signal extraaxial collection *(arrowheads)* consistent with a left temporal subdural hematoma.

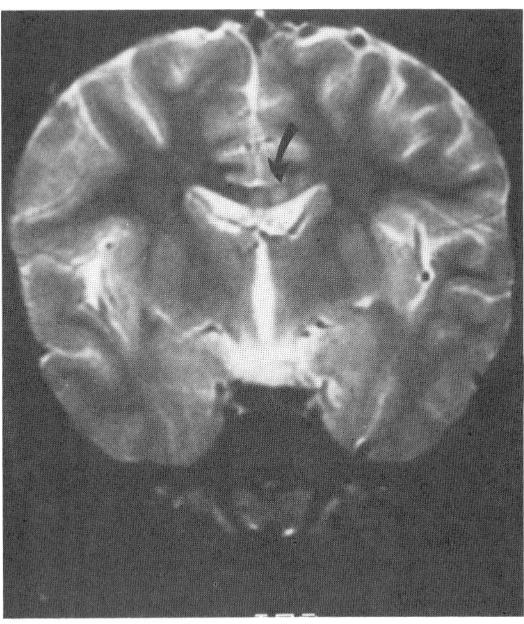

Figure 22–46 Five-year-old injured in a motor vehicle crash. Initial CT scans were normal. Coronal T2 weighted image demonstrates bright signal lesions in the corpus callosum *(arrow)*, consistent with shearing injury.

In the past, the use of MRI in evaluation of a child with an acute condition was limited. Ferromagnetic materials could not be placed in the scanner room, thus preventing examination of children on life support equipment. The availability of MRI-compatible life support systems now allows for these children to be studied.[63] Several problems remain however. Sedation is generally required because of prolonged acquisition periods. MRI proton imaging does not detect signals from bone, making it difficult to evaluate for bone fragments and depressed fractures. The high cost and limited number of scanners available restrict its use as a screening examination in acute trauma.

MRI offers several advantages in the evaluation of the injured child. Because of the unique signal characteristics of blood and the capability of MRI to image the brain in multiple planes, MRI is superior to CT in detecting subdural, epidural, and parenchymal hemorrhage.[29,35,126] Small superficial hemorrhagic contusions often missed on CT appear clearly in MRI. MRI is more sensitive in identifying small subdural hematomas, particularly when they are located beneath the temporal and parietal lobes (Fig. 22-45).[126] Subacute and chronic subdural hematomas that are isodense in CT remain high in signal intensity in MRI.[122]

Diffuse axonal injuries often missed in CT are clearly demonstrated in MRI (Fig. 22-46). This is attributable to the high water content at sites of axonal disruption. Hemorrhage need not be present for the demonstration of these injuries.[28]

MRI is superior to CT in the detection of brainstem injuries[27]; the beam-hardening artifact that interferes with CT images is absent. Demonstration of hematoma and contusion is easy because of their unique signal characteristics and the ability to examine the brain in sagittal and coronal planes.

MRI is the best modality for assessing spinal soft tissue damage. Contusion, intramedullary hemorrhage, and spine transection are clearly evident on MRI.* The finding of acute hemorrhage within the cord indicates a poor neurologic outcome, as compared with hemorrhages whose signal intensity indicates only edema (Fig. 22-47).[14,24,37,54] Epidural hematoma and disc herniation are also easily detected. MRI is useful in the evaluation of hyperextension injury of the cervical spine, because identification of ligamentous disruption is possible.[32] Major vascular injuries that accompany spine trauma are also evident on MRI.

---

*References 24, 32, 33, 47, 64, and 107.

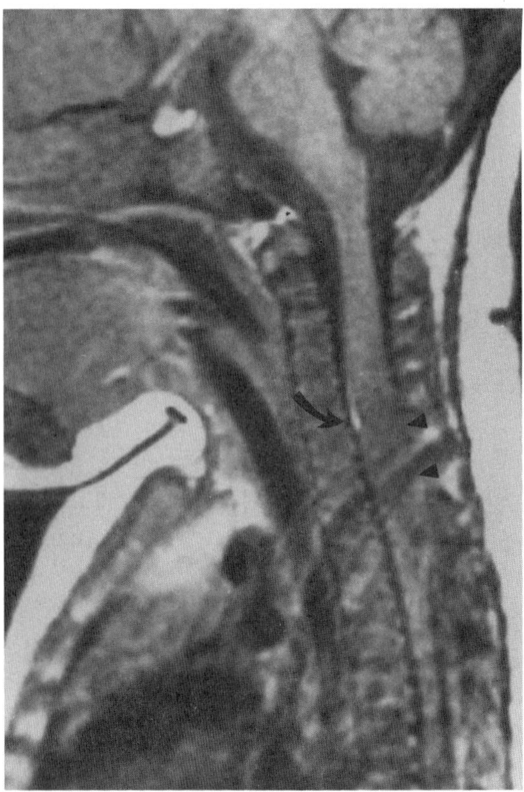

Figure 22–47 One-month-old status following motor vehicle crash. Sagittal T1 weighted image of the cervical thoracic spine demonstrates a region of low signal intensity consistent with edema *(arrowheads)*. An adjacent small region of high signal represents blood. Infant remains paraplegic.

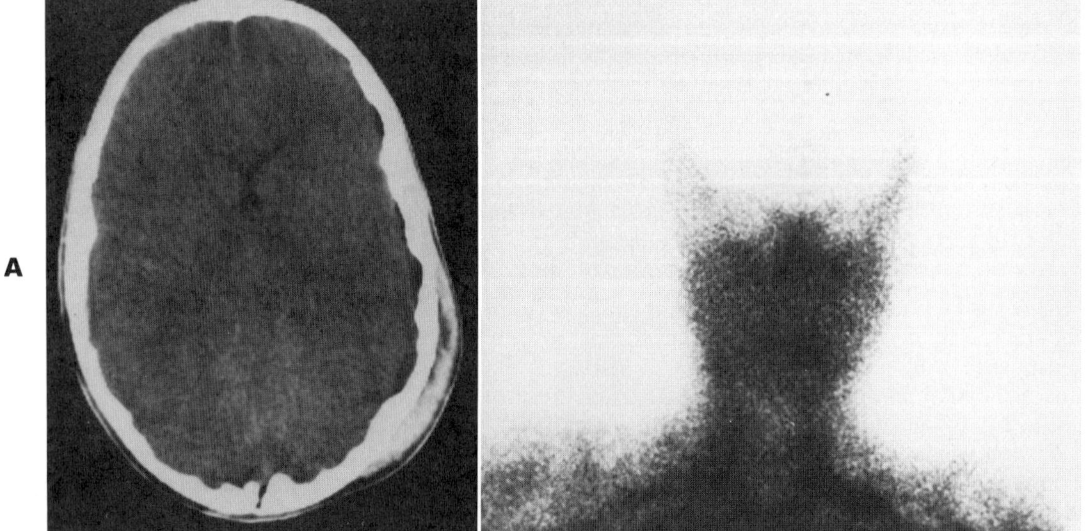

Figure 22–48 Twelve-year-old injured in a motor vehicle crash. **A,** CT demonstrates diffuse edema with loss of grey and white matter differentiation. **B,** Technetium 99 m pertechnetate scan demonstrates no cerebral blood flow. Findings are consistent with brain death.

MRI has several limitations in the evaluation of intracranial injury. Cortical bone, which contains little hydrogen, is not visible in MRI. Thus, depressed bone fractures and fragments are difficult to identify. Subarachnoid hemorrhage is also poorly shown in MRI. Other disadvantages, including high cost and prolonged scanning time, limit its use in the acute evaluation of cranial trauma. Presently, MRI is most useful when a child's status does not correlate with CT findings, and is usually reserved for follow-up evaluation of the trauma patient.

Radionuclide imaging

Radionuclide brain scanning enhances the evaluation of brain death in severely injured children. A radiopharmaceutical, most commonly technicium 99 m sodium pertechnetate, is injected intravenously. Immediate and delayed images of the brain are obtained. Virtually no cerebral radioactivity will be present in cases of brain death (Fig. 22-48).[5,53,72]

Cerebral angiography

Arteriography following trauma is limited to the evaluation of vascular injury such as dissection, rupture, pseudoaneurysm, or fistula.[19] The examination is invasive, time-consuming, and requires sedation of the child. The technique requires placement of a catheter into the femoral artery and then advancing it to the region of injury. Contrast material is injected and multiple films are obtained. Radiation exposure is high, and there is the additional risk of reaction to intravenous contrast material.

Intentional injury

Both CT and MRI are essential in the evaluation of children with head trauma resulting from intentional injury.[15,91,109,127] Child abuse often involves the child's being shaken, which causes shearing of the parenchyma, rupturing of the bridging veins, and consequently, the formation of subdural hematoma. Computed tomography is most effective in identifying subarachnoid hemorrhage and skull fracture (Fig. 22-49).[6,87] MRI, however, is superior in demonstrating white matter injury, as well as subdural collections.[3,6,87] Because the signal characteristics change with time, MRI can estimate the age of a subdural collection (Fig. 22-50). The finding of several lesions of varying ages may provide proof that the child has been repeatedly injured.

Follow-up imaging

Many children with severe head injury evidence no abnormality upon initial examination.[57,58,66,80] In-

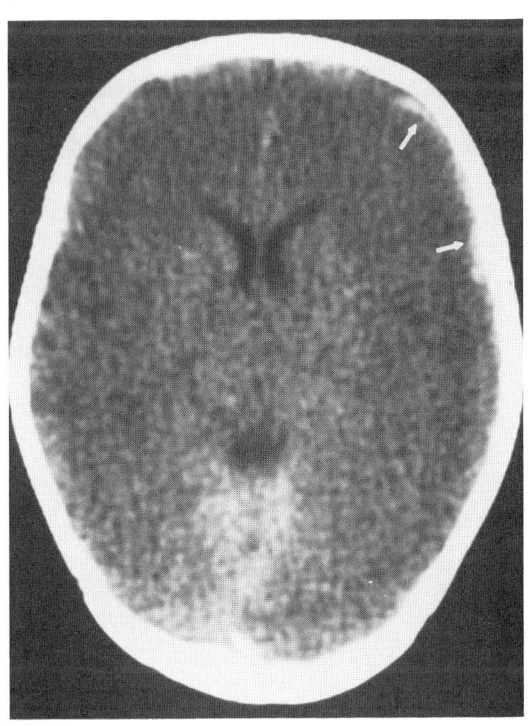

Figure 22–49 Seven-month-old victim of abuse. CT demonstrates homogeneous low attenuation of the cerebrum consistent with cerebral edema. A thin layer of subarachnoid blood is present along the left frontal lobe *(arrows)*.

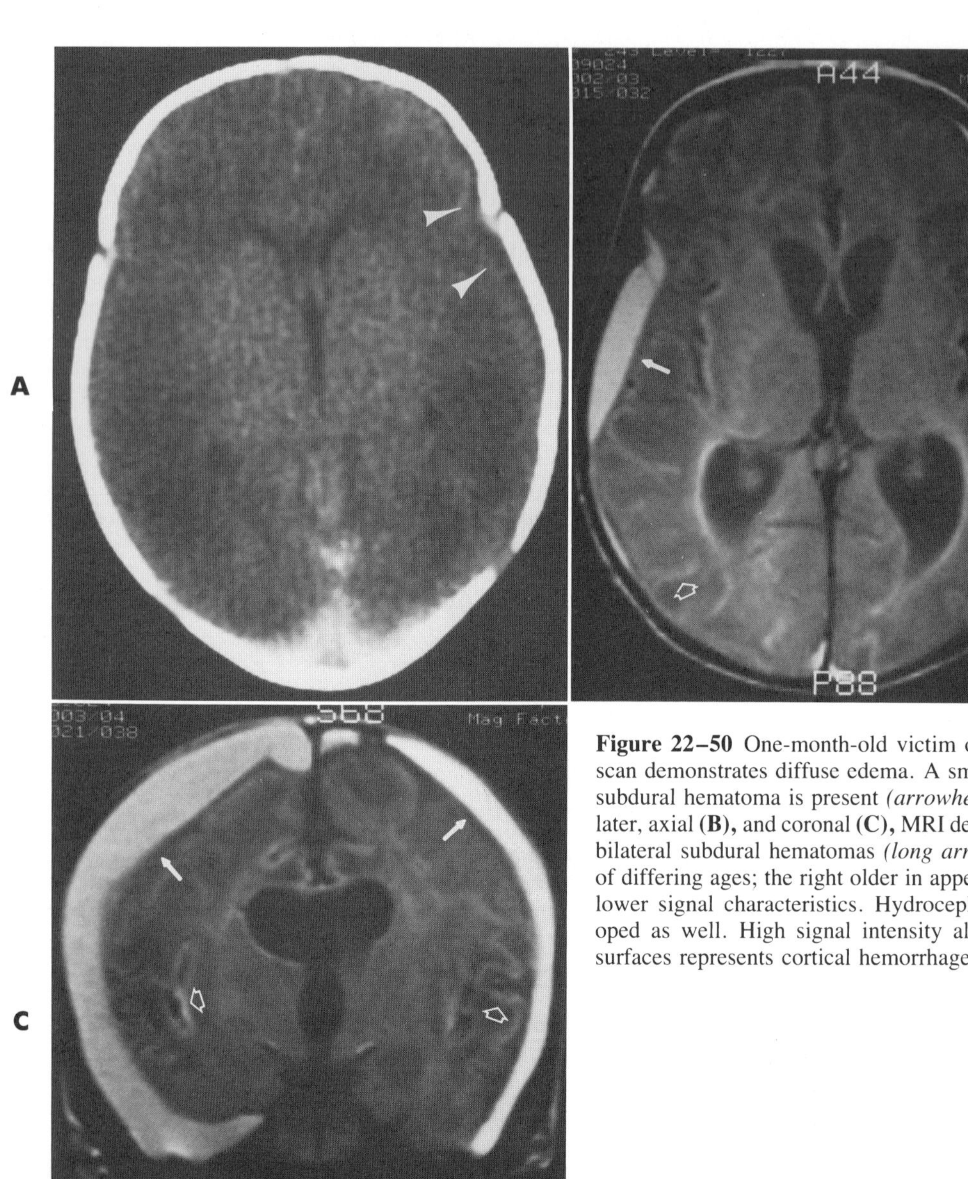

Figure 22–50 One-month-old victim of abuse. **A,** CT scan demonstrates diffuse edema. A small left isodense subdural hematoma is present *(arrowheads)*. One week later, axial **(B),** and coronal **(C),** MRI demonstrates large bilateral subdural hematomas *(long arrows)*. These are of differing ages; the right older in appearance owing to lower signal characteristics. Hydrocephalus has developed as well. High signal intensity along the cortical surfaces represents cortical hemorrhage *(short arrows)*.

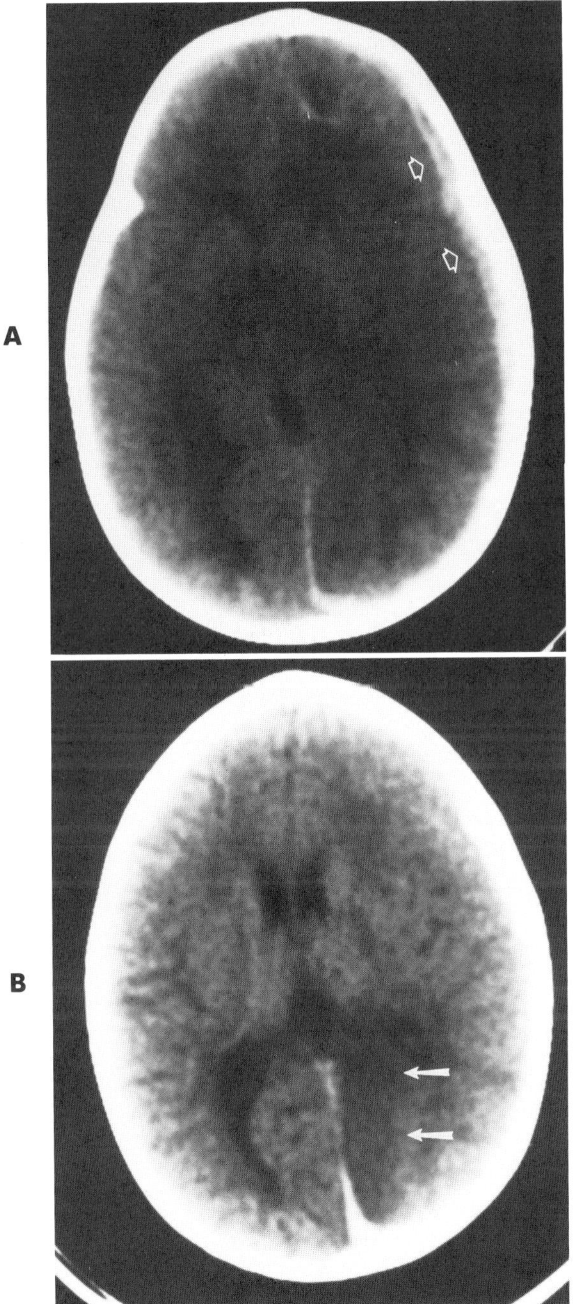

Figure 22–51 Posttraumatic infarct. **A,** Sixteen-month-old child with left subdural hematoma *(arrows)* following trauma. There is mass effect with shift of midline structures to the right. **B,** At follow-up 10 days later a low attenuation area is present in the distribution of the left posterior cerebral artery *(arrows)*, indicative of an infarct.

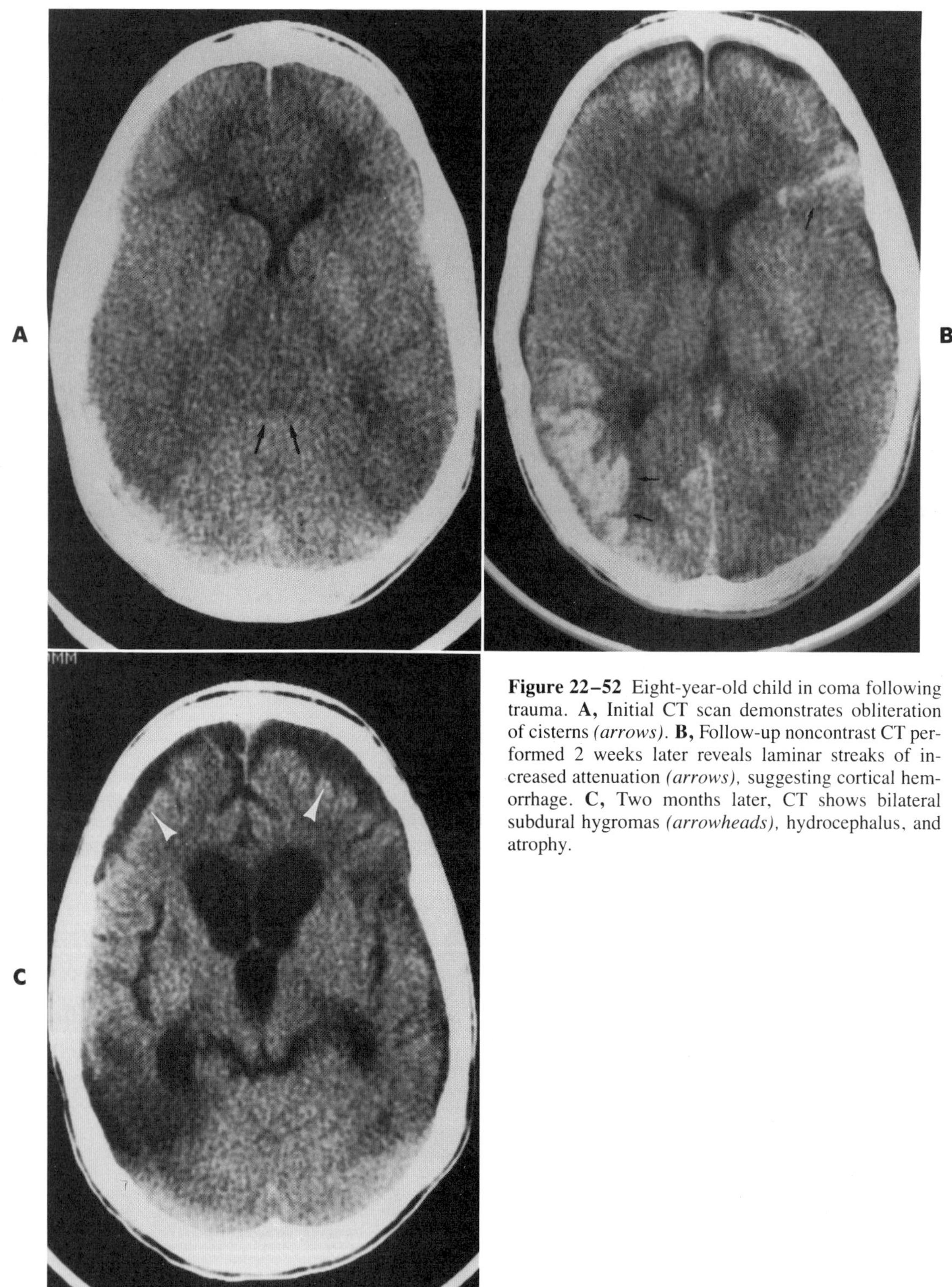

Figure 22–52 Eight-year-old child in coma following trauma. **A,** Initial CT scan demonstrates obliteration of cisterns *(arrows)*. **B,** Follow-up noncontrast CT performed 2 weeks later reveals laminar streaks of increased attenuation *(arrows)*, suggesting cortical hemorrhage. **C,** Two months later, CT shows bilateral subdural hygromas *(arrowheads)*, hydrocephalus, and atrophy.

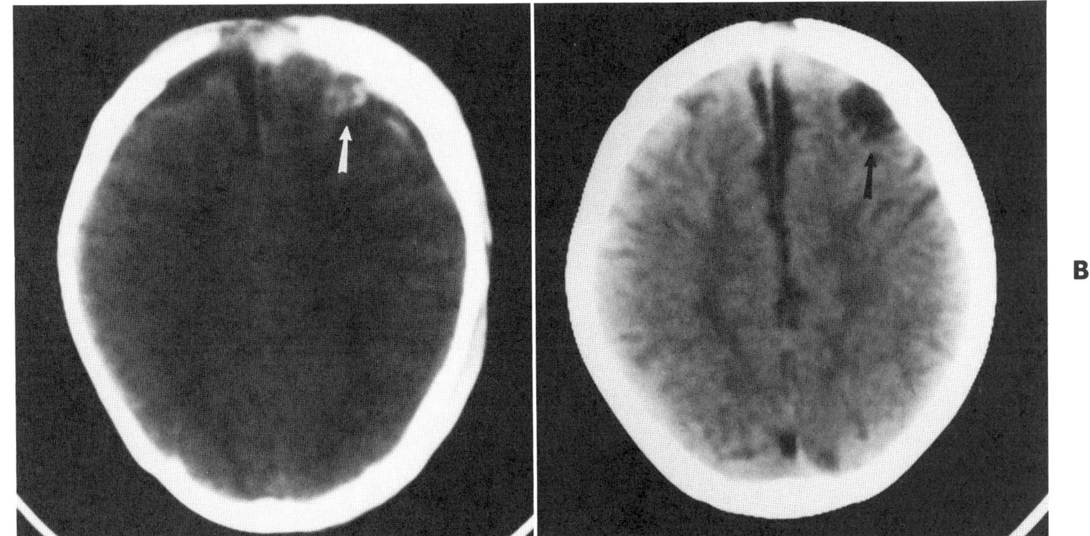

Figure 22–53 Three-month-old child injured in a motor vehicle crash. **A,** Left frontal hemorrhagic contusion *(arrow)* with adjacent subarachnoid blood is present. **B,** Follow-up CT 4 months later demonstrates a focal region of encephalomalacia *(arrow)*.

farction, hematoma, intraventricular hemorrhage and hydrocephalus may be first noted in follow-up examination (Fig. 22-51). Clinical neurologic deterioration following admission is an indication for urgent repeat CT scanning. For children with residual neurologic impairment, MRI is the imaging modality of choice. MRI is superior to CT in identifying subacute and chronic lesions.[59,71,122]

Follow-up imaging studies of children with intraparenchymal injury demonstrate encephalomalacia, or loss of brain tissue (Figs. 22-52 and 22-53). If tissue loss is severe, porencephaly results, with cystic cavities communicating with the ventricles or subarachnoid space. There is a high incidence of permanent disability in injured children with cerebral atrophy 6 months following the initial insult.[58]

CONCLUSIONS

The choice of imaging modality following brain or spinal cord injury depends on the clinical setting. In the acute phase, when the child is unstable and cooperation is limited, CT is the examination of choice for rapid identification of possible life-threatening intracranial lesions. If a spinal injury is suspected, however, MRI is the study of choice. MRI has also become the modality of choice in subacute and chronic follow-up evaluation of intracranial injury.

REFERENCES

1. Acheson M, Livingston R, Richardson M et al: High-resolution CT scanning evaluation of cervical spine fractures: comparison with plain film examinations, *AJR* 148:1179-1185, 1987.
2. Adams JH, Graham DI, Murray LS et al: Diffuse axonal injury due to nonmissile head injury in humans: an analysis of 45 cases, *Ann Neurol* 12:557-563, 1982.
3. Alexander RC, Schor DP, Smith WL: Magnetic resonance imaging of intracranial injuries from child abuse, *J Pediatr* 109:975-979, 1986.
4. Anderson MJ, Schutt AH: Spinal injury in children: a review of 156 cases seen from 1950 through 1978, *Mayo Clin Proc* 55:499-504, 1980.
5. Ashwal S, Smith AJK, Torres F et al: Radionuclide bolus angiography: a technique for verification of brain death in infants and children, *J Pediatr* 91:722, 1977.
6. Ball WS: Nonaccidental craniocerebral trauma (child abuse): MR imaging, *Radiology* 173:609-610.
7. Berland LL, Van Dyke JA: Decreased splenic enhancement of CT in traumatized hypotensive patients, *Radiology* 156:469-471, 1985.
8. Bond SJ, Gotschall CS, Eichelberger MR: Predictors of abdominal injury in children with pelvic fracture, *J Trauma* (in press).
9. Brant-Zawadski M, Miller EM, Federle MP: CT in the evaluation of spine trauma, *AJR* 136:369, 1981.
10. Bruce DA, Alavi A, Bilaniuk L et al: Diffuse cerebral swelling following head injuries in children: the syndrome of malignant brain edema, *J Neurosurg* 54:170-174, 1981.
11. Bulas DI, Taylor GA, Eichelberger MR: The value of CT in detecting bowel perforation in children after blunt abdominal trauma, *AJR* 153:561-564, 1989.
12. Cass A, Ireland G: Bladder trauma associated with pelvic fractures in severely injured patients, *J Trauma* 13:205, 1973.

13. Cattell HS, Filtzer DL: Pseudosubluxation and other normal variations in the cervical spine in children, *J Bone Joint Surg Am* 47:1295-1309, 1965.

14. Chakeres DS, Flickinger F, Bresnahan JC et al: MR imaging of acute spinal cord trauma, *AJNR* 8:5-10, 1987.

15. Cohen RA, Kaufman RA, Myers PA et al: Cranial CT in the abused child with head injury, *AJR* 146:97-102, 1986.

16. Cook DE, Walsh JW, Vick CW et al: Upper abdominal trauma: pitfalls in CT diagnosis, *Radiology* 159:65-69, 1986.

17. Corriere JN Jr, Harris JD: The management of urologic injuries in blunt pelvic trauma, *Radiol Clin N Am* 19:187, 1981.

18. Cywes S, Rode J, Millar AJW: Blunt liver trauma in children: nonoperative management, *J Pediatr Surg* 20:14-18, 1985.

19. Davis JM, Zimmerman RA: Injury of the carotid and vertebral arteries, *Neuroradiol* 25:55-69, 1983.

20. DeSmet AA, Fryback DG, Thornbury JR: A second look at the utility of radiographic skull examination for trauma, *AJR* 132:95-97, 1979.

21. de Villansante JM, Taveras JM: CT in acute head trauma, *AJR* 126:765-768, 1976.

22. Federle MP: CT of upper abdominal trauma. *Semin Roentgenol* 19:269-279, 1984.

23. Fesmire FM, Luten RC: The pediatric cervical spine: developmental anatomy and clinical aspect, *J Emerg Med* 7(2):133-142, 1989.

24. Flanders AE, Schaefre DM, Doan HT et al: Acute cervical spine trauma: correlation of MR imaging findings with degree of neurologic deficit, *Radiology* 177:25-33, 1990.

25. Gennarelli TA, Thibault LE, Adams JH et al: Diffuse axonal injury and traumatic coma in the primate, *Ann Neurol* 12:564-574, 1982.

26. Gentry LR, Godersky JC, Thompson BH: MR imaging of head trauma: review of the distribution and radiopathologic features of traumatic lesions, *AJNR* 9:101, 1988.

27. Gentry LR, Godersky JC, Thompson BH: Traumatic brain stem injury; MR imaging, *Radiology* 171:177-187, 1989.

28. Gentry LR, Thompson B, Godersky JC: Trauma to the corpus callosum: MR features, *AJNR* 9:1129-1138, 1988.

29. Gentry LR, Godersky JC, Thompson BH et al: Prospective comparative study of intermediate-field MR and CT in the evaluation of closed head trauma, *AJR* 150:673-682, 1988.

30. Gillespie JE, Isherwood I, Balu GR et al: 3-D reformations of CT in the assessment of fascial trauma, *Clin Radiol* 38:523, 1987.

31. Glancy KE: Review of pancreatic trauma, *West J Med* 151:45-51, 1989.

32. Goldberg AL, Daffner RH, Schapiro RL: Imaging of acute spinal trauma: an evolving multi-modality approach, *Clinical Imaging* 14:11-16, 1990.

33. Goldberg AL, Rothfus WE, Deeb ZL et al: The impact of magnetic resonance on the diagnostic evaluation of acute cervicothoracic spinal trauma, *Skeletal Radiol* 17:89-95, 1988.

34. Reference deleted in proof.

35. Gomori JM, Grossman HI, Goldberg HI et al: High field magnetic resonance imaging of intracranial hematomas, *Radiology* 157:87-93, 1985.

36. Greene R: Lung alterations in thoracic trauma, *J Thorac Imaging* 2:1-11, 1987.

37. Hackney DB, Asato R, Joseph PM et al: Hemorrhage and edema in acute spinal cord compression: demonstration by MR imaging, *Radiology* 161:387-390, 1986.

38. Halimi P, Doyan D, Bekal F et al: Contribution of CT to the radiologic study of craniofacial injuries, *J Neuroradiol* 13:253, 1986.

39. Han BK, Towbin RB, De Courten-Myers G et al: Reversal sign on CT: effect of anoxic/ischemic cerebral injury in children, *AJR* 154:361-368, 1990.

40. Harbedo JE, Nilsson B: Hemodynamic changes in brain caused by local infusion of hyperosmolar solutions in particular relation to blood-brain barrier opening, *Brain Res* 181:45-49, 1980.

41. Harris JH, Edeiken-Monroe B: The radiology of acute cervical spine trauma, Baltimore, 1978, Williams & Wilkins, pp 31-34.

42. Hayman LA, Evans RA, Bastion FO et al: Delayed high dose contrast CT: identifying patients at risk of massive hemorrhagic infarction, *AJNR* 2:139-147, 1981.

43. Holliday PO, Kelly DL, Ball M: Normal computed tomograms in acute head injury: correlation of intracranial pressure, ventricular size and outcome. *Neurosurgery* 10:25-28, 1982.

44. Hubbard DD: Injuries of the spine in children and adolescents, *Clin Orthop* 100:56-65, 1974.

45. Reference deleted in proofs.

46. Jeffrey RB, Federle MP, Crass RA: Computed tomography of pancreatic trauma, *Radiology* 147:491-494, 1983.

47. Kalfas I, Wilberger J, Goldberg A et al: Magnetic resonance imaging in acute spinal cord trauma, *Neurosurgery* 23:295-299, 1988.

48. Kane NM, Cronan JJ, Dorfman GS et al: Pediatric abdominal trauma: evaluation by computed tomography, *Pediatrics* 82:11-15, 1988.

49. Karp MP, Cooney DR, Pios GA et al: The non-operative management of pediatric hepatic trauma, *J Pediatr Surg* 18:512-518, 1983.

50. Kaufman R, Towbin R, Babcock DS et al: Upper abdominal trauma in children: imaging evaluation, *AJR* 142:449-460, 1984.

51. Kjos BO, Brant-Zawadski M, Young RG: Early CT findings of global CNS hypoperfusion, *AJNR* 4:1043-1048, 1983.

52. Koo AH, Laroque RL: Evaluation of head trauma by CT, *Radiology* 123:345-350, 1977.

53. Korein J, Maccario M: On the diagnosis of cerebral death: a prospective study on 55 patients to define irreversible coma, *Clin Electroencephal* 2:178, 1971.

54. Kulkarni MV, McArdle CB, Kopanicky D et al: Acute spinal cord injury: MR imaging at 1.5 T, *Radiology* 164:837, 1987.

55. Levin HS, Amparo E, Eisenberg HM et al: Magnetic resonance imaging and computerized tomography in relation to the neurobehavioral sequelae of mild and moderate head injuries (ab), *Radiology* 166:590, 1988.

56. Lewis CA, Castillo M, Hudgins PA: Cervical prevertebral fat stripe: a normal variant simulating prevertebral hemorrhage, *AJR* 155:559-560, 1990.

57. Lipper ML, Kishore PR, Girevendulis AK et al: Delayed intracranial hematoma in patients with severe head injury, *Radiology* 133:645-649, 1979.

58. Lobato RD, Sarabia R, Rivas JJ et al: Normal computerized tomography scans in severe head injury: prognostic and clinical management implications, *J Neurosurg* 65:784, 1986.

59. Mark AS: MRI in evaluation of cerebral trauma, *MRI Decisions* 26, 1989.

60. Masters SJ: Evaluation of head trauma: efficacy of skull films, *AJR* 135:539, 1980.

61. Mauser HW, van Nieuwenhuizen O, Veiga-Pires JA: Is contrast-enhanced CT indicated in acute head injury? *Neuroradiology* 26:31-32, 1984.

62. Mavroudis C, Roon AJ, Baker CC et al: Management of acute cervicothoracic vascular injuries, *J Thorac Cardiovac Surg* 80:342, 1980.

63. McArdle CB, Nicholas DA, Richardson CJ et al: Monitoring of the neonate undergoing MR imaging: technical considerations, *Radiology* 159:223-226, 1986.

64. McArdle CB, Wright JW, Prevost WJ et al: MR imaging of the acutely injured patient with cervical traction, *Radiology* 159:273, 1986.

65. McCort JJ: Caring for the major trauma victim: the role of radiology, *Radiology* 163:1-9, 1987.

66. McMicken DB: Emergency CT head scans in traumatic and atraumatic conditions, *Ann Emerg Med* 15:274-279, 1986.

67. Meyers MA: *Dynamic radiology of the abdomen*, ed 2, New York, 1982, Springer-Verlag, pp 20-104.

68. Mirvis SE, Whitley NO, Gens DR: Blunt splenic trauma in adults: CT based classification and correlation with prognosis and treatment, *Radiology* 171:33-39, 1989.

69. Mirvis SE, Geisler FH, Jelinek JJ et al: Acute cervical spine trauma: evaluation with 1.5 TMR imaging, *Radiology* 166:807-816, 1988.

70. Mirvis SE, Whitley NO, Vainwright JR et al: Blunt hepatic trauma in adults: CT based classification and correlation with prognosis and treatment, *Radiology* 171:27-32, 1989.

71. Mirvis SE, Wolf AL, Numaguchi Y et al: Post traumatic cerebral infarction: diagnosis by CT, *AJR* 154:1293, 1990.

72. Mishkin F: Determination of brain death by radionuclide angiography, *Radiology* 115:135, 1975.

73. Moore EE, Shackford SR, Pachter HL et al: Organ injury scaling: spleen, liver and kidney, *J Trauma* 29:1664-1666, 1989.

74. Newman KD, Bowman LM, Eichelberger MR et al: The lap belt complex: intestinal and lumbar spine injury in children, *J Trauma* 30:1133-1138, 1990.

75. Oldham KT, Gulce KS, Ryckman F et al: Blunt liver injury in childhood: evolution of therapy and current perspective, *Surgery* 10:542-549, 1986.

76. Osborn AG, Anderson RE, Wing SD: The false falx sign, *Radiology* 134:421-425, 1980.

77. Pang D, Wilberger JE Jr: Spinal cord injury without radiographic abnormalities in children, *J Neurosurg* 57:114-129, 1982.

78. Peyster RG, Hoover ED: CT in head trauma, *J Trauma* 22:25-38, 1982.

79. Rachesky I, Boyce WT, Duncan B et al: Clinical prediction of cervical spine injuries in children, *ADJC* 141:199, 1987.

80. Rivara F, Tanaguchi D, Parish RA et al: Poor prediction of positive computed tomographic scans by clinical criteria in symptomatic pediatric head trauma, *Pediatrics* 80:579, 1987.

81. Rizzo MJ, Federle MP, Griffith BG: Bowel and mesenteric injury following blunt abdominal trauma: evaluation with CT, *Radiology* 173:143-148, 1989.

82. Rose SC, Moore EE: Emergency trauma angiography: accuracy, safety, and pitfalls, *AJR* 148:1243, 1987.

83. Rose SC, Moore EE: Angiography in patients with arterial trauma: correlation between angiographic abnormalities, operative findings, and clinical outcome, *AJR* 149:613, 1987.

84. Sandler CM, Hall JT, Rodriguez MB et al: Bladder injury in blunt pelvic trauma, *Radiology* 158:633-638, 1986.

85. Sandler CM, Harris JH Jr, Corriere JN Jr et al: Posterior urethral injury after pelvic fracture, *AJR* 137:1233-1237, 1981.

86. Sandler CM, Phillips JM, Harris JD et al: Radiology of the bladder and urethra in blunt pelvic trauma, *Radiol Clin North Am* 19:195-211, 1981.

87. Sato Y, Yuh WTC, Smith WL et al: Head injury in child abuse: evaluation with MR imaging, *Radiology* 173:653-657, 1989.

88. Sclafani SJA, Cooper R, Shafran GW et al: Arterial trauma: diagnostic and therapeutic angiography, *Radiology* 161:165, 1986.

89. Sherck JP, Oakes DD: Intestinal injuries missed by computed tomography, *J Trauma* 30:1-5, 1990.

90. Shigeru E, El-Khoury GY, Sato Y: Cervical spine injury in children: radiologic manifestations, *AJR* 151:1175-1178, 1988.

91. Sinai SH, Ball MR: Head trauma due to child abuse: serial CT in diagnosis and management, *South Med J* 80:1505-1512, 1987.

91a. Sivit CV, Ingram JD, Taylor GA et al: Postraumatic adrenal hemorrhage in children, *Am J Radiol* 158:1299-1302, 1992.

92. Sivit CJ, Peclet M, Taylor GA: Life-threatening intraperitoneal bleeding: demonstration with CT, *Radiology* 171:430, 1989.

93. Sivit CJ, Taylor GA, Eichelberger MR: Chest injury in children with blunt abdominal trauma: evaluation with CT, *Radiology* 171:815-818, 1989.

94. Sivit CJ, Taylor GA, Eichelberger MR: Visceral injury in battered children: a changing perspective, *Radiology* 173:659-661, 1989.

95. Sivit CJ, Taylor GA, Bulas DI et al: Blunt trauma in children: significance of peritoneal fluid, *Radiology* 178:185-188, 1991.

96. Sivit CJ, Taylor GA, Newman KD et al: Safety belt injuries in children with lap-belt ecchymosis, *AJR* 157:111-114, 1991.

97. Stauffer ES, Mazur JM: Cervical spine injuries in children, *Pediatr Ann* 11:502-511, 1982.

98. Swischuk LE: *The cervical spine in childhood: current problems in diagnostic radiology*, vol 2, 1984, Yearbook Medical Publishing, p 40.

99. Taylor GA, Eggli KD: Lap-belt injuries of the lumbar spine in children: a pitfall in CT diagnosis, *AJR* 150:1355-1358, 1988.

100. Taylor GA, Eichelberger MR: Abdominal CT in children with neurologic impairment following blunt trauma, *Ann Surg* 210:229-233, 1989.

101. Taylor GA, Eichelberger MR, Potter BM: Hematuria: a marker of abdominal injury in children after blunt trauma, *Ann Surg* 208:688-693, 1988.

102. Taylor GA, Fallat ME, Eichelberger MR: Hypovolemic shock in children: abdominal CT manifestations, *Radiology* 164:479-481, 1987.

103. Taylor GA, Eichelberger MR, O'Donnell R et al: Indications for computed tomography in children with blunt abdominal trauma, *Ann Surg* 213:212-218, 1991.

104. Taylor GA, Fallat ME, Potter BM et al: The role of computed tomography in blunt trauma in children, *J Trauma* 28:1660-1664, 1988.

105. Taylor GA, Guion CJ, Potter BM et al: CT of blunt abdominal trauma in children, *AJR* 153:555-559, 1989.

106. Taylor SB, Quencer RM, Holzman BH et al: CNS anoxic-ischemic insult in children due to near drowning, *Radiology* 156:641-646, 1985.

107. Tarr RW, Drolshagen LF, Kerner TC et al: MR imaging of recent spinal trauma, *J Comput Assist Tomogr* 11:412-417, 1987.

108. Toutant SM, Klauber MR, Marshall LF et al: Absent or compressed basal cisterns on first CT scan: ominous predictors of outcome in severe head injury, *J Neurosurg* 61:691-694, 1984.

109. Tsai FY, Zee CS, Apthorp JS et al: CT in child abuse head trauma, *CT* 4:277-286, 1980.

110. Umlas SL, Cronan JJ: Splenic trauma: can CT grading systems enable prediction of successful nonsurgical treatment? *Radiology* 178:481-487, 1991.

111. Vandemark RM: Radiology of the cervical spine in trauma

patients: practice pitfalls and recommendations for improving efficiency and communication, *AJR* 155:465-472, 1990.

112. van Donger KJ, Braakman R, Gelpke GJ: The prognostic value of computerized tomography in comatose head injured patients, *J Neurosurg* 59:951-957, 1983.

113. Virapongse C, Shapiro M, Gnitro A et al: Three-dimensional computed tomographic reformation of the spine, skull, and brain from axial images, *Neurosurgery* 18:53-58, 1986.

114. Walker RH, Burton DS: Computed tomography in assessment of acetabular fracture, *J Trauma* 22:227-231, 1982.

115. Weir DC: Roentgenographic signs of cervical injury, *Clin Orthop* 109:9, 1975.

116. Wolk DJ, Sandler CM, Corriere JN Jr: Traperitoneal bladder rupture without pelvic fracture, *J Urol* 134:1199-1201, 1985.

117. Yock DH Jr, Marshall WH: Recent ischemic brain infarcts of CT, appearances pre and post contrast infusion, *Radiology* 117:599-608, 1975.

118. Young JWR, Resnik CS: Fracture of the pelvis: current concepts of classification, *AJR* 155:1169-1175, 1990.

119. Young JWR, Burgess AR, Brumback RJ et al: Pelvic fractures: value of plain radiology in early assessment and management, *Radiology* 160:445-451, 1986.

120. Zimmerman RA, Bilaniuk LT: CT in pediatric head trauma, *J Neuroradiol* 8:257-271, 1981.

121. Zimmerman RA, Bilaniuk LT: Computed tomographic staging of traumatic epidural bleeding, *Radiology* 144:809, 1982.

122. Zimmerman RA, Bilaniuk LT: MRI in subacute head injury, *Neuroradiology* 28:363-370, 1986.

123. Zimmerman RA, Bilaniuk LT, Gennarelli T: Computed tomography of shearing injuries of the cerebral white matter, *Radiology* 127:393-396, 1978.

124. Zimmerman RA, Bilaniuk LT, Bruce D et al: Computed tomography of pediatric head trauma: acute general cerebral swelling, *Radiology* 126:403, 1978.

125. Zimmerman RA, Bilaniuk LT, Dolinskas C et al: Computed tomography of acute intracerebral hemorrhagic contusion, *CT* 1:271, 1977.

126. Zimmerman RA, Bilaniuk LT, Hackney DB et al: Head injury: early results comparing CT and high field MR, *AJR* 147:1215-1222, 1986.

127. Zimmerman RA, Bilaniuk LT, Bruce D et al: CT of craniocerebral injury in the abused child, *Radiology* 130:687-690, 1979.

128. Zimmerman RD, Russell EJ, Yurberg E et al: Falx and interhemispheric fissure on axial CT. II. Recognition and differentiation of interhemispheric subarachnoid and subdural hemorrhage, *AJNR* 3:635-642, 1982.

129. Zinreich SJ, Wang H, Abdo F et al: 3-D CT improves accuracy of spinal trauma studies, *Diagn Imag* p 102-107, 1990.

PART FIVE

General Considerations

Blood Use and Coagulation

Ramesh I. Patel

PATHOPHYSIOLOGY

The leading cause of morbidity and mortality in injured children is deprivation of oxygen delivery to vital organs. Oxygen delivery to the tissue is impaired if there is a severe decrease in cardiac output, hemoglobin concentration, or oxygen saturation. In an injured child, all three may be decreased. The body tries to compensate by redistributing blood flow from the skin, muscle, and splanchnic bed to vital organs such as the heart and brain. If hemorrhage continues, however, reduction in blood volume and in oxygen-carrying capacity occurs. The body is then unable to compensate, and tissue perfusion and oxygen delivery to the organs are seriously impaired. Establishment of the airway and improvement of the oxygen saturation of the hemoglobin will improve the oxygen content (oxygen carried per gram of hemoglobin) of the blood. Yet because of the loss of a large volume of blood (that is, red blood cells), impairment of cardiac output and hemoglobin concentration continues.

The most useful guide in estimating the impact of blood loss in acute hemorrhage is the systolic blood pressure. If blood pressure is less than 80 mm Hg for a child under 5 years of age, or less than 90 mm Hg for a child over the age of 5, suspect significant hemorrhage. Pulse rate is not a reliable guide to assess blood volume in injured children.

FLUID THERAPY

Expansion of blood volume, which leads to increased cardiac output and better tissue perfusion, by infusing crystalloids is the first principle of transfusion therapy. The need for massive transfusion of fluids and blood requires insertion of at least two large-bore intravenous catheters. Use of 24-gauge catheters with microdrip chambers in such situations is counterproductive. Rapid infusion of lactated Ringer's solution or Normosol is necessary until vital signs return to acceptable range or until administration of packed red blood cells (PRBC) is possible. Avoid the use of Dextran, which impairs platelet function and interferes with subsequent cross match of blood. The use of colloids during initial volume resuscitation in injured children is controversial. Routine use of hypertonic saline solution is not currently recommended, in spite of its efficacy in treating hemorrhagic shock.

MONITORING

The second important principle of fluid therapy is monitoring the child's response to transfusion. An indwelling intraarterial catheter allows the clinician to monitor rapid changes in blood pressure and establishes a port for drawing blood samples for analysis of acid-base balance, electrolytes, hemoglobin, and coagulation values. To assess for hypothermia, measure body temperature continuously. Urine output provides a measure of intravascular volume and can offer clues to such events as reactions to blood transfusion. Central venous pressure monitoring is useful in assessing changes in blood volume.

BLOOD THERAPY: CRITERIA FOR TRANSFUSION

When oxygen saturation is restored following establishment of ventilation, and cardiac output improves after infusion of crystalloid, the only uncorrected parameter is decreased hemoglobin concentration. This is corrected by infusing PRBC which contain hemoglobin.

What is the minimal or optimal hemoglobin concentration? Cardiac output rises in compensation for low oxygen delivery, but it does not increase in healthy adults until hemoglobin values fall below 7 g/dl. Current experience suggests that otherwise healthy patients with hemoglobin values of 10 g/dl or greater rarely require blood transfusion; however, the combination of hypovolemia and anemia may result in severe morbidity and mortality.[7]

Blood and blood products must be administered when needed, but a conservative approach is best to avoid the risks associated with transfusion of blood products. This is especially important in the treatment of injured children in whom autologus transfusion or directed donor blood is not an option. It is important to make every effort to conserve as much blood as possible through meticulous attention to hemostasis and by acceptance of lower hemoglobin values.

The decision to transfuse a specific child takes into consideration the initial hemoglobin concentration, extent of surgery, intravascular blood volume, probability of massive blood loss, and physical conditions such as impaired pulmonary function and inadequate cardiac output.

The best predictor of the need for blood in adult trauma patients is the trauma score (TS). In one study, 91% of patients with a TS of more than 14 did not require transfusion, whereas 70% of those with a TS of 14 or less required transfusion.[22] All patients with a TS of 14 or less should have immediate crossmatch of blood equal to at least two units of PRBC or half the estimated blood volume (that is, approximately 4 to 6 units of PRBC in adults). Communication to the blood bank of the expected need for massive transfusion, and of its urgency, is important. Fundamental to the efficient treatment of injured children is the ability to provide large quantities of blood products on short notice day or night. Rapid results of laboratory tests are essential for prompt therapy, including complete blood count, electrolytes, platelet count, prothrombin time, partial thromboplastin time, fibrinogen level, thrombin time and fibrin split product tests.

Estimates of blood loss and replacement requirements in children are calculated as milliliters per kilogram (ml/kg) and expressed as a fraction of total blood volume. For a given quantity of blood, this fraction varies significantly between an adult and a child. For example, a blood loss of 500 ml in an adult with a blood volume of 5000 ml is only a 10% decrease in blood volume; a loss of one unit of blood. By contrast, in a 20-kg, 5-year-old child with a blood volume of 1400 ml, a blood loss of 500 ml is equal to 25 cc/kg, or nearly one-third total blood volume. Physiologic compensation for a 10% blood loss is common, whereas compensation for a 33% loss will not be adequate. Therefore it is extremely important to refer to blood loss/replaced in terms of ml/kg or to compare the loss with the total blood volume.

Estimated blood volumes in children are as follows: neonates, 100 cc/kg; 1 month to 2 years, 80 cc/kg; 2 years to adult, 70 cc/kg. As a general guideline:

1. Transfusion of 1 ml of PRBC per kilogram of body weight increases the hematocrit by 1%, or
2. 3 ml/kg of PRBC raises the hemoglobin level by 1 g/dl.

SELECTION OF BLOOD PRODUCTS
ABO group

Administration of group O PRBC is best for children who need immediate transfusion; for others, provide group-specific, screened PRBC, or cross-matched blood. *Type and cross match* is a laboratory process in which donor cells are mixed with recipient serum to determine the potential for serious transfusion reaction. *Type and screen* is a process in which recipient serum is mixed with commercially supplied red cells (instead of donor cells) that are specifically selected to contain an optimal number of common red cell antigens. Donor serum is also screened for unexpected antibodies to prevent their introduction into the recipient serum. The differences between the two processes are becoming increasingly less significant. A type-and-screen unit of blood is more than 99.9% effective in preventing incompatible transfusion reactions resulting from unexpected antibodies.[15]

Group O blood is usually available within a few minutes, whereas type-specific, nonscreened, immediate phase cross-matched blood requires 15 minutes. Type-specific blood that has been screened for antibodies is usually available within 45 minutes. Unfortunately, complete cross match of blood requires 60 to 75 minutes.

Technically, there are no universal donors or recipients, since transfusion of separated blood components is the usual practice. Group O donors are universal donors for PRBC, and Group AB donors are universal donors for fresh frozen plasma (FFP). Group O recipients should receive exclusively group O PRBC but may receive FFP, platelets, and cryoprecipitate of any group. Group A children should receive group A or O red cells, or group A or AB FFP. Group B children can receive group B or O red cells, or B or AB FFP. Group AB patients can receive PRBC from anyone, but preferably FFP and platelets from a group AB donor. In general, platelets and cryoprecipitate are given without regard to ABO group.

In neonates Hb F comprises 60% to 80% of total hemoglobin. By the time the child is 6 to 12 months of age, Hb F generally is no longer present. Hb F has high affinity for oxygen, which decreases the release of oxygen to tissues in the newborn. Neonates in the first 4 months of life do not possess alloantibodies nor do they produce them in response to transfusion, owing to the immaturity of the immune system; therefore, administration of uncross-matched blood is possible in infants up to the age of 4 months.

If a group A, B, or AB child receives more than 2 units, or half the blood volume, of group O PRBC, it is best to continue transfusion of group O cells. The anti-A, anti-B agglutinins in group O donor plasma can cause major hemolysis if the child subsequently receives group-specific blood. It is best to withhold transfusion of group-specific blood for 14 days, or until anti-A, anti-B agglutinins disappear from the blood.

Rh-negative women of childbearing age should receive only Rh-negative blood; all other patients (including children) can receive Rh-positive blood. Seventy-five percent of Rh-negative recipients who receive Rh-positive products produce anti-D antibodies. Because of the presence of red cells, platelets should always be Rh-specific.

ADMINISTRATION

Adequate venous access is extremely important. Mix each unit of PRBC with about 100 cc of 0.9% saline solution to decrease viscosity. Avoid the use of lactated Ringer's solution, which contains calcium, or of glucose-containing solutions to dilute PRBC. A standard 170-μm filter must be used for proper administration of the blood product.[10] The use of 40-μm filters is controversial. The administration system must also warm the blood before infusion in the child. Such devices must have the capacity to quickly warm a large volume of fluid and a thermistor to prevent excessive temperature elevation, which can harm the blood products. Avoid the use of unmonitored water baths and microwave ovens to warm blood. Vital signs, urine output, color of the skin, pulse oximetry, and serially measured hemoglobin-hematocrit levels provide useful information about the total blood volume and oxygen-carrying capacity.

AVAILABLE PRODUCTS
Packed red blood cells (PRBC)

One unit of PRBC has a volume of 250 ml and a hematocrit of 60% to 70%. A single unit of PRBC can be divided into two or four smaller aliquots for use in neonates and infants. Each unit of PRBC has 60 ml of preservative CPD-A (citrate, phosphate, dextrose, and adenine). Citrate chelates the calcium and prevents coagulation; dextrose and phosphate provide the necessary nutrients; and adenine maintains the high intracellular adenosine triphosphate (ATP) concentration necessary for cell viability. The shift in the United States in 1972 from acid citrate dextrose (ACD) to citrate phosphate dextrose (CPD) solution as a blood preservative allows for retention of higher levels of 2,3 DPG for longer a time. PRBC with CPD permit storage for up to 21 days, whereas those containing CPD-A increase storage time to about 35 days. Storage of PRBC at 1° to 6° C decreases the rate of glycolysis so that the cells survive without excessive nutrient consumption. Stored blood must maintain viable cells during storage, and at least 75% of the red cells must survive at least 24 hours after transfusion.[16] Even though 2,3 DPG level is low in stored blood, it rises to 25% of normal

within 8 hours of transfusion and is fully functional by 24 hours.

Plasma pH decreases during storage of PRBC owing to production of lactate by glucose metabolism. The inhibition of the Na-K pump at 1° to 6° C leads to hyperkalemia and hyponatremia in stored blood. Plasma hemoglobin increases due to enhanced osmotic fragility of cells. Levels of 2,3 DPG and activity of factors V and VIII decrease during storage of blood.

Modified preparations

Modified preparations of PRBC include leukocyte-poor RBC, washed cells, frozen deglycerolized cells, and irradiated cells. Leukocyte-poor cells are indicated for children with allergic reactions to white blood cells (WBC) and for prevention of febrile nonhemolytic transfusion reactions. Because the cytomegalovirus (CMV) is harbored exclusively in white cells, reducing the number of leukocytes decreases the risk of CMV in neonates and children with compromised, immature systems. To be labeled "leukocyte poor," at least 70% of the original leukocytes have to be removed from cells. This is done via in-line filters or by washing red cells, which removes 70% to 90% of leukocytes, plasma, platelets, and microaggregates. Washed red cells do not have excess extracellular potassium and are therefore useful in neonates. Frozen ($-8°$ C), deglycerolized red cells are also free of WBC, platelets, plasma anticoagulants, and microaggregates. Both washed and frozen cells must be used within 24 hours of release. Because the methods used in preparation of modified red cell components require additional time, emergency transfusion of such products is not feasible.

Irradiation of red cells is the only method currently available to decrease the activity of lymphocytes that cause transfusion-associated graft-versus-host disease (TA-GVHD). Prolonged storage of irradiated PRBC may increase the free plasma hemoglobin and potassium levels; blood administered to neonates and children should therefore be irradiated just prior to its use.

Fresh frozen plasma (FFP)

Plasma is separated from whole blood and stored at $-18°$ C within 8 hours of collection. Once thawed, it must be transfused within 24 hours when stored at 4° C. A National Institutes of Health (NIH) Consensus Conference, which has evaluated the indications for use of FFP, recommends that it not be used as a volume expander because of the risk of transfusion-transmitted diseases.[8]

Because FFP contains anti-A and anti-B antibodies, it should be ABO compatible. Rh type is not considered, and cross match with recipient blood is unnecessary. FFP provides factors II, V, VIII, IX, X, and XI and antithrombin III. Following massive transfusion of stored PRBC, deficiency of factors V and VIII occurs; administration of FFP corrects such deficiency. Following massive transfusion, however, the serum levels of clotting factors are not related to the total number of units of blood administered[5]; consequently, transfusion of FFP based on number of PRBC used is inappropriate. Clinical evidence of a bleeding diathesis after transfusion of more than one blood volume of PRBC is a strong indication for use of FFP. Usually 30% to 50% of normal clotting factor activity is sufficient for hemostasis; this degree of activity is present after transfusion of 20 to 30 ml/kg of FFP. Laboratory values (PT, PTT, thrombin time) and clinical assessment should guide further transfusion therapy. A 170-μm micron filter is used to transfuse FFP. Any blood product dispensed in syringes must be prefiltered by the blood bank.

Platelets

Centrifugation and recentrifugation of whole blood produce a unit of random donor platelets, which are then suspended in 50 to 75 ml of plasma and stored at 22° C on a mechanical rotator. It is preferable to administer ABO-matched platelets. They should be administered through 170-μm filters. Avoid transfusion of Rh-positive platelets to an Rh-negative woman of childbearing age.

The decrease in platelet count following massive hemorrhage is less than that predicted by the standard washout formula, suggesting mobilization of platelets from the bone marrow and spleen. In a child who receives massive transfusion, dilution thrombocytopenia, defects in platelet function, or both occur before clotting factor deficiencies develop. The need to transfuse platelets arises before the need to administer FFP. Following one volume replacement of PRBC, 35% to 40% of platelets remain in circulation.[6] Prophylactic administration of platelets during massive transfusion does not prevent microvascular nonmechanical bleeding.[11,18] As the PRBC transfusion increases during massive blood loss, however, the platelet count decreases.[5] Cote and associates[9] concluded that during massive blood transfusion in children a platelet count of less than 100,000/mm^3 suggests impending coagulopathy and that a decrease to less than 50,000/mm^3 after massive transfusion requires platelet administration. Transfusion of 0.3 unit/kg of platelets was required before abnormal oozing ceased.[9] The initial dose of 0.1 unit/kg of platelets will raise the platelet count by about 40,000/mm^3.

Cryoprecipitate

Refreezing the insoluble portion of plasma produces cryoprecipitate, which is used to increase the levels of fibrinogen and factor VIII during massive transfusion. Each 20- to 40-ml bag provides 80 units of factor VIII, 100 to 350 mg of fibrinogen, factor XIII, von Willebrand factor, and fibrinectin. The initial recommended dose of cryoprecipitate is 0.1 unit/kg. ABO-compatible cryoprecipitate is preferable, and Rh type and cross match are not necessary. The use of cryoprecipitate should be carefully monitored, since administration of large doses in a patient with normal fibrinogen may produce thrombosis and disseminated intravascular coagulation (DIC).

Alternative therapy

Two types of products have been developed as alternatives to PRBC. Stoma-free hemoglobin does not transmit diseases, does not require cross match, and has a long shelf life. However, its short plasma life and increased oxygen affinity limit its peripheral off-loading capability. Perflurochemicals (for example, Flurosol-DA) contain solvents to dissolve oxygen, but recent studies show no practical use. Neither product has yet been used in injured children.

In injured children the cell-saver technique for autotransfusion is useful. Autotransfusion techniques are safe in children[21] and in adults.[13,20] The blood obtained through the cell-saver technique is type- and group-specific, warm, fresh, rich in 2,3 DPG, and devoid of risk of infection. It also provides additional platelets and clotting factors, but lacks fibrinogen. Several systems are available, all of which can be assembled quickly. Contraindications to autotransfusion include contamination of the abdomen with feces and presence of tumor cells.

TECHNIQUES TO REDUCE BLOOD LOSS

A meticulous surgical technique is of unequaled value in reducing blood loss. Aprotonin, a protease inhibitor, has been shown to decrease blood loss in cardiac surgery.[2] Although it mitigates platelet dysfunction and inhibits fibrinolysis, its usefulness in injured children has not been determined. Desmopressin acetate also decreases bleeding by improving platelet function in patients with uremia and in those undergoing cardiopulmonary bypass. It is of little benefit in children under maximum stress of injury.

RISKS OF TRANSFUSION

The risks of blood transfusion are outlined in Table 23-1.

Incompatibility

Manifestations of minor incompatibility caused by platelets, plasma proteins, and WBC are limited to fever, chills, and urticaria. Incompatibility in the

Table 23–1 Risks of transfusion

Routine transfusion
Incompatibility
    Minor: plasma protein, WBC, and platelets
        act as antigens
    Major: ABO/Rh and other RBC antigens
Infection
    Viral: non-A, non-B hepatitis, CMV, human
        immunodeficiency virus (HIV)
    Bacterial
    Parasites: malaria
Foreign-body contamination
Transfusion-associated graft-versus-host disease
    (TA-GVHD)

Massive transfusion
Risks mentioned above
Volume overload
Hypothermia
Coagulopathy
Metabolic: hyperkalemia, hypokalemia, hypo-
        calcemia, acidosis
Microaggregates
Respiratory distress syndrome (ARDS)

ABO system, however, is the most common cause of fatality secondary to blood transfusion.[17] The incidence of hemolytic transfusion reaction is 1:4000 to 1:6000, and the incidence of fatal reactions is 1:100,000; most of these reactions are a result of clerical error. The best safeguard against such mishaps is direct issuance of blood from the blood bank and identification of each child by an approved wristband. Signs and symptoms of a mismatched-transfusion reaction are fever, chills, bronchospasm, chest pain, rash, hypotension, and hemoglobinuria. Transfusion must be stopped immediately when a reaction is suspected. In this event, levels of plasma and urine hemoglobin, serum haptoglobin, and direct antiglobulin are assessed. Treatment consists of alkalinization of urine, diuresis, and supportive therapy.

Infection

Each unit of blood is tested for the following: HIV; non-A, non-B hepatitis or hepatitis C virus; hepatitis B core antigen; human T-cell lymphotrophic virus (HTLV-I); syphilis; alkaline aminotransferase (ALT); and ABO and Rh groups. In addition, evaluation for the presence of CMV in the blood of neonates and immunosuppressed children is important.

Hepatitis

The incidence of hepatitis B is 1:1000 units. Non-A, non-B hepatitis or hepatitis C occurs in about 1:100 units, although most have nonicteric hepatitis. Ninety percent of posttransfusion hepatitis is due to hepatitis C virus. The recent introduction of a test to detect hepatitis C will certainly decrease the incidence of hepatitis following transfusion.

Human immunodeficiency virus (HIV)

Even though all units of blood are tested for HIV, the critical window of incubation still makes it possible to contract HIV following transfusion. The incidence of HIV infection following transfusion is 1:40,000 to 1:1,000,000.

Cytomegalovirus (CMV)

CMV is harbored in the circulating leukocytes. The risk of CMV is greatest in neonates and immunosuppressed children. These children should receive blood only from CMV-negative donors or washed or deglycerolized PRBCs.

Transfusion-associated graft-versus-host disease (TA-GVHD)

TA-GVHD may occur in newborns and immunocompromised children. When such children receive lymphocytes from an immunologically competent donor, the transfused T lymphocytes proliferate and engraft in the tissues because the recipients are incapable of rejecting foreign cells. Irradiation of the blood product eliminates T-cell lymphocytes and the risk of TA-GVHD.

COAGULOPATHY

A thorough knowledge of the coagulation and anticoagulation systems (Fig. 23-1) is essential to understand the coagulopathy associated with massive transfusions. There are three components to hemostasis: vascular, platelet, and coagulation cascade. An interruption of vascular integrity is a major cause of bleeding during injury. Damage of the vascular endothelium activates a coagulation cascade, and platelet aggregates plug the injured vessel. Platelet release and aggregation are mediated by ADP. Increased concentration of ADP stimulates platelet aggregation, and a decreased level has an inhibitory effect.[19] Release of ADP is increased by thromboxane A_2, which is found in platelets, and decreased by prostacyclin PGI_2, which is stored in the vascular endothelium. Platelet factor III (PF III), released from platelets, is responsible for platelet aggregation and activation of coagulation cascade.

The anticoagulation mechanisms that prevent continuous formation of clots are (1) blood flow decreasing the procoagulants, (2) hepatic clearance of factor X, (3) inhibitors such as antithrombin III, and (4) plasmin, which causes fibrinolysis. Specific anticoagulants are antithrombin III, heparin, alpha-2 globulin, and fibrin split products. Lysis of blood clots occurs through plasmin or through fibrinolysin, whose precursors are plasminogen or profi-

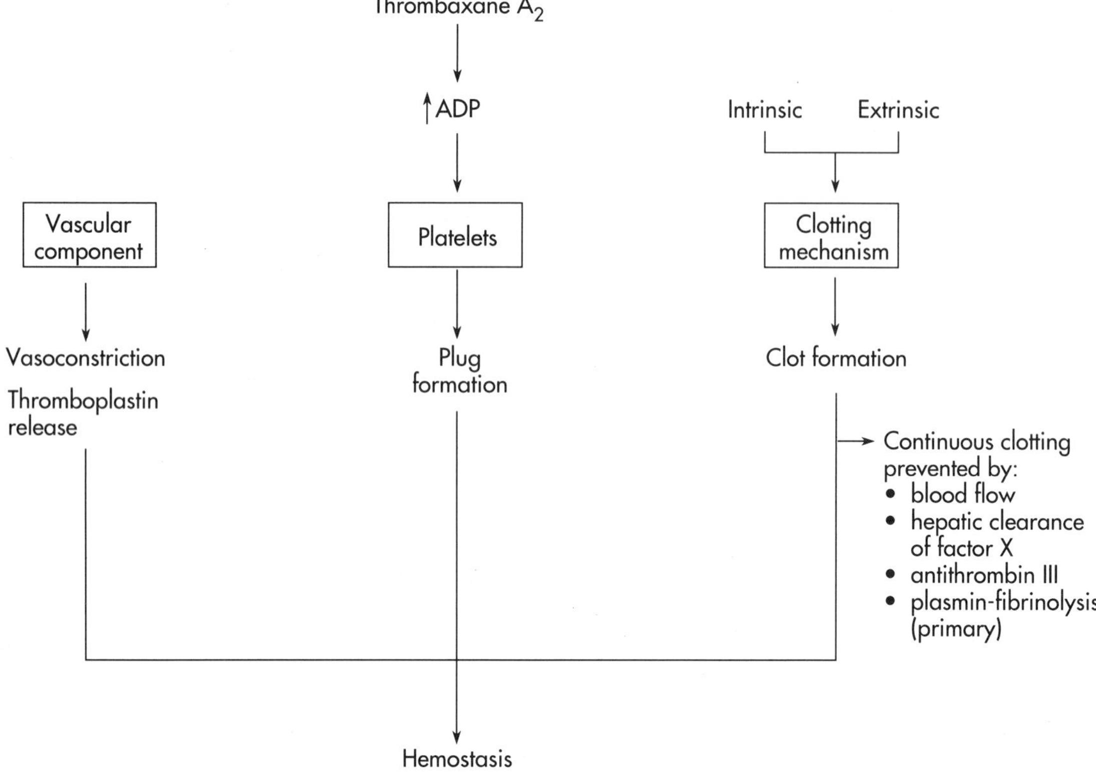

Figure 23–1 Normal hemostasis.

brinolysin, which are activated by thrombin, streptokinase, lysomal enzymes from tissues, and factor XIIa.

Massive transfusion is defined as administration of more than one and a half times the child's estimated blood volume.[14] Coagulopathy is rarely observed until more than two blood volume transfusion occurs. Bleeding diathesis (medical bleeding) does not occur until prothrombin or partial thromboplastin time (PT or PTT) is prolonged to 1.5 to 1.8 times the control level (Table 23-2) and the clotting factors are decreased to less than 25% of normal.

Coagulopathy occurs following massive transfusion as a consequence of a decrease in platelets and clotting factors. This decrease is due to hemodilution and consumption (Fig. 23-2). Thrombocytopenia generally appears after transfusion of PRBC equivalent to two blood volumes. Dilutional thrombocytopenia is due to transfusion of stored blood, which has low platelet activity. Similarly, levels of factors V and VIII decrease following massive transfusion as a result of hemodilution. Extensive tissue damage associated with trauma triggers a coagulation cascade because of the release of tissue thromboplastin, which causes widespread coagulation, consuming platelets and most

Table 23–2 Tests performed to assess coagulation

Platelet count: >100,000
Prothrombin time: 11 to 13 sec (evaluates extrinsic and final pathway)
Partial thromboplastin time: 25 to 38 sec (evaluates intrinsic and common pathway)
Thrombin time: 9 to 12 sec (evaluates final pathway)
Bleeding time: 4 to 6 min (evaluates platelet function)
Fibrinogen level: 200 to 400 mg/dl (minimum acceptable: 100 mg/dl)
Fibrin split products: <10 μg/ml
Dimer test (D-dimer test): normal <500 μg/ml (a sensitive test for DIC)

---

of the clotting factors. Depletion of platelets, fibrinogen, and factors I, II, V, VIII, and XIII results in consumptive coagulopathy. Consumptive coagulopathy is called *disseminated intravascular coagulopathy* (DIC); it is a paradox because bleeding and thrombosis occur simultaneously. The hypercoagulable state not only depletes platelets and coagulation factors but also interrupts blood flow in microvessels through fibrin deposition. The fibri-

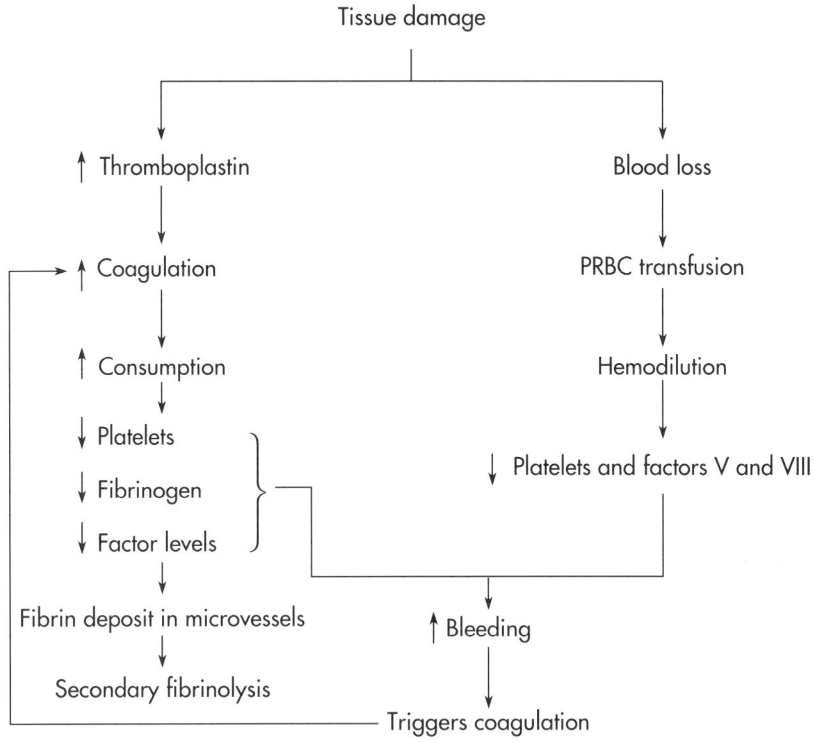

Figure 23–2 Coagulopathy following massive injury.

nolytic system is activated to combat the hypercoagulable state. Plasmin converted from plasminogen causes fibrinolysis, which releases fibrin split products. Children with good perfusion do not develop coagulopathy, but a hypotensive child who requires massive transfusion is likely to develop consumption and dilutional coagulopathy. Clotting abnormalities following head injuries have been described. DIC complicating isolated cerebral trauma is related to release of large amounts of thromboplastin into the circulation. DIC is self-limited when definitive therapy for the primary problem is accomplished.

Treatment of DIC consists of resolving the primary event and providing coagulation factors and platelets. Heparin is used to stop the cycle of hypercoagulability, depletion of clotting factors, and bleeding. The dose of heparin administered to prevent consumption is about 20 units/kg. Its use, however, is controversial.

METABOLIC DERANGEMENTS
Hyperkalemia

Potassium levels are as high as 30 mEq/L in a unit of blood stored for 21 days. Rapid transfusion of a large volume of blood in infants may lead to hyperkalemia, hypokalemia and hypocalcemia. In a study of 121 adults who had received more than 20 transfusions, 25% had hyperkalemia, 60% had normal potassium levels, and 15% had hypokalemia.[23] In adults, hyperkalemia developed only when the rate of transfusion of stored blood exceeded 0.4 ml/kg/min.[12] In children, a combination of massive rapid blood transfusion and low cardiac output is associated with hyperkalemia.[3,4] Hypokalemia is also known to occur during massive transfusion.

Hypocalcemia and citrate toxicity

Citrate present in the anticoagulant CPD-A binds with calcium. Citrate is rapidly metabolized in the liver, after which the ionized calcium level returns to normal. The serum calcium level in children is stable when the transfusion rate is less than 30 ml/kg/hr.[1] Calcium concentration decreases with a more rapid transfusion but returns to normal within 5 to 10 minutes.[1] Calcium administration may be of benefit in situations in which combined hyperkalemia and hypocalcemia reduce myocardial performance.[12]

Acid-base abnormalities

The pH of blood is 7.16 after collection and decreases to 6.7 during storage. This is due to the acidic preservative solution, increased pCO_2, and release of lactic and pyruvic acid by the red blood cells. However, empiric administration of bicarbonate is not helpful. An increase in pH occurs following blood transfusion because of improved tissue perfusion and metabolism of citrate and lactate.

Hypothermia

Infusion of blood products stored at 4° C causes hypothermia. Blood must be warmed before infusion, particularly in children who are prone to hypothermia.

Microaggregates

Deposits of microaggregates from blood transfusion may cause ARDS. The microaggregates range in size from 10 to 164 μm. Transfusion of a large volume of bank blood through the standard 170-μm filters results in delivery of a large number of microaggregates to the circulation. However, the role of such microaggregates in organ dysfunction is not yet clear.

In essence, blood therapy is like any other treatment. Side effects and risk of potential complications have to be considered before initiation of therapy, but treatment should never be withheld when needed. An estimated volume of blood product is administered, and response is monitored to assess the need for further therapy.

REFERENCES

1. Abbott TR: Changes in serum calcium fractions and citrate concentrations during massive blood transfusions and cardiopulmonary bypass, *Br J Anaesth* 55:753-760, 1983.
2. Blauhut B, Gross C, Necek S et al: Effects of high dose Aprotonin on blood loss, platelet function, fibrinolysis, complement and renal function after cardiopulmonary bypass, *J Thorac Cardiovasc Surg* 101:958-967, 1991.
3. Brown KA, Bissonnette B, McIntyre B: Hyperkalemia during rapid blood transfusion and hypovolemic cardiac arrest in children, *Can J Anaesth* 37:747-754, 1990.
4. Brown KA, Bissonnette B, MacDonald M et al: Hyperkalemia during massive blood transfusion in pediatric craniofacial surgery, *Can J Anaesth* 37:401-408, 1990.
5. Counts RB, Haisch C, Simon TL et al: Hemostasis in massively transfused trauma patients, *Ann Surg* 190:91-99, 1979.
6. Consensus Conference: Platelet transfusion therapy, *JAMA* 257:1777-1780, 1987.
7. Consensus Conference: Perioperative red blood cell transfusion, *JAMA* 260:2700-2703, 1988.
8. Consensus Conference: Fresh frozen plasma: indications and risks, *JAMA* 253:551-553, 1991.
9. Cote CJ, Liu LMP, Szyfelbein SK et al: Changes in serial platelet counts following massive blood transfusion in pediatric patients, *Anesthesiol* 62:197-201, 1985.
10. Durtschi MB, Haisch CE, Reynold L et al: Effect of micropore filtration in pulmonary function after massive transfusion, *Am J Surg* 138:8-14, 1979.
11. Harrigan C, Lucas CE, Ledgewood AM et al: Serial changes in primary hemostasis after massive transfusion, *Surgery* 98:836-844, 1985.
12. Linko K, Saxelin I: Electrolyte and acid base disturbances caused by blood transfusion, *Anesthesiol Scand* 30:139-144, 1986.
13. Mattox K, Walker LE, Beall AC et al: Blood availability for the trauma patient—autotransfusion, *J Trauma* 15:663-669, 1975.
14. Miller RD: Complications of massive blood transfusions, *Anesthesiol* 39:82-93, 1973.
15. Miller RD, Brzica SM: Blood, blood products, colloids and autotransfusion therapy. In Miller RD, editor: *Clinical anesthesia*, ed 2, New York, 1986, Churchill Livingstone, pp 1329-1367.
16. Moroff G, Sohmer PR, Button LN: Proposed standardization of methods determining the 24 hour survival of stored red cells, *Transfusion* 24:109-114, 1984.
17. Myhre BA: Fatalities from blood transfusion, *JAMA* 244:1333-1335, 1980.
18. Reed RL, Ciavarella D, Heimach DM et al: Prophylactic platelet administration during massive transfusion, *Ann Surg* 203:40-47, 1986.
19. Shattil SJ, Bennett JS: Platelets and their membranes in hemostasis: physiology and pathophysiology, *Ann Intern Med* 94:108-118, 1990.
20. Stehling LC, Zauder HL, Rogers W: Intraoperative autotransfusion, *Anesthesiol* 43:337-345, 1975.
21. Wesson DE, Ein SM, Vallamater J: Intraoperative autotransfusion in blunt abdominal trauma, *J Pediatr Surg* 15:735-736, 1980.
22. West HC, Jurkovich G, Donnell C et al: Immediate prediction of blood requirements in trauma victims, *South Med J* 82:186-189, 1989.
23. Wilson RF, Dulchavsky SA, Sobllier G et al: Problems with 20 or more blood transfusions in 24 hours, *Am Surg* 53:410-417, 1987.

24 Nutrition

Catherine A. Musemeche and *Richard J. Andrassy*

Once the acute phase of resuscitation and treatment of a child's traumatic injury has been successfully completed, attention is turned to the support of the child through the stress and vulnerability of the recovery period. One of the major advances in trauma care in the past decade has been the recognition and therapy of the metabolic response to trauma and the increased nutritional needs that accompany it. Effective nutritional support during this period of critical illness and recovery can increase resistance to infection, improve wound healing, prevent organ failure, and reduce mortality. An individual plan of nutritional therapy must be formulated and instituted early in the course of trauma management, as major nutritional deficiencies can develop early and progress quickly in the critically injured child.

NUTRITIONAL REQUIREMENTS IN TRAUMA

The metabolic response to injury or stress has been studied extensively in the adult. Stress mediators and hormonal changes modulate the metabolic consequences of injury. The stress response is initiated when afferent neural signals from the wound reach the hypothalamus and the pituitary is stimulated to release ACTH, which then acts on the adrenal cortex to produce cortisol. In conjunction with glucagon and catecholamines, cortisol stimulates tissue catabolism, resulting in mobilization of amino acids from skeletal muscle. Amino acids provide substrates for wound healing and serve as precursors for the hepatic synthesis of acute-phase proteins and glucose. The sympathetic nervous system activates the adrenal medulla to elaborate epinephrine and norepinephrine. These catecholamines, which play an important role in maintaining hemodynamic stability in times of stress, also have potent metabolic effects. They are essential in the stimulation of hepatic glycogenolysis, fat mobilization, and gluconeogenesis. To summarize the classic description of the neuroendocrine response to trauma, there is a rise in catecholamines, glucagon, and glucocorticoids with an inappropriately low serum insulin. The net effect is an elevation of glucose, free fatty acids, and ketones, and a decrease in amino acid levels.[1] Interventional pharmacologic and nutritional therapy may modulate these responses.

Extensive urinary nitrogen losses occur in all children suffering major injuries. It has been established that these losses result from a generalized breakdown of muscle protein.[33] Nitrogen loss and muscle catabolism are potentiated in children treated with systemic corticosteroids for head injuries.[6] Profiles of the mobilized amino acids are not the same as the composition of muscle protein. Alanine and glutamine constitute 50% to 60% of the amino acids released, whereas each makes up only about 6% of muscle protein.[27] The branched-chain amino acids make up approximately 6% of the released amino acids but comprise nearly 15% of muscle protein. Oxidation of branched-chain amino acids by skeletal muscle is accelerated following injury, which may account for their diminished release in trauma. Glutamine and alanine are of major importance in the transfer of nitrogen from skeletal muscle to visceral organs. Glutamine is also taken up by the gastrointestinal tract and serves as an oxidative fuel.[34] Gut enterocytes convert glutamine to ammonia and alanine, which are released into the portal blood. Ammonia removed by the liver is converted to urea or glutamine, and alanine removed by the liver serves as a gluconeogenic precursor.[29]

Physiologic responses of the child are similar to the adult's, but there are some important differences that leave children at a significant nutritional disadvantage in times of stress. In addition to increased caloric demands, there is usually a decrease in caloric intake during times of severe illness. Nutritional stores in a child younger than 1 year of age are considerably less than in an adult because of the child's lower percentage of body fat and protein. In a premature baby, fat constitutes approximately 1% of body weight, whereas in a 1-year-old 20% of body weight may be fat[8] (21% in adults). Children have an increased need for calories because their basal metabolic rate is higher than that of adults (55 versus 35 kcal/kg/h). Children also have increased requirements because they are growing and because metabolic organs com-

"

Table 24–1 Energy requirements (kcal/kg/24 hr) for various ages at basal, maintenance, growth, and illness levels

	1 Year	5 Years	10 Years	16 Years
Basal	55	45	38	27
Maintenance	83	75	56	42
Growth	89	77	78	43
Illness	95	78	66	45

Adapted from Briglia FA, Pollock MM: Fluid and nutritional therapy in the critically ill child, *Indian J Pediatr* 54:819-829, 1987.

pose a greater percentage of their body weight.

Determining energy requirements begins with a knowledge of the basal metabolic rate (BMR) for infants and children. The BMR is derived from a measurement of heat production in a resting-fasting state. Maintenance requirements are 120% to 150% of BMR. Growth requirements are an additional 5 kcal per gram of weight gained. An approximation of energy needs during critical illness is 150% to 200% of BMR (Table 24-1). These increased needs can vary according to the traumatic illness, for example, burns increase metabolic rate up to 100%, sepsis by 50%, and long bone fractures by 20% (Table 24-2).[33]

The caloric requirements of patients with head injuries vary and seem to show a correlation with the severity of brain injury.[25] Brain injury may also produce increased metabolic demands that are seemingly out of proportion with the degree of obvious trauma. There are two reasons for this: (1) brain trauma may increase the metabolic response to injuries that occur in other parts of the body and (2) steroid treatment for a brain injury may increase the hypermetabolic response to trauma.[13]

It is especially important to maintain adequate nutritional support in the child who has been receiving ventilator therapy for longer than a week. During this time, muscle mass decreases and the diaphragm and intercostal muscles become weak. This deficit impairs the patient's respiratory efforts and makes weaning from the ventilator difficult. Overfeeding of carbohydrates is to be avoided during the weaning period as it may increase the respiratory quotient and lead to increased carbon dioxide production.[21] If hypercapnia is persistent during the weaning period despite adequate pulmonary mechanics, it is advisable to lower the percentage of calories administered as glucose and administer a greater percentage of fat.[18]

The protein requirements of an injured child depend on the patient's age, the type of traumatic wound, and the protein source that is used to support the child. In infants less than 6 months of age, protein requirements are 2 to 3 g/kg/day to main-

Table 24–2 Percent increase in caloric expenditure resulting from traumatic injury

Type of injury	Percent increase
Head trauma	25%-100%
Burns	100%
Sepsis, peritonitis, severe cellulitis	25%-50%
Single long bone fracture	20%
Open wound	20%-50%

tain normal growth and development. This decreases to 1.5 to 2.0 g/kg/day in infants more than 6 months old, and to 1 to 2 g/kg/day in older children. Children with large open wounds, burns of large areas of body surface, or severe diarrhea may have even greater protein requirements owing to increased losses.

The amount of protein required depends on its essential amino acid content. Essential amino acids should constitute 40% of an infant's protein intake, 30% of a child's protein intake, and 20% of an adult's protein intake.[9] The availability of the protein provided in enteral diets is also of issue. A free amino acid solution may allow for greater nitrogen absorption than do oligopeptide or whole protein diets, partly because the free amino solution requires no digestion. Amino acids, dipeptides, and tripeptides are considered elemental; that is, they can be absorbed without digestion. Larger peptides must be digested into dipeptides and tripeptides or amino acids before absorption.[5]

Critically ill children require protein intake in greater amounts to achieve positive nitrogen balance. Twenty-four-hour urine collections and nitrogen determinations can aid in calculating what is needed. In general, no more than 30% of calories should be provided in the form of protein.[9,26]

Essential fatty acid requirements (linoleic acid) may be met by supplying 4% to 8% of the daily caloric requirements with fat,[8] but on average fat is used to provide 20% to 30% of total calories.

Table 24–3 Calcium and phosphorous requirements in infants and children

Age	Calcium	Phosphorous
<6 mo	80 mg/kg/day	1-2 mM/kg/day
6 mo-2 yr	40 mg/kg/day	1 mM/kg/day
2 yr-10 yr	400 mg/day	10-30 mM/day
>10 yr	600 mg/day	15-20 mM/day

In light of recent evidence that high levels of polyunsaturated fatty acids have an immunosuppressive effect in burn patients, these limits should not be exceeded.[3] There remains considerable controversy on whether omega 6 or omega 3 polyunsaturated fatty acids are best for the critically ill or traumatized patient. Studies have demonstrated that younger animals require more fat in the diet than adult animals for normal healing and immune functions.[23] During severe sepsis, because of impairment in fat utilization, not more than 10% of dietary energy requirements should be fat.

Complete nutritional support requires adequate amounts of vitamins, minerals, and trace elements. Vitamins are especially important in wound healing and immunity. Thiamine, riboflavin, niacin, and vitamin B_6 are components of enzymes and coenzymes used to metabolize carbohydrate, fat, and protein. Animal studies suggest that deficiencies in vitamins A and D, ascorbic acid, thiamine, folic acid, and others may reduce host resistance to infection.[7] The administration of vitamin supplements depends on the child's preinjury nutritional status. In children not previously deficient, supplements are approximately two to three times minimum daily requirements.[2] Excesses of fat-soluble vitamins (A, D, and E) can be toxic in large quantities and should be limited to recommended allowances. Selenium is an essential element in infants and children that provides antioxidant protection in concert with vitamin E.[20] Long-term total parenteral nutrition (TPN), which provides very little selenium, has been demonstrated to result in low serum levels and leg muscle pain in severe cases.

Calcium and phosphorus supplementation is especially important in infants and children because of the increased requirements for bone growth (Table 24-3). Hypophosphatemia can cause red blood cell and leukocyte dysfunction, encephalopathy and myopathy.[17] Hypomagnesemia can cause nausea, anorexia, neuromuscular irritability, and encephalopathy. Magnesium requirements are 1 to 2 mEq/kg/day for infants less than 6 months old and 0.5 mEq/kg/day for older infants and children.

NUTRITIONAL ASSESSMENT

The nutritional assessment provides a baseline of the child's nutritional state and aids in decisions regarding timing and selection of route of support. It begins with the dietary history, which defines the chronicity of the nutritional deficiencies (weight change, previous illness) and documents gastrointestinal complaints (vomiting, diarrhea, or food intolerance).

Objective data include anthropometric measurements and results of biochemical testing. The most common anthropometric measure, weight, is not reliable in critically injured children who undergo fluid resuscitation. This is because fluid shifts affect weight and may result in an underestimation of the actual loss of body mass. The triceps skinfold thickness is usually not affected by edema and is a more reliable estimate of total body fat. Protein stores are determined by estimating skeletal muscle mass from mid-arm muscle circumference. The excretion of creatinine, a by-product of creatine (muscle protein) can also be used to estimate total body muscle mass. Normal daily creatinine excretion (mg/kg/day) is equal to $15 + \frac{1}{2}$ age in years.[28]

Laboratory markers of visceral protein depletion are albumin and transferrin. Hypoalbuminemia is associated with increased mortality in all patients.[30] Albumin has a half-life of 20 days, so there is a delay in the measured decrease in protein malnutrition. An albumin level <3.0 mg/dl is indicative of either protein malnutrition or liver dysfunction. Low transferrin levels (<150 mg/dl) may indicate visceral protein depletion. Transferrin has a shorter half-life, 9 days, and is a more reliable indicator of recent protein depletion. Total lymphocyte count, derived from the differential white blood cell count, may be a function of protein malnutrition. Prothrombin level may be used as an indicator of vitamin K deficiency in the absence of liver disease.

ENTERAL FEEDINGS

There are definite physiological and economic advantages to enteral feedings, and they are preferred if a child's gastrointestinal tract is functioning. An understanding of the effects of critical illness on the gastrointestinal tract can explain when enteral feedings can be tolerated.

There are alterations in gastrointestinal enzymes and in the structure of intestinal villi in the critically ill child. Animal studies have shown that this gastrointestinal dysfunction is most likely to occur with parenteral nutrition and after a large burn injury.[10,16,19,22] Ileus can be due to any of a number of causes, including abdominal surgery, intraabdominal sepsis, head or spinal injury, and metabolic disturbances. Postoperative ileus does not affect the entire gastrointestinal tract uniformly. The stomach may be nonfunctional for 2 to 3 days. The motility of small bowel, however, usually returns within 24 hours.[31] Colonic function may take 3 to 5 days before returning to normal.[35] Prolonged ileus may be secondary to bowel wall edema, which can result from a low tissue oncotic pressure caused by an albumin deficit.[12] Albumin deficit can be calculated by this formula:

Albumin replacement = [3.0 g/dl − serum albumin (g/dl)] × [wt (kg) × 3]

The deficit is replaced with 25% albumin in three divided doses daily.

Enteral nutrition has been shown to be superior to parenteral nutrition in maintaining gastrointestinal integrity and gut hormonal balance. Food ingestion stimulates growth and replication of enterocytes and secretion of mucus.[4] In studies of the nutritional requirements of the gut itself, glutamine has been found to be a major energy source and nutrient. The gut uptake of glutamine exceeds that of any other amino acid. After severe injury, glutamine concentration in blood and skeletal muscle decreases and intestinal glutamine uptake increases. Current parenteral solutions contain no glutamine, and this may partly explain the villous atrophy in patients receiving long-term TPN. Preserving the gut-mucosal barrier through enteral nutrition may also affect the incidence of bacterial translocation from the gut to the systemic circulation. In a critically ill child with a compromised immune system, this can be of major concern.

Enteral nutrition preserves the normal physiologic sequence of nutrient absorption and metabolism. Feeding stimulates secretion of bile salts and results in decreased cholestasis. The safety of enteral nutrition versus parenteral nutrition has been debated. Clearly, the complications of central line insertion, such as pneumothorax, hydrothorax, hemothorax, and catheter embolus are avoided in enteral feedings. There are, however, inherent risks to enteral alimentation also, such as vomiting, aspiration, and diarrhea.

Enteral feeding can be instituted orally if the patient is awake and cooperative, but in the head-injured or critically ill child this is not usually an alternative. A nasoenteral tube is a traditional option. To avoid the hazards of reflux and aspiration, the tip of the tube should be positioned in the duodenum. A Dobhoff tube (weighted with mercury) is designed to be passed through the pylorus. Nasogastric or gastrostomy tube feedings, if tolerated without reflux, allow the choice of bolus feedings at some point. Children who require laparotomy or other operative interventions are candidates for placement of a needle catheter jejunostomy at the time of the operation.[24] Intestinal feedings should be given by continuous infusion. These should begin with small volumes (1 ml/kg/h) of half-strength formula. If this is well tolerated during the first 24 hours, volume can be increased by 0.5 ml/kg/h until the desired volume is being delivered. Once the required volume has been achieved, the concentration can be increased. If enteral feedings are delivered into the stomach, bolus feedings can be initiated by delivering 2 ml of formula per kilogram of body weight every 3 to 4 hours, starting with half-strength formula on the first day. If gastric residuals are not substantial, the volume can be gradually increased. The strength of the formula can be increased after the first day if diarrhea does not ensue. If stool output becomes unmanageable at any point in the tube feeding regimen, both strength and volume of the tube feeding can be decreased until it is tolerated.

The formula chosen for enteral feedings depends on the child's digestive activity, as well as on individual metabolic restrictions. The formulas can be thought of in three broad categories: formulas requiring normal digestion, elemental diets, and caloric additive or "modular" formulas (Table 24-4). Normal digestion formulas are composed of protein hydrolysates, glucose polymers, and long-chain fatty acids. They require intact lipolytic and proteolytic activity for digestion.

Elemental diets are available for children who have limited digestive ability. These are solutions of short-chain peptides (<3) or amino acids and simple sugars. They are usually low in fat. Elemental diets provide the advantage of easy and complete absorption in the upper small intestine with minimal residue. These are hyperosmolar, and gradual introduction is necessary to minimize osmotic diarrhea. Elemental diets are particularly useful for early postoperative feeding via jejunostomy and in the management of gastrointestinal fistulas.

Caloric additive diets are designed to provide extra calories or to supplement a specific nutrient. They also allow for possible mixing of separate sources, that is, "modules" for protein, carbohydrates, and fat.

TOTAL PARENTERAL NUTRITION

When use of the gastrointestinal tract is precluded because of severe acute illness and intestinal dysfunction, TPN can be instituted. Since 1968, when Dudrick demonstrated that central venous alimentation is life sustaining, this technique has been particularly valuable in infants and children in whom nutritional reserves are limited.[32]

Table 24–4 Composition of enteral formulas

	Calories (cal/ml)	Osmolality (mOsm/L)	Carbohydrate (g/L)	Fat (g/L)	Protein (g/L)
Normal digestion					
Ensure	1.0	450	145	37.0	37
Isocal	1.0	300	132	44.0	34
Pregestamil	0.67	350	90	27.0	18
Citrotein	0.71	495	130	1.7	44
Pediasure	1.0	310	108	49.0	29
Elemental					
Vivonex	1.0	550	231	1.0	22
Criticare HN	1.0	650	222	3.0	38
Modular components					
Polycose	2.0	850	500		
MCT oil	7.7	N/A		933	

TPN can be implemented by either a peripheral or a central route. Peripheral TPN offers the advantage of a lower incidence of catheter-related complications; however, it is difficult to achieve full nutritional support through the peripheral route. Peripheral infusion of glucose in concentrations of greater than 10% to 12% produces damage to the intima of veins, which can result in phlebitis and sclerosis. The peripheral administration of fat emulsions greatly augments the caloric value of peripheral nutrition. However, lipid intake (3 to 4 g/kg/day) is on average limited to 30% of total caloric requirements. In addition to caloric restraints, peripheral TPN prevents the use of hyperconcentrated glucose and amino acids, which are valuable when fluid restriction is indicated. Peripheral TPN may serve its greatest role as a supplement to an enteral diet in a child who will not or cannot eat enough to meet caloric needs.

Critical illness frequently precludes enteral feeding, and central TPN then becomes the best option for complete nutritional support. This is particularly appropriate when the need for prolonged support is anticipated and peripheral venous access is limited. The technique of central venous cannulation varies, depending on the size of the child, previous sites of insertion, and the child's injuries. In infants and young children the apex of the lung is high and the subclavian and jugular veins are small. Central venous lines in these children are usually inserted in the operating room by cutdown on the external or internal jugular vein. Older children or those weighing more than 10 kg can, generally, safely undergo percutaneous subclavian catheter placement.

Although perenteral nutrition in children has been used for about 20 years, data on the specific intravenous nutrient requirements are still very limited. There is large variation in TPN solution formulations.

Dextrose is the predominant carbohydrate source in parenteral solutions. In infants and children, a final solution containing 20% to 25% dextrose is usually sufficient if intralipid is also used. This hyperosmolar solution must be infused centrally where it is rapidly diluted.

All of the amino acid solutions contain the eight known essential amino acids plus histidine, which is considered essential in children.[36] There is much variability in the provision of "nonessential" amino acids. Some feel that all 20 amino acids used in protein synthesis should be provided in these formulations, but they often are not, usually for technical reasons.[15] Of the total amino acids provided, 40% to 50% are essential amino acids. Amino acids are available in 3% to 10% solutions. In infants, metabolism is more sensitive to varying mixtures of amino acids, and the content of methionine cysteine, phenylalanine, tyrosine, and glycine is of particular concern.

The high caloric density of lipid (9 kcal/g) has made it an excellent caloric supplement. It is available in 10% or 20% solutions, either of which may be infused centrally or peripherally. As previously mentioned, fat generally constitutes approximately 30% of total caloric intake. Intravenous fat solutions should be initiated in children at a slow rate and gradually increased if a child is having no reaction and if the serum triglyceride does not exceed 150 mg/dl. Above these levels, the lipoprotein-lipase enzyme system that metabolizes fat emulsions is saturated. The total daily amount of fat should be infused over at least 8 hours and bolus infusion avoided. Fat emulsions are now stable in hypertonic glucose solutions, and it is possible to infuse the two simultaneously.

The addition of electrolytes and minerals to the TPN solutions depends on the maintenance needs and ongoing losses of the child. Calcium (see Table 24-3) in the form of gluconate or chloride, phosphorous as sodium or potassium phosphate, and magnesium sulphate should be added. Trace elements (zinc, copper, manganese, and chromium) are routinely provided on a daily basis but are not actually required for several weeks after TPN is instituted.

Difficulty in maintaining intravenous access in infants and children may necessitate the concomitant administration of medications while the TPN solution is infusing. The list of drugs compatible with TPN includes ampicillin, cefazolin, clindamycin, cloxacillin, gentamicin, tobramycin, cimetidine, furosemide, heparin, hydrocortisone, regular insulin, and phenobarbital.[11] Intravenous lipid should be discontinued when drugs are administered because it is unstable when in contact with most additives.

COMPLICATIONS OF TOTAL PARENTERAL NUTRITION

Complications of TPN can be divided into technical complications resulting from catheter insertion, infectious complications, and metabolic complications. Most complications of central line insertion are related to the percutaneous approach to the subclavian. Pneumothorax, hemothorax, chylothorax, and brachial plexus injury can occur upon insertion of a subclavian line.

Late complications in the use of a central venous catheter include venous thrombosis in up to 20% of children, thromboemboli caused by the catheter tip, air embolism, and catheter erosion. Central line infections are usually the result of contamination during blood drawing or medication infusion. If possible the catheter should be limited to TPN infusion only, to minimize the risk of infection.

There are many potential metabolic complications of TPN. One of the most common is hyperglycemia secondary to glucose overinfusion. This may be of acute concern in children with diabetes, sepsis, or stress-related insulin resistance. Hypoglycemia can accompany a rapid cessation of TPN therapy, especially in neonates and infants. It is therefore important to wean children from TPN gradually if at all possible.

A wide variety of fluid, electrolyte, and mineral abnormalities can also result from TPN administration. Hyponatremia, especially in young infants, can result from dehydration and the inefficient urine concentration capacity of the kidney. Hyponatremia, on the other hand, is likely to result from water retention secondary to an impaired ability to excrete free water. Serum potassium may decrease, depending on gastrointestinal and renal losses, and should be replaced as necessary. Hyperkalemia is a possible danger in children with severe catabolism or acidosis, or after extensive muscle injury.

Intrahepatic cholestasis is a well-documented complication of prolonged TPN administration in infants. Jaundice and elevation in liver enzymes are typically seen. This is a condition that may be alleviated or prevented by cycling the TPN intermittently throughout the day. Severe cases have progressed to cirrhosis and liver failure.

Hypertriglyceridemia secondary to excessive intravenous fat administration should be prevented. Recent data on neonates have shown that intravenous fat infusion can inhibit polymorphonuclear leukocyte and platelet function.[14]

MONITORING THERAPY

Monitoring of TPN therapy has two purposes. The first is to ensure safe and accurate therapy through biochemical measurements that fluctuate acutely. The second is to measure the success or failure of therapy by assessing weight gain, muscle mass, and fat stores.

Biochemical factors are measured more frequently at the beginning of therapy. Initially, a complete baseline determination of blood count and blood chemisty is obtained. During the first 1 to 2 weeks, levels of serum electrolytes, blood urine nitrogen (BUN), creatinine, and glucose are obtained daily. The urine is checked each nursing shift to assess glucose levels. Complete blood count (CBC), prothrombin (PT), partial thromboplastin time (PTT), liver function studies, and calcium, phosphorous, and magnesium levels are obtained two to three times a week. After therapy has been adjusted to the child's metabolic needs and no further acute changes in formulations are expected, laboratory studies, including serum electrolytes, glucose, creatinine liver function tests, and CBC are performed once or twice a week. Blood cultures are prepared only if there is a clinical suspicion of infection, but not as a routine measure.

One of the most useful indicators in determining response to nutritional intervention is nitrogen balance, a measure of net changes in total protein mass. A positive nitrogen balance of 4 to 6 g is optimum. In calculating nitrogen balance, nonurinary nitrogen losses (through skin, stool, and hair) must be estimated and subtracted from the total nitrogen balance. When a formula is changed, at least 48 hours should elapse before nitrogen balance is recalculated. If there is persistent diarrhea of unknown etiology, it may be useful to perform a malabsorption workup that includes a fecal fat study, D-xylose test, Schilling test, and lactose tolerance test.

SUMMARY

Technologic and pharmaceutic advances have made possible a sophisticated array of nutritional support modalities. Adequate and early nutritional intervention can affect outcome in the management of injured children. There is no question that a child's nutritional status affects wound healing and competency of the immune system. In the future, nutritional support will be increasingly well tailored to fit the individual child's specific deficiencies in these areas.

At the present time, the available nutritional tools should be applied in a logical and consistent manner that follows basic physiologic principles. When possible, the enteral route is preferred. If gastrointestinal function is compromised, parenteral nutrition is available as a life-saving technology.

REFERENCES

1. Abbott WC, Echenique MM, Bistrian BR et al: Nutritional care of the trauma patient, *Surg Gyn Obstet* 157:585-597, 1983.
2. Alexander SJW: Nutrition and surgical infection, *Manual of surgical nutrition*, 1975, American College of Surgeons Committee on Pre and Post Operative Care p. 393.
3. Alexander JW: Nutrition and infection: new perspectives for an old problem, *Arch Surg* 121:966-972, 1986.
4. Alverdy J, Chi HS, Sheldon GF: The effect of parenteral nutrition on gastrointestinal immunity: the importance of enteral stimulation, *Ann Surg* 202:681-684, 1985.
5. Andrassy RJ: Choosing the right diet: amino acid vs peptide formulas, *Excerpta Medica Symposia Reporter* 14:1, 1990.
6. Andrassy RJ, Dubois T: Modified injury severity scale and concurrent steroid therapy: independent correlates of negative nitrogen balance in pediatric trauma, *J Pediatr Surg* 20:799-802, 1985.
7. Andrassy RJ, Nirgiotis JG: Preserving the gut and enhancing the immune response: the role of enteral nutrition in decreasing sepsis, *J Japanese Soc Pediatr Surg* 26:1057-1071, 1990.
8. Briglia FA, Pollock MM: Fluid and nutritional therapy in the critically ill child, *Indian J Pediatr* 54:819-829, 1987.
9. Dominioni L, Trocki O, Fang C et al: Enteral feeding in burn hypermetabolism: nutritional and metabolic effects of different levels of caloric and protein intake, *J Parenter Enteral Nutr* 9:269-229, 1985.
10. Eastwood GL: Small bowel morphology and epithelial proliferation in intravenously alimented rabbits, *Surgery* 82:613-620, 1977.
11. Fargo S: Compatibility of antibiotics and other drugs in total parenteral nutrition solutions, *Can J Hosp Pharm* 34:43, 1983.
12. Ford EG, Jennings LM, Andrassy RJ: Serum albumin (oncotic pressure) correlates with enteral feeding tolerance in the pediatric surgical patient, *J Pediatr Surg* 22(7):597-599, 1987.
13. Gadisseux P, Ward JD, Young HF et al: Nutrition and the neurosurgical patient, *J Neurosurg* 60:219-232, 1984.
14. Herson VC, Block C, Eisenfeld L et al: Effects of intravenous fat infusion on neonatal neutrophil and platelet function, *J Parenter Enteral Nutr* 6:620-622, 1989.
15. Jackson AA: Amino acids: essential and nonessential? *Lancet* VI (8332):1034-1036, 1983.
16. Johnson LR, Copeland EM, Dudrick SJ et al: Structural and hormonal alterations in the gastrointestinal tract of parenterally fed rats, *Gastroenterol* 68:1117-1183, 1975.
17. Krochel JP: The pathophysiology and clinical characteristics of severe hypophosphatemia, *Arch Intern Med* 137:203-220, 1977.
18. Kudsk KA, Stone J, Sheldon GF: Nutrition in trauma, *Surg Clin North Am* 61:671-679, 1981.
19. Levine GM, Dren JJ, Steiger ET et al: Role of oral intake in maintenance of gut mass and disaccharide activity, *Gastroenterol* 67:975-982, 1974.
20. Litou RE, Combs GF Jr: Selenium in pediatric nutrition, *Pediatrics* 87:339-351, 1991.
21. McCarthy MC: Nutritional support in the critically ill patient. *Surg Clin North Am* 71:831-841, 1991.
22. Mochizuki H, Trocki O, Dominioni L et al: Mechanism of prevention of postburn hypermetabolism and catabolism by early enteral feeding, *Ann Surg* 200:297-310, 1984.
23. Nirgiotis JG, Hennessey PJ, Andrassy RJ: The effects of an arginine free enteral diet upon wound healing and immune function in the post-surgical rat, *J Pediatr Surg* 26:936-941, 1991.
24. Page CP, Carlton PK, Andrassy RJ et al: Safe, Cost-effective postoperative nutrition: defined formula diet via needle-catheter jejunostomy, *Am J Surg* 138:939-945, 1979.
25. Rapp RP, Young B, Tyman D et al: The favorable effect of early parenteral feeding on survival in head-injured patients, *J Neurosurg* 58:906-912, 1983.
26. Reimer SL, Michener WM, Steiger E: Nutritional support of the critically ill child, *Pediatr Clin North Am* 27:647-660, 1980.
27. Ruderman NB: Muscle amino acid metabolism and gluconeogenesis, *Ann Rev Physiol* 37:245-258, 1975.
28. Siegler RL: Nutritional support. In Mayer TA, editor: *Emergency management of pediatric trauma*, ed 1, Philadelphia, 1985, WB Saunders, pp 125-138.
29. Souba WW, Smith RJ, Wilmore DW: Glutamine metabolism by the intestinal tract, *J Parenter Enteral Nutr* 9:608-617, 1985.
30. Sullivan M: Monitoring nutritional status of critically ill patients, *Excerpta Medica Symposia Reporter* 14:5, 1990.
31. Wells C, Tinkler L, Rawlinson K et al: Postoperative gastrointestinal motility, *Lancet* i:4, 1964.
32. Wilmore DW, Dudrick SJ: Growth and development of an infant receiving all nutrients exclusively by vein, *JAMA* 203:860, 1968.
33. Wilmore DW, Aulick LH, Mason AD Jr et al: The influence of the burn wound on local and systemic responses to injury, *Ann Surg* 186:444, 1977.
34. Windmueller HG: Glutamine utilization by the small intestine, *Advances in Enzymology* 53:202-237, 1982.
35. Woods JH, Erickson LW, Condon RE et al: Postoperative ileus: a colonic problem, *Surgery* 84:527, 1978.
36. Zlotkin SH, Stallings VA, Pencharz PB: Total parenteral nutrition in children, *Pediatr Clin North Am* 32:381-400, 1985.

25 Infection

Bernhard L. Wiedermann and William J. Rodriguez

Infectious complications of trauma are an important cause of morbidity and mortality in children. Survivors of the early posttrauma period are at increased risk for infection, related both to the secondary immunodeficiency from significant stress and trauma and to the complications of critical care, including the use of blood products, surgical procedures, and artificial devices such as vascular lines, urinary catheters, nasogastric and endotracheal tubes, and intracranial pressure–monitoring devices. Use of broad-spectrum antibiotics and parenteral hyperalimentation are further risk factors for the development of infection, particularly with multiply resistant organisms.

Infections following penetrating injuries are common, stab wounds being somewhat less likely to develop infection than trauma produced by projectiles. Several factors appear to be related, including the presence of a foreign body (bullet, shrapnel, clothing fragments) in the tissue, the extent of devitalized tissue produced (greater with high-velocity missiles and fragments), and the extent of internal organ disruption. Infections following nonpenetrating trauma are most common in burn patients. In children with blunt trauma, those with multiple organ trauma, and trauma to the esophagus, liver, or pancreas are more likely to develop infection.

This chapter addresses the practical aspects of preventing and managing infections in the injured child. Because many clinical situations do not fit well into standardized management protocols, it is most important to reassess the child and the treatment regimen continually, making adjustments as needed. Once the acute posttrauma period is over, the clinician must attempt to "wean" the patient from broad-spectrum antibiotics, indwelling devices, and other infectious hazards as soon as feasible to prevent new infectious complications.

USE OF THE MICROBIOLOGY LABORATORY

Appropriate use of the diagnostic services of a clinical laboratory is essential for optimal management of infection in injured children. Frequently, antibiotic therapy is begun on an empiric basis, but rapid test results, such as from Gram-stained smears of exudate or other specimens, are valuable aids in the selection of antimicrobial therapy. Although these tests cannot provide certain confirmation of a specific organism, they often permit the clinician to predict the types of organisms involved and, therefore, to make a more judicious therapeutic decision. In addition, the absence of bacteria on Gram-stained purulent material is sometimes a clue that other organisms, for example, fungi or mycobacteria, are the causative agents.

Proper use of culture materials can aid in diagnosis. Many pathogenic organisms are quite sensitive to the effects of heat, cold, oxygen, or drying, and specimens require special handling to ensure optimal recovery of organisms. It often happens that a large abscess is drained surgically, but only a single (often dry) swab of the material is sent for processing to the laboratory. It is optimal to provide a large quantity of material for culture and stain, ensuring laboratory personnel a sufficient amount of material for all appropriate tests. Specimens for anaerobic culture require anaerobic transport media, which should be available in all surgical suites and wards. Separate specimen containers for fungal and mycobacterial cultures are also necessary for proper culture potential. Similarly, viral cultures require specialized transport media and laboratory handling, depending on the specific virus suspected. Direct communication between the clinician and laboratory personnel is most helpful and prevents misunderstandings and errors in specimen collection.

PRINCIPLES OF ANTIMICROBIAL THERAPY

In general, the less antimicrobial therapy an injured child receives, the less likely the risk of superinfection with multiply resistant bacteria or opportunistic organisms. Therefore, one begins antibiotic therapy with clear goals that delineate a definite end point to limit therapy. The use of the term *prophylactic therapy* is misleading in reference to infection in the injured child, because most of the wounds are contaminated and antibiotic treatment is considered therapeutic rather than a prophylactic intervention. Still, in many instances of trauma, antibiotic therapy is initiated immediately following the injury, without clear-cut evidence of infection but with a high risk of infection. In many instances, however, it is difficult to prove a benefit for antibiotic treatment, because the infection risk is still relatively low. In other clinical presentations, such as compound fractures, the benefit is more readily apparent. Table 25-1 lists some situations in which this type of "prophylactic" therapy is probably useful. In keeping with principles of appropriate use of prophylaxis, the clinician should direct antimicrobial therapy not at all potential pathogens but at the most likely organisms capable of causing infection.

For established infections, Table 25-2 summarizes the common etiologic agents and recommendations for initial therapy. Table 25-3 provides a broader listing of antibiotics by class, with suggested pediatric dosages.

Table 25-1 Traumatic conditions usually requiring antimicrobial therapy

Open fractures
Ruptured gastrointestinal viscus with spillage
Penetrating trauma with foreign body
Any intracranial projectile injury

Table 25-2 Common etiologic organisms and drugs of choice for initial therapy* of trauma-related infections

Type of injury	Common organisms	Empiric therapy
Head and neck		
Intracranial (penetrating)	*Staphylococcus* species, Gram-negative enterics	Vancomycin plus 3rd gen. ceph.†
CSF leak	Pneumococcus, *Haemophilus*	3rd gen. ceph., ± vancomycin
Eyelid	*S. aureus,* group A *streptococcus*	Oxacillin
Cornea	Gram-positive, gram-negative	Ampicillin, penicillin, or clindamycin, others prn
Orbit	*B. cereus, S. epidermidis,* many others	Broad-spectrum multidrug (vancomycin, gentamicin, others)
Sinus-related	*S. aureus,* respiratory flora, nosocomial organisms	Cefuroxime or vancomycin plus 3rd gen. ceph.† if nosocomial
Mouth-related	Anaerobes, group A *streptococcus*	Penicillin or clindamycin
Chest	*S. aureus,* respiratory flora	See sinus above
Abdomen, pelvis	Anaerobes, gram-negative enterics	Cefoxitin, or clindamycin plus gentamicin
Contaminated wounds		
Soil	Multiple bacteria and fungi	Ticarcillin plus clavulanic acid
Salt water	*Aeromonas, Vibrio*	Aminoglycoside or 3rd gen. ceph.†
Fresh water	*Aeromonas, Pseudomonas, Mycobacterium marinum, Erysipelothrix*	Aminoglycoside
Bites		
Human	*Eikenella corrodens,* anaerobes, staphylococci	Ticarcillin plus clavulanic acid
Dog, cat	*Pasteurella multocida,* anaerobes, staphylococci	Ticarcillin plus clavulanic acid
Reptile	Mixed gram-positive, gram-negative, anaerobes	Ampicillin
Marine	See salt water, plus anaerobes	Ticarcillin plus clavulanic acid
Burns	*Staphylococci, streptococci, Pseudomonas*	Vancomycin plus aminoglycoside

*Therapy of established infections.
†Third-generation cephalosporin.

Table 25–3 Pediatric dosages for parenteral use of commonly used antimicrobial agents*

Drug	Daily dosage per KG	Dosing interval
Penicillin G	100,000-200,000 U	4-6 hr
Ampicillin	150-200 mg	4-6 hr
Oxacillin, nafcillin	100-150 mg	4-6 hr
Ticarcillin	150-300 mg	4-6 hr
Cefazolin	100 mg	6-8 hr
Cefoxitin	160 mg	8 hr
Cefuroxime	180 mg	8 hr
Cefotaxime	150-200 mg	8 hr
Ceftriaxone	50-75 mg	12-24 hr
Ceftazidime	100 mg	8 hr
Gentamicin†	5-7.5 mg	8 hr
Tobramycin†	5-7.5 mg	8 hr
Amikacin†	15-20 mg	8 hr
Clindamycin	25-40 mg	6-8 hr
Trimethoprim-sulfamethoxazole	6-12 mg (of trimethoprim)	12 hr
Chloramphenicol†	50-75 mg	6 hr
Vancomycin†	30-45 mg	6-8 hr
Metronidazole	30 mg	8 hr

*Doses given are for noncentral nervous system infections.
†Serum drug levels should be monitored during therapy.

INFECTIONS OF THE EYE AND PARANASAL SINUSES

Penetrating injuries can affect the eyelid, the orbital cavity, and the orbit, either singly or in combination. The depth of penetration and the nature of involvement (that is, whether the orbital septum is involved) determines the severity of the process. Whenever the septum is intact after superficial trauma, microorganisms such as *Staphylococcus aureus* and group A streptococci occur predominantly. Thus, initial antimicrobial therapy should include coverage for at least those two pathogens.

Infection of the lens is usually an insidious process, and a high level of suspicion on the part of the clinician is necessary for early diagnosis and institution of therapy. Gram-positive organisms from the skin or conjunctival sac, such as *Propioni bacterium,* contaminate the wound. Corneal ulcers occur following blunt injury to the eye from a baseball. Among others, *Pasteurella multocida,* a ubiquitous microbe usually associated with animals and birds, may be present in some cases. This finding emphasizes the need to obtain bacterial cultures early to help guide therapy, because *P. multocida* is very susceptible to penicillin and ampicillin but is less susceptible or resistant to other antimicrobial agents.

Penetrating injury to the orbit permits access of a variety of pathogens. *Bacillus* organisms are by far the most common agents recovered, particularly from injuries associated with penetrating metallic objects.[1] These bacteria produce gas and destroy the intravitreal contents of the eye. Consequently, it is imperative to use diagnostic vitrectomy for cultures as well as for administration of subconjunctival and intravitreal antibiotics such as clindamycin or vancomycin and gentamicin, while providing systemic infusion of the drugs. The duration of therapy is very controversial because of a lack of adequate clinical studies of this condition; a minimum of 5 days is necessary.

Osteomyelitis of facial bones, such as the maxilla, is a rare occurrence which causes facial and palatal swelling. Although one expects gram-positive bacteria, such as *S. aureus* and *Staphylococcus epidermidis,* gram-negative bacteria including the *Enterobacteriaceae* or *Pseudomonas* species do cause the infections. Additionally, this infectious process is sometimes polymicrobial in nature. *Pseudomonas aeruginosa* also causes osteomyelitis of the maxilla secondary to a vertical root fracture of the maxillary lateral incisors. In instances in which penetration of the oral mucosa occurs, expect mouth flora including anaerobic organisms. When they are present, necrotizing fasciitis may result, especially in cases of mandibular fracture. Obtaining appropriate cultures to establish etiology is critical in determining definitive antimicrobial therapy.

Even nasotracheal intubation in children without preceding head trauma results in paranasal (predominantly maxillary) sinusitis.[9] *S. aureus* is the predominant organism, followed by facultative gram-negative aerobes such as members of the *En-*

terobacteriaceae, and anaerobic flora such as *Bacteroides* species. An aggressive diagnostic approach, preferably using computerized tomography (CT) of the sinuses with bone window settings and supplemented by aspiration of the affected sinus contents for Gram stain and culture is optimal. Initial empiric antimicrobial therapy should be directed to cover the common nosocomial pathogens of the individual hospital. However, removal of the nasal tubes and administration of nasal decongestants tend to speed up the recovery process. Bacteremia has been found to be extremely rare in this situation.

INFECTIONS OF THE CENTRAL NERVOUS SYSTEM

Infections of the central nervous system occur in association with approximately 10% of trauma cases. Disruption of the dura mater resulting in cerebrospinal fluid (CSF) leak is a common mode of intracranial infection; meningitis followed by ventriculitis and brain abscess also occurs. When confronted with meningitis without obvious intracranial penetration, assume the presence of cranial (temporal bone) or cribriform plate fracture with resultant CSF leak. Obvious leaks that persist more than 8 weeks require surgical repair. The bacteriology associated with infections following these traumatic events reflects the portal of entry. Hence, cribriform plate fractures, or those with close association to mucosal respiratory flora, are associated with traditional respiratory pathogens such as *Streptococcus pneumoniae, Haemophilus influenzae,* and, occasionally, *S. aureus.* Gram-negative enteric bacteria and anaerobes infect the region infrequently. The growth of *P. multocida* in the CSF of immunocompromised children who have sustained trauma rarely occurs without obvious intracranial trauma. In these cases, the respiratory tract provides the portal of entry.

When the injury is caused by penetrating projectiles, such as lawn darts or gunshots, skin surface flora and soil organisms predominate. Occasionally, unusual pathogens, such as *Pseudomonas paucimobilis,* are recovered. An abscess develops early, usually within 4 to 6 weeks after injury. Delays in recognition of the condition and definitive treatment result in high mortality and morbidity.

Central nervous system infection can also occur as an undesirable side effect of technologic advances, such as insertion of intracranial monitoring devices that measure intracranial pressure.[8] Unfortunately, the system provides bacterial access into the subarachnoid space or ventricle; nosocomial bacterial infection occurs particularly when the device remains in place longer than 5 days.

Table 25–4 Penetration of selected antimicrobial agents through inflamed meninges

Antibiotic	Approximate % penetration*
Cephalothin†	15
Cefuroxime†	15
Cefoxitin†	50
Ceftazidime	20
Cefotaxime	10
Ceftriaxone	5
Clindamycin†	Nil
Chloramphenicol	50-100
Metronidazole	50-100
Penicillin G	5-18
Ampicillin	5-14
Oxacillin, nafcillin	9-20
Mezlocillin	3-20
Piperacillin	8-30
Ticarcillin	20-40
Rifampin	30
Sulfisoxizole	80-100
Trimethoprim	30
Vancomycin	20
Amphotericin B	Nil‡

*Expressed as a percentage of concomitant serum levels.
†Not recommended for use in central nervous system infections.
‡Higher levels have been recorded in premature infants, and amphotericin B may accumulate in meningeal tissue.

In attempting to formulate therapy against significant potential pathogens, consider the intracranial nature of the infection, the predisposing factors, the suspected identity of the pathogen, and the ability of the antibiotic to enter brain tissue or CSF. Table 25-4 shows generally the CNS penetration by various antimicrobial agents. The beta lactam antibiotics (with extended gram-negative spectra), along with an antimicrobial drug with a reasonable gram-positive spectrum, such as vancomycin, provide adequate treatment during the wait for definitive bacterial identification and organism susceptibility results. Aggressive evacuation of any identifiable accumulation of pus is mandatory.

It is of interest that even fungal agents such as *Coccidioides immitis* can cause meningitis following head injury with open skull fracture and contaminated wounds. In those cases, initial treatment with amphotericin, followed by long-term therapy with fluconazole or other antifungal agents, may be necessary.

Subgaleal infections, which occur in association with trauma and minor scalp wounds, may develop into extensive abscesses with progression to fatal necrotizing fasciitis. Furunculosis of the scalp is also possible as a consequence of facultative gram-negative bacilli and *Clostridium perfringens* infection. A third-generation cephalosporin and penicillin constitute effective treatment. Additionally, necrotizing fasciitis associated with scalp wounds occurs with infection by staphylococci and group A streptococci. Meticulous attention to aggressive debridement and drainage frequently prevents death.[18]

Fractures of the skull have also been complicated with gas gangrene caused by *C. perfringens,* either singly or in association with *Escherichia coli.* This complication appears within 24 hours after compound depressed skull fracture.[16] A high level of suspicion, appropriate aggressive debridement, and treatment with penicillin (for *C. perfringens*) and antibiotic medication for gram-negative bacteria, are therapeutic.

Trauma to the spinal cord results in a variety of infectious processes. Following dislocation of the atlantoaxial joint, group A β-hemolytic streptococcal peripharyngeal abscess may develop.[4] In individuals with longstanding spinal cord injury who have a fever of unknown origin, *S. aureus* and gram-negative enteric bacteria cause a primary pyomyositis of the thigh musculature. After fracture of the spinal column, osteomyelitis secondary to *Serratia marcescens* (or, rarely, fungi) occurs in immunosuppressed individuals. A high level of suspicion is necessary to detect infection in children with spinal cord trauma. Initial antimicrobial drug coverage effective against both gram-positive and gram-negative bacteria is reasonable. Appropriate bacterial culture guides definitive therapy in conjunction with evacuation of purulent collections.

CHEST INFECTIONS

Approximately one third of children who sustain trauma to the thorax will develop pneumonia. Prolonged hospitalization permits colonization of their respiratory tracts by hospital flora. Colonization by enteric bacteria is a step that often leads to subsequent development of gram-negative bacterial pneumonia. Moreover, endotracheal intubation accelerates this process. *S. pneumoniae, S. aureus* and *Haemophilus* species are common pathogens, as are *Klebsiella* species and other gram-negatives such as *Pseudomonas.* Children with *Pseudomonas* species colonization have a high risk for secondary bacteremia and for increased mortality.

Infection of the mediastinum along with sternal osteomyelitis secondary to *S. aureus* infection occurs in association with closed cardiac compression during resuscitation. Sternal fracture and subsequent bacteremia may explain the pathogenesis of this rare infection.

Children who manifest a pneumothorax that requires placement of a thoracostomy tube can develop empyema with gram-negative bacteria, such as coliforms and *Pseudomonas* species. In those cases in which hemothorax is extant, *S. aureus* is the predominant organism.

Following thoracotomy, infection caused by gram-positive aerobic bacteria, facultative gram-negative rods, *Pseudomonas* species, or anaerobic bacteria is possible. Hence, vancomycin combined with either an aminoglycoside or a third-generation cephalosporin is reasonable for initial therapy of infectious conditions that involve the mediastinum. If anaerobic bacteria are detected, clindamycin or metronidazole is useful. It is important to remember that metronidazole is not effective against gram-positive anaerobes.

In anticipation of the need for antimicrobial intervention, obtain a Gram stain and culture of the endotracheal secretions, if they are particularly increased or thickened, to detect bacterial flora and to determine drug susceptibility. In symptomatic children, a specimen brush and quantitative culture are useful in establishing a diagnosis of nosocomial pneumonia.

The prophylactic use of antibiotics is controversial, and the degree of contamination caused by the trauma determines the need for presumptive treatment during the wait for culture confirmation of specific identification of the pathogenic organisms. Antimicrobial therapy directed against gram-positive bacteria, especially staphylococci, and gram-negative bacteria, generally constitutes sufficient initial treatment. Gram stains and cultures are indispensable in determining treatment.

INTRAABDOMINAL INFECTIONS

Contamination of the peritoneal cavity by intestinal contents or foreign bodies is the primary mode of acquisition of intraabdominal infection in the injured child. Occasionally, abdominal infections are attributable to contiguous spread from other infected sites, such as the pleural space, skin, or bone.

In cases of penetrating trauma, spillage of gastrointestinal contents usually results in polymicrobial infection and eventual abscess formation. Commonly involved are *S. aureus, Enterobacteriaceae* such as *E. coli* and the *Klebsiella-Enterobacter* groups, *Pseudomonas aeruginosa,* and anaerobes such as *Bacteroides fragilis, Peptostreptococcus,* and other organisms. Early antibiotic therapy lessens the chance of major infectious complications in this patient group, but discontinuation of therapy within 5 days is indicated, especially in the absence of clinical infection. Published trials that com pare antibiotic regimens for abdominal injury do not establish the best combination. However, we prefer the use of a regimen with adequate coverage for the common organisms found, particularly anaerobes and the *Enterobacteriaceae*.[3,10]

Abscess formation is usually accompanied by persistent fever, abdominal pain, and peritoneal signs. Most abscesses develop in the pelvic gutter, in the subphrenic or subhepatic space, or in the lesser sac. Abdominal CT scan and sonogram are valuable diagnostic aids, although it may be difficult to distinguish abscess from hematoma or inflammatory tissue mass on the basis of these studies. Use of a gallium scan is less helpful, because false-positive findings may occur as a consequence of the injury. Reexploration with drainage of purulent material or percutaneous drainage of the abscess is essential. Antibiotic therapy should continue until clinical evidence of infection resolves.

Blunt trauma to the abdomen may also cause intraabdominal infection, even in the absence of overt signs of bowel perforation, and bacteremia may develop. There is no clear evidence that early antibiotic therapy is useful in this situation. It may serve only to select out resistant organisms, allowing them to cause a nosocomial infection. Therefore, antibiotic therapy in the absence of spillage of intestinal contents is unnecessary.

GENITOURINARY INFECTION

Most urinary tract infections in injured children are related to the use of indwelling urinary catheters. Fortunately, the sequelae are usually mild and urosepsis is uncommon. The *Enterobacteriaceae* such as *E. coli* and *Klebsiella* are the common pathogens in the urinary tract, but *Pseudomonas* and *Candida* infections are also seen, the latter particularly with long-term use of broad-spectrum antibiotics. Diagnosis may be difficult because most children with long-term indwelling urinary catheters manifest bacteriuria, which usually represents colonization of the catheter rather than a true infection of the bladder. The presence of pyuria or systemic signs of infection are indicators of a true urinary tract infection. For children who require long-term bladder catheterization, it is helpful to perform a routine urinalysis and urine culture. Proper surveillance permits early identification of infection.

Treatment of catheter-associated urinary tract infections is possible by removal of the catheter, especially for the child who does not show signs of systemic infection. If subsequent urine culture 24 to 48 hours later shows presence of the pathogen, systemic antimicrobial therapy (oral or parenteral) is therapeutic. Treatment for 5 to 7 days is sufficient for infection confined to the bladder, but upper urinary tract involvement may require 10 to 14 days of antimicrobial therapy. Therefore, exclusion of upper urinary tract disease by renal sonogram or by renal scan with 99 m Tc-dimercaptosuccinic acid is helpful. In the special case of bladder candidiasis, bladder washout with amphotericin B may be curative without resorting to systemic therapy. Infusion of amphotericin B (10 μg/mL) into the bladder in a volume sufficient to fill the viscus and maintenance of the solution within the bladder for 90 minutes is a useful maneuver to treat the candidiasis. This regimen is repeated over a period of 5-to-7-days and is usually sufficient to eradicate bladder infection. If cultures remain positive for *Candida* after treatment, further exploration for other foci of infection is indicated.

SEPSIS

Bacteremia is a frequent complication of severe injury, associated particularly with multiple-system trauma and with shock. Major factors that cause infection by pathogenic organisms are direct contamination of the vascular space, a viscus rupture, and central venous access. Infections associated with bacteremia also reflect the overall gravity of the injury.[14]

Some organisms are more likely than others to cause vascular contamination and septicemia. For example, *S. aureus* is a common cause of bacteremia, as are *Klebsiella* species, *E. coli*, and *Enterobacter* species. *P. aeruginosa* is also frequently seen in infections involving the respiratory or the gastrointestinal tract.[14]

Because it is difficult to recognize infection in sedated or comatose children in whom fever may be the sole clinical finding, the peripheral white blood cell count is often useful. Also helpful is measurement of the platelet count, BUN, creatinine, and blood culture from any indwelling vascular catheters and from a peripheral vein. Initial antimicrobial therapy is most appropriate when information is available about the common nosocomial pathogens in a particular care unit. Further modification is possible if blood culture precedes initiation of therapy. Generally, empiric therapy early in a child's hospitalization involves an agent with antistaphylococcal activity combined with an aminoglycoside or a third-generation cephalosporin. For nosocomial infection, when multiply resistant organisms are more suspect, antistaphylococcal agents, such as vancomycin, and an appropriate gram-negative antimicrobial drug are indicated. An aggressive diagnostic effort to identify the pathogen is critical. Once culture-specific information is available, appropriate modification of the initial plan of therapy is possible.

INFECTIONS OF SKIN AND SUBCUTANEOUS TISSUE

Injuries that disrupt the skin surface produce dirty wounds. Although chances for development of infection and for morbidity are great, wound infection does not contribute significantly to mortality.

Overall, gram-positive bacteria are the most common causes of infection of skin and subcutaneous tissue in injured children; *S. aureus* and *Streptococcus pyogenes* (group A *Streptococcus*) are the most important. *S. aureus*, the most common cause of wound infection, also results in bacteremia, osteomyelitis, abscess, and complications related to toxin production, such as toxic shock syndrome, scarlet fever–like syndrome, and scalded skin syndrome in infants. Group A streptococcal infections may typically produce rapidly spreading cellulitis (erysipelas) and cause bacteremia, osteomyelitis, and distant abscess. More recently, pyogenic toxin-producing strains of group A *Streptococcus* have been associated with a "toxic strep syndrome," often resulting in septic shock and other serious complications.[13] Gram-negative bacilli are also common causes of skin infection, usually developing later in the course of care.

Other organisms causing cutaneous infections are associated with specific mechanisms of injury.[2,5,7,12] For example, cat bite wounds result in a rapidly progressing cellulitis because of the presence of *P. multocida*. Wounds contaminated with saltwater result in infection by *Vibrio* species such as *Vibrio vulnificus*. Deep infections following puncture wounds of the foot almost always involve *Pseudomonas aeruginosa*, sometimes in combination with *S. aureus*. In these special situations, it is often helpful to notify the bacteriology laboratory so that technologists may focus attention upon isolation and identification of these unusual organisms.

An open fracture presents a special case of skin and subcutaneous tissue infection, in that osteomyelitis is a dreaded possible complication. The fracture is usually contaminated with bacteria before institution of any specific therapy. The risk of development of osteomyelitis parallels the degree of soft tissue damage occurring with the injury. A fracture associated with a clean, small (<1 cm) laceration is relatively unlikely to develop infection, whereas a laceration greater than 1 cm that has extensive soft tissue damage, such as in a farm-related injury, a neglected injury, or a gunshot wound, is more likely to develop significant infection.[6] The organisms complicating such an open fracture are similar to those that cause soft tissue infection. Duration of therapy for osteomyelitis accompanying such an injury, however, requires several weeks. Diagnosis of osteomyelitis is difficult and usually requires histologic confirmation because radiologic assessment is misleading in the presence of a fracture.

Two serious forms of wound infection merit special attention because of their severity. Clostridial myonecrosis, or gas gangrene, occurs in situations of local trauma in which the site is contaminated with *C. perfringens* or, occasionally, other clostridial species. There are significant pain locally, swelling, crepitus, and often patches of bullae and necrosis present. Fever, toxic appearance, and rapid course are common. Deep surgical drainage, debridement of necrotic tissue, and administration of high-dose penicillin G are essential. Hyperbaric oxygen therapy is a useful adjunct. More common than myonecrosis, however, is clostridial cellulitis, in which the process is confined to the skin and to the subcutaneous tissue without involvement of deep fascia or muscle. Progression is usually not as rapid as in myonecrosis, and bullae are usually absent; nevertheless, treatment is the same.

Necrotizing fasciitis is another serious soft tissue infection that carries a high mortality. Onset is gradual, over a period of 3 to 7 days, with development of cutaneous erythema "tissue swelling" and a shiny appearance to the skin surface. The wound is usually exquisitely tender, and the infected child manifests systemic toxicity. Eventually, areas of cutaneous necrosis appear, and the area becomes anesthetic following interruption of neural and vascular supply to the site. Successful treatment requires early recognition and aggressive surgical debridement. Histologic findings on tissue biopsy, which may consist of superficial fascial necrosis with acute inflammatory infiltration and small vessel inflammation with thrombi, are helpful both in making a diagnosis and in ensuring that debridement has removed all involved tissue. Multiple debridement procedures are often needed. A number of organisms, including *S. aureus*, group A *Streptococcus* and other streptococci, the *Enterobacteriaceae*, and anaerobes such as *Bacteroides* and *Peptostreptococcus* species cause this process. Therefore, initial therapy with broad-spectrum drugs to cover anaerobic, gram-positive, and gram-negative bacteria is essential. Even with optimal therapy, mortality approaches 12%.[15]

INFECTIONS IN BURN PATIENTS

Children with extensive burns are very prone to infection, owing to both the extensive disruption of the protective dermal layer and serious compromise of normal host defense mechanisms. Unfortunately, 50% of all mortality resulting from burns is associated with infection. Therefore, prevention and early recognition of burn wound infection is important for effective management.

The use of prophylactic systemic antibiotic therapy for children with serious burns is not beneficial. However, systemic antibiotic therapy is a helpful adjunct during grafting procedures or extensive debridement. The choice of agents depends on the predominant flora in the child and the burn center.

Use of topical antimicrobial agents, early excision of burn wounds, and early wound coverage with skin grafts have reduced the incidence of serious infection-complicated burns. Other measures that enhance therapy and reduce infection are enteral (rather than parenteral) nutrition and avoidance of long-term indwelling vascular catheters.

Silver sulfadiazine (Silvadene) is the most popular topical antimicrobial agent. It is active against gram-negative bacteria and yeasts, but not against gram-positive bacteria. It does not penetrate the eschar well and can occasionally cause neutropenia and hypersensitivity reactions such as urticaria or anaphylaxis. Mafenide acetate (Sulfamylon) is active against gram-positive and gram-negative bacteria and yeasts. Unfortunately, treatment is painful and causes hypersensitivity reactions. Some centers prefer to alternate these topical agents to discourage the development of resistant pathogenic bacteria. Mupirocin (Bactroban), active only against gram-positive bacteria, is useful as topical treatment for methicillin-resistant *S. aureus* cutaneous burn infections.[11] Routine replacement of indwelling vascular catheters every 3 days reduces septicemia. Use of oral nystatin to decrease yeast colonization in the intestinal tract lacks proof of efficacy.

Surface cultures of wounds are not as helpful as punch skin biopsy specimens for histology or quantitative culture to allow diagnosis of burn wound infection. Demonstration of tissue invasion by bacteria or fungi, or growth of greater than or equal to 10^5 organisms per gram of tissue, correlates well with a poor outcome.[17]

A change in the appearance of the burn eschar or purulent wound drainage is clinical evidence of burn wound colonization; surgical debridement or a change in topical therapy is indicated. Systemic signs of illness, such as hypotension, tachycardia, ileus, oliguria, altered mental status, thrombocytopenia or other hematologic changes, and unexplained metabolic acidosis indicate current or impending sepsis. Institution of parenteral antimicrobial therapy, after appropriate cultures are obtained, is essential. Fever is a relatively unreliable sign of infection in burned children, because extensive tissue destruction stimulates a febrile reaction for many days even in the absence of infection. Cytomegalovirus infection is a common cause of fever in burned children but seldom causes significant morbidity or mortality.

SYSTEMIC TOXIN-RELATED DISEASES ASSOCIATED WITH TRAUMA
Rabies

Rabies is caused by rhabdoviruses transmitted in the saliva of infected animals. Any bite or scratch from an infected animal that causes a break in the skin can result in transmission of the virus. Risk factors for the disease are type of animal, whether the attack was provoked or unprovoked, and the prevalence of the disease in the geographic area. A local health department can provide information on prevalence. Raccoons, foxes, bats, skunks, and woodchucks are typical carriers of the rabies virus. Domestic animals in the United States, such as dogs and cats, are seldom infected, particularly if immunized. Bites from lagomorphs and rodents including rats, rabbits, and squirrels rarely need prophylaxis for rabies. When an animal is infected, it usually becomes symptomatic within 3 days. Diagnosis of rabies is accomplished by immunofluorescent staining of infected tissue.

Acute treatment of any wound inoculated with saliva contaminated with the virus includes local wound care, human antirabies immunoglobulin treatment, and human diploid cell–strain vaccine. Wound care consists of a soap scrub to cause bleeding, and water irrigation. Application of iodine solutions, alcohol, or quaternary ammonium is helpful but not superior to the use of soap. If these agents are used, however, they should be applied after removal of soap, which could inactivate them. Administer human antirabies immunoglobulin (20 IU/kg) by injecting half around the wound and half intramuscularly. Provide human diploid-cell rabies vaccine as soon as possible, preferably as soon as the rabid status of the animal is proven or strongly suspected. Five doses (1 ml/dose) are given, one initially, then at 3, 7, 14, and 28 days. Injection in the deltoid muscle is preferable for adults because some have had lower antibody response when injected in the gluteal area. Delay primary closure of the wound and debride deep puncture wounds. Isolate children suspected of having rabies, including the use of barriers against aerosolized saliva. Tranquilization, sedation, and anticonvulsant medication are important adjuncts, as are routine supportive care and measures to reduce cerebral edema. There is, however, no effective treatment for rabies, and survival is quite rare.

Tetanus

Tetanus, also referred to as "lockjaw," has been well known since biblical times. The disease is mediated by the exotoxin released by the spore-forming organism, *Clostridium tetani*. This microbe can be recovered from the stool of humans and animals and from the environment. Introduction of the spores into injured tissue and anaerobic wounds lead to generation and release of the toxin. Conditions that can encourage the disease range from contamination of the umbilical stump of neonates, either accidentally or by unsanitary delivery

Table 25–5 Use of adult diphtheria-tetanus vaccine (Td) and tetanus immune globulin (TIG) for tetanus prophylaxis*

	Type of wound			
	Minor, clean		Other wounds†	
Past medical history	Td‡	TIG	Td‡	TIG
Status unknown or incomplete primary series	+	−	+	−
Primary series completed or more§	− #	−	− ‖	−

* Modified from the report of the Committee on Infectious Diseases of the American Academy of Pediatrics, ed 21, 1988.
† Puncture wounds, wounds caused by penetrating projectiles, thermal wounds, crushing injuries, wounds contaminated by dust, soil, saliva, fecal matter.
‡ For patients older than 7 years; younger patients use DT or DTP.
§ A fourth dose of absorbed toxoid is recommended beyond the first three doses.
# Patients who received the last dose over 10 years ago should be given a booster.
‖ If the last booster was given more than 5 years ago, please give another dose.

practices, to contamination of wounds (even surgical wounds) by stool or dirt where the spores are found. Tetanus is a preventable disease, and the routine immunization practices recommended by the American Academy of Pediatrics along with recall immunization every 10 years are sufficient to preserve immunity. This recommendation is applicable to minor clean wounds. For any injury in which there is gross contamination (such as with stool, saliva, or dirt) that occurs 5 years or more after the preceding dose of tetanus vaccine, another booster dose of 0.5 ml is imperative.

Specifically, if the history of immunization is unknown or not up to date, for minor wounds administer only adult tetanus and diphtheria toxoid (Td). Major wounds in children with uncertain or incomplete immunization history, particularly those associated with crushing, missile, thermal, or puncture injuries should have Td and tetanus immunoglobulin (TIG) 250 U given intramuscularly. Tetanus antitoxin (TAT) can be used if TIG is unavailable. Injured children whose tetanus immunizations are up to date do not need reimmunization unless the injury is major and more than 5 years have elapsed since the last tetanus shot (Table 25-5).

For children with clinical manifestations of disease, debridement of the wound is imperative. Tetanus immunoglobulin (500 to 3000 U) is injected, half intramuscularly and half around the wound. If no TIG is available, administer TAT in a dose of 50,000 to 100,000 U (after first testing the child for hypersensitivity). Penicillin G (100,000 U/kg/day) is provided for 10 to 14 days. Tetracyclines can also be used for children 9 years of age and older. Sedation, reduction of environmental stimuli, and preservation of the airway are mainstays of supportive care for children with this disease.

Diphtheria

Diphtheria is an extremely rare disease in the United States, but more common in tropical climates. Initially, the area of skin inoculated with *Corynebacterium diphtheriae* becomes ulcerated and has well-defined borders. The base may show a gray, dense membrane similar to that seen in other forms of the disease. If the strain involved produces diphtheria toxin and the host is not immune, signs of intoxication such as neuritis or myocarditis develop. However, this is less likely to occur in a wound than with diphtheria involved in other sites. In individual cases, it may be difficult to determine whether a *C. diphtheriae* isolate from a wound is just a commensal organism or is actually causing cutaneous disease. Treatment is with penicillin; antitoxin does not appear to have any benefit in cutaneous diphtheria.

CONCLUSIONS

Infections in the injured child are significant causes of morbidity and mortality. Proper management requires knowledge of the major pathogens associated with different types of trauma and an understanding of the use of laboratory results and proper antibiotic therapy. Even with optimal management, infections will continue to occur in injured children. Trauma prevention will provide the most significant advances in reducing the impact of disease on children.

REFERENCES

1. Affeldt JC, Flynn HW, Foster RK et al: Microbial endophthalmitis resulting from ocular trauma, *Ophthalmology* 94:407-413, 1987.
2. Brennan SR, Rhodes KH, Peterson HA: Infection after farm machine-related injuries in children and adolescents, *Am J Dis Child* 144:710-713, 1990.
3. Brook I: Management of infection following intra-abdominal trauma, *Ann Emerg Med* 17:626-632, 1988.
4. Clark WC, Coscia CM, Acker JD et al: Infection-related spontaneous atlantoaxial dislocation in an adult; case report, *J Neurosurg* 69:455-458, 1988.
5. Dellinger EP, Wertz MJ, Miller SD et al: Hand infections: bacteriology and treatment: a prospective study, *Arch Surg* 123:745-750, 1988.
6. Gustilo RB, Gruninger RP, Davis T: Classification of type III (severe) open fractures relative to treatment and results, *Orthopedics* 10:1781-1788, 1987.
7. Huiming T, Deng G, Huang M et al: Quantitative bacteriologic study of the wound track, *J Trauma* 28(suppl 1):S215-216, 1988.
8. Kanter RK, Weiner LP, Patti AM et al: Infectious complications and duration of intracranial pressure monitoring, *Crit Care Med* 13:837-839, 1985.
9. Linden BE, Aguilar EA, Allen SJ: Sinusitis in the nasotracheally intubated patient, *Arch Otolaryngol Head Neck Surg* 114:860-861, 1988.
10. Nichols RL, Smith JW, Klein DB et al: Risk of infection after penetrating abdominal trauma, *N Engl J Med* 311:1065-1070, 1984.
11. Rode H, Hanslo D, de Wet PM et al: Efficacy of mupirocin in methicillin-resistant *Staphylococcus aureus* burn wound infection, *Antimicrob Agents Chemother* 33:1358-1361, 1989.
12. Semel JD, Trenholme G: *Aeromonas hydrophila* water-associated traumatic wound infections: a review, *J Trauma* 30:324-327.
13. Stevens DL, Tanner MH, Winship J et al: Severe group A streptococcal infections associated with a toxic shock-like syndrome and scarlet fever toxin A, *N Engl J Med* 321:1-7, 1989.
14. Stillwell M, Caplan ES: The septic multiple trauma patient, *Critical Care Clin* 4:345-373, 1988.
15. Sudarsky LA, Laschinger JC, Coppa GF et al: Improved results from a standardized approach in treating patients with necrotizing fasciitis, *Ann Surg* 206:661-665, 1987.
16. Sutcliffe JC, Miller JD, Whistle IR et al: Gas gangrene occurring after compound depressed skull fracture. *Acta Neurochir* (Wien) 95:53-56, 1988.
17. Taddonia TE, Thomson PD, Tait MJ et al: Rapid quantification of bacterial and fungal growth in burn wounds: biopsy homogenate Gram stain versus microbial culture results, *Burns Incl Therm Inj* 14:180-184, 1988.
18. Wiley JF, Sugarman JM, Bell LM: Subgaleal abscess: an unusual presentation, *Ann Emerg Med* 18:785-787, 1989.

26 Care of Traumatic Wounds

Robert M. Arensman, Geoffrey C. Fenner, William A. Loe, Jr., and Daniel J. Ledbetter

Trauma is the most important illness of childhood and is the primary cause of death. A wound may be defined as a disruption of normal dermal anatomic relationships resulting from injury. Whether traumatic wounds are the consequence of isolated soft tissue injuries or major, multisystem injuries, optimal treatment follows basic and biologic surgical principles.

Skin has many biologic functions and physical properties. Within an individual, each dermatologic segment has a unique set of characteristics based on the quantity, quality, and interactions of collagen, elastin, and the ground substance. Important principles of wound healing and surgical repair are based on visoelastic properties, skin tension and extensibility, inflammation, and collagen synthesis. Practical surgical repair of wounds encompasses a broad, yet basic, protocol based on a knowledge of the extent and mechanism of injury.

ASSESSMENT

Overall care of a child with a soft tissue injury must begin with a complete evaluation of the child and history of the accident. The mechanism of injury, wound location, depth, size, degree of contamination, and the time elapsed since the accident are important variables. In addition, individual factors, including age, nutrition, presence of diabetes, steroid use, and peripheral vascular disease or coagulopathy have great impact on the eventual treatment of an injury.

After initial routine assessment and resuscitation, a history should be obtained from the child or reliable witnesses. Was a motor vehicle accident, fall, stab, or gunshot the mechanism of injury? Did the wound result from a handgun of large or small caliber, of high or low velocity, or from a short-range sawed-off shotgun? Was a fork, jackknife, or machete employed? Was a clean plate-glass window, a grimy drill press or a carnivorous assailant the cause of injury? What degrees of blood loss, shock, and resuscitation were recorded or required? This information will guide the physician in selecting subsequent radiologic studies, specialty consultations, antibiotic therapy, type of closure, length of observation and admission, and frequency of outpatient follow-up.

The initial contact between the physician and child is often stressful. First of all, the injury is likely to be recent and still painful. In addition, the clinical environment is terrifying, either because it is strange or because it stirs memories of previous similar experiences. A simple initial observation of the injury in an apprehensive child, therefore, will serve to calm the child and permit observation of neuromuscular function indicative of intact tendons and nerves.[73] Prior to the formal physical examination, time spent in reassuring the child of the physician's good intentions will often be worthwhile. The physician's hands should be empty and movements should be slow. As many of the required tests as possible should be performed before the dressing is removed. If pain must be inflicted, it should be withheld until the end of the examination, because all cooperation will cease at that point. Children, if very fearful, can sometimes be calmed by the firm promise that they will be warned if they are to be hurt at any stage. Remember that deception dispels the trust of children forever.

Proper systematic physical examination is imperative for proper wound management. Such examination is dependent upon lighting, instrumentation, anesthesia, and the maturity of the patient. First, the skin should be inspected for the location and nature of any contusions, abrasions, or wounds. Contusions or abrasions may indicate damage to the underlying skeleton. The site of an open wound is often significant, but its size is not. A wound of any size that gapes and reveals a dark blood clot usually covers deep damage.

To be aware of the significance of a particular site, the surgeon must have a thorough knowledge of the underlying anatomy. Location of the wound raises suspicion of which regional vital structure of adnexa may be injured. Furthermore, location predicts the extent of the local blood supply. Adequate blood flow helps in estimating the potential of local defense mechanisms in contaminated wounds, rate of wound healing, and length of necessary suture apposition. For instance, the excellent blood supply to the face and scalp provides more inherent resistance to a bacterial inoculum than is present in the lower extremities and pannicular regions (abdomen, buttocks).[50]

The depth and extent of injury is physically assessed by the degree of hemodynamic, functional, or neurologic compromise, by the degree of gross skeletal deformity, or by direct exploration. Accurate anatomic appraisal will guide radiologic surveys, angiographic studies, and eventual repair by an appropriate surgeon or surgical subspecialist. The true extent of soft tissue injury with respect to location and visoelastic properties will determine whether closure by primary or secondary intention, skin grafting, or use of complex musculocutaneous or composite grafts will be necessary.

Finally, the circumstances of wounding, nature of inoculum, and time elapsed since injury are important factors obtained in the history and physical examination. Lacerations caused by broken windshields and glass windowpanes instill a small inoculum in surgical-type wounds and may be confidently closed. In contrast, wounds from human bites, from soiled or greased instruments, or those more than 6 hours old require debridement, topical and systemic antimicrobials, and frequent dressing changes for optimal outcome.

The successful treatment of a simple or complex would is dependent upon historical, anatomic, and bacteriologic evaluation, which dictate individual treatment and appropriate surgical or multidisciplinary referral. The injured child is at greatest risk for undeserved long-term functional, cosmetic, psychosocial, and economic disability. For these reasons, such a child warrants prompt, high quality medical and surgical care.

PRECAUTIONS

In an era of pervasive blood-borne diseases, when government legislation may direct the occupational course of HIV-infected health care workers, it is imperative to standardize and document patient contact precautions, the infectious status of high-risk children, and accidental exposures to blood, blood products, or other body fluids. The incidence of HIV and hepatitis infection in emergency rooms of American hospitals is thought to be much higher than in the general population.[68] Other communicable diseases such as hepatitis and cytomegalovirus (CMV) are also likely to be found in children who frequently visit emergency departments.[68]

Since March 1985 all blood donors in the United States have been screened for HIV via a commercially available anti-HTLV III antibody. Of the 0.25% of donors found to be positive for HIV infection, 98.9% are adults, 94% are male, 90% are between 20 and 49 years old, 60% are white, 25% black, and 14% Hispanic.[35] A positive serology for HIV is not necessarily diagnostic of AIDS, in that only 1 in 50 to 100 persons infected with HIV demonstrate overt active disease. Stated another way, the projected attack rate of HIV infected persons is 1% to 2%.

The Centers for Disease Control have identified specific high-risk groups. Of those persons who are HIV antibody positive, 73.4% are homosexual, 17% are intravenous drug abusers (IVDAs), 1.4% are transfusion recipients, 0.7% are hemophiliacs, 0.8% have had documented heterosexual contact with an infected partner, and 6.7% are of various other sources, including those of Haitian origin.[20] It is believed that 1 : 100,000 transfusions results in the transmission of clinically active AIDS.[11]

In comparison, although less a therapeutic dilemma, hepatitis infection is of much higher prevalence and, therefore, an occupational risk. An estimated 200,000 persons, primarily young adults, are infected each year, and 5% of all healthy adults have evidence of previous infection with hepatitis B virus.[16] The estimated lifetime risk of infection for members of high-risk groups (homosexuals, IVDAs) is almost 100%, and between 6% and 10% of adults actively infected with hepatitis B become chronic carriers.[15]

The documented risk of posttransfusion hepatitis is 3% for those patients receiving 1 to 5 units of blood.[4] Hepatitis B accounts for 5% to 10%, and non-A, non-B hepatitis for 90% to 95% of posttransfusion hepatitis (including factor XIII and IX concentrates). Compared with a 3.5% prevalence among volunteer blood donors, 19% of physicians have antibodies to hepatitis B. Among physicians, surgeons were found to have the highest prevalence (28%) of anti-HBsAg. The prevalence of antibodies increases with age and with the number of years in practice.[16]

There are currently two vaccines available for active immunization; Heptovax, an inactivated live virus, the Recombivax, produced using recombinant DNA technology. Primary vaccination costs approximately $100 and consists of three IM injections, one initially, then subsequently at 1 and 6 months. This is 80% to 95% effective in preventing infection in susceptible persons.[11]

Hepatitis B immunoglobulin is also available for immediate passive immunization. It should be considered if there is (1) sufficient evidence of perinatal exposure of an infant born to an HBsAg-positive mother or (2) accidental percutaneous or permucosal exposure to HBsAg-positive blood.[12] The CDC recommendations for hepatitis B prophylaxis following percutaneous exposure are shown in Table 26-1.[12]

Table 26–1 Hepatitis B prophylaxis

Source	Unvaccinated	Vaccinated
HBsAg positive	1. HBIG × 1 immediately 2. Initiate HB vaccine series	1. Test exposed person for anti-HBsAg. 2. If Ab's inadequate give HBIG × 1 and HB vaccine booster dose.
High risk	1. Initiate HB vaccine series 2. Test source for HBsAg. If +, give HBIG × 1	1. Test source for HBsAg. 2. If person exposed is vaccine nonresponder and source is +, give HBIG × 1 and HB booster.
Low risk	Initiate HB vaccine series	Nothing
Unknown	Initiate HB vaccine series	Nothing

HBsAg = Hepatitis B surface antigen; HBIG = Hepatitis B immunoglobulin; Ab's = Antibodies.

One should assume that all children are potential sources of infection and standardize precautions appropriately. Universal precautions are imperative in the treatment of all children:

1. Gloves are mandatory if hands will be in contact with blood, bodily fluids, or wet body surfaces (for example, mucosa).
2. Gowns, masks, and protective goggles are indicated if aerosolization or spattering of body fluids is possible.
3. Hands and other skin surfaces must be washed immediately if contaminated with body secretions.
4. Management of sharp items and contaminated trash must be done according to CDC guidelines.
5. If a health care worker is injured by a contaminated needle or otherwise exposed to possible infection, every effort is made to protect him or her by ascertaining the risk of HIV transmission by immunization. The local infectious disease specialist should be consulted.[68]

WOUND CLASSIFICATION

Accurate wound classification implies an understanding of causal mechanisms, anatomy and function, and wound bacteriology. A child's ultimate functional and aesthetic results depend on individual assessment and visualization of the underlying structures.

Examination

Satisfactory anesthesia must often be provided to ensure the child's comfort during wound assessment and treatment.[68] The age and mental status of the child, as well as the extent of the wound, dictate whether a local, regional, or general anesthetic is preferable.[68] Frequently, a sedative supplemental to local or regional anesthesia may be useful and necessary in the very anxious child.

Adequate lighting, functional instruments, and retraction, irrigation, and suction capabilities should be readily available for complete wound evaluation. Overlying clot or debris commonly conceals underlying neurovascular disruption, exposed bone, or fascial penetration in deeply penetrating or complicated avulsion-type wounds. Therefore, to avoid missed injury, foreign body retention, and subsequent sepsis, optimal controlled examination under appropriate anesthesia is essential.

The skin should be inspected for the location and nature of any contusions, abrasions, or wounds.[50] Contusions or abrasions may indicate damage to the underlying skeleton.[50] The cardinal signs of fracture—deformity, swelling, tenderness, abnormal movement, and loss of distal function—may be observed singly or in any combination. Of these signs, only tenderness and swelling will almost always be present. Swelling may be found without fracture, however, and is an unreliable sign of fracture in the young.[50] Much depends on the radiologic evaluation, which must be adequate both in selection of views and in the surgeon's ability to read them.

Neurologic injury, unfortunately, is often discovered after examination, when the child notices atrophy or even trophic ulceration. Sensory testing of children can produce very unreliable findings. A child's attention is hard to retain, and answers are often erroneous. Sharp objects must never be used: approaching any child with a needle is tantamount to a declaration of war. Requests for comparison of sensation are preferable to absolute, abstract demands. "Does this feel different from that?" is often more successful than "Do you feel that?" Interactive participation rarely works with the younger child. Rather, the detection of sweating, or its absence, in comparison with an area known to be sensate, is preferred. This can be done simply by comparing the friction present between the skin and the barrel of a plastic pen. In warm surroundings, sweating will be appreciably reduced in denervated regions. Motor testing of children can often be similarly unrewarding. Placing an uninjured limb in the posture produced by the muscle under test and having the child keep it in that position will demonstrate whether the child can understand. Repeating the maneuver on the injured limb may reveal intact muscles. Failure to maintain a particular posture is not irrefutable proof of injury, whereas ability to do so is proof of an intact nerve supply.[50]

Vascular injuries may be open, such as those caused by a laceration, or closed, such as those caused by a fracture. Open injury, if partial, constitutes an acute emergency. A partially transected artery cannot contract and arrest hemorrhage as can one that is completely divided. Thus, partially severed arteries are the only potentially fatal injury of the upper extremity and the only reason for the use of an upper arm tourniquet.[50]

Tissue injury is caused by mechanical forces. Shear, distraction, and compressive forces alone or in combination produce predictable patterns of tissue injury.[68] Knowledge of the nature and magnitude of the mechanical forces employed to produce the injury allows the surgeon to predict the extent of tissue damage. The predictability of certain injury patterns has allowed classification of wounds into specific categories: abrasion, laceration, contusion, avulsion, amputation, and bursting injury.[68] In approximately 80% of soft tissue injuries, a shearing force has been applied to tissue by a piece of glass, a metal edge, or a knife.

Closed wounds

Contusion. Contusion, or bruise, results from injury to the capillaries and adjacent tissue by a blow or fall that does not break the skin. Such wounds are painful and rapidly become discolored because of capillary bleeding into the tissue. Cold compresses or ice packs should be applied within the first hour of injury. After 12 to 24 hours, heat may hasten reabsorption of the blood, but if it is used too early, it can add to the amount of hemorrhage and fluid extravasation.[72]

Hematoma. A hematoma, a discrete collection of blood, may develop if bleeding is sufficient to disrupt the cleavage planes of the traumatized tissue or if the bleeding is in continuity with a preexisting bursa or fascial plane.

If the hematoma is fluctuant, aspiration with a 16- to 18-gauge needle may reduce pain and hasten healing. Great care must be taken not to infect the hematoma. Occasionally, because of its large size or because clotting has occurred, incision and drainage under local or general anesthesia is re-

quired. If the hematoma becomes secondarily infected, it must be drained by means of an adequate incision with complete evacuation and subsequent packing.[72]

Open wounds

Puncture wound. A puncture wound is caused by a nail, knife, gun shot, glass, or other sharp objects. The danger of a puncture wound is infection, particularly clostridial tetanus. The closed nature of the wound allows anaerobic growth of bacteria found on the embedded foreign material. The wound edges are debrided by excision of several millimeters around the opening. The wound is irrigated and left open under a sterile dressing. Tetanus toxoid should be administered.[72]

Laceration. Lacerations result from shear forces applied to the skin by sharp objects. Relatively little energy is required to produce such lacerations, and a minimal amount of the tissue is injured. Consequently, the general demands for wound healing are easily satisfied and wound infections are relatively infrequent. The techniques of primary closure, delayed primary closure, and healing by secondary intention depend largely on the risk or estimate of infection.

Through the technique of primary closure the tissues of the wound are carefully approximated after thorough cleansing and debridement of foreign material and devitalized tissue. Most incisions are managed in this fashion, and the technique may be applied to many clean accidental injuries in which the risk of infection is small. Closure may be by suture or by Steri-strips. Primary healing produces minimal scarring, deformity, or functional impairment.

Delayed primary closure is applicable to many dirty wounds. The technique may be used with excellent results when the degree of contamination or the delay between injury and treatment is such that the risk of infection appears high. The wound is debrided and irrigated as in primary repair, but instead of being closed immediately it is carefully packed open and a sterile dressing applied. If by the third or fourth day after injury there is no evidence of infection and the entire wound appears healthy, without any necrosis or debris, closure is accomplished by skin approximation. Because closure is accomplished prior to the proliferative phase of healing, no delay in healing is measurable. If infection or necrotic debris persists, the technique of delayed primary closure should be abandoned.

Healing by secondary intent is employed in grossly infected or contaminated wounds. It should also be used in wounds that have been closed and later become infected. Healing is accomplished through wound contraction, granulation tissue formation, and epithelialization. Although ultimate results may be quite good, considerable delay in healing and formation of excess granulation tissue can be anticipated.

Avulsion. Tensile forces can tear soft tissue. When tensile force exceeds the elastic yield of the tissue, stretching and eventual separation of the dermis and its associated elements occur. The amount of energy absorbed by the soft tissue is great, leading to intimal damage of surrounding blood vessels and subsequent thrombosis and ischemia. The structural integrity of the nerves, muscles, ligaments, and tendons may also be disrupted. Such an injury, an avulsion, places a greater demand on the biologic process of repair, decreases wound defense mechanisms, and enhances susceptibility to infection.[68]

In avulsion injuries a segment of skin, or skin and subcutaneous tissue, is torn from its bed, occasionally supplied by a tenuous vascular pedicle. It often contains foreign material and requires careful debridement and irrigation before closure. Management is essentially the same as that for lacerations. If the edges are viable, suturing the skin back to its original position suffices. Large U-shaped avulsion flaps usually cannot be sutured back successfully because of inadequate marginal blood supply. Interrupted sutures, working from the base outward, help prevent subsequent wound contracture. If significant tissue loss occurs, a split-thickness skin graft may be used to cover the exposed space.

Crush injury. Soft tissue compression between two opposing forces results in the greatest amount of tissue damage. When the mechanism is compression, tissue failure occurs at energy levels of 2.52 joules/cm^2.[9] The level of energy is comparable to that encountered by the soft tissues overlying the cranium striking the dashboard in a high-speed automobile accident. Wounds caused by impact injuries are 100 times more susceptible to infection than those caused by shear forces. In these injuries immediate antibiotic therapy is clearly beneficial.[21]

Bursting injury. Firearms are of two basic types: rifled firearms and shotguns. A rifled firearm, which includes pistols and rifles, has spiral grooves in its barrel and discharges hot gases, soot, powder grains, and a bullet. Missiles that are classified as low-energy depositors include .22 rimfire bullets and all handgun bullets, with the exception of the .44 magnum, and expend less than 400 joules of kinetic energy into the wound. Low-energy deposit projectiles cause injuries similar to simple stab wounds, the tissue destruction being confined to the wound tract. They usually do not require

debridement and may be treated conservatively inasmuch as the profile of the wound tract is narrow and unlikely to be contaminated by debris drawn in from the outside. In contrast, bullets classified as high-energy depositors transfer 400 or more joules of kinetic energy into the wound and include all center-fire rifle bullets, as well as .44 magnum pistol bullets. Because they result in tissue destruction that extends beyond the permanent wound tract, extensive tissue debridement of devitalized tissue in the operating room is necessary. The magnitude of tissue destruction is extensive and difficult to ascertain soon after injury, therefore, the wound is left open and reexamined daily to debride any residual necrotic tissue.[21]

Shotguns differ from rifles and pistols in that they have a smooth barrel that discharges hot gases, a wad, and either multiple projectiles or a single projectile. Shot charges containing multiple projectiles spread out from the muzzle in a conelike pattern. The distance from the muzzle of the shotgun to the point of impact is a key indicator of the magnitude of injury. At short range, less than 7 meters, the shot charge containing multiple projectiles results predominantly in a single hole inshoot wound (with a diameter less than 6 cm) that communicates with a deep, underlying wound with massive tissue destruction. When the impact range exceeds 7 meters, the multiple projectiles result in multiple discrete wounds that are not associated with underlying massive tissue destruction.

When the range is less than 45 meters, shotguns can discharge rifled slugs that are high depositors of energy. Although rifled bullets maintain their velocity over 45 meters, the rifled slugs experience a marked decrease in velocity over that distance (approximately 25%). This rather dramatic inverse relationship between the velocity of the slug and the deposited energy affects the impact energy and the ultimate tissue injury.

Wound bacteriology

The humoral and cellular defense mechanisms of the body are usually sufficient to control infection and promote wound healing. However, they cannot function efficiently in an environment of debris, necrotic tissue, hematoma, and virulent and numerous bacteria. In all these circumstances, bacteria may compete effectively with phagocytes, fibroblasts, endothelial cells, and epithelium and produce infection and delayed wound healing. In addition, some children are especially susceptible to infection because of impaired host defenses. Individuals who are diabetic, have cancer, or have sustained major trauma or surgery all have decreased host defenses.[31]

The major advance in the prevention and management of infections in soft tissue has been the understanding that the presence of microorganisms in a wound is less important than the level of bacterial growth. A wealth of clinical and experimental data have shown that a level of bacterial growth of greater than 10^5 organisms per gram of tissue is necessary to cause a wound infection and create the potential for invasive bacterial sepsis.[52] Only the β-hemolytic *Streptococcus* appears capable of routinely causing infection at levels of less than 10^5 organisms per gram of tissue.[49]

Infections can be prevented by maintaining the host's defense at peak efficiency. The effect of the interaction between the bacteria and the host, although under systemic influence, is ultimately determined by local factors in the wound.[48] Among these are necrotic tissue, decreased local wound perfusion, foreign bodies, hematoma, and dead space. The surgeon plays a significant role in eliminating the local deterrents to effective host defense in the wound. If they are not controlled, equilibrium is upset and circumstances are such that a normally subinfectious innoculum of bacteria may multiply to levels sufficient to produce infection.

The bacterial count of the skin is normally quite high. Bacteria reside both on the surface of the skin and deep in the hair follicles and sweat glands. The amount of bacteria normally present in the recesses is 1000 organisms per gram of tissue.[52] Even wounds that appear to be clean may harbor organisms with sufficient frequency that their presence can be suspected in every case. All traumatic wounds are contaminated at least to the extent that bacteria can always be identified by cultures performed on tissue biopsies of the specimens. Mechanical contamination in the form of debris, necrotic tissue, or sutures provides a further nidus for multiplication of initially small numbers of bacteria to significant levels of growth. In a study on infections, Elek has shown that the presence of a single silk suture will reduce by 10,000 times the number of *Staphylococcus* necessary to cause a wound infection[25]; however, the initial inoculum into a wound may be so massive that the local defense mechanisms are overwhelmed from the outset.[50]

Wounds may be classified according to the expected level of bacterial contamination into the following categories: clean, potentially contaminated (clean-contaminated), or contaminated. A thyroidectomy incision produced under sterile operating room conditions is a clean wound. Examples of clean-contaminated wounds include stab wounds with a kitchen knife, lacerations with glass or other relatively clean objects, or wounds in which a hollow viscus, such as the gall bladder, stomach, trachea, ureter, or appendix, has been entered but gross spillage controlled. Contaminated wounds contain quantitative bacterial counts exceeding 10^5 bacteria per gram of tissue. A puncture wound from a dirty nail or human bite, a wound with uncontrolled spillage from a hollow viscus, and any wound over 6 hours old are examples of contaminated wounds. The diagnosis of the degree of contamination is dependent on clues obtained when taking the history. For example, the bacterial inoculum from the bite of a non–meat eating dog may be low and allow primary closure, whereas the inoculum from a human bite (up to 10^8 bacteria per gram of tissue), a source usually heavily contaminated with facultative species and obligate anaerobes, creates a high rate of risk for infection.[21,50]

The location of a wound reflects the potential of local defense mechanisms to withstand contamination. A facial wound, with its excellent blood supply, is more resistant to an inoculum for a longer period of time than a pretibial wound, where a poor blood supply may allow bacterial growth with even minimal contamination.[50]

Time is also an important historical factor in determining the potential for wound contamination. In a 1987 study, Robson demonstrated that the mean time since injury was 2.2 hours for patients with less than 10^2 bacteria per gram tissue in their wounds; 3 hours for the group with 10^2 to 10^5 bacteria per gram tissue, and 5.17 hours for those wounds with more than 10^5 bacteria per gram tissue.[29] Only those patients in the last group developed infections that prevented primary healing.[50]

For prognostic purposes, superficial wounds may be classified as tidy or untidy (Table 26-2). Tidy wounds are caused by sharp objects, result in minimal tissue injury and contamination, and can usually be closed under favorable circumstances. Untidy wounds, however, are manifested by extensive soft tissue injury or contamination and require major intervention to allow satisfactory healing.

In the emergency room, when a wound of potential or questionable contamination is presented and primary closure is desired, a wound biopsy for quantitative rapid slide determination (Table 26-3) will provide objective data reinforcing appropriate wound care. In this technique, a specimen is removed from the wound, weighed, diluted, and homogenized. An aliquot of the suspension is then placed on a glass slide and Gram stained. If a single organism is seen on HPF magnification, the bacterial count is greater than 10^5 bacteria per gram of tissue, prohibiting wound closure. If other injuries require hospital admission, tissue cultures may provide more exact wound counts, bacterial identification, and antibiotic sensitivities within 24 to 36 hours. The identification of *Streptococcus* and *Clostridia* species (*tetani* and *perfringens*) in contaminated wounds is important to prevent premature closure and mandate radical debridement.

Tetanus Prophylaxis

Two thirds of recent tetanus cases in the United States have followed laceration, puncture wound, or crush injury.[29] The indications and guidelines for tetanus prophylaxis after such injuries are standardized and based on recommendations by the Committee on Trauma of the American College of Surgeons (Table 26-4).[13] The need for tetanus prophylaxis is based on two conditions: previous immunization history and whether the wound is tetanus prone. Tetanus-prone wounds are those (1) containing devitalized tissue, such as those caused by crushing or gunshot wounds and/or (2) more than 6 hours old. The only contraindication to tetanus and diphtheria toxoids is a history of neuro-logic or other hypersensitivity reactions after administration of a previous dose.[36] Local reactions such as erythema and induration without tenderness are common and not contraindications. If the use of a tetanus-toxoid–containing preparation is contraindicated, passive immunization against tetanus should be considered in a tetanus-prone wound.

ANESTHESIA

There are special concerns regarding anesthesia in the treatment of a child. Modern agents and techniques now make it possible to anesthetize a non-premedicated, struggling, screaming child within a few minutes.[58] As a result, premedication has assumed more value in the emotional protection of the child than as an adjunct to anesthesia.[26] Most authors state that if a child has been properly prepared, premedication is not necessary,[17,63] or even desirable, if it prolongs recovery and delays dis-

Table 26–2 Wound classification

Wound type	Treatment
Tidy wounds	
1. Lacerations	Clean, suture.
2. Contusions	Ice, elevate with wrap.
Untidy wounds	
1. Abrasions	Clean, debride (remove tattooing), dress; allow to heal by secondary intent.
2. Lacerations	Clean, debride. Consider delayed primary closure, except on face or scalp when primary is indicated.
3. Puncture wounds	Clean, dress. Allow to heal by secondary intent.
4. Crush wounds	Clean, debride, dress. Consider closure, skin grafting, flaps, or whatever is necessary at delayed closure.
Dirty wounds	
1. Bites	Animal bites may be cleaned, debrided, and, if they involve the face, primary closure may be considered. Antibiotics are indicated. Human bites are cleaned, debrided, and dressed. Primary closure is contraindicated. Delayed primary closure may be considered. Antibiotics are indicated.
2. Grossly contaminated	Clean, debride, and dress. Delayed primary closure may be considered versus healing by secondary intent.
3. Wounds over 6 hr old	Clean, debride, and dress. Closure by delayed primary closure or secondary intent.
Complicated wounds	
1. Open fractures	Clean, debride, immobilize. Specialist consultation is mandatory. Antibiotics are indicated.
2. Perineal/perianal	Clean, debride. Generally allow to heal by secondary intent. Rule out rectal perforations. Antibiotics are indicated.
3. Intraoral lacerations	Clean, minimally debride. Often may be left to heal by secondary intent or closed with absorbable suture if large. Full-thickness lip lacerations are closed in three layers (mucosa, muscle, and skin). Approximate vermillion border exactly.

Table 26-3 The "rapid slide" bacterial quantitative assay

1. Clean the surface of the wound biopsy area with 70% isopropyl alcohol.
2. Obtain the biopsy specimen with a 3 or 4 mm dermal punch or with a scalpel. No anesthesia of the patient is required for treatment of an open wound.
3. After the tissue is weighed, flamed, and diluted 1:10 with thioglycolate (1 ml/g), it is homogenized.
4. Spread exactly 0.02 ml of the suspension with a 20-λ Sahli pipette on a glass slide. The inoculum is confined to an area 15 mm in diameter.
5. Oven dry the slide for 15 min at 75° C.
6. Stain the slide, using either Gram's stain or the Brown and Brenn modification for tissue staining, to accentuate the gram-negative organisms.
7. Read the smear under 1.9-mm (magnification × 97) objective and examine all fields for the presence of bacteria.
8. The presence of even a single organism is evidence that the tissue contains a level of bacterial growth greater than 10 bac/g of tissue.

charge to home.[6,46,61] Others believe that some form of anesthesia is advantageous. The age, mental status of the child, and extent of the wound dictate whether a local, regional, or general anesthetic is preferable. For the anxious, struggling child sedation is often a prerequisite to allow proper examination, debridement, and closure of wounds.

Narcotic analgesics have been widely used for pediatric sedation for many years. It has been stated that morphine is unsurpassed for its analgesic and euphoric actions, as well as its predictability.[67] Narcotic analgesics, however, produce significant respiratory depression, especially in younger infants, and the incidence of postprocedure vomiting may be increased by the use of these drugs. Infants are especially sensitive to the respiratory depressant effects of morphine, possibly because of the distribution of the drug across the blood-brain barrier.[69] Therefore, morphine must be carefully ordered for infants under 1 year of age or of less than 10 kg body weight. Meperidine (Demerol), a synthetic narcotic analgesic, has also been commonly used as a sedative. The usual dose is 1 to 1.5 mg/kg. It results in less sedation, euphoria, and respiratory depression than morphine. Although morphine and meperidine can be reversed by antago-

Table 26-4 Sedatives

Name	Dose	Comments
Narcotics		
Morphine	0.1-0.2 mg/kg IM/IV	Standard
Meperidine	1-1.5 mg/kg IM/IV	
Fentanyl	1-2 μg/kg IV	Drug of choice in infants
Pentazocine	1.5 mg/kg	
Barbiturates		
Pentobarbitol	2-3 mg/kg PO	
	2-4 mg/kg PR	
	3-4 mg/kg IM	
Benzodiazepines		
Diazepam	0.3-0.5 mg/kg Im	Good for child >3yr
	0.75 mg/kg PR	
Midazolam	80 μg/kg IV	PR excellent for child 1-3yr
	0.2-0.3 mg/kg PR	
	0.8 mg/kg PO	
Others		
Methohexitol	25-30 mg/kg PR	Approx. 8 min induction
Pentothal	40 mg/kg PR	
Chlorpromazine	1.5 mg/kg IM	Good for mentally retarded child
Ketamine	1-2 mg/kg IV	CV stability and burn patients

nists such as naloxone, their effects last 3 to 4 hours, which may be longer than desired, and reversal results in immediate onset of pain and discomfort. A currently favored approach is the use of a short-acting narcotic analgesic such as fentanyl (1 to 2 µg/kg).[57] Intravenous use allows more accurate titration of the dose to the individual child and avoids the use of "standard" dosage based on weight.

Pentazocine (Talwin), a benzomorphan derivative introduced as a nonnarcotic analgesic, produces sedation similar to that produced by morphine, with similar side effects, and is administered in doses of 1.5 mg/kg IM. Pentazocine has not been widely adopted as a premedicant as it has no clear advantage over other narcotic analgesics and may produce the additional complications of hallucinations, seizures, and bronchospasm.

The short-acting barbiturate drugs are widely used for pediatric sedation. Pentobarbitol may be given orally (2 to 3 mg/kg), rectally (2 to 4 mg/kg), or IM (3 to 4 mg/kg). For children up to 3 years of age, the rectal route of administration is usually preferred. It is well known that barbituates have no analgesic properties and, consequently, in children with pain, they may cause excitation and irrational behavior.

The neuroleptic drug droperidol (Inapsine), originally used because of its antisialagogue and antiemetic effects, has been essentially abandoned owing to its effects of restlessness, anxiety, and motor disturbances.[19,40] Diazepam (Valium) has been advocated as a premedicant, although studies show variable results. Absorption and, therefore, the anxiolytic effect is better achieved through the GI tract than the IM route.[5] The usual oral dosage is 0.3 to 0.5 mg/kg given 1 hour prior to a procedure.

Midazolam (Versed), a benzodiazepine derivative, has hypnotic, anxiolytic, and amnesiac effects.[14] In children, midazolam has been used via IM injection for premedication. It is reported to allay anxiety and to facilitate a smooth induction of anesthesia, causing less postoperative vomiting than narcotics.[47] Excellent results have been seen in children when given midazolam via the oral route at 0.8 mg/kg (mixed with apple juice, for instance), if administration allows approximately 45 minutes before the time of wound repair.

Rectal sedatives take a little longer to induce anesthesia than those given by the intravenous route, but not much, and the benefits to a frightened child are great.[32] Children fall asleep within approximately 8 minutes after administration of methohexital (Brevitol; 25 mg/kg). Recovery from sedation is not prolonged. Children are as awake and alert 30 minutes after anesthesia, and are as ready for discharge, as those anesthetized with halothane and NO_2 alone. There are multiple advantages to giving methohexital rectally. First, sleep can be induced while the child is in the parent's arms. This alleviates separation anxiety. Second, the induction is smooth and does not require inserting needles or placing a mask over the child's face. Third, the drug can be used in mentally retarded or frightened children. Fourth, children accustomed to rectal thermometers are less threatened by rectal insertion of a small plastic catheter. There is only one disadvantage: occasionally a child has a bowel movement as the drug is injected. This may be prevented by holding or taping the buttocks together for several minutes and concentrating the drug dose in a small volume.

Rectal thiopental sodium (Pentothal 40 mg/kg) is just as effective as methohexitol; however, children recover from the latter more quickly.[71] Diazepam can also be given rectally, but sleep is rarely induced by this drug in these doses (.75 mg/kg). Use of rectal midazolam (0.2 to 0.3 mg/kg) often causes sleep to occur within 5 to 10 minutes (unpublished data).[32]

When drugs are given rectally, they should be administered below the dentate line if possible, because they will go to the central nervous system (CNS) before they go to the liver. If drugs are given above the dentate line, they go to the liver first and part of the drug is metabolized before its distribution to the CNS.

Anesthesia can be induced with various IM medications. The chief advantage of sedation through this route are ease of administration and rapidity of onset of anesthesia. However, there are disadvantages, which include pain at the injection site, occasional sterile abscess formation, and slow and variable uptake of the drug from the tissue, especially in the presence of reduced peripheral perfusion. Induction is helpful in children with behavior problems, mental retardation, poor veins, or congenital heart disease. Children usually lose consciousness in 30 to 45 seconds, at which point IV access may be obtained. Midazolam and methohexitol are also effective and quick acting via the IM route.

Ketamine was introduced in 1970 and was initially considered a major anesthetic advance because it was said to preserve laryngeal competence and respiratory drive, and to provide somatic analgesia and excellent cardiovascular stability. Further experience with ketamine has demonstrated numerous disadvantageous properties, including increased salivary secretion, increased airway reflexes (causing laryngospasm), and an increase in intracranial pressure. Currently, its use is limited to induction of children at high risk of cardiovascular instability, sedation of mentally retarded or

Table 26–5 Local anesthetics: ester linked

	Procaine (Novocaine)	Chloroprocaine (Nesacaine)	Tetracaine (Pontocaine)
Concentrations	0.25%	1.0%	1.0%
	0.5%	2.0%	2.0%
		3.0%	
No epinephrine	5-8.5 mg/kg	11 mg/kg	Particularly effective on oral mucosa; swab lightly until surface is insensate
Total dose	350-600 mg	800 mg	
Epinephrine	14 mg/kg	14 mg/kg	
Total dose	1000 mg	1000 mg	

poorly behaved children, and sedation of burned children during repeated dressing changes and debridements.

The simplest practical technique of anesthetizing most wounds is infiltration anesthesia. The anesthetic agent may be infiltrated directly into the wound to reduce the discomfort associated with injection. Pain associated with cutaneous injection is due, in part, to the stretching of sensory nerve endings in the dermis and may be minimized by using smaller, concentrated volumes with slower infiltration rates with small (27g) needles. The least amount of anesthetic that will produce adequate anesthesia should be employed to minimize distortion of important landmarks and optimize anatomic approximation. Initial hemostasis resulting from vessel vasospasm, platelet plugging, and fibrin clot formation may be disrupted by the vasodilatory effects of some local anesthetics. The addition of epinephrine to anesthetic solutions in a concentration of 1:200,000 optimizes vasoconstriction, improves hemostasis, decreases regional clearance and, therefore, systemic toxicity. Epinephrine-containing solutions may compromise local wound defense mechanisms by their vasoconstrictive effect and should not be used in heavily contaminated wounds. They are also contraindicated in regions supplied by end-arteries, such as the digits, ears, nose, and penis.

Signs of anesthetic toxicity, which are remarkably absent in the use of the different local anesthetic solutions, are always dose-related and include numbness, tingling, diplopia, mental confusion, and convulsions. Although allergies to ester-linked local anesthetics are well documented in adults, toxicity and allergy are rare in adults, and even more rare in children.

Among the amide local anesthetics (Tables 26-5, 26-6), xylocaine (Lidocaine) has been extensively studied, and recommended maximum dosages for children are similar to those for adults on a kilogram basis (up to 4.5 mg/kg uncombined,

Table 26–6 Local anesthetics: amide linked

	Lidocaine (Xylocaine)	Bupivacaine (Marcaine)
Concentrations	0.5%	0.25%
	1.0%	0.50%
	1.5%	0.75%
	2.0%	
No epinephrine	4.5 mg/kg	2.0-2.5 mg/kg
Total dose	300 mg	175 mg
Epinephrine	7.0 mg/kg	3.0 mg/kg
Total dose	500 mg	225 mg

and up to 7 mg/kg with epinephrine).[66] Bupivicaine (Marcaine) has achieved great popularity as a neural blockade for postoperative pain because of its prolonged duration of action. In addition, the use of concentrate (0.25%) produces greater block for sensory fibers than for motor fibers and thus preserves function. Allergy to amide-linked local anesthetics is virtually nonexistent, and most reported reactions are vagovagal in nature. If a toxic reaction should occur after infiltration with local anesthesia, the physician must be prepared to hyperventilate the child, administer diazepam to increase the seizure threshold, and place the child in the Trendelenburg position to maintain adequate cerebral blood flow.

Lidocaine and most other local anesthetics do not provide adequate local anesthesia in areas of established infection. Local anesthetics, which are weak bases, are inactivated by the acidic environment found in areas of infection. In addition, diffusion of local anesthetic solution is hampered by loculations and other physical barriers present in infected wounds. If adequate anesthesia of an infected wound cannot be attained via local or regional anesthesia, general anesthesia may be indicated.

Certain wounds are particularly adapted to regional anesthetic techniques. Such techniques may

Table 26–7 Regional anesthetics

Region		Target site	Injection site
Spinal/subarachnoid		T2-S5	Sitting or lateral decubitus position Newborn, conus at L3, dural sac at S3 One-year-old, conus at L1, sac at S1
Caudal/epidural		T4-S5	Prone or lateral decubitus position 22g through sacral hiatus through sacro-coccygeal ligament
Hand			
	Median n.	Palmar aspect of lateral 3.5 fingers	Between tendons of flexor carpi radialis and palmaris longus at proximal volar skin crease
	Ulnar n.	Ulnar palm, little finger, and ulnar aspect of ring finger	Between ulnar artery and flexor carpi ulnaris
	Superficial radial n.	Radial dorsum of hand	Raise a subcutaneous ring of anesthetic at level of flexor carpi radialis and extending radially dorsal to styloid process
	Digital n.	Digit	Midportion of base of proximal lateral phalanx. Should blanch skin on palmar surface of web space
Foot			
	Saphenous	Proximal medial half of foot	Near saphenous vein anterior to medial malleolus
	Post. tibial	Medial aspect of sole of foot	Between medial malleolus and Achilles tendon just posterior and deep to posterior tibial artery
	Sural n.	Lateral foot and little toe	Cuff from lateral malleolus to Achilles
	Deep peroneal	Adjacent joints and skin between first and second toes	Lateral to extensor hallucis longus at distal tibia
	Supfl. peroneal	Dorsum of foot	Cuff extending from lateral malleolus extensor hallucis longus
	Hallux		Collar ring block beginning at dorsilateral aspect of base of toe
Head			
		Scalp	Line circling head just above ear through occiput and glabella
	Supra-orbital	Forehead	Supraorbital notch
	Infra-orbital and alveolar n.	Lower eyelid, lateral nose, upper lip, mucus membranes of mouth, upper cuspid and incisor	Infraorbital foramen
	Lingual nerve	Anterior 2/3 tongue, floor of mouth and gums	Intraoral: medial to body of mandible, 1 cm above occlusive surface of third molar
	Mental nerve	Lower lip, central mucous membranes and submental area	Intraoral: junction of lower lip and lower gum just posterior to first premolar tooth
Arm	Brachial plexus		Lateral to brachial artery until pop through plexus sheath
Leg			
	Femoral n.	Anterior thigh	Lateral to femoral artery, 1-1.5 cm below inguinal ligament
	Lateral fem. cutaneous n.	Lateral thigh	Medial and inferior to anterior superior iliac spine below inguinal ligament
	Sciatic n.	Posterior thigh and leg to dorsum of foot	Intersection of line from midpoint of line connecting greater trochanter and posterior iliac spine, and midpoint of line from greater trochanter to tip of coccyx
Penis	Dorsal penile		Through Buck's fascia immediately inferior to lower border of symphysis pubis

allow more extensive exploration and debridement than possible with local blocks. In addition, regional anesthesia avoids local distortion of tissues and allows precise alignment in complicated wounds. Table 26-7 lists potential avenues to achieve regional anesthesia.

Although infiltration and regional anesthesia are the most common anesthetic techniques for treating lacerations, topical anesthesia is increasing in popularity. Skin lacerations may be anesthetized by a topical solution containing 0.5% tetracaine, 1:2000 epinephrine solution, and 11.8% cocaine (TEC or TAC). In a randomized prospective study involving a relatively small number of patients, TEC, as compared with 1% xylocaine infiltration, reduced both discomfort and tissue swelling, but provided adequate hemostasis secondary to vasoconstriction.[45]

PREPARING THE WOUND FOR CLOSURE
Skin antisepsis

The *sine qua non* of any wound is closure, and in all instances it must be determined whether the wound is ready for closure. Criteria for closure include an acceptable bacterial level, absence of nonviable or potentially nonviable tissue, and absence of any clot or foreign debris.[50] To minimize bacterial contamination of the wound, various antiseptic techniques for skin have been developed to decrease the bacterial counts on the surgeons hands, within the wound, and on the surrounding skin. Care must be taken to avoid exposing the wound to materials that lead to further tissue injury or impede the wound's defense mechanisms. The clinician should avoid placing anything in the wound that would not be placed into the conjunctival sac.

Nonirritating soaps, fat solvents (degreasers), and ionic soaps may be used to clean the surrounding skin. After application to intact skin, these surgical scrubs should be rinsed away, removing gross contaminants, transient microflora, and coagulated blood.[72] Degerming agents, including iodine, hexachlorophene, and alcohol, may next be applied to the intact skin. Povidone-iodine (Betadine) has a rapid onset of action, a broad antimicrobial spectrum, is inexpensive, and is the most popular disinfectant. These solutions reduce the number of resident and contaminating bacteria on the intact skin surface. Care should be taken with Betadine application. If it is allowed to bathe an open wound, free iodine may be absorbed and result in high serum levels. In addition, this solution may destroy cells responsible for local defense and tissue repair.

Hair removal

Skin hair is a source of contamination and is usually removed from wound edges.[18] Furthermore, removal of hair facilitates closure by preventing it from becoming entangled in the sutures and the wound during closure. Although a razor is convenient to use, the infection rate after razor preparation was found by one study to be 5.6%, as compared with 0.6% after preparation with a depilatory.[59] In another 5-year prospective study of 23,649 wounds, the infection rate was 2.3% in patients shaved and only 0.9% in patients not shaved or clipped.[15] Shaving, or even clipping, may destroy some of the natural integumentary defenses and may produce multiple superficial lesions containing exuded tissue fluids that favor bacterial growth. Thus, current recommendations are, if feasible, to leave hair alone or to paint inconvenient hair away from the wound with antiseptic, sterile gel lubricants, or antibiotic ointments.[72] If necessary, excess hair can be removed by electric clippers immediately prior to surgery.[1]

Hair removal by depilatories does not increase the risk of infection; however, care must be taken to avoid wound contact, as these compounds can give rise to inflammation or dermatitis and delay wound healing.[2] Lacerations through the eyebrow or hairline signal absolute contraindications to hair removal. Accurate cosmetic approximation of the wound edges is dependent on visualization of the juncture of hair and non–hair bearing areas.

Debridement

Pierre-Joseph Desault (1744–1795), the chief surgeon at the Hotel Dieu in Paris, coined the term *debridement*. A World War I physician, H. W. Orr, treated open fractures of the lower extremity by incising the wound to ensure drainage and then placing the leg in a plaster cast.[42] More recently, in the Spanish Civil War (1935-1938), J. Trueta performed true surgical debridement and noted a significant reduction in military infection rates.[65] Sharp debridement today remains the most efficient way to prepare a traumatic wound for closure and prevent major wound complications.[50]

Debridement removes a large portion of the contaminating bacteria and impaled foreign bodies, and aids alignment of complex or stellate wounds. Retrieval of radiolucent foreign bodies (wood) may be a difficult challenge, resulting in exploration in the operating room with optimal lighting, instruments, and anesthesia.[72] Radiopaque foreign bodies may often be localized with multiple x-rays, flouroscopy, or xerography.[72] Deep road burns may result in a permanent tattoo. To prevent this may require tedious debridement under general anesthesia shortly after the injury.

Guidelines for determining tissue viability must be based on careful wound evaluation and sound clinical judgment. If the viability of tissue remains in question after debridement, intravenous fluorescein can be given and the wound tissue inspected under ultraviolet light. Tissue fluorescence, or sufficient levels attained with the digital fluorometer, suggests viability.[8,50] Trauma surgeons often base their judgment of tissue viability on the color and consistency of exposed or wounded tissue, the degree of wound edge bleeding, and the functional stimulated contraction of involved underlying muscle.[50] Alternatively, when tissue of questionable viability remains after initial debridement, a second look 24 to 48 hours later may reveal overt demarcation, allowing appropriate excision and utilization of initially marginal tissue.

Avulsed or amputated tissue will become necrotic unless the part can be converted to a graft or the blood supply reestablished. Unless cellular destruction has occurred, avulsed skin can frequently be debrided, defatted, and reapplied successfully as a free graft.

An exception to the general principle of debriding all devitalized tissue is made in treating specialized tissues that perform important physical functions, regardless of their viability. Tissues such as dura, fascia, and tendon may survive as free grafts without living cells if they are immediately covered by healthy pedicle flaps.

Irrigation is an important adjunct to sharp debridement. Up to 90% of a bacterial inoculum may be removed via irrigation, but its efficacy is related to hydrostatic pressure. Low-pressure gravity flow and Asepto irrigation do not adequately reduce the bacterial concentration.[72] A pulsating jet lavage, available in many emergency rooms, has had documented success in reducing the bacterial level to below 10^5 organisms per gram tissue, resulting in significantly fewer wound infections. Pulsating lavage delivers a stream of water that alternatively produces compression and interpulse decompression. This allows soft tissue, with its inherent elasticity, to rebound, thus loosening contaminating particles.[34] If pulsating lavage is not available, it has been shown that saline lavage, achieved with a 35-ml syringe and 19-g needle, generates a pressure of 7 to 10 lb per square inch, and is far superior to standard low-pressure wound irrigation.[62]

The preliminary irrigation should allow the surgeon to identify all injured structures and formulate a systematic plan of repair.[73] Debridement must never be done hurriedly and in some cases may actually consume more time than the subsequent repair.[73]

Hemostasis

In addition to obscuring underlying injury, a blood clot acts as a foreign body and provides excellent culture media for bacteria within wounds. A clot shifts the osmotic gradient toward the extravascular space, and eventual expansion impairs capillary perfusion of overlying skin flaps and grafts. Therefore, every effort must be made to obtain meticulous hemostasis prior to wound closure, application of a skin graft, or flap reconstruction.

Vasoconstriction and the primary platelet plug are responsible for the initial, tenuous hemostasis of acute wounds. Subsequent motion, debridement, infection, or fibrinolysis may weaken this plug and result in significant hemorrhage. All visible vessels traversing a wound should therefore be explored, regardless of the presence or absence of bleeding.[72] Hemostasis in most wounds is achieved by direct pressure. Vessels larger than 2 mm may require suture ligation, a clip, or electrocoagulation. Ligation and application clip should include only the specific vessel, with a short distal segment to minimize the amount of devascularized or necrotic tissue. It should be remembered that sutures and clips are foreign bodies that increase the wound's susceptibility to infection. Fine, absorbable (polyglycolic acid, polygalactin, or catgut) sutures are recommended for use in suture ligation in acute wounds. In addition, it is recommended that indiscriminate electrocoagulation, which can result in charred, necrotic tissue, be avoided in order to minimize infection.

Antibiotic therapy

The relative success of antibiotics in the prevention of infection is dependent on the timing of administration, the mechanism of injury, and the bacterial count of the wound.[21] Prophylactic antibiotics significantly decrease the risk of postoperative sepsis if adequate tissue levels are reached before the bacteria arrive in the wound.[72] Such prophylaxis would be unusual in the case of an emergency room patient; however, a single IV dose administered promptly in the emergency department is indicated, especially for children with blast, crush, cellulitic, or contaminated wounds with $<10^9$ bacteria per gram tissue. Systemic antibiotics have potential value only if therapeutic levels are achieved within the first 4 hours after the child has been injured.[50] After that period, as demonstrated by J. F. Burke, bacterial lodgement is not influenced and infection rates are significantly higher.[7]

Most wounds contain less than 10^2 bacteria per gram of tissue at the time an injured child arrives in the emergency room.[50] Quantitative bacterial studies, as previously mentioned, demonstrate that the critical factor in predicting wound sepsis is the number of bacteria at the time of closure, not the type of bacteria. Infection will occur if wounds with more than 10^5 bacteria per gram of tissue are closed without adjunctive measures.[50] Blast and crush injuries commonly contain more devitalized tissue, foreign debris, bacteria, and blood clots; however, if the extent of tissue injury does not contraindicate closure, prophylactic antibiotics may allow primary, uncomplicated wound closure and healing after standard debridement and irrigation.

Wounds with more than 10^9 bacteria per gram of tissue caused by contamination with pus, saliva, feces, or vaginal secretions will suppurate despite administration of antibiotics. These wounds should be debrided and left open with application of topical antimicrobials. The magnitude of bacterial contamination is estimated through experience with treatment of various wounds, their mechanisms, and appearance. A more definite assessment is obtained through quantitative bacterial assays; that is, the rapid slide technique. These values, available in 15 minutes, help the clinician to prevent unwarranted wound morbidity when dealing with wounds of questionable contamination.

In most trauma centers, a cephalosporin such as cefazolin (Ancef) or penicillin is administered for prophylaxis as soon as conveniently possible after primary evulation. Further antibiotic treatment is controversial. In questionable wounds, especially after crush of impact injuries, many clinicians prescribe 3 to 7 days treatment with oral cephalexin (Keflex), penicillin, or ampicillin-clavulonic acid (Augmentin).[50]

Chronically contaminated wounds, as opposed to acute, potentially contaminated wounds, all contain tissue bacterial flora. The characteristic of such wounds is granulation tissue, likened to a pyogenic granuloma, and, by definition, they are contaminated with bacteria. Successful closure of chronic wounds is dependent on the ability to limit bacterial contamination to less than 10^5 organisms per gram tissue by meticulous surgical technique and judicious use of topical antimicrobials.[48] Frequent debridement and surgical cleansing are critical. Enzymatic debridement may be beneficial in small wounds, especially those of the hands and extremities; however, the potential for bacterial proliferation in larger wounds, such as burns of more than 20% total body surface area (TBSA), can lead to overwhelming sepsis if a concurrent topical antimicrobial is not used.[38]

Systemic antibiotics are not indicated in the treatment of chronic soft tissue wounds because of their lack of effect on the wound bacterial count.[53] Topical antimicrobials, however, do penetrate the depths of such wounds and directly affect bacterial growth. Use of 0.5% silver nitrate, Sulfamylon, and Silvadene became popular in the 1960s. Silvadene (silver sulfadiazene) is the antimicrobial of choice in many emergency rooms and most burn centers; it has a broad spectrum of coverage. There is a low incidence of the development of resistant strains during its use, and its application is relatively pain free.[54] Silvadene may be easily applied as a thin layer over the wound once or twice daily. It should be removed by irrigation or gentle debridement prior to each reapplication. Disadvantages include its tendency to develop a coagulum with time, its expense, and a known incidence of systemic hypersensitivity resulting in neutropenia.

Sulfamylon (mafenide) is useful in suppressing bacterial proliferation through eschars. It has greater wound penetration than Silvadene and is therefore indicated in infected wounds, wounds secondary to electrical injury, and wounds with exposed fascia, tendon, ligament, cartilage, or bone. Its disadvantages are that it is painful upon application and it is a carbonic anhydrase inhibitor, leading to metabolic and acid-base disturbances.[54]

Antibiotic treatment is also indicated for injured children with minor lacerations prone to develop infectious endocarditis.[37] In addition, children with wounds occurring in lymphedematous extremities should routinely receive prophylactic antibiotics, regardless of the mechanism of injury or the degree of contamination.[21]

WOUND CLOSURE

Wound closure may be classified as primary, delayed primary (tertiary), or spontaneous (secondary intention). Primary repair undertakes immediate reapproximation of wound layers, can be accomplished through a variety of techniques, and provides the most aesthetically pleasing result. If after adequate exploration, debridement, and irrigation there is no contraindication, the various anatomic layers are reapproximated through gentle surgical technique and optimal suture selection. Gentle surgical technique means the use of a minimal amount of sutures to achieve coaptation without tension or strangulation.

After appropriate debridement, wounds that cannot be closed primarily because of contamination or tissue loss can undergo delayed closure or be allowed to close spontaneously. The optimal time of delayed closure has been shown to be on or after the fourth day following injury.[24] Treatment of the soft tissue should be initiated during the open-wound period so as to hasten the decrease in bacterial levels. The debrided wound may be dressed with sterile fine-mesh gauze, a moist or greasy dressing to prevent wound desiccation, and topical antimicrobials. The rationale for delayed primary closure is that the healing open wound gradually gains sufficient resistance to infection to permit an uncomplicated closure. Resistance is gained as capillaries and young fibrous tissue, referred to as granulation tissue, proliferate. Quantitative biopsies after the fourth day help to dictate the subsequent wound treatment: further debridement, adjunctive antimicrobials, more frequent dressing changes, or closure.

Spontaneous closure, on the other hand, is necessary for chronically infected or complex wounds and is facilitated by wound contracture and epithelialization from wound margins and cutaneous adnexa.

Methods of closure

Once it is decided to close the wound, a closure technique must be selected that provides accurate and secure approximation of the skin edges. The decision requires an understanding of the objectives of the repair, as well as of the materials implemented to effect such a repair. The ultimate goal of any closure is to achieve precise, tensionless alignment of the injured parts, restoring prompt function and cosmetic appearance.

The choice of appropriate material for wound closure is based on its biologic and mechanical properties, as well as the character of the tissue being approximated. Although the clinician's armamentarium includes a variety of sutures, staples, and tapes, it should be remembered that choice of material is less important than proper surgical technique. Each suture should be precisely placed and tied without undue tension, in order to avoid ischemia of the wound margins. The smallest size and amount of suture that will adequately approximate the tissue should be employed, especially in contaminated wounds.

Sutures that undergo rapid degradation in tissue, losing their tensile strength within 60 days, are considered absorbable sutures.[22] Those that maintain their tensile strength longer than 60 days are nonabsorbable sutures. Absorbable sutures (catgut, chromic, polyglycolic acid, polydoxane) are easily handled, knot securely when properly tied, and, because of their absorption, may be indicated in contaminated wounds.[44] The synthetic absorbable sutures (polyglycolic acid, polygalactin, and polydoxane) have several advantages over catgut: improved initial tensile strength, predictable rate of strength loss and absorption, and less tissue reaction. The nonabsorbable sutures may be classified according to their origin. Natural fibers include silk, cotton, and linen. Metallic sutures are derived from stainless steel. Synthetic materials include polyamides (nylon), polyesters (Dacron), and polyolefins (polyethylene, polypropylene).

The necessity to close individual layers of the wound is based on knowledge of local wound stresses, the presence of dead space, and the necessity for accurate approximation of tissues. The dense connective tissues (dermis, fascia, ligaments, tendons) represent the strength layers, heal slowly, and are therefore best approximated with synthetic, nonabsorbable monofilament sutures. Muscle and adipose tissue are often approximated to minimize infection associated with dead space resulting from tissue loss. When necessary, dead space should be approximated with a minimum number of loosely tied absorbable sutures.

The technique of suture closure of the skin can be divided into two methods: percutaneous and dermal. The choice of method depends on location of the wound, its direction, and local stress factors. In the first method, the sutures are passed through the epidermal and dermal layers. In the latter method, also called subcuticular, the sutures reapproximate the divided edges of the dermis without penetrating the epidermis.

Wounds that are oriented in the direction of skin wrinkles are subjected to less tension during healing and consequently produce a more favorable scar. Wounds that cross the lines of maximal stress are subjected to increased tension during healing and have a propensity to widen and hypertrophy with time. The degree of gaping prior to epidermal reapproximation reflects the potential width of the scar. Particularly in areas of high skin tension, layered wound closure is indicated. Because skin wounds are subjected to considerably less stress than fascial wounds and need support for only short periods of time, the least reactive absorbable sutures should be utilized.

The everting interrupted suture is the most frequently employed type of suture in plastic surgery (Fig. 26-1). The needle penetrates the tissue close to the incision line, diverging from the edge of the wound in order to encircle a larger amount of dermis and tissue in the depths of the wound than at the surface.[41] In this manner the suture everts as well as approximates. Subcuticular buried sutures are placed on the undersurface of the dermis, with the knot downward beneath the dermis. These are useful approximating sutures if tension is present and a widened scar is feared.[41]

Vertical mattress sutures are useful to evert the wound edges or maintain the skin coapted to the underlying fascial layer (Fig. 26-2). The horizontal mattress suture with a dermal component is also a useful stitch if tension is present. This suture is helpful in scalp lacerations, in flap approximation, and in situations in which there is a discrepancy in thickness between two opposing skin edges. In some areas, as satisfactory an approximation can be obtained by a carefully inserted continuous running suture as that produced by interrupted sutures. The removable continuous intradermal is of particular value in children, whose skin is normally under greater tension than that of adults and in

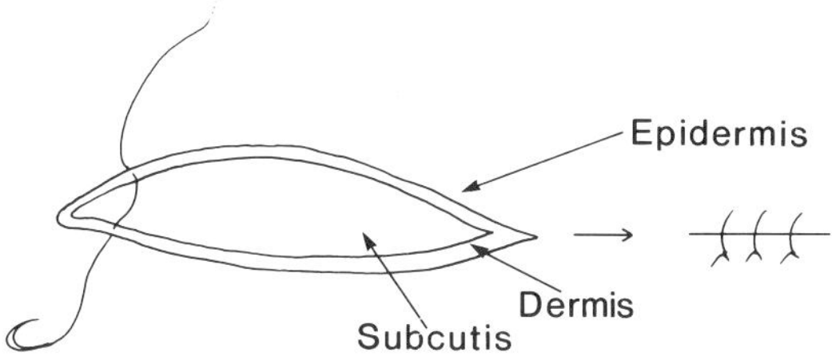

Figure 26–1 Simple everting suture technique for skin closure to achieve coaptation and an everted closure.

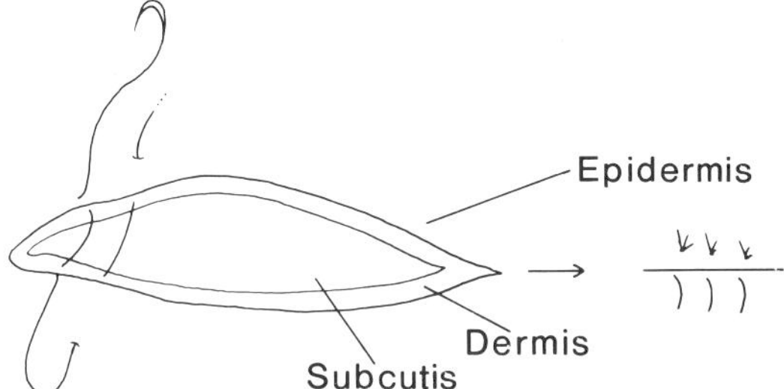

Figure 26–2 Vertical mattress suture technique for skin closure under slight tension.

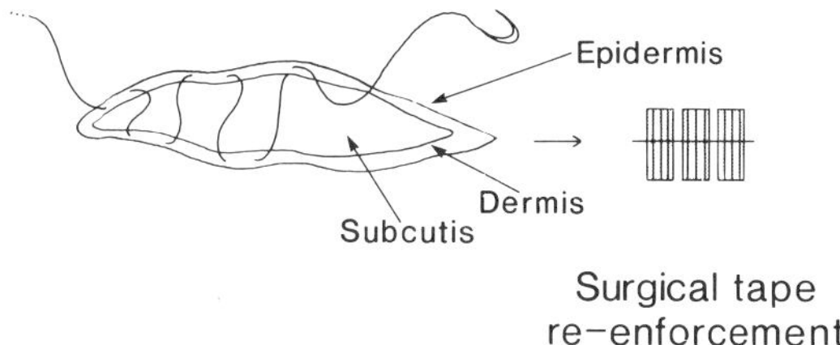

Figure 26–3 Continuous dermal or subcuticular suture technique, which can be left in place for extended periods of time and eliminates suture removal in small children.

whom suture marks are apt to occur. The continuous subcuticular suture may be left in place for a longer period, thus ensuring maturation of the collagen in the wound without danger of producing suture marks.

Following closure of the dermis, the strength layer of the wound, the epidermal layer can be adjusted with fine, nonabsorbable, monofilament sutures or surgical tape. This method of wound closure is designed to produce the least noticeable scar and is most appropriate for facial lacerations. An alternative measure to reduce the static skin tensions on the wound is to undermine wound edges before closure.

In special circumstances, continuous dermal sutures are preferable to precutaneous sutures (Fig. 26-3). Infants frightened by the prospects of suture removal, noncompliant children, and vagrant children, who may fail to return for wound inspection, are candidates for subcuticular closure, thus avoiding the inconvenience of suture removal. Subcuticular closure is also advisable for children susceptible to keloids, to avoid promoting keloid formation through epithelialization of suture tracts. Sutures should be removed before the seventh day to avoid epithelialization of suture tracts and the resultant objectionable erythematous "railroad track" scar. Sutures may be removed as soon as the second to fourth day in well-perfused regions with high visibility such as the face.

In the past, stainless steel sutures, skin clips, and staples have been used because of their presumed inertness. Studies have demonstrated actually slightly increased infection rates with these materials (compared with nylon or polypropolene), probably owing to mechanical irritation associated with their inherent rigidity. Staples, if removed prior to the seventh postoperative day, are acceptable, produce an everted skin closure, and reduce closure time—advantages in the treatment of a debilitated, multiply injured child.

Surgical tapes also have some advantages. They do not require anesthesia nor do they cause pain during closure—aspects attractive in caring for the pediatric population. Moreover, taped wounds have the least propensity for infection.[23] Tapes are quick to apply, cause minimal skin reaction, and prevent puncture scars. In certain situations, one may close the deeper layers of the wound with sutures and coapt the epidermis with tape, thus avoiding suture removal at a later date. Adherence is enhanced if moisture is minimized, the skin is defatted with freon or acetone, and benzoin is applied. Disadvantages of surgical tape use includes lack of precise anatomic approximation, absence of an everted edge, and the potential for scar widening.

Dressing

After wound closure, an adequate dressing is applied to the wound. Functions of dressings include (1) protection, (2) absorption, (3) compression, (4) immobilization, and (5) aesthetics. Protection from mechanical injury of the wound edges, desiccation, and exogenous bacterial contamination is necessary. Experimental studies have shown that closed wounds can be infected by surface bacterial contamination within the first 2 to 3 days.[55] Following this period, sutured wounds gain considerable resistance to infection and dressings no longer play a protective role. The dressing should keep the wound surface free of excess fluids to minimize maceration and prevent associated bacterial proliferation while avoiding desiccation. To accomplish such protection, a variety of materials may be used. The inner layer in contact with the wound should be fine-mesh gauze, either plain (Telfa) or impregnated (Xeroform or petroleum). The purpose of impregnating gauze is not to prevent its sticking to the wound (macerating amounts of impregnate would be necessary to accomplish this); rather, it provides a coating to the fibers and thereby promotes drainage through to the absorptive layers of the dressing. Absorbancy is caused by the capillary forces of attraction exerted by the capillary spaces between the dressing fibers. The beneficial effects of absorbancy are that the bacteria contained within the absorbant fluid are removed, the exudate itself is removed, depleting the wound of bacterial nutrients, and tissue maceration is prevented. High absorbancy is incompatible with nonadhesion because the serous exudate forms a powerful and coherent glue as it dries. Removal of an absorbant dressing, if not used in conjunction with a coated contact layer, disrupts the fibrinous scab and any granulation tissue that has become entrapped in the dressing. Absorbant dressings are, therefore, useful in the debridement of open wounds. Plain gauze tends to entrap the drainage and form a coagulum at the innermost layer. Commercially impregnated gauze must be "wrung out" because its heavy impregnation tends to prevent drainage and macerate tissue. Fluffed gauze sponges, mechanic's waste, and bulk cotton may be added next as an absorptive layer to allow the dressing to conform to the desired shape and to provide immobilization of the wounded part. Nonstretchable, firm, roller gauze bandage and adhesive tape complete the typical occlusive dressing.

Immobilization of the site of injury is essential in the management of contaminated wounds because lymphatic flow is thus diminished, minimizing the spread of wound microflora. Immobilization also places the wound at rest, decreasing pain and metabolic demands of the tissue. In addition, immobilization may protect the newly formed capillaries from disruption, thus preventing formation of small clots and allowing the wound to heal more expeditiously.

Elevation is essential to minimize edema and its deleterious effects. Edema has been called "the mother of scar," as it slows repair and increases fibrous tissue proliferation. Elevation of the wounded part above the level of the heart is the simplest method of limiting the amount of edema. Carefully applied, uniform, distal-to-proximally applied compression may add to the benefits of elevation.

Finally, a dressing should be esthetically acceptable, because it is the portion of wound management that a surgeon first presents to the patient and others—the signature on a surgeon's work.

REFERENCES

1. Alexander JW, Fisher JE, Boyajian M et al: The influence of hair removal methods on wound infections, *Arch Surg* 118:347, 1983.
2. Almersjo D, Hulten L, Rhoberg B et al: Wound healing after depilation with a keratolytic cream: a tensiometric and histologic study in rats, *Acta Chir Scand* 133:355, 1967.
3. Altemeier WA, Gibbs EW: Bacterial flora of fresh accidental wounds, *Surg Gynecol Obstet* 78:164, 1944.
4. Aoch RJ, Lander JJ, Sherman LA et al: Transfusion-transmitted viruses: interum analysis of hepatitis among transfused and nontransfused patients. In Vyas GN, Cohen SN, Schmid R, editors: *Viral hepatitis*, Philadelphia: 1978, Franklin Institute Press.
5. Assaf RAF, Dundee JW, Gamble JAS: The influence of the route of administration of the clinical action of diazepam, *Anesthesiology* 30:152, 1975.
6. Bezustowicz RM, Nelson DA, Betts EK et al: Efficacy of oral premedications in children for outpatient surgery, *Anesthesiol* 55:328, 1981.
7. Burke JF: The effective period of preventitive antibiotic action in experimental incisions and dermal lesions, *Surgery* 50:161, 1961.
8. Bongard FS, Elings VB, Maricson RE: New uses of fluorescence in the management of necrotizing soft tissue infection, *Am J Surg* 150:261, 1985.
9. Cardant CR, Rodeheaver G, Thacker J et al: The crush injury: a high risk wound, *J Am Coll Emerg Phys* 5:965, 1976.
10. Carson IW, Moore J, Balmer JP et al: Laryngeal competence with ketamine and other drugs, *Anesthesiology* 38:128, 1973.
11. Centers for Disease Control: Adult immunization. Recommendations of the Immunization Practices Advisory Committee (ACID), *MMWR* 33:15, 1984.
12. Centers for Disease Control: Recommendations for protection against viral hepatitis, *MMWR* 34:314, 1985.
13. Commission on Trauma of the American College of Surgeons: Prophylaxis against tetanus in wound management, *Bull Am Coll Surg* 69 (10):22, 1984.
14. Conner JT, Katz RI, Pagano RR et al: RO 21-3981 for IV surgical premedication and induction of anesthesia, *Anesthesiology* Analg 57:1, 1978.
15. Cruse PJE, Foord R: A 5-year prospective study of 23,649 surgical wounds, *Arch Surg* 107:206, 1973.
16. Denes AE, Smith JL, Maynard JG: Hepatitis B infections in physicians, *JAMA* 239:210, 1978.
17. Desjardins R, Ansara S, Charest J: Preanesthesia medications in pediatric day-care surgery, *Can Anaesth Soc J* 28:141, 1981.
18. Dineen P, Drusin L: Epidemics of post operative wound infections associated with hair carriers, *Lancet* 2:1157, 1973.
19. Dudre LJ, Stieglitz P: Extrapyramidal syndromes after premedication with droperidol in children, *Br J Anaesth* 52:831, 1980.
20. Editorial: Blood transfusion, hemophilia and AIDs, *Lancet* ii:1433, 1984.
21. Edlich RF, Rodeheaver GT, Thacker JG: Wounds, bites, and stings. In Mattox KL, Moore EE, Feliciano DJ: *Trauma*. East Norwalk, 1988, Appleton and Lange.
22. Edlich RF, Panek PH, Rodeheaver GT et al: Physical and chemical configurations of sutures in the development of surgical infections, *Ann Surg* 177:697, 1973.

23. Edlich RF, Rodeheaver GT, Kuphal J et al: Technique of closures: contaminated wounds, *J Am Coll Emerg Phys* 3:375, 1974.
24. Edlich RF, Rogers W, Kasper G et al: Studies in the management of the contaminated wound. I. Optimal time for closure of contaminated open wounds. II. Comparison of resistance to infection of open and closed wounds during healing, *Am J Surg* 117:323, 1969.
25. Elek SD: Experimental staphylococcal infections in the skin of man, *Ann NY Acad Sci* 65:85, 1956.
26. Epstein BS, Hannallah RS: Outpatient anesthesia. In Gregory GA, editor: *Pediatric anesthesia,* 1989, Churchill Livingstone.
27. Farmer CB, Mann RJ: Human bite infections of the hand. *South Med J* 59:515, 1966.
28. Filston HC, Moylan JA: Management of the acutely injured pediatric patient. In Serafin D, Georgiade NG, editors: *Pediatric plastic surgery.* St Louis, 1984, Mosby.
29. Fraser DW: Preventing tetanus in patients with wounds, *Ann Intern Med* 84:95, 1976.
30. Gibson T: Physical properties of skin. In McCarthey JB: *Plastic and reconstructive surgery,* 1990, Mosby–Year Book.
31. Gordon H, Sasaki GH, Krizek TJ: Biology of tissue injury and repair. In Georgiade NG, Georgiade GS, Riefkohl R et al, editors: *Essentials of plastic, maxillofacial, and reconstructive surgery,* Baltimore, 1987, Williams & Wilkins.
32. Goresky GV, Steward DJ: Rectal Methohexatone for induction of anesthesia in children, *Can Anaesth Soc J* 26:213, 1979.
33. Gregory GA: Induction of anesthesia. In Gregory GA, editor: *Pediatric anesthesia,* 1989, Churchill Livingstone.
34. Hamer ML, Robson MC, Krizek TJ et al. Quantitative bacterial analysis of comparative wound irrigations, *Ann Surg* 181:819, 1975.
35. Howard RJ: Hospital acquired infections in surgical patients. In Howard RJ, Simmons RL: *Surgical infectious diseases,* 1988, Appleton & Lange.
36. Immunization Practices Advisory Committee (ACIP): Supplementary statement of contraindications to receipt of pertussis vaccine, *MMWR* 33:169, 1984.
37. Kaplan EL, Anthony BF, Bisen A et al: Prevention of bacterial endocarditis, *Circulation* 56:1399, 1977.
38. Krizek TJ, Robson MC, Groskin MG: Experimental burn wound sepsis: evaluation of enzymatic debridement, *J Surg Res* 17:219, 1974.
39. May JW, Hansen RH: Soft tissue reconstruction of the upper extremity in children. In Serafin D, Georgiade NG, editors: *Pediatric plastic surgery,* St Louis, 1984, Mosby–Year Book.
40. McGarry PMF: A double blind study of diazepam, droperidol and meperidine as premedications in children, *Can Anaesth Soc J* 17:157, 1970.
41. McCarthey JG: Introduction to plastic surgery. In McCarthey JG, editor: *Plastic surgery,* Philadelphia, 1990, WB Saunders.
42. Orr HW: *Osteomyelitis and compound fractures and other infected wounds,* St Louis, 1929, CV Mosby Co.
43. Peacock EE, Van Winkle W Jr: *Wound repair,* Philadelphia, 1970, WB Saunders.
44. Postlethwait RW: Sutures and suturing. In Wolcott MW, editor: *Ambulatory surgery and the basics of emergency surgical care,* Philadelphia, 1988, JB Lippincott.
45. Pryor GJ, Kilpatrick WR, Opp DR: Local anesthesia in minor lacerations, topical: TEC vs lidocaine infiltration, *Ann Emerg Med* 9:568, 1980.
46. Rita L, Seleny FL: Pediatric outpatient anesthesia: premedication vs no premedication and the choice of anesthetic agents, *Anesth Rev* 1:9, 1974.
47. Rita L, Seleny F, Mazurek A et al: Intramuscular midazolam for pediatric preanesthesic sedation: a double-blind controlled study with morphine, *Anesthesiology* 63:528, 1985.
48. Robson MC: Infection in the surgical patient: an imbalance in the normal equilibrium, *Clin Plast Surg* 6:493, 1979.
49. Robson MC, Heggers JP: Surgical infections. II. The beta hemolytic streptococcus, *J Surg Res* 9:289, 1969.
50. Robson M, Zachary L: Repair of traumatic cutaneous injuries involving the skin and soft tissue. In Georgiade, Georgiade, Riefkohl et al: *Essentials of plastic, maxillofacial and reconstructive surgery,* 1987, Williams & Wilkins.
51. Robson MC, Duke WF, Krizek TJ: Rapid bacterial screening in the treatment of civilian wounds, *J Surg Res* 14:426, 1973.
52. Robson MC, Krizek TJ, Heggers JP: Biology of surgical infections. In *Current problems in surgery,* Chicago, 1973, Yearbook Medical Publishers.
53. Robson MC, Edstrom LE, Krizek TJ et al: The efficacy of systemic antibiotics in the treatment of granulating wounds, *J Surg Res* 16:299, 1974.
54. Salisbury RE: Thermal burns. In McCarthy JG, editor: *Plastic surgery,* Philadelphia, 1990, WB Saunders.
55. Schauerhamer RA, Edlich RF, Panek P et al: Studies in the management of the contaminated wound. VII. Susceptibility of surgical wounds to post-op bacterial contamination, *Am J Surg* 122:74, 1971.
56. Schecter WP: Occupationally acquired HIV infection and workers compensation, *Resident and Staff Physician* pp 51-55, Aug 1991.
57. Schmidt KF, Garfield JM, Korten K: The pharmacology of agents used in outpatient anesthesia, *Int Anesth Clin* 14:15, 1976.
58. Seawall K: Preoperative medication for children, *Surg Clin N Am* 50:775, 1970.
59. Seropian R, Reynolds BM: Wound infections after pre-op depiliation vs razor preparation, *Am J Surg* 121:251, 1971.
60. Sethna NF, Berde CB: Pediatric regional anesthesia. In Gregory GA, editor: *Pediatric anesthesia* 1989, Churchill Livingstone.
61. Shah CP, Robinson GC, Kinnis C et al: Day care surgery for children: a continuing study of medical complications and parental attitudes, *Medical Care* 10:437, 1972.
62. Stevenson TR, Thacker JG, Rodeheaver GT et al: Cleansing the traumatic wounds by high pressure syringe irrigation, *J Am Coll Emerg Phys* 5:1, 1976.
63. Steward DJ: Outpatient pediatric anesthesia, *Anesthesiology* 43:268, 1975.
64. Steward DJ: Psychologic preparation and premedication. In Gregory GA, editor: *Pediatric anesthesia* 1989, Churchill Livingstone.
65. Trueta J: *Treatment of war wounds and infections,* New York, 1940, Paul B Hoeber.
66. Tucker GT, Mather LE: Pharmacokinetics of local anesthetic agents, *Br J Anaesth* 47:213, 1975.
67. Vivori E: Preparation of surgery and premedication. In Gray TC, Rees GJ, editors: *Modern trends in pediatric anesthesia,* London, 1981, Butterworth.
68. Walton R, Chick L, Bunkis J: Wounds. In Trunkey DD, Lewis FR Jr: *Current therapy of trauma,* Philadelphia, 1991, BC Decker.
69. Way WL, Costley EC, Way EL: Respiratory sensitivity of the newborn infant to meperidine and morphine, *Clin Pharm Ther* 6:454, 1965.
70. Warden GD: Management of infections and wounds. In Wolcott MW, editor: *Ambulatory surgery and the basics of emergency surgical care,* Philadelphia, 1989, JP Lippincott.
71. Whitham JG, Manners JM: Clinical comparison of thio-

pentone and methohexatone, *Br Med J [Clin Res]* 1:1663, 1962.
72. Wolcott MW: Soft tissue injuries and foreign bodies. In Wolcott MW, editor: *Ambulatory surgery and the basics of emergency surgical care*, Philadelphia, 1988, JP Lippincott.
73. Wolff TW, Lister GD: Surgical treatment of the acutely injured upper extremity. In Serain D, Georgiade N, editors: *Pediatric plastic surgery*, St Louis, 1984, Mosby–Year Book.

27 Guidelines for Determination of Brain Death

Dennis L. Johnson

The death of an injured child occurs unexpectedly and without recompense. Children are the wellspring of precious innocence, the embodiment of our hopes and dreams, and the future of society. The death of a child brings parents to the depths of despair, engenders anguish in the hearts of caregivers, and saps the strength of our society.

The determination of brain death is a personal and societal tragedy that has important ramifications. Homicide, inheritance, and life insurance benefits are medicolegal issues that demand a precise determination of death. In an era of increasing costs, the timely determination of death allows a more equitable distribution of limited resources. Moreover, vital organs are best donated as soon as possible after brain death in order to transplant them in optimal physiologic condition. Although organ donation is death's gift for the renewal and continuation of life, the determination of death must be separated from and not influenced by the pressure to save and preserve another life.

Physicians hold sacred the health and well-being of children. They also acknowledge the need to minister to the family of a sick or dying child. The determination of brain death cannot be arrogated by the physician, and yet should not unnecessarily encumber the family. Even though parents will participate in the decision-making process, they should not bear the full burden of guilt associated with discontinuing life support. The determination of brain death requires the skills and humanity of an experienced clinician, complemented by the spiritual comfort offered by a pastoral caregiver and the emotional and logistical support of a social worker.

The process of declaring a child dead can be divided into four phases. In the assessment phase the severity of the injury is appraised; the parents' reaction is characterized by shock and disbelief. During the recognition phase the diagnosis of brain death is made by the physician and conveyed to the family. The family's hope for recovery fades to the despair of death. Guilt and anger may surface as hostility toward caregivers. In the third phase the family accepts the death of their child. A "time out" to say good-bye is often necessary for the family to adapt to their loss. In the last phase the details of the child's disposition are clarified. The child's care is turned over to a transplant team, or the cardiopulmonary support systems are discontinued.

PHASE I: ASSESSMENT

The assessment phase begins when the child is brought to the emergency room. Arrest at the scene of the accident or full cardiopulmonary arrest upon arrival are strong indications that a child will die. Once a child is resuscitated from shock and the airway cleared, a quick assessment of neurologic status provides important clues to survival. Dilated pupils that do not constrict or react to a bright light, and that are not associated with direct orbital injury give the single most reliable sign of cerebral herniation and impending brain death. Hypothermia must be corrected. Coincident drug intoxication should be considered, but is seldom at issue in a child less than 12 years of age who comes from the scene of an accident with external signs of trauma. Flaccid muscle tone and lack of response to painful stimuli are also important clues. A high cervical spine injury can be concealed by coma in cases of severe head injury, which makes the outlook even more ominous. In addition to cervical spine x-rays being taken in the emergency room, a CT scan must be obtained as soon as possible. Generalized swelling, the salt-and-pepper appearance of severe contusion, intraventricular hemorrhage, pneumocephalus, acute subarachnoid or subdural hemorrhage, hypodense areas in the basal ganglia, and the lack of basal cisterns (Fig. 27-1) are all important signs of severe brain injury (which must be correlated with findings of the neurologic examination). The single most ominous radiographic sign of severe brain injury is a uniformly hypodense cerebral cortex associated with relatively hyperdense tentorium, cerebellum, and brainstem. Primary hypoxia resulting from apnea at the scene of the accident or ischemia related to

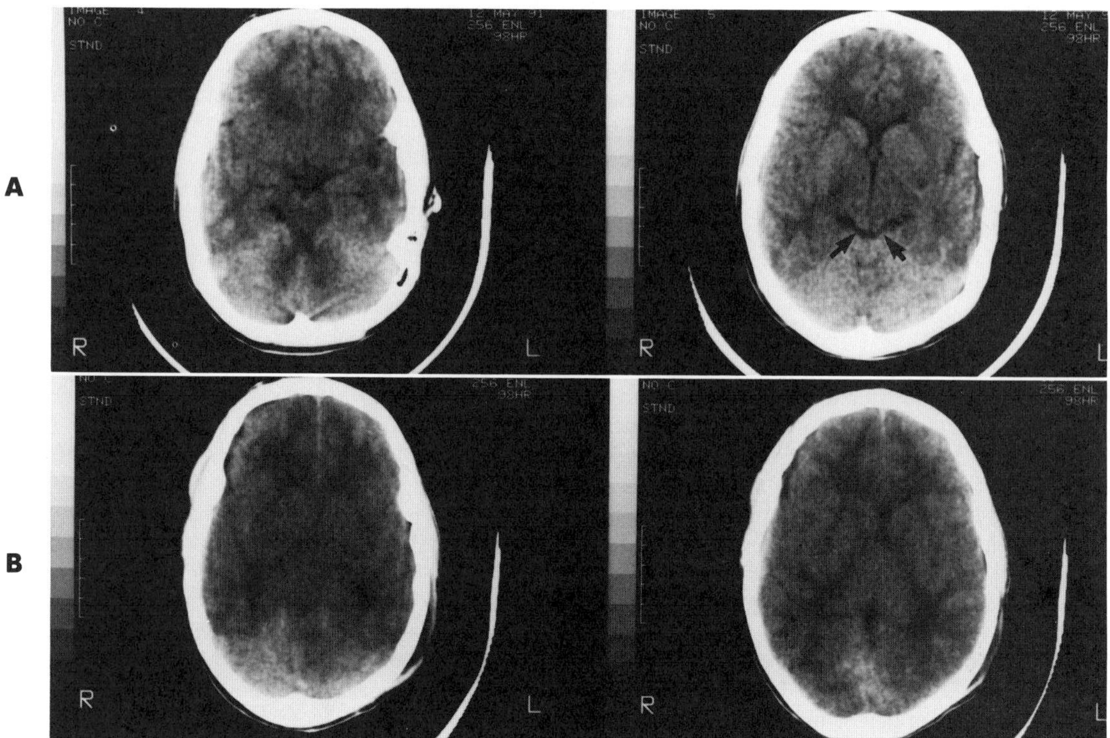

Figure 27–1 12-year-old boy struck by a car. **A,** Normal CT scan upon admission with well-defined perimesencephalic cistern *(arrows);* **B,** Diffuse cerebral edema on second day of hospitalization with obliteration perimesencephalic cistern.

severe intracranial hypertension is the most probable cause of this phenomenon.

During this assessment phase of the child's care, parents are often in a state of shock and disbelief. It is important to develop a reasoned expectation of survival and to share the known facts with the family. Both parents deserve full attention, even if one takes control and acts as the spokesperson for the couple. Family, especially grandparents, can be a tremendous resource for parents as they come to grips with their tragedy. On the other hand, if not well informed, they can be a source of discordant opinion and make parents' decisions more agonizing. Although the primary communication should be between the parents and the attending physician, periodic involvement of the entire family in open discussion can be helpful. The family's questions center on prognosis and the likelihood of the child's dying. An honest yet sensitive response emphasizes the seriousness of the injury and the uncertain prognosis. Pastoral caregivers and social workers are invaluable in providing solace to the entire family during this phase.

PHASE II: RECOGNITION

Even with evidence of a severe irreversible brain injury, concurrent drug intoxication or high cer-

vical spine injury is possible. For a child who has been transferred from another institution following resuscitation, the effect of anticonvulsant medication and pharmacologic muscle paralysis must also be taken into account. A barbiturate level in the low therapeutic range (phenobarbitol <10 μg/ml, pentobarbital <2 μg/ml, thiopental <5 μg/ml) is necessary before brain function can be assessed. Neurologic examination of a brain-dead child reveals no response to pain, no spontaneous movements, no pupillary response, no corneal reflex, no cough or gag, no oculocephalic reflex (doll's eye phenomenon), and no oculocervical response. Moreover, the blood pressure and pulse do not change with stimulation. One of the most reliable clinical signs of brain death is a cold forehead in a child who is otherwise normothermic; brain death is associated with lack of cerebral perfusion and thus no mechanism for warming the head. A core temperature within 2° of normal, blood pressure within the normal range,[2] and normal serum electrolytes and liver enzymes are mandatory. As long as the tympanic membranes are intact, cold caloric stimulation is performed. The head of the bed is elevated 30 degrees, and each external auditory canal is irrigated with 100 ml of ice-cold water. A 20-cc syringe attached to a 16-gauge intravenous catheter is a well-tested means of introducing the water into the external canal. In a comatose patient, the normal response is conjugate deviation of the eyes to the side of the cold irrigation. No response during the 5 minutes following irrigation confirms the absence of brainstem function. Five minutes are allowed to elapse before the other canal is irrigated.

If the child's cardiopulmonary status warrants, an apnea test should be performed. The patient is preoxygenated with 100% oxygen for 10 minutes at a PCO_2 of 35 to 40. The ventilator is stopped for 10 minutes, but oxygen should be continued by cannula into the endotracheal tube at 6 L/minute. Oxygen can be delivered to the carina through a suction catheter or by continuous positive airway pressure (CPAP). The PO_2 should not fall below 200 torr, and PCO_2 should rise to at least 60 to assure adequate respiratory stimulation; PCO_2 rises about 4 torr during the first minute, and then 3 torr each minute thereafter.[1] The test is aborted if the child's blood pressure falls when ventilation is withdrawn.

This sequence confirms the physician's diagnosis that the child is dead. The law in the District of Columbia and in many states mandates simply that the attending physician certify death. Death is defined as irreversible loss of brain and brainstem function in accordance with accepted medical standards.[4] If the attending physician is uncertain or insecure about the findings, another opinion from an experienced clinician is helpful. Test results confirming the diagnosis of brain death, as they become available, should be shared with the parents. Periodic counseling sessions with the entire family are helpful to avoid misunderstanding and to manage disputes that may arise among family members. The parents' response remains one of disbelief, mixed with anger and hopeful, but fragile, optimism. No purpose is served nor advantage gained by insisting that the parents accept the death of their child. Acceptance comes in time. The parents will perceive that the physician is acting in their child's best interest because his or her actions and concern reflect a deep commitment to their child.

The importance of the social worker and pastoral caregiver as sources of emotional support is revealed as they assist the parents through this agonizing experience. The social worker guides the family through the maze of the health care system and alerts the team to sources of miscommunication. Pastoral caregivers remain a buttress of spiritual strength.

The question, "Is my child dead?" is answered: "Yes, I am certain that your child's brain has died and that we have done everything humanly possible to save him."

PHASE III: ACCEPTANCE

Although an attending physician cannot change a child's condition, he or she remains ethically bound also to attend to the family. It is essential to resist the temptation to turn away and leave the determination of death to other caregivers or to a fashionable ancillary test that confirms death.

The transition from recognition to acceptance of death is not always smooth. Depending on their fund of knowledge and understanding, the family may remain unconvinced of their child's death. Confirmation of the clinical diagnosis by EEG, cerebral angiography, MRI angiography, isotope angiography, or determination of cerebral blood flow may be helpful to the family. An equally effective and less costly method to confirm brain death for the benefit of the family is a repeat clinical examination in 12 to 24 hours, complete with cold caloric stimulation and apnea test. Observation periods, also recommended in published guidelines, are longer for infants than for children 1 year and older.[3] Such an interval allows parents to adjust and see for themselves that their child is not responsive and is indeed dead. This is the time for the family to say good-bye to their child and to begin the mourning process. If given sufficient time and enough information, most parents will accept the diagnosis and be ready to move on to the next phase.

Impulsive decisions by parents to withdraw support suggest that the child's death has not been truly accepted. Alert clinicians provide time for discussion and acceptance. Occasionally, recalcitrant parents distrust or disbelieve the physician because they cannot or are unwilling to accept the child's death. Frequently, a resistant parent says, "You want me to tell you to pull the plug, and I am not going to do that because there may be a chance that she will recover." Arguing with or cajoling the parent may produce an adversarial relationship, which is a disservice to both the parent and the child. Under these circumstances it is preferable to embrace the family and reassert the commitment to the child and the child's well-being, rather than to step back and withdraw. The pastoral caregiver, social worker, and supportive family members can be instrumental to the parents' coming to grips with the child's death. In these exceptional cases time will often clear the confusion of emotions and facts. Lack of sophistication, ignorance, or mental illness within the family will require that more time, individual attention, and support be given to family members by caregivers.

PHASE IV: CONCLUSION

The conclusion phase is as critical as any other and deserves delicate and sensitive planning. Despite the most careful explanation, however, the family will often focus on the removal of the ventilator as the event marking the death of the child. In our institution the parent must consent to removing the life support system. Many parents cannot bear this final burden. I have found it useful to explain the process and make the simple statement, "Unless you object, I will remove your child's body from the support system." Thus the responsibility is not borne solely by the parents but is shared with the physician.

Once brain death is accepted by the family, the concept of organ transplantation is introduced. The determination of death must be kept separate from the discussion of transplantation in order to avoid any conflict of interest. Although the family's decision may be facilitated by the attending physician, a detailed discussion of transplantation is left to the transplant coordinator. Once the decision is made either to donate organs or to withdraw life support, a timetable is provided to the parents. If they choose to withdraw support or if organs are not suitable for donation, the parents may wish to stay with the child after the ventilator is withdrawn and the heart continues to beat. The physician can conclude his or her commitment to the child and parents by accompanying the body to the morgue. If permission for transplantation is granted, the child's care is entrusted to the transplant team.

Pastoral caregivers are invaluable in ministering to the family's spiritual needs, and the social worker provides not only emotional support but very meaningful practical advice and guidance in regard to day-to-day activities, managed care utilization, temporary monetary support, and funeral arrangements. The social worker translates medical jargon into lay terms that can be easily understood by the family and can promote organ transplantation.

Determination of death cannot be relegated to a videotape or to the void of a "team" approach. The physician cannot depend on a "canned" response, but must face each individual case with genuine concern and sincerity.

The determination of death is a classic story that remains the longest running play in history. The actors change but the content of the play should not. The play's reception and critical review by the audience will depend on the quality and commitment of the company.

REFERENCES

1. Ashwal S, Schneider S: Brain death in children, Part I, *Pediatr Neurol* 3:5-11, 1987.
2. Blumenthal S, Epps RP, Heavenvich R et al: Report of the task force on blood pressure control in children, *Pediatrics* 59(suppl):797-820, 1977.
3. Guidelines for the determination of brain death in children: report of the medical consultants on the diagnosis of death to the President's Commission for the Study of Ethical Problems in Medicine and Biomedical and Behavioral Research, *Neurology* 32:395-399, 1982.
4. President's Commission for the Study of Ethical Problems in Medicine and Biomedical and Behavioral Research: Guidelines for the determination of death, *JAMA* 246:2184, 1981.

28   Organ Procurement

Margaret J. Schaeffer

Approximately 25,000 people (700 of whom are infants or children) in the United States are currently waiting for an organ transplant.[5] They are at home, in dialysis units, in critical care units, on beepers, waiting by the telephone. Their waiting began only after weeks, months, perhaps years of illness and debilitating disease. The cause of the failing organ may be genetic (polycystic kidney disease or diabetes), infectious (cardiomyopathy due to viral infection), or congenital (abnormality such as biliary atresia).

Successful solid organ transplantation began with a kidney transplant between identical twins by Dr. Joseph Murray in Boston in 1954. It was advanced by the pioneering work of Dr. Thomas Starzl with liver transplantation and Dr. Norman Shumway's accomplishments with heart and heart-lung transplants. Today, at multiple medical centers, in the hands of countless talented and dedicated surgeons and transplant team members, the 700 infants and children are being given a chance to live through transplantation. These transplant "miracles" often have their beginnings in the emergency departments and critical care units of pediatric trauma centers.

Topics included in this chapter are the identification of a potential donor, the referral and evaluation process, the proper approach to a potential donor family and the consent process, legal considerations, donor management, surgical removal and preservation of solid organs, and the present system of allocation. Tissue donation is also briefly discussed.

IDENTIFICATION AND CRITERIA FOR DONATION

For 20 years the potential for donation has been estimated between 20,000 and 25,000 donors annually in the United States. That estimate by the Centers for Disease Control (CDC) was based on the number of deaths reported in categories thought to be appropriate for donation. Recent information from actual chart reviews in hospitals around the country show that the original estimates may have been too high. The 1987-1988 Pennsylvania Donor Study, a combined effort of the Delaware Valley Transplant Program and the Pittsburgh Transplant Foundation, found the number of potential donors to be closer to 12,000 to 15,000 per year, and the 1989 survey of the Association of Organ Procurement Organizations substantiated the lower number.[1]

Whatever the real potential is, the fact remains that it has never been approached in actual donations. Although the number of donations increased during the early 1980s, there was no further increase of potential donors in the late 1980s, and in the best year there were only 4000 donors. There are several approaches to potential donors that may increase that number. The first relates to the issue of identification of a potential donor in the early stages of a patient's hospitalization.

Traditionally, donors have been found among patients who have sustained trauma that has produced serious head injury. The most common forms of trauma causing such an injury in children are motor vehicle accidents in which the child was an unrestrained passenger or a pedestrian struck by a vehicle. Any child with a potentially fatal head injury should be considered as a possible organ donor. Other sources of donors include the child who has an extensive anoxic incident secondary to a drowning, anaphylaxis, status epilepticus, or asthma; the child who has a ruptured arteriovenous malformation with extensive bleeding or who has hydrocephalus and a malfunctioning ventriculo-peritoneal shunt; and the child with a primary brain tumor.

Age criteria for donation are widely accepted now as *newborn to 70 years* of age. The newborn, although difficult to diagnose as dead through brain-death criteria, is a valuable resource, as there are many in the newborn and infant population in need of a heart or a liver.

Untreated systemic infection is a contraindication to donation. However, antibiotic therapy for 72 hours with resultant negative blood cultures, normothermia, and a normal white blood count (WBC) renders a donor acceptable. A potential donor should not be considered infected because of increased body temperature or an elevated WBC alone, as these are also indicative of the body's

"

response to neurologic trauma and may not indicate infection at all.

Extracranial malignancy is a contraindication to donation. A patient with a primary brain tumor, malignant or benign, without metastasis may be accepted for donation. In situations in which the malignancy is extracranial, donation of the eyes or corneas should be considered.

These are only general criteria for consideration of a child as an organ donor. Each donor situation and each organ system should be evaluated by an organ procurement specialist before a decision of suitability is made. Therefore, early recognition of the potential donor is important so that proper evaluation can be performed.

REFERRAL AND EVALUATION

There are approximately 70 organ procurement organizations (OPO) in the United States. Some are hospital or transplant center based. The majority are independent organizations. The federal government oversees these OPOs through a private nonprofit network, the United Network for Organ Sharing (UNOS). Each OPO has been given a specific geographic area within which its services are required for organ donor referral and evaluation. Every hospital has an OPO to whom referrals are made. (Information about contacting regional OPOs is available from the United Network for Organ Sharing, 1-800-24DONOR.)

The OPO specializes in organ donation. Its coordinators are prepared with up-to-date information regarding criteria and need. When called early in the management of a potential donor, they do their evaluations from an inconspicuous position, either in the unit or over the telephone, whichever is more appropriate.

Evaluation begins with the immediate medical history of the patient. Cardiac arrest with resuscitation is *not* a contraindication to donation. The duration of the arrest and the subsequent treatment modalities (e.g., defibrillation and vasopressor/inotropic support) are noted and their impact on the organ function considered. Such evaluation is made for all organs, including the heart.

Trauma, especially blunt trauma to the abdomen, crush injuries, and electrical injuries may have effects on the kidneys, liver, and pancreas. The damage is assessed by laboratory values that reflect renal, hepatic, and pancreatic function.

The status of the heart and lungs also depends on the extent of any thoracic trauma. The use of chest tubes does *not* preclude donation of either heart or lungs. A history of aspiration does affect the lungs and should be reported to the coordinator. Laboratory studies that are important for determination of heart and lung function include arterial

blood gases, CPK with isoenzymes, and a sputum Gram stain. A 12-lead ECG and the results of an echocardiogram are also helpful in this evaluation. Readings of chest x-rays from admission and the most recent films may also be requested. If a Swan-Ganz line is present, pressure readings are helpful for determination of cardiac function.

For evaluation of all organs, the patient's blood group and weight are needed. The OPO coordinator also needs to know the transfusion history, the need for vasopressor/inotropic support, and the use of antibiotics or steroids.

Any information about the patient's previous medical history is valuable. In particular, the coordinator looks for history of infection, drug use, alcohol use, cigarette smoking, hypertension, diabetes, pancreatitis, seizures, use of birth-control pills, and prior surgeries.

During this evaluation phase, the OPO coordinator or specialist is a valuable investigator. Based on his or her findings, a recommendation is made for or against moving ahead with the consent process. Because of the amount of information to be reviewed, an early referral, even prior to the final declaration of death, is reasonable. This review usually takes place once the child's poor prognosis has been identified and the mechanisms for determination of brain death have been begun.

APPROACH, REQUEST, AND CONSENT

The traumatic death of a child is a devastating event, emotionally exhausting to everyone involved in that child's life: parents, siblings, friends, and all health care team members who worked to save that life. The sadness and despair derive from the finality of the event. Modern medicine has found a way to ease the finality, however, to continue life even in the face of death. Although we cannot return a child who has died to his parents, we can offer them some solace through the life-giving organ donation process. Studies have revealed that 79% of families who donated the organs of a loved one felt that the donation helped them in their grieving process, and 89% said they would donate again if the situation arose.[2]

The professionals whose involvement in organ donation is essential, physicians in the neurosciences and intensive care unit (ICU) nurses, also report positive attitudes about donation. More than 90% in each category strongly approve of donation, and an equal percentage would consider donating their own organs or those of a loved one.[4]

There is, however, a wide discrepancy between these attitutes and actual donation numbers. Of the potential donors each year, be they 12,000 or 20,000, many are lost through lack of identification. Many more, perhaps as many as one third to one half of the total potential, are lost somewhere in the consent process. The most difficult part of the donation process is the period of approach and consent; it is difficult for both the child's family and the health care team. Because of the difficulties encountered, this is the most likely point for the process to fall apart.

It is well documented that sudden trauma and sudden unexpected death cause tremendous stress to a family, which is particularly disabling when the lost one is a child. The unexpected incident shocks the family. The control of their lives and of their child are taken over by others. They become powerless in a foreign setting, having to rely on the knowledge and communication of people they do not know. For these reasons, information given to family members must be consistent and not misleading. For example, a ventilator should be referred to as just that, not as *life support*. Using the term *brain death*, instead of simply *death*, may also be confusing and make the family think that their child is not really dead. The family must be supported by the health care team with factual information about the child's condition and given time to absorb and understand what they have been told. This is most important when death by brain criteria is expected and then diagnosed. *No family should ever be approached about organ donation until it is certain that they understand and accept the fact that their child has died.* The concept of donation should not be used to convince them that death has really occurred.

In an ongoing study at four sites around the country, the Partnership for Organ Donation reports that separating or "decoupling" the discussion of death from the discussion of organ donation results in a consent rate three times higher than that achieved when the diagnosis of death and the concept of organ donation are presented together.[3]

Death, especially the death of a child, also puts the health care team under tremendous stress. Dealing with death declared by brain-death criteria requires solid education, understanding, and acceptance of the concept of brain death by physicians, nurses, social workers, and pastoral caregivers. The concept of donation need not be agreed upon by all, but recognition of the family's right to form their own opinion and make their own decisions is imperative. No member of a health care team should feel pressured to approach a family about donation if he or she has ambiguous feelings. Similarly, uneasiness or fear of this discussion should be taken seriously, and someone with training and experience in the request process should lead the way. This may be a physician, nurse, social worker, pastoral caregiver, or, ideally, an OPO coordinator. This specialist is a resource that a hospital team should not overlook. When brought on site early in the process, the donation coordinator can help the team decide when, how, and who is to approach the family. If the OPO coordinator is to make the initial approach, it is important for someone from the team, with whom the family is familiar, to introduce the coordinator to the family.

In addition to identifying the proper time and person to seek consent for organ donation, the technique of the request is also critical. The conversation should be held in a quiet, private place if at all possible. This affords the family an opportunity to feel free to ask questions and voice concerns. A comfortable opening statement might be, "There are some decisions that you will need to make at this time. One will be the choice of a funeral director to assist you with your preparations. We would also like to offer you the opportunity to discuss organ or tissue donation. Would you like to speak with someone?"

The person making the request should be prepared to answer questions on a number of issues that are commonly raised. These include the surgical procedure itself, the use of the organs or tissues, the cost to the family for the donation, and the information they will receive about the fate of the organs.

Families may be assured that an open-casket funeral will be possible after the donation. None of the surgical procedures change the outward appearance of the body. This is true even in the cases of eye and bone donation, as prosthetics replace the donated tissue. Transplantation is the goal of all donation procedures. If the organs cannot be placed for transplant, however, the OPO will want to place them for research. The family may state a wish not to donate for research, and this should be documented on the consent form.

There is no cost to the donor family for the donation. Expenses incurred before the declaration of death will be passed on to them, but all costs after the time of death will be billed to the OPO. If the family receives a bill that they feel is in error, they should contact the OPO immediately.

The identity of the donor family remains confidential, as does the identity of recipients. The OPO sends a letter to the donor family, if they desire, informing them of the general outcome of the donation (for example, "a 13-year-old boy received the heart"). Some OPOs have established donor family after-care programs. The donor family is approached in the first few months after the donation with information on support groups available to them near their homes.

To meet the legal requirements for informed consent, the OPO, or other person making the request, must inform the family that the donor will be tested for infectious diseases such as HIV and hepatitis. This is usually stated on the form. In addition, it is imperative to avoid misunderstanding by listing on the form the exact organs or tissues being donated. This can be done sensitively, without making the form appear like a shopping list, by interjecting the use and need for each organ or tissue. The order of legal priority to give consent for organ donation is the same as that required for any major procedure in a hospital:

Spouse
Adult child (no order of priority is given by age)
Parent (either, preferably both)
Sibling (no order of priority is given)
Legal guardian of the decedent
Any person authorized and obligated to dispose of the body

It may also be necessary to have the family sign an autopsy permit. This depends on the scope of the donation and the needs of the family or institution. Be prepared to explain and have this consent form signed also. It is disconcerting for a family to be asked continually to sign papers, especially if it means that they must return to the hospital after they have said their good-byes.

Above all else, remember that the approach in discussing donation must be done with sensitivity to the individual needs of a particular family and with compassion for their loss.

LEGAL ISSUES OF ORGAN DONATION

The Uniform Anatomical Gift Act of 1968 established the legality of donating a deceased individual's organs or tissues for transplantation or other uses. This law protects the health care team from potential liability arising from the donation. In 1980 the Uniform Determination of Death Act recognized that brain death is death. It defined brain death as the complete and irreversible cessation of all functions of the entire brain. In 1986 many states and, eventually, the federal government mandated "required request." These laws state that a hospital must have protocols to identify donors, must be affiliated with a federally designated OPO, and must ensure that the families of potential donors are given the option to donate.

Other legal concerns may relate to donor cases that fall within the jurisdiction of the local coroner or medical examiner. Deaths caused by accidents, homicide, suicide, or any unknown etiology are usually cases that involve a medical examiner or coroner. There is a misconception held by many physicians and nurses that children cannot act as donors under these circumstances. Because of this misunderstanding, they will not refer any patient for donation who has died under questionable circumstances. Most OPOs have close working re-

lationships with local medical examiners, and so such cases should be referred to the OPO. The donation specialist works with the police department and the medical examiner's office to be sure that their requirements are met. On occasion, a local medical examiner accompanies the donation team into surgery to make certain that the final report is accurate relative to the solid organs that have been donated.

DONOR MANAGEMENT AND ORGAN ALLOCATION

Once a family has signed consent for a donation of organs, they are encouraged to say their good-byes and leave the hospital. At this time the care and maintenance of the donor becomes the responsibility of the OPO. The coordinator or donation specialist, who is usually on site, writes all orders for care. In some rural areas where this arrangement is not possible, nurses have been trained to manage donors with direction from the OPO coordinator over the telephone. In either case, the ICU nurse will be critical in the labor-intensive process of donor management, which may last from 2 to 12 hours.

Now an entire change of direction is needed. No longer is the team caring for the life of a patient. That patient has died. The team has before it a body that houses the organs to be given to others before the body is buried. This transition in mental and emotional attitude is often very difficult. Attention and care are now directed to maintaining the delicate vital organs and bring them to optimum function for the sake of many lives. In essence, care has shifted from one person to a potential six or more persons.

Because of the nature of the causes of death that produce donors, almost every case involves the same problems to be addressed. Care of children with head injuries requires dehydration and chemical interference in the process of cerebral swelling. Once a patient has died, however, a reversal of these treatments is necessary to preserve the organs. The objective of management is to restore the organs to as normal a physiologic state as possible prior to surgical removal. The following is a list of common conditions found in donors, their causes, and the interventions necessary.

Hypovolemia

Hypovolemia is caused by therapeutic dehydration, hemorrhage, diabetes insipidus (resulting from loss of hypothalamic function and ADH secretion caused by brain death). Treatment should produce a CVP of 6 to 12 cm H_2O. Crystalloid and colloid infusion through large bore lines is needed, with attention to electrolyte imbalances. Packed red blood cells may be used if the hematocrit is <24 and/or hemoglobin is <8. Until the CMV status of the donor is known, it is advisable to transfuse only CMV negative blood or use a special filter to avoid passing the CMV to the donor and, ultimately, to the organ recipient. CMV infection may be fatal to a recipient. Diabetes insipidus may be diagnosed by a urine output >2cc/kg/hr. If the output can be matched with fluid replacement, that may be sufficient. If not, aqueous vasopressin may be used. It is preferably given as a continuous intravenous infusion, as opposed to nasal or subcutaneous administration, because absorption is quicker and deleterious effects are more easily reversed.

Hypotension

Hypotension is caused by decreased cardiac output resulting from hypovolemia and/or peripheral vasodilatation caused by loss of brain-controlled vasomotor tone. Treatment is the same as for hypovolemia. In addition, the use of vasopressors may be needed, with dopamine as the drug of choice; however, dobutamine may also be effective. If further inotropic support is necessary, epinephrine or norepinephrine may be used. Overall, these medications may be necessary only until the fluid imbalance is corrected. If they cannot be withdrawn, the cardiac system is likely deteriorating and a recognition of time limitations is essential.

Hypertension

Hypertension is caused by continuing increased intracranial pressure or fluid overload. Hypertension may damage the heart and ineffectively perfuse other organs. Administration of a small dose of Furosemide will quickly relieve the effects of fluid overload. Nitroprusside may be used, in a continuous intravenous infusion, to bring the pressure within normal limits (90 to 100 mm Hg systolic blood pressure).

Hypoxia

Hypoxia is caused by loss of the respiratory center function and underventilation and oxygenation by the ventilator. Accurate placement of the endotracheal tube and aggressive pulmonary toilet are essential. An FiO_2 that maintains a PAO_2 >100 torr is adequate. The potential for pulmonary toxicity in the lung donor is greater if the FiO_2 is above 0.5. Positive end-expiratory pressure (PEEP), usually at a level of 5 cm H_2O is desired to increase alveolar ventilation. Tidal volumes should range from 10 to 15 cc/kg. Neurogenic pulmonary edema can be a problem, in which case, increased FiO_2 and PEEP, along with administration of Furosemide, will be necessary.

Hypothermia

Hypothermia is caused by loss of the hypothalamus, which controls body temperature. Once the body becomes hypothermic, dysrhythmias, changes in cardiac contractility, decreased glomerular filtration, and changes in arterial blood gases (ABG) may be seen. The best treatment is prevention. Covering the head, use of warming blankets, heat lights, warmed and humidified oxygen, and warmed IV fluids are good interventions. If the body needs to be warmed quickly, continuous lavage via a nasogastric tube with warmed normal saline is very effective.

Hyperthermia

Hyperthermia may be caused by a response to trauma, damage to the central nervous system, or infection. Most cadaver donors have sustained conditions that would make them good candidates for infection, such as open wounds and large-bore intravenous lines placed in the field. These infections usually manifest themselves with a slow and continuous increase in the WBC and body temperature. Hyperthermia, which occurs as a sudden spike at the time of herniation or most extreme brain trauma along with a similar sudden increased WBC, may indicate a response to trauma. The latter usually reverses itself without treatment over the course of a few hours. All donors are covered with broad spectrum antibiotics (for example, 25 mg/kg Cefazolin q8h [up to 1 g maximum]), and the use of Tylenol suppositories is reasonable. The more important issue here is to be sure to retrieve serum for cultures of blood, urine, and sputum before antibiotic therapy is begun. If bacterial growth is detected later, the recipients of organs can then be treated appropriately.

While the ICU team, under the guidance of the organ recovery coordinator, is treating these disturbances and imbalances, there must be continuous assessment of the condition of the organs. The same laboratory tests used in the evaluation phase are often repeated two or three times during donor management to determine whether function has improved or deteriorated.

Simultaneously, organ allocation is begun. Once the donor specialist has information regarding the donor's blood group, weight, height, and recent laboratory results, he or she will place a call to the United Network for Organ Sharing (UNOS) and register the donor. The list of all patients in the United States who are waiting for organs is matched with the donor information. Based on blood group and size compatibility, urgency of need, distance from the donor, and time waiting, all possible recipients of extrarenal organs acquire points. The donor specialist receives a list of patients in order of greatest need and will then call the transplant surgeons of those patients. The donor situation is discussed, and the surgeon makes the final decision of acceptance or refusal for a particular patient. When recipients have been found for all extrarenal organs, a time can be set with the operating room when all the donor teams will be present.

Kidneys are placed similarly, but additional points are included for tissue type match between the donor and the recipients. They are usually not placed until after nephrectomy, as they can withstand time outside the body longer than the other organs, up to approximately 48 hours.

Time spent on donor management and organ allocation may vary from as little as 2 hours to as much as 12 to 16 hours. The goal is always to ensure the best and safest organs for all recipients. The shorter time frames may be a result of donor instability. If the donor becomes hemodynamically unstable, CPR will be instituted to maintain perfusion until at least the kidneys can be removed. Donor management may take longer than 12 hours when organs are difficult to place or there is a delay in the availability of a donor team to remove them.

Donor management can be an exciting and challenging experience. Overall, these hours are spent in an intense use of human and material resources. Sometimes the ICU staff may be resentful that a "bed is taken up by a dead body." Once again, it is important to remember that the lives of several unseen persons are at stake. The expertise and dedication to the saving of life is just as important now as before the donor died.

ORGAN RETRIEVAL AND PRESERVATION

The multiorgan donor operating room can be quite chaotic. In the past, surgical teams of three to six persons flew in from all over the country for each organ to be removed. At any one time as many as 25 people could be in the room, vying for position. Furthermore, because of the delicate dissection of the liver, the procedure could last 6 to 8 hours.

Today the multiorgan donor operating room is much more orderly. Dissection times have been reduced by experience, and a complete case may take only 3 to 4 hours from incision to completion. Fewer participants are the norm, owing to the increase in small local teams experienced at removing all abdominal organs (liver, pancreas, kidneys). Modern transplant centers facilitate the removal of the organs, which are then shipped by air to the locations of the recipients. Current methods of preservation enhance this practice by allowing some organs to travel by commercial carrier, and even to be held for scheduled surgical time the

following morning. Besides settling the atmosphere in the donor operating room, costs have been lowered and the implanting team faces the job well rested and alert for the task at hand.

Just as in the ICU, the staff of the donor hospital are key players in the operating room, led and coordinated by the OPO recovery specialist. A circulator, a scrub nurse or technician, and anesthesia personnel are also needed.

The duties of the scrub nurse and circulator are no different from those in any other major abdominal case. The room set-up is basically the same, with some additional equipment. Two cautery machines, several rolling IV poles, a warming blanket on the table, and several large suction canisters are necessary. For an extensive abdominal case, certain instrumentation is needed. If the thoracic organs are to be removed, a sternal saw is required. Each organ to be removed necessitates a small back table for packaging. These tables should be draped and equipped with a round basin to hold slush solution, small scissors and pickups, and some type of measuring device.

Anesthesia personnel are required in the donor operating room to maintain the hemodynamics that have been so diligently managed in the ICU. Adequate oxygenation and blood pressure support, as well as continued good urine output, are essential throughout the procedure. The administration of drugs (mannitol, Lasix, heparin) is also requested of the anesthetist. Anesthetizing drugs are not administered, although a muscle relaxant may be requested upon incision. When all organs are dissected and ready to be removed, at cross-clamp of the aorta, the anesthesiologist is asked to discontinue the ventilator and may then leave the room.

To ready the donor for organ removal, the body is placed in a supine position with arms wrapped at the sides. A standard chin-to-groin, bed-to-bed scrub with an antibacterial preparation is performed. The incision is midline from the suprasternal notch to the symphysis pubis. First the thoracic organs, and then the abdominal organs, are dissected and visualized. The cavities are explored for previously undetected disease or trauma. After dissection of all organs that are to be donated, there follows simultaneous clamping of the aorta and flushing in situ with cold preservation solutions through cannulas in the aorta and portal vein. The heart and lungs are removed first, followed by the pancreas, liver, and kidneys. In addition, the spleen and multiple lymph nodes are removed for tissue typing, as are the iliac veins and arteries for possible reanastomosis during liver transplant.

Techniques of preservation, cold storage, and solutions that arrest cellular metabolism allow the heart and lungs to be preserved for 4 to 6 hours, the pancreas up to 8 hours, the liver up to 24 hours, and the kidneys up to 48 hours.

Once the organs are removed, if there is also to be a donation of corneas, skin, or bone, the tissue technicians begin their surgery. If there is to be no tissue donation, the OPO coordinator assists the operating room scrub nurse and circulator with closing the body, wrapping it, and transporting it to the morgue.

The challenges in the donor operating room are no less than those in the ICU. Professional surgical staff will find they have the skills that are needed. Once again, the difficulties encountered may stem from the issue of death. Surgical staff members do not deal with death routinely. In donor cases, they may find they are assisting with a body of a child who only 2 days before was in their operating room for a craniotomy and did well. This experience can be disconcerting and stressful. Once again, the key is to remember the lives of those who are to receive the transplants.

TISSUE DONATION

Although this chapter is primarily about solid organ procurement, it would be incomplete without at least a mention of tissue donation. Most deaths in the pediatric setting are declared at the cessation of cardiac function. The percentage of deaths declared through brain-death criteria is very small in comparison, but almost every patient who dies may be a potential donor.

There is a great need for human heart valves and corneal tissue for transplantation in children. Unless there has been trauma or disease associated with those tissues, every pediatric death holds the potential for donation of corneas and heart valves. There is also a need for allograft bone and skin for reconstructive surgery. Donors of these tissues are to be found in the older pediatric population. Bone donors must be over the age of 14 and skin donors must weigh more than 110 pounds.

As in solid organ donation, the key is early recognition of a potential donor, a sensitive, compassionate approach to the family, and the involvement of a resource person from either a local OPO or tissue bank.

SUMMARY

The death of a child is painful and tragic. The donation of a child's organs and tissues is a complex concept, and some may find the process too distressing to participate. Yet, if we are willing to see beyond the tragedy of the donor's situation, we may save the life, health, and even the laughter of other children.

More than any other field of medicine, donation requires the expertise and cooperation of *all* members of a health care team. There must be an understanding and acceptance that the death of one child need not be so final. There must be a commitment to the life and health of other children, even those unseen by the team. Finally, there must be courage to not walk away from the potential recipients of solid organ and tissue transplants.

REFERENCES

1. Delaware Valley Transplant Program and the Pittsburgh Transplant Foundation: *Pennsylvania Donor Study,* 1989, and Association of Organ Procurement Organizations (AOPO): *1989 Data Survey.*
2. Gallup Survey: *Americans and organ donation: current attitudes and perceptions,* October 1990, The Partnership for Organ Donation.
3. The Partnership for Organ Donation: *Solving the organ donor shortage,* 1991, the Partnership.
4. Prottas, Batten: *Attitudes and incentives in organ procurement,* I, Report to the health care financing administration, April 1986.
5. United Network for Organ Sharing (UNOS), public information department, October 1991.

29 Vascular Trauma

Philip C. Guzzetta

The epidemiology of vascular trauma in children continues to evolve as inner-city violence claims an ever-increasing number of young victims. Iatrogenic injury, usually following cardiac catheterization, traditionally has been the most common type of vascular injury in children. Prior to 1988, the most common causes of noniatrogenic vessel injury in children treated at the Children's National Medical Center (CNMC) in Washington, D.C., were accidental laceration of an extremity vessel by a fall through glass or damage to a vessel by a fracture fragment. After 1987, penetrating trauma by gunshot wound or stab wound became the major cause. This change in etiology of injury affects the age of the children treated, the severity of the injury, and the location of the injured vessels.

A review at CNMC revealed 45 children admitted between January 1, 1985, and October 1, 1991, with an injury to a major vessel, proximal to the hand or foot, or to the heart. The locations of those injuries were primarily in the extremities, with one third occurring in the neck or torso (Table 29-1). In 2 children injury was to the heart; in 7, to a vein only; in 28, to an artery only; and in 8, to both a major artery and a major vein.

Table 29–1 Location of vascular injury

Neck/chest	8
Abdomen	8
Upper extremity	15
Lower extremity	14
TOTAL	45

Table 29–2 Cause of vascular injury, 1985-1991

Gunshot wound	9
Stab wound	9
Motor vehicle accident–pedestrian	8
Fall onto sharp object	7
Motor vehicle accident–passenger	5
Other	7
TOTAL	45

In the years 1985 to 1987, 17 children were admitted with major vascular injury (5.7 per year), with a median age of 9 years. During that period, three children were admitted with stab wounds and none with gunshot wounds; only 17.6% of the vascular injuries, therefore, were due to nonaccidental penetrating trauma. There were two deaths (11.8%), both involving children who were pedestrians struck by a vehicle. In the years 1988 to 1991, 28 children were admitted with vascular injury (7.0 per year), with a median age of 14 years. During this recent period, six patients had stab wounds and seven gunshot wounds, representing a 46.4% incidence of penetrating trauma as the etiology of the vascular injury. There were six deaths (21.4%); four children succumbed to penetrating trauma and two were pedestrians struck by a vehicle. The cause of injury for all patients in the 7 years is listed in Table 29-2.

In March 1991, the Health and Human Services' National Center for Health Statistics revealed that in the United States, a black male was three times more likely to die from a bullet than from a disease, and for the first time the firearm death rate for both black and white teenagers exceeded the mortality from all natural causes.[5] The recent increase in serious vascular injuries resulting from stab wounds and gunshot wounds in the CNMC confirms the impact of these sobering statistics on an urban children's hospital.

Equally devastating is the number of children accidentally killed or seriously injured while playing with guns. According to the Center to Prevent Handgun Violence, in 1991, on average, one child was killed and 10 others were injured each day in the United States by accidental gunshots. The prevalence of firearms in the home and the disrespect for the value of human life have fostered these senseless injuries and deaths.

INITIAL MANAGEMENT OF CHILD WITH VASCULAR INJURY

Initial resuscitation of children with vascular injury is usually begun in the field and consists of compression of the bleeding vessel, when possible, volume resuscitation, and oxygen administration.

Once a child arrives at the hospital, airway management and rapid administration of blood to treat shock are of first priority while the operating room is being prepared. In children with an arterial injury caused by a fracture, it is vital to obtain orthopedic consultation immediately so that reduction of the fracture may possibly release a "trapped," rather than lacerated, artery and restore arterial flow. In the alert child, it is mandatory to assess neurologic function of the injured limb because of the high incidence of concurrent nerve and vessel injuries, particularly in an injury of an upper extremity.[8] General management of the child in hypovolemic shock is covered in detail in Chapter 18.

BLUNT INJURY TO EXTREMITY VESSEL

In children with multisystem trauma and multiple fractures, careful evaluation of distal pulses in all injured extremities is a part of the secondary survey assessment. Although venous injury may cause significant blood loss, particularly with an open fracture, only rarely is isolated venous bleeding an indication for surgical exploration. Assessment of the arterial status must precede any manipulation of a limb with a fracture, and such an assessment must be clearly documented on the chart. If the child is hypotensive upon arrival at the emergency room, pulses must be reevaluated once hemodynamic stability is achieved.

Any arterial evaluation must be repeated following reduction of the fracture. Return of a normal pulse after fracture reduction confirms arterial patency; in this case, no arteriogram is necessary. Failure of the pulse to return to normal after fracture reduction should not be ascribed simply to arterial spasm, which is usually transient and in a well perfused, warm child should abate within 10 minutes. Repeated physical examination by the same examiner is the best means to ascertain adequacy of arterial flow. In children with poor distal pulses by palpation but triphasic arterial signals by Doppler, a period of several hours of observation with repeat examinations is appropriate. As evidence is accumulating that intimal injury with good distal pulses is safely managed nonoperatively[3] there is no need for angiography on every fractured extremity with a temporary pulse deficit; however, this approach increases the importance of the careful reassessment of these children after fracture fixation.

When fracture reduction is not associated with return of the pulse to normal, an immediate arteriogram is indicated to confirm the arterial injury and locate the exact site of damage. Most fracture-related arterial injuries occur in the distal femoral or proximal popliteal arteries and are associated with a distal femur fracture or posterior dislocation of the knee (Fig. 29-1). Brachial artery injury just proximal to the elbow is the next most common injury and occurs with supracondylar humerus fracture. Repair of the arterial injury must occur within 6 hours—ideally, within 4 hours of the time of injury—to minimize ischemic sequelae. If angiography will substantially delay repair of the injury, it is preferable to explore the vessel and perform arteriography by direct arterial injection in the operating room to confirm the area of injury if it is not immediately apparent by direct observation. In the experience of CNMC, every arterial thrombosis or laceration associated with a fracture was within 2 cm of the fracture and was easily visualized upon exploration.

After a child is fully evaluated to rule out the presence of other life-threatening injuries, attention is directed to correction of the vascular injury. Following induction of anesthesia in the operating room, the injured extremity is prepared circumferentially. An uninjured leg is prepared from the foot to the knee in anticipation that use of the saphenous vein may be necessary to bridge a long gap of

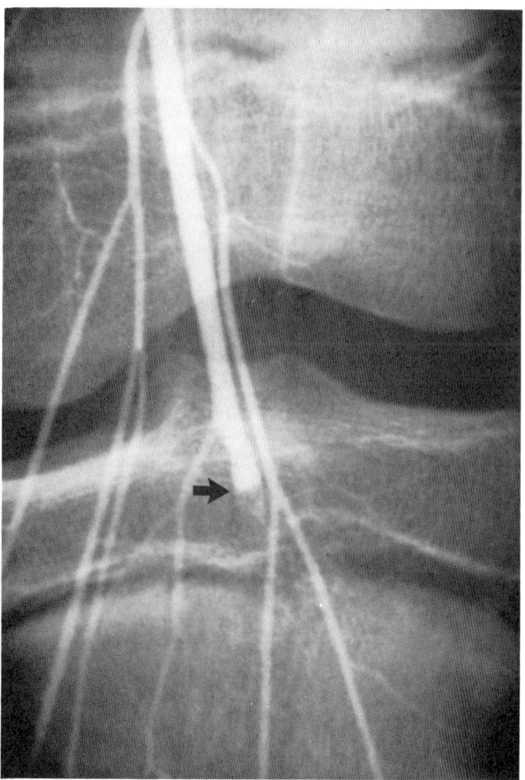

Figure 29–1 Angiogram of a right popliteal artery occlusion *(arrow)* in a 10-year-old girl with a tibial plateau fracture and posterior dislocation of the knee following a motor vehicle–pedestrian accident.

damaged vessel. The saphenous vein from the injured leg is never used, because of the substantial risk of deep venous injury from the fracture, which would place a large burden on the superficial saphenous vein to act as the main route of venous return for the leg. When the injured artery is the distal superficial femoral or popliteal artery, the injured leg is flexed about 30 degrees and the hip externally rotated so that the vessel can be approached medially in the area of the adductor canal or distally, as needed.

The orthopedic team must be available in the operating room at the onset of the procedure. In injuries to the femoral artery with femur fratures, fracture stabilization usually precedes repair of the artery. This approach is the most expeditious, eliminates the risk of anastomotic disruption during fracture fixation, and allows accurate assessment of the length of injured artery that needs to be repaired or replaced. Once the injury is confirmed surgically, the child is heparinized with 150 units of heparin/kg body weight, unless there is a contraindication, such as evidence of an intracerebral hemorrhage.

Occasionally there may be a long delay between the time of injury and arrival in the operating room, as may happen when a child is seen first at another hospital and then transferred for definitive care. In this situation, it is best to explore the artery, heparinize the child, and place an intravascular temporary shunt around the injured arterial segment. The orthopedic surgeons can then fix the fracture in an unhurried fashion while the leg is perfused. After fixation, the arterial repair is performed. This approach has been necessary only once in the last 10 years at CNMC.

Of six children with femoral or popliteal artery injury associated with fractures seen at CNMC, three required saphenous vein interposition for a tension-free anastomosis and three required repair by resection of the damaged segment and end-to-end anastomosis; all repairs remained patent. When the saphenous vein is needed, even in children less than 5 years of age, the distal saphenous is usually large enough to use as a free graft. In children of less than 10 kg, the proximal saphenous vein is more appropriate for use as an interposition graft.

In small children, repair is accomplished with interrupted 6-0 or 7-0 polydioxone suture (PDS) to allow for later growth. In teenagers, repair is done with two continuous sutures of 6-0 PDS or Prolene. Prior to repair, the proximal and distal arteries are cleared with Fogarty catheters. For children with excellent flow following repair, no intraoperative angiogram is necessary, nor do they require heparin or dextran postoperatively. Distal fasciotomy is used liberally.

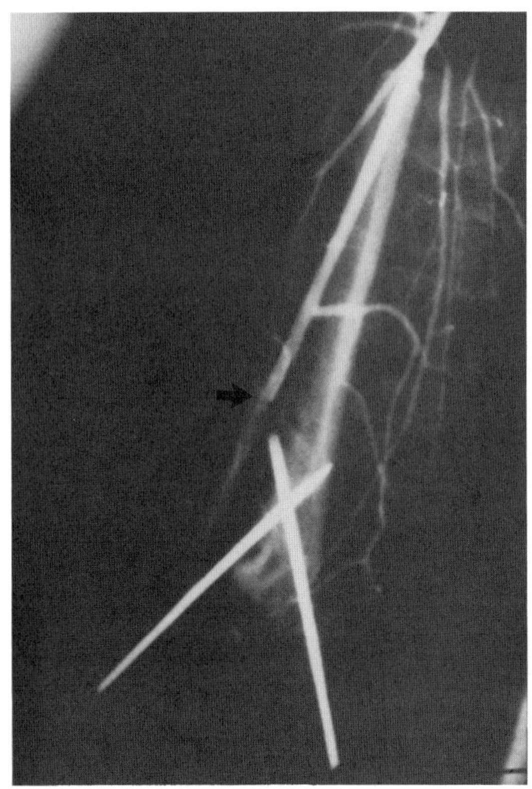

Figure 29–2 Angiogram of a left brachial artery occlusion *(arrow)* following a fall by a 7-year-old boy that resulted in a supracondylar humerus fracture. The radial pulse was lost after pin reduction.

The approach to brachial artery injury with a supracondylar fracture also emphasizes fracture fixation followed by arterial repair. Primary repair, without the need for saphenous vein interposition graft, was accomplished without difficulty in two children with this injury complex, although the distal ankle was prepared. The incision for the brachial artery injury is on the medial side of the arm between the biceps and triceps muscles with an extension into the midportion of the antecubital space. Fasciotomy is rarely necessary, unless there has been a long delay between the time of injury and repair. Elevation of the extremity is essential after humeral fracture and brachial artery repair.

The outcome for children with fracture and arterial injury is excellent unless significant delay precedes repair. Two children required amputation following arterial injury caused by a fracture. A 12-hour delay in the repair of the common iliac artery, because of stabilization at another hospital following a massive crush of the left pelvis in an auto accident, eventually necessitated left hip disarticulation in a 9-year-old girl.

The other child had a complex open femur and tibia-fibula fracture with posterior knee dislocation, significant soft tissue loss, femoral nerve damage, and popliteal vein damage. Despite a functioning arterial repair, the child eventually required an above-the-knee amputation. Another child with a supracondylar humerus fracture was transferred to CNMC several hours after pin fixation of the fracture, which resulted in loss of the radial pulse. Subsequent angiography confirmed complete occlusion of the brachial artery (Fig. 29-2). Surgical exploration revealed that the artery was trapped by the fracture fragments that had been reduced. The arterial injury was repaired and the hand preserved, but there was some ischemic damage to the forearm muscles with resultant hand dysfunction (Volkmann's contracture). One child with a lethal head injury and a femoral artery occlusion resulting from a femur fracture died. All other children with an extremity fracture and an arterial injury that were repaired survived their hospitalization.

PENETRATING INJURY TO EXTREMITY VESSEL

In the experience of the CNMC staff, an equal number of penetrating injuries to the upper extremity injured the brachial, ulnar, and radial artery. Despite impressive bleeding following the injury, only 1 of 12 children with a penetrating injury to an upper extremity arrived at the emergency room with hypotension. Because of the proximity of the brachial artery to the median nerve, careful preoperative evaluation of the distal neurologic function was imperative.[8] Three children with complete transection of the brachial artery treated since 1985 also had transection of the median nerve. The arterial injury was repaired first, and then the nerve during the same procedure.

The approach to artery repair in this case is similar to that for brachial artery repair following humerus fracture. In all cases we have been able to primarily repair the artery after proximal and distal mobilization, and we have not needed to perform a saphenous vein interposition graft. In all these children, the vessel injury was obvious and there was no need for angiography. Repair was accomplished with 6-0 or 7-0 PDS or Prolene interrupted sutures. Distal fasciotomy was not necessary, but elevation of the extremity was mandatory following surgery.

All four children with penetrating trauma to the femoral artery were in shock when admitted to the emergency room, but the one child who had a femoral vein injury without an artery injury was stable upon admission. Prompt volume resuscitation with Ringer's lactate and uncross-matched blood while maintaining direct pressure on the injured vessel in the emergency room rapidly restores blood volume and improves tissue perfusion. One must resist the urge to rush the hypotensive child with a lower-extremity vessel injury to the operating room before resuscitation is complete. Preparation of the operating room proceeds while the resuscitation of the child is under way in the emergency room.

Direct manual pressure on the medial side of the leg to compress the vessel against the femur is usually effective in controlling hemorrhage. Placement of any clamps into the depths of the wound is injudicious. In the face of obvious life-threatening hemorrhage from a gunshot wound, the only necessary diagnostic study is an x-ray of the extremity to determine the presence of a fracture and to evaluate the path of the bullet. Once the child is taken to the operating room, an assistant controls bleeding with direct pressure while the extremity is prepared and the procedure begun.

Proximal and distal control of the injured vessel prior to direct visualization of the injury is essential. Injury often occurs to both the superficial femoral artery and the superficial femoral vein. It is critical that the saphenous vein on the side of the injury be preserved to minimize venous stasis after vascular repair, particularly in those children with venous injury. We routinely prepare the distal lower extremity of the uninjured leg if injury to the femoral or popliteal vessels is suspected. It is rarely necessary to place a saphenous vein interposition graft for a stab wound to these vessels; however, an interposition graft was necessary in two children at CNMC with gunshot wounds because of the blast injury to the vessel.

Positioning of the child is the same as that for femoral vessel injury due to a fracture. Once the injured vessel is controlled, the child is heparinized with 150 units of heparin/kg of body weight and the proximal and distal ends are cleared of any clots with a Fogarty catheter. Arterial repair is performed in large teenagers with two continuous sutures of 6-0 PDS or Prolene, and in smaller children with 7-0 PDS as interrupted sutures. Repair of the concurrent venous injury is best performed by lateral venorraphy or end-to-end anastomosis, if possible, because of the high incidence of venous thrombosis when a vein graft is necessary to bridge a venous defect.[6] Soft tissue coverage of the vascular repair is sometimes challenging when a high-velocity bullet or a shotgun blast was the mechanism of injury, but use of a local muscle flap is usually possible.

Indications for fasciotomy in lower-extremity penetrating vascular trauma include prolonged time from injury to repair (greater than 4 hours), concurrent vein and artery injury, and profound hypotension upon admission. Because most children in the CNMC group with femoral or popliteal artery injury had at least one indication, fasciotomy was commonly performed. The preferred technique for four-compartment fasciotomy is that recommended by Mubarak and Owen.[7] Using one posteromedial skin incision 2 cm posterior to the edge of the tibia, approximately 15 cm long, the superficial posterior compartment and deep posterior compartment can be decompressed with extension of the fascial incisions proximally and distally beneath the skin. A second anterolateral skin incision is made 2 cm anterior to the fibula, also 15 cm long, and the anterior and lateral compartments are widely opened again beneath skin.

Partial resection of the fibula during fasciotomy can be done, but excessive bleeding postoperatively and prolonged morbidity often result with this procedure. The edges of the fasciotomy skin incisions can usually be closed with steristrips 5 days after surgery. In those with massive swelling, a skin graft can be placed on the site prior to discharge.

The children are not maintained on heparin or dextran postoperatively. Thrombosis of the vascular repair usually occurs early, if at all, and pulse should be checked hourly for the first 24 hours. Slight elevation of the foot and knee will minimize foot edema, particularly in a child with a venous injury. One child with a saphenous vein graft repair of a superficial femoral artery gunshot wound required reexploration several hours after surgery for successful revision of the repair. All other children had patent arterial repairs as defined by normal distal pulses. Routine evaluation of the venous repairs was not done and thus the long-term patency rate of those repairs is unknown. All children retained a functioning extremity. There were no deaths in this group even though several children sustained cardiovascular collapse.

BLUNT INJURY TO VESSELS OF TRUNK

Blunt injuries to vessels of the trunk can be classified as thoracic or abdominal. Vascular injuries of the chest due to blunt trauma almost invariably are caused by a severe deceleration force, such as might happen to an unrestrained passenger in a head-on collision or a pedestrian struck by a vehicle. Because the rib cage is very pliant in young children, it is common to see major intrathoracic injury without rib fractures. When children present with rib fractures, they commonly have severe associated injuries. In a recent study 42% of children with rib fractures died and 71% of children with rib fractures and a head injury died.[4] The two vascular chest injuries due to blunt trauma in our experience were rupture of the descending aorta.

In one child who had a ruptured aorta, there was evidence of a widened mediastinum on the chest x-ray and a pleural effusion on the left side. These children had a concurrent head injury and underwent a computed tomography (CT) scan evaluation of the head and chest. CT scan of the chest is not diagnostic for an aortic tear, although it may show fluid adjacent to the aorta. When a chest x-ray or CT suggests an aortic tear, aortography is essential. As in adults, the site of injury in children is invariably just distal to the ligamentum arteriosus.

Exsanguination is prevented by containment of bleeding from the aortic adventitia. One of the children had complete transection of the aorta, but the adventitia served as an adequate vascular conduit for a few hours until the aorta was successfully repaired. In some cases, repair can be performed without cardiopulmonary bypass, but this procedure should be immediately available during exploration. Repair may be performed with either direct anastomosis or a prosthetic graft, depending on the size of the tear and condition of the adjacent aorta. The youngest child in our experience with this condition was a 2-year-old struck by a car.

Recent legislation mandating seat-belt restraint has been a double-edged sword for children. Because the rear seat usually does not have three-point restraint belts and because the lap belt rests on the abdomen instead of the hips, there have been several intraabdominal vascular injuries as part of the "lap-belt complex" (see Chapter 44). Children have sustained injuries to the superior mesenteric vein, portal vein, or the hepatic artery as a component of their lap-belt complex, which emphasizes the tremendous compression and shearing forces responsible for this injury. Three children were treated with blunt trauma to the renal vessels, which in each case resulted in nephrectomy or nonfunction of the involved kidney. Similarly, penetrating trauma to the renal vessels almost invariably necessitates nephrectomy.[2]

PENETRATING INJURY TO VESSELS OF TRUNK

As "street guns" have become more powerful, an ever-increasing number of children are brought to our emergency room with CPR in progress because of gunshot wounds to the chest. Despite aggressive resuscitation, four of the eight deaths in children with vascular injury since 1984 have been due to penetrating trauma to the chest, two with cardiac injury and two with aortic injury. It is a credit to the local emergency medical technicians and a testimony to the resiliency of youth that some of these patients survived despite having arrived at the emergency room without a heart beat. In the last

7 years, emergency room thoracotomy has resulted in no survivors when the injury was to the aorta, but one child did survive a stab wound to the heart initially managed with emergency room thoracotomy, resulting in a 20% survival rate for this patient population. This poor survival rate is similar to that reported from other pediatric trauma centers.[1]

When a major vessel is injured, penetrating abdominal trauma has a much better outcome than chest trauma. Even with aortic perforation, most children can be resuscitated and the injury repaired. Major venous injury, particularly to the inferior vena cava and portal vein, is more problematic, but generally patients with these injuries also survive. Repair of the aortic injury may require the use of a prosthetic graft when primary closure of a large defect would significantly narrow the aorta. Although the use of prosthetic material when intestinal injury has occurred carries a risk of serious infection, the goal of restoring aortic continuity without stenosis must be met, even if that means placing an aortic graft.

One of the most challenging injuries confronting the surgeon is a penetrating injury to the retrohepatic inferior vena cava. Our experience with temporary bypass of the inferior vena cava by a transatrial catheter has not been good, and we would recommend a combined thoracoabdominal incision to obtain control of the injury and rapid mobilization of the liver to visualize and repair it.

SUMMARY

Children have a remarkable capacity to tolerate an insult to a major vessel and the associated physiologic derangements. The normal vessels lend themselves to a variety of repair methods, but all must be done in a manner that allows for the child's expected growth. It is hoped that in the future fewer children will need care for those vascular injuries inflicted intentionally.

REFERENCES

1. Beaver BL, Colombani PM, Buck JR et al: Efficacy of emergency room thoracotomy in pediatric trauma, *J Ped Surg* 22:19-23, 1987.
2. Carrol PR, McAninch JW, Klosterman P et al: Renovascular trauma: risk assessment, surgical management, and outcome, *J Trauma* 30:547-554, 1990.
3. Frykberg ER, Crump JM, Dennis JW et al: Nonoperative observation of clinically occult arterial injuries: a prospective evaluation, *Surgery* 109:85-96, 1991.
4. Garcia VF, Gotschall CS, Eichelberger MR et al: Rib fractures in children: a marker of severe trauma, *J Trauma* 30:695-700, 1990.
5. Guns and youth: HHS's grim statistics, *The Washington Post*, p 1, section A, March 14, 1991.
6. Meyer JP: Improvements in the management of civilian vascular trauma, *Surg Ann* 21:1-25, 1989.
7. Mubarak SJ, Owen CA: Double-incision fasciotomy of the leg for decompression in compartment syndromes, *J Bone Joint Surg* 59:184-187, 1977.
8. Wolf YG, Reyna T, Schropp KP et al: Arterial trauma of the upper extremity in children, *J Trauma* 30:903-905, 1990.

30 Penetrating Injuries

M. Margaret Knudson

EPIDEMIOLOGY

In 1988, nearly 4000 children (ages 1 to 19) lost their lives as the result of injuries by firearms.[3] The risk of death from these injuries increased with age, from a low of 1:100,000 population at ages 1 to 4 to 17.7:100,000 population at ages 15 to 19. Of the 4000 pediatric deaths caused by firearms, 3200 were among teenagers, accounting for 20% of all teenage deaths. The circumstances of injury varied with the age of the child. Among the youngest children (ages 1 to 9), homicide accounted for 56% of firearm injuries, and unintentional injuries for 43%. For children 10 to 14 years old, homicide and unintentional firearm injuries each accounted for about 35% of the deaths, with 24% resulting from suicide. The rate of firearm deaths also varied with race. In children 1 to 9 years of age, the firearm homicide rate for black males was four times the rate for white males. For black females 10 to 14 years of age, the firearm death rate more than doubled between 1987 and 1988.

Penetrating injuries resulting from stabbings are also on the rise (Fig. 30-1). At the trauma center of San Francisco General Hospital, stab wounds and gunshot wounds are increasing in equal numbers in the pediatric population and are currently responsible for 35% of all pediatric trauma admissions. Gang violence and drug trafficking have produced similar increases in penetrating injury rates among children at many other urban trauma centers. Because of these dismal statistics, it is obvious that all surgeons caring for injured children must be knowledgeable in the treatment of penetrating injuries.

PENETRATING NECK WOUNDS
Initial evaluation and resuscitation

Of immediate concern in any child with a penetrating neck wound is the status of the airway. An expanding hematoma or a direct injury to the larynx can result in severe respiratory compromise and require the immediate attention of a physician skilled in airway management. If a child with a major penetrating neck injury is ventilating without difficulty, manipulation of the airway should be minimized until the time of definitive treatment in

the operating room, as misdirected manipulation may result in airway obstruction. When emergency endotracheal intubation is required, the surgeon must remain in attendance, gloved and ready to provide a surgical airway should oral intubation fail. The preferred *emergency* surgical airway is affected by a temporary needle cricothyroidotomy, followed by jet ventilation, until establishment of a more formal airway in the operating room. Attempted tracheostomy in a child with a neck wound in the emergency department without proper lighting and equipment places the child at great risk. Occasionally, tracheal intubation is possible directly through the entrance created by the wounding instrument, with the use of a cut-off endotracheal or tracheostomy tube.

Once the airway is secured, the child must be thoroughly examined. Subcutaneous air that is palpated or visualized in a lateral neck x-ray can be associated with injuries either to the airway (trachea or larynx) or to the pharynx or esophagus. Hoarseness is another sign of airway injury, and hemoptysis suggests pharyngeal penetration. A thorough neurologic examination must be recorded, as injuries to the carotid vessels or cranial nerves may be present. The size, nature, and location of any neck hematoma should also be noted. Chest x-rays may reveal an associated hemothorax or pneumothorax. Apical caps or a widening of the mediastinum seen on chest films suggests involvement of the great vessels at the base of the neck. Fractures of the cervical spine, also possible following bullet injury, require careful assessment.

Following the initial examination, further diagnostic studies are dictated by the location of the penetrating injury. For clinical purposes, the neck can be divided into anterior and posterior halves. The anterior neck is anterior to the transverse processes of the cervical vertebrae and can be further subdivided into three zones (Fig. 30-2). Zone I encompasses the base of the neck and extends from the clavicle to the cricoid cartilage. Zone II includes the midneck between the cricoid cartilage and the angle of the jaw or the hyoid bone. Zone III extends from the suprahyoid region to the base of the skull. The structures in Zone II are easily

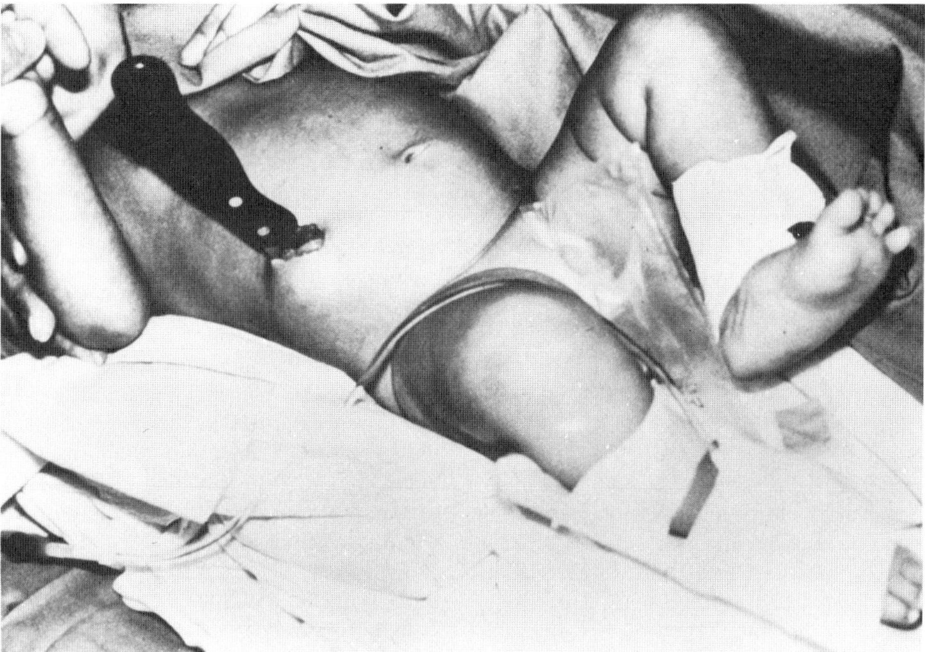

Figure 30–1 Penetrating trauma in an infant.

approached operatively, and most penetrating injuries to Zone II that extend through the platysma muscle are explored surgically without further diagnostic studies. In contrast, injuries at the base of the neck (Zone I) may involve the proximal carotid artery, esophagus, lung, trachea, subclavian artery, or other major thoracic vessels. Repair of these injuries may require a median sternotomy, thoracotomy, or a combined neck and chest approach. Therefore, in the stable child, a careful preoperative evaluation including arteriography, bronchoscopy, esophagoscopy, or contrast esophagogram, or both, should be performed first to facilitate the choice of operative approach. Likewise, the area in Zone III is difficult to expose, and preoperative evaluation should include angiography. Vascular injuries in Zone III may be amenable to angiographic embolization. If the diagnostic evaluation of children with Zone I or Zone III penetrating wounds fails to reveal significant injuries, these children are safely observed without surgical exploration. The posterior neck (that is, posterior to the transverse cervical processes) contains no major structures, and children with penetrating injuries isolated to this area can similarly be observed without surgery.

Operative treatment

Penetrating neck wounds are usually best approached through a lateral neck incision along the

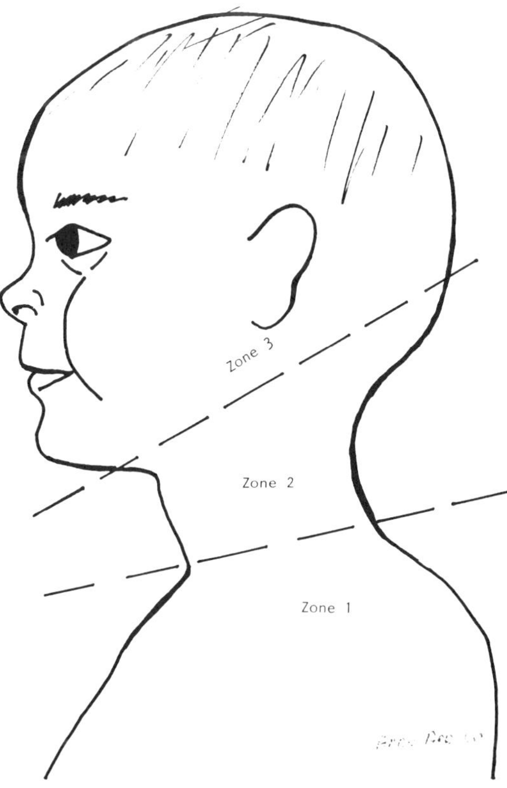

Figure 30–2 The three zones of the anterior neck.

anterior border of the sternocleidomastoid muscle, similar to the incision made for carotid surgery. If the injury involves both sides of the neck, a transverse supraclavicular incision may be more cosmetic. In either case, once the platysma muscle is transacted, the carotid sheath is opened at the base of the neck and the carotid artery gently encircled with a vascular loop for proximal vascular control, should it be required. The vagus nerve and internal jugular vein are also inspected. Venous injuries are treated by either ligation or repair, depending on the condition of the child. Transacted nerves may also be repaired primarily by debridement of the injured portion and reapproximation of the perineurium. If primary repair is not possible, the nerve should be tagged for later reconstruction.

If a carotid injury is suspected, both proximal and distal vascular control must be obtained prior to opening the hematoma and exposing the underlying injury. Injuries to the external carotid artery can be either ligated or repaired, again depending on the stability of the child. Treatment of injuries to the common and internal carotid is more controversial. Most surgeons agree that the carotid artery requires repair if the child is neurologically normal on presentation. However, if the child already has a dense hemiparesis or is comatose, ligation is generally recommended. Repair of the carotid artery requires debridement or resection, or both, of the injured segment. Primary repair may be accomplished by either lateral arteriorrhaphy or direct end-to-end repair with fine vascular sutures (6-0 or 7-0 monofilament). Patch grafts using the saphenous vein or interposition grafts with the adjacent external carotid artery have also been used.

Injuries to the carotid or vertebral artery at the base of the skull are extremely difficult to control. If they are recognized preoperatively, angiographic intervention may be possible. If they are encountered in the operating room, control may be accomplished by the introduction of a small balloon-tipped Fogarty catheter into the distal stump. This catheter can be left in place until the vessel undergoes thrombosis. Exposure and control of the internal carotid at the base of the skull may also be accomplished by anterior dislocation of the jaw.

After control or repair of any vascular injury present, the trachea and larynx should be inspected. Injuries to the trachea can usually be repaired primarily with a single layer of monofilament absorbable suture. These simple injuries do not require tracheostomy after repair. More severe tracheal or laryngeal injuries, especially those resulting from large-caliber bullets, may require extensive reconstruction and tracheostomy.

Finally, a routine neck exploration following penetrating trauma should include visualization of the cervical esophagus. This dissection can be facilitated by placement of a nasogastric tube. Once the esophagus is identified, the nasogastric tube can be partially withdrawn to the level of the injury, and air, saline, or methylene blue injected into the tube to identify sites of perforation. Direct repair of esophageal injuries with two layers of sutures is possible in most cases. Occasionally, diversion of the cervical esophagus and later reconstruction may be required.

Postoperative care

In the early postoperative period, both the airway and results of neurologic examinations must be carefully monitored, generally in an intensive care unit. Prior to extubation, a direct inspection of the vocal cords for position and of the trachea for hematoma is essential. Closed-suction drainage of cervical wounds is recommended, but the drains can generally be removed after 24 hours unless an esophageal injury is present. Antibiotics are used only perioperatively. The majority of children with penetrating neck injuries that do not involve the spinal cord can be expected to recover fully.

PENETRATING THORACIC INJURIES

Injuries to the thoracic cavity from a stabbing or gunshot wound can range from simple chest wall trauma needing no intervention, to lethal wounds to the heart or great vessels. The degree of injury incurred depends on the nature of the wounding instrument and the location of the penetration. Injuries to the thorax may also involve the neck, spinal cord, abdomen, or the hemithorax opposite the entrance site, and these areas must not be overlooked during initial evaluation.

Initial evaluation and resuscitation

When a child arrives *in extremis* with a penetrating chest wound, emergency department thoracotomy is indicated. A recent review of emergency thoracotomy encompassing a 10-year period at San Francisco General Hospital has helped in formulating new guidelines for determining which patients will benefit most from this heroic procedure. If a child with penetrating chest trauma arrives without *vital signs,* but with a clear history of *signs of life* at the scene (for example, pupillary reflexes, agonal respirations), emergency department thoracotomy is performed. The highest salvage rate following emergency department thoracotomy is accomplished in children with stab wounds that result in pericardial tamponade. However, there has been some success following a gunshot wound to the heart as well. A description of emergency department thoracotomy technique follows.

Children who arrive with vital signs following

penetrating chest trauma must first be quickly assessed for adequacy of the airway and for any respiratory compromise resulting from the injury. Intravenous catheters are inserted and blood drawn for hematocrit, hemoglobin, and arterial blood gas analysis. During the initial evaluation, blood pressure, pulse, and oxygen saturation as measured by pulse oximetry are continually monitored. If a pneumothorax is obvious by examination, a thoracostomy tube of appropriate size for the child can be inserted prior to x-ray evaluation. (Chest tube size is 12-18Fr for a newborn, 14-24Fr for a toddler, 28-38Fr for adolescents.) Similarly, if a sucking chest wound is apparent, the wound can be partially occluded with a gauze dressing and a chest tube inserted. The initial chest x-ray may reveal the presence of a pneumothorax or hemothorax, or the presence and location of bullet fragments. (Note: the entrance and exit sites of bullets should be marked with paper clips before obtaining the chest film.) Air seen in the mediastinum should alert the surgeon to the possibility of an esophageal injury. Massive subcutaneous emphysema is most likely due to disruption of a major bronchus, and is accompanied by a large pneumothorax and a pleural effusion. Apical thoracic caps seen on an x-ray raise the possibility of large vessel injury, as does the presence of a widened mediastinum.

Wounds medial to the midclavicular line, either anterior or posterior, should always be suspected of producing a cardiac injury. Occult cardiac penetration in a stable child can be quickly detected by cardiac echocardiography in the emergency department, in a search for fluid in the pericardium. In stable children with wounds in close proximity to the heart, central venous monitoring should be considered in order to detect early changes in pericardial pressure.

After initial evaluation and resuscitation, including the placement of chest tubes as required, further diagnostic studies may be indicated. Evaluation of the heart and pericardium is performed using Doppler ultrasound techniques. Bronchoscopy, esophagoscopy, and contrast esophagoscopy should be performed if injuries to the bronchial tree or esophagus are suspected. Angiography of the aorta and great vessels is performed if a pleural cap or a widened mediastinum is evident on plain films. Even if the initial chest x-ray findings are normal, radiography should be repeated within the first 6 hours, as a later evaluation may demonstrate a pneumothorax or the presence of a hemothorax not evident in the first examination.

Operative treatment

The majority (approximately 85%) of children with penetrating thoracic injuries require either no invasive procedure or a simple tube thoracostomy. Indications for thoracotomy following penetrating chest trauma include massive hemothorax (the initial return of 20% of the child's estimated blood volume or the continued bleeding of 1 to 2 ml/kg/hr from the chest tube) or the presence of injuries identified by the studies outlined previously.

Emergency department thoracotomy should be performed on children who arrive *in extremis* following penetrating thoracic trauma, but with a history of *signs of life* at the scene or en route to the hospital. The thoracotomy is performed at approximately the fifth intercostal space anterolaterally in the left chest. After opening the pleura, a pediatric rib spreader is inserted. If there is evidence of pericardial tamponade, the pericardium is quickly opened in a longitudinal direction in order to avoid injury to the phrenic nerve, and the cardiac wounds are rapidly controlled with the use of a skin stapler (Fig. 30-3). If pericardial tamponade is not present or shock persists after the release of tamponade, the aorta should be quickly cross-clamped with a vascular clamp. If a pulmonary hilar injury is identified, it should also be immediately clamped in order to avoid air embolism. If the child does not respond to these measures, resuscitative efforts should be terminated. Those who do respond to resuscitative thoracotomy should then be taken immediately to the operating room.

The choice of operative incisions for thoracic wounds depends on the condition of the child and the nature of the wound. As in all trauma cases, the clinician must anticipate the need for extending or changing any incision and drape the child from the base of the skull to the knees bilaterally. For cardiac wounds, if a left anterolateral thoracotomy has not been performed emergently, the selection of either a median sternotomy or left anterior thoracotomy incision is reasonable. The median sternotomy is preferred by many, as it offers the best exposure of the right ventricle, the area of the heart most likely to be injured in penetrating trauma. If a left thoracotomy incision is used and exposure is inadequate, however, it can be easily extended across the sternum into the right hemithorax. Wounds of the right atrium are best repaired with simple or horizontal mattress sutures, whereas those of the right ventricle are especially suitable for cardiac stapling. Cardiovascular sutures that are pledgeted may be required for extensive right or left ventricular wounds. The pericardium is generally left open after the repair, and the mediastinum drained with chest tubes.

Aside from the heart, the most likely source of massive hemothorax following penetrating trauma is a severed intercostal vessel. Thus, for lateral chest wounds requiring thoracotomy for hemor-

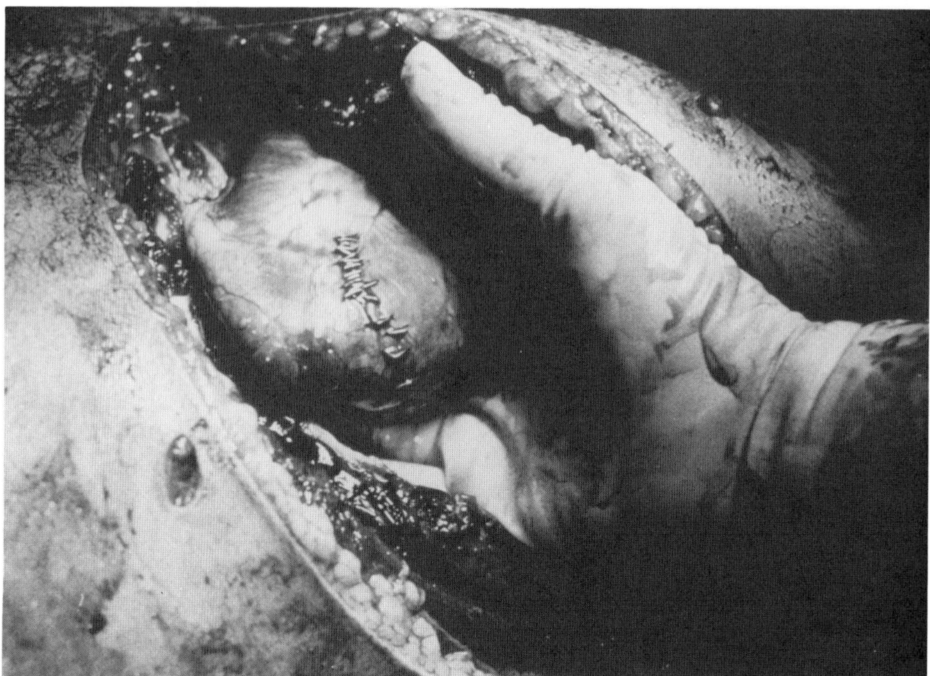

Figure 30–3 Penetrating wounds to the heart are rapidly controlled with use of a skin-stapling device. (Photograph by John Burgess.)

rhage, a left posterolateral thoracotomy incision is often used. The injured intercostal artery is then suture-ligated by encircling the adjacent rib with sutures on both sides of the artery. Injuries to the peripheral lung encountered at thoracotomy can usually be easily controlled with limited resection of the involved segment with a stapler. An extensive hilar injury may require resection of the involved lobe, but formal pneumonectomy is rarely indicated following penetrating trauma.

Esophageal injuries are generally approached through a right posterolateral thoracotomy unless the injury is known to be near the gastroesophageal junction, which is more accessible through the left chest. The injured esophagus should be debrided and closed in two layers if possible. The repair is buttressed with a pleural or intercostal muscle flap in an attempt to prevent postoperative leak. If the wound is extensive, or there has been a delay prior to surgery, esophageal exclusion and later interposition repair may be necessary. In either case, extensive drainage of the area is indicated. Penetrating injuries to the mainstem bronchus, which are rare, are also best approached via a right posterolateral thoracotomy. Selected intubation of the opposite bronchial tree with a double lumen tube can greatly facilitate the operation. These injuries are repaired primarily with a single layer of interrupted absorbable suture.

Ideally, the location of the injuries to great vessels will be appreciated preoperatively so that the surgical approach can be tailored to the injury. The right subclavian artery may be approached via a right supraclavicular incision, but if control of the base of the artery is required, this incision must be extended into a median sternotomy. Control of the left subclavian artery may require a "trap door" incision, which includes a left supraclavicular incision, a median sternotomy, and a limited left anterior thoracotomy in the fourth intercostal space. The descending aorta is approached through a left posterolateral incision. Most penetrating arterial injuries can be repaired directly with standard vascular techniques. Occasionally, by-pass procedures are required, and either saphenous vein or artificial graft material (Dacron or PTFE) can be used, depending on the size of the vessel.

Postoperative care

Complications following penetrating thoracic trauma are common. Surprisingly, wound infections are uncommon, even when the thoracotomy has been performed in the emergency department. Pneumonia is a common complication, however, especially if prolonged mechanical ventilation is required. Attention to pulmonary toilet and adequate pain control help to prevent pulmonary infections. Antibiotics should be used only in the immediate perioperative period unless an infection is identified. Chest tubes should not be removed until they have served their purpose of completely expanding the involved lung and evacuating the chest of blood. After the lung is reexpanded on suction, a trial on water seal before removal of the chest tube will help to avoid residual pneumothorax. Occasionally, children require thoracotomy because of incomplete evacuation of blood from the chest, which leads to a clotted hemothorax. Empyema may also result from residual hemothorax. Nutritional support is important early in cases requiring prolonged ventilation or in the presence of an esophageal injury. Children with cardiac wounds must be examined daily for the development of new cardiac murmurs signaling valvular involvement or the presence of a ventricular-septal defect. Echocardiography can be helpful in the evaluation of the heart postoperatively. Chest pain, fevers, and the presence of pericardial fluid weeks after surgery are typical of the postpericardiotomy syndrome, which generally responds to antiinflammatory agents. The long-term physical outcome following a stabbing or a gunshot wound to the chest is generally favorable, but it has been noted that most children who sustain such injuries have psychological problems that are best addressed soon after the injury.

PENETRATING ABDOMINAL TRAUMA
Initial evaluation and resuscitation

Any penetrating injury to the torso from the level of the nipples through the pelvis has potential for causing intraabdominal injury. More than 90% of gunshot wounds to this area cause significant injuries, and there is little need for extensive preoperative evaluation. When a child with a gunshot wound to the abdomen arrives in the emergency department, a primary survey is quickly performed, intravenous catheter access established, and blood obtained for type and cross match. A chest x-ray is obtained to evaluate potential involvement of the thoracic cavity. Intravenous radiographic contrast material can be injected before obtaining an abdominal film (a "one-shot" intravenous pyelogram [IVP]), so that the function of both kidneys is known preoperatively. Tetanus toxoid is given if needed, and a broad-spectrum antibiotic with anaerobic coverage, such as a second-generation cephalosporin, is administered. The child can then be taken directly to the operating room.

The approach to stab wounds to the abdomen has been modified, based on the fact that these low-velocity wounds have a much lower potential than gunshot wounds for causing significant injury. Children who are in shock after stab wounds or who present evidence of ongoing hemorrhage or peritonitis should be taken directly to surgery. Those without obvious injury can be treated selectively, either by serial abdominal examinations and repeated laboratory studies (WBC, amylase) or by further evaluation through diagnostic peritoneal lavage. If peritoneal lavage is used, the diagnostic criteria for a "positive" count must be lowered to reflect the fact that most stab wounds involve hollow viscus organs rather than solid organs, and these tend to bleed less. In general, a red blood cell count of $>25,000/mm^3$ or a white blood cell count of $>500/mm^3$ on the lavage aspirate is considered an indication for celiotomy following stab wounds.

Stab wounds to the flank also can be approached selectively, as many of these wounds do not enter the peritoneal cavity. The retroperitoneal structures at risk can be evaluated with the use of triple contrast computed tomography (CT) scanning (using IV, oral, and rectal contrast). Injuries to the colon may be missed with this approach, however, and children with this type of injury still deserve close observation after the study if laparotomy is not indicated initially.

Operative treatment

Children undergoing abdominal exploration for penetrating wounds must be prepared widely, including the chest, abdomen, and upper thighs in the event that saphenous vein is needed. Perioperative sigmoidoscopy should be performed if blood is present upon rectal examination and the injury involves the pelvis. Children with suspected rectal injuries are best placed supine in the lithotomy position. A midline laparotomy incision is performed for all penetrating injuries. If bleeding is encountered upon opening the peritoneum, the four quadrants of the abdomen are packed with laparotomy sponges and the anesthesia staff is alerted to the fact that blood transfusion may be required. Cell-saver devices can be used if there is no gross fecal contamination. While hemorrhage is being controlled with packs, a thorough and systematic evaluation of the abdomen is undertaken, including an inspection of both diaphragms, the spleen, liver, stomach, small and large intestines, pancreas, and central retroperitoneal structures.

Diaphragm, stomach, small bowel, and small intestine. Diaphragmatic injuries are easily overlooked unless the assessment is specific. They are also easily repaired with large sutures of absorbable suture placed in a figure-eight fashion. A chest tube is left in place in the involved chest when a diaphragmatic penetration is present. Penetrating wounds of the stomach often bleed vigorously. These injuries are usually simply debrided and closed in two layers, with an absorbable running suture in the mucosa for hemostasis and an outer layer of silk or a longer-lasting absorbable suture (Maxon or PDS) on the seromuscular layer. It is important to carefully inspect the posterior wall of the stomach by dividing the gastrocolic omentum in order to identify a second hole. The small bowel is then inspected from the ligament of Treitz to the cecum, ensuring visualization of both sides of the wall and the entire mesentery. Most perforations of the small intestine can be debrided and closed in either one or two layers (usually one layer in very small children). More extensive injuries require segmental resection and primary anastomosis, especially if the mesentery to the injured segment is involved as well.

Colon and rectum. The treatment of penetrating injury to the colon has changed much over the past several years. Many trauma surgeons, including those at San Francisco General Hospital, debride and close these injuries even if the left colon is involved. In some circumstances when primary closure is not possible, segmental resection and reanastomosis can be performed safely with a relatively low risk of the postoperative anastomotic breakdown that has been the feared complication of primary treatment. Diverting colostomy is indicated if the injury is extensive, if the child is too unstable for primary repair, or if the rectum is involved. Children with penetrating rectal injury should undergo diverting sigmoid colostomy with the creation of a mucous fistula, distal rectal washout, and presacral drainage.

Spleen. Penetrating injuries to the spleen are usually managed easily with local hemostatic techniques. More extensive gunshot wounds may necessitate segmental resection. In children, all attempts are made to preserve at least 50% of the spleen. Splenectomy after penetrating trauma is reserved for unstable patients with extensive injuries or for those in whom the vascular pedicle is severely compromised.

Liver. Penetrating wounds of the liver, particularly bullet wounds, remain a great challenge to the trauma surgeon. If the wound is not bleeding at the time of surgery, it should simply be drained. Extensive debridement of the bullet tract is not indicated if there is no active hemorrhage. In children with continued hemorrhage from a liver wound, finger fracture of the involved segment is performed and all bleeding vessels encountered are suture-ligated directly. If massive hemorrhage results from a penetrating injury to the liver, a Pringle maneuver is performed by applying a vascular clamp to the portal triad. Failure of the Pringle maneuver to control hemorrhage indicates that the bleeding is of venous origin. In children with this

injury, the incision is quickly extended into the mediastinum and an atrial-caval shunt made from an endotracheal tube is quickly placed to control the hemorrhage before any further dissection. Fortunately, extensive resection of the liver following penetrating injury is rarely required. Clinicians have noted progressive healing of the tracts created by missile wounds over time, and although bile drainage from the wounds may persist for several weeks, a second operative procedure is rarely required (Fig. 30-4). The status of the gallbladder and gastrohepatic ligament must be ascertained as well. An injured gallbladder should be removed and the duct drained with a T tube in the adolescent. Common duct injuries should be repaired if possible.

Duodenum and pancreas. Penetrating injury to the duodenum or pancreas implies high morbidity and mortality. Mortality is associated with the vascular injuries often present in this area, whereas morbidity derives from postoperative small bowel and pancreatic fistula and intra-abdominal infections. Simple lacerations of the duodenum are closed in a transverse fashion so as not to narrow the lumen. The repair is drained with closed suction drains. More extensive duodenal wounds may require resection and reconstruction with a duodenal jejunostomy. Combined injuries to the duodenum and pancreatic head can be "diverticularized," a process that includes stapling off the pylorus, creating a gastrojejunostomy, draining the common duct with a T tube, placing a tube duodenostomy distal to the repaired duodenum, and draining the pancreas extensively. Pancreaticoduodenectomy is rarely indicated following penetrating trauma. Isolated pancreatic injuries that do not involve the pancreatic duct can simply be drained. The entire length of the pancreas must be visualized, a process that involves an extensive Kocher maneuver, and a direct view must be obtained after the gastrocolic omentum is taken down. Distal pancreatectomy with preservation of the spleen is possible when the pancreatic injuries are confined to the area to the left of the mesenteric vessels.

Vascular system. Abdominal vascular injuries may also result from penetrating trauma. Any retroperitoneal hematoma should be suspected of harboring major vascular injuries and must be carefully explored. The extrahepatic vena cava can usually be visualized directly via an extended Kocher maneuver with rotation of the right colon, duodenum, and pancreatic head medially. The injury will bleed readily when encountered and is best controlled with direct pressure via sponge sticks. Lateral venorraphy is usually successful with the use of cardiovascular suture materials.

Injuries to the aorta distal to the superior mes-

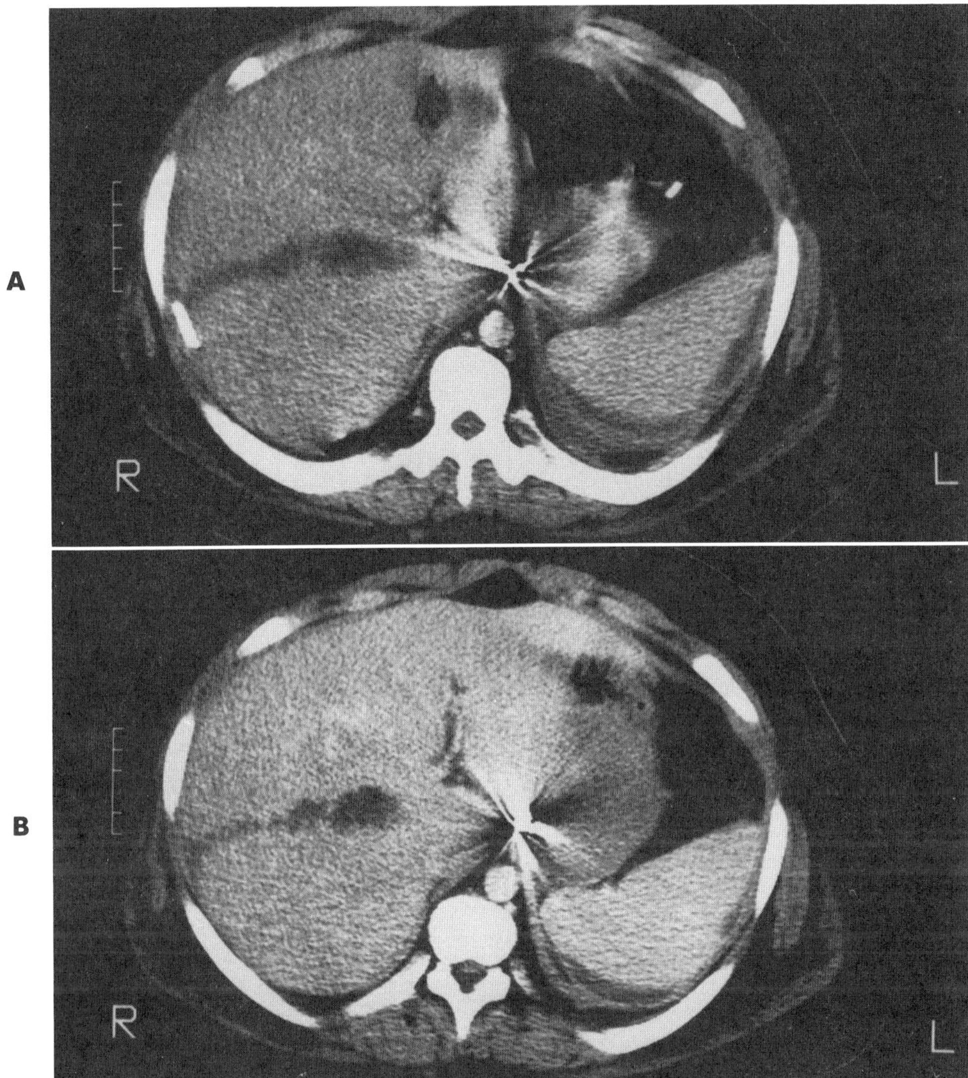

Figure 30–4 A, A CT scan of a young male with a gunshot wound to the abdomen. Note the tract through the right lobe of the liver created by the bullet. **B,** A repeat CT scan of the injury after 5 days. Note that there are already signs of spontaneous resolution of the injury.

enteric artery can be approached directly by opening the midline retroperitoneum over the aorta, after evisceration of the small bowel and superior retraction of the transverse mesocolon. The retroperitoneal incision is extended to the level of the left renal vein, where the proximal control is obtained with a vascular clamp. Distal control is accomplished with relative ease at the level of the aortic bifurcation, and simple aortorraphy can usually be performed. If there is a through-and-through aortic injury, the posterior wall can be repaired through the anterior hole. On occasion, a patch graft may be required.

If a supramesocolic hematoma is encountered,

the suprarenal aorta, celiac axis, proximal renal artery, or proximal superior mesenteric artery may be involved. Control and exposure of the aorta at this level is difficult but can be accomplished by medial rotation of the left colon, spleen, tail of the pancreas, and the left kidney, if needed. This approach allows exposure of the entire abdominal aorta.

A hematoma in the lateral pelvis suggests the presence of injuries in the iliac artery or vein. These can be approached by opening the retroperitoneum over the aortic bifurcation, maintaining digital pressure on the area of injury until proximal and distal control can be secured. Iliac artery injuries should be repaired, and iliac veins can be either sutured or ligated.

Postoperative care

Early complications following gunshot or stab wounds to the abdomen in children are primarily related to continued bleeding from the injuries not controlled with initial surgery. This may be particularly likely in liver injuries, or if the child has been hypotensive during the procedure and bleeding resumes when normal blood pressure is restored. Later complications relate to anastomotic failures (which are rare) and to intraabdominal abscesses (which are common). In clinical experience, most of the abscesses that developed in children following penetrating injuries were readily drained percutaneously under CT guidance and rarely required reoperation. Complete recovery is possible in the great majority of children who survive initial surgery.

PENETRATING INJURIES TO THE GENITOURINARY SYSTEM
Initial evaluation and resuscitation

Penetrating injuries may involve the kidney, renal vasculature, ureter, bladder, or urethra. Although the hallmark of urinary injury is hematuria, it may be absent, particularly in the case of renal artery injury. Preoperative visualization of the kidney and ureters with a limited IVP can be extremely helpful in planning the approach to these injuries. Should nephrectomy be considered, the presence and function of the opposite kidney must be ascertained. Abdominal CT scanning with intravenous contrast material is an excellent method of staging renal injuries.

Operative treatment

When a lateral retroperitoneal hematoma is encountered at laparotomy, a renal injury should be suspected. After the other abdominal injuries are addressed, vascular isolation of the kidney on the involved side should be obtained prior to opening the hematoma. The transverse colon and small bowel are lifted to the right to expose the retroperitoneum, where an incision is made directly over the aorta. As the aorta is exposed, the left renal vein is identified as it crosses the aorta just below the duodenum. By gentle traction on the left renal vein, the artery can usually be identified posteriorly. In a similar fashion, the right renal artery is controlled, but the right renal vein is very short and is found using a right lateral approach at its junction with the vena cava.

Renal injury resulting from penetrating trauma can frequently be debrided and repaired through either primary suture repair or partial nephrectomy

followed by the application of Dexon mesh or omental patches to the residual renal surface (Fig. 30-5). Renal arterial or venous injuries should be repaired if possible, reserving nephrectomy for unstable children with significant renovascular injuries. Stab wounds to the ureter are relatively rare and may be difficult to demonstrate at the time of surgery. If the ureter is bruised but no perforation can be identified, the area should be drained and any drainage fluid tested for creatinine in the postoperative period. Gunshot wounds to the ureter are generally more readily identified. Ureteral injuries are debrided or resected and repaired through ureteroureterostomy with fine interrupted absorbable sutures. Near the bladder, ureteral reimplantation with a submucosal technique is preferred. Successful ureteral repairs depend on the creation of a tension free, spatulated anastomosis that is watertight and well drained. Ureteral stenting should be considered when there is extensive devascularization of the ureter.

Injuries to the bladder resulting from a transpelvic gunshot wound are debrided and repaired in two layers with absorbable suture. In the unfortunate circumstance of penetrating trauma to the urethra, the preferred initial management is urinary diversion via a suprapubic cystostomy, with a delayed reconstruction at a later date, once the extent of the injury is fully delineated.

Postoperative care

Complications following penetrating genitourinary trauma are rare, but may include urinary tract infection, ureteral fistulas or stricture, and the development of hypertension as the result of segmental renal infarction. The outcome of penetrating genitourinary trauma in pediatric patients has generally been favorable.

PENETRATING EXTREMITY TRAUMA
Initial resuscitation and evaluation

Injuries to the extremities of children caused by stabbings and gunshot wounds are assessed for the presence of fractures and neurovascular damage. X-rays are obtained and reviewed to locate the bullet, if present, and to determine the presence of fractures. The neurologic examination of the involved extremity is carefully recorded. Similarly, the initial vascular examination is recorded and the ankle brachial index (ABI) determined for wounds to the lower extremity. (Normally, the ABI is greater than 1). Pulseless extremities or those with expanding hematomas are explored without further delay, as the point of vascular injury is usually determined easily. Children with abnormal ABIs, but without obvious vascular injury, should undergo arteriography of the involved extremity. Ar-

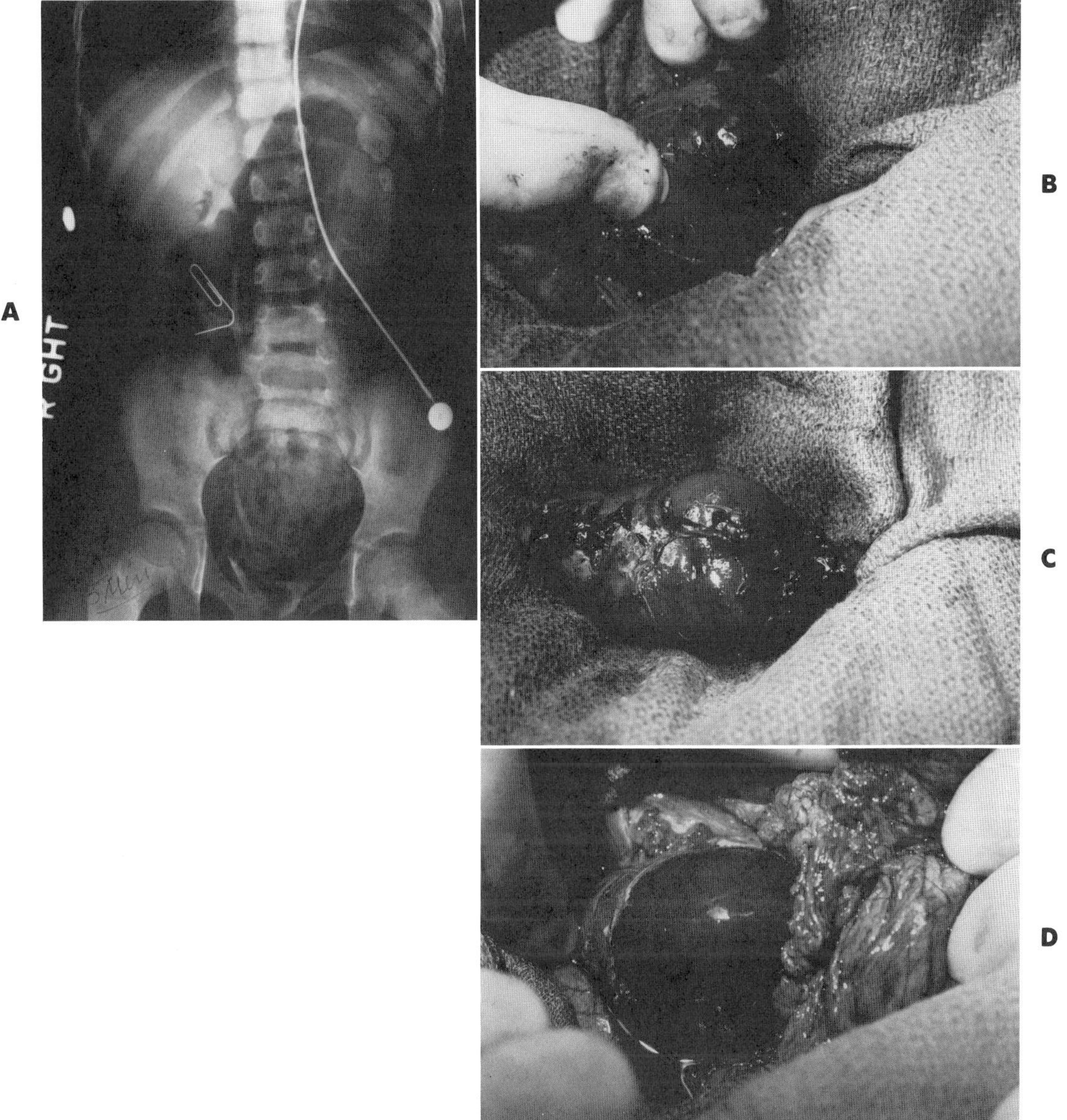

Figure 30–5 A, A preoperative IVP on a 5-year-old with a gunshot wound to the abdomen. Note the delayed visualization of the left kidney. **B,** The injury to the lower pole of the kidney as visualized at surgery. **C,** The kidney after resection of the lower pole. **D,** Omental patch applied after partial nephrectomy. (**B** to **D** provided courtesy of Dr. J. McAninch.)

teriography is not performed for potential injuries in proximity to a vessel if the vascular examination is normal, but Doppler ultrasound examination of these extremities may be helpful in excluding occult injuries.

Operative treatment

Fractures following penetrating trauma are debrided and irrigated. Primary fixation may be indicated, depending on the nature of the fracture. Vascular injuries are repaired either primarily or with a conduit of saphenous vein if possible. Once again, proper positioning and preparation of the patient should anticipate the vascular repair, as well as the harvest of the vein. After the repair, a completion arteriogram is essential to evaluate the repair and the flow distal to the repair. Nerve injuries encountered during the initial surgery should be repaired primarily, if feasible, or tagged for a later repair. Indications for fasciotomies of the involved extremity include the presence of extensive soft tissue injury accompanying the fracture or vascular repair, and delayed vascular repair (generally, longer than 6 hours). For extensive arterial repairs or arterial repairs delayed until after fracture fixation, an arterial shunt is inserted to maintain flow down the extremity.

Postoperative care

Complications following penetrating injury to an extremity include residual neurologic deficits, osteomyelitis resulting from infection of the open fracture, and the late development of pseudoaneurysms or arterial-venous fistulas after arterial injury. Many of the initial neurologic symptoms may be attributed to neuropraxia, but an electromyogram (EMG) study may suggest permanent neurologic injury. Children with such injury should be considered for nerve grafts if the defect limits function of the extremity. Osteomyelitis requires at least prolonged intravenous antibiotics and, if not recognized, may inhibit fracture healing. Most arterial injuries that are repaired go on to heal without complications, but missed injuries or those initially thought to be insignificant may threaten the limb if the delayed complications of pseudoaneurysms or arteriovenous fistulas are not recognized and promptly treated.

COST, OUTCOME, AND PREVENTION OF PENETRATING INJURIES

The cost to society of each pediatric death resulting from firearm injury is estimated at $373,500.[2] This figure reflects the loss of lifetime earnings caused by premature death. The average cost for each hospitalized child following firearm injury is $33,000, and there is a cost of $460 per gunshot wound that does not require hospitalization. Overall, firearm injuries are the third most costly cause of injury in all age groups in the United States. These cost estimates do not include the tremendous emotional expense of the families touched by these tragedies.

With modern trauma care, most children who arrive at the hospital with signs of life following penetrating trauma will survive. The trauma staff at San Francisco General Hospital recently compared their results in the treatment of pediatric trauma to those in the population of trauma patients included in the "Major Trauma Outcome Study."[4] Using the methodology developed by this study (TRISS methodology), actual deaths can be compared with predicted deaths based on the degree of anatomic injury and the physiologic status of the patient on arrival at the hospital. Interestingly, the majority of those children who were predicted to die by criteria of the study but who actually survived at San Francisco General Hospital were victims of penetrating trauma who arrived at the hospital *in extremis*. The staff postulated that the young patient is most likely to benefit from the aggressive care provided in a well-organized trauma center.

Despite these good results, however, there are still far too many children whose lives are wasted by violent crimes. Increased efforts are imperative in the effort to prevent penetrating trauma, which currently takes a heavy toll on our nation's children.

REFERENCES

1. Blaisdell FW, Trunkey DD, editors: *Trauma management*, vol 2, Urogenital trauma, New York, 1985, Theime-Stratton.
2. Center for Injury Prevention, San Francisco: *Injury prevention network newsletter* vol 7, 1990.
3. Centers for Disease Control: Monthly vital statistics report Vol 39, March 14, 1991.
4. Champion HR, Copes WS, Sacco WJ et al: The major trauma outcome study: establishing national norms for trauma care, *J Trauma* 30:1356, 1990.
5. Moore EE, Mattox KL, Feliciano DV, editors: *Trauma*, ed 2, Norwalk, Conn, 1991, Appleton & Lange.

PART SIX

Neurologic Injury

General Characteristics of Neurologic Injury

Thomas G. Luerssen

BRAIN INJURY

Within the spectrum of childhood trauma, injury to the brain is a major factor influencing treatment outcome. Several studies of childhood accidents indicate that perhaps as many as three quarters of all deaths of children attributable to mechanical trauma are the direct result of brain injury. Furthermore, for the survivors, the morbidity caused by severe brain injury can be devastating. It is now clear that a child has a better likelihood of surviving a brain injury than a similarly injured adult. There are several reasons for this, including what appears to be a primary effect of age. There is really no indication, however, that a child can recover more completely from a diffuse brain injury than an adult. In contrast, many studies have shown that brain-injured children may be indeed more vulnerable to lasting cognitive and behavioral disturbances than adults. Remarkably, even the magnitude of injury necessary to impart permanent sequelae to a child is not known. Whereas it appears that the vast majority of adults can recover completely from a mild, concussive type of brain injury, there are studies that suggest that permanent cognitive sequelae may be imparted to a child by a mild head injury if the injury occurs before the age of 4 years.

Only about 5% of all head-injured children die from their injuries. Almost all who die are severely injured and have profound neurologic and systemic disturbances at the time of presentation. Nevertheless, there is a small group of head-injured children who ultimately die from their injuries who are not in coma at the time of presentation. These are children who have survived the initial "primary" injury, only to succumb to a "secondary" brain injury. Many of the elements of the secondary brain injury are preventable or can respond to appropriate therapy. Accordingly, the major objective for the physician is to identify early and correctly the head-injured child at risk for death or deterioration so that appropriate interventions can be instituted to protect the patient from further injury. The specifics of management of brain and spinal cord injury are the focus of subsequent chapters. The purpose of this chapter is to provide a general overview of pediatric neurotrauma, emphasizing the clinical presentations and the generally expected outcomes.

Clinical characteristics of head injury in children

Multiple clinical factors influence the outcome in pediatric head injury, and many of these factors are so closely related that the individual impact of any single one is difficult to ascertain. Most studies of outcome in head injury have shown that the major clinical factors relating to outcome are the patient's age, the mechanism of injury, the initial degree of neurologic dysfunction, and the additional impact of complicating systemic factors that result in hypoxia and/or hypotension.

Age and outcome. Mortality resulting from head injury varies continuously with age, but the relationship is not direct (Fig. 31-1). Unlike the adult population wherein increasing age is associated with increased mortality, the general relationship of age to outcome is just the opposite for the pediatric age group: infants have the highest mortality from head injury; early adolescents have the lowest.[12] This trend is related partially to mechanism of injury, the interaction of systemic injuries, and the developmental state of the brain. However, multifactorial analyses have almost universally found that age itself is an independent factor affecting the outcome in brain injury. This age-related mortality trend is reversed at about age 15, when the adult pattern of increasing age associated with increasing mortality begins. Late adolescence heralds the beginning of the "trauma-prone" years, and the initial slope of this portion of the age-mortality curve is very steep at its beginning, which is probably related to the older adolescent's access to motorized transportation and alcohol.

Epilepsy. Posttraumatic epilepsy appears to be a slightly more common occurrence in children than in adults. Furthermore, children with "early" epilepsy generally experience seizures earlier than adults with early epilepsy. These impact-related seizures that occur commonly in young children are not usually associated with significant brain injury. In adults, however, early epilepsy is very often a sign of significant brain injury.

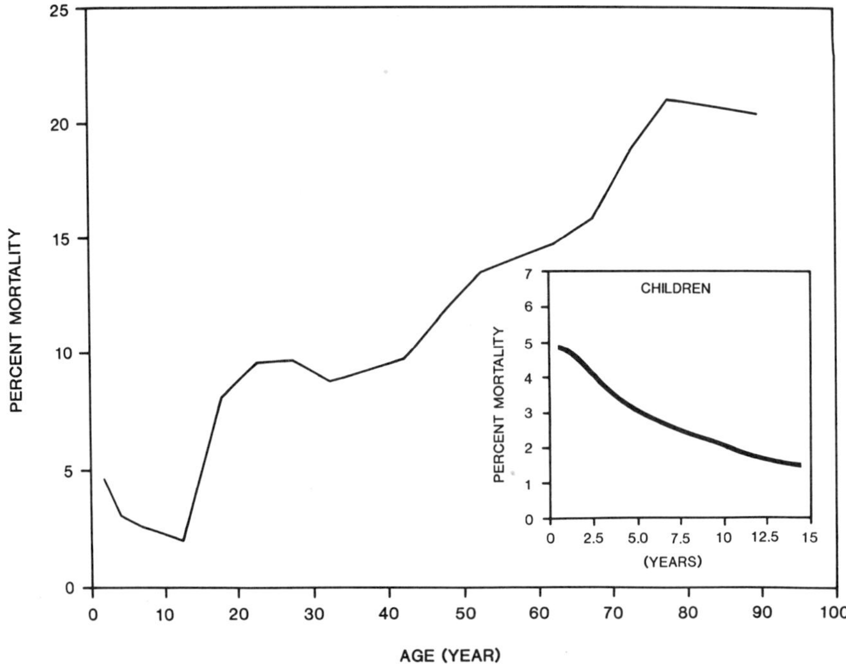

Figure 31–1 Relationship of age to mortality resulting from head injury. The overall trend for children *(inset)* shows decreasing mortality with increasing age. The trend for adults begins in early adolescence and shows a positive relationship of age and mortality. These trends are not explainable by changes in mechanism, injury severity, or surgical masses or complications, and support the idea of an independent effect of age on the outcome of head injury. (Adapted from Luerssen TG, Klauber MR, Marshall LF: Outcome from head injury related to patient's age: a longitudinal prospective study of adult and pediatric head injury, *J Neurosurg* 68:409-416, 1988.)

Mechanisms. The major mechanisms of childhood brain injuries are also age related. In the youngest children, serious head injury is caused by four major mechanisms: falls, motor vehicle accidents, bicycle accidents, and assaults. The incidence of falling as a mechanism of injury declines with increasing age, and bicycle accidents become a significant cause of head injury in older children. Although falls are the most common cause of head injury in children, the overall mortality from falls appears to be quite low. Moreover, bicycle accidents are common occurrences, but a life-threatening head injury resulting from a bicycle accident usually involves collision with a motor vehicle. Therefore, the majority of lethal accidental head injuries occurring in childhood involve a motor vehicle accident, with the child either as a passenger, as a pedestrian, or on a bicycle.

Abuse and neglect are important causes of brain injury, especially in younger children. The overall contribution of abuse to head injury statistics is confounded by the fact that a history of a fall is frequently put forth for severely head-injured infants who are ultimately found to have been shaken or beaten. Significant brain injury in an infant is frequently the result of abuse, and this mechanism must be considered when subdural or subarachnoid hemorrhage is detected. Brain-injured infants must be examined for retinal hemorrhage. This ocular finding is a strong indicator of a shaking injury. Older children frequently avoid giving a correct history. Abuse should be suspected when multiple injuries are detected in the absence of motor-vehicle–related trauma. Finally, a child with injuries of differing ages or in unusual locations is very likely to have been abused.

Neurologic grade. It has been known for some time that the outcome in head injury is related to the degree of neurologic dysfunction seen early after the injury. Prior to the mid-1970s it was extremely difficult for investigators to characterize reproducibly the neurologic examination of acutely head-injured patients so that outcomes (and all factors that might be related to outcome) could be reliably compared.[11] A major step toward a solution to this problem was the development and clinical testing of the Glasgow Coma Scale (GCS) score. This scale is essentially a numeric descriptor of the level of consciousness of a brain-injured patient. Admittedly, there are substantial problems with any clinical scoring system,[19] but the GCS has undergone extensive study and critical analysis and it is now very clear that both the short- and long-term outcomes in head injury can be correlated to the admitting coma sum score.

Some investigators feel that the GCS has certain drawbacks that limit its accuracy as a predictor of outcome. One complaint is that the coma sum score includes categories that may be arbitrary at best and unreliable at worst, as well as not reproducible because of the inability to assess the true level of eye-opening or speech function (for example, in an intubated patient or a very young child). It has been suggested that the full scale score is, by definition, inaccurate for young children. Accordingly, a variety of brain injury scoring systems have been developed that are aimed at improving upon the predictability of the clinical examination. Despite the continued development of these "improved" brain injury scales, the GCS has withstood the test of time and critical analysis. Furthermore, it still completely fulfills the requirements of a brain-injury scoring system by (1) providing a common language to describe the level of consciousness for head-injured patients, (2) providing comparable series of patients between centers, eras, or treatments, and (3) providing a general prediction of the outcome from a head injury. The vast majority of head-injured patients currently being studied and reported in the literature are categorized by GCS scores. Therefore, although individual and more specific brain-injury severity scales are useful for individual institutional or particular study purposes, it seems reasonable to use the GCS for head-injured children because of the broad comparability it provides.

Other arguments against using the GCS in children are less compelling. Although it is true that areas assessing the eye and speech in the GCS can be difficult to assign in young children, it has been demonstrated that these two elements are the least important parts of the scale. For head-injured patients of all ages, the motor score element is the most predictive of outcome. It is also the element of the examination that can be reproducibly assigned to a patient of any age. If a physician wishes to use the clinical examination only to predict the ultimate outcome of a head-injured patient in order to direct management and to counsel families, he or she can refer to several studies that have shown that the motor score examination, the number of reactive pupils, the systolic blood pressure, and the patient's age are the major factors associated with a prediction of mortality in head injury.[2,3,10]

There is still some variation in the literature about the timing of coma scoring after head injury. This factor becomes important in trying to compare the outcomes of similarly injured patients. Early work with the GCS used coma scores assigned 6 hours after head injury. With improved transport and triage, most head-injured patients have undergone medical or surgical therapy well before 6 hours have elapsed. Furthermore, head-injured patients who are hypotensive or hypoxic can exhibit an artificially increased neurologic deficit owing to these systemic alterations, and correction of these conditions can improve the neurologic function dramatically, thereby increasing the GCS sum score. For this reason, most of the recent prospective studies of head injury have chosen to obtain the neurologic scoring as soon after the head injury as possible, but also after the systemic alterations have been corrected with volume replacement, ventilation, and, possibly, diuretic therapy.

Radiologic correlates of head injury

The radiographic findings for head-injured children are also generally age related. Although the incidence of skull fracture is roughly the same in children and adults, within the pediatric age group itself the occurrence of skull fracture is age related, and is more common in younger children. Surgical mass lesions (that is, extradural, subdural, and intracerebral hematomas that require operative evacuation) are more common in adults, whereas isolated brain swelling appears to be more common in children. Like clinical findings, these radiographic diagnoses are related to the mechanism and severity of injury and to each other.

Skull fractures. It has been known for some time that the presence of a skull fracture in an adult is an indication of a more severe head injury and is also associated with abnormalities seen on CT scans upon admission.[14] Studies have now been extended to include the pediatric age group, and it appears that the finding of a skull fracture in a head-injured child does not carry the same prognostic significance as for an adult. Even though it appears that the relative risk of intracranial hematoma is less for children with skull fractures than for adults with skull fractures, however, the absolute risk of intracranial complication in both age groups is significantly higher if a skull fracture is present.[18] These studies indicate that the detection of an acute skull fracture, either clinically or on plain skull radiographs, is sufficient indication for hospital admission, computed tomography (CT) scanning, or both. In contrast, it appears that the risk of intracranial hematoma in a normally conscious child with normal skull radiographs is only about 1:13,000 cases. There is at present little question that skull radiography is a useful screening tool for

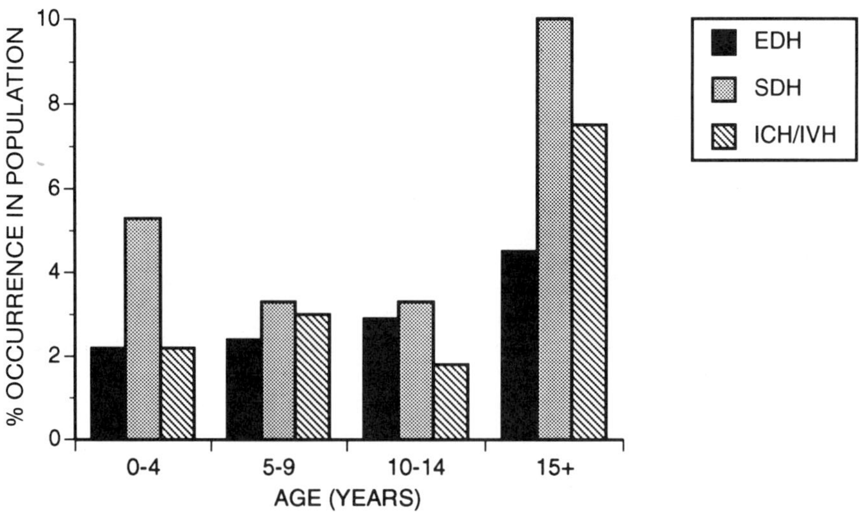

Figure 31–2 Incidence of hemorrhagic lesions grouped by age. There is general decline in the incidence of subdural hematoma (SDH) in childhood. There is also a change from the so-called infantile subdurals to the true unilateral hemispheric lesions seen in adults. The incidence of extradural hematoma (EDH) increases slightly with increasing age in childhood. Intracerebral hematomas (ICH) and intraventricular hemorrhage (IVH) are rare in children as compared with their occurrence in adults. (Adapted from Luerssen TG, Klauber MR, Marshall LF: Outcome from head injury related to patient's age: a longitudinal prospective study of adult and pediatric head injury, *J Neurosurg* 68:409-416, 1988, including some unpublished data from the study.)

head-injured children and adults, and a variety of guidelines for obtaining skull films after head injury have been put forth.[13,16] It is important to emphasize, however, that the improved outcomes in head injury reported in the past 15 years have been directly related to the availability and routine use of CT scanning. With the wide availability of CT scanners in the United States, the practical utility of skull radiography as a screening tool after head injury has been debated.[5] Therefore, rather than trying to identify a set of guidelines for obtaining skull radiographs in head-injured children, the clinician can generally summarize all of the present guidelines by saying that a CT scan of the brain is indicated if there is any concern at all about the possibility of a brain injury, arising either from clinical examination or from findings in skull radiography.

Surgical mass lesions. The occurrence of subdural hematoma in childhood, as well as the significance of this lesion, are age related (Fig. 31-2). The subdural hematoma of infancy is well described, as is its now clear relationship to non-accidental injury. The more classic unilateral hemispheric subdural hematoma occurs in children, especially over the age of 2, and these lesions are markers of a severe brain injury. With the exception of the infantile subdural hematomas, subdural hematomas in children carry essentially the same prognosis as those occurring in young adults, in

whom the mortality is about 40%. Extradural hematomas are more likely to occur in older children and are almost invariably associated with a skull fracture. Extradural hematomas in children tend to occur more posteriorly, that is in the parietal region, rather than in the frontotemporal region customary in adults. Furthermore, children harboring extradural hematoma generally present at the higher levels of GCS than adults, are usually treated before deterioration into coma, and, therefore, have significantly better outcomes than adults. Perhaps as many as half of the children with surgically significant extradural hematoma have no neurologic deficit at the time of presentation, which is another indication of the importance of early CT scanning for brain-injured children.

Cerebral swelling. Acute diffuse swelling of one or both cerebral hemispheres after a closed head injury has been generally found to be more common in children than in adults. The pathophysiology of generalized swelling is not clear, but cerebrovascular congestion appears to be the best explanation at present. Some investigators have indicated that the outcome of patients shown to have swelling on initial CT scans is better for children than for adults. However, recent studies have indicated that there is no difference in outcome related to age for this particular finding on a CT scan. In one study, diffuse swelling carried a mortality of over 40%.[1] The finding of cisternal compres-

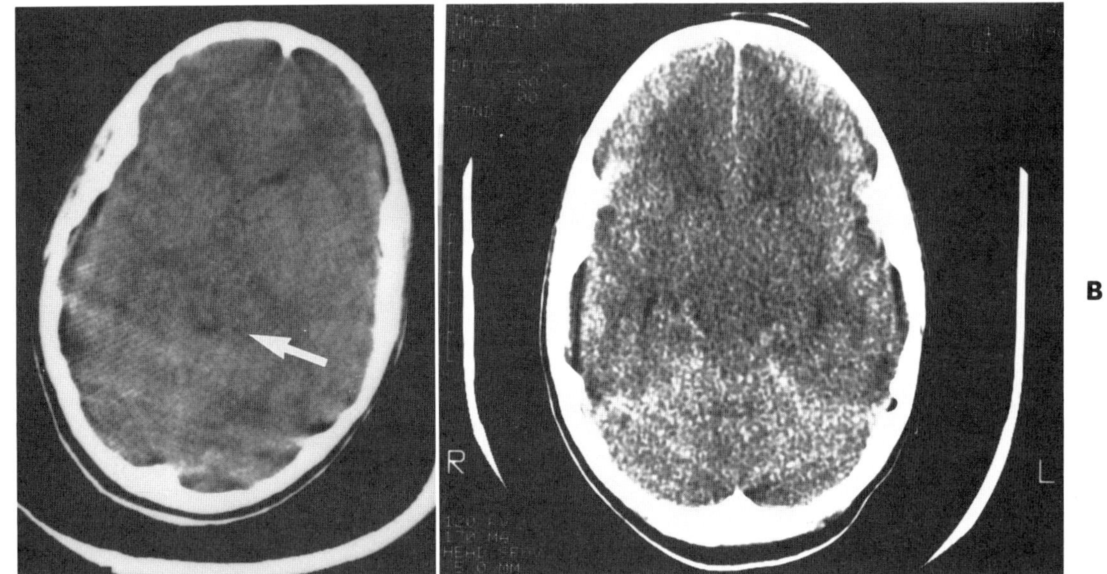

Figure 31–3 Series of CT scans of the brain of a 9-year-old child struck by an automobile. No loss of consciousness was observed, but she was intermittently combative and confused. She progressively improved neurologically during transport to the hospital. GCS score on admission and after medical stabilization was 13. **A,** Admitting CT scan shows early compression of the quadrigeminal cistern *(arrow),* portending problems with elevated intracranial pressure (ICP). **B,** CT scan 6 hours later shows diffuse swelling. Control of elevated ICP required intensive therapy.

sion, swelling, or shift on the initial CT scan is a strong indicator of the future development of elevated intracranial pressure. In some cases, these radiologic indicators predate any clinical change (Fig. 31-3).

Pathophysiologic responses to injury and therapy

All of the factors previously discussed, the distribution of injury, susceptibility to certain mechanisms of injury, the occurrence of intracranial hemorrhages, and the increased tendency for cerebral swelling, suggest strongly that there are some differences between children and adults in the dynamic responses of the brain to injury and to the various therapies required in the management of their injuries. A young child's brain and skull are undergoing a variety of changes that must have some effect on the primary and secondary responses to injury. The skull is undergoing changes in thickness and elasticity. The brain is undergoing a decrease in the water content of gray and white matter and an increase in myelinization. Brain metabolism is increasing, and the cerebral blood flow is becoming regional and coupled to metabolism. Some of these processes may be protective, but others may cause the brain to be more reactive in response to injury or more resistant to certain therapies.

It is now clear that there is less buffering capacity for volume change in the intracranial space in a young child than in an adolescent or an adult. Remarkably, the presence of skull fontanelles or expandable cranial sutures does not add acute buffering capacity. It appears that the young child's overall smaller volume of cerebrospinal fluid, especially in the spinal axis, is the major factor. This factor is important at the clinical level because it means that the brain-injured child may be at greater risk for early decompensation and secondary ischemia with relatively small changes in cerebral blood volume, cerebral tissue volume, or additional intracranial mass resulting from hemorrhage.

SPINAL CORD INJURY

Spinal cord injury is uncommon in the pediatric age group. Children account for less than 10% of all spinal cord injuries reported. It appears that the risk for spinal cord injury increases with increasing age, and some large series seem to show a bimodal distribution to the injury pattern, with one proportion of the injuries occurring in very young children and the other in early adolescence. Younger children tend to have injuries above the level of the fourth cervical segment, whereas older children tend to exhibit a pattern more like adults', with lower cervical cord injuries and thoracolumbar injuries. This distribution appears to be based mainly on the anatomic and biomechanic differences of the younger developing spine supporting a relatively large head, compared with the older, more "adult" spine of the adolescent.

The very young child's spine is much more mobile than that of an older child or adult. Cervical muscles do not become supportive until puberty, and the immature ligaments and joint capsules are more flexible in the child. The facet joints of the immature spine are horizontal, allowing more forward displacement during flexion. The facets begin to assume the more vertical adult orientation beginning at about the age of 4. These anatomic features of a young child's spine allow the kind of mobility that results in the normal and well-described "pseudosubluxation" of childhood.[4] The fulcrum of motion of a child's spine occurs in the upper cervical levels. This, coupled with a child's relatively larger head size, results in the tendency for spinal cord injuries to occur above the level of the third cervical segment. As the age of the child increases, however, the biomechanic properties of the spine become more like those in the adult. Therefore, the majority of cervical spinal cord injuries in older children occur at the fifth or sixth cervical level.

The mechanism of injury also affects the type and location of cord injuries in children. Very young children are most frequently injured as pedestrian victims in motor vehicle accidents, as passengers in motor vehicle accidents, and as victims in a fall, either from a substantial height or in a complicated pattern, such as down a flight of stairs while in a walker. Older children are more likely to be injured during recreational activities and sports.

Diagnosis of spinal cord injury in children can be difficult. About two thirds of young children who suffer a spinal cord injury present no evidence of vertebral fracture or subluxation. This entity has been termed "spinal cord injury without radiographic abnormality" (SCIWORA),[15] but in the era of magnetic resonance imaging one can frequently detect intradural or intramedullary hemorrhage, or swelling of the spinal cord in the acute phase (Fig. 31-4). Nevertheless, the plain spine films and CT scans obtained immediately do not show bony disruption, hence the utility of the term "without radiographic abnormality." Because of this specific injury, which is peculiar to young children, a normal lateral cervical spine film does not rule out the possibility of spinal cord injury or spinal instability in a child.

Some children with SCIWORA can show the delayed onset of neurologic deficits, hours to days after an injury. Almost all of them experience some

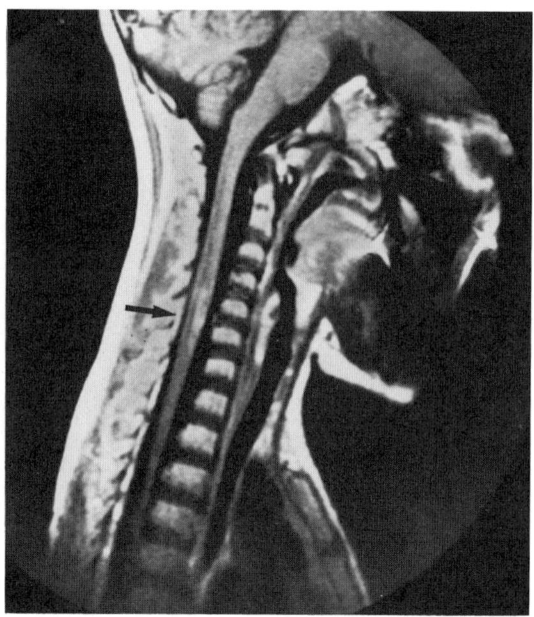

Figure 31–4 Magnetic resonance imaging (MRI) of the cervical spinal cord in an 8-year-old boy who fell from a trampoline. He immediately complained of neck and back pain and developed a mild quadriparesis. Plain films of the cervical spine and CT scan of the head and spine were normal. MRI showed swelling and increased signal consistent with edema at the C5-6 level *(arrow)*. This child was treated with cervical immobilization and recovered completely over several weeks.

transient paralysis or sensory disturbance immediately following injury. It is likely that these children have suffered a ligamentous injury and that the resulting spinal instability places them at risk for delayed injury to the spinal cord. Therefore, a careful history and a meticulous examination may be the only means of identifying an injured child at risk for deterioration.

Most recent studies reporting the outcomes of spinal cord injury in children indicate a good prognosis, except for those children suffering complete physiologic transection. In a large study of patients treated at one institution, almost 90% of partial cord injuries improved. The mortality for this series was less than 3%, occurring exclusively in patients with complete injuries.[9]

Thoracolumbar injuries seem to be the second most commonly occurring spinal injury in children, especially in young children. These injuries are frequently associated with improperly positioned lap belts and high-speed motor vehicle collisions. Intraabdominal injuries are very common with this particular spine injury, a relationship that must be remembered during the evaluation of a child with a neurologic deficit at the level of the thoracic cord, conus medullaris, or cauda equina.

PERIPHERAL NERVE INJURY

Little has been written specifically addressing the characteristics of peripheral nerve injuries in children. In large studies discussing the management and outcome of nerve injuries, it appears that about 10% of the reported populations are children. Throughout the literature, one concept seems to be universally accepted: children with peripheral nerve injuries, even those that require grafting to repair, recover faster and more completely than adults with similar injuries. This phenomenon is apparently inversely related to increasing age.

With the exception of birth injuries, peripheral nerve injuries in children are commonly associated with skeletal fractures and dislocations, or injection injuries. The vast majority of nerve injuries in continuity associated with a long bone fracture recover spontaneously. One exception to this finding is a fracture occurring between the middle and distal third of the humerus, which has a high incidence of nerve disruption or entrapment.

Children seem to be particularly susceptible to medication-injection injuries. The tendency for a child to move abruptly at the time of injection increases the risk of nerve injury. The sciatic nerve is the most frequently involved in injection injuries, and trauma to this nerve is usually related to a misplaced gluteal injection. This type of nerve injury can be due to direct mechanical trauma from the needle or from intraneural hemorrhage, or as the result of the toxic effects of the injected agent. Some drugs are clearly neurotoxic when applied closely to a peripheral nerve, but it does not appear that early operation for neurolysis or irrigation provides any added benefit to the patient.[6] Partial injuries improve with time, and it is only the rare and very severe injection injury that merits operative exploration. The most important aspect of injection injuries is their preventability by thoughtful selection of sites for intramuscular injections.

BIRTH INJURIES

Injuries to the central and peripheral nervous system can occur as the result of birth. At one time birth trauma was relatively common and responsible for 2% of all neonatal deaths, but recent reviews indicate that although about 3% of all live-born infants suffer major trauma at birth, the mortality rate is now vanishingly low.[8,17] The incidence of birth injury has progressively declined over the years because of improvements in the diagnosis and management of complicated pregnancies, the realization of the risks of certain obstetric techniques, and a marked increase in the use of cesarean section. After clavicular fracture, the most common birth injury is injury to the brachial plexus.

Brachial plexus injuries occur in about 1:1000 live births. The major factors associated with this injury are shoulder dystocia and macrosomia. The vast majority of these injuries are stretch injuries in continuity, and therefore complete or nearly complete recovery is the rule. The lesion usually affects the roots and trunks of the upper portion of the plexus. Although very few babies with such injuries ultimately require surgery, failure to show any recovery after 4 months should prompt further investigation. When operative reconstruction or grafting is performed, infants generally respond well.

Spinal cord injuries at birth are usually the result of traction on the spinal column and are associated with fetal position at birth. The breech presentation has been noted in 60% to 75% of cases. These are also stretching injuries. Most commonly, multiple segments are involved, usually in the cervical spinal cord or at the cervicomedullary junction. Spinal fractures are generally not seen. Mortality in this injury may be as high as 50%.[7]

In the modern age, significant brain injury as a result of birth is exceedingly rare. With current obstetric techniques, depressed fractures of the skull are extremely unusual. The most common intracranial lesion detected after birth (even uncomplicated birth) is subarachnoid hemorrhage, but this is rarely associated with subsequent complications.

REFERENCES

1. Aldrich EF, Eisenberg HM, Saydjari C, et al: Diffuse brain swelling in severely head injured children: a report from the Traumatic Coma Data Bank, *J Neurosurg* 76:450-454, 1992.
2. Born JD, Albert A, Hans P et al: Relative prognostic value of best motor response and brainstem reflexes in patients with severe head injury, *Neurosurgery* 16:595-601, 1985.
3. Braakman R, Gelpke GJ, Habbema JDF et al: Systematic selection of prognostic features in patients with severe head injury, *Neurosurgery* 6:362-370, 1980.
4. Cattell HS, Filtzer DL: Pseudosubluxation and other normal variations in the cervical spine in children, *J Bone Joint Surg(Am)* 47:1295-1309, 1965.
5. Feuerman T, Wackym PA, Gade GF et al: Value of skull radiography, head computed tomographic scanning, and admission for observation in cases of minor head injury, *Neurosurgery* 22:449-453, 1988.
6. Gentili F, Hudson AR, Hunter D: Clinical and experimental aspects of injection injuries of peripheral nerves, *Can J Neurol Sci* 7:143-151, 1980.
7. Godersky JC, Menezes AH: Optimal management for children with spinal cord injury, *Contemp Neurosurg* 11:1-6, 1989.
8. Gresham EL: Birth trauma, *Pediatr Clin North Am* 22:317-328, 1975.
9. Hadley MN, Zabramski JM, Browner CM et al: Pediatric spinal trauma: review of 122 cases of spinal cord and vertebral column injuries, *J Neurosurg* 68:18-24, 1988.

10. Klauber MR, Marshall LF, Luerssen TG et al: Determinants of head injury mortality: importance of the low risk patient, *Neurosurgery* 24:31-36, 1989.

11. Luerssen TG, Klauber MR: Outcome from pediatric head injury: on the nature of prospective and retrospective studies, vol 9. In Marlin AE, editor: *Concepts in pediatric neurosurgery*, Basel, 1989, Karger, pp 198-210.

12. Luerssen TG, Klauber MR, Marshall LF: Outcome from head injury related to patient's age: a longitudinal prospective study of adult and pediatric head injury, *J Neurosurg* 68:409-416, 1988.

13. Masters SJ, McClean PM, Arcarese MS et al: Skull x-ray examinations after head trauma: recommendations by a multidisciplinary panel and validation study, *N Engl J Med* 316:84-91, 1987.

14. Mendelow AD, Teasdale G, Jennett B et al: Risk of intracranial haematoma in head injured adults, *Br Med J [Clin Res]* 287:1173-1176, 1983.

15. Pang D, Wilberger JE: Spinal cord injury without radiographic abnormalities in children, *J Neurosurg* 57:114-120, 1982.

16. Royal College of Radiologists: Patient selection for skull radiography in uncomplicated head injury, *Lancet* i:115-118, 1983.

17. Salonen IS, Uusitalo R: Birth injuries: incidence and predisposing factors. *Z Kinderchir* 45:133-135, 1990.

18. Teasdale GM, Murray G, Anderson E et al: Risks of acute traumatic intracranial haematoma in children and adults: implications for managing head injuries, *Br Med J [Clin Res]* 300:363-367, 1990.

19. Wasson JH, Sox HC, Neff RK et al: Clinical prediction rules: applications and methodological standards, *N Engl J Med* 313:793-799, 1989.

32 Head Trauma

Derek A. Bruce

Head injuries account for 70% of traumatic deaths in children, and thus early care of the traumatized child must focus on treatment that can minimize the destructive pathology in the brain. To understand the interrelationship of medical care to the underlying pathology, it is important to consider the pathologic changes produced by traumatic brain injury. Current knowledge divides these changes into two separate categories consisting of primary and secondary injuries, and focal and diffuse injuries.

PATHOPHYSIOLOGY

Primary brain injury is the result of events that take place during the few milliseconds of an actual occurrence of injury to the head. Damage resulting in dysfunction occurs to neurons, axons, and blood vessels, as well as to scalp and skull. The events that take place in the neurons and synaptic apparatus are poorly understood and are not yet amenable to any therapy. Diffuse axonal injury (DAI) appears to be the substrate of acceleration-deceleration forces to the brain. These forces can produce a functional disturbance of the white matter, with no permanent or identifiable pathology (a state that is reversible); disruption of the myelin sheaths, resulting in longer-lasting and greater disturbance of brain function as the forces are increased (this, too, is often reversible over time as the oligodendrocytes remake the myelin sheaths); and, finally, an actual tearing of the axons. Even this latter process may be reversible in some situations, but it takes many months to years. The distribution of the diffuse white matter damage is variable, depending on the actual profile of the injury, but usually involves the corpus callosum, corona radiata, internal capsule, thalamus, superior cerebellar peduncle, and brainstem. This type of injury has been referred to as "brainstem injury," a useless term inasmuch as the pathology is diffuse and not just in the brainstem. Moreover, the term *brainstem injury* has, in the past, often carried with it the connotation of being untreatable. Children with DAI are at risk to develop the same secondary injuries that occur in those without DAI and thus need appropriate intensive care to prevent them.

Other primary injuries are (1) skull fractures, (2) vascular injuries resulting in hematoma (intracerebral, subdural, epidural), (3) brain contusion or laceration, and (4) subarachnoid hemorrhage.

A secondary injury is the result of events precipitated by the trauma that produce damage to the brain minutes, hours, or even days after the initial event. Major pathophysiologic events are the result of systemic hypotension, hypoxemia, hypercarbia, or intracranial hypertension. All of these are at least potentially avoidable, depending on how long after the initial injury they occur and the severity of the primary brain injury. In addition, vasospasm, seizures, meningitis, and hydrocephalus may all produce secondary injury.

Focal injuries are usually the result of impact trauma that produces skull fractures, extracerebral hematomas, coup or contrecoup contusions, as opposed to the diffuse damage typified by DAI that results from acceleration injuries. It is common for both types of injuries to exist simultaneously (for example, after an impact to the freely mobile head). Both diffuse and focal injuries may be associated with secondary damage.

Secondary injury resulting from the processes described can often be prevented, and current management of the head-injured child requires an understanding of the cause of the secondary injury. Hypoxia and hypercarbia may result from an inadequate airway resulting from traumatic unconsciousness, with loss of airway reflexes, or the position of the patient, or both; vomiting and aspiration; primary chest and lung injury; or inadequate ventilation owing to traumatic unconsciousness or spinal cord injury. Hypotension is rarely caused by a primary brain injury, and other causes of bleeding should always be sought; the site is most frequently intraabdominal. Injury to the medulla oblongata may produce dysfunction of the medullary blood pressure centers, resulting in hypotension, as may injury to the cervical spinal cord. Systemic hypotension can result in decreased cerebral perfusion, which can be aggravated if cerebrovascular autoregulation has been damaged. Inadequate circulation must be corrected as soon as possible.

Intracranial hypertension occurs in 50% to 75% of children with severe head injuries (Glasgow Coma Scale [GCS] score <8) as a result of disturbed intracranial pressure (ICP) volume relationships. Inside the cranium are blood in the arteries and veins (10% of intracranial volume), cerebrospinal fluid (CSF) in the ventricles and subarachnoid space (10%), and the cerebral tissue itself (80%). Normally, when one of these compartments expands, the others are decreased, resulting in no net rise in ICP. However, after head injury all three of the components may experience an increase in volume, which results in a rise in ICP.

Cerebral blood volume

An increase in cerebral blood volume (CBV) can be the result of hypoxia or hypercarbia, each leading to an increase in cerebral vasodilatation and thus blood volume. The effect of arterial hypoxemia on cerebral blood flow and volume does not begin until the Pao_2 drops below 50 torr. The effects of an alteration in $Paco_2$ are immediate with a change in flow of 1.5 to 2.0 ml/100 g of brain per 1 torr change in $Paco_2$ and are extremely important during the early phase of resuscitation. Diffuse brain swelling, which appears to be mainly due to vasodilatation, is found in up to 50% of children with a GCS score of 8 or less; diffuse brain swelling is another cause of increase in blood volume.

Cerebrospinal fluid

An increase in CSF can occur because of obstruction of the outflow by subarachnoid hemorrhage, distortion of the ventricular system by a mass effect resulting in compression of the foramen of Munro, or brain shift or herniation resulting in occlusion of the subarachnoid pathways.

Brain volume

Intracranial hematoma takes up volume in the cranium, and contusion or edema increases the volume of the brain itself. Thus all three compartments may experience an increase in volume simultaneously or serially, the buffering capacity is lost, and intracranial hypertension results. The deleterious effects of elevated ICP are due to the brain distortion and herniation that results from focal or diffuse vascular compression and the resulting brain ischemia.

CLINICAL EVALUATION

The aim of neurologic examination following head trauma is to evaluate the severity of the cerebral injury, to assess the injury within the central nervous system, and to define the course of any neurologic changes that are found. A single neurologic examination is much less important than serial examinations, because it is the course of the disturbance of consciousness that dictates the urgency and degree of resuscitation and investigation. The child who is briefly unconscious but recovers in a few minutes requires quite a different response than the child with an initially mild alteration of consciousness who develops severe headache and a rapid decrease in consciousness. The GCS, although a little difficult to apply to the very young infant, has been demonstrated to be a reliable tool in evaluation of level of consciousness and in heightening sensitivity to changes in the level of consciousness. Simple modifications of the scoring system make it applicable across age groups, and because the motor score seems to carry as much weight as the compound score it can be used alone. In addition to speech, pain response, and motor response, it is necessary to evaluate brainstem function. This involves pupil size and response to light, cold caloric responses (doll's eye maneuver), and gag and ventilatory activity and pattern. (Examination of the external ear canal must be done to exclude hemorrhage in the canal or laceration with CSF leakage.) Abnormal pupil responses are indicative of either third nerve compression, direct injury to the third nerve, carotid artery injury, or midbrain dysfunction; cold caloric responses measure pontine function, and gag and ventilation medullary function. As motor response is examined, it is necessary to record whether both sides of the body are equally active and whether responses in the legs are equal to those in the arms. A side-to-side difference may indicate focal brain dysfunction. If the arms are more responsive than the legs, spinal cord injury should be suspected. When a painful stimulus is used, it should be applied to both an extremity and a central trunk site. In the presence of total brain dysfunction (brain death) spinal cord reflexes can produce a withdrawal response that can easily be misinterpreted as a sign of higher cerebral function. Examination of the central nervous system (CNS) can be done during resuscitation and takes very little time. A general physical examination complements the CNS examination.

Once the level of consciousness is established and the airway, breathing, and circulation (ABC) stabilized, the scalp and back can be examined for lacerations or evidence of depressed skull fractures. The concern for associated spinal cord trauma is ever present, but whereas the incidence of head trauma in children is 300:100,000 per year, the incidence of spinal cord trauma is 1.8:100,000 per year. In addition, 25% to 60% of children with spinal cord injuries have normal spine x-rays (spinal cord injury without radiological abnormality

[SCIWORA]). Thus, although it is routine to obtain a lateral spine x-ray before endotracheal intubation, *adequate resuscitation should never be postponed because such an x-ray is unavailable.* The immediate risk of hypoxic or hypercarbic injury greatly outweighs the small risk of spinal cord injury. The level at which spinal cord injury occurs varies with age. In children younger than 8 years, injuries are predominantly at the upper cervical region C1-3, whereas after 8 years the pattern is like that in adults, with injury in the lower cervical region. Although a soft cervical collar may help to remind the trauma team to be careful with the neck during movement of the child, use of a collar is contraindicated for distraction injuries of the upper spine. Consequently, not all children should have a collar placed after trauma. In small children the collar is rarely in the right position because of mismatch between the size of the child and the size of the collar. A collar may function only to give false assurance of the stability of the spine. Children in whom the history of the trauma implies a high risk of spinal cord injury are those to whom a collar should be applied.

The best radiologic study for evaluation of the brain is the computerized tomography (CT) scan. Current scanners are fast and give excellent detail of significant skull injuries (for example, depressed fractures, intracranial hematomas, contusions, brain swelling, brain shifts, CSF spaces, and areas of ischemia). It is rare that skull films are also required. All children with a GCS score of 14 or less require a CT scan. Children who have a GCS score of 8 or less, or who have decreasing level of consciousness, require a scan as soon as they are stable, because the sooner surgically treatable mass lesions are identified and removed, the better the outcome. CT of the spine gives a good view of bony damage but is of little value in visualizing the spinal cord; for this, magnetic resonance imaging (MRI) is needed.

THERAPY

Children are unconscious after head injury because of the primary head injury. There are currently no therapeutic maneuvers available to reverse traumatic unconsciousness and, therefore, no reason for giving the unconscious child mannitol or steroids as a routine. Therapy follows the perceived pathophysiology discussed earlier. The pathology is not static; therefore what is appropriate therapy on day 1 might be quite inappropriate on day 3 or day 10. Brain swelling may be replaced by brain edema, which may in turn be replaced by hydrocephalus. Each of these developments can produce intracranial hypertension and each requires different therapy.

Airway and ventilation

The primary concern in treatment of the unconscious child is to establish a good airway and adequate ventilation. The former is done by cleaning out the mouth, ensuring that the tongue is not blocking the airway, suctioning the pharynx, and, if necessary, inserting an oral airway. Unless there is serious facial trauma, ventilation is usually adequate once the airway is clear; indeed, spontaneous hyperventilation generally occurs because of CSF acidosis and subarachnoid hemorrhage. If ventilation is inadequate, moderate hyperventilation is performed by bag and mask in the sniffing position. Gentle pressure on the cricoid cartilage can prevent regurgitation of gastric contents and prevent air from entering the stomach and producing abdominal distention. Poor ventilatory effort despite a patent airway suggests medullary dysfunction or high spinal cord injury. In addition, children are generally placed with the head elevated 15 to 20 degrees (if blood pressure is stable) and in the neutral position to avoid jugular compression. In general, children with a GCS score of less than 8 require endotracheal intubation to ensure adequate hyperventilation, to maintain ventilation during transport to and from the scan, and to protect them from aspiration and obstruction. Ideally, intubation should be done as it would be in the operating room for a child with elevated ICP or reduced intracranial compliance:

Hyperventilation with 100% O_2

Nondepolarizing muscle relaxant (for example, vencuronium)

Sodium pentothal or a similar rapid-acting anesthetic agent

The insertion of the endotracheal tube can then be done with the least risk of increasing the ICP and the best control of the airway. The initial Pa_{CO_2} target is 25 torr. A CT scan can now be obtained without movement, and the abdomen or chest can be scanned at the same time without concern for the airway or ventilation while the child is in the scanner. The loss of neurologic assessment for the short period required to obtain the scan is of no concern. If the child's neurologic state is rapidly worsening or there is concern that the ICP is high, then an ICP monitor can be inserted in the emergency room after intubation. The Camino fiberoptic monitor is currently preferred because it allows ICP to be monitored in the scanner and during transport through the hospital.

Fluid therapy

Fluid therapy in the child with a pure head injury or in the child who is not in shock begins with two-thirds maintenance with either ½ normal saline or Ringer's lactate. Except in the infant under 6 months of age, sugar is not necessary at this point; indeed, many children with head injuries have elevated blood sugar as a result of the high circulating catecholamine levels. There is experimental evidence that the pathologic effects of ischemia are aggravated under conditions of hyperglycemia. If a child is in shock or has multiple traumatic injuries requiring additional fluid volume, the clinician should administer fluids carefully, using isotonic solutions and aiming to keep the serum osmolality as close to 300 mOsm as possible. In a child in shock or with a GCS score of 6 or less, it is helpful to place the ICP monitor in the emergency room and monitor ICP during resuscitation. This allows the cerebral perfusion pressure to be monitored. Commonly, ICP rises with blood pressure, resulting in no cerebral perfusion. With use of the ICP monitor, rising ICP can be identified and treated. There is no contraindication to giving blood for resuscitation if it is required. At all times the goal of resuscitation is to achieve and maintain a stable blood pressure.

Surgical intervention

If the CT scan shows a mass lesion, a decision must be made as to whether surgery is required. Only 20% to 30% of children with severe head trauma require surgery. Intracerebral hematoma is rarely large enough to require evacuation. Subdural hematoma is usually associated with severe brain injury and, unless the hematoma is large, surgery is often not necessary and indeed may result in increased swelling or cerebral laceration, causing even more swelling and more difficulty in controlling ICP postoperatively. Most epidural hematomas require surgical evacuation but, again, this depends on the state of the child and the size and location of the hematoma.

Compound depressed skull fractures or penetrating injuries of the brain or spinal cord require surgical exploration, debridement of the brain, and dural closure. It is usual in the treatment of children to save all bone fragments, soak them in betadine solution (1:4), and reconstitute the bone after dural closure. Every effort should be made to close the dura to prevent continued cortical herniation out of the dural defect as brain swelling occurs.

Following acute trauma in children, neurosurgery, usually necessitates a craniotomy. Acute blood in the epidural or subdural spaces clots rapidly. For the first few days after injury the hematoma is solid, making evacuation via a burr hole an unsatisfactory procedure that rarely achieves complete drainage of the clot. In the rare case of a chronic subdural hematoma with fresh hemorrhage, burr-hole evacuation is effective. In children this situation is most commonly seen in the first

year of life, and the fluid mass can be drained by a fontanelle tap. In adults, acute drainage through a twist drill hole or burr hole can be lifesaving in the face of rapidly progressive herniation with pupillary dilatation. This is an uncommon situation in children and there is no evidence supporting the use of this approach. In a situation in which a neurosurgery specialist is unavailable, an epidural hematoma is expected, and herniation occurs, insertion of a twist drill hole or burr hole is reasonable. This should not be done without the availability of suction and cautery. If CT scan has not been performed, there are two major problems likely to surface at this point:

1. In children, rapid deterioration is more frequently associated with diffuse brain swelling than with epidural hematoma.
2. In children less than 5 years old the epidural hematoma is often in the high or midparietal area rather than in the low temporal area. Thus, placing the typical temporal burr hole in a child runs a risk of missing the hematoma. In this setting, skull x-rays can be helpful because if a fracture is present, the most likely place for an epidural hematoma is at the center of the fracture line.

Thus, except in rare circumstances, emergency burr holes in the emergency room are not indicated for children with head trauma.

Acute surgical intervention is usually performed for a large subdural or epidural hematoma. Both these lesions require formal craniotomy which, in the case of subdural hematoma, may need to be large. Craniotomies should be performed in an operating room equipped for neurosurgery and, ideally, with an anesthesiologist who understands the physiology of children and the problems of acute head injury. Several critical points in the evacuation procedure can make the difference between a good and a bad outcome. The children usually have significant intracranial hypertension at the time of surgery and may, in addition, have experienced some degree of fluid restriction through an effort to avoid aggravation of ICP. Many of these children will also have received mannitol, producing further dehydration. The increase in ICP results in increased peripheral resistance, which keeps the blood pressure at a normal or elevated range. When ICP is suddenly lowered by removal of the clot or the opening of the dura, the drop in ICP can lead to an acute drop in peripheral resistance and blood pressure. If the anesthesiologist is unprepared for this event, profound hypotension or, occasionally, cardiac arrest can result. Because the location of the epidural hematoma is often different in the child, obtain a CT scan prior to any surgery. Usually, after the removal of an epidural hematoma, the underlying dura matter is flaccid. If it is not, or if it becomes tense, suspect an acute subdural hematoma; make a small opening of the dura to rule this out.

It is rare that surgery is required for children with intracerebral hematoma. Craniotomy with resection of contused brain (for example, temporal or frontal lobe) is rarely indicated in children because the brain is often capable of recovery, and if it is resected no recovery can occur. Thus, in children with contusions the initial management approach is to control ICP by medical means and to consider surgery only if this effort is failing.

Brain swelling

The early cause of elevated ICP and reduced intracranial compliance appears to be an excess of blood within the vessels of the brain. This brain swelling is different from brain edema, which is an increase in water content of the brain tissue. Brain edema can be extracellular or intracellular. Extracellular or vasogenic brain edema occurs 24 hours or more after trauma and results from plasma filtrate entering the brain through areas of disruption of the blood-brain barrier. Intracellular brain edema occurs because of disturbed cellular metabolism and is primarily the result of ischemic or hypoxic brain injury. This type of edema can take several days to reach a peak after injury or can be seen on initial CT scan as loss of definition between the gray matter and the white matter. When seen on an early CT scan this is a sign of brain ischemia or hypoxia associated with high ICP and it implies a poor prognosis.

Because the early pathology is swelling of the brain, the best therapy is to lower $Paco_2$ through hyperventilation and maintain Pao_2 at about 100 torr. If ICP remains above 20 torr despite $Paco_2$ in the low 20s, muscle paralysis, sedation, and the use of such drugs as fentanyl can be employed. If, despite these therapies, ICP remains above 20 torr, the use of barbiturates, usually pentobarbital, may decrease brain metabolism blood flow and volume and, therefore, ICP. The barbiturate is not used as a brain-protective agent but purely to help lower ICP. If blood pressure is adequate, a test of the value of barbiturates may be done by giving the child sodium pentothal. If this lowers ICP transiently, the use of a longer-acting agent is likely to have a similar and more prolonged effect. There is no evidence that the use of fentanyl or other narcotics has any direct effect on ICP, and they should not be relied on to lower ICP. If therapy is being given to treat elevated pressure, then the pressure should be monitored. This is the only way to know whether the pressure is high, whether the treatment being given has lowered the pressure,

and when, assuming pressure does decrease, it rises again. A variety of ways to monitor ICP are available, and most of them can be inserted at the child's bedside or in the intensive care unit.

If, despite hyperventilation as low as 15 to 18 torr, muscle paralysis, and barbiturates or sedation, ICP remains above 25 torr, ICP waves are occurring or there are changes in pupil size with the increases in pressure, other therapy is needed. If the ventricles are not slit-like, a ventricular catheter can be placed and CSF drained. Usually, the CSF reservoir is rapidly exhausted and no further drainage can be obtained, making this of little benefit. Despite the absence of true brain edema at this early stage, mannitol can often lower ICP and is therefore worth trying. The smallest dose required to obtain the desired ICP is best, beginning at 0.5 g/kg. If the serum osmolality is checked, it can often be found to be well below 300 mOsm, and the use of colloid and crystalloid plus furosemide can help to raise the osmotic pressure and prevent shifts of water from the blood to the brain. It is better to prevent ICP from increasing to the 30 to 40 torr range through early therapy than to try to treat it once it is high.

Despite early therapy and preventive measures, ICP may remain over 25 torr. The question is then how much to push therapy (for example, pentobarbital, mannitol, or manipulation of the osmolality is an attempt to maintain an ICP below 20 torr). As the levels of these agents are increased, the side effects multiply: hypotension, electrolyte imbalance, dehydration, alkalosis. At some point a decision must be made as to what level of ICP is acceptable at what level of therapy. If pupil function is intact and the pupils do not dilate with an ICP of 30 to 35 torr, it may be advisable to accept that level of pressure in order to moderate the amount of therapy and to have a reserve if pupil function should change or ICP should increase. Because of the variability of injury in head trauma and the variable state of cerebral autoregulation, there is no single ICP level that is ideal. Children may herniate at an ICP of 20 torr or fail to herniate at much higher ICP levels. The perfusion pressure (as defined below) is:

Cerebral perfusion pressure (CPP)
    = mean arterial pressure (MAP) − ICP

In normal adult humans and in many adult animals, there is a low threshold of 50 torr, below which a decrease in cerebral blood flow occurs. The blood flow in the healthy animal and human, however, is maintained above 50% of normal (adequate to supply substrate and prevent ischemia) until a CPP of 25 to 30 torr is reached. The levels for infants and children are not known. Moreover, if there is a variable loss of autoregulation, the CPP adequate for perfusion in one area may be quite different in another. As a result, the clinician should put less reliance on CPP and aim for as normal an ICP as possible, plus a normal or slightly elevated MAP for the age of the child. In a few children, despite all available therapy, ICP will rise inexorably and death will result.

When the pressure has been easily controlled for a day or more but starts to rise again, a CT scan is required to ensure that there is no delayed hematoma, to evaluate the status of the brain swelling, and to be sure that hydrocephalus has not developed. Control of ICP may be required for as long as 2 to 3 weeks in some cases. In addition, whenever there is a change in ability to control ICP, check the following:

Blood gases
Ventilator settings
Chest x-ray
Electrolytes and serum osmolality
Reliability of the monitor, temperature, and CBC findings

After the first 2 to 3 days brain swelling is less but brain edema is more likely; thus, hyperosmolar therapy can be of greater value at this point. Either mannitol or glycerol may be used. After 7 to 10 days, increasing ventricular size and some extracerebral collections of CSF can be seen on the CT scan. If ICP is still elevated and requiring therapy, then drainage of CSF may be a useful mode of treatment. If there is no mass effect and the cisterns are open, then CSF may be safely removed by the lumbar route. Often a single lumbar puncture will suffice to reestablish CSF circulation and no further therapy is required. If there is evidence of noncommunicating hydrocephalus, an unusual situation, the CSF should be drained by ventricular puncture and a shunt may be required.

The finding of extracerebral collections is common at about 10 to 14 days posttrauma. In my experience these rarely produce pressure, despite apparent distortions of the underlying brain and, unless ICP is still elevated, it is best to leave them alone. In such cases, in which the collections have been drained, there has been a 60% incidence of seizure occurring within 48 hours after drainage and, in general, no sign of the collections' being under pressure. In addition, some children have developed rapidly progressive hydrocephalus after drainage of these lesions so that a CSF shunt was necessary. It is my opinion that these collections represent a build up of CSF at the arachnoid villi as a result of elevated outflow resistance and that, when removed, the subarachnoid space collapses with resultant hydrocephalus.

Diabetes insipidus

Acute diabetes insipidus is rare after head injury. When seen acutely, it is most often associated with brain death and severe intracranial hypertension. This situation is associated clinically then with fixed dilated pupils, flaccid motor examination, and apnea. The only reason for treatment in this case is to keep the child's physiologic state sufficiently stable to permit organ donation.

In slow deforming injuries of the head, as in a child whose head is run over, fractures occur that cross the base of the skull through the optic foramen and pituitary fossa, resulting in potential damage to the pituitary stalk and pituitary gland. Diabetes insipidus in this case is often postponed for 24 to 48 hours and may be preceded by a period of inappropriate antidiuretic hormone (ADH) secretion. This latter situation must be watched more closely to ensure that dramatic drops in serum sodium do not occur. In general, children are likely to have somewhat elevated levels of ADH and are at risk to develop acute drops in serum sodium. This necessitates frequent measurement of serum electrolytes, hourly urine output, and urine specific gravity. When diabetes insipidus occurs there are usually associated clinical clues related to the fractures crossing the skull base. Most likely are Horner's syndrome resulting from carotid artery injury, visual loss owing to optic nerve or chiasm injury, and problems with temperature control resulting from hypothalamic damage. Diabetes insipidus usually requires treatment with IV desmopressin acetate (DDAVP) or subcutaneous aqueous pitresin. Both of these drugs have a short half-life and the risk of overreplacement and resultant hyponatremia is less in IV administration than in using either nasal DDAVP or pitresin in oil. In children with severe head injury, the risks to the brain for increased edema and increased ICP are considerably greater as the result of overtreatment of diabetes insipidus than as the result of undertreatment. Thus the aim is to maintain serum sodium above 135 mEq/L. Similar disturbance of pituitary stalk function can be seen without such fractures, and the therapy for diabetes insipidus in this case is the same. The course of posttraumatic diabetes insipidus is variable, but in up to 50% of children it may be permanent. Delayed posterior pituitary or hypothalamic dysfunction can occur months after injury. Dysfunction is rarely total, however, and there is often a cyclical picture associated with aggressive behavior, overeating, and overdrinking. Any child receiving therapy for posttraumatic diabetes insipidus should be studied for pituitary hypothalamic axis function 3 to 6 months posttrauma to identify other areas of pituitary dysfunction.

Disseminated intravascular coagulation

In adults a correlation has been shown between the early signs of coagulopathy and final poor outcome after trauma. In general, disseminated intravascular coagulation (DIC) is found in patients with polytrauma and, usually, shock. There are few studies examining this condition in children. My experience is that the incidence is very low in children with pure head injury. When seen, it is usually in association with multiple trauma and extensive blood loss. Large cerebral contusions can be associated with release of brain thromboplastins and result in the production of DIC. It is important to check PT, PTT, and platelets upon admission. If a child needs surgery, the studies should be repeated immediately prior to surgery. Treatment of the disturbed clotting factors is treatment of the shock state. Symptomatic correction can be achieved with fresh frozen plasma in doses of 50 ml/kg and platelet transfusions of 0.2 to 0.4 U/kg. When the source of DIC is cerebral injury, the clotting factors may become acutely disturbed during the surgical procedure (usually for removal and repair of depressed skull fracture with brain laceration). If excess oozing is noted during the operation, repeat clotting studies are needed. Currently, no study showing correlation with bad outcome and the presence of clotting disturbance exists.

Seizures

Seizures occur with approximately 6% of mild and moderate head injuries and 35% of severe injuries. The majority of these seizures occur in the first 24 hours, many of them in the first hour. A single seizure occurring at the time of trauma or within the first hour after trauma usually does not need treatment, but repeated seizures or ongoing seizures to require therapy. The selection of a drug depends on the age of the child, the neurologic state, and the ICP if it is known. In a child whose GCS score is less than 8 for whom therapy for elevated ICP is likely, phenobarbital is probably the drug of choice. It is easy to obtain a rapid rise to good blood levels; in those children who require endotracheal intubation there is no concern about any sedative effect. Although Dilantin has less sedative effect, it is notoriously difficult, in children, to achieve and maintain therapeutic levels. If Dilantin is used, blood levels should be assessed frequently to ensure that drug levels are therapeutic. In children whose seizures are frequent or difficult to control it may be necessary to monitor the child via electroencephalogram (EEG) while in the intensive care unit to be sure that seizures have stopped. In paralyzed sedated children it can often be difficult to identify ongoing seizures. The only

clues may be alterations in heart rate, pupil function, or respiration, which can just as easily be due to changes in ICP or to primary brain injury. For the child in status epilepticus, Lorezepam is the drug of choice; phenobarbital is a next option. Dilantin may be used once seizures are controlled in a child with a GCS score above 8 to avoid the sedating effects of phenobarbital; frequent assessment of blood levels is required to ensure appropriate therapeutic levels.

Nursing care

For the child with elevated ICP following severe head injury there are several points in nursing care that require emphasis. The child is frequently in the supine position, with pressure on the back of the head, yet the child is not being moved because of concern about increasing ICP. It is all too common to find a pressure sore or areas of alopecia over the occipital region. This can be prevented by using a pressure-dispersing system (foam padding) under the occiput and by altering the head position frequently.

In children who are receiving hyperventilation it is necessary to continue hyperventilation during periods of suctioning, since the CO_2 level rises rapidly, resulting in an increase in ICP. This is easily done by using a bagging technique with only short breaks for suctioning. The procedure may require more than one nurse. In addition, the child should receive manual hyperventilation to reach the presuctioning CO_2 level before being reconnected to the ventilator. This will prevent the rise in ICP that can occur during the period it takes for the ventilator to establish the prior level. It is also important to begin early passive range of motion therapy and good joint positioning during this early stage. In addition, a quiet and loving atmosphere can help to produce a level of calmness even in an unconscious child.

CHILD ABUSE: INTENTIONAL TRAUMA

A special category of childhood trauma is typified by the child under 2 years of age whose injury is produced not by accidental trauma but by another person, usually one who is "caring" for the child at the time of injury. Many intentional injuries are the result of a momentary loss of control attributable to an adult's frustration because of an infant's uncontrollable crying or conflict with an older child about potty training. In many cases the intent is not to harm the child. Such episodes can produce fear and guilt in the person responsible for the trauma, resulting in failure to obtain immediate medical attention. The child is often put to bed in the hope that he or she will recover. Recovery rarely happens, and soon after the injury the child may suffer a respiratory arrest or a seizure, which then triggers the call for emergency help. Upon the child's arrival at the hospital it is usual for clinicians to receive no history of trauma or a history of minor trauma. Thus further time is spent in trying to determine a diagnosis while the child may be suffering further damage as a result of elevated ICP. In some cases of child abuse there is obvious evidence of external trauma and diagnosis is easily made. Homicide is the most common cause of death in children aged 1 month to 1 year (17%). Child abuse accounts for about 10% of trauma in children under 2 years of age, and for 80% of deaths.

To determine a diagnosis of child abuse requires a high level of suspicion. Any child under 2 years of age who is seen in the emergency department with an altered level of consciousness and either no history of trauma or a history of minor trauma (for example, "fell off the couch") should be considered to be a possible victim of intentional trauma. The examination should begin with an immediate look at the optic fundi. The presence of retinal hemorrhage in this setting is pathopnemonic of nonaccidental trauma. All children in whom this condition is seen require a CT scan and careful observation for seizures or delayed deterioration of consciousness. In a child who has a tight fontanelle, decerebrate posturing, or dilated pupils, a tap of the fontanelle after a good airway is established can be acutely helpful. Typically, 10 cc of bloody CSF may be obtained from the subdural space bilaterally, thus lowering ICP. This will allow time for a CT scan to be obtained with reduced ICP. Unless the child has been struck on the face, it is rare that an operative lesion is found. The scan typically shows brain swelling, subdural along the falx, and subarachnoid hemorrhage. These problems relate to high ICP, brain ischemia, and systemic hypoxia, which in many cases have occurred prior to the child's being hospitalized. In those children admitted who have a GCS score of 5 or less, mortality and morbidity are high (70%). Many of these children have uncontrollably elevated ICP, which is the cause of death. The general pathophysiology and therapy in cases of intentional trauma are little different from those in other types of trauma, except that significant brain ischemia and hypoxia have often occurred, and a serious second injury has resulted before the child is ever seen for medical attention. Thus therapy to prevent secondary injury is considerably less effective in this setting. It appears that the only way to improve outcome is either to prevent injury from occurring or to be sufficiently supportive of caregivers so that

when injury occurs they do not hesitate to seek medical attention. Success of the later strategy seems unlikely; therefore, the only hope of forestalling this wastage of our children is prevention.

The outcome in childhood head injury appears to be good if only mortality and morbidity are examined. Mortality rates of 10% to 20% in all children with GCS scores or 8 or less have been found in most recent studies. In several series the mortality rates for children with GCS scores of 5 or greater is very low, varying from 0% to 10%. Mortality rates for children with scores below 5 vary from 50% to 70%. In all categories of GCS scores the presence of shock significantly worsens outcome. The incidence of the persistent vegetative state in children is only 1% to 3%. Unfortunately, as children who have recovered from severe head injury are more carefully followed, there is clearly a high incidence of social, behavioral, educational, and psychiatric disturbances in their lives. Significant educational or behavioral disturbances can be expected in 30% to 50% of children who had GCS scores of 8 or less. Follow-up MRI in these children shows lesions in the frontal lobe and corpus callosum, which may have a correlation with functional disturbances. It is clear that despite apparently good neurologic recovery the subtle remaining dysfunctions of the brain are as frequent in children as in adults. Thus it is important to appreciate that head-injured children warrant careful follow-up and active rehabilitation, not only for physical and occupational recovery, but for cognitive function as well.

REFERENCES

1. Adams JH, Mitchell DE, Graham DI et al: Diffuse brain damage of immediate impact type: its relationship to primary brainstem damage in head injury, *Brain* 100:489-502, 1977.
2. Alberico AM, Ward JD, Choi SC et al: Outcome after severe head injury: relationship to mass lesions, diffuse injury and ICP course in pediatric and adult patients, *J Neurosurg* 67:648-656, 1987.
3. Bruce DA: Management of cerebral edema, *Pediatr Rev* 4:217-224, 1983.
4. Bruce DA: Scope of the problem: early assessment and management (chap 35). In Rosenthal M, Griffith ER, Bond M et al, editors: *Rehabilitation of head injured patients,* Philadelphia, 1990, FA Davis.
5. Bruce DA, Zimmerman RA: Shaken impact syndrome, *Pediatr Ann* 18:482-494, 1989.
6. Bruce DA, Alavi A, Bilaniuk LT et al: Diffuse cerebral swelling following head injury in children: the syndrome of "malignant brain edema," *J Neurosurg* 54:170-178, 1981.
7. Bruce DA, Raphaely RC, Goldberg AI et al: Pathophysiology, treatment and outcome following severe head injury in children, *Child's Brain* 5:174-191, 1979.
8. Gennarelli TA, Thibault LF, Adams JH et al: Diffuse axonal injury and traumatic coma in the primate, *Ann Neurol* 12:564-574, 1982.

9. Graham DI, Ford I, Adams JH, et al: Ischemic brain damage is still common in fatal, non-missile head injury, *J Neurol Neurosurg Psychiatry* 52:346-350, 1989.

10. Hahn YS, Fuchs S, Flannery AM et al: Factors influencing posttraumatic seizures in children, *Neurosurgery* 22:864-867, 1988.

11. Kollevold T: Immediate and early cerebral seizures after head injuries. I. *J Oslo City Hosp* 26:99-114, 1976.

12. Leursen TG, Melville RK, Marshall LF: Outcome from head injury related to patients age, *J Neurosurg* 68:409-416, 1988.

13. Leursen TG, Huang JC, McLone DG et al: Retinal hemorrhages, seizures and intracranial hemorrhages: relationships and outcome in children suffering traumatic brain injury, *Concepts Pediatr Neurosurg* 11:87-94, 1991.

14. Muizelaar JP, Marmarou A, DeSalles AA et al: Cerebral blood flow and metabolism in severely head injured Children. I. Relationship with GCS, outcome, ICP and PVI. II. Autoregulation. *J Neurosurg* 71:63-76, 1989.

15. Pang D, Wilberger JE Jr: Spinal cord injury without radiographic abnormalities in children, *J Neurosurg* 57:114-129, 1982.

16. Walker ML, Mayer TA, Storrs BB et al: Pediatric head injury: factors which influence outcome, *Concepts Pediatr Neurosurg* 6:84-97, 1985.

17. Wilkinson WS, Han DP, Rappley MS et al: Retinal hemorrhage predicts neurological injury in the shaken baby syndrome, *Arch Ophthalmol* 107:1472-1474, 1989.

33 Spinal Trauma

Curtis A. Dickman and Harold L. Rekate

The unique biomechanical and structural properties of the immature vertebral column predispose children to distinct patterns of injury. This chapter provides a comprehensive analysis of vertebral column and spinal cord trauma in children. The diagnostic evaluation, clinical characteristics, and therapeutic alternatives for management of childhood spinal injuries are emphasized.

EPIDEMIOLOGY

More than 1065 children sustain spinal cord injury each year in the United States, and a much higher number sustain injury to the vertebral column.[5,10] Although pediatric spinal injuries are not rare, few medical centers treat large numbers of victims. Children in the first decade of life have the lowest incidence and prevalence of spinal cord injury among all age groups.[5,7,10] There is a fourfold difference between the injury rates in children and those in young adults. Between 1970 and 1977, the occurrence rate of hospitalization for spinal cord injury was 21.2 per million population per year among children under 19 years of age, as compared with 68.0 per million population per year in the 20 to 24 year age group.[5] As in all forms of trauma, males tend to sustain the preponderance of spinal injuries (a 2:1 male-to-female ratio).[5,10]

Motor vehicle crashes are the leading cause of spinal cord injury in children, as they are for all age groups. In addition to passenger-related automobile injuries, pedestrian-vehicular and bicycle-vehicular crashes account for a significant proportion of injuries in young children. Alcohol or drugs often contribute to motor vehicle crashes involving adolescents and young adults; substance abuse has been implicated in 25% of injuries. Injuries related to recreation and sports occur principally among adolescents, but are rare among young children. Falls and child abuse are other important mechanisms of spinal injury in young children.

Pediatric spinal injuries are underestimated and underreported for a variety of reasons.[5] Children with either very mild or fatal injuries are usually not included in clinically based studies of spinal trauma. Rather, these reports tend to assess the incidence of hospitalization for spinal cord injury.

Half of all children with spinal cord injury die immediately or within the first hour of injury, and another 20% of survivors succumb to complications within 3 months. Birth-related injuries, autopsy data, and cervical strain or whiplash injuries have received little attention. Although data are rapidly accumulating as pediatric spinal injuries are subjected to analysis, comprehensive sources are currently unavailable.

Bias inherent in reporting methods and classification patterns of pediatric injuries has contributed to the problems of accurate epidemiological analysis.[5] Variation among classification schemes is the dominant factor limiting the comparative analysis of data. Well-defined age categories have not been employed consistently among the reporting systems, and the nonuniform age intervals cannot be compared reliably. Most of the available conclusions have been drawn from series based on sharply circumscribed clinical experiences.

MECHANISMS OF PEDIATRIC SPINE INJURIES

Vertebral column maturation is a continuous, dynamic process; however, developmental patterns and injury patterns among children are best divided into two categories: young children (birth through age 8) and adolescents (ages 9 through 16).[1,3,5-8,10,11] The phases of maturation and patterns of injury differ between these groups. During the first 8 years of life, spinal maturation is characterized primarily by alterations in the geometric configuration of vertebrae, development of ossification centers, closure of epiphyseal plates, alterations in ligamentous and soft tissue characteristics, and changes in osseous strength and integrity. The anatomic, physiologic, and pathologic features of spinal injury change after the age of 8.

Excessive spinal mobility, incomplete ossification, and structural weakness at epiphyseal plates provide substrates for injury in young children. Hypermobility of the vertebral column occurs because of its wedge-shaped, cartilaginous vertebral bodies, horizontally oriented facets, underdeveloped paraspinous muscular strength, highly elastic ligaments, and the child's disproportionately large head.

Among young children, most spinal cord injuries occur in the cervical spine, particularly in the occiput through C3. Spinal cord injury without radiographic abnormality (SCIWORA), ligamentous dislocation injury, growth plate injury, and a tendency to sustain severe neurologic injury are patterns characteristic of the first 8 years of life.[1,5,8,10-12]

Hypermobility of the child's spine is the single most important determinant of injury.[3,5-7] It appears to protect the spinal cord from injury, allowing the absorption of energy by dispersing force over multiple vertebral levels. Hypermobility accounts not only for the low incidence of spinal injury in the young but also for the patterns of injury. When spinal cord injury does occur, it is typically severe. Spinal cord injury results in complete loss of function more often in young children than in any other age group.

As the vertebrae ossify and enlarge and the ligaments and muscles become stronger and less elastic during adolescence, injury patterns begin to approach the patterns seen in adults.[1,5,8,10,11] However, adolescents sustain intermediate, transitional patterns of injury between those of young children and adults. Adult morphologic characteristics and patterns of injury become fully manifest only after the age of 15. In contrast to children, adolescents tend to sustain "true" fractures rather than ligamentous and growth plate injuries. However, compared with adults, adolescents have a higher proportion of ligamentous injuries such as subluxations without fractures and fracture-dislocations.[5,7,8]

INITIAL RESUSCITATION

Successful management of pediatric spinal injury begins with the assumption that any child with a head injury or with multiple traumatic injuries has a spinal cord injury—until proven otherwise. Immediate immobilization of the spine in a neutral position is a priority, concurrent with initiation of respiratory and cardiovascular resuscitation.

The acute phase in management of pediatric spinal cord injury begins early with aggressive "field" resuscitation and spinal stabilization. A large proportion of all spinal cord injuries are incomplete. If care is taken to protect the spine and spinal cord with full immobilization, recovery can be maximized. Spinal immobilization of a young child with a standard backboard can be hazardous. Young children have disproportionately large heads. If a child is positioned on a flat surface, the head may be forced forward, causing flexion of the neck and spinal cord injury. A standard backboard can be modified by using a recess to lower the occiput or a doubled mattress pad to raise the chest.

Spinal restraint systems designed specifically for children are also commercially available.

The treatment of *any* and *all* life-threatening injuries remains the initial priority of management. Specific attention to hypotension is urgent during the initial resuscitation. Hypotension should be assumed to result from hemorrhage until it is proven otherwise, even if a neurologic injury exists. Acute hypotension is rarely caused by neurologic injury alone. If the cause of persistent hypotension is uncertain, evaluate the child, if possible, with a pulmonary artery catheter (Swan-Ganz). It should, however, be used only after elimination of other probable causes.

The hallmarks of neurogenic shock, which often occurs with complete upper spinal cord injury, are hypotension, bradycardia, and hypothermia. These conditions are manifestations of the interruption of sympathetic outflow from the cervicothoracic region of the spinal cord. A loss of vasomotor tone accompanies spinal cord injuries in these cases, which can be treated effectively with alpha-adrenergic stimulation (Neo-synephrine).

Spinal shock differs from the physiologic syndrome of neurogenic shock. Spinal shock refers to the temporary but complete loss of all segmental reflex activity after a severe spinal cord injury. Children with spinal shock also have neurogenic shock and flaccid, areflexic limbs with no sensory or sphincteric function; priapism may also be present. After 7 to 21 days, the segmental reflex function returns, accompanied by signs and symptoms of spasticity.

Physical examination of the injured child provides important clues about the presence of spinal injury. A complete examination of the neck and back is necessary to evaluate for evidence of trauma. Abrasions or ecchymoses of the abdomen caused by "lap" seat belts may be clues to a lumbar fracture. Ecchymosis, abrasion, deformity, swelling, and tenderness of the spine are signs of injury.

Multiple injuries should alert the clinician to the possibility of spinal injury. Trauma to the face or head transmits forces to the neck, with a resultant high incidence of associated injury. Thoracic fractures are often associated with rib fractures, and lumbar fractures can occur with a significant retroperitoneal injury or intestinal perforation.

Spinal cord injury is detected through meticulous attention to the neurologic examination. Complete testing of the motor, sensory, and reflex functions of all extremities is necessary. Sacral and sphincteric function and pathological reflexes should also be evaluated. Sensory testing of the older child should include sharp-dull discrimination with a pin, light touch, proprioception, vibratory sense, and

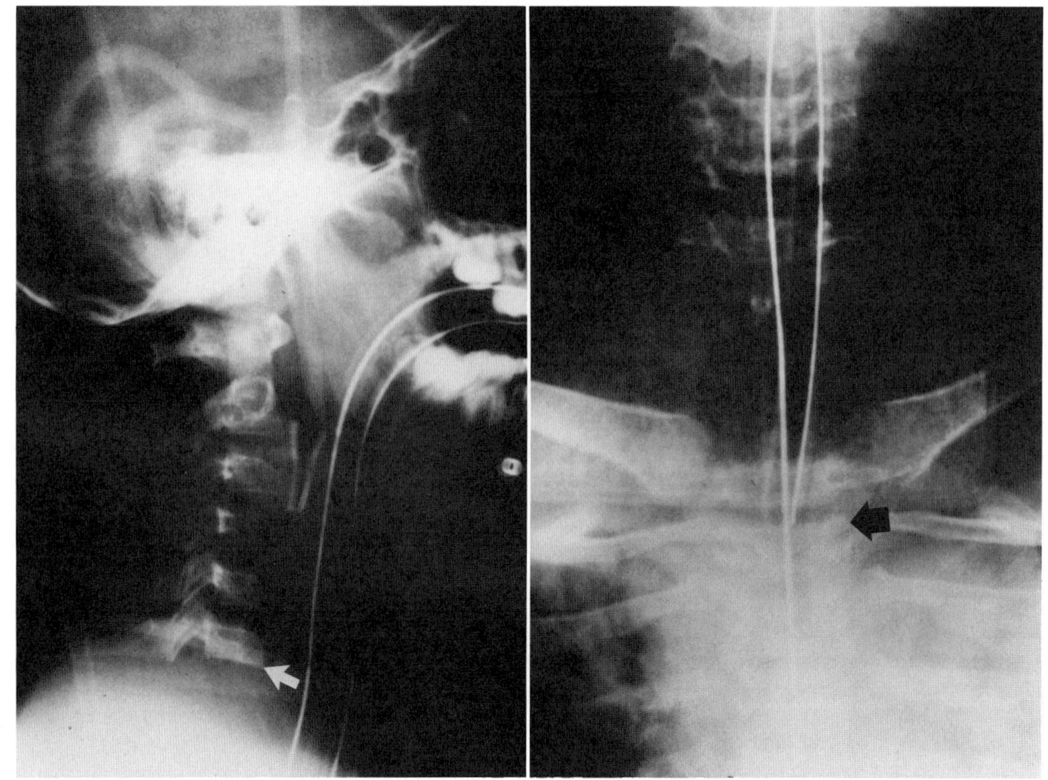

Figure 33–1 A, Lateral and **B,** anteroposterior cervical spine radiographs demonstrate a distraction injury of C6 (**A,** *arrow*) and C7. This dramatic dislocation illustrates the importance of fully assessing the cervicothoracic junction (**B,** *arrow*) with plain radiographs prior to "clearing" the cervical spine.

deep pain. Such an examination of a young child may be difficult, particularly when the child is afraid of being restrained, and the initial examination may be of limited benefit. Avoid the use of a hypodermic needle during examination because although full penetration of the skin with minimal pain is possible, it can lead to bleeding. A safety pin or disposable pin made for such a purpose is optimal. Begin distally and move proximally, using gentle pressure. Record the sensory level, if present, as the lowest area of perception of pain. Reassuring the child enhances a reliable examination. Determination of a sensory level is helpful in localizing the site of a spinal cord injury. Motor testing involves full examination of all muscle groups, including evaluation and grading of volitional strength. Sacral testing should include rectal tone, perianal sensation, saddle sensation, and the bulbocavernous and cremastic reflexes.

The young or unconscious child's inability to communicate symptoms verbally or to cooperate with the examination makes assessment difficult. Careful and repeated systematic examinations of neurologic function may be needed to exclude injury. In the presence of altered consciousness, significant neck or back pain, neurologic deficits, or neurologic symptoms, assume instability of the spine. If there is doubt, protect the spine with appropriate immobilization techniques.

RADIOLOGIC EVALUATION

A complete plain spinal radiographic analysis helps in assessment for injury of the spine in children. Any child with a head injury of multiple injuries must be evaluated for spinal injury. Between 10% and 20% of children with a spinal fracture have a second, noncontiguous level of spinal injury.[5,7,8] Complete radiographic assessment, including anteroposterior and lateral views of the cervical, thoracic, and lumbosacral spine, is indicated for children with preexisting head or spinal cord injuries. Cervical spine films must include the cervicothoracic junction (Fig. 33-1); visualization of the C7-T1 alignment improves by gentle caudal traction on the child's arms or by obtaining a "swimmer's view" of the cervical spine.

Dynamic flexion and extension views are used in the assessment of spinal stability. Reserve these

Table 33–1 Normal variations in the cervical spine in children

---

Hypermobility of the spine

1. Increased distance between the odontoid process and anterior arch of the atlas during flexion
2. Overriding of the anterior arch of the atlas on the odontoid process in extension
3. Pseudosubluxation
4. Angular or translational motion appearing in excess of normal

Variations in the curvature of the cervical spine that may resemble muscle spasm or ligamentous injury

1. Absence of uniform angulation between adjacent vertebrae with the neck in flexion
2. Absence of normal cervical lordosis in the neutral position
3. Absence of a flexion curve between C2 and C7 with flexion

Variations related to skeletal growth centers resembling fractures

1. Epiphyseal variations
   a. Apical odontoid epiphysis
   b. Secondary ossification of spinous processes
   c. Basilar odontoid synchondrosis
2. Incomplete ossification
   a. Subdental synchondrosis
   b. Apparent anterior wedging of the vertebral body

From Dickman CA, Sonntag VKH, Rekate HL, et al: Pediatric spinal trauma: vertebral column and spinal cord injuries in children, *Pediatr Neurosci* 15:237-256, 1989.

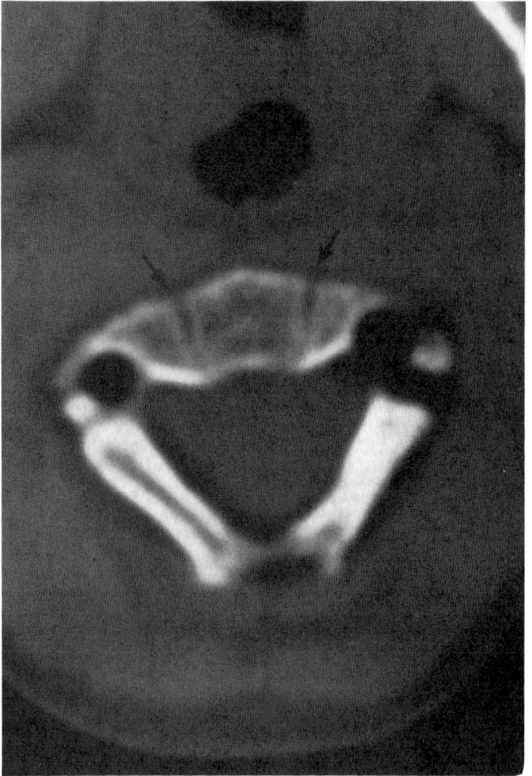

Figure 33–2 Computed tomography of C3 vertebral body in a 3-year-old child. The neurocentral synchondroses are visualized *(arrows)*. The smooth contours of the synchondroses and characteristic location differentiate these from fractures.

radiographs for alert, cooperative children without extensive fractures, subluxations, or neural injuries. Fluoroscopy is useful in assessing spinal stability in uncooperative or comatose children. If further evaluation is necessary (e.g., plain radiography is suggestive of a fracture), tomography and thin-section computed tomography (CT) detail osseous abnormalities best. In children with definite neurologic and spinal cord injury, myelography and magnetic resonance imaging (MRI) permit visualization of neural structures to assess compressive pathology.

In the normal child, skeletal and ligamentous immaturity produces radiographic peculiarities that may raise suspicions about the presence of injury (Table 33–1).[3,5] Epiphyses and synchondroses may resemble fracture lines (Fig. 33-2). The subdental synchondrosis is present in all children at 3 years and in half at 5 years; it usually disappears by 7 years. The normal subdental synchondrosis resem-

bles an odontoid fracture. Epiphyseal separation of this region occurs in the development of the os odontoideum.[3,5]

Pseudosubluxation; variations in the curvature of the cervical spine; and a wide, mobile atlantodental interval are normal radiographic manifestations of hypermobility of the cervical spine (Fig. 33-3).[3,5] Pseudosubluxation occurs at the C2-3 level in half of all children at age 7 and can also occur at the C3-4 level. Pseudosubluxation never exceeds 4 mm and should reduce completely with extension. Spinolaminar alignment as seen on flexion and extension x-rays is preserved with pseudosubluxation, and prevertebral soft tissue swelling is usually absent. The space between the dens and the ring of C1 (i.e., the atlantodental interval) is normally less than 5 mm in children and 3 mm or less in adults on lateral radiographs.[3,5]

Because a large proportion of pediatric spinal injuries are ligamentous or involve the growth plates, radiographic evaluation of the paravertebral soft tissues is important. A general guideline is that the prevertebral soft tissues should not exceed two

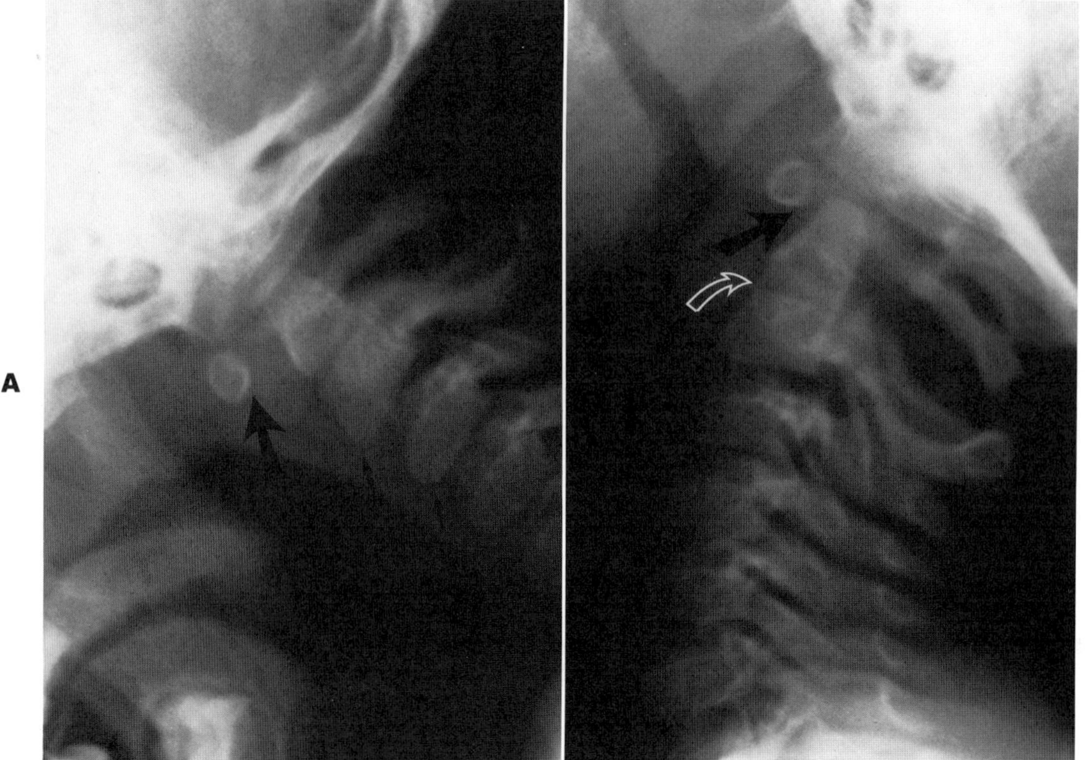

Figure 33–3 A, Flexion and **B,** extension lateral cervical spine radiographs in a 2 ½-year-old male. The atlas is mobile *(large arrows)*. Observe the pseudosubluxations at C2-3 and C3-4 that reduce with extension *(small arrows)*. The subdental synchondrosis is prominent as a lucency between the dens and the body of C2 *(open arrow)*.

thirds of the width of the vertebral body of C2. This principle is applicable only to a quiet child, as the soft tissue relationships change with forced respiration. Even with full radiographic and imaging evaluation, a significant proportion of children with spinal cord injury manifest a normal radiographic study.* Therefore, a meticulous clinical diagnostic evaluation is mandatory. The clinician must maintain a suspicion of spinal cord injury in children even if all spinal radiographs are normal.

SPECIFIC INJURIES AMONG CHILDREN
Birth injury

Birth-related injuries do not usually produce any radiographic abnormalities; however, these injuries are not usually classified as traumatic. Autopsy studies document that spinal cord damage contributes to 10% of all neonatal deaths, but incidence of this phenomenon has decreased with improve-

ments in prenatal evaluation and obstetrical techniques.[5,6]

In birth injury, the upper cervical spine or the cervicothoracic junction is typically affected; however, any spinal level is at risk.[5,6] Injury usually accompanies breech presentation. A third of the cases occur with cephalic birth canal presentations or in infants in the transverse position. These cases can occur following mechanical injury such as traction or ischemia of the spinal cord. Autopsy of newborns with spinal cord injury reveals transection, contusion, infarction, laceration, dural disruption, vertebral artery injury, and epidural and subdural hematoma.

The absence of radiographic findings makes diagnosis of birth-related spinal cord injury difficult. Severe injury causes death immediately. Incomplete neurologic injury results in death within the neonatal period or, at times, permits survival. Mild or moderate spinal cord injury may be accompanied by respiratory distress, a low Apgar score, or hypotonia (floppy infant syndrome). These injuries have often been mistakenly ascribed to congenital abnormality.[5,6]

---

*References 1, 5, 7, 8, 11, 12.

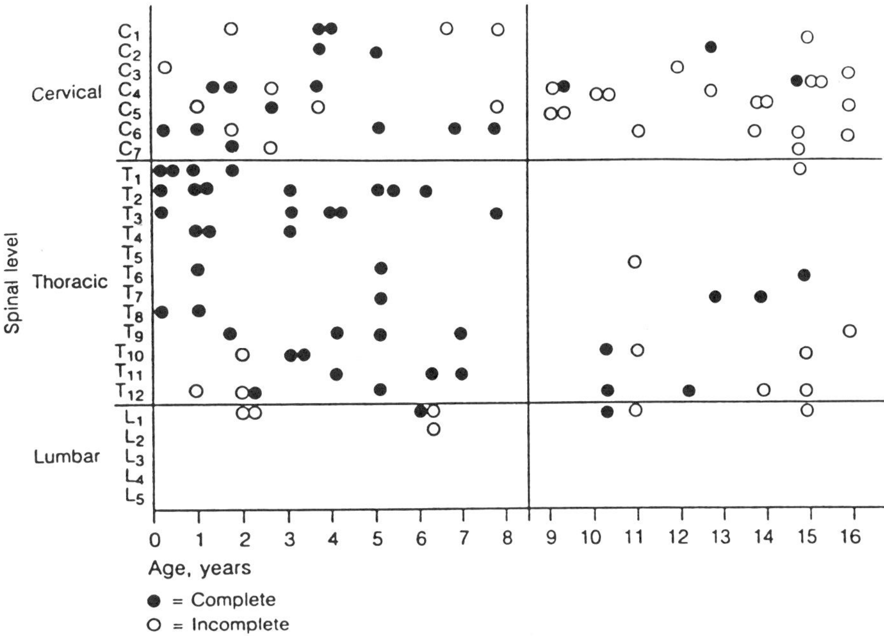

Figure 33–4 Age, spinal level, and neurologic status among SCIWORA injuries. (From Dickman CA, Sonntag VKH, Rekate HL et al: Pediatric spinal trauma: vertebral column and spinal injuries in children, *Pediatr Neurosci* 15:237-256, 1989.)

Child abuse

Intentional injury is manifested by severe neurologic dysfunction resulting from either intracranial or spinal injury.[5,7] Head injury is characterized by retinal hemorrhages, cerebral edema, intracranial hemorrhages, and profound neurologic impairment. Concurrent vertebral column injury results from a variety of traumatic mechanisms. Multiple vertebral fractures, soft tissue injuries, or SCIWORA also occur. Violent and forceful shaking of an infant causes cervical spinal cord contusion or cervical epidural and subdural hematomas in addition to intracranial injury.

SPINAL CORD INJURY WITHOUT RADIOGRAPHIC ABNORMALITIES

SCIWORA has been defined using plain radiographic studies, dynamic plain radiographic views, plain tomography, and CT. Although all of these studies can be normal, myelography or MRI finding can be abnormal in 5% to 70% of all pediatric spinal cord injuries.[1,5,11,12] If referral bias and the introduction of newer radiologic techniques are considered, SCIWORA accounts for 15% to 25% of all pediatric spinal cord injury.

SCIWORA occurs almost exclusively among children; two thirds of cases are seen in children aged 8 years or younger. SCIWORA is less common in adolescents and rare among adults. Al-though central cord injury occurs in middle-aged and elderly patients, spondylotic changes can create spinal cord injury without fracture or demonstrable osseous injury. However, the mechanisms of injury and clinical course in these older patients are distinct from those seen with SCIWORA.

In SCIWORA, injury to the cervical and thoracic spinal levels occurs with equal frequency, whereas the lumbar levels are rarely involved (Fig. 33-4). The cervical spine is overrepresented in this type of injury, considering its length and number of vertebrae. Of all reported injuries, about half are complete and half are incomplete neurologically. Thoracic lesions tend to be complete, whereas cervical and lumbar injuries are incomplete.

These are important differences between the young group (birth to 8 years) and adolescents (9 to 16 years) with SCIWORA. Young children sustain two thirds of all SCIWORA and have a higher proportion of complete neurologic injury. In this age group, 75% of all injuries are complete and 25% are incomplete. In adolescents the opposite pattern is evident (73% incomplete, 27% complete). Spinal cord "concussion-type" injury is more common in adolescents; myelopathy recovers within 48 hours.

The onset of severe neurologic deficit in SCIWORA following initially "trivial" symptoms occurs up to 4 days after injury in as many as 22%

of cases.[11,12] Brief sensory or motor deficits, such as shocklike sensations or rapidly clearing weakness, are often noted initially. Affected children can progress to complete neurologic injury and have a poor prognosis. Another phenomenon, recurrent injury,[12] also occurs among children with mild initial deficits. These children resume normal activities too early and disregard their immobilization devices. Recurrent injury is typically more severe than initial injury and can have permanent sequelae. The institution of more rigid cervical braces, the strict limitation of activity, and close follow-up help prevent the serious risk of recurrent injury.

MRI or myelography and dynamic radiographs are indicated for children with SCIWORA in assessment for spinal instability or compressive lesions.[5] Widening of the spinal cord, partial or complete blockage, and a normal plain radiographic study have been the most common findings in myelography. Extravasation of dye, presumably from traction injury, is a particularly poor prognostic finding. Thin-section CT, two vertebral levels above and below the neurologic level of injury, is indicated. MRI, which has been used only occasionally with SCIWORA, shows spinal cord contusions, cord widening, or normal spinal cord anatomy.[5]

Operative exploration of SCIWORA rarely reveals a treatable lesion.[5] Surgery of the spine has revealed spinal cord contusion, necrosis, atrophy, edema, infarction, transection, epidural hematoma, and spinal instability. Autopsy studies of children with fatal spinal cord injury, whose radiographs are normal, reveal muscular and ligamentous disruptions, growth plate avulsion, epiphyseal separation, spinal instability, and subdural or epidural spinal hematomas. The most common autopsy finding is a growth plate avulsion injury.

Ligamentous flexibility and the elasticity of the immature spine play a major role in the pathogenesis of SCIWORA.[5,6,11,12] A young child's vertebral column may withstand traction and torsion without evidence of deformity while the spinal cord tears. In longitudinal traction, the cadaveric infant spine is able to withstand up to 2 inches of stretch without disruption, whereas the spinal cord ruptures after only ¼ inch of stretching. This mismatching partially accounts for the neural injury seen in normal radiographic vertebral anatomy. Other mechanisms include reversible disk protrusion, vasospasm, vascular occlusion, and transient subluxation (Table 33-2).

Children with a complete spinal cord lesion, delayed onset of deficits, delayed deterioration of function, and recurrent injury usually have a poor

Table 33–2 Mechanisms of SCIWORA

Direct spinal cord traction
1. Longitudinal spinal cord traction
2. Root traction/avulsion

Direct spinal cord compression
1. Transient compression
   a. Ligamentous bulging
   b. Reversible disk protrusion
   c. Transient subluxation of vertebrae
2. Persistent compression*
   a. Occult fracture with spinal cord compression
   b. Spinal epidural hematoma
   c. Persistent disk herniation
   d. Occult subluxation/instability

Indirect spinal cord injury
1. Transmission of externally applied kinetic energy to spinal cord (spinal cord concussion)

Vascular/ischemic injury
1. Vascular occlusion, dissection, spinal cord infarction
2. Vasospasm
3. Hypotension, impaired spinal cord perfusion

*Potentially requires operative intervention.

prognosis. However, the overall prognosis for children with SCIWORA directly relates to the severity of the initial spinal cord injury.

Cervical injuries[1,4-8,11,12]

Ligamentous elasticity, osseous immaturity, and hypermobility in young children provide the basis for a tendency to sustain vertebral column soft tissue injury rather than a true fracture. These injuries manifest as SCIWORA, dislocation, subluxation without fracture, epiphyseal separation, or avulsion of the growth plate. These characteristics account for the high incidence of immediate and early death following injury and for the apparent higher incidence of complete injuries in young children.

Congenital malformation, segmentation abnormality, inflammation, or a neoplastic process affecting the spine can predispose young children to injury. Nontraumatic atlantoaxial subluxation that occurs with cervical lymphadenitis is referred to as Grisel's syndrome.

Most spinal injuries in the first decade of life involve the cervical region, mainly the occiput through C3. Sixty percent to 80% of vertebral injuries in young children affect the cervical spine, as compared with 30% to 40% of all adult vertebral injuries. Data on cervical sprains, probably the

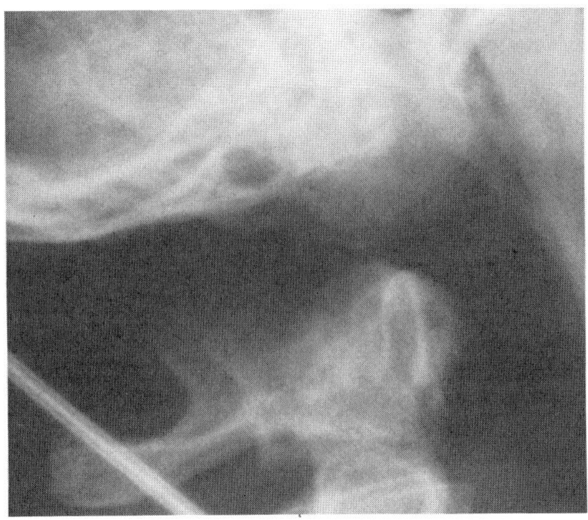

Figure 33–5 Lateral radiograph showing a craniovertebral junction dislocation. The occipital condyles are longitudinally distracted and displaced anteriorly in relationship to the atlas.

most common form of spinal injury, are poorly documented. Cervical sprains account for as many as a third of all hospital admissions for pediatric neck injury.

Although young children are prone to dislocation without fracture at all vertebral levels, serious ligamentous injuries most frequently occur in the upper cervical spine. Atlantooccipital dislocations are often fatal, owing to neural or arterial injury at the cervicomedullary junction (Fig. 33-5). Biomechanically, these dislocations are highly unstable because of ligamentous avulsion. To prevent further distraction in injured children, avoid the use of traction with tongs. Internal fixation is indicated in the presence of salvageable neurologic function; halo immobilization is inadequate to maintain proper alignment in these injuries.

A variety of ligamentous injuries occur at the C1-2 level. Anterior atlantoaxial subluxation occurs with injury to the transverse ligament. Posterior subluxation can occur only with a dens fracture, an incomplete C1 ring, or separation of the subdental synchondrosis. The latter is thought to be the cause of os odontoideum. Anterior subluxation is present if the predental space is greater than 5 mm in a child or greater than 3 mm in an adolescent. Neurologic injury is rare with C1 subluxation, which is better tolerated than subluxation at lower cervical levels because the spinal canal is more capacious at the C1 level.

The presenting symptoms of atlantoaxial rotatory subluxation are neck pain and torticollis (Fig. 33-6). A rotatory dislocation is unstable only if associated with transverse ligament rupture.

The treatment of atlas, axis, and lower cervical fractures depends on several factors: (1) the extent of osseous displacement, (2) the extent of ligamentous damage, (3) the presence of neurologic injury, and (4) the presence of additional contiguous spinal fractures. Minor, nondisplaced, or minimally displaced atlas fractures are treated with a Philadelphia collar, a Yale brace, or a sternal-occipital-mandibular immobilizer (SOMI). C1 fractures with wide displacement of bone (more than a 7-mm displacement of the lateral masses in open-mouth views) or disruption of the transverse ligament are initially treated with a halo brace for 12 weeks (Fig. 33-7).

Most C2 fractures (odontoid, hangman's, and miscellaneous fractures) are managed effectively with a halo brace; however, minor fractures are treated with less rigid immobilization (Fig. 33-8). Odontoid type II fractures with more than a 5-mm displacement of the dens have a high risk of nonunion and are candidates for early operative management with internal fixation.

The discovery of an atlas or axis fracture should raise the suspicion of additional injury. C1 and C2 fractures often occur together (Fig. 33-9). CT is indicated to fully delineate areas of suspected injury. Most combination fractures can be treated effectively with a halo brace for 12 weeks. However, compulsive follow-up is mandatory for all cervical spinal injuries. Flexion and extension radiographs are typically necessary after an orthosis has been removed, to detect nonunion and persistent instability.

Lower cervical spinal injuries in young children are treated according to similar treatment principles. Ligamentous instability may become evident only after muscular spasm subsides; therefore, late dynamic x-rays help in assessment of stability in children with pain, stiffness, or torticollis after trauma. The treatment of fractures of lower cervical levels must be individualized.

THORACIC AND LUMBAR SPINE INJURIES[5,7-10]

Thoracic and lumbar fractures resulting from hyperflexion are the most common injuries to the young, immature thoracolumbar spine. These injuries usually involve multiple vertebral bodies (in 50% to 75% of cases) and occur in the midthoracic or midlumbar regions in young children. Adolescents tend to sustain fractures between T10 and L2 at the thoracolumbar junction. This hinge region between the relativity rigid thoracic spine and the mobile lumbar spine is particularly susceptible to injury after complete ossification and closure of epiphyseal plates.

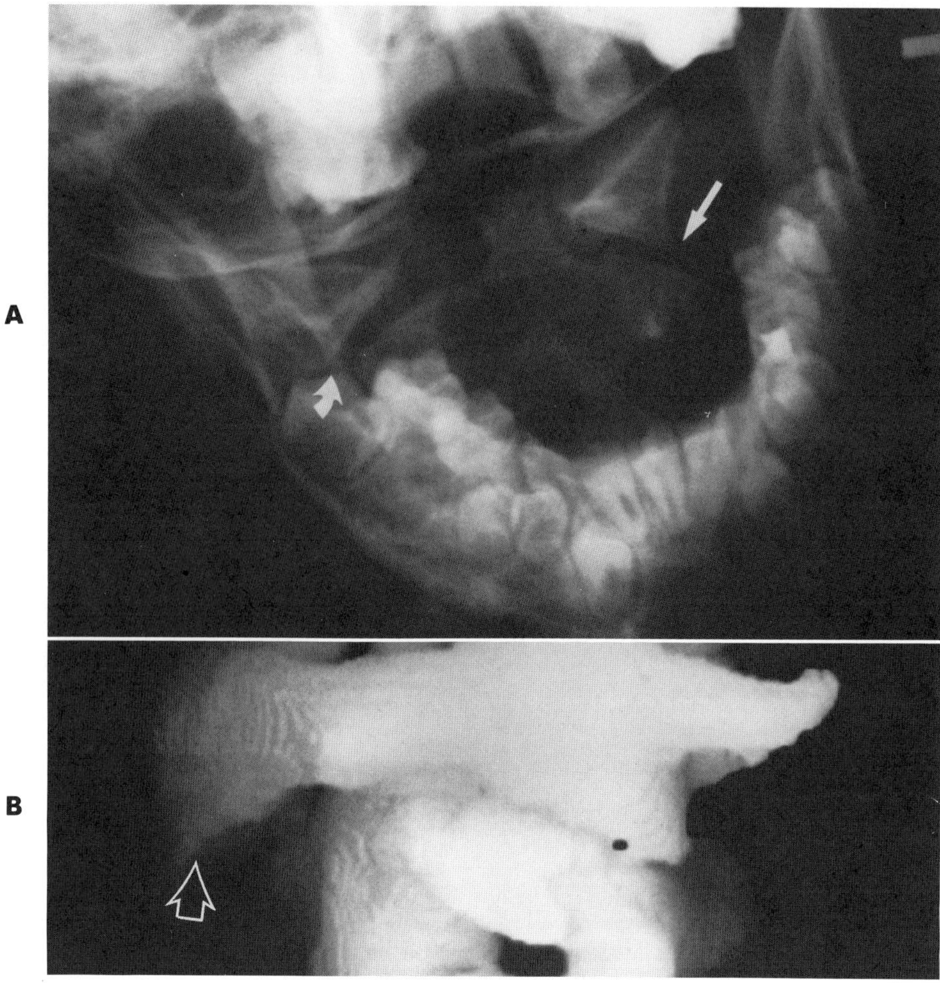

Figure 33–6 Atlantoaxial rotatory dislocation. **A,** Open-mouth anteroposterior roentgenogram (straight arrow indicates C2 articular facet; curved arrow indicates displaced C1 lateral mass), and **B,** three-dimensional CT reconstruction. The C1 lateral mass is displaced anteriorly *(open arrow)*.

The treatment of thoracic and lumbar spinal injuries depends on the presence of pain, spinal deformity, or neurologic deficit, and the characteristics of the fracture. Children with extensive vertebral body compression (more than 50% of the height of the vertebral body), translocation, spinal instability, kyphotic deformity, or severe intractable pain require open reduction and internal fixation. Children with incomplete neurologic deficits resulting from compression of neural elements are candidates for surgical decompression of the spinal cord and/or nerve roots. Despite decompression of the spinal cord, children who experience complete neurologic deficits do not tend to recover function.

Compared with spinal cord injuries, compression of the cauda equina must be considered a special case. The nerves are "peripheral nerves" and can regenerate. Therefore, surgical decompression of the cauda equina may be considered even when profound neurologic deficits exist.

Lap-belt injuries of the lumbar spine[9]

Lap-belt injuries are associated with midlumbar spinal fractures resulting from deceleration front-end-impact motor vehicle crashes. Postural abnormalities and poorly developed anterosuperior iliac spines cause children to wear seatbelts around the abdomen rather than the pelvis, which accounts for the injury. External belt-shaped abrasions across the lower abdomen are important clues to this injury. Thirty percent of affected children have associated visceral injury. These flexion-distraction injuries occur with fractures and/or ligamentous avulsion. Vertebral injuries are usually centered between the second and fourth lumbar vertebrae.

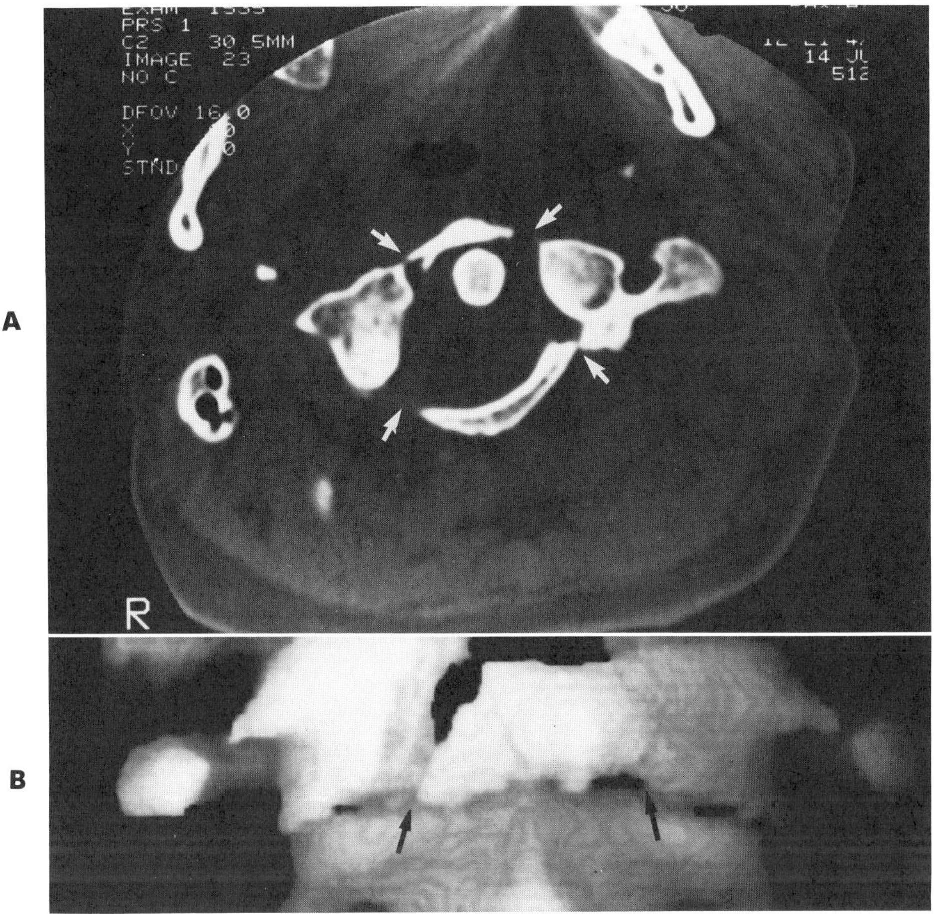

Figure 33–7 Atlas fracture with "burst" pattern. **A,** Thin-section CT image; **B,** three-dimensional computed tomography (posterior view). *(Arrows indicate fractures.)*

PRINCIPLES OF TREATMENT OF CHILDHOOD SPINAL INJURIES

The only truly effective way to ensure intact neurologic function is injury prevention. Educational efforts to prevent injury are crucial. An important national spinal injury prevention program has been implemented. The American Association of Neurological Surgery and Congress of Neurological Surgeons have jointly established an educational program to prevent head and spinal cord injuries, entitled "Think First." The Think First Foundation has been formed as a nonprofit organization to raise and expend funds and to supervise the function of the injury prevention program. Similarly, the practice of driving while intoxicated has been subjected to increasing social and legal consequences.

The principles of treatment of vertebral column or spinal cord injury are based on preservation of existing neurologic function and prevention of further neurologic injury. Strict and continuous im-

mobilization of the entire spine is mandated while the presence of spinal injuries is assessed clinically and radiographically. If injuries to the spine or spinal cord are present, immobilization is maintained and treatment rapidly instituted.

Systemic hypotension can cause spinal cord ischemia, which can further compromise spinal cord function. Specific attention must be given to maintaining a mean blood pressure at normal levels with fluid resuscitation and pressor agents, if needed. Intravenous Neo-synephrine (50 mg in 250 ml of 5% dextrose in water titrated at 50 to 100 µg/hr) is particularly useful for hypotension caused by a loss of sympathetic tone resulting from neurogenic shock syndromes. Adequate resuscitation of the intravascular volume is the initial priority; pressors should be reserved until euvolemia is attained.

Pharmacologic intervention to limit secondary spinal cord injury has focused on biochemical, systemic, and cellular mechanisms. An intravenous

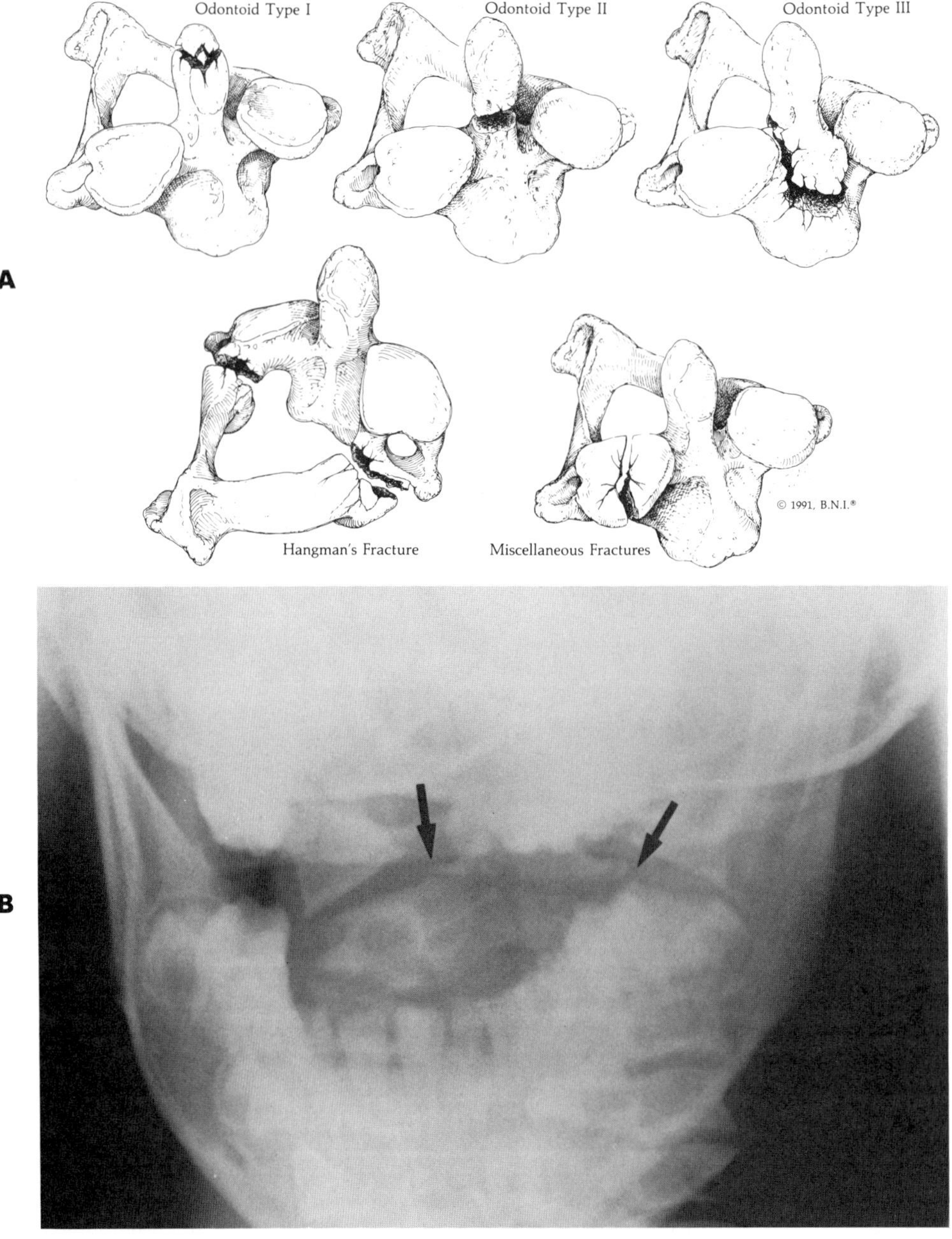

Figure 33–8 Axis fractures. **A,** Classification scheme for types of C2 fractures. **B,** Anteroposterior cervical radiograph of an odontoid type III fracture *(arrows)* in a 6-year-old male.

bolus dose of methylprednisolone (Solumedral) (30 mg/kg) followed by an intravenous dose at 5.4 mg/kg/hr for 23 hours has been advocated for acute spinal cord injuries. This regimen has a significant benefit if begun within 8 hours of injury.[2]

There is an urgent need to correct malalignment by reducing the spine in children with spinal subluxation or dislocation.[5] Early external reduction and realignment of spinal subluxations is advocated for "decompression" of the spinal cord. Reduction of cervical dislocations in children requires consideration of skull thickness and spinal ligamentous elasticity. Traction in infants to reduce subluxation is possible with the use of Holter traction or bilateral burr holes and wires. Weight should be limited to 2 pounds. In children with thicker skulls, Gardner-Wells tongs or a halo ring permits appropriate traction. During attempted external reduction,

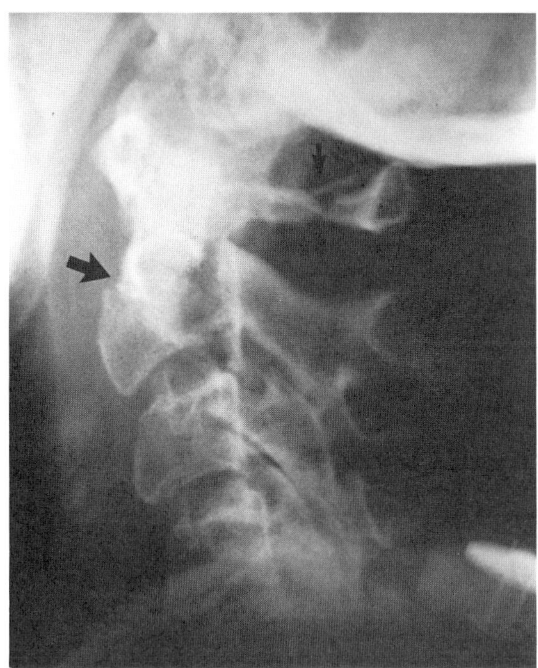

Figure 33–9 Lateral radiograph of combination atlas-axis fractures *(arrows)*.

careful evaluation of the child is necessary. If any deterioration in neurologic function occurs, abandon external reduction of the spine and proceed to internal reduction. Thoracic or lumbar fracture with deformity frequently improves alignment on a flat bed (Stokes bed). Subluxation refractory to reduction with external traction requires surgical reduction with internal fixation. Surgical repair of the spine is necessary for unstable fractures that cannot be maintained with external orthoses or for fractures with a high risk of nonunion.

ORTHOSES[5,7]

The use of external orthotic devices after an acute injury depends on the type of injury and the age of the patient. A soft cervical collar or a Philadelphia collar restricts cervical motion minimally. These devices are used for muscular injuries and certain instances of atlantoaxial rotatory subluxation and nondisplaced atlas fracture. Yale, SOMI, and four-poster braces provide an intermediate range of immobilization of the cervical spine. Unfortunately, these orthoses may cause malocclusion or mandibular deformity in young children.

The halo apparatus has the best immobilization characteristics of any orthosis for the cervical spine. It completely fixes the head to the thorax and allows no rotation, lateral displacement, or sagittal plane motion of the upper cervical spine.

However, minimal motion of lower cervical spine segments may occur. The halo is dependable and is particularly suited for uncooperative or unreliable children.

The use of the halo brace in children requires special attention (Fig. 33-10). This device has been used successfully in children as young as 7 months, although it is preferable to use it in children of 3 years or more. Calvarial thickness should be assessed with a CT scan before halo application. A thin skull limits pin pressure to 1 to 2 inches per pound of torque and requires insertion of 6 to 10 pin sites to distribute the forces evenly in order to prevent skull penetration. In the infant, a custom halo ring and a lightweight vest are necessary. A custom lightweight thermoplastic Minerva jacket is an alternative to the halo brace.

External immobilization is effective for a displaced atlas fracture, most C2 fractures, and certain middle and lower cervical fractures. Selection of a particular brace depends on the individual clinical and radiographic circumstances of each child. A molded plastic body jacket, which is well tolerated by children, is appropriate for stable thoracic, thoracolumbar, or lumbar fractures (Fig. 33-11).

OPERATIVE INTERVENTION[5,7]

Surgery is indicated for an unstable fracture, irreducible dislocation, progressive neurologic deficit with an incomplete spinal cord injury, debridement of a compound wound, persistent instability despite the use of external orthoses, or progressive spinal deformity. Atlantooccipital dislocation injury, atlantoaxial rotatory fixation, atlantoaxial subluxation, compression burst fracture, and fracture-dislocation are usually unstable injuries that frequently require surgical stabilization. The decision to perform surgery and the choice of operative approach must be individualized. Evoked potential monitoring of the somatosensory and motor pathways during surgery can detect changes in the physiologic integrity of the spinal cord.

Skeletal development affects options for surgical treatment of spinal injury in children. Vertebral fusion is effective if limited to unstable segments to preserve physiologic mobility and growth. Extensive fusion at a young age shortens trunk height, because the bony fusion mass does not elongate. Multilevel laminectomy in children risks spinal deformity, a result that should be prevented. Surgical exposure of incompletely developed vertebral cartilage and of ossification centers may cause a widespread fusion or "creeping fusion." Children's bone is highly osteogenic; consequently, insertion of wire is not always necessary for fusion. Onlay bone grafts are adequate to fuse the cervical spine. However, a spinal fusion that employs bone secured by

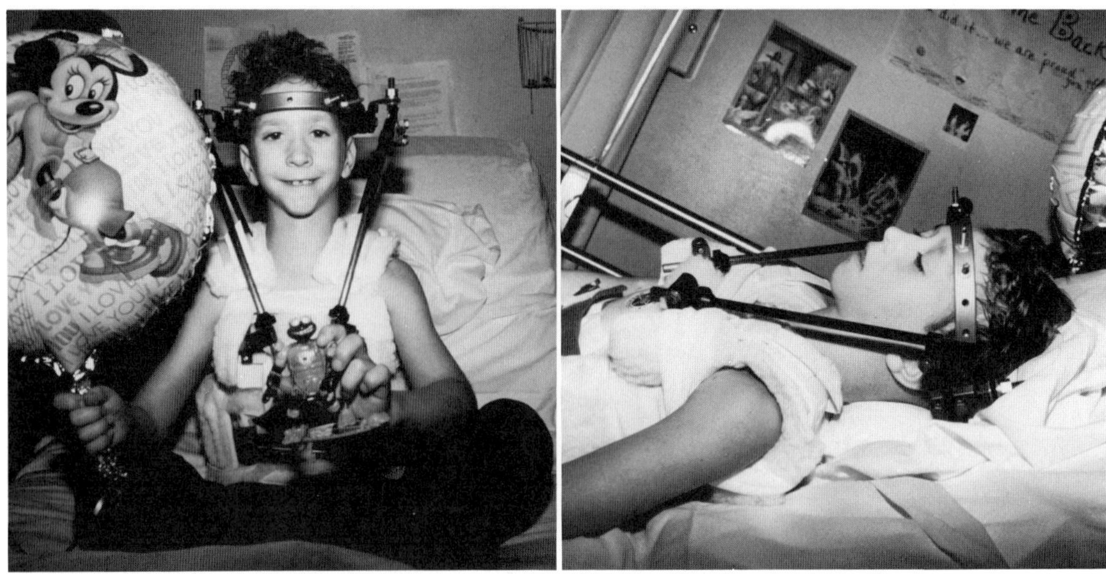

Figure 33–10 Photograph of a 7-year-old boy in a halo brace.

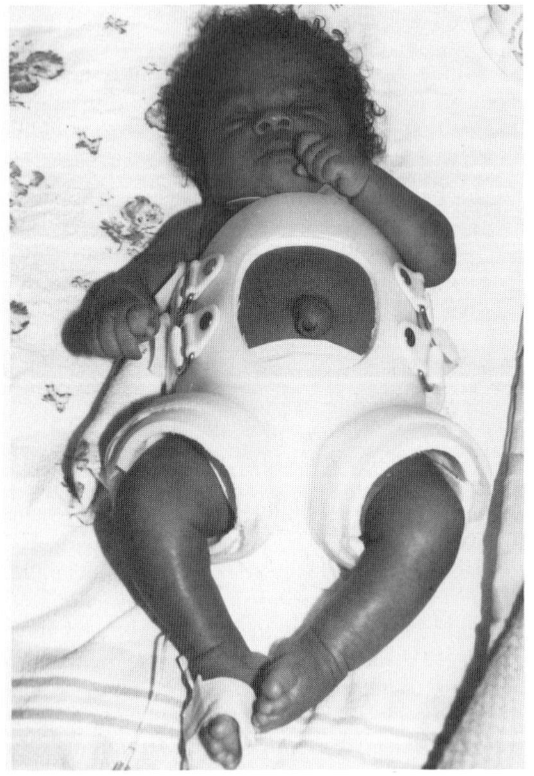

Figure 33–11 Lightweight custom-molded thoracolumbar jacket for an infant.

wire to the facets or laminae is optimal for long-term stability in children. The use of wire alone is hazardous, because it may tear through the cartilaginous, incompletely ossified bone. Without bone grafting, wire does not produce long-term stability, because the wire will break with spinal growth.

For internal fixation of the thoracic or lumbar spine, instrumentation in conjunction with bone grafting is usually indicated. A variety of options for fusion are available. In the very young child, rib grafts provide struts for fusion (Fig. 33-12). In older children, Cotrel-Dubousset, Luque, or Harrington rod systems are available for internal fixation.

OUTCOME[5,8-12]

Half of all children with spinal cord injury die at the site of injury or shortly thereafter. Among the initial survivors, 20% die within 3 months because of complications of the injury. In contrast, children who survive the first 3 months after injury have a greater chance of surviving 5 years, as compared with other age groups with spinal cord injury. Life expectancy diminishes with increasingly severe neurologic injury. The high initial mortality suggests that pediatric trauma victims sustain more severe neurologic injury or tolerate multiple severe injuries more poorly than older victims.

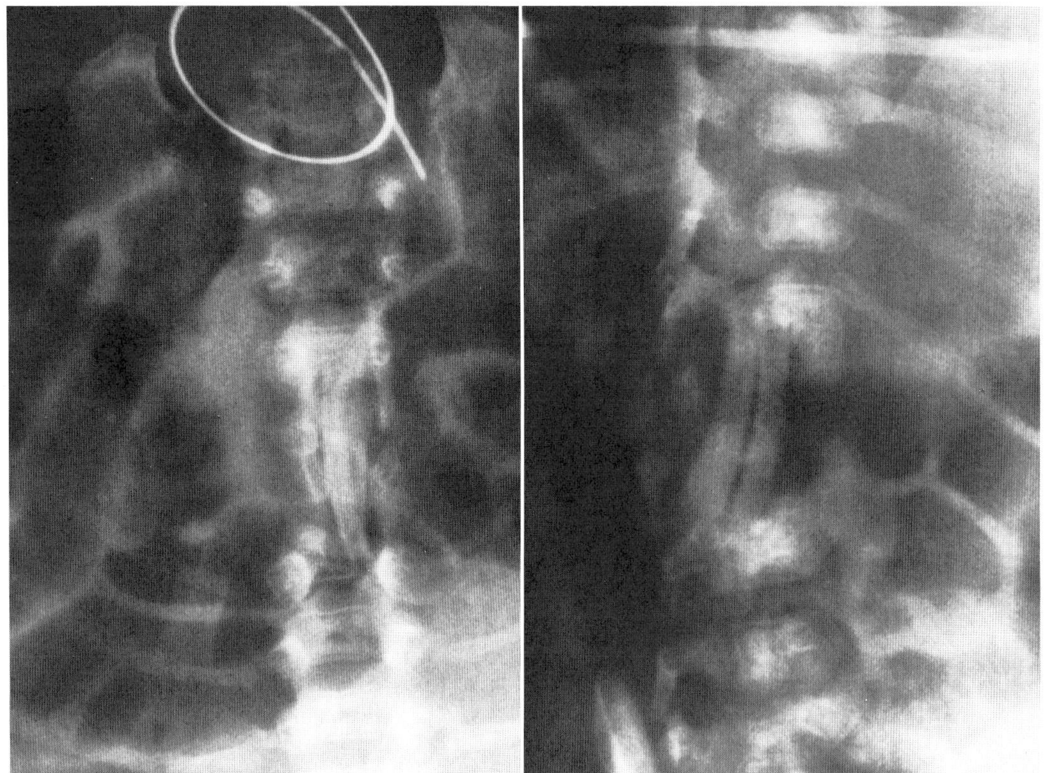

Figure 33–12 Rib strut grafts placed for fusion of the midlumbar vertebral segments in a 4-month-old infant. **A,** Anteroposterior and **B,** lateral radiographic views.

A high percentage of spinal cord injuries in young children are complete injuries. This trend appears to be particularly relevant to young children (birth through 8 years) with ligamentous injuries or SCIWORA. The very young tolerate spinal cord injury poorly. In contrast, adolescents (ages 9 to 16) sustain injuries of a severity intermediate between young children and adults.

Prognosis for recovery of neurologic function after pediatric spinal cord injury is uncertain. Opinions regarding prognosis often conflict. Some suggest that children with incomplete spinal cord injury may recover more function than adults with comparable deficits. The hypothesis that the immature spinal cord possesses greater "plasticity" and is capable of greater functional recovery is unconfirmed. In contrast, some suggest that children generally have a poor prognosis after spinal cord injury.

A review of the literature indicates that the prognosis for recovery among children with neurologic injury appears to be directly related to their functional neurologic status following initial injury. Children with complete spinal cord injury have a limited prognosis for functional recovery that ranges between 0% to 10%. Those with incomplete spinal-cord injuries have a better prognosis; the degree of recovery correlates directly with the severity of loss of motor function.

COMPLICATIONS[5,7]

Progressive vertebral column deformity occurs in a large proportion of children with spinal cord injury. These deformities include scoliosis, kyphosis, and lordosis. The predisposition to develop a progressive vertebral column deformity occurs secondary to damage of growth plates, an imbalance between pelvic and paraspinous muscles, and unequal bone growth after fracture. The younger the patient at injury and the higher the level of the neurologic injury, the worse the deformity will be. The relationship of injury to growth phase is critical. More than 90% of children sustaining paraplegia before the adolescent growth spurt develop spinal deformity. Children sustaining vertebral column fracture or neurologic injury before this growth spurt are at high risk for spinal deformity and should be followed carefully. Early immobilization with an external orthosis is initially indicated. Instability, progression of a neurologic deficit, or progressively worsening deformity indicates a need for internal fixation. Another delayed complication of spinal cord injury is posttraumatic syringomyelia, which is characterized by progressive pain, spinal deformity, increasing neurologic dysfunction or all three. Both drainage of the syrinx and correction of the spinal deformity are helpful.

Other complications associated with spinal cord injuries include deep venous thrombosis, decubitus ulcer, urinary infection, respiratory insufficiency, neurogenic bladder, bowel dysfunction, spasticity, pain syndromes, and psychosocial dysfunction. These complications require the comprehensive attention of a *team* consisting of a pediatrician, neurosurgeon, pediatric neurologist, orthopedist, psychiatrist, and urologist during the acute and rehabilitative phases following injury.

Deep venous thrombosis is exacerbated by limb paralysis and bed rest. Although unusual in young children, its occurrence and incidence may be minimized with subcutaneous, prophylactic, minidoses of heparin (5000 U two or three times a day) and sequential air-compression or elastic-compression stockings. Even low doses of heparin cause thrombocytopenia; therefore, platelet count monitoring is routine. Sequential air-compression stockings are indicated to prevent deep venous thrombosis of the lower extremities in order to reduce the incidence of pulmonary embolus.

Respiratory insufficiency can follow either direct injury of the cervical spinal cord or peripheral nerve injury. The outflow of the phrenic nerve originates from the third, fourth, and fifth cervical segments. Spinal cord injury at or above these levels causes diaphragmatic paralysis. Children with acute cervical spinal cord injury who have intact ventilatory function require close assessment (every 8 to 12 hours) and sequential respiratory measurements (for example, tidal volume, negative inspiratory force, forced vital capacity) to detect a decompensation in pulmonary function. Delayed intubation is often needed in children with lower-level cervical cord injury. If nerve conduction and electromyographic examinations demonstrate that the phrenic nerve outflow is intact, pacing of the phrenic nerve with an implantable system is possible. Respiratory insufficiency resulting from impaired thoracic and intercostal excursion can also occur when the spinal cord is injured below the level of phrenic outflow. Early physical mobilization and aggressive pulmonary physiotherapy help minimize complications. Tracheostomy is needed for patients who require prolonged mechanical ventilation.

Neurogenic bladder and bowel dysfunction require acute and chronic treatment. Urinary retention predisposes children to chronic infection and bladder cancer. An indwelling Foley catheter is initially placed during the acute injury phase and changed to long-term, intermittent clean catheterization. Pharmacologic therapy is instituted as indicated by urodynamometric studies.

Loss of rectal sphincter tone and volitional control is treated with stool softener, substances to add bulk to the stools, and local anal dilatation. These treatments stimulate a reflexive contracture of the sigmoid to train the bowel to empty. A Dulcolax suppository every day or every other day with dilatation is very successful.

Pain syndromes, spasticity, and psychological sequelae are the most difficult chronic problems to treat in children with spinal cord injury. No therapy is uniformly successful, and all of these conditions may require a combination of medical, surgical, and pharmacologic treatment.

CONCLUSION

Spine injuries in children are often accompanied by devastating neurologic injury with permanent sequelae. Protection of the vertebral column and prevention of injury are of paramount importance. Meticulous clinical and radiographic assessment is necessary in children with suspected spinal injury. Flexibility and elasticity of the immature spine predispose children to spinal injuries with normal radiographs (SCIWORA), ligamentous injury, and severe spinal cord injury. The operative and nonoperative management strategies must be individualized, based upon the patient's age, the characteristics of the vertebral column injury, and the severity of associated neurologic deficits. Prognosis depends directly on the functional neurologic status following injury. Children with an incomplete spinal cord syndrome have a relatively good prognosis for recovery of neurologic function. Diligent follow-up and multimodality rehabilatative services are essential to assess and treat the sequelae following injury.

REFERENCES

1. Birney TJ, Hanley EN Jr: Traumatic cervical spine injuries in childhood and adolescence, *Spine* 14:1277-1282, 1989.
2. Bracken MB, Shepard MJ, Collins WF et al: A randomized, controlled trial of methylprednisolone or naloxone in the treatment of acute spinal-cord injury, *New Engl J Med* 322:1405-1411, 1990.
3. Cattell HS, Filtzer DL: Pseudosubluxation and other normal variations in the cervical spine in children: a study of one hundred and sixty children, *J Bone Joint Surg* 47A:1295-1309, 1965.
4. Dickman CA, Hadley MN, Browner C et al: Neurosurgical management of acute atlas-axis combination fractures: a review of 25 cases, *J Neurosurg* 70:45-49, 1989.
5. Dickman CA, Rekate HL, Sonntag VKH et al: Pediatric spinal trauma: vertebral column and spinal cord injuries in children, *Pediatr Neurosci* 15:237-256, 1989.

6. Glasauer FE, Cares HL: Biomechanical features of traumatic paraplegia in infancy, *J Trauma* 13(2):166-170,
1973.
7. Godersky JC, Menezes AH: Optimal management for children with spinal cord injury, *Contemp Neurosurg* 11:1-6,
1989.
8. Hadley MN, Zabramski JM, Browner CM et al: Pediatric
spinal trauma: review of 122 cases of spinal cord and vertebral column injuries, *J Neurosurg* 68:18-24, 1988.
9. Johnson DL, Falci S: The diagnosis and treatment of pediatric lumbar spine injuries caused by rear seat lap belts,
Neurosurgery 26:434-441, 1990.
10. Kewalramani LS, Kraus JF, Sterling HM: Acute spinal-
cord lesions in a pediatric population: epidemiological and
clinical features, *Paraplegia* 18:206-219, 1980.
11. Pang D, Wilberger JE Jr: Spinal cord injury without radiographic abnormalities in children, *J Neurosurg* 57:114-
129, 1982.
12. Pollack IF, Pang D, Sclabassi R: Recurrent spinal cord
injury without radiographic abnormalities in children, *J
Neurosurg* 69:177-182, 1988.

34 Peripheral Nerve Injury

Dennis L. Johnson

Peripheral nerve injuries are uncommon in children and easy to overlook because they may be obscured by other injuries, or by a child's inability to articulate symptoms or apprehensive lack of cooperation. Indeed, a peripheral nerve injury may be difficult to differentiate from the immobility of a painfully fractured leg of a frightened, crying child. Nevertheless, early recognition is essential, and timing critical to successful management of nerve injuries.

Neurologic examination can identify the muscles that have been affected by a nerve injury. The closest muscle to the injury is the "target muscle" and is the first to be reinnervated. Reinnervation of the target muscle is the initial clinical sign of regeneration (see Table 34-1). If the injured nerve is concussed and only temporarily dysfunctional, movement will recover within a few weeks. Most nerve injuries are treated for the first few weeks in anticipation of early return of function. If recovery has not occurred within 6 weeks, regeneration in an anatomically intact nerve can be confirmed and traced electrophysiologically. As successive muscles are reinnervated, movement and then function are restored. If the nerve is severed, torn, or crushed, surgical reanastomosis is the only hope for recovery. However, if spontaneous regeneration or surgical anastomosis do not permit the nerve to reach a muscle within 6 to 12 months, fibrosis of the muscle and myoneural function will prevent reinnervation.

PATHOPHYSIOLOGY

The discussion will focus on the motor neuron and the motor unit, which consists of the neuron and the muscles that the neuron innervates. The sensory neuron provides essential input to the final common motor pathway and provides protective sensation to weight-bearing surfaces; however, assessing sensation is problematic in children. The approach to nerve repair must consider not only the anatomy and physiology of the motor nerve, but also the innervated muscles and the surrounding connective tissue.

The basic unit of the peripheral nerve is the nerve fiber. Each nerve fiber consists of an axon, its myelin sheath, and a Schwann cell which produces the myelin. These components are bundled together by *endoneurium*. Multiple nerve fibers are bound together by *perineurium* to form a fascicle, which in turn is wrapped with other fascicles by *epineurium* to form a nerve. The endoneurium, perineurium,

Table 34–1 Neurologic examination

Nerve	Motor	Autonomous sensory zone*
Median	Opposition of thumb	Tips of thumb and index finger
Ulnar	Straightening ring and little finger; adduction and abduction of little finger	Tip of little finger
Radial	Wrist extension (forearm fractures); arm extension (humeral fractures)	Back of the hand
Peroneal (lateral popliteal)	Dorsiflexion of foot	Middorsum of foot
Tibial (medial popliteal)	Plantar flexion of toes	Weight-bearing surface, bottom of foot

*Although the surface area supplied by a nerve and the amount of overlap with adjacent nerves varies from one individual to another, the *autonomous* zone is the most dependable area of sensory loss.

378

and epineurium are the connective tissues of the nerve and provide the strength and substance of the anastomosis (Fig. 34-1, *B*).

The neuronal cell body is the point of origin of the axon. The biochemical apparatus for repair resides in the central cell body, which, in motor nerves, is within the spinal cord and, in sensory nerves, in the dorsal root ganglion, just outside the cord (Fig. 34-1, *A*). If the central cell body is damaged directly, the mechanism for repair is also destroyed. If the axon is injured, the process of Wallerian degeneration is activated; the axoplasm distal to the injury disintegrates. Schwann cells phagocytize their own myelin, and transmitter materials decrease. In the cell body, deoxyribonucleic acid (DNA) is transformed to ribonucleic acid

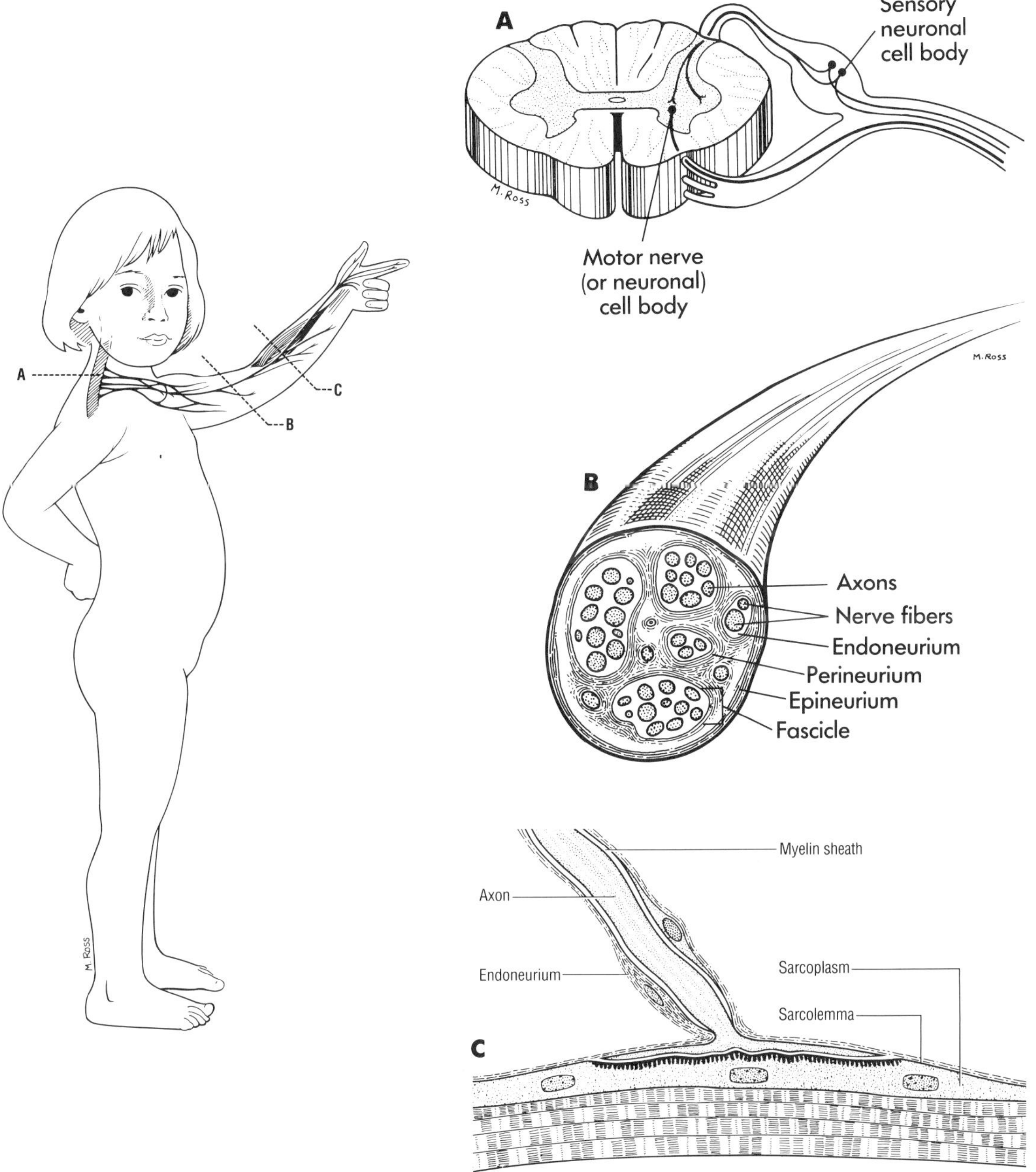

Figure 34–1 A, Cross section through cervical spinal cord. **B,** Cut section of nerve showing endoneurium surrounding several axons to form nerve fiber, several nerve fibers bound together by perineurium to form a fascicle, and fascicles interwoven by epineurium. **C,** Myoneural junction showing axonal endplate.

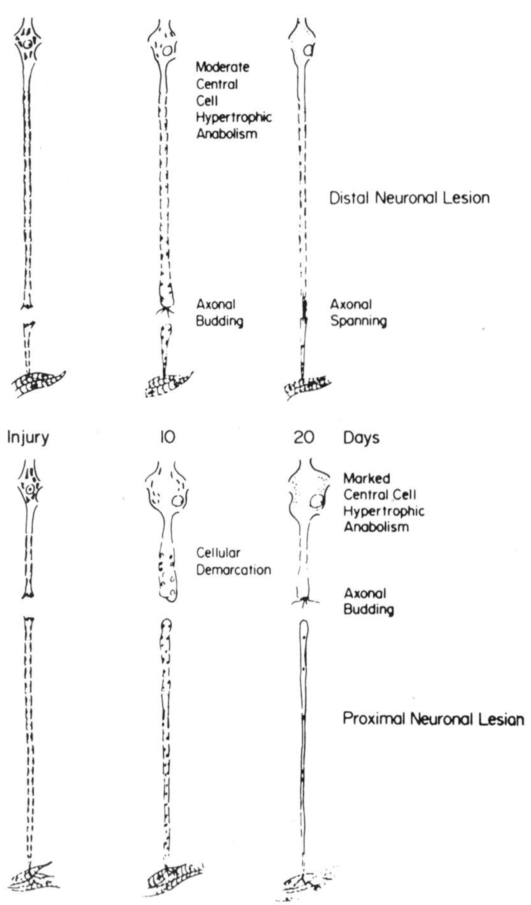

Figure 34–2 Timing of nerve repair. (From Ducker TJ: The metabolic background for peripheral nerve surgery, *Neurosurgery* 30:274, 1969.)

(RNA) to produce polypeptides for protein repair of the axoplasm. Denervated muscles release trophic factors to stimulate regeneration, but dead and necrotic tissues produce antitrophic substances that impair regeneration. Within 24 hours of the injury a "growth cone" 1 cm in length is produced at the proximal cut end (Fig. 34-2). After 7 days axonal sprouting begins a few millimeters proximal to the injury, and at 7 to 21 days axon buds advance across the injury site. Regeneration then proceeds down the lattice of intact axons at 1 mm/day or 1 inch/month.[4]

Within 48 hours of the injury the epithelial cells of the endoneurium, epineurium, and perineurium begin to proliferate connective tissue. If the nerve has been crushed or severed, the axon buds advance to the injury site and encounter a barricade of newly proliferated connective tissue. In a parallel process, denervated muscle cells begin to shrink and their connective tissue sheaths thicken. The regenerating

axon must reach the muscles that it innervates before the muscle sheath becomes too thick for endplate formation and reinnervation (Fig. 34-1, *C*).

Several simple axioms follow from this discussion of pathophysiology. If the nerve cell body is destroyed, no regeneration will occur. *If a nerve is avulsed from the spinal cord, no recovery will occur* unless an adjacent, functional nerve root is surgically transposed to the avulsed nerve. Moreover, *regeneration cannot proceed without axonal continuity* and a path along which the nerve can regenerate. Although these principles are elementary, their clinical interpretation is complex. *The quality of recovery from nerve injury depends on the competing forces of nerve regeneration and connective tissue proliferation.*

The complexity of peripheral nerve repair has been simplified by Seddon's classification of nerve injury: neuropraxia, axonotmesis, and neurotmesis.[16]

Neuropraxia describes the nerve that is temporarily dysfunctional but has suffered no permanent injury. Function usually recovers within 2 weeks.

In *axonotmesis* recovery of nerve function is possible. The biochemical apparatus is damaged and must be replaced, but the anatomic structure is left intact. The principal limitation to functional recovery is the time required for the regenerating nerve to reach the muscles it innervates. Connective tissue proliferation in denervated muscles proceeds apace as the regenerating nerve advances toward the muscle. If the distance is too great, the connective tissue surrounding the targeted muscles will be too thick for satisfactory endplate formation. Examples include compression damage caused by adjacent fractures and chemical injury caused by injection. The key clinical axiom is that *spontaneous repair is better than surgical repair* because the existing anatomic framework is better than any surgical match that could be made.

Neurotmesis characterizes the nerve injury in which anatomic continuity has been lost. If anastomosis of the nerve does not occur surgically, the nerve buds will not have an anatomic path to follow and the nerve fibers will become hopelessly entangled. The resulting neuroma has little or no connection to the distal segment. To complicate recovery even further, it may happen that only part of a nerve is disrupted and entangled in the neuroma. Although the neuroma may appear to be in continuity with the rest of the nerve, excision of the injured nerve is imperative. The cut ends of the nerve must be free of connective tissue and the severed fascicular bundles reapproximated for there to be any hope of successful repair. If the distance from the site of injury to the target muscles is too great, then the perimysium will be too thick for endplate formation when the regenerating nerve arrives. Neurotmesis may apply to only a portion of the nerve or, depending on the mechanism, irreparable injury may extend over a great length of the nerve. A crush or stretch injury to the nerve results in extensive axonal degeneration, as well as anatomical disruption of the nerve. Although the nerve may appear grossly intact, its internal structure has been disrupted, and no framework for regeneration exists. These *lesions in continuity* are the most difficult to assess and repair.[12] Without resecting the damaged nerve and inserting nerve graft, functional recovery will not occur. Timing is the key to successful management of all nerve injuries.

If a nerve is neuropraxic, repair is unnecessary; if the injury is axonotmetic, repair is meddlesome; but if the injury is neurotmetic, then functional recovery depends on expeditious repair. Delay in repair means continued connective tissue proliferation in the muscles to be innervated. The critical judgments are how long to wait for anticipated recovery and when to repair the nerve. Although surgical technique is beyond the scope of this chapter, the critical issue of timing will be discussed within the context of the clinical examination: neurologic examination, electrophysiologic studies, and intraoperative monitoring.

CLINICAL EXAMINATION
Neurologic examination

Injuries to the major peripheral nerves can be best diagnosed in children by studying spontaneous and voluntary movement. Sensory examination of the young child is often not reliable and may provoke anxiety and resistance to further examination (Table 34-1).

Injured nerves in the arm are the axillary, radial, medial, and ulnar nerves. The axillary nerve innervates the deltoid muscle and is responsible for abduction or winging of the arm. The radial nerve serves elbow extension and wrist extension. A "drop wrist" implies an injury to the radial nerve above the elbow. If the drop wrist is accompanied by an inability to push the examiner away (elbow extension), then the radial nerve has been damaged at the head of the humerus.

The median nerve provides pronation of the arm, flexion of the wrist, flexion of the fingers, and opposition of the thumb to the palm. The pathognomonic sign of median nerve injury is an inability to flex the index finger. A "benediction" hand is typical of median nerve injury (Fig. 34-3). When the arm is raised, the index finger cannot be flexed and the middle finger is only partially flexed, as a clergyman's hand in benediction.[9] In wrist injuries the benediction posture can be mim-

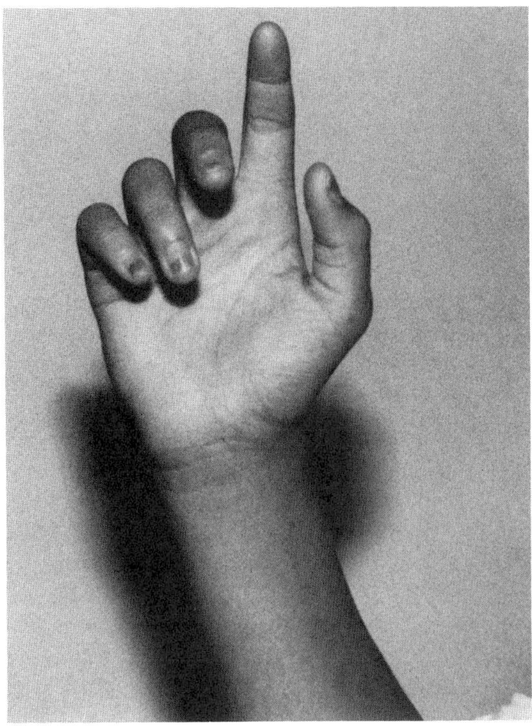

Figure 34–3 Benediction posture of median nerve injury.

icked by laceration of the deep flexors of the index finger. Injury of the median nerve at the wrist preserves arm pronation and finger flexion, although thumb opposition is absent.

The ulnar nerve allows fingers to be spread apart (abduction) and pressed together (adduction). The pathognomonic sign of an ulnar nerve injury is an inability to abduct the fifth digit. The hand eventually assumes the posture of a claw, which is produced by extension of the metacarpophalangeal joints and flexion of the interphalangeal joints. The clawed hand at rest resembles the hands of a piano player poised to begin play (Fig. 34-4). The ulnar nerve is also responsible for adduction of the thumb through innervation of the adductor pollicis. The function of thumb adduction can be substituted by the flexor pollicis longus, which is supplied by the median nerve. Adduction is necessary for holding a card between the thumb and the index finger. When the ulnar nerve is injured, the card is held by the pincer grasp of the flexor pollicis longus instead of the adductor pollicis (Foment's sign) (Fig. 34-5).[9]

In the lower extremities, the femoral nerve supplies the muscles of the anterior thigh and thus provides extension at the knee. Just above the knee, the sciatic nerve divides into the medial popliteal

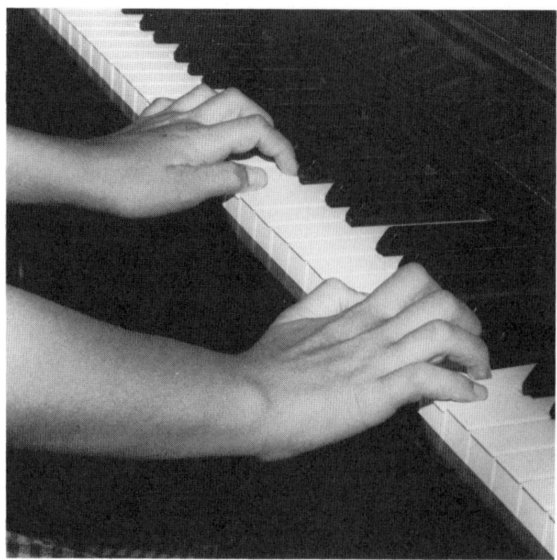

Figure 34–4 Piano player poised to begin play.

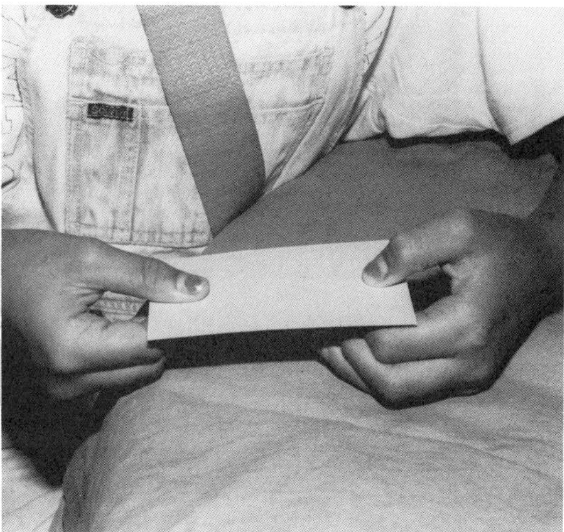

Figure 34–5 Foment's sign. Right hand pinching card in manner characteristic of ulnar nerve injury.

and the lateral popliteal nerves. The medial popliteal nerve, or tibial nerve, lies lateral to the popliteal artery and vein, supplies the posterior aspect of the leg, and is responsible for plantar flexion and internal rotation of the foot. The lateral popliteal nerve branches at the level of the head of the fibula into the anterior tibial nerve, which provides dorsiflexion of the ankle and extension of the great toe, and the musculocutaneous nerve, which targets external rotation of the foot.

Electrophysiologic studies

The neurologic examination is complemented by electrophysiologic tests.[2] Electrophysiologic changes of nerve recovery anticipate and precede physical signs of recovery. Electromyogram (EMG) and evoked responses to sensory and motor nerve stimulation provide information that confirms denervation in a target muscle and can be used to monitor reinnervation. Figures 34-6 to 34-8 illustrate the nerves in the front of the arm, back of the leg, and anterior thigh.

Conventional EMG derives information from the insertion of electrodes into the muscle (insertional activity), when the muscle is at rest with the electrodes in place (denervation potentials), and when the muscle is voluntarily contracted (volitional activity). Although EMG of the muscle at rest is feasible in children, too many artifacts are created by withdrawal movements to study insertional activity, and a frightened child does not always cooperate for volitional muscle studies. The denervated muscle at rest is characterized by fibrillations, (spontaneous discharges of single muscle fibers of short duration [0.5 to 3 msec] and of small amplitude [50 to 150 μV] and positive sharp waves (PSWs) (spontaneous potentials measuring 10 to 100 msec in duration and 50 μ to 1 mV in amplitude). Normal muscles do not have fibrillations or PSWs. They appear 10 to 14 days after the muscle has been denervated while Wallerian degeneration is taking place. Reinnervation is characterized by a decrease in fibrillation potentials, the appearance of nascent motor potentials (small amplitude, short duration potentials), polyphasic action potentials, and then normal action potentials.

A response can be evoked and measured from an intact nerve. For example, nerve conduction across a neuropraxic injury will be present despite the absence of clinical function. The nerve distal to an axonotmetic lesion may conduct for up to 24 hours, but by that time all axoplasmic flow has ceased. In the normal muscle, stimulation at the motor point (the anatomic point where the nerve enters the muscle) with direct current produces a visible twitch at threshold. As the current is increased above threshold, tetanus occurs. The tetanus-twitch current ratio in normal muscle is 3.5 to 6.5. In denervated muscle the ratio is 1. If the amount of current is graphed on semilog paper against the duration of stimulation, the amount of current of infinite duration required to evoke a minimal contraction can be determined. This value, reported in milliamperes, is known as *rheobase*. Most muscles are not excited by currents under 2.5 × rheobase. Rheobase is used to calculate chronaxie, which is a useful measure of denervation and reinnervation. Chronaxie is the duration of stimulation that will cause minimal contraction by a current 2 × rheobase. Each muscle has its own

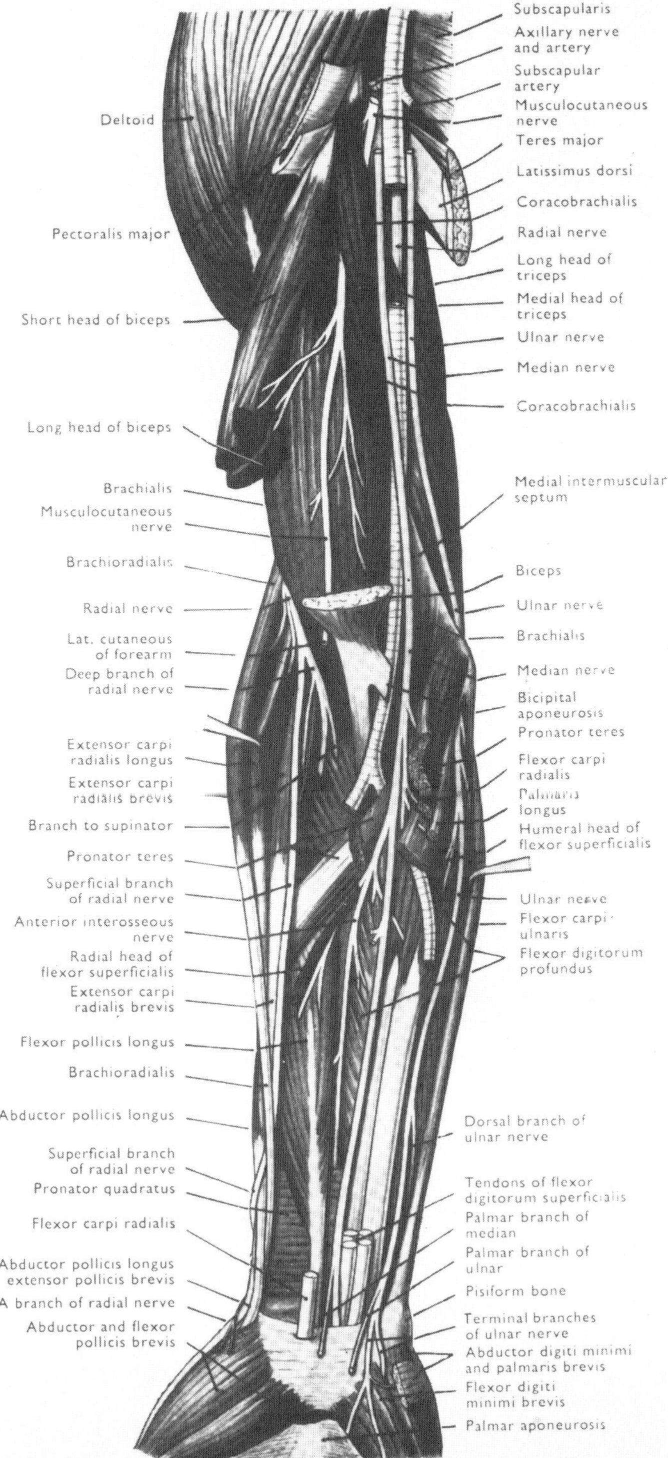

Figure 34–6 Nerves in front of arm. (From Romanes GJ, editor: *Cunningham's textbook of anatomy,* ed 10, New York, 1964, Oxford University Press, p 728, by permission of Oxford University Press.)

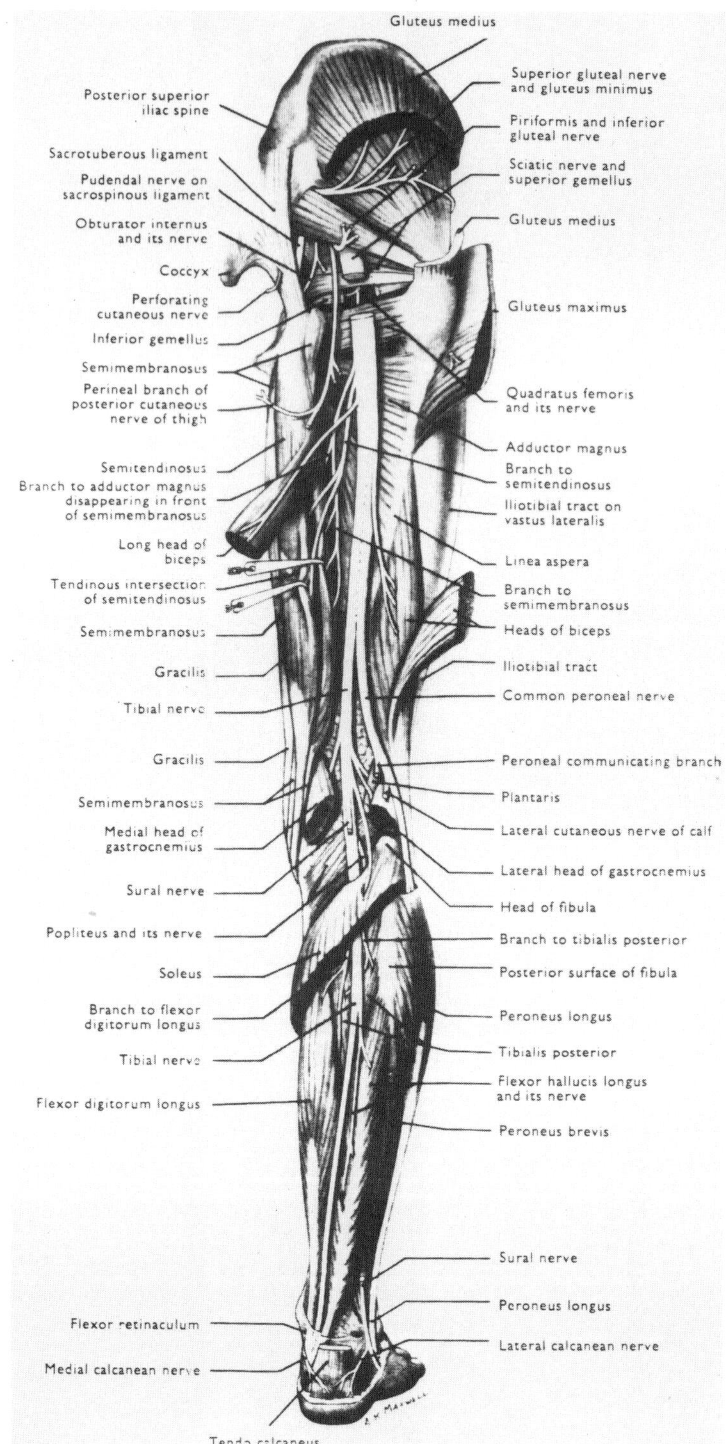

Figure 34–7 Nerves in back of leg. (From Romanes GJ, editor: *Cunningham's textbook of anatomy,* ed 10, New York, 1964, Oxford University Press, p 750, by permission of Oxford University Press.)

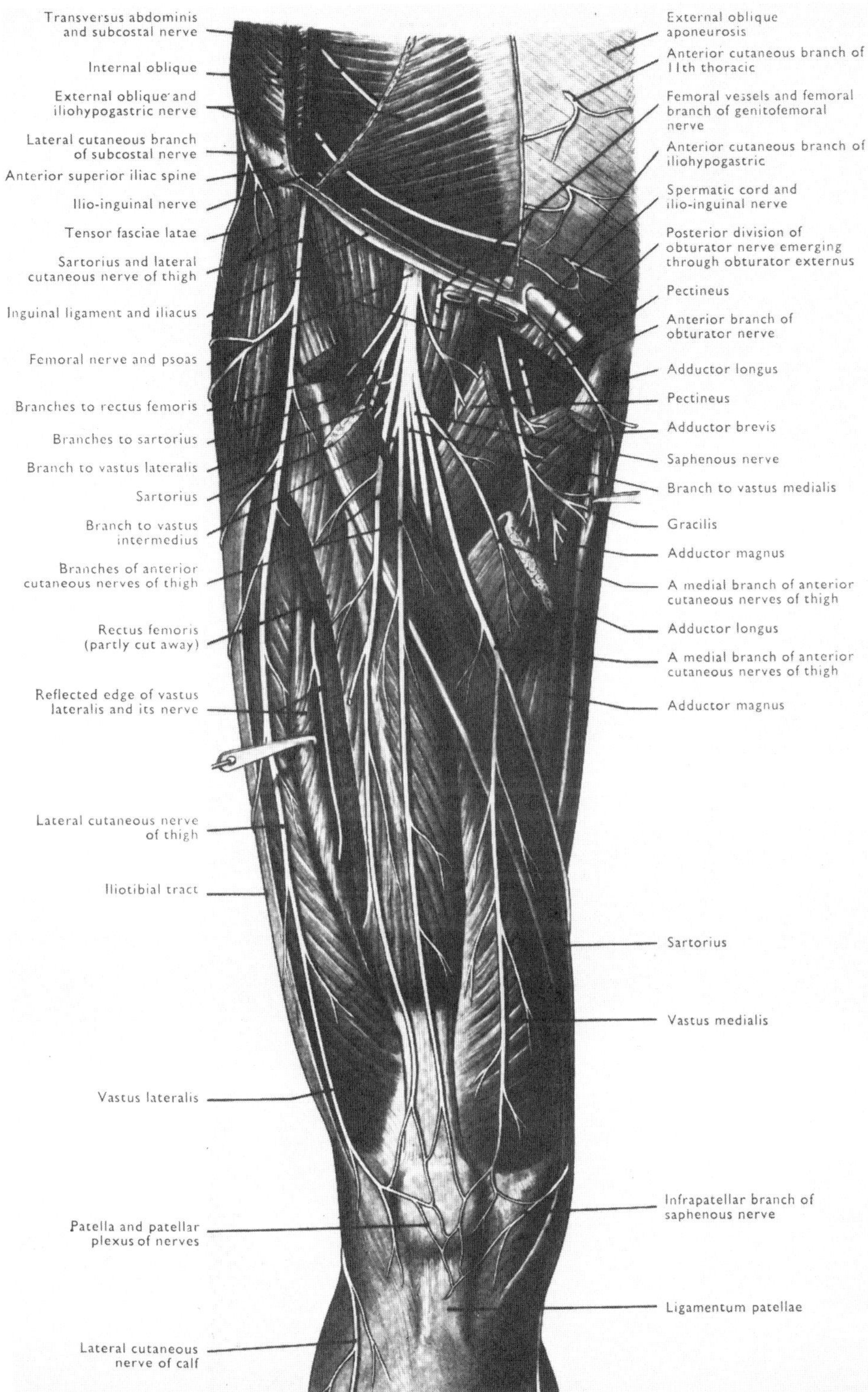

Figure 34–8 Nerves in anterior thigh. (From Romanes GJ, editor: *Cunningham's textbook of anatomy,* ed 10, New York, 1964, Oxford University Press, p 750, by permission of Oxford University Press.)

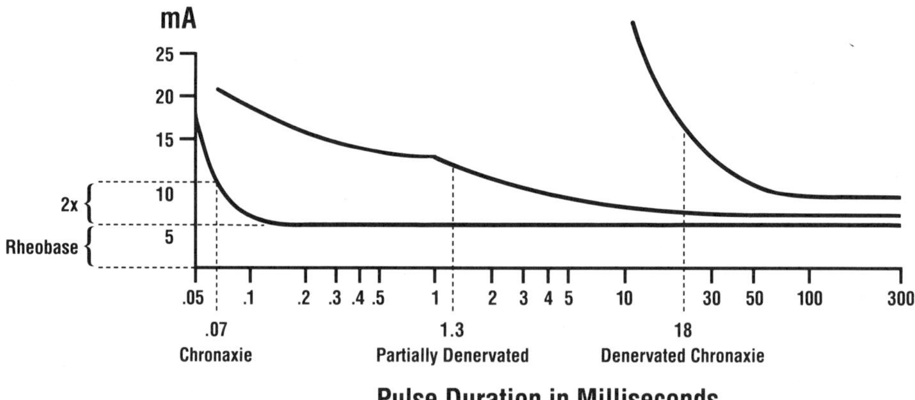

Pulse Duration in Milliseconds

Figure 34–9 Strength-duration curves showing chronaxie of normal muscle *(left)* and denervated muscle *(right)*.

chronaxie. A chronaxie of less than 1 msec is probably normal, and a value of 18 msec indicates complete denervation. The strength-duration curve is far to the right in the denervated muscle and moves to the left with reinnervation (Fig. 34-9).

At 10 to 14 days after injury, the normal brisk twitch of direct current stimulation at the motor point is replaced by a slow vermicular (wormlike) response. Stimulation of a muscle at the motor point with alternating current, as contrasted with direct current, normally produces a tonic contraction. About a week after denervation, the response to alternating current disappears.

Evoked sensory responses can be helpful in localizing an injury and in predicting recovery of the mixed nerve (a nerve with both sensory and motor fibers).[11] Normal sensory-evoked responses (SERs) in a child without sensibility indicates that the sensory pathways to the spinal cord are intact, and recovery can be anticipated. Absence of SER implies interruption of the sensory pathway, whether it be preganglionic (central to the dorsal root ganglion) or postganglionic (peripheral to the ganglion). For example, fibrillations and PSWs in the cervical erector spinae muscles indicate involvement of the roots or, more precisely, the nerves prior to exit of the posterior ramus nerves that supply the erector spinae muscles, as when the roots are avulsed from the cord. An absence of fibrillations or PSWs in the paraspinal musculature indicates that the injury is distal to take-off of the posterior ramus and is more characteristic of nerve root rupture.

SPECIAL MECHANISMS OF NERVE INJURY
Brachial plexus injury or obstetrical palsy

In the first decade of life, brachial plexus injuries are seen almost exclusively as a result of obstetrical delivery. In older children and adolescents they are most commonly caused by gunshot wounds and motorcycle crashes.

Obstetrical paralysis, which is a brachial plexus injury associated with delivery of an infant, occurs in less than 1 in 1000 live births. Shoulder dystocia, high birth weight, and a breech presentation are major risk factors (Fig. 34-10). Upper brachial plexus injuries are much more common than lower plexus injuries. Injury occurs after the head has emerged from the birth canal and is being used to deliver the rest of the infant. The upper elements of the plexus are stretched and injured when the head presents and is used to distract the impacted shoulders or when the arms are used to extract the after-coming head (breech delivery). If the arms remain abducted over the after-coming head, the lower brachial plexus is stretched more than the upper.

The spinal nerves C6, C7, and C8 are the principal input to the plexus. A variable contribution is also made by the C5 and T1 nerve roots.[17] If C5 makes a substantial contribution to the plexus, the contribution from T1 is minor. The upper trunk then makes up more than one half of the posterior cord, and the lateral cord does not receive a contribution from C8. Conversely, if a more substantial contribution is made from T1, the input from C5 is limited. The lower trunk will dominate the posterior cord and C8 will contribute to the lateral cord. Upper brachial plexus injury or Erb's palsy is usually associated with *rupture* of the C4, C5, and C6 nerve roots, whereas lower brachial plexus injury or Klumpke's paralysis is due to *avulsion* of the C7 and C8 nerve roots from the spinal cord.

Although their patterns of innervation overlap and intertwine, C6 is basically responsible for the shoulder, C7 the arm, and C8 the hand. To provide their pattern of innervation, the roots join to form

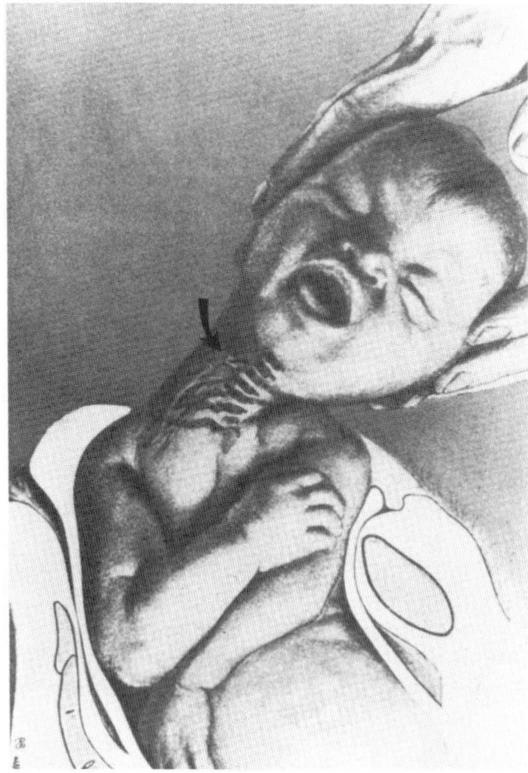

Figure 34–10 The mechanism of obstetrical palsy associated with shoulder dystocia. The *arrow* indicates ruptured roots in the upper brachial plexus. (From Brown KLB: Review of obstetrical palsies. Nonoperative treatment, *Clin Plast Surg* 11:182, 1984.)

trunks in the supraclavicular region of the neck. The trunks divide into divisions, which in turn divide and rearrange themselves into cords below the clavicle. Divisions of the cords are then regrouped in the axilla of the arm to form the major nerves of the arm. The number of fascicles increases, and their pattern becomes more complex in passage from roots to trunks to cords to peripheral nerves. The spinal nerves or roots are monofascicular; their cross section consists of one large fascicle surrounded by perineurium and epifascicular epineurium. The divisions of the upper trunk and the posterior division of the lower trunk are monofascicular and bifascicular, respectively. The origin of the suprascapular nerve and the musculocutaneous nerve are also monofascicular. The remaining components of the brachial plexus are polyfascicular. Moreover, fascicles branch or merge as often as every 5 mm.[18] The ability to approximate fascicles is critical to achieving a successful nerve repair and is most easily done at the level of roots and trunks.

Electrical and burn injuries

The nervous and vascular systems are paths of least resistance to electrical shock from lightning or a high-voltage line. The neurovascular bundle undergoes both ischemic and coagulative necrosis. Devastating injury also occurs to the muscles supplied by the neurovascular bundle. Because the injured muscles release antitrophic substances that inhibit regeneration and long spans of nerve are destroyed, the prospects for repair and recovery are poor.

Injection injuries

The nerves most commonly injured by direct injection are the sciatic nerve in the buttock and the radial nerve in the upper arm, but drug abuse and nursing error can also cause injury to the median, ulnar, and lateral femoral cutaneous nerves. The needle itself causes little damage, and if only saline is injected, no injury occurs. The severity of the injury correlates with the toxicity of the substance injected, and the injection must be intrafascicular, not simply near the nerve. Dexamethasone causes the least injury. Benzylpenicillin, diazepam, tetanus toxoid, triamcinolone, hexacetonide, dimenhydrinate, hydrocortisone, procaine hydrochloride, and tetracaine hydrochloride cause the most severe injuries. Gentamycin, cephalothin, chloramphenicol, triamcinolone acetonide, methylprednisolone, and lidocaine hydrochloride (with or without epinephrine) produce intermediate injuries.[10] Fortunately, in modern pediatric practice the buttock is almost never used for injection (the vastus lateralis muscle of the upper thigh is preferred).

PRINCIPLES OF TREATMENT

Treatment is dictated by anatomic continuity, supervised by electrophysiologic monitoring, directed by the pathophysiologic principles of repair, and produced by appropriate timing.

The ideal nerve repair joins together the nerve ends and matches the internal fascicular pattern of the nerve. Because the fascicular pattern can change dramatically along a given centimeter of the nerve, anastomosis of a nerve after a segment of damaged nerve is excised may not result in proper fascicular alignment. If long segments of the nerve are damaged, anatomic approximation becomes even more problematic. Although perineurial fascicle-to-fascicle anastomosis is theoretically sound, no practical difference has been found between epineurial nerve-to-nerve and perineurial fascicle-to-fascicle suture[5,13] (Fig. 34-11). Because no surgical nerve repair can perfectly line up each nerve fiber within each fascicle, the repaired nerve will always function less well than the original anatomically intact nerve.

Spontaneous regeneration associated with axonotmesis is far better than nerve suture. Neuropraxic or axonotmetic injuries can be identified early by frequent neurologic examination and elec-

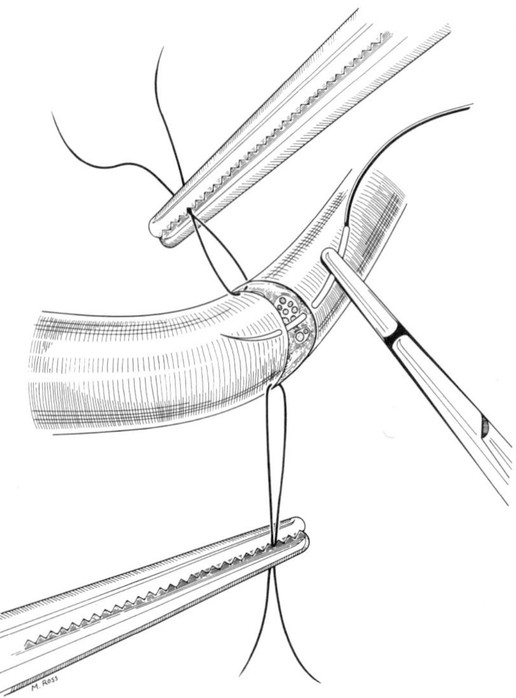

Figure 34–11 Reapproximation of cut nerve ends with epineurial suture.

trophysiologic monitoring of the target muscle or of the first muscle to be reinnervated (Tables 34-2 and 34-3). Tinel's sign (an electrical sensation along the distribution of the nerve caused by percussing the injury site) is of no value unless it advances on sequential examinations along the course of the regenerating nerve. If no evidence of regeneration is apparent in 6 weeks, nerve exploration should be considered. A surgical anastomosis of the median nerve at the elbow that is delayed 3 months will not deliver useful motor function to the hand. If the total time to reinnervation, whether axonotmetic regeneration or diagnostic delay plus regeneration after repair, exceeds 1 year, the function of the muscle will be poor. For regeneration times of 2 years or more there is no hope for motor return, but sensation in the hand or on the plantar aspect of the foot is a laudable goal. The exceptions to these general rules include lacerations, brachial plexus injuries, burns and electrical injuries, and injection.

Obvious lacerations should be urgently explored and the nerve ends tagged with small 7-0 stainless steel wire sutures so that they can be identified by radiography and easily found at the time of delayed repair. Because of contusion to the cut ends of the nerve, which inevitably accompanies nerve lacer-

ation, repair is best delayed 1 or 2 weeks to allow the contusion to mature and the irreversibly damaged ends to demarcate. If opposing sutures are placed in the epineurium of the cut ends of the nerve as it lies in anatomic position, correct alignment of the fascicular bundle at the time of delayed repair is more likely. At the time of secondary repair, the nerve ends are trimmed of necrotic tissue and excess connective tissue. A sharp "tendon cutter" shaves the nerve back until well-defined fascicles can be seen on frozen section.

For brachial plexus injuries, timing is particularly important because of the long distance over which the nerve must regenerate to reach the muscles that it innervates, especially the muscles of the hand. In older children, hand function after plexus repair should not be anticipated. In contrast, hand function can be expected after surgical repair in *infants* with obstetrical palsy. The first priority in treatment of children is to stabilize the shoulder by repairing the nerve to the supraspinatus muscle. The second priority is innervation of the biceps so that the hand can be brought to the mouth and, finally, reinnervation of the median nerve for sensation to the hand in anticipation of reconstruction of the hand and arm to achieve useful function. In both total obstetrical paralysis and lower plexus injuries, the C8 and T1 roots of the plexus are usually avulsed from the spinal cord and give no hope of regeneration because the nerve cell bodies are destroyed. The upper roots of the plexus are usually not avulsed but ruptured, and repairs can be made to preserve the supraspinatus nerve or anastomosis performed to the distal portions of lower avulsed nerves to provide innervation to the entire arm. *If biceps function is not recovered by 3 months, the final unrepaired functional result will be poor.*[7] If a repair is attempted 9 or more months after the birth injury, the result will be equally poor. However, repairs in a child between 3 and 6 months of age can result in useful hand function. In a typical case of total obstetrical paralysis of the arm and hand, avulsions of C8 and T1 are confirmed by evoked potentials. Because the upper paraspinal musculature is not denervated, C5, C6 and C7 have not been avulsed and their ruptured ends are found at surgical exploration to be bound into a neuroma in continuity. Rupture is confirmed by stimulation across the neuroma with nerve action potentials. The proximal stumps of C5, C6, and C7 are dissected free of the neuroma and used to "neurotize" or reinnervate the three trunks of the plexus, as well as the suprascapular nerve. The gaps between the stumps and the trunks are bridged with cable grafts taken from the sural nerve.

Electrical or burn injuries are debrided aggres-

Table 34–2 Recovery targeting in arm

Nerve	Mechanism	Injury site	Target muscle
Median	Fractures	Upper arm	Pronator teres
		Proximal forearm	Flexor pollicis longus
		Middle third of forearm	Pronator quadratus
		Distal forearm	Abductor pollicis brevis and opponens pollicis
Radial	Neurofibromatosis*; often associated vessel injury; crutch palsy	Proximal to triceps branch	Triceps
	Humeral fracture	Midhumerus	Brachioradialis (nerve arises 3 in below midhumerus) and extensor carpi radialis (wrist extension)
	Humeral fracture	Distal third of humerus	Extensor digitorum longus
	Radial head fracture, gunshot wound	Proximal forearm (posterior interosseus)	Abductor pollicis longus and extensor pollicis longus
Ulnar		Axilla to elbow	Flexor carpi ulnaris (motor point is 1 in proximal to elbow)
		Proximal forearm	Flexor digitorum profundi, little finger
		Midforearm to wrist	Abductor digitorum quiniti and opponens digiti quiniti
	Entrapment in Guyon's canal; glass or knife wound, often with ulnar artery bleeding	Below wrist	First dorsal and palmar interossei; adductor pollicis

sively, and cut nerve ends marked with steel sutures. Secondary ischemia is heralded by pain, and continuing nerve damage produced by ischemia is prevented by fasciotomy and by releasing any circumferential eschars. Elevation of the extremity and fluid resuscitation are added to the list of supportive measures.

Injection injuries are almost always axonotmetic, and a full 3 months should lapse before the nerve is explored. Immediate exploration to open the nerve longitudinally and flush out the toxic substances is not worthwhile.[6]

REHABILITATION

Rehabilitation begins within days of the injury to prevent contractures and to maintain range of motion while the nerve recovers. Although electrical stimulation maintains muscle bulk, connective tissue proliferation continues at the myoneural junction and is the principal stumbling block to reinnervation, especially when distance is great and regeneration time is prolonged. Occupational therapy can provide sensory reeducation once touch has returned in the distribution of the injured nerve, especially if recovery is incomplete.[3] Thumb sensibility can be achieved by transplanting existing areas of full sensibility on a neurovascular pedicle, for example, the ulnar-innervated lateral aspect of ring finger or the dorsal surface of the middle finger, which is innervated by the superficial radial nerve. Sensory pads can also be transferred from the toes to the fingers.

Table 34–3 Muscle targeting in leg

Nerve	Mechanism	Site of injury	Target muscle
Ilioinguinal	Hernia surgery	Superficial inguinal ring	None (sensation over symphysis pubis and dorsum penis)
Femoral	Gunshot wound, neuro-fibromatosis	Above inguinal ligament	Iliopsoas
	Knife; gunshot wound; glass	Below ligament	Quadriceps femoris
Obturator	Pelvic fracture	Within pelvis	Adductor magnus
Pudendal	Gunshot wound	Within pelvis	External sphincter anus and bladder
Sciatic	Dislocation of hip; injection injury	Above gluteal crease	Gastrocnemius; medial hamstrings*
Peroneal	Fracture and dislocation, knee	Popliteal fossa	Tibialis anterior and extensor hallucis longus
	Fracture of fibula while skiing	Head fibula	Evertors ankle and foot
Tibial	Dislocation of knee	Below knee	Tibialis posterior; flexor digitorum longus
	Neurofibromatosis; ankle fracture; tendon transfer	At the ankle	Toe spreading and curling

*Nerve to hamstring muscles is medial and usually not injured in hip dislocation and injection injuries.

Tendon transfers should be considered when there is no hope for recovery of innervation. If no function returns to the shoulder after 1 year, or below the elbow after 2 years, tendon transfers are in order.

OUTCOME

The majority of blunt nerve injuries are neuropraxic and recover without surgical intervention. Axonotmetic injuries recover if the distance from the injury to the motor point of the paralyzed muscle is less than 18 inches. For example, the chance for recovery of hand function in axonotmetic injuries of the ulnar and median nerves in the upper arm is poor, but the prognosis for recovery of these same nerves in the forearm or wrist is good. Axonotmetic injuries to the peroneal nerve at the fibular head do well.

Recovery of neurontmetic injuries depends not only on regeneration distance and time but also on the fascicular complexity of the nerve. Mixed nerves, such as the peroneal nerve, consist of multiple motor and sensory fascicles twisted in a complex cable. Recovery after repair of this nerve is generally poor because too few fibers find their way to the motor point. Burns and electrical injuries have the poorest chance of spontaneous recovery because long segments of the nerves must be replaced with cable grafts; moreover, the muscles are invariably damaged as well.

Monofascicular nerves, which are composed of a single fascicle, are more amenable to repair, although distance may compromise the ultimate functional result. The radial nerve, for example, is predominantly a motor nerve and largely monofascicular; functional repairs are commonplace even in the upper arm.

The ulnar nerve at the medial humeral epicondyle, the radial nerve in the spiral groove, the axillary nerve in the axilla, the C5, C6, C8, and T1 spinal nerves, the suprascapular and musculocutaneous nerves at their origins, and the upper trunk of the brachial plexus and its divisions are all monofascicular and more amenable to repair.

More than 80% of children with obstetric palsies also recover completely, although the figure from the collaborative perinatal study is higher (95%)[8] the figure from series in rehabilitation units is lower (6% to 13%).[5] All arms that are destined to recover completely show improvement in 1 to 2 weeks, and functional recovery in 1 month. Horner's syndrome, total paralysis, and lower plexus injuries have poor prognoses for spontaneous, nonsurgical recovery. Despite avulsion of the involved nerve roots, hand function can be achieved with well-timed surgical repairs.[14]

REFERENCES

1. Brown KLB: Review of obstetrical palsies: nonoperative treatment. In Terzis JL, editors: *Microreconstruction of nerve injuries*, Philadelphia, 1987, WB Saunders, pp 499-511.
2. Delagi EF: Electrodiagnosis in peripheral nerve lesions. In Omer GE, Spinner M, editors: *Management of peripheral nerve problems*, Philadelphia, 1980, WB Saunders, pp 30-43.
3. Dellon AL: Functional sensation and its re-education. In Terzis JL, editor: *Microreconstruction of nerve injuries*, Philadelphia, 1987, WB Saunders, pp 181-190.
4. Ducker TB: Pathophysiology of peripheral nerve trauma. In Wilkins RH, Rengachary SS, editors: *Neurosurgery*, New York, 1985, McGraw-Hill, pp 1812-1816.
5. Eng GD, Koch B, Smokvina MD: Brachial plexus palsy in neonates and children, *Arch Phys Med Rehabil* 59:458-464, 1978.
6. Gentili F, Hudson AR, Kline DG, et al: Early changes following injection injury of peripheral nerves, *Can J Surg* 23:177-182, 1980.
7. Gilbert A, Tassin JL: Reparation chirurgicale du plexus brachial dans la paralysie obstetricale, *Chirurgie* 110:70-75, 1984.
8. Gordon M, Rich H, Deutschberger J et al: The immediate and long-term outcome of obstetric birth trauma. I. Brachial plexus paralysis, *Am J Obstet Gynecol* 117:51-56, 1973.
9. Haymaker W, Woodhall B: *Peripheral nerve injuries*, ed 2, Philadelphia, 1953, WB Saunders.
10. Hudson AR: Nerve injection injuries. In Terzis JK, editor: *Microreconstruction of nerve injuries*, Philadelphia, 1987, WB Saunders, pp 173-179.
11. Jones SJ: Diagnostic value of peripheral and spinal somatosensory evoked potentials in traction lesions of the brachial plexus. In Terzis JK, editor: *Microreconstruction of nerve injuries*, Philadelphia, 1987, WB Saunders, pp 463-471.
12. Kline DG, Hackett ER: Management of the neuroma in continuity. In Wilkins RH, Rengachary SS, editors: *Neurosurgery*, New York, 1985, McGraw-Hill, pp 1864-1871.
13. Kline DG, Hudson AR, Bratton BR: Experimental study of fascicular nerve repair with and without epineurial closure, *J Neurosurg* 54:513-520, 1981.
14. Laurent JP, Shenaq S, Lee R et al: Upper brachial plexus birth injuries: a neurosurgical approach, *Concepts Pediatr Neurosurg* 10:156-178, 1990.
15. Orgel MG, Terzis JK: Epineurial vs perineurial repair: an ultrastructural and electrophysiologic study of nerve regeneration, *Plast Reconstr Surg*, 60:80-91, 1977.
16. Seddon HJ: *Surgical disorders of the peripheral nerves*. Edinburgh, 1972, Churchill Livingstone.
17. Slingluff CL, Terzis JK, Edgerton MT: The quantitative microanatomy of the brachial plexus in man: reconstructive relevance. In Terzis JK, editor: *Microreconstruction of nerve injuries*, Philadelphia, 1987, WB Saunders, pp 285-324.
18. Sunderland S: *Nerves and nerve injuries*. Edinburgh, 1972, Churchill-Livingstone.

PART SEVEN

Maxillofacial Injury

35 Maxillofacial Injury

Michael J. Boyajian

Facial injury involves superficial abrasions, lacerations, and multiple fractures of the facial bone. The pediatric facial skeleton is lighter, has less pneumatization, and is more protected than its adult counterpart. It is therefore no surprise that only 10% of maxillofacial injuries occur in the younger age groups. Facial lacerations, in contrast, are quite common in children. This chapter deals with the special aspects of soft tissue and skeletal injuries in children. Restoration of function and of appearance is essential to outcome.

MECHANISM OF INJURY: GENERAL

The etiology of facial trauma in children varies from that in adults. The two most common causes are motor vehicle crashes and falls. Collision with a playmate or blunt object, such as a baseball bat or a rock, results in injury. Laceration results from blunt or sharp penetrating trauma. Laceration caused by blunt trauma results when a shear stress exceeds the elasticity of the skin. Penetrating trauma frequently takes the form of laceration from windshield glass and animal or human bites. Birth trauma can also result in a variety of facial injury, although it is usually mild.

The frequency of facial fracture in children is 1.4% to 10% of the frequency in adults. Considerable force is necessary to generate such injury in children because (1) the facial skeleton of a child is relatively elastic as a consequence of incomplete calcification and incomplete suture closure, (2) the cranium is large as compared wtih the face and provides a protective canopy, (3) the facial skeleton is not as weakened by the development of air-filled sinuses as an adult's, and (4) the neck of the condyle of the mandible resists fracture because it is short and thick.

CLINICAL ASSESSMENT OF INJURY: GENERAL

The natural orifices for respiration are in the face, and they are at risk for obstruction caused by direct collapse, blood, soft tissue swelling, and loss of anterior tongue support. The generous vascularity of the face predisposes the child to profuse hemorrhage, even from relatively small wounds. A history of the extent of blood loss at an injury scene is useful, although it is often either exaggerated or underestimated. A relatively small blood loss, however, can result in shock in a child.

The frequency of associated injuries with significant maxillofacial fracture exceeds 50%. These are often more critical than the obvious facial injury. Cervical spine injury can result from any force sufficient to cause maxillofacial injury. During evaluation of the child for maxillofacial fracture, always consider the presence of a cervical spine injury.

Laryngeal injury results from blunt trauma to the neck during hyperextension of the head, which fixes the trachea against the spine. Suspect this injury whenever there is an anterior cervical contusion, a change (usually lowering) in the voice pitch, subcutaneous emphysema, or loss of thyroid cartilage prominence. Emergency laryngoscopy defines the injury, guides temporary orotracheal intubation, and reveals the need for surgical exploration.

IMMEDIATE MANAGEMENT OF MAXILLOFACIAL INJURY

The priorities for treatment are preservation of an adequate airway, establishment of the mechanics of respiration, and control of hemorrhage. Definitive treatment of facial fracture or laceration is seldom an emergency.

Airway

Blood clot, vomitus, or tooth displacement into the nose, mouth, or pharynx compromises the airway if unrecognized; removal by manual extraction or by suction is essential. The prone position is very useful, if moving the child will not compromise the cervical spine. Soft tissue swelling can obstruct the airway, usually in the presence of significant fracture.

Mandibular fracture with displacement of the tongue, particularly in an obtunded child, also causes airway obstruction. Forward traction of the tongue or mandible helps to open the airway; a towel clip, gauze pad, or hemostat may facilitate tongue manipulation. Endotracheal intubation stabilizes the airway; however, this procedure should be avoided in the presence of laryngeal fracture. In addition, nasotracheal or nasogastric tube placement should be delayed in the presence of a midface fracture because it can result in cribriform plate injury. Half of all children with fracture of the midface require tracheostomy. It is preferable to perform elective tracheostomy as part of the initial treatment.

Hemorrhage

Bleeding from an injury to the face may be substantial. Direct pressure to an open wound is an effective means of hemostasis. Occassionally, insertion of an anterior or posterior nasal pack is necessary to control bleeding from the nasopharynx. Topical agents, such as 0.4% cocaine or 0.5% Neo-synephrine, can produce vasoconstriction of superficial vessels.

Major uncontrolled hemorrhage from a midface injury requires emergency fracture reduction or external carotid artery ligation. Shock, as the result of isolated facial fracture, is unusual; if present, evaluate the child for concomitant intraabdominal or intrathoracic trauma.

Clinical examination

The clinical examination of facial injuries is the keystone of the evaluation and more important than a radiographic study. Wound inspection without exploration precedes definitive treatment. During an orderly assessment, consider the size and character of the wound, including the possible damage to underlying structures, such as the skeleton, branches of the facial nerve, parotid gland, and nasolacrimal apparatus. Facial asymmetry and muscle weakness are important observations; contour defect, contusion, or edema heralds deep or skeletal injury. Palpation and intraoral examination provide further information about structural injury.

The bony surface of the forehead is a good place to begin confirmation of the integrity of the superior orbital rim. A single finger is used to palpate the lateral and inferior orbital rim for a step deformity of focal tenderness. Palpate the nasal bone for irregularity, depression, or tenderness. Also evaluate the symmetry of the bilateral malar prominences, the smoothness of the anterior maxillary, and the integrity of the midface. Intraoral examination includes inspection of the teeth, evaluation of occlusion, palpation of the mandible and maxilla, and observation of any intraoral mucosal ecchymosis, which is highly suggestive of fracture. An eye examination is an essential part of the evaluation and should include a test of visual acuity.

The occipitomental (Waters's) view is the most useful single radiographic screening study in eval-uation of the maxilla, zygomata, and frontal sinuses. Specific radiologic evaluation depends on clinical indications such as local tenderness, instability, edema, contour defects, and mucosal ecchymosis.

CLINICAL DIAGNOSIS: SPECIFIC INJURY
Nasal fracture

Fracture of the nasal bones is the most common facial fracture in children. Ecchymosis, swelling on the dorsum of the nose, and palpation of bony irregularity or asymmetry after direct trauma are diagnostic. Swelling may interfere with the examination if it is not detected immediately after the injury. An intranasal examination is essential to determine the presence of a septal hematoma or dislocation. Radiographic studies of the nasal bones usually reveal the fracture, but clinical assessment is more important for diagnosis and management.

Mandibular fracture

The prominence of the lower jaw accounts for the frequency of its fracture, which is second only to that of the nose. More than half of all mandibular fractures are multiple fractures because of the jaw's closed-loop arrangement. Common patterns of fracture combination include (1) the cuspid (canine tooth) area and the opposite mandibular angle in the area of the third molar, (2) the cuspid area and opposite condyle, (3) the symphysis and opposite angle, and (4) the symphysis and one or both condyles. Whenever one fracture site is known, familiarity with these patterns helps to identify a second site. The hallmark of a mandibular fracture is malalignment of the teeth. There is almost always local pain and usually a contusion or laceration over the fracture; often the fracture penetrates the oral mucosa. Ecchymosis in the floor of the mouth is nearly pathognomonic of mandibular fracture, implying a tear in the periosteum above and below the mylohyoid insertion. Placement of the small finger in the child's ear permits palpation of condylar movement of the jaw; absence of this finding suggests fracture or dislocation of the condyle.

The appropriate x-ray views for suspected mandibular fracture are oblique, lateral, and posterioanterior mandible and Townes' view; the best single study is a panorex.

Zygomatic complex fracture

The common term "tripod fracture" is a misnomer. The zygoma articulates not only with the frontal, maxillary, and temporal bones but also with the greater wing of the sphenoid bone and with the palatine bone. The zygoma forms at the lateral rim and much of the inferior rim of the orbit and serves as the attachment of the lateral canthus. The tem-

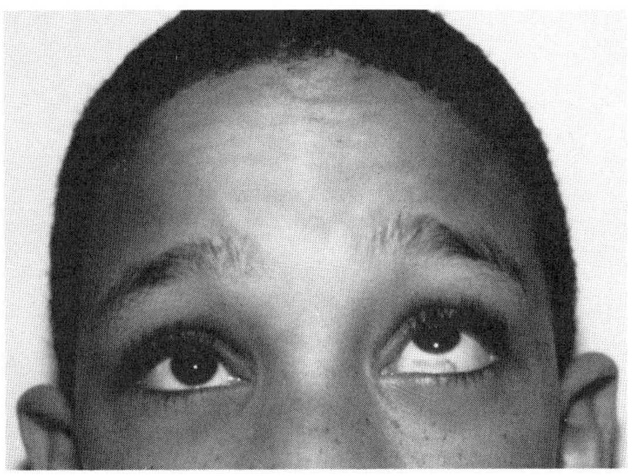

Figure 35–1 Entrapment due to blowout fracture.

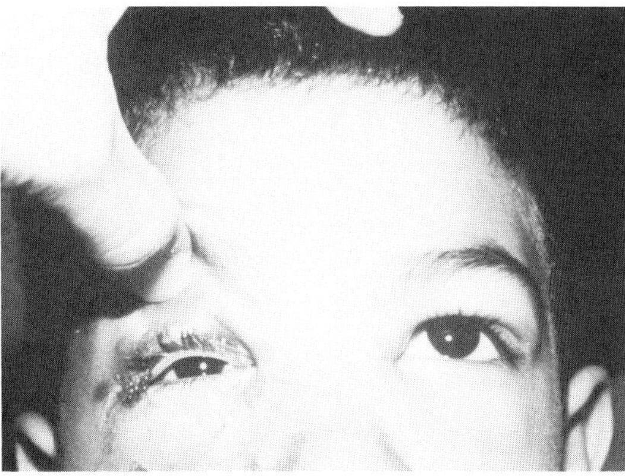

Figure 35–2 Enophthalmus due to zygomatic complex fracture.

poralis muscle and the coronoid process of the mandible are deep to the zygoma. The hallmark of zygomatic fracture is flatness of the malar prominence, best viewed from above. Displacement of the fracture inhibits movement of the coronoid process, causing limitation of mandibular excursion, which is a diagnostic sign. Other common signs include anesthesia of the lateral upper lip and teeth and of the distribution of the intraorbital nerve, unilateral nosebleed, and palpable step deformity with tenderness at the inferior or lateral orbital rim.

Ocular and periorbital signs, including periorbital ecchymosis and empyema, subconjunctival hemorrhage, and canting of the palpebral fissure (tilting of the lid opening) may be prominent; these suggest zygomatic fracture. A classic finding is diplopia on upward and downward outward gaze. Entrapment of the periorbital tissue within the fracture of the orbital floor limits the excursion of the inferior oblique and inferior rectus muscles (Fig. 35-1). Direct ophthalmologic inspection is necessary to define hyphema, blood in the anterior chamber of the eye. A test of visual acuity and an ophthalmology consultation are essential.

The appropriate x-ray views for suspected fracture of the zygoma are the submental-vertex and the Waters views. It is important to assess for asymmetry of the orbital inlet and the maxillary sinus and for displacement of the zygoma of the frontozygomatic suture or inferior orbital rim.

Blow-out fracture of the orbital floor

An orbital floor fracture is a common component of the zygomatic complex fracture, but may be an isolated injury. In this form it is usually the result of blunt trauma to the eye that causes an acute increase in intraorbital pressure and a fracture in the very thin floor or, less frequently, in the medial wall of the orbit. Indicative of this injury are diplopia, downward displacement of the globe or enophthalmus, and retrodisplacement of the globe (Fig. 35-2). The ocular and periorbital signs discussed previously characterize this fracture. An x-ray film (Waters view) and a computed tomography (CT) scan are appropriate radiographic studies. Upon examination, the floor appears fragmented, and soft tissue herniation into the partially blood-filled maxillary sinus creates the appearance of a "tear drop."

Midface fracture

Fractures of the middle third of the face, which are the result of a distortion force to the maxillae, naso-orbital complex, and zygomata, follow the classic patterns described by LeFort (Fig. 35-3).

The Lefort I fracture is a displacement, often of a single fragment, of the maxilla at the level of the nasal floor. The Lefort II (or pyramidal) fracture fragment includes, in addition to the maxilla, the nasal bones, medial orbits, and maxillary antra. The Lefort III fracture, or craniofacial disjunction, is the LeFort II fragmentation including the zygomata. Associated problems, especially with the LeFort III fracture, are airway compromise, intracranial injury, cerebrospinal fluid leak, and loss of ocular support. These injuries are usually caused by high-speed motor vehicle crashes.

Characteristic of any midface fracture is distortion of the facial proportions. The face appears lengthened and the midface flat. The teeth do not align properly and there is evidence of molar impingement or an open-bite deformity. Telecanthus, a widened distance between the medial canthi, results from any comminution that involves the attachments of the medial canthal tendons; pain, tenderness, ecchymosis, and swelling are usually present. The diagnosis is evident by movement of the entire midface with gentle superior and inferior

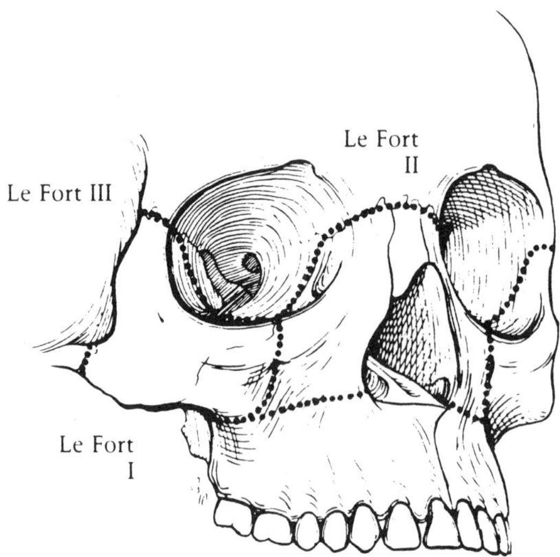

Figure 35–3 Le Fort fractures. Le Fort I, a horizontal or transverse fracture, separates the maxillary alveolus at the lower margin at the piriform aperture and extends through the maxillary sinus. Le Fort II fracture separates a pyramid-shaped segment from the upper craniofacial structures. The fracture lines extend from the Le Fort I level upward through the inferior orbital rims and across the bridge of the nose in either a high or a low fashion. Le Fort III fracture separates the cranial from the facial bones. It is a "craniofacial disjunction" with fracture lines separating the frontal bone from the zygoma and orbits. The fracture lines extend across the floor of the orbit and up through the nasofrontal area. If this area is comminuted, a nasoethmoidal orbital fracture may be produced. (From Smith JW, Aston SJ, editors: *Grabb and Smith's plastic surgery;* ed 4, Boston, 1991, Little Brown, p 374.)

traction applied to the maxillary incisor teeth. Palpation of the frontozygomatic and frontonasal sutures at the inferior orbital rim and intraorally at the zygoma is important. Mucosa ecchymosis in the area of the zygomaticomaxillary buttress is nearly pathognomonic of midface fractures.

Radiologic evaluation begins with a lateral cervical spine view and a skull series; appropriate facial views are submental-occipital and Waters's. A CT scan is usually helpful.

Nasoorbital fracture

Blunt trauma to the area between the eyes may result in disruption of the entire complex and detachment of the medial canthal tendons. The injury is characterized by a triad: (1) widened nasal bridge, (2) telecanthus greater than 34 mm, and (3) almond-shaped palpebral fissures. The Waters view, orbital tomography, and CT scan are appropriate radiographic studies.

Soft-tissue injury

Soft-tissue injuries range from a bruise or abrasion to extensive laceration and avulsion. With any superficial injury, the presence of related, specific deep soft-tissue injury is possible.

Nasolacrimal apparatus laceration. Tears are produced by the lacrimal gland in the lateral upper lid. The nasolacrimal apparatus passes medially across the cornea and drains by the way of the puncta of both lid margins into the canaliculi, which leads to the nasolacrimal sac and then into the nasal cavity. Any laceration of the medial third of the lid, particularly the major draining lower lid, raises the suspicion of injury to the canaliculus. Diagnosis requires direct visualization of the white tubular structure by passing a lacrimal duct probe or Silastic tube from the puncta into the wound while the child is under general anesthesia.

Parotid duct laceration. The parotid duct passes from the parotid gland to the meatus near the first maxillary molar. A laceration of the cheek that crosses the middle third of a line drawn from the tragus of the ear to the oral commissure should raise suspicion of an injury to this structure. Diagnosis is made by passing a probe or cannulas through the intraorbital meatus while the child is under general anesthesia.

Facial nerve injury. With any significant laceration to lateral areas of the face, injury to the facial nerve or its branches is possible. Inspection for symmetry of animation is essential; ask the child to raise the eyebrows, tightly close the eyelids, smile, and expose the lower teeth. Microsurgery permits repair of any facial nerve injury lateral to a perpendicular line from the lateral canthus; the more medial, finer branches usually do not require repair.

TREATMENT

After evaluation of the child, treatment depends on the severity of individual injuries. Facial fracture is usually not an emergency. Repair of small lacerations in a cooperative child is possible with adequate sedation and local anesthesia in the operating room. Complex laceration, fracture, and underlying soft-tissue injury are best treated in the operating room while the child is under general anesthesia. Evaluate the child's tetanus immunization status. Administration of an antibiotic for open fracture and for contaminated wounds, particularly from bites, is important. Specific antibiotics are selected according to probable contaminating organisms, such as oxacillin and penicillin for intraoral wounds and a cephalosporin for skin contamination of an open fracture. This treatment is started as soon as practical.

Bites

Most animal bites are inflicted by dogs and occur in children 5 to 10 years of age. The prevention of wound infection, tetanus, and rabies is an important consideration. Copious irrigation with saline is an essential therapy. Small wounds are best treated by complete excision and closure, and the margins of larger wounds require sharp debridement of the exposed cutaneous surfaces before closure. Small puncture wounds are best left open after irrigation. Wide-spectrum antibiotics, such as cephalosporin, are started as early as possible; the most common organism in a dog's mouth is *Staphylococcus*. Clinical infections are often the result of other organisms, such as *Pasteurella*. A combination of penicillin and oxacillin provides coverage for most oral organisms.

In contrast to animal bites, human bites are even more heavily inoculated with virulent organisms. The treatment for a human bite is similar to that for an animal bite, but human bites are commonly left open.

Lacerations

Every wound is potentially contaminated. Because the risk of infection increases with time, a wound is ideally closed within 12 hours. There is, however, no "golden" period for closure of a minimally contaminated wound of the face. For example, closure of a clean laceration a day after injury is possible if treatment consists of appropriate irrigation and debridement.

A child who is to be treated requires a gentle, personal, but firm approach and, above all, understanding and patience. Administration of an intramuscular mixture of sedatives (e.g., Demerol, 1 mg/kg; Thorazine, 2 mg/kg; and Phenergan, 1 mg/kg) is a useful adjunct but is not a substitute for proper emergency room manner. It is essential to wait at least 30 to 45 minutes after intramuscular sedation before beginning treatment. Avoid the use of physical restraints or a papoose board if at all possible. Lidocaine (0.5%) with epinephrine (1:200,000) usually provides adequate local anesthesia and hemostasis; a more concentrated solution is of no increased value.

Preparation of the wound is at least as important as the suture technique. Cleanse the wound with copious saline irrigation. Betadine or Hibiclens solution provides useful surface antisepsis, but vigorous chemical internal wound lavage should be avoided. Debride devitalized tissue conservatively because questionable tissue on the face often proves to be viable. Also remove any dirt in the laceration or abrasion to prevent the formation of a scar tatoo; a dirty abrasion requires a thorough scrub after adequate anesthesia. Trim the wound with a scalpel to square the edges, and release the wound margins to reduce tension on the closure.

A stellate laceration presents a difficult treatment problem. Debridement and suture closure must be meticulous to achieve a satisfactory result; a triangulation stitch helps to prevent flap-tip necrosis. All complex wounds require treatment in the operating room. Because the goal is primary healing, and conservatism is the rule, preserve as much tissue as possible. Excellent hemostasis is essential.

Deep suture of absorbable material permits restoration of muscle continuity and supports a tension-free skin closure. If possible, avoid the use of subcutaneous fat sutures to close dead space, because they increase, rather than decrease, the incidence of wound infection. Sutures of fine Vicryl or Dexon in the dermis or dermosubcutaneous junction placed with the knot buried will relieve skin tension and allow early suture removal; the skin edge apposition and eversion is best achieved with 6-0 nylon. Eversion of the skin edges is accomplished by passing the needle so that a wider bite of tissue is taken deeply rather than superficially; skin edges that are not everted can result in dermal depression when the scar contracts. The correct number of sutures in the skin is the minimum necessary to ensure accurate edge closure; placement of the sutures 3 to 5 mm apart is usually adequate.

A special problem is an avulsion flap, which may form a "trapdoor" scar as it contracts over time. If possible during initial treatment, excision and linear closure are best. Complete tissue avulsion often requires release of the skin edges to permit advancement. Large defects require placement of a skin graft, but not on the day of injury. Sometimes an occlusive sterile dressing is the best initial therapy.

Ear or nose. When ear or nose cartilage is disrupted, a minimum number of stabilizing sutures placed in the perichondrium help to maintain the normal position. Adequate skin closure is extremely important. Exact alignment of a margin, such as the edge of the nostril or the edge of the ear lobe, is essential, inasmuch as any step deformity in these structures is noticeable.

The lip. A major consideration in lip laceration is proper alignment of the skin edges, particularly of the vermilion border. After mucosal closure with a fine chromic suture, the muscle is repaired with Vicryl or Dexon. The closure of the skin begins with accurate restoration of the mucocutaneous junction or vermilion border. To improve visualization of the junction of the red and white lip, avoid the use of epinephrine-containing solutions. A small step deformity is noticeable and difficult to correct. Prophylactic treatment with systemic penicillin is helpful to reduce the incidence of infection.

Oral mucosa or tongue. Small lacerations of the oral mucosa or of the tongue do not require suture approximation, as they will heal rapidly. The healing time of a gaping laceration may be shortened by loose closure with chromic sutures.

Parotid duct. In the evaluation or repair of parotid duct division, cannulate the oral opening opposite the second maxillary molar with a polyethylene tube; magnification permits primary repair with the use of fine nylon suture. The tube is left in place as a stent and a layered closure of the overlying soft tissue then follows.

Facial nerve. Facial nerve injury lateral to the lateral canthus requires repair under the operating microscope with 9-0 or 10-0 nylon sutures. If this is not possible in a contaminated avulsion, mark the nerve end with a suture for secondary reconstruction.

The eyelid. Treatment of laceration of the eyelid requires closure of several layers: (1) conjunctiva and tarsal plate, with a pull-out nonabsorbable suture, (2) muscle, with an absorbable suture such as Vicryl, and (3) skin, with 6-0 nylon. It is necessary to place sutures so that the loose ends cannot irritate the cornea. Repair a lacrimal duct injury using a surgical microscope and provide a stent for the duct, brought out through the nose.

Wound dressing

A simple wound dressing is best. Cover small wounds with an adhesive bandage strip. The indications for application of a dressing are the need to splint the skin edges, absorb drainage, or protect the wound from the child. Application of an antibiotic ointment such as bacitracin can enhance wound asepsis.

Postoperative care

Facial wounds are generally sealed to external contamination by 24 hours. Wounds that are adequately closed will certainly tolerate soap and water by 48 hours; nevertheless, they should be examined early and routinely for any signs of infection. Early suture removal prevents the cross-hatching suture marks that complicate an otherwise good result; removal is done as early as 3 days or as late as 5 days after placement.

The maturation of the scar is a 6-month process for the average wound; during this time the wound may become erythematous and indurated before it slowly softens and flattens. Scar remodeling improves by application of Steri-strips to splint the wound, by a pressure-massage regimen, and by protection from the sun.

REFERENCES

1. Manigha AJ, Kline SN: Maxillofacial trauma in the pediatric age group, *Otolaryngol Clin N Am* 16, 1983.
2. Kaban LB, Mulliken JB, Murray JE: Facial fractures in children: an analysis of 122 fractures in 109 patients. Paper presented at the annual meeting of the American Association of Plastic Surgeons, Atlanta, Georgia, May 12, 1976.
3. Riefkohl R, Georgiade NG: Facial fractures in children, *Pediatr Plast Surg* 2:518-530, 1984.

36 Ocular Trauma

David S. Friendly and Mohamad S. Jaafar

Three common types of pediatric eye injury are traumatic hyphemas, those secondary to physical child abuse, and orbital wall fractures. Inner-city children with these types of eye injuries have been referred to the Children's National Medical Center (CNMC) in Washington, DC, a tertiary trauma center, over the course of many years. The authors have developed specific concepts and plans for the treatment of such patients. This chapter discusses our specific approaches to these relatively common types of pediatric eye trauma.

TRAUMATIC HYPHEMA
Definition

The presence of blood in the normally optically empty space between the cornea and the anterior surface of the iris constitutes a hyphema (Figs. 36-1 and 36-2). Most hyphemas are readily visible with an ordinary flashlight, but some may be microscopic in size, requiring the high magnification of the slitlamp to detect the brownish-colored red blood corpuscles suspended in the clear aqueous humor that fills the optically empty space between the iris-lens plane and the endothelium of the cornea. Gross hyphemas settle inferiorly by gravity. Hence, they are generally seen in the inferior chamber angle and have a curvilinear inferior border and a flat superior border. Hyphemas are traditionally divided between traumatic and nontraumatic types. The latter are quite rare, as they are caused in children by such unusual disorders as juvenile xanthogranuloma, retinoblastoma, and leukemia. On the other hand, traumatic hyphemas are relatively common.

Etiology

The major causes of traumatic hyphema in children are missiles, fisticuffs, sports injuries, motor vehicle crashes, stick injuries, and physical abuse. At CNMC belt injuries resulting from parents' attempts to discipline their children constitute a common cause. Not surprisingly, boys are more frequently affected than girls, and traumatic hyphema is rarely bilateral.

A contusion injury to the eye produces a pulse of increased pressure in the aqueous humor, which in turn tears the ciliary body tissue in the region of the iris insertion to this structure. The blood emanates from fine vessels in the ciliary body, not from the iris. The amount of blood that appears in the anterior chamber following a blunt contusion injury is quite variable and, in fact, ranges from a microscopic amount to an amount that completely fills the space occupied by the aqueous humor (Figs. 36-1 and 36-2).

Diagnosis

The emergency room physician or pediatrician who first examines a child with a history or with signs or symptoms suggesting eye trauma must keep in mind the possibility of traumatic hyphema during the eye examination. The color contrast between a darkly pigmented iris and immediately adjacent blood is not great. If the anterior chamber is not carefully observed with direct illumination—as with a pocket flashlight—the diagnosis may easily

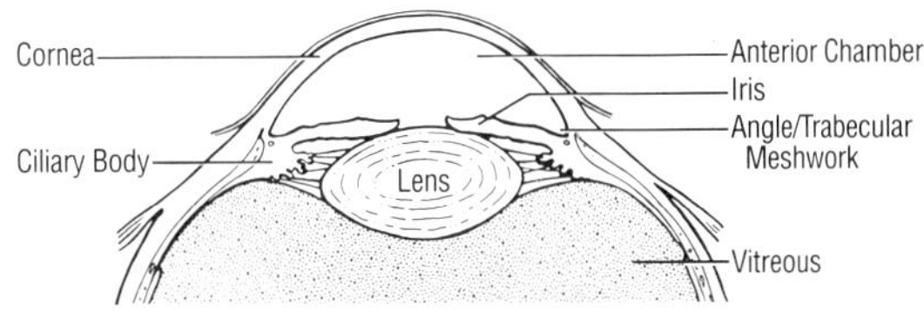

Figure 36–1 Anatomy of the anterior segment of the eye.

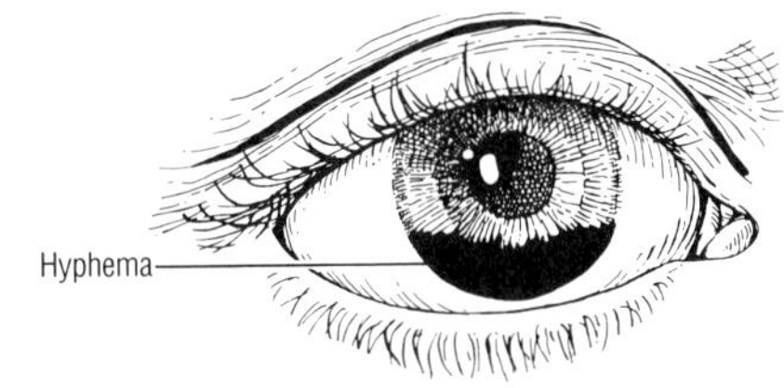

Figure 36–2 Appearance of traumatic hyphema.

be missed. The maroon-colored blood is much more visible against a lighter background; thus diagnosis is considerably easier in blue-eyed individuals.

Secondary hemorrhages

The clots that normally form in the torn fine vessels of the ciliary body are apparently quite fragile. Secondary hemorrhages from these vessels occur in a significant percentage of cases. The prevalence of spontaneous rebleeding, which varies greatly in the literature, may possibly be influenced by racially inherited factors; the frequency of rebleeding is stated to be higher in black individuals than in whites. We assume a 20% rate of secondary hemorrhages in the largely inner-city population served by the CNMC. The cause of secondary hemorrhages is not well understood, but may relate to clot dissolution. They typically occur on the third or fourth day following injury. Secondary hemorrhage is primarily associated with the dreaded complications of traumatic hyphema, specifically glaucoma (increased pressure within the eye) and bloodstaining of the cornea. There are several mechanisms responsible for the rise in pressure within the eye, but mechanical blockage of the outflow passages leading from the anterior chamber towards Schlemm's canal by the red corpuscles is a common one. Corneal bloodstaining is due to the presence of blood and blood products in the corneal stroma. Damage to the corneal endothelium at the time of injury or increased pressure within the eye (or combinations of both mechanisms) allow the blood products to penetrate into the corneal stroma. Naturally, vision is adversely affected by the blood-induced opacification of the cornea. In young children (particularly those under 6 years of age) such visual deprivation can lead to amblyopia and strabismus. Both glaucoma and corneal bloodstaining are uncommon in the absence of secondary hemorrhages. However, an exception to this rule is a primary hemorrhage that completely fills the anterior chamber. Total hyphema is sometimes referred to as "black-ball" or "eight-ball" hemorrhage because the deoxygenated blood has a dark appearance. Such hemorrhage is associated with these complications because of their large size.

Associated pathology

It is important to realize that visible blood in the anterior chamber may signal a significant problem. There may also be unseen damage to the interior of the eye. Orbital fracture, intraocular foreign body, traumatic retinopathy (particularly to the macula), traumatic cataract, lens subluxation, late-developing glaucoma, pupillary occlusion, vitreous hemorrhage, choroidal tears, scleral rupture, and optic atrophy are just some of the more serious conditions that can also be present or may subsequently occur.

Clinical management

Historical assessment relevant to evaluation of blunt ocular trauma includes the circumstances of the injury, previous treatment, the child's general health (including ocular health), use of medications (particularly aspirin), presence of a bleeding tendency or coagulopathy, hemoglobinopathy, current pregnancy, and past adverse reactions to general anesthesia or to previously administered topical or systemic medications. A thorough general physical examination complements the eye examination. The latter should be done by a physician experienced in evaluating ocular injury. Some of the necessary data includes the visual acuity of both eyes, the results of a slitlamp examination, the intraocular pressure, and the appearance of the fundus, if it is visible by direct or indirect opthalmoscopy. If the interior of the eye is not visible, a B-scan ultrasound evaluation is indicated. On rare occasions, a computed tomography (CT) examination or magnetic resonance imaging (MRI) of the eye is useful. Laboratory studies in addition to the routine complete blood count (CBC) and urinalysis include a sickle hemoglobin screening test for black patients which, if positive, should be followed up by hemoglobin electrophoresis.

Hospitalization of a child who has sustained blunt ocular trauma is in the child's best interest because it is difficult to assure compliance with medical instructions and follow-up on an outpatient basis. Because of the possibility of secondary hemorrhage, hospitalization for 6 to 7 days posttrauma is advisable. Treatment consists of bed rest with bathroom privileges, a metallic or plastic shield over the injured eye and elevation of the head of the bed. The latter causes the blood to settle by gravity into the relatively less important inferior portion of the anterior chamber, thereby sparing the visual axis. Permit television viewing but not reading, because of its associated rapid eye movements. The long-term bedside presence of family members, usually the child's mother in particular, helps to control anxiety and activity levels better than oral sedatives. Encourage listening to the radio and to stories read aloud by others.

Topical medications are kept to a minimum so as to prevent unnecessary eyelid manipulation and additional trauma to the eye. If the hyphema covers the pupil, 1% atropine drops are instilled once each day to enlarge the pupillary opening and reduce posterior synechiae, adhesions between the back of the iris and lens. Some practitioners recommend topical steroid drops to reduce intraocular inflammation. Topical antiglaucoma medication such as Timoptic or Betoptic drops are used twice each day if intraocular pressure is elevated.

Amicar (aminocaproic acid), an antifrinolytic compound, reduces secondary hemorrhage by delaying the dissolution of blood clots. Rare side effects associated with Amicar in the recommended dosage include abdominal pain, nausea and vomiting, diarrhea, hypotension, dizziness, tinnitus, headache, and skin rashes. Amicar is given 50 mg/kg q4h to a maximum of 5 g q4h for 5 days by mouth. Contraindications to the use of Amicar include pregnancy, renal disorders, clotting disorders, and a thrombotic history.

Diamox tablets are given every 6 hours if intraocular pressure is elevated and the child does not have a hemoglobinopathy. If the child has sickle-cell disease, Neptazane is substituted for Diamox to prevent the associated decrease in pH in the aqueous humor that enhances sickling. Avoid the use of dehydrating agents such as oral glycerine or intravenous Manitol in children with abnormal hemoglobin; these agents are occasionally useful in other children with elevated intraocular pressure. Unfortunately, decreases in intraocular pressure obtained with such medications are usually transient. The brief duration of their effect limits their usefulness. Aspirin and aspirin-containing medications are contraindicated.

Daily ocular examination is indicated. Question the child regarding eye pain, because this may be the first indication of secondary glaucoma. Also important are assessment of visual acuity, evaluation of applanation pressure, and slitlamp examinations. Record the extent of the hyphema and any presence of bloodstaining of the cornea. Avoid application of excessive force to the injured eye, as this may cause or aggravate a secondary hyphema. During a child's hospitalization, exclude such procedures as Schiotz tonometry, in which a weighted pressure-measuring instrument is applied to the cornea to determine introcular pressure; scleral indentation, in which an instrument depresses the sclera to visualize the retinal periphery by indirect ophthalmoscopy; and gonioscopy, in which a corneal contact lens is applied to the eye to enable visualization of the anterior chamber angle.

Because management of traumatic hyphema is complicated by the presence of multiple clinical variables, and because of the rapid turnover of house officers at our institution, CNMC uses an original computer program that requests input of such information as the child's weight, applanation pressure, extent of hyphema, and race; it prints out a checklist of contraindications to the use of Amicar, a list of appropriate laboratory tests, suggested hospital admission orders, including dosage of all medications, and a list of all desired daily observations. The program is written in Basic for the Apple IIe and compatible computers.

Occasionally, despite best efforts, a child may require surgical removal of blood from the anterior chamber of the eye under general anesthesia. Results are improved with the use of a surgical microscope. It is important to explain to parents that this type of intraocular surgery is not predictable and that serious complications sometimes occur, including bleeding from the ciliary body during or after surgery. Indications for surgery include sustained elevation of intraocular pressure, blood-staining of the cornea, and persistence of a clot for more than 9 days. Children with sickle-cell disease or trait require more aggressive management because they are more likely to sustain optic nerve infarction. In these children, a small hyphema causes higher than expected intraocular pressure and thrombotic closure of blood vessels occurs at relatively low levels of intraocular pressure.

Children are reexamined in an outpatient setting 1 month after discharge from the hospital. At this time the anterior chamber angle is visualized for evidence and extent of recession indicating a tear in the ciliary body. This is an important observation because of the association between circumferentially large recessions and late glaucoma. Severely affected children require lifelong periodic ophthalmologic observation to detect and subsequently treat increased intraocular pressure. This type of glaucoma may occur several years after trauma. In addition, the retinal periphery should be examined by indirect ophthalmoscopy and scleral depression at the initial outpatient visit. If peripheral retinal breaks are identified, the child should be referred to a retinologist for assessment and possible treatment to avoid retinal detachment.

CHILD ABUSE
Prevalence

A common variety of eye injury is due to physical child abuse. Not only can vision become impaired by direct and indirect ocular injury, it can also become impaired by injury to the visual pathways and visual cortex of the brain, as well as by damage to the motor centers and motor pathways that subserve ocular positioning and movement. In other words, the entire visual system is quite vulnerable to physical abuse. In a series of patients studied at CNMC, the finding of eye injuries in physically abused children varied from 25% to 41%.

In our experience, the most common reason for failure to make a correct diagnosis has been naivete of the physician. Physical abuse is still not recognized because of a lack of emphasis on this disorder in medical school curricula, as well as a lack of willingness on the part of some physicians to recognize its possibility. Violence to children is so foreign to the experience or comprehension of many physicians that it is simply dismissed as a possibility. It is important to realize that physical abuse is not always willful, as in the cases of some infants with shaken baby syndrome who suffer whiplash injuries during misguided resuscitation efforts, and that parties other than parents may be responsible, such as siblings or adult surrogate caregivers.

Within all jurisdictions of the United States, the law requires the reporting of suspected cases of physical child abuse to an appropriate local agency. Reporting physicians are protected from being sued if the report is made without malicious intent. Failure to initiate a report can result in legal action against the responsible physician.

About 10% to 15% of all hospital emergency room visits are due to physical child abuse, which is associated with a mortality of up to 10%. There is a 30% to 50% incidence of recurrent trauma in affected children. Eye injury is the presenting sign of physical child abuse in up to 6% of all cases.

History

An inadequate explanation for an injury should alert the physician to the possibility of physical child abuse. For example, a fall from a bed or from a highchair is insufficient to account for a skull fracture in a normal infant.

Most physically abused children are under 3 years of age, and many are premature at birth. The parents themselves frequently have been victims of childhood abuse and often display antisocial tendencies, such as evidenced by arrest records, alcoholism, and other forms of drug abuse. Separation, divorce, and other signs of parental discord are common. Although abuse occurs in all strata of society, most reported cases come from the lower socioeconomic segments of the population. Many parents responsible for child abuse are emotionally immature and have difficulty with impulse control. A careful history and subsequent investigation may reveal that a child has been admitted to the same or another health care facility for similar problems in the past. Registries, if available, can be of great value in piecing together the medical history of the child.

Examination

Direct trauma to the eyes may produce such findings as retinal and vitreous hemorrhage, periorbital hemorrhage, retinal detachment and scarring, lens opacity and dislocation, and subconjunctival hemorrhage. Anterior chamber hemorrhage, traumatic hyphema, resulting from belt-buckle injury, occurs

in older children. Indirect trauma to the eyes is often part of the shaken baby syndrome. Infants have disproportionately large heads and lack the neck muscular control necessary to prevent the development of violent acceleration and deceleration during episodes of shaking. The exact mechanism by which such whiplash head movements result in retinal hemorrhages is uncertain. Greenwald suggests that acceleration produces lens-vitreous body displacement.[9] Attachments of the vitreous to the retina transmit the force generated by the product of lens-vitreous mass and acceleration to the inner retinal layers. This results in retinal splitting, retinoschisis, with associated intraretinal hemorrhage. There is some clinical, histopathologic, and electrophysiologic evidence to support this theory. Large retinal hemorrhages can break through the inner retinal membrane and cause vitreous opacification. The shaken baby syndrome consists of retinal hemorrhage, intracranial hemorrhage, and fractures of long bones. Victims of this syndrome may show little or no external manifestations of physical abuse. Hence it is no exaggeration that the examining physician must have a high level of suspicion and routinely request ophthalmologic consultation when confronted with infants with unexplained seizures, unusual irritability, altered mental status, hydrocephalus, or in whom the diagnosis is suspected because of other clues in the child's history or physical examination. Imaging studies of the brain and long bones are helpful in making the diagnosis. Up to 80% of abused children have retinal hemorrhage. For obscure reasons, retinal hemorrhage occasionally occurs in the fundus of just one eye. The hemorrhage may be of any type and size. White-centered hemorrhages are occasionally seen in physically abused infants, but their presence does not usually require investigation—as would be necessary in children and adults—for sepsis, subacute bacterial endocarditis, leukemia, and anemia. White-centered hemorrhages are commonly seen in infants with intracranial hemorrhage. The finding of retinal hemorrhage of any type in a physically abused child almost always indicates the presence of intracranial hemorrhage. Accidental head trauma, such as results from a motor vehicle crash, very rarely causes retinal hemorrhage.

The differential diagnosis of retinal hemorrhage requires consideration of such entities as hypertension, bleeding disorders, vasculitis, meningitis, sepsis, and leukemia. However, the main problem in differential diagnosis is birth trauma. A reasonably safe rule is that retinal hemorrhage seen 6 weeks or more after parturition is very rarely due to the birth process.

Fundus examination by indirect ophthalmoscopy

Table 36–1 Diagnostic features of the battered child syndrome

1. Affected children generally 3 years old or younger
2. Fractures and soft-tissue injuries in different stages
3. Disproportionate degree of soft-tissue injury
4. Parents' or guardians' account of history incompatible with injury
5. Multiple admissions to different hospitals
6. No fresh lesions during hospitalization

Modified from Harcourt B, Hopkins D: *Brit Med J* 3:398, 1971.

requires prior instillation of cycloplegic and mydriatic drops to obtain pupillary dilation. However, pupillary light reflexes should be examined before drop instillation. The examining ophthalmologist should discuss the necessity of eye drop instillation with the physicians responsible for the child's care. The written ophthalmology report should clearly state that dilating drops were used. Only rarely is a child's neurologic condition so precarious that pupillary dilation is contraindicated.

Traumatic cataracts are common after severe blunt eye injury. They vary greatly in appearance and cannot be differentiated from cataracts of other causes on the basis of morphology alone. A portable slitlamp is extremely useful in determining the location, size, shape, and density of the opacification. The eyes of battered children may have partially displaced lenses. There is nothing pathognomonic about these lens subluxations, and they must be differentiated from those associated with genetic disorders. The latter are usually bilateral but may be asymmetric in severity. Associated findings and laboratory studies are helpful in differential diagnosis.

There is no substitute for a high level of suspicion. For example, an infant was presented to the CNMC with what initially appeared to be unilateral primary congenital glaucoma. More careful ophthalmologic examination with the portable slitlamp through the enlarged and cloudy cornea revealed an iris sphincter tear in the affected eye, a defect virtually indicative of direct trauma and not compatible with the original clinical diagnosis. Bone surveys requested subsequent to this new finding revealed posterior rib fractures. Repeat questioning of the infant's parent produced a history of child battering.

Various mechanisms may produce glaucoma. Damage to aqueous humor outflow passages associated with tears in the ciliary body is common. These tears maybe visualized by gonioscopy, a diagnostic procedure that requires heavy sedation or general anesthesia in a young child.

Optic nerve injury is occasionally present in battered children and is usually a late finding. It may be due to increased intracranial pressure and papilledema or to pressure on the nerve from sheath hemorrhages. Alternately, central retinal artery occlusion or direct injury to the nerve as it traverses the bony canal may be responsible. In some cases the optic nerve pallor may be secondary to extensive retinal damage (retinoschisis) or possibly a result of retrograde transsynaptic degeneration. Occasionally, there is damage to the visual cortex and oculomotor nerves. Strabismus of both the paretic and nonparetic varieties are common in affected children. Table 36-1 lists diagnostic features of the battered child syndrome.

Management

Management of children who have suffered physical abuse requires a multidisciplinary approach. We are fortunate in having at CNMC a team of physicians, social workers, and attorneys who together handle the associated medical, social, psychological, and legal aspects of these cases. The role of the ophthalmologist is limited but important. The well-being of each child requires prompt diagnosis, and thorough investigation of each case by specialists from all relevant disciplines is essential. Careful follow-up of all known and suspected cases by child protective agencies is likewise mandatory if further abuse is to be prevented.

ORBITAL WALL FRACTURES

The orbital bones are of delicate, eggshell-like consistency. The proximity of the paranasal sinuses, nerves, vessels, eyeball, extraocular muscles, and other orbital structures predispose them to a wide variety of possible damage from injury-producing orbital fractures.

Pathophysiology

A blow-out fracture occurs when an object larger than the anterior orbital opening strikes the eyeball or orbital rim. Offending objects include a fist, tennis ball, snowball, baseball, and door knob. The mechanism of blow-out fracture is controversial.[11] Two main theories dominate the literature. In 1957 Smith and Reagan described the "hydraulic theory": the fracture is caused by transmission of the force striking the globe to the thin orbital floor via an increase in intraorbital pressure. In approximately half of affected children, there is a concomitant fracture of the lamina papyracea, nasally, which is commonly asymptomatic. Less frequently, there is also a fracture of the orbital roof. The blow to the globe causes an increase in intraorbital pressure that produces bone fractures in which orbital soft tissues become entrapped. In 1974 Fujino proposed a second hypothesis. He speculated that most orbital fractures are the result of "buckling" forces transmitted to the floor by transient deformity of bones produced by a direct blow to the rim. In these instances, the rim does not infracture.

Clinical findings

Blow-out fractures are more common in males (male-female ratio = 5:1). Children present acutely with pain and tenderness at the impact site, lid edema, ecchymosis, epistaxis, orbital emphysema, exophthalmus or enophthalmus, diplopia, hypophthalmus, hypoesthesia in the distribution of the infraorbital nerve, and associated ocular injuries.

Ecchymosis and edema of the eyelids are variable with orbital wall fracture. A significant "black eye" may or may not be associated with an orbital wall fracture. Of more importance is that an orbital wall fracture can exist without severe external signs. Epistaxis and orbital emphysema are due to a fracture of the lamina papyracea, which permits communication between the ethmoid sinus and the orbital content. Palpating the eyelids demonstrates the subcutaneous air causing crepitance. Acute symptoms in children with orbital wall fracture include exophthalmus secondary to intraorbital hemorrhage and edema. However, when a large orbital fracture is present, with prolapse of orbital tissue into the maxillary sinus and a large fracture of the medial orbital wall, enophthalmus may also be present. The globe may actually fall inferiorly into the bony defect, resulting in hypophthalmus. In rare instances, total eye displacement occurs through the fracture into the maxillary sinus. Progressive enophthalmus occurs days to weeks after an injury as a result of resorption of orbital edema and hemorrhage, necrosis and atrophy of the orbital fat, and fibrosis and shortening of the entrapped ocular muscles. When enophthalmus is present, narrowing of the palpebral fissure and pseudoptosis may be evident. Any fracture involving the infraorbital canal affects the infraorbital nerve and may cause hypoesthesia or anesthesia of the lower eyelid, cheek, and lateral side of the nostril and may extend down to the upper lip and ipsilateral upper teeth.

One of the most dramatic symptoms in children with blow-out fracture is double vision. Diplopia has essentially two primary mechanisms: (1) a mechanical entrapment of the inferior rectus muscle, the inferior oblique muscle, and/or orbital fibrous connective tissues in the fracture site, and (2) a paralytic component wherein injury to the inferior

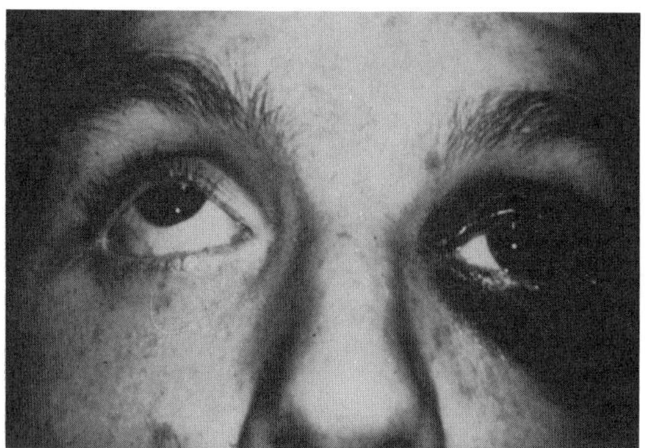

Figure 36–3 A thirteen-year-old girl, 2 days following trauma to the left eye resulting in ecchymosis of eyelids, orbital floor fracture, and severe restriction to elevation of the left globe.

division of the third cranial nerve, which innervates both the inferior rectus and inferior oblique muscles, may cause a paresis of these muscles. The paresis is usually, but not invariably, transient in nature. Hemorrhage or edema within the extraocular muscle may also cause transient paresis. A third but much less common etiology for diplopia is a phoria that decompensates into a frank tropia because of the trauma and interruption of fusion. The motility findings thus vary according to the nature of the fracture, its size and location, and the specific tissues displaced and caught within the fracture site (Fig. 36-3 and Fig. 36-4). Hypophthalmus, which is a downward displacement of the globe, rarely causes diplopia. In the absence of eye muscle involvement, a minimum of 15 mm displacement of the eyeball is needed for the development of diplopia.

There are, however, other causes of restricted eye movement besides entrapment. They include orbital edema, hemorrhage, and muscle intrasheath hematoma. These conditions usually clear within the first 10 to 14 days after injury.

Orbital wall fracture is probably due to increased hydrostatic pressure within the rigid confines of the bony orbit, which is relieved when a wall fracture occurs. A blow-out fracture may thus act as a safety valve in protecting the globe itself from rupture. Although rupture of the globe is uncommon in blow-out fracture, intraocular injuries are present in up to 50% of cases. These include corneal and scleral rupture, hyphema, iritis, iris sphincter rupture, iridodialysis, angle recession, subluxated lens, cataract, glaucoma, vitreous hemorrhage, choroidal rupture, optic nerve damage, and retinal hemorrhage, edema, scar, hole, and detachment. A partial or complete visual loss may result from direct damage or secondary compression of the optic nerve, or from interruption of its vascular sup-

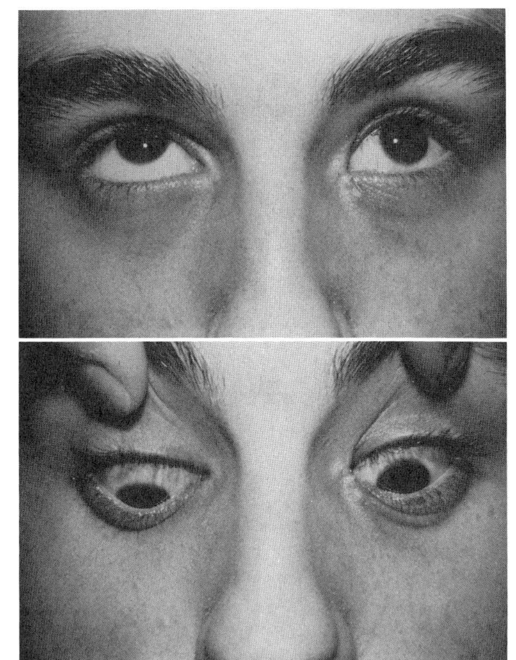

Figure 36–4 A 15-year-old boy, 3 weeks after a fist injury to the left orbit resulting in orbital floor fracture. **A,** Limited elevation of the left eye secondary to entrapment of inferior rectus muscle. **B,** Limited depression of the left eye secondary to inferior rectus muscle paresis.

ply. The presence of reduced vision, subconjunctival hemorrhage, decreased intraocular pressure, or a relative afferent pupillary defect raises the possibility of an associated ocular injury. Initial clinical evaluation must detect ocular damage, which is a true emergency.

An aid to the evaluation of children with orbital wall fracture is to remember the mnemonic HEADER, which emphasizes that affected children are usually young, active male fighters, who are predisposed to this type of injury.

*H*yphema: Evaluate the child for bleeding into the anterior chamber and for other intraocular injury.

*E*mphysema: Eyelid crepitation.

*A*nesthesia: Anesthesia or hypoesthesia along the distribution of the infraorbital nerve.

*D*iplopia: Double vision secondary to trauma to the extraocular muscles with paralytic or myogenic component.

*E*nophthalmus: Enophthalmus or exophthalmus.

*R*estriction: Entrapment of extraocular muscles and orbital tissue in the fractured wall(s).

As a consequence of the thinness of the bone, the medial wall (lamina papyracea) and the orbital floor (roof of the maxillary antrum) are the surfaces most frequently damaged. Medial wall fractures seldom produce any functional disturbance, such as diplopia, and may be overlooked. They may, however, cause expansion of the orbital volume and secondary enophthalmus. Orbital floor fracture usually involves the weak posterior medial orbital floor in the maxillary bone and is of much greater importance, both functionally and cosmetically. Orbital roof fractures are uncommon. Because of the secondary involvement of the levator and superior rectus muscles, the child may have ptosis and hypotropia. This is partially due to the hematoma that involves the superior orbit with, or without, the superior rectus–levator-muscle complex. Roof fractures are not usually associated with vision reduction, permanent motility defects, or lid dysfunction. Superior displacement (blow-out) and inferior displacement (blow-in) roof fractures are equally uncommon.[2,9] When orbitral roof fracture is suspected, the child should undergo CT scan of the orbits and brain and should be followed for the development of an encephalocele. Fractures of the lateral wall of the orbit are usually not associated with any significant morbidity and may show only transient paresis of the lateral rectus muscle. Any of the four walls of the orbit may be fractured individually or in combination with one another.

Evaluation

Evaluation of children with orbital floor fracture depends on the clinical findings. The mnenomic HEADER again serves as as a convenient checklist. The ocular adnexa, eyeball, and ocular motility require evaluation. Document visual acuity in each eye at presentation and at each subsequent examination. Follow-up of the child with diplopia is greatly enhanced by serial drawings of the binocular fields of single vision (Fig. 36-5). Attention is drawn to the field of vision where the child's perception is single. The most important gaze positions for daily function and for reading are straight ahead and down.

Use of the forced duction test is valuable to elucidate the mechanism of a motility disturbance and to differentiate between the mechanical restrictive group and the neurogenic-myogenic–decompensated phoria groups. Perform forced duction by anesthetizing the conjunctiva and sclera near the inferior rectus insertion in both eyes with a cotton applicator soaked in topical anesthetic. Grasp the sclera with forceps and ask the child to move the eye into the limited-gaze position. Increased resistance to passive movement is a "positive" forced duction test, implying restriction. Forced duction test results must be interpreted in conjunction with CT scan findings, because hemorrhage, edema, or fibrosis can cause a false-positive result. Treatment

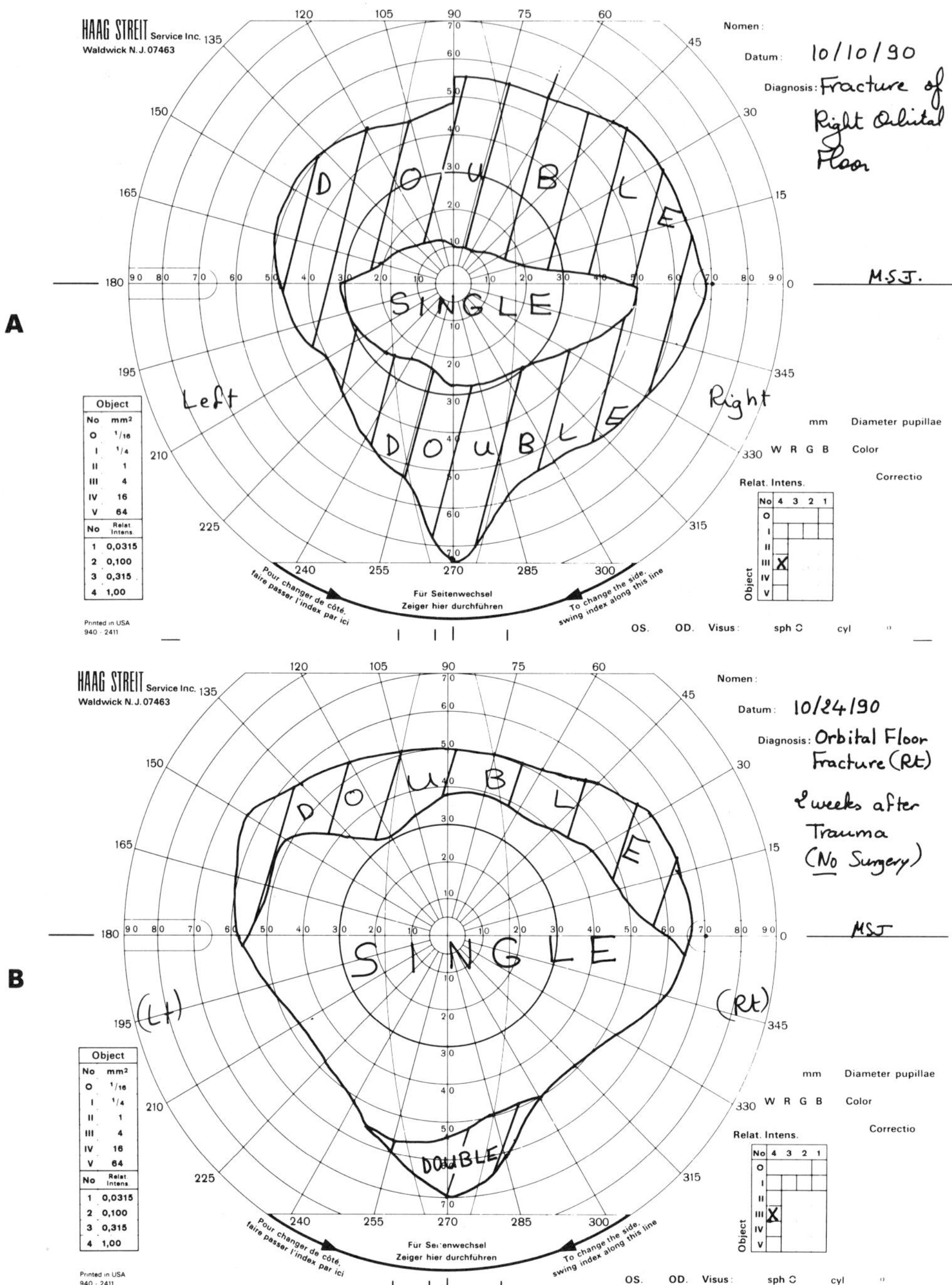

Figure 36–5 Fields of single binocular vision plotted with the Goldmann perimeter. **A,** Thirty-six hours after injury, only a small island of single binocular vision is demonstrated in primary gaze, and up to 27 degrees in downward gaze. **B,** Two weeks after injury, the field of single binocular vision has expanded spontaneously with resolution of orbital edema and hemorrhage. Diplopia was still demonstrable in extreme upward and downward gaze.

of the child with systemic steroids for 6 days (prednisone 1 mg/kg by mouth per day for 2 days, 0.66 mg/kg for 2 days, and 0.33 mg/kg for 2 days) occasionally facilitates resolution of restriction secondary to orbital edema and hemorrhage. If motility restriction is secondary to true entrapment of the extraocular muscles or orbital tissues, however, steroid therapy produces only minimal improvement in diplopia.

Evaluation of the orbit includes recognition of

globe displacement. The exophthalmometer is useful in determination of anterior globe displacement. Estimation of hypophthalmus or vertical displacement is possible by noting displacement of the center of the pupil from a straight edge from one lateral canthus. Medial displacement is determined by placing a ruler on the bridge of the nose and measuring the distance of each pupil from the center of the nose.

The clinical examination and CT assessment of the orbit provide the basis for determination of injury to both bone and soft tissue. A cloudy sinus is suggestive, but not diagnostic, of an orbital wall fracture. The opaqueness is caused by accumulation of blood or prolapsed orbital tissue. High resolution CT scans yield information on fracture patterns, muscle relationships, and displacement of bone and soft tissues. The optic nerve and the extraocular muscles are all easily visualized in multiple planes, such as the longitudinal axis of the optic nerve. Scans of true axial and coronal sections (3 mm intervals) must be obtained (Figs. 36-6 and 36-7). In 1985, Gilbard[7] emphasized the prognostic significance of CT scan in predicting enophthalmus and diplopia. Half of the children with "large" orbital defects were found to develop enophthalmus. Those in whom the inferior rectus muscle lay adjacent to bone fragments on both sides were at high risk for persistent diplopia. Small orbital fractures were more likely to incarcerate extraocular muscles than large fractures; this resulted in muscle infarction secondary to a "compartment syndrome." A small fracture with an entrapped muscle may thus be an indication for immediate surgical exploration. Children who had a free inferior rectus muscle on CT scan showed no persistent diplopia. With contusion, the extraocular muscle manifests a rounded appearance on CT scan.

Management

The management of orbital fractures is still controversial. In a recent article, Dutton and colleagues[5] reviewed the two schools of thought and elucidated the indications and the results of early versus late surgical repair of orbital blow-out fractures.

Indications for early surgery (within 1 to 2 weeks) are symptomatic diplopia with positive forced-duction test results, CT evidence of muscle entrapment, and lack of clinical improvement over 1 to 2 weeks; early enophthalmus of 3 mm or more; significant hypophthalmus; a large orbital wall defect likely to result in late enophthalmus; and associated rim or facial fractures. The indications for conservative observation without treatment are diplopia in extreme lateral and vertical gaze, with

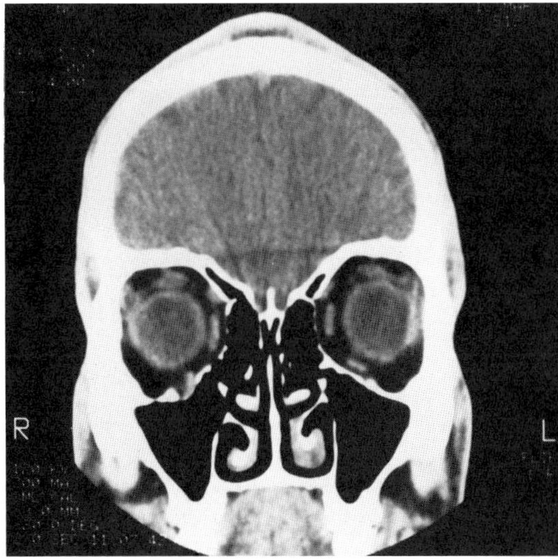

Figure 36–6 Coronal CT scan showing fracture of floor of right orbit with entrapment of inferior rectus muscle. Maxillary antrum is translucent as CT scan is taken 4 weeks after injury.

good motility that shows evidence of clinical improvement over several weeks, and without CT evidence of muscle entrapment; absence of significant enophthalmus or hypophthalmus; and small bony defects not likely to result in late enophthalmus. The decision becomes more difficult in marginal cases in which there is slow but steady resolution of diplopia with slight changes in enophthalmus or hypophthalmus. In this group of cases, frequent measurements of extraocular muscle motility, diplopia, enophthalmus, and hypophthalmus are necessary. Systemic steroids can speed up the improvement in those children without entrapped muscles.

Operative repair of a blow-out fracture is directed toward freeing the orbital tissues and entrapped extraocular muscles and restoring the integrity of the orbital wall. The best results derive from early liberation of the incarcerated tissue from the fracture. In the treatment of enophthalmus and hypophthalmus, restoration of the eye position depends primarily on the anatomical restoration of the shape and volume of the bony orbital cavity. If identification of the infraorbital nerve is possible at the time of surgery, bony fragment decompression is helpful. Sensation may return as late as 1 year following an orbital fracture.

Immediate surgical intervention is usually not necessary. Some delay is advantageous in that it allows the traumatic edema and ecchymosis to subside. Even though failure to diagnose fractures that require early treatment may result in complications owing to fibrosis, contracture, and unsatisfactory

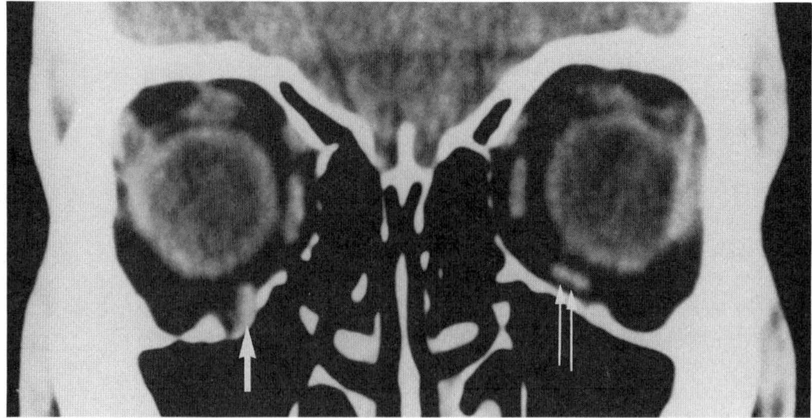

Figure 36–7 Magnified view of coronal CT scan. Arrow shows the right inferior rectus muscle vertically rotated and displaced inferiorly. Double arrow shows the normal orientation of the left inferior rectus muscle, tangential to the globe. Bone fragments of the orbital floor surround the right inferior rectus muscle both nasally and temporally.

union, it is usually possible to treat a fracture as an acute condition for up to 3 weeks following injury. During the first 3 weeks, the surgeon may evaluate the progress of spontaneous recovery by monitoring the child's visual acuity, ocular motility, diplopia in the primary and reading positions, and exophthalmometry every few days. Surgery is indicated if enophthalmus begins to develop or ocular motility does not improve significantly during this period.

The presence of crepitation—a sign of communication between the ethmoid sinus and the subcutaneous and orbital tissues—requires antibiotic therapy against nasal and paranasal flora.

Blow-out fractures can be approached surgically through either the orbit or the maxillary sinus. Advantages of the orbital approach include direct visualization of the fracture, ability to free entrapped tissue, and exploration and protection of the ocular contents. Visualization of the fracture permits gentle removal of incarcerated tissue. Repair of bony defects is best achieved with the use of synthetic material, such as Silastic or Teflon, or by autografts with iliac bone and rib cartilage.

Extraocular muscle surgery is performed in most children with visually handicapping diplopia that persists longer than 3 weeks after injury. This usually consists of recession of the inferior rectus muscle until the eye can move upward freely in a forced duction test; 3 to 6 months later, a transposition procedure of the medial and lateral rectus muscles to 3 mm behind the original insertion of the paralytic inferior rectus muscle is performed.

Residual enophthalmus or diplopia several months after a blow-out fracture must be approached differently. Late repair of orbital fractures is usually disappointing in regard to improvement of motility defects. Efforts are directed to achieve single binocular vision in the primary and reading positions by operating on the extraocular muscles of the involved eye, as well as those of the contralateral eye.

REFERENCES

1. Agapitos PJ, Noel LP, Clarke WN: Traumatic hyphema in children, *Ophthalmology* 94:1238-1241, 1987.
2. Antonyshyn O, Gruss JS, Kassel EE: Blow-in Fractures of the Orbit, *Plast Reconst Surg* 84:10-20, 1989.
3. Bloom JN: Traumatic hyphema in children, *Pediatr Ann* 19:368-375, 1990.
4. Deutsch TA, Weinreb RN, Goldberg MF: Indications for surgical management of hyphema in patients with sickle cell trait, *Arch Ophthalmol* 102:566-569, 1984.
5. Dutton JJ, Manson PN, Iliff N et al: Management of blow-out fractures of the orbital floor. *Surv Ophthalmol* 35:279-98, 1991.
6. Friendly DS: Ocular manifestations of physical child abuse, *Trans Am Acad Ophthalmol* 75:318-332, 1971.
7. Gilbard S, Mafee M, Lagouros P et al: Orbital blowout fractures, *Ophthalmology* 92:1523-8, 1985.
8. Goldberg MF: Antifibrinolytic agents in the management of traumatic hyphema, *Arch Ophthalmol* 101:1029-1030, 1983.
9. Greenwald MJ, Boston D, Pensler JM et al: Orbital roof fractures in childhood, *Ophthalmology* 96:491-497, 1989.
10. Greenwald MJ, Weiss A, Oesterle CS et al: Traumatic retinoschisis in battered babies, *Ophthalmology* 93:618-625, 1986.
11. Kersten RC: Blowout fracture of the orbital floor with entrapment caused by isolated trauma to the orbital rim, *Am J Ophthalmol* 103:215-220, 1987.
12. Levin AV: Ocular manifestations of child abuse, *Ophthalmol Clin N Am* 3:249-264, 1990.
13. Palmer DJ, Goldberg MF, Frenkel M et al: A comparison of two dose regimens of epsilon aminocaproic acid in the prevention and management of secondary traumatic hyphemas, *Ophthalmology* 93:102-108, 1986.

37 Dental Trauma

Lezley P. McIlveen and Donald J. Forrester

DENTOALVEOLAR INJURY
Epidemiology of dental trauma

Injury to the permanent dentition is twice as common in males as in females and is usually the result of a fall, fight, motor vehicle crash, or sports injury. In the primary dentition this ratio is reduced, but males are still more likely to sustain a dental injury than females. Falls are the main etiology of dental trauma in the primary dentition. Other less common causes of dental trauma include seizures and child abuse. In both primary and permanent dentitions the teeth most commonly affected are the maxillary central incisors, followed by the mandibular central incisors and maxillary lateral incisors. Luxation injuries tend to be more common in the primary dentition, whereas crown fractures predominate in the permanent dentition. There is also a seasonal variation in the frequency of traumatic injuries, such that an increased number of cases occur during the warmer months. Individuals with protruding upper incisors and insufficient lip closure are at increased risk for dental trauma. Orthodontic correction of this malocclusion should be initiated as soon as possible. Protective mouth guards have been shown to reduce significantly the incidence of sports-related dental trauma and are indicated for use during all active contact sports.

Dentoalveolar injuries can be classified in the following categories (Fig. 37-1): (1) hard tissue and pulp injuries, (2) injuries to periodontal tissues, and (3) alveolar fractures.

Injury to the hard tissue and pulp. These injuries are classified as complicated or uncomplicated, depending on whether the dental pulp is exposed (complicated, Fig. 37-2) or not (uncomplicated, Fig. 37-3). In the former case, bacterial contamination of the dental pulp can lead to infection and necrosis. The prognosis is more favorable for an uncomplicated fracture.

Many uncomplicated fractures involve the enamel only. If the fracture is more extensive, however, the dentin is exposed. A common complaint with this type of injury is sensitivity to cold liquids or air. Management of this type of uncomplicated fracture is aimed at protecting the exposed sensitive dentin. A protective base of calcium hydroxide is placed over the exposed dentin as soon as possible. This provides thermal and chemical insulation and is followed by a temporary restoration. An esthetic restoration is placed at a later date. The prognosis for uncomplicated fracture is usually favorable.

Complicated fractures by definition involve the dental pulp. Prognosis depends on the size of the exposure and the length of time the pulp has been exposed. To preserve pulp vitality therefore, therapy should be instituted as soon as possible. Primary teeth with this type of injury are generally extracted. In light of the potential for pulpal necrosis following such injuries, periodic evaluation by a dentist familiar with their management is recommended.

Root fracture involves the dentin, pulp, and cementum and is more common in the maxillary central incisor area of patients between 11 and 20 years old. In the younger age group, incomplete root formation of permanent teeth coupled with their various stages of eruption is associated with luxation injuries (Fig. 37-4). In the primary dentition, root fractures are more likely to occur in children

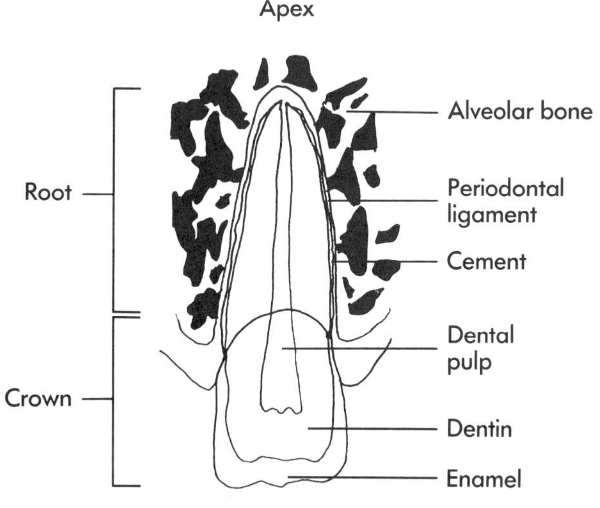

Figure 37–1 Basic dental anatomy.

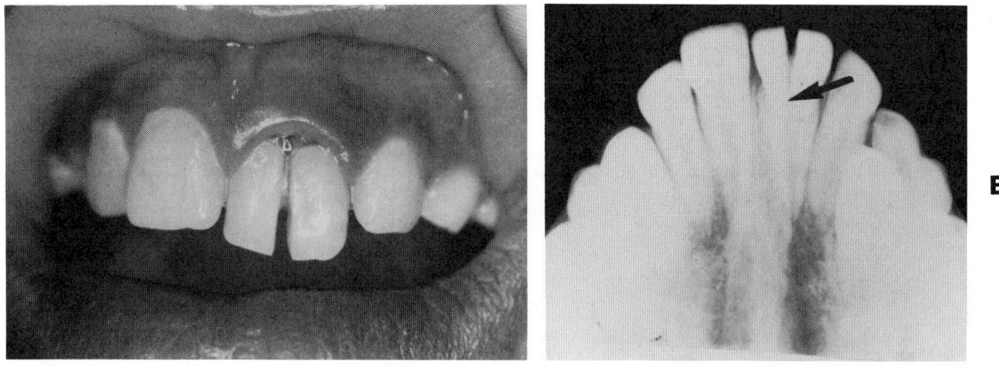

Figure 37–2 A, Complicated fracture of maxillary permanent central incisor. **B,** Intraoral dental radiograph demonstrating fracture and pulpal involvement.

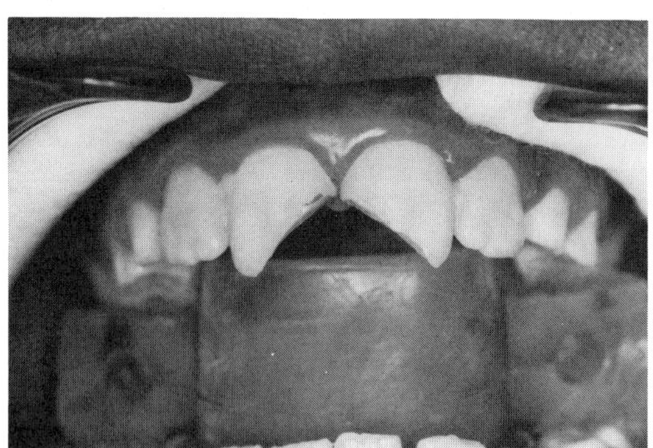

Figure 37–3 Uncomplicated fracture of maxillary central incisors.

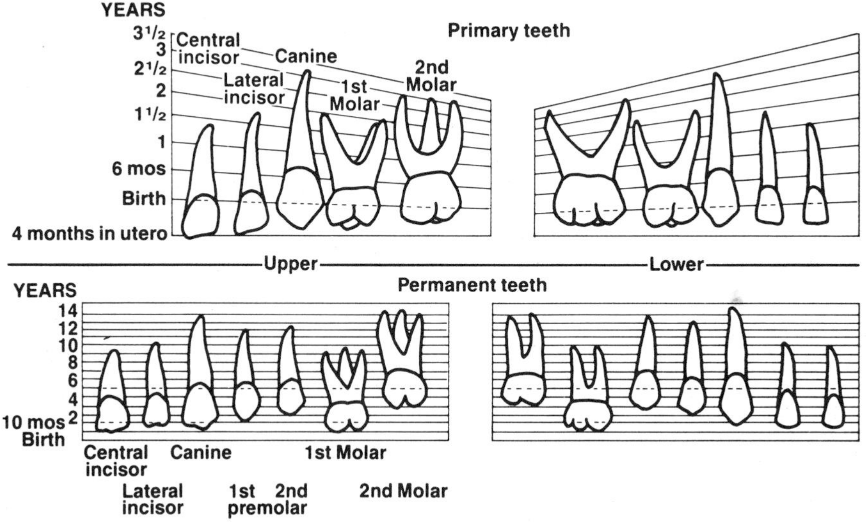

Figure 37–4 Chronology of tooth development in gross labial view. (From Glick PL: Mineralization of the teeth: prenatal and postnatal nutrient requirement. In Wei SHY, editor: *Pediatric dental care: an update for the pediatrician,* New York, 1978, Medcom.)

aged 3 to 4 when physiologic root resorption has commenced and resulted in a weakening of the root (Fig. 37-5). The location of the fracture determines the degree of mobility of the coronal fragment; for example, fractures in the coronal half of the root show greater mobility and displacement than fractures in the apical segment. The affected tooth tends to be lingually displaced and extruded. However, wide individual variation in tooth position and eruption can mask crown displacement and complicate diagnosis of root fractures. As a result, root fractures are easily overlooked during clinical evaluation. Intraoral dental radiographs are required for determination of the exact location of the fracture—most root fractures are located in the middle third of the root. If this type of injury is suspected the dental service should be consulted immediately.

Permanent teeth require rigid fixation with an acid-etch resin splint for a period of 2 to 3 months, coupled with radiographic observation and pulp vitality tests to detect pulpal necrosis. Primary teeth with root fractures and minimal dislocation can be preserved, and subsequent normal exfoliation is the rule. If displacement is severe, the coronal fragment should be extracted in light of the potential for pulp necrosis and damage to the permanent tooth bud. The apical root fragment should be left in place to prevent trauma to the permanent tooth bud; physiologic resorption of this fragment will occur.

Injury to the periodontium. The tooth is supported in the socket by the periodontal ligament, which consists of elastic collagen fibers. These fibers can be broken by trauma to the tooth, which results in increased mobility, displacement, or heightened sensitivity.

Luxation injuries represent 15% to 40% of traumas to the permanent dentition and 60% to 70% of injuries to the primary dentition. The most commonly involved teeth are the maxillary incisors. The force and direction of impact and the age of the patient significantly influence the type of luxation injury. Wide variation in individual tooth position and eruption can complicate diagnosis of displacement injuries.

Concussion. The periodontal ligament sustains only minor injury, so that no loosening or displacement occurs. The tooth may be sensitive, and a marked reaction to percussion can be elicited from the patient. Affected teeth do not generally require any intervention; however, because of the potential for pulpal necrosis, they should be monitored radiographically for 1 year.

Subluxation. This type of injury generally results in abnormal mobility and sensitivity to percussion and occlusal forces, although normal position in the dental arch is retained. Hemorrhage may be observed at the gingival margin and is a result of damage to the periodontal tissues (Fig. 37-6). Teeth showing minimal mobility generally do not require splinting. If considerable mobility of a tooth is detected during clinical examination, however, an injury of this type should be referred for immediate therapy. An acid-etch splint should be placed to immobilize the tooth and facilitate healing of the periodontal tissues. The tooth should also be monitored radiographically for 1 year.

Intrusive luxation. In injuries of this type teeth are displaced into the alveolar bone, which leads

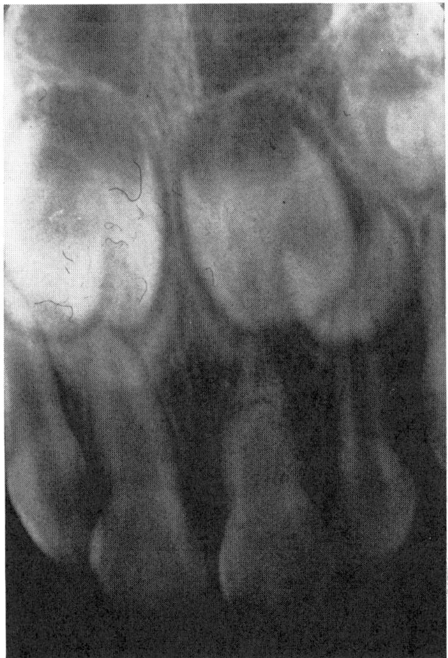

Figure 37-5 Dental radiograph demonstrating apical third root fracture of maxillary primary left central incisor.

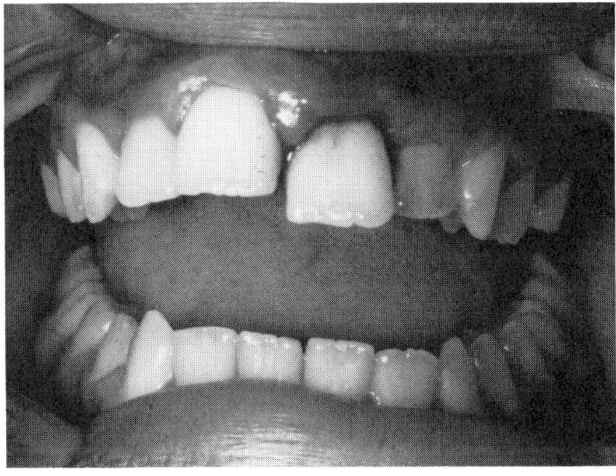

Figure 37-6 Hemorrhage at gingival margin secondary to subluxation of maxillary left central incisor.

to comminution or fracture of the socket. If a tooth is completely intruded, it may give the appearance of being avulsed. To rule out the possibility of avulsion and confirm intrusion, an intraoral dental radiographic examination is required. Intruded primary teeth must be evaluated radiographically to determine their position relative to the developing permanent teeth (Fig. 37-7). Intruded primary teeth usually reerupt spontaneously within several months. However, if the apices of the primary teeth are displaced toward the permanent sucessor (and the crown displaced labially) and a dental radiograph indicates that the apex is in close proximity to the crown of the permanent sucessor, the primary tooth should be extracted. Intrusive luxation injuries have a very poor prognosis, especially if root formation is complete. Revascularization is more easily established in teeth with an open apex, thus increasing the probability of pulp survival. Therefore, waiting for spontaneous reeruption of intruded permanent teeth is contraindicated. Immediate dental consultation and orthodontic repositioning are necessary.

Extrusive luxation. In extrusive luxation injuries teeth are partially displaced out of the socket, appearing elongated and lingually displaced upon

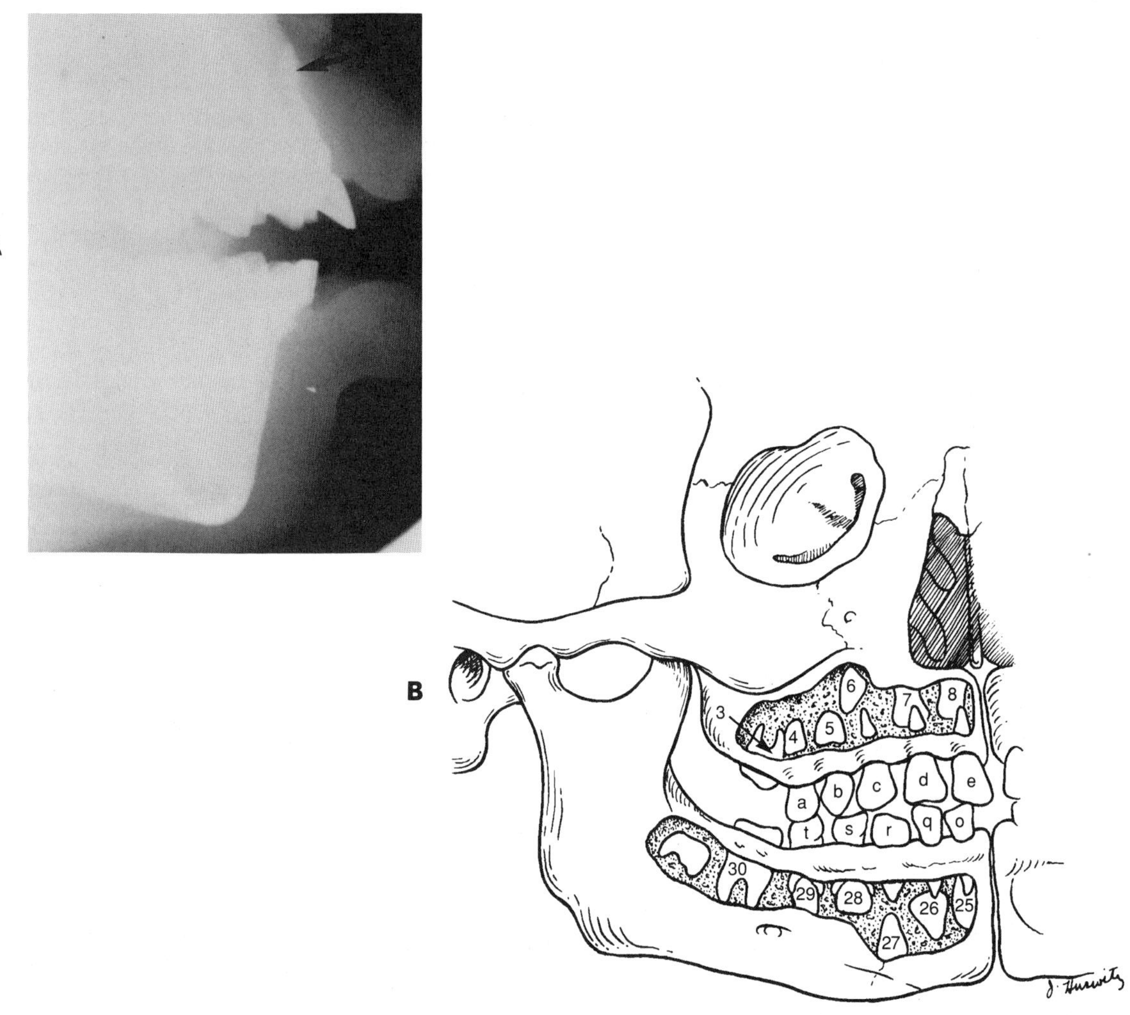

Figure 37–7 A, Dental lateral radiograph used to determine location of the apex of an intruded primary relative to the permanent tooth. In this film the apex of the primary tooth has been displaced labially (away from the permanent successor). **B,** Relative position of primary and permanent teeth in a 6-year-old child, demonstrating the close relationship of the developing permanent teeth and roots of the primary teeth. Letters are used to identify primary teeth, and numbers to identify permanent teeth.

clinical examination. Hemorrhage around the gingival margin is also noted (Fig. 37-8). Primary teeth with this kind of injury are usually extracted, but permanent teeth can be repositioned by digital pressure and immobilized—if the patient seeks immediate medical or dental attention. Otherwise, the teeth become consolidated in their new positions. They should be repositioned orthodontically or allowed to align spontaneously. Early dental intervention and close follow-up is essential, as many of these teeth undergo pulpal necrosis. Prognosis is more favorable if root formation is incomplete.

Lateral luxation. In this type of injury the tooth is displaced in a direction other than axially. The crown is usually displaced lingually, and an associated fracture of the socket wall is present. In individuals with rotations and unusual inclination of the maxillary incisors, evaluation of lingual displacement is often difficult. Management of such injury is similar to that of intrusive luxation. Prognosis, however, is more favorable.

Avulsion. This term describes all injuries in which a tooth is completely displaced from the alveolus (Fig. 37-9). The teeth most commonly affected are the maxillary incisors. The age group most commonly affected includes children 7 to 10 years old. The loosely attached periodontal ligament fibers around erupting teeth makes them prone to avulsion. Reimplantation of teeth has been considered a temporary measure because many of these teeth develop root resorption and are eventually lost, although they can remain functional for many years. The prognosis of this type of injury is significantly affected by two factors: (1) the length of the extraalveolar period and (2) the conditions under which an avulsed tooth has been stored.

Chances for a good prognosis are considerably reduced if the extraalveolar period is greater than 2 hours, in that 95% of the teeth show resorption. However, if the time is reduced to less than 30 minutes, only 10% of the teeth will show root resorption. The manner in which a tooth is stored is also significant. It is essential that the tooth be kept moist; drying of the periodontal ligament fibers is associated with a less favorable prognosis. An appropriate storage medium is milk or saline. If neither of these are available, saliva can be used. Removal of the periodontal tissue also worsens the prognosis. Therefore, parents should be instructed not to scrub the root surface. As in intrusion injuries, teeth with incomplete root formation have a better prognosis.

Reimplantation of primary teeth is not recommended because of the significant potential for damage to the permanent successors. If parents do not want to reimplant the tooth themselves,

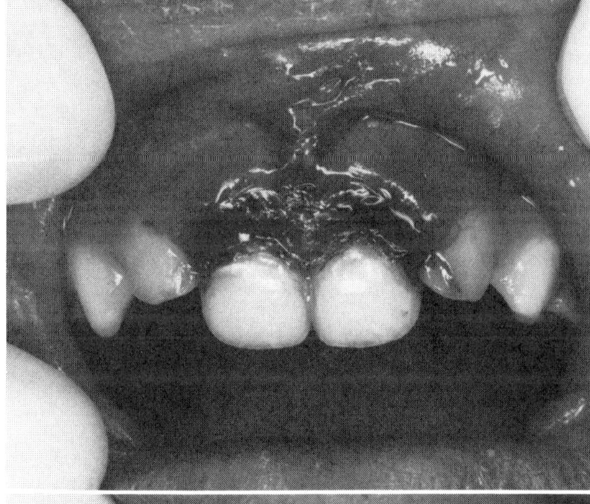

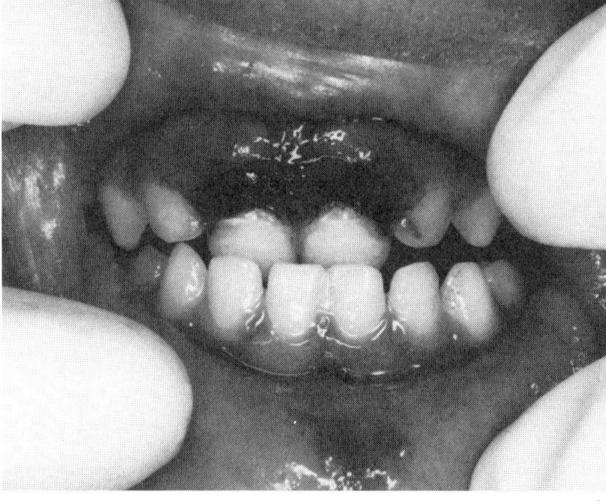

Figure 37–8 A, Extrusion of maxillary primary central incisors. **B,** Disruption of occlusion is often associated with displacement injuries.

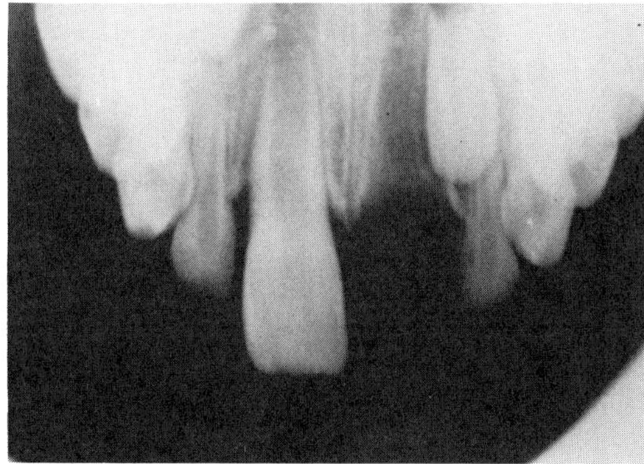

Figure 37–9 Dental radiograph confirming avulsion of maxillary left permanent central incisor.

Table 37–1 Management of avulsed teeth

1. Find the tooth.
2. Hold the tooth by the crown.
3. Clean the tooth by rinsing under gently running water (put the plug in the sink) or by agitating in milk or water. *Do not scrub the tooth.*

   If parents feel comfortable in doing so, they should be instructed to reimplant the tooth as follows:
4. Insert the tooth in the socket, using digital pressure. Check that the tooth is correctly oriented buccolingually.
5. Have the child bite on a large gauze pad or on a towel to hold the tooth in position.
6. Go *immediately* to a hospital emergency room or to a dentist.

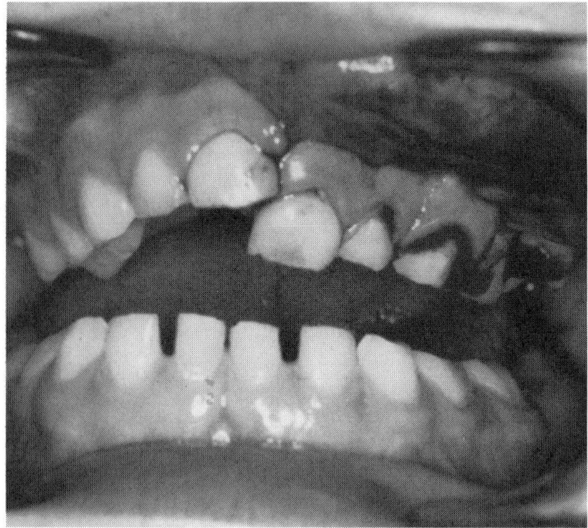

Figure 37–10 Alveolar fracture. (Courtesy of Gerber Products Co.)

they should be instructed to place the tooth in milk and seek medical or dental care immediately (Table 37-1).

If the tooth cannot be located, the possibility of aspiration should be considered. Tetanus prophylaxis should also be considered inasmuch as many avulsed teeth and concomitant wounds are soil contaminated. Ater reimplantation, an acid-etch splint should be placed as soon as possible. Dental follow-up is essential inasmuch as complex pulpal therapy is generally required.

Alveolar fracture. This injury tends to be more common in the adult population and is often associated with other dental injuries, such as extrusive or lateral luxations and root fractures. A fracture located apical to the apices of the teeth often involves the alveolar socket (Fig. 37-10). Clinical diagnosis of this injury is relatively simple, owing to displacement of the fragment. In addition, when mobility of a single tooth is tested, adjacent teeth are seen to move simultaneously. Radiographic examination may not reveal the fracture in spite of strong clinical evidence.

Alveolar fractures of the primary dentition are encountered prior to eruption of the primary dentition as there is little or no support in the lateral segments.

Treatment of an alveolar fracture involves the placement of an acid-etch splint for 4 weeks; this period can be reduced to 3 weeks in children. An acid-etch splint or arch bars are used for fixation. In the young child with teeth inadequate for splinting it may be necessary to use an acrylic splint and perimandibular wiring. If the fracture can be reduced to a stable position, the splinting procedure can be omitted and the patient restricted to a soft or liquid diet.

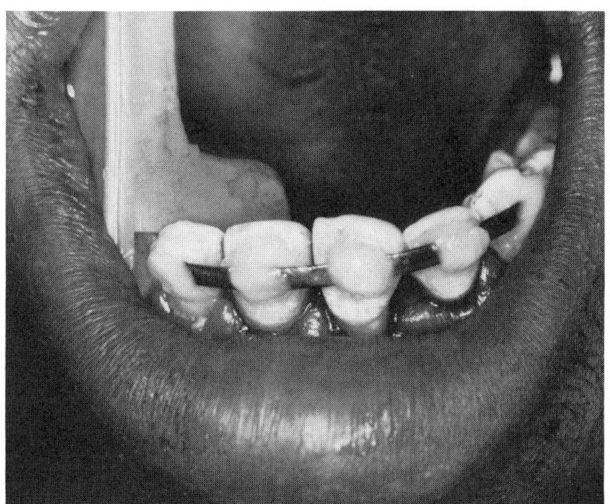

Figure 37–11 Acid-etch splint.

Splinting modalities. Methods of stabilization have traditionally consisted of arch bars, wire, or acrylic splints. More recently, use of the acid-etch technique has allowed the development of a splinting technique that closely approximates the ideal (Fig. 37-11). Other splinting modalities have significant disadvantages. Interdental wiring has a distinct disadvantage in that during tightening of the wires, extrusion of mobile teeth can occur. If an arch bar is used, correct positioning of the teeth may not be achieved, owing to difficulties in exact adaptation of the bar to the dental arch. Acrylic splints are useful if there are insufficient adjacent teeth for support; however, the impression technique required to fabricate this splint further traumatizes the periodontium. A useful alternative is the suture splint (Fig. 37-12), especially in cases

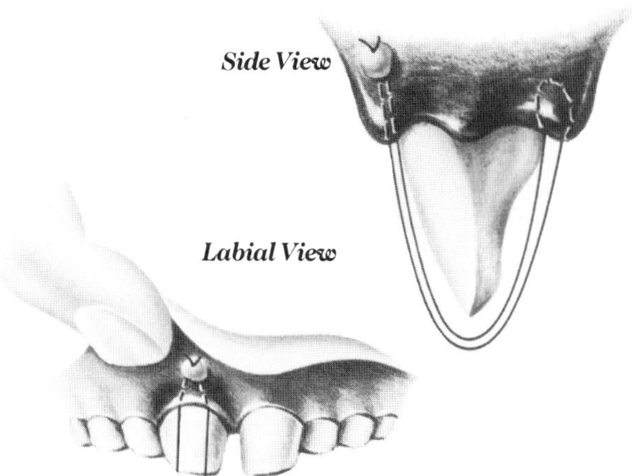

Figure 37–12 Suture splint. (From Dentoalveolar trauma, *AAOMS Surg Update,* winter, 1987-88.)

in which a partially erupted tooth presents an inadequate area for etching.

MANDIBULAR FRACTURE

Fractures of the facial skeleton are relatively uncommon in children as compared with adults. Fractures of the nasal bones and the mandible account for the great majority of facial fractures in the pediatric population. In an analysis of 1088 facial fractures, Hall found that 46.6% involved the nasal bones and 24.2% involved the mandible.[5] Common sites of mandibular fracture include the condyle, the angle, and the subcondylar region. Symphysis and parasymphysis fractures are more common in children than in adults, and body fractures are rare. The most commonly reported etiologies of facial fractures in children are falls, motor vehicle crashes, and sports injuries. The possibility of child abuse should also be considered.

Diagnosis

Clinical evaluation. The signs and symptoms of mandibular fracture are described below.

Change in facial contour. Although swelling and ecchymoses can mask changes in facial contour, the mandibular arch form should be inspected for any change in contour or symmetry. The locations of contusions should be noted, as these can provide information about the direction and force of the trauma and the site of a fracture. Palpation should progress bilaterally from the condylar region along the lower border of the mandible. The presence of point tenderness or a step deformity is pathognomic of a fracture.

Crepitus. If no obvious displacement is noted, manual palpation should be performed. The forefingers of each hand should be placed on the oc-

clusal surfaces of the mandibular teeth, and the thumbs on the inferior border of the mandible. Starting at the right retromolar area and maintaining a space of several teeth between the fingers, the hands are moved around the arch. An alternate up-and-down movement is performed. Abnormal mobility or crepitus is elicited across the fracture site.

Parasthesia. Changes in sensation in the lower lip may be associated with lip and chin lacerations. However, parasthesia or anesthesia in the distribution of the inferior alveolar nerve is strongly indicative of a fracture distal to the mandibular foramen (Fig. 37-13).

Abnormal mandibular movement. Limitation of opening due to muscle spasm or pain is a common finding. Certain mandibular fractures are associated with specific abnormal mandibular movements. For example, as a result of unopposed lateral pterygoid muscle function, unilateral subcondylar fractures show mandibular deviation toward the side of the fracture. If bilateral subcondylar fractures are present, the patient will show mandibular retrognathia and open bite because of the resultant short ramus and depressor action of the suprahyoid muscles. Inability to open the mandible may be caused by the coronoid process impinging on the zygoma, as the result of either a coronoid or ramus fracture or a zygomatic arch fracture.

Change in occlusion. A wide range of occlusal disharmonies can occur as a result of mandibular fractures. Inspection of the occlusal plane may reveal the presence of a step deformity at the fracture site. Anterior alveolar process fracture or parasymphyseal fractures may produce premature tooth contact that is manifested as a posterior open bite.

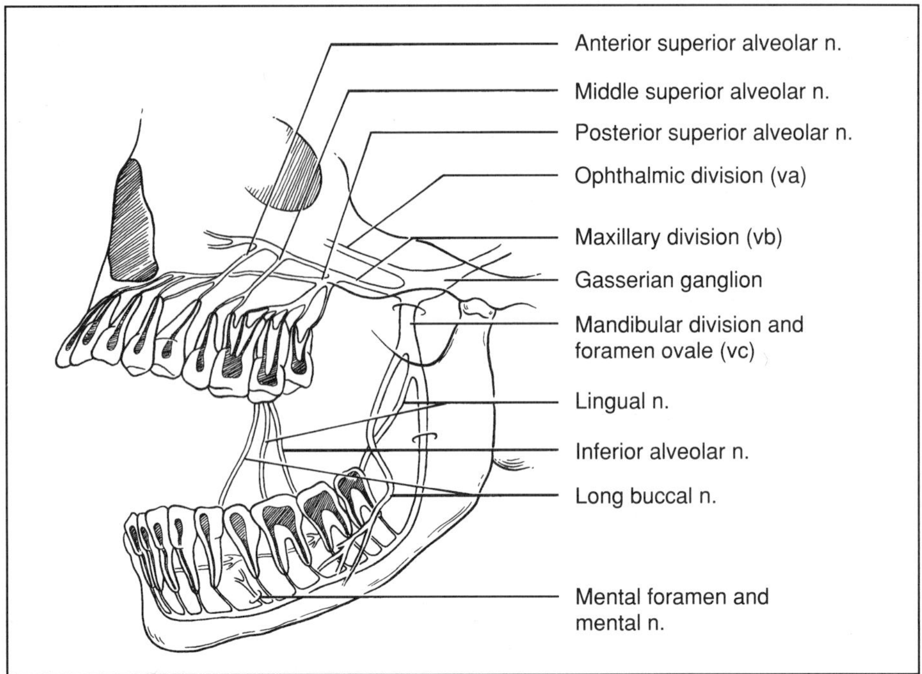

Figure 37–13 Innervation of the dentition and the supporting structures. (From Cooke-Waite Laboratories: *Manual of local anesthesia in dentistry,* ed 3, Rochester: Eastman Kodak, 1980, p 26.)

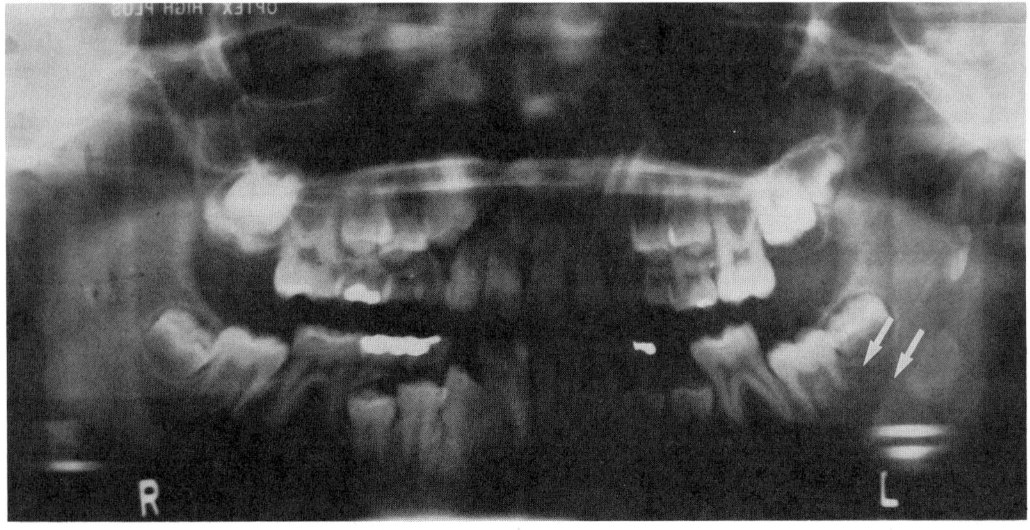

Figure 37–14 Panoramic radiograph. Left angle fracture of the mandible in an 11-year-old male.

In general, any change in occlusion should be considered strongly suggestive of a mandibular fracture.

Hematoma. The presence of a hematoma in the buccal sulcus may follow a blow to the lower jaw that was insufficient to cause a fracture. However, if it is located in the floor of the mouth, a hematoma indicates a fracture of the mandibular body or symphysis.

Radiographic examination. The views recommended for radiographic examination of mandibular fractures are described below.

Panoramic. This is the single most informative view of the mandible (Fig. 37-14). The main disadvantage is that the patient needs to be upright and that buccolingual displacement or medial condyle displacement is difficult to appreciate. If a

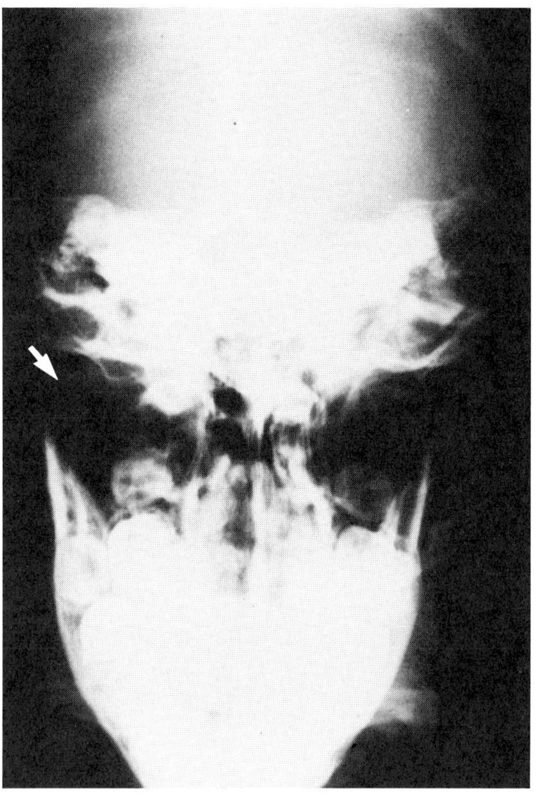

Figure 37–15 Towne's view demonstrating fractured and medially displaced fractured condyle.

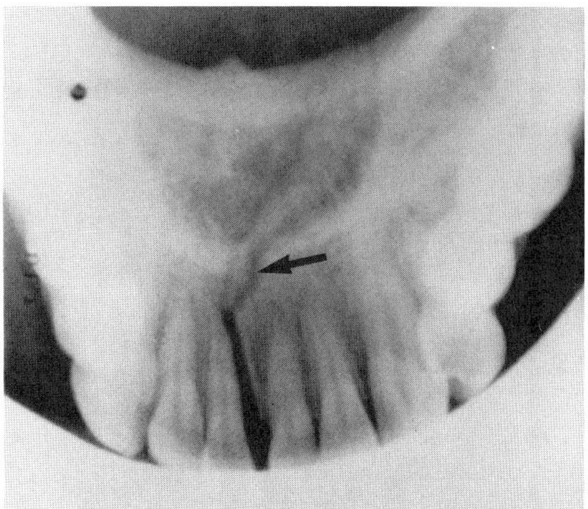

Figure 37–16 Mandibular occlusal radiograph.

panoramic view is combined with a posteroanterior view, further radiographs are not required and the radiation dose to the patient is therefore minimized.

Lateral oblique. This view demonstrates fractures of the ramus, angle, and posterior body of the mandible. The condylar, symphysis, and bicuspid regions are obscured.

Posteroanterior. Displacement of the body and angle are well demonstrated in this view. However, the condyle area is obscured.

Reverse Towne's. This view is used to show medial displacement of the condyle and condylar fractures (Fig. 37-15).

Mandibular occlusal. This intraoral view demonstrates fractures in the symphysis area, the relationship of teeth to the fracture site, and the damage to the teeth themselves (Fig. 37-16).

Considerations in the management of mandibular fractures in children

Anatomic variation, patient cooperation, the potential for disruption of mandibular or dental development, and rapidity of healing in the child are all factors that need to be taken into account when managing mandibular fractures. Treatment should

be carried out as soon as possible after the injury. The high osteogenic potential of the periosteum and the increased metabolic rate in the child result in early union. Consequently, bone fragments may become partially united in 4 days and stable in 7 days. The period of immobilization is also reduced in treatment of the child patient. If at the initial evaluation the fracture is firm, even though the fragments are not ideally reduced, refracturing the mandible is not indicated. Continued growth and development of the mandible and dentition will often compensate for imperfect reduction of fracture in a child.

Greenstick fractures are more common in this age group owing to the elasticity of the developing bone. These fractures tend to be long and oblique and extend down and forward from the upper body of the mandible. Multiple unerupted permanent teeth occupy large areas of the body of the mandible and are frequently located in the line of fracture. These teeth should be retained. However, disturbed formation has been reported in 72% of immature teeth involved in the line of fracture. Placement of intraosseous wires, plates, or pins can also traumatize developing tooth buds and lead to failure of eruption of permanent teeth and atrophy of the alveolar ridge.

Immobilization techniques require modification depending on the age of the child and the stage of dental development. If the primary teeth are unerupted or few primary teeth are present, an acrylic splint is fabricated (Gunning splint). Perimandibular wires are used to retain the splint. Intermaxillary fixation is used if the fracture cannot be adequately immobilized by the splint alone; that is, if the fracture is located in the posterior region of the body beyond the maximum possible extension of the splint.

Condylar fracture has been reported to result in disturbance of mandibular growth and development, thus leading to facial asymmetry. Most studies indicate that growth abnormalities are rare and tend to be associated with prolonged immobilization or crush injuries to the condyle. The majority of condylar fractures can be treated conservatively with analgesics and a liquid diet for 5 to 7 days. If mandibular deviation is present, training elastics or midline opening exercises are recommended. In children, remodeling of the fractured and displaced condyle occurs to a greater extent than in adults and postpubertal adolescents, so that the ramal height on the fractured side may exceed that of the nonfractured side. Even in cases of bilateral fracture a reconstituted condyle is frequently located in the glenoid fossa.

Crushing injury of the condylar cartilage in young children may result in ankylosis. The condylar cartilage in the young child shows greater vascularity than in the adult. Crushing injury to this area may be associated with considerable hemorrhage, disturbance of the remodeling process, ossification of the hematoma, and ankylosis. Close follow-up of injuries of this type is essential, as surgical intervention may be indicated to minimize or prevent significant facial deformity. Children who have a history of trauma to the chin should be carefully evaluated for this type of injury, as it is easily overlooked and early intervention is essential for a favorable prognosis.

REFERENCES

1. Andreasen JO: *Traumatic injuries of the teeth*, Philadelphia, 1981, WB Saunders.
2. Banks P: *Killey's fractures of the mandible*, London, 1991, Wright.
3. Bruce R, Fonseca RJ: Mandibular fractures. In Fonseca RJ, Walker RV, editors: *Oral and maxillofacial trauma*, Philadelphia, 1991, WB Saunders.
4. Cameron YS, McCullom C, Blaustein DI: Pediatric chin injury: occult condylar fractures of the mandible, *Ped Emerg Care* 7:160-163, 1991.
5. Hall RK, Thomas G, Buzowski G: *Ten-year survey of traumatic injuries to the face and jaws of children, 1970 to 1979: a computer analysis.* Paper presented at the eighth International Conference on Oral Surgery, Berlin, 1983.
6. Hurt TL, Fisher B, Peterson BM et al: Mandibular fractures in association with chin trauma in pediatric patients, *Ped Emerg Care* 4:121-123, 1988.
7. James D: Maxillofacial injuries. In Row NL, Williams JL, editors: *Maxillofacial injuries*, New York, 1991, Churchill Livingston.
8. Kaban LB: *Pediatric oral and maxillofacial surgery*, Philadelphia, 1990, WB Saunders, pp 242-260.
9. Perez R, Berkowitz R, McIlveen L et al: Dental trauma in children, *J Endod Dent Traumatol* 7:1-2, 1991.

Otolaryngologic Injury

38 Otolaryngologic Injury

Gregory Milmoe

If one views the head and neck region as the intake organ of the body for respiration, alimentation, and sensation, then injuries in this area assume relevance to the extent that they affect these functions. The aesthetic and communicative aspects of facial and cervical injuries are also important.

In the immediate management of otolaryngologic injury, airway, mechanics of breathing, and circulation are primary in importance. Ability to secure the airway by a variety of means is an essential attribute of a trauma facility. This is all the more important in the treatment of children, given the smaller limits of tolerance for the pediatric airway. Hemorrhage, particularly epistaxis, can complicate the task of stabilizing the airway.

Injury to other otolaryngologic structures commonly accompanies cerebral trauma and facial skeleton injuries. Often these injuries are not life-threatening, but they can pose a large obstacle to successful rehabilitation if overlooked. Frequently, such injury is a clue to more threatening problems (e.g., hemotympanum, retropharyngeal air). For this discussion, topics will be presented by region.

EAR

Trauma to the ear can be divided by anatomic site of injury to the pinna, canal, drum and middle ear, and inner ear and temporal bone.

For the pinna, mechanism of injury leads to further subdivision. Blunt trauma can result in an auricular hematoma, producing a cauliflower ear deformity. In addition, structural collapse occurs when an abscess results in perichondritis, which causes the elevation of the perichondrium away from the cartilage, thus depriving it of a blood supply. The appropriate acute treatment is needle aspiration of the blood and application of a pressure dressing, which pads both the lateral and medial aspects of the ear lobe so that a child will tolerate the dressing. Administration of an antibiotic and repeated aspiration are often necessary for effective care. Through-and-through drainage is reserved for extensive injury, especially for injuries that accompany laceration. Frequent dressing change permits inspection over the course of 7 to 10 days, usually every other day.

Mechanisms of penetrating trauma include lacerations and bites, either human or animal. Careful debridement is important to preserve cartilage and to prevent tattoo formation. Meticulous suture technique is required to avoid a step-off deformity, which is easily visible on the helical rim. Animal and human bites place a severe limitation on the extent of primary repair as a consequence of the saliva-induced bacterial contamination. Administration of an appropriate antibiotic helps reduce the complications of infection. Loss of tissue can be overcome to some degree along the helical rim, but often secondary reconstruction is necessary.

Thermal injury at both extremes is devastating. Both scalding and flame burns will destroy cartilage readily; topical care helps to prevent unsightly deformity. Management of frostbite to the pinna is similar to the approach to cold injury to the extremities: gradual warming and protection from barotrauma.

TRAUMA TO THE CANAL AND TYMPANIC MEMBRANE

Self-inflicted injury is the most common type of injury to the ear canal. Children often insert various objects into the ear canal, either spontaneously or in imitation of a parent's attempt at wax removal. Pain and bleeding usually ensue. Fortunately, the external canal is angled so that objects ordinarily strike the posterior canal wall before engaging the tympanic membrane and the middle ear. The immediate pain eliminates further manipulation.

In other penetrating injuries, perforation of the tympanic membrane and damage to the ossicular chain are areas of concern. Barotrauma can also cause a blast injury to the drum. External pressure from a cupped hand against the ear, a firecracker, or blunt trauma to the head against a surface can tear the tympanic membrane. Excess internal pressure resulting from submersion during an underwater dive can also rupture the drum. If there is no acute vertigo or profound deafness, then management is conservative. Instillation of antibiotic drops is helpful if there is gross contamination. However, if vertigo or extreme hearing loss is present, assume inner ear damage. Moreover, tympanic membrane perforation or hemotympanum is a clue to the presence of basilar skull fracture. A blow to the mandible can also produce an ear canal laceration, with or without a drum tear, by displacing the mandibular condyle posteriorly.

Temporal bone fracture is a subset of basilar skull fracture. In fact, bloody otorrhea is taken as evidence for a basilar skull fracture until proven otherwise. One must obtain as detailed a history as possible of how the accident occurred, particularly if there had been loss of consciousness. Associated physical findings can include disorientation, mastoid battle sign, raccoon eyes, facial paralysis, nystagmus, gross cerebrospinal fluid (CSF) leak, deep lacerations, convulsions, and midface distortion.

In general, fracture of the temporal bone is grouped into two general categories with some overlap: longitudinal fracture and transverse fracture. The possible consequences in either type include sensorineural and conductive hearing loss, vertigo, facial paralysis, CSF leak, and subsequent meningitis. Longitudinal fractures are more common; they occur along the long axis of the petrous temporal bone and are accompanied by external canal laceration, a mild to moderate hearing loss, and the likelihood of normal facial nerve function. The less common transverse fractures are generally accompanied by only a hemotympanum, although a tear within the canal can occur. There is a 50% chance of both facial nerve injury and a profound hearing loss.

In all children arriving at the emergency room with blood or cerebrospinal fluid coming from the ear, minimize instrumentation of the canal. This will lessen the risk of bacterial contamination and additional disruption or bleeding. Intravenous antibiotic administration is no substitute for sterile care; a sterile dressing will keep bacteria and rough hands out. Following an appropriate computed tomography (CT) scan, an otolaryngologist should examine the ear under sterile conditions with a microscope and suction. Appropriate auditory assessment will exclude a sensorineural hearing loss.

Facial paralysis can be immediate or delayed, partial or complete, peripheral or central. Often there is no chance to observe whether the onset was immediate, and, fortunately, many cases recover spontaneously. However, to avoid overlooking the case that would require surgical decompression, it is imperative to assess children with facial paralysis early. A child who manifests a complete, peripheral, indeterminate, or immediate onset facial paralysis requires a CT scan, utilizing a thin slice of the temporal bone, and electrophysiologic testing. If the child is cooperative, behavioral au-

diometry is in order; otherwise, an evoked response test is performed.

EPISTAXIS

Facial trauma frequently results in epistaxis. Usually it is of short duration and requires no active intervention, but sometimes the nasal bleeding is profuse and persistent. Measures to stop or reduce flow should proceed swiftly.

Examination of the pharynx is the first step. Significant amounts of blood can be swallowed with little evidence at the nares. The degree of midface fracture is also important. Unfortunately, a catheter or nasal pack can end up in the cranial cavity. One must identify several features of the nasal bleeding; most important is to determine which naris is involved and to what relative depth in the nose.

Before insertion of a nose pack, the surgeon must protect the airway and establish intravenous access. Airway protection may range from simply maintaining the child in the upright position and performing proper suctioning, to placing an endotracheal tube or tracheostomy. Epistaxis is more threatening as an airway risk than as a blood loss problem. Intravenous access allows continued fluid replacement and provision for necessary medications.

Several materials are available to pack the nose. The most readily obtainable are a Foley catheter and gelfoam strips (absorbable collagen). They are also the easiest to use and can be quickly and safely placed to control a nosebleed. Frequently, this will reduce but not eliminate the bleeding. One places the catheter in the side with the brisk bleeding far enough back to see the tip just below the palate. The balloon is then inflated to block the nasopharynx; most often a 5 cc balloon is sufficient for all but the largest children. At this point, more blood is coming from the front of the nose and one must quickly place several 5 cm-long strips of gelfoam alongside the catheter to stop the flow. The remaining leakage can be plugged by a cotton ball coated with antibiotic ointment or surgical lubricant. The catheter itself must be secured with a hemostat or umbilical clip. This cinches the balloon up against the back end of the septum. It is also wise to interpose a gauze sponge between the clip and the anterior nose; this avoids undue pressure on the cartilage, as well as its attendant pain and risk of necrosis. The pack is left in place for 2 to 3 days and antibiotics are administered.

If a more secure packing is necessary, the otolaryngologist will need to employ ribbon gauze, using proper lighting, suction, restraint, and equipment. It is unsafe and cruel to a child to allow free head movement. Additional personnel can provide restraint of the child and help with suctioning, both of which can have a calming effect. With a headlight, the otolaryngologist can then use a speculum to visualize the deeper structures of the nose, localize the bleeding, and apply a firmer packing by layering the ribbon gauze in long pieces from the back to the front. This may be preceded by placing a balloon catheter if posterior tamponade is required. The gauze should be coated with an antibiotic ointment. One major disadvantage of the ribbon gauze technique is the requirement to remove it. This procedure produces its own irritation, the possibility of bleeding, and some discomfort.

The presence of pressure necrosis makes commercial epistaxis balloons a less favorable choice. In addition, their points of pressure do not always coincide with the trauma-induced points of bleeding.

REFERENCES

1. Mitchell DP, Stone P: Temporal bone fractures in children, *Can J Otolaryngol* 2:156-162, 1973.
2. Myer CM III, Orobello P, Cotton RT et al: Blunt laryngeal trauma in children, *Laryngoscope* 97:1043-1048, 1987.
3. Parisier SC: Injuries of the ear and temporal bone. In Bluestone CD, Stool SE: *Pediatric otolaryngology,* ed 2, Philadelphia, 1990, WB Saunders.

39 Tracheobronchial Injury

Itzhak Vinograd and *Raphael Udassin*

Rupture of the tracheobronchial tree, although described well over 100 years ago, is very much a modern hazard. In children, in whom penetrating chest trauma is rare, tracheobronchial rupture is associated mainly with blunt chest trauma, often sustained in high-speed vehicle crashes, and with iatrogenic injury caused by modern diagnostic or therapeutic airway equipment. It is accepted that the incidence of traumatic airway rupture has increased at least tenfold over the past 20 years. Nevertheless, the overall incidence of this lesion remains low in comparison with other intrathoracic injuries. The trachea *does not frequently* sustain blunt or penetrating trauma. The sternum, mandible, vertebral column, and cervical musculature all serve as protection. The mobility and compressibility of the trachea further reduce the likelihood of injury should this area be subjected to deforming forces. The *true incidence* of tracheal trauma is probably somewhat greater than reported. First, many affected children suffer grave injuries and die before they arrive at the hospital, so that diagnosis is not made. Second, some victims of tracheal injury do not develop signs or symptoms until weeks or even months after they are first seen.

Although penetrating chest injuries are dramatic in presentation, blunt airway injuries are not always obvious and are easily overlooked, especially in children. Early recognition and prompt treatment can save lives; improper management or delayed diagnosis can result in long-term disability or even death.

This chapter limits itself to tracheal and bronchial trauma.

MODES OF TRAUMA AND MECHANISM OF INJURY

The trachea can be injured by internal or external agents. *Internal* injury can result from intubation, inhalation, or aspiration of a foreign body, *external* injury from either blunt or penetrating trauma. It is not clear which form of injury is more frequent (Figure 39-1).

Iatrogenic perforation of trachea

One of the most frustrating injuries is iatrogenic perforation of the trachea during bronchoscopy, especially when the trachea is inflamed secondary to the presence of a foreign body. During multiple insertions of a rigid bronchoscope, a perforation may occur. Blood seen during bronchoscopy should raise the suspicion of trauma to the trachea, and every attempt should be made to visualize all involved areas. The postbronchoscopy chest x-ray requires a thorough assessment for extratracheal air (Figure 39-2). A long-standing foreign body may produce severe inflammation sufficient to cause an acquired tracheoesophageal fistula.[9] This is possible, for example, when the object is a disc battery which may erode rapidly into the tracheal wall.

Tracheal injury may also occur during neonatal repair of congenital tracheoesophageal fistula when the separation of the esophagus is too close to the trachea, resulting in a narrowing of the trachea. Leave 1 or 2 mm of esophageal fistula attached to the tracheal wall to prevent such sequelae.

Rupture of a major airway as a result of *tracheal intubation* for anesthesia is rare. The inexperience of an operator, the intubation stylets used, and multiple attempts at intubation may all lead to rupture, regardless of the nature of the tube. Many endotracheal tubes have high-pressure cuffs, which, when overinflated, can produce tracheal rupture; and if the cuff inflates asymmetrically, as many of them do, it may also drive the tip of the tube into the trachea. Overdistension may occur when excessive volumes of air are injected in an attempt to obtain a good cuff seal or by diffusion of nitrous oxide into the balloon during prolonged anesthesia. The newer, softer polyvinyl chloride tubes with low-pressure concentric cuffs assume the high-pressure characteristics if more than 3 ml of air is used to inflate the balloon. Neonates, as well as young children, have been affected, although the premature infant is at greatest risk. Avoid the use of cuffed tubes up to a size no. 4 in all children. A catastrophe rarely seen is the *explosion of anesthetic gases* within the tracheobronchial lumen.

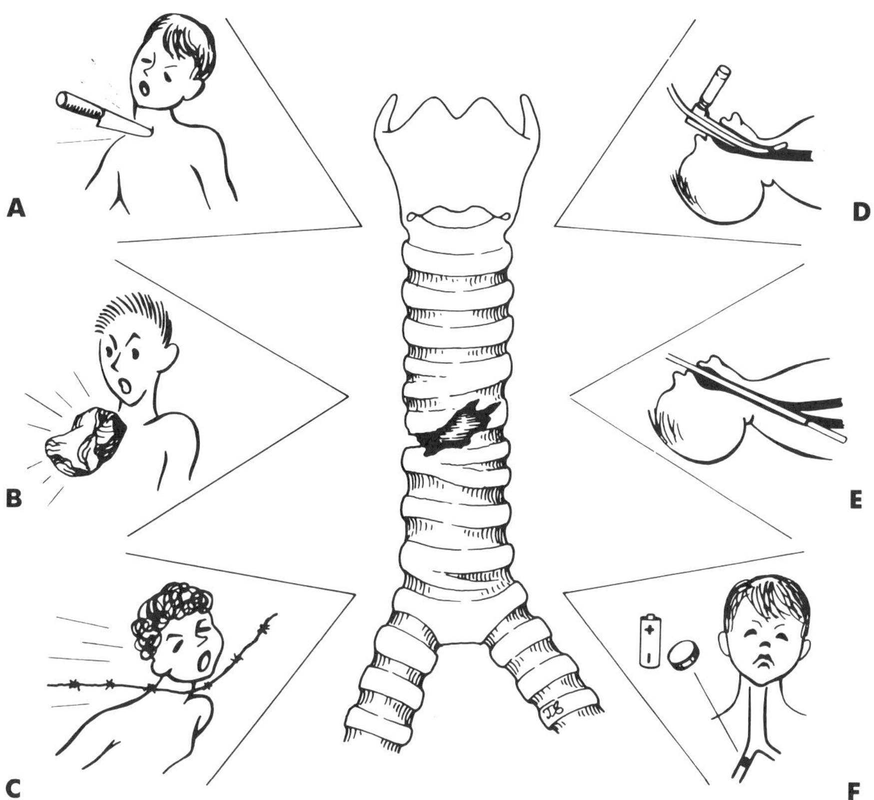

Figure 39–1 The most common causes for airway injury: external agents (**A–C**) and internal (**D–F**). In children, it is not clear which is more frequent.

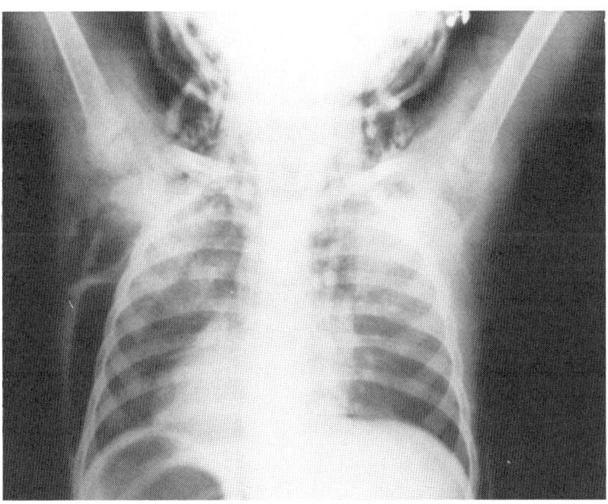

Figure 39–2 Chest x-ray of an 8-month-old girl with rupture of the right main bronchus secondary to an attempted removal of a foreign body. Note the massive amount of extratracheal air, and mediastinal and subcutaneous emphysema.

Application of *vigorous suction* with a catheter inserted too far into the endotracheal tube is yet another cause of tracheobronchial trauma in small infants. Iatrogenic bronchial perforation is suspected in an infant who deteriorates following endotracheal tube suction, who has a bloody endotracheal aspirate, or who has an air leak that is unresponsive to chest tube insertion. A *nasogastric tube* can cause the same injury when inadvertently passed into the trachea.

Expulsion of foreign body

Another mode of internal injury includes the violent backward fling of the head during an extremely strong cough to expel a *foreign body,* which may cause avulsion of the larynx and cricoid cartilage from the trachea. Such a strong cough may also cause a pressure gradient between the alveoli and interstitium, with resultant air dissection along the perivascular sheaths toward the mediastinum and pneumomediastinum.

Burn inhalation injury

Children who sustain a major flame burn in a closed space are exposed to direct injury to the tracheobronchial tree from the smoke. Trauma to the upper airway, including the supraglottic region, is much more likely than trauma to the lower airway. The natural cooling capacity of the upper airway mucosa absorbs the heat of the gases before they reach the trachea. Hot fumes will also cause a reflex closure of the glottis, affording excellent protection to the trachea and lungs. Steam injury is a major exception because the heat-carrying capacity of water-laden air is many times greater than that of dry air. Apparently inconsequential steam inhalation can cause severe lower airway damage prior to reflex glottic closure.

Penetrating injury

Penetrating injury, which is less common in children, can be caused by a gunshot, knife, or projectile object such as a stone. Children may also be injured by *impalement upon a sharp object* such as a stick or the edge of a brick. That penetrating trauma usually involves other adjacent organs adds to the complexity of the condition.

Direct blunt trauma

Blunt trauma may be direct to the cervical trachea or indirect to the thoracic tracheobronchial tree. External trauma to the larynx and cervical trachea in children is unusual, but the *use of minibikes and motorcycles* by young children is changing existing patterns of injury. A minibike is lower than a motorcycle, and the rider's neck is unprotected with the chin slightly elevated and the neck in extension. If the rider runs into an unseen wire or cable, it may compress the larynx and trachea against the cervical vertebrae. Transection of the trachea, recurrent nerves, and esophagus is possible even without laceration of the skin. Direct trauma to the laryngotracheal area compresses the trachea against the vertebral bodies, which results in a crush injury.

Hyperextension of the neck causes an avulsion injury by pulling the larynx away from the distal trachea, which is restricted in its excursion by surrounding tissue and by the left main stem bronchus which passes beneath the aortic arch. *Striking the neck against an unseen wire or chain while riding a motorcycle or snowmobile accounts for a number of such injuries.* The *padded dashboard syndrome* results when a passenger's head hits the windshield of a vehicle, the neck is hyperextended, and the exposed cervical trachea strikes the dashboard; the compression causes a fracture of contusion of the trachea.

Strangulation

Accidental hanging occurs in infants who become entangled in their clothing or bed linen. Unfortunately, hanging may also be the result of violent crime, including *child abuse.* Death by ligature strangulation, or garroting, involves the constriction of the neck by a ligature that is pulled tight by an assailant's hands, rather than by the victim's body weight. *Throttling,* or manual strangulation, is the compression of the neck by human hands.

Thoracic blunt trauma

Thoracic blunt trauma is still the most common cause of tracheobronchial injury in children. Perhaps the most unusual feature of the child with respect to thoracic trauma is the amazingly compliant thorax. The bony and cartilaginous structures are extremely flexible. It is common for a child to sustain major internal injury by compression of the chest without fracture of the bony thorax. Another major difference in the small patient that has significant physiologic consequences is found in the free movement of the mediastinum. The mediastinum of children, and particularly of infants, is capable of wide shifts with dislocation of the heart, with angulation of the great vessels, with compression of the lung, and with angulation of the trachea. The elasticity of the ribs in children reduces the frequency of recognized rib fractures in cases of blunt trauma, but there can still be severe damage to the intrathoracic contents, and to the liver, spleen, and kidneys within the abdomen.

The mechanism and pathophysiology of the tracheobronchial injury in blunt trauma are speculative, but most agree that at least two mechanisms are present. The first is a sudden, crushing anteroposterior compression of air in the tracheobronchial tree against a closed glottis (similar to traumatic asphyxia). This results in a lateral side-to-side widening of the lumen with subsequent disruption, distraction, and stretching in the area of the tracheobronchial carina. Second, contributing to the injury is a shear force between the bronchus and posterior vertebral column.

Anatomy and mechanism of injury

Knowledge of the anatomy of the mediastinum in the region of the tracheal bifurcation is important in understanding the mechanism of injury to the tracheobronchial tree. The distal trachea lies in the superior mediastinum. Uncomplicated tracheal or bronchial rupture or bronchial avulsion is caused by the relative fixation of the trachea, by the greater mobility of the tracheal bifurcation and major bronchi, and by an increase in intratracheobronchial pressure. That the distal trachea and right main bronchus overlie the vertebral bodies increases the likelihood of injury, because the immovable vertebral body thus becomes an anvil at the time of injury. Rupture of the great vessels may well be associated with tracheobronchial injury.

With a severe blow to the anterior thoracic wall, the anterior-posterior diameter of the chest is abruptly decreased, and several events take place simultaneously. As the anterior-posterior diameter of the chest is decreased, the transverse diameter is increased. Associated with this phenomenon is separation of the lungs and consequent stretching of the major bronchi, thus putting tension on the carina. If this force exceeds the elasticity of the tracheobronchial tissue, rupture occurs. The intrapleural and intrapulmonary pressure is increased significantly, which narrows the mediastinum and increases the intratracheal and intrabronchial pressure. Rupture of the bronchus usually occurs within 2.5 cm of the tracheal bifurcation, the area of junction between the fixed segment of the trachea and the freely mobile segment of the distal trachea and the bronchi. Extension of the neck at the time of injury pulls the tracheal bifurcation higher into the mediastinum and increases its fixation. Closure of the glottis, preventing escape of air from the tracheobronchial tree, further increases the intraluminal pressure, which dilates and stiffens the extrathoracic segment of the trachea.

At the time of tracheobronchial injury, there are a variety of mechanical forces also at work. These include acceleration, deceleration, torsion, compression, and shear. Different rates of deceleration for different organs, or even for parts of organ systems, may complicate the mechanics of injury. In any specific situation one or more of these forces may predominate and produce the major part of the injury.

SURGICAL PATHOLOGY

Injury to the trachea occurs as a laceration, through-and-through perforation, transection, tangential tear, or avulsion. Penetrating injury may be single, tangential, or coupled wounds, depending on the *trajectory* of the missile or blade. Blunt injury can lead to a tear that is transverse, longitudinal, complete, or incomplete. Cervical tracheal injury is usually a transverse fracture between tracheal rings, whereas thoracic tracheal injury is commonly a longitudinal tear in the posterior membranous wall within a few centimeters of the carina.

The site and extent of an injury of the trachea and bronchi are related to the nature of the trauma. In penetrating wounds, any part of the tracheobronchial tree can be involved by a single, tangential, or coupled wound, depending on the *trajectory*. In blunt trauma, the most likely point of injury occurs at the main bronchi or trachea at or within a few centimeters of the carina. The character of the lesion in blunt trauma varies from a small laceration to an extensive linear tear involving the trachea, main bronchi, and branch bronchi, or to complete separation. When rupture and separation of trachea or bronchus occur, continuity persists as a consequence of the loose peritracheal or peribronchial tissue. Associated injury of the parenchyma of the lung, of the large vessels of the hilus, or of the esophagus is a less frequent complication.

Very few cases (mostly in adults) of traumatic, nonpenetrating tracheoesophageal fistula have been reported. Most such injuries result from a "steering wheel type" mechanism and are thought to be a consequence of a compression of the trachea and esophagus between the sternum and the vertebral body. As a result, a partial tracheal laceration occurs, which heals rapidly. Concomitantly, the esophagus is damaged anteriorly, resulting in impairment of its blood supply and subsequent necrosis of the contused area. The site of injury is usually at the level of the carina in half the cases, and in the cervical area in 10 percent of cases. The late sequelae of partial rupture of a main bronchus are eventual chronic, fibrous stricture and bronchopulmonary suppuration with saccular bronchiectasis, atelectasis, and fibrosis. In complete rupture separation with complete obstruction of a main bronchus, the tributary lung is totally atelectatic and unaffected. This favorable pathologic condition offers the possibility of later reconstruction of the bronchus and of the lung. After a period of collapse as long as 15 years, some lungs have reexpanded subsequent to reconstruction.

CLINICAL MANIFESTATION AND DIAGNOSIS

Major intrathoracic tracheobronchial injury produces symptoms and signs identical to more common conditions that result from penetrating or blunt trauma of the airway and chest. Associated injuries that also require urgent attention frequently occur.

Thus, when a tracheobronchial injury is present, it is often not recognized, so that diagnosis requires a high level of suspicion. Intrathoracic tracheobronchial injury must be considered in all penetrating injuries to the lower neck and upper chest. Moreover, children with evidence of violent blunt injury to the upper chest, particularly when pneumothorax and subcutaneous emphysema are present, require close evaluation. These clinical signs, especially following endoscopy or a difficult endotracheal intubation, clearly suggest tracheal injury.

Mediastinal and suprasternal emphysema appear in the majority of children with injuries of the thoracic trachea and major bronchi. The emphysema spreads rapidly into the neck and face and down to the shoulders and arms. The finding of xyphosternal crunch, or Hamman's sign, and tension pneumothorax strongly suggest the presence of intrathoracic injury.

An air leak and pneumothorax that persists following thoracostomy tube insertion, and persistent lung collapse following application of suction to the chest tube are reliable signs that major intrathoracic injury is present. Rupture of the cervical trachea is associated with subcutaneous emphysema in the anterior aspect of the neck; pain on swallowing, hoarseness, and hemoptysis are other characteristic features.

With a small airway laceration, the cough is hacking and nonproductive; subcutaneous emphysema is delayed. With extensive laceration, severe cough with hemoptysis and massive mediastinal and cervical emphysema develop rapidly. In children with these conditions, dyspnea and cyanosis occur and are not relieved by oxygen treatment; airway obstruction may be present. If one of the major pulmonary vessels is injured, bleeding may be severe. Pneumothorax and bleeding complicate tension pneumothorax and worsen respiratory distress. In blunt trauma to the chest, the pulmonary vessels usually escape injury because of their elasticity and low intraluminal pressure.

Chesterman and Santsangi[2] have reviewed the immediate clinical features in 200 patients, most of them adults. Nearly 10% of the patients were symptomatic; however, 75% had dyspnea and 30% had cyanosis. These findings are consistent in blunt trauma in children, but minor airway laceration in a child, particularly following iatrogenic injury, may remain asymptomatic for several days.

If a child survives the initial stage of acute injury without surgical treatment, symptoms of respiratory distress following a tracheal injury appear up to 2 weeks later as a consequence of ingrowth of granulation tissue, of displacement of the tracheal wall segment, and of the surrounding hematoma. If injury occurs to the main stem bronchus, atelectasis and mediastinal shift to the ipsilateral side become evident.

Radiologic signs that indicate the presence of major airway trauma include rib fracture, soft tissue air, pneumothorax, pneumomediastinum, hyoid bone elevation (indicating tracheal transection), air surrounding the bronchus, and obstruction of an air field bronchus (Figure 39-3). The widening of the right paratracheal strip, the interface between the lung and the right lateral wall of the trachea in the supraazygos recess, is significant in children, but seldom appears. The vast majority of children with intrathoracic airway injury do not have rib fracture, consistent with the compliant and flexible chest wall of the young. Another important sign occurs following transection of a main bronchus: the affected collapsed lung drops down onto the diaphragm following loss of suspension from the upper tracheobronchial tree. This is in contrast to the usual finding in simple pneumothorax, in which the lung collapses toward the mediastinum. Tomography is an excellent noninvasive method of excluding complete bronchial avulsion.

Rigid bronchoscopy is the best means to establish a diagnosis and to determine the location and extent of an injury. It is important that the examination be performed early in the clinical course. Evaluation of the tracheobronchial tree with a flexible bronchoscope is best when injury to the head, face, or cervical spine is present. Diagnosis depends on observation of mucosal disruption, of cartilaginous intrusion of the lumen, or of defects in the posterior, membranous part of the trachea. Evacuation of blood and debris enhances visual assessment of the airway. The bronchoscope should not pass the site of injury, to avoid extension of the injury during instrumentation. When the location of the injury is identified, surgical repair is possible.

Esophagoscopy complements bronchoscopy during evaluation of tracheal injury or unexplained mediastinal emphysema. Aortography is imperative if chest radiography demonstrates a widening of the mediastinal shadow and opacification of the thoracic apex, or if penetrating injury occurs to the neck and upper chest. Because of the general condition of the child after trauma, bronchography is usually contraindicated. Moreover, bronchography may miss a small laceration.

CLINICAL APPROACH

The definitive clinical approach depends on the following criteria:

1. The respiratory stability of the child

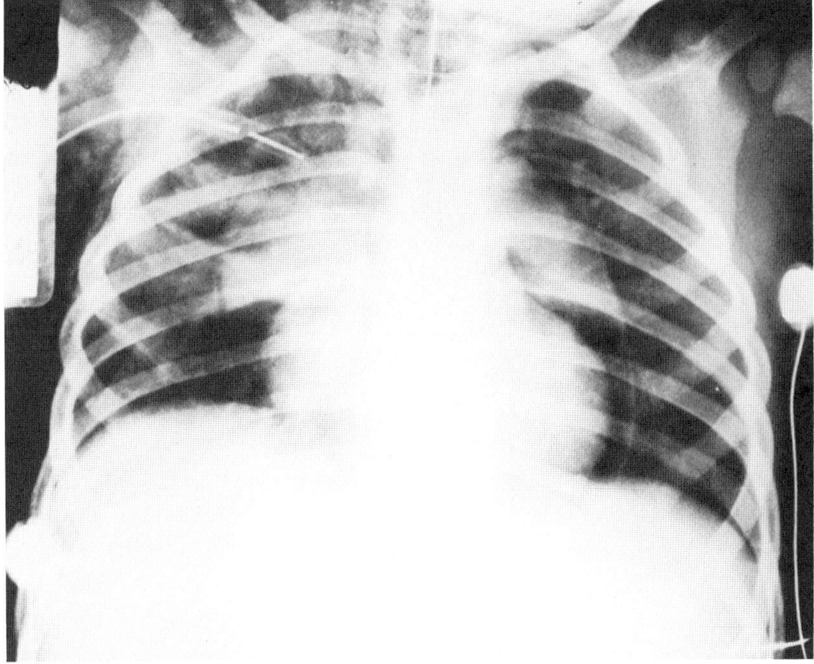

Figure 39–3 Severe pneumomediastinum owing to a small laceration of the trachea, following severe blunt trauma in 9-month-old infant. Note the air surrounding the thymus and the heart.

2. Associated trauma
3. The extent and site of airway injury
4. The clinical progression of the injury

There are basically three clinical patterns of airway injury in children who survive an initial insult. The first is found in children who rapidly decompensate because of severe airway compromise or hemorrhage from associated injury; they arrive at the hospital alive but require an immediate operation. The primary concern here is adequate control of the airway. If tracheal disruption is suspected, bronchoscopy is an essential procedure. Perform bronchoscopy in the operating room so that immediate surgical repair is possible. In addition, control of an injured, unstable airway is possible through visualization of the disruption and by passage of the bronchoscope distal to the injury to permit ventilation; placement of the bronchoscope through the endotracheal tube facilitates its insertion.[8] If bronchoscopy is not immediately possible, attempt endotracheal intubation with care to avoid further injury or disruption of the tenuous airway. Placement of a long endotracheal tube beyond the injury or into the normal lung can provide single-lung ventilation.[7]

If endotracheal intubation is unsuccessful, surgical tracheostomy or cricothyroidotomy is essential. Complete transection of the trachea can result in retraction of the distal portion of the trachea into the mediastinum; unfortunately, sufficient exploration is necessary to secure the distal tracheal segment in order to permit a direct intubation. Once the airway is secure, definitive diagnostic and surgical procedures should follow without delay.

The second pattern of airway injury is found in children who are not easily stabilized. This group includes children who have persistent air leak or lung collapse in spite of thoracostomy tube drainage. These children require prompt bronchoscopy in the operating room, followed by surgical repair.

The third pattern is seen in injured children who respond appropriately to initial therapy and easily stabilize. Therefore, the presence of bronchial injury is unsuspected until stenosis or occlusion from stricture at the site of injury occurs; as the airway narrows, dyspnea occurs. Airway occlusion is due to the ingrowth of granulation tissue into the lumen. Bronchography or flexible bronchoscopy is useful to delineate the location of bronchial deformity prior to surgery. Reconstructive operation, rather than local excision of the granulation tissue, is indicated at this stage if the lesion is in the trachea or main stem bronchus; simple dilatation is ineffective. Pulmonary function is best following early surgical reconstruction[1]; late repair is associated with a less favorable result.

SURGICAL TREATMENT

Surgical repair is the most effective treatment for airway injury. Nevertheless, a nonoperative approach is acceptable under two circumstances. The first includes a longitudinal tear that involves only a short length of posterior tracheal membrane and a minimal leak of air into the soft tissues. The second circumstance is the presence of a bronchial laceration that is less than one third the circumference of the bronchus and the complete reinflation of the lung without an air leak. Close follow-up is necessary to detect either an early complication that would demand repair or the later development of a stricture. A case in point is that of a child who was treated nonoperatively for a small tear in the membranous trachea. Three weeks following injury, the child required repeated bronchoscopy to excise granulation tissue that occluded the trachea.

Surgical repair of tracheobronchial injury requires excellent anesthesia, as well as the close cooperation of the surgeon and anesthesiologist. If the lesion is in the cervical trachea, exposure of the injury is best achieved through a transverse cervical incision that can be extended down over the sternum to expose the superior mediastinum by an inverted-T sternotomy. In a child with a small laceration no tracheostomy is indicated; an endotracheal tube can be left as a stent for a few days. In older children with a complete rupture-separation, tracheostomy complements the surgical repair. Tracheostomy helps to prevent an increase of the intraluminal pressure to minimize the leak of air through the laceration repair.

For intrathoracic tracheal injury, a right posterolateral thoracotomy provides the best access to the proximal left main bronchus and right main bronchus (Figure 39-4). A left thoracotomy is necessary for injuries to the distal left main bronchus. A median sternotomy is used only to repair a combined injury to the proximal innominate artery and anterior tracheal wall. An anterior tracheal injury is easily managed through a right thoracotomy.

During repair of a tracheobronchial injury, the surgeon passes a sterile, flexible connecting tube from the operating field to the anesthesiologist. The repair is possible by intermittently removing the tube and placing individual sutures. Alternatively, insertion of the posterior row of sutures occurs with a sterile tube in place; subsequently, sterile tube is replaced with an endotracheal tube, which passes through the anastomosis prior to final closure of the anterior row of sutures. The anesthesiologist then withdraws the orotracheal tube so that the tip lies proximal to the repair. In very small children or in children with proximal tracheal laceration,

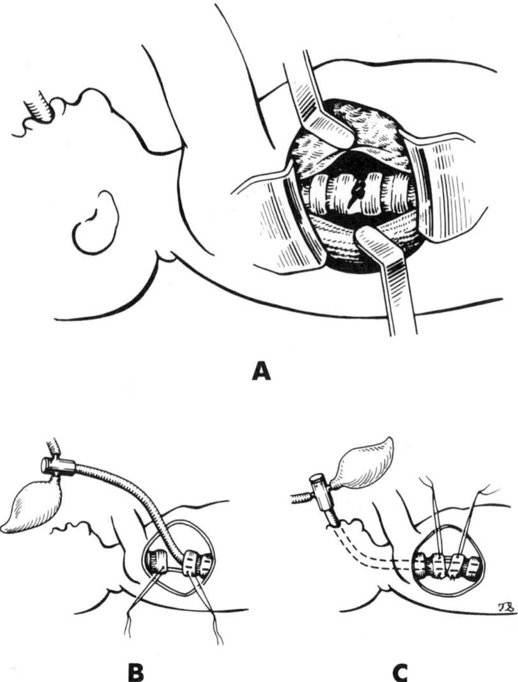

Figure 39–4 Right-sided thoracotomy enables the best exposure for right main bronchus and thoracic tracheal lacerations (**A**). A flexible sterile tube passed into the distal segment via the operative field (**B**). Reinsertion of transoral endotracheal tube after completion of the posterior layer sutures (**C**).

the use of the endotracheal tube as an internal stent for a few days is best.

In a child with a small laceration of the trachea or bronchus, interrupted monofilament polygluconate 910 (Vicryl) with a knot tied on the outside is recommended for repair. Successful repair is also possible with silk, polygalactin, and other sutures. Occasionally, children require operative bronchoscopy to remove silk sutures, which stimulate a granulation reaction.[4] Reinforce the suture line with adjacent tissue if possible; muscle, pericardium, or pleura help to prevent fistula in injured vessels or the esophagus.

When tracheal injury is more extensive, repair requires debridement, resection of the fractured rings, and elimination of the shredded margins. Conservation of viable tracheal tissue is important to avoid the need for extensive reconstruction. When tracheal damage is severe, a resection of the separated segment and end-to-end anastomosis is the treatment of choice. Because of the possible need for extended resection, useful techniques include bronchoplasty, laryngeal release, and pulmonary resection. An important maneuver following long tracheal segment repair is immobilization of the trachea with the neck in flexion; this decreases tension on the tracheal repair.

An alternative method for tracheal or bronchial repair is use of a free cartilage graft to increase the airway lumen and to avoid partial airway resection or total excision of the lung. This approach is mainly used in the repair of congenital airway stenosis. The technique is especially useful when the lesion is very distal to the carina and close to the main bronchial division. When the fracture is located at the carina, resection and end-to-end anastomosis is practically impossible. The limit of tracheal resection and end-to-end anastomosis in adults is a maximum 6.6 cm; the limit in children is unknown. The greater flexibility and elasticity of immature tissue, however, allow resection of a larger percentage of trachea in very young children. Longaker[6] has reported a successful outcome in a 16-month-old boy with congenital stenosis following resection and anastomosis of more than half of the trachea.

Various types of free graft tissues are useful to repair airway defects: rib cartilage, pericardial patch, and periosteum. Most experience with these tissues results from repair of congenital tracheal stenosis. A free tibial periosteal graft was used in an 8-month-old boy and in a 1-year-old girl, both with tracheal injury following instrumentation. A longitudinal incision over the narrow tracheal segment permitted placement of a custom-fit graft of periosteum. The graft was sutured to the margins of the defect with interrupted 5-0 Vicryl sutures with the osteogenic layer facing toward the tracheal lumen, and the endotracheal tube left in place as an internal stent for 1 week. Postoperatively, granulation growth into the tracheal lumen required reoperation in one child and excision of granulation through the bronchoscope in the other. The pericardial patch graft, which is less likely to produce granulation tissue, has been used only in children with congenital stenosis.[3] Hembra[5] reported on balloon tracheoplasty in 37 children. Although the results are promising, only four of the children had acquired tracheal lesions, three resulting from caustic and smoke inhalation and one from external trauma.

Following trauma, the main problems that reduce the tracheal lumen are formation of granulation tissue, edema, and fibrosis. Free graft or balloon dilatation may certainly increase the tracheal lumen, but only resection of the involved segment and end-to-end anastomosis gives the definitive solution. In the future, the use of the laser technique in combination with free grafting may prove to be a better solution for dealing with the late sequelae of airway injury.

REFERENCES

1. Carter R, Wareham EE, Brewer LA III: Rupture of the bronchus following closed chest trauma, *Am J Surg* 104:177-183, 1962.
2. Chesterman JT, Santsangi PN: Rupture of the trachea and bronchi by closed injury, *Thorax* 21:21-27, 1966.
3. Cosentino CM, Backer CC, Idriss FS et al: Pericardial patch tracheoplasty for severe tracheal stenosis in children: intermediate results, *J Pediatr Surg* 26:879-885, 1991.
4. Ein SH, Friedberg J, Shandling B et al: Traumatic bronchial injuries in children, *Ped Pulmonary* 2:60-64, 1986.
5. Hebra A, Powell DD, Smith CD et al: Balloon tracheoplasty in children: results of a 15-year experience, *J Pediatr Surg* 26:957-961, 1991.
6. Longaker M, Harrison MR, Adzick NS: Testing the limits of neonatal tracheal resection, *J Pediatr Surg* 25:790-792, 1990.
7. Mathisen DJ, Grillo HC: Laryngotracheal trauma, *Ann Thorac Surg* 43:254-262, 1987.
8. O'Neill MJ Jr, Myers JL, Brown AR: Avulsion of the innominate artery from the aortic arch associated with a posterior tracheal tear, *J Trauma* 22:56-59, 1982.
9. Szold A, Udassin R, Seror D et al: Acquired tracheo-esophageal fistula in infancy and childhood, *J Pediatr Surg* 26:672-675, 1991.

PART NINE

Thoracic Injury

40 Patterns of Thoracic Injury

Michael J. Allshouse and *Martin R. Eichelberger*

The leading cause of childhood injury and death in the United States is blunt trauma. Our streets and highways are the most dangerous environments for children—whether as passengers, pedestrians, or cyclists—and are where most childhood thoracic injury occurs.[36,40,41,48] Traffic-related injuries are associated with 30% of all admissions to the trauma service at the Children's National Medical Center (CNMC).[40] Institutions that serve children in large urban areas experience a greater incidence of penetrating injury.[33]

The patterns of thoracic injury documented in 2086 children consecutively admitted to the trauma service at CNMC are representative of urban, suburban, and rural populations less than 15 years of age.[41] In stark contrast to the low incidence of thoracic injury in children (104 of 2086 patients, 4.4%) is the high overall mortality (26%) in this group[41]; this includes victims who were dead on arrival at the emergency department. Three distinct groups categorize the mechanisms of thoracic injury: pedestrian-vehicular, passenger-vehicular, and penetrating[41]; pedestrian injuries are most common (37%). Children injured as passengers in crashes constitute the second largest group (31%). The mean age of this group of children is 6.2 years, and roughly half of them are less than 4 years of age.[41]

SEVERITY OF INJURY

The study of thoracic injury in children correlates severity and mechanism of injury. The most striking observation is the association of chest trauma with a multisystem injury pattern that occurs in approximately 80% of cases. Comparison of injured children with and without thoracic injury reveals significant differences. Children with chest injury had lower mean Trauma Scores (TS = 10.8 vs. 14.8) and Revised Trauma Scores (RTS = 5.5 vs. 7.5), indicating greater degrees of physiologic derangement. Increase in an anatomic indicator of severity among children with chest injuries is evident from higher mean Injury Severity Scores (ISS 26.7 vs. 7.3). Children with thoracic injury require critical care unit admission more frequently, but the mean length of stay is not longer. The dramatic difference in mortality rates between children with thoracic injury (26%) and those without thoracic injury (1.5%) reinforces the clear association of thoracic trauma with severe and multisystem injury.[41]

Motor vehicle-related thoracic injury resulted in a mean TS of just under 11, a mean ISS of approximately 30, and a mortality of just under 30%. Penetrating injury from gunshot and stab wounds resulted in a mean TS of 9.5 with a mean ISS of 18.1 and a mortality of 25%. The most dismal statistics relate to victims of child abuse; this group of children had a mean TS of 8 and a mortality of 50%.[41] Children who sustain chest injuries in falls are typically the least severely injured; no child in the group studied died as the result of chest injury sustained in a fall.

The number and type of thoracic injuries, plus the association with injury of other body regions, have a profound impact on the mortality rate. There is an inverse correlation with age; the youngest children have the highest mortality rate.[48] In the experience of the CNMC, the mortality rate for children with thoracic injury was 26%. Other pediatric centers report mortality rates between 7% and 15% for chest injury.[36,48] Among various thoracic injuries, the highest mortality rates occur with heart and great vessel injury (75%), followed by hemothorax (53%), lung laceration (43%), and rib fracture (42%). The mortality rate for children with isolated chest injury is 5%. Addition of abdominal injury raises this rate to 20%, and the addition of head trauma escalates it to 35%. Unfortunately, 58% of children with chest injury also have concomitant head injury[41]; the majority of deaths in this group of children are due to head injury. In a large series of adults with blunt thoracic injury, 43% had concomitant head injury and the overall mortality was 15.5%.[46] Because outcome analysis of blunt trauma shows no significant difference between children and adults below the age of 54,[13] the higher incidence of head injury in children negatively impacts mortality figures.

Analysis of the CNMC data by the Trauma and Injury Severity Scores (TRISS) method reveals that the probability of survival (Ps) is less (0.701 vs.

0.977) for children who have thoracic trauma as a component of their pattern of injury.[41] Death from thoracic injury occurs early in children, most often within the first 3 days. In adults, many more deaths (20%) are delayed, owing to a higher incidence of sepsis, adult respiratory distress syndrome (ARDS), and multiple system organ failure syndrome.[46]

There are several notable differences between childhood and adult patterns of chest injury. Blunt trauma to the chest produces rib fracture in 70% of adults,[46] as compared with a 30% to 50% incidence in children.[36,41,48] Pulmonary contusion is more common in children, occurring at a rate of approximately 50% versus 30% in adults.[33,36,41,46,48] Flail chest is quite rare in children. Pneumothorax is common in both groups, but the rate of tension pneumothorax is surprisingly high in children.[36,41]

ANATOMIC CONSIDERATIONS

Within the human thorax lie the body's life-support systems, the target of the *ABC*s (*A*irway, *B*reathing, and *C*irculation) of resuscitation. The effective management of airway and ventilation are the most crucial aspects of pediatric trauma resuscitation.[58] Children with chest injuries must have these derangements identified and treated as a priority in their management.

Certain characteristics of thoracic injury in children result from static and dynamic differences in the chest of the child as compared with that of the adult. Static differences include small size, decreased thoracic anterior-posterior diameter, small cross-sectional diameter of the airway, less skeletal ossification, and underdeveloped musculature. Dynamic differences include greater elasticity of the bony and cartilaginous chest wall structures and greater mediastinal mobility.

Smaller size and a large surface area/mass ratio create unique problems in intravenous access and thermoregulation. In the hypovolemic child, percutaneous intravenous access is initially attempted. If this is unsuccessful, saphenous or antecubital cutdown should be performed to obtain rapid and reliable access for fluids and medications. Intraosseous infusion is an alternative option in small children.[58] The internal diameter of the trachea is small and is easily compromised by even small amounts of edema or obstruction. Failure to appreciate differences in size and distance relationships of anatomic structures (that is, tracheal length) in children results in higher rates of iatrogenic injury.

The elastic thoracic cage of the child transmits kinetic energy more readily to underlying parenchyma. The high incidence of pulmonary contusion relative to rib fracture and flail chest reflects this

phenomenon. The mediastinum in infants and in children may shift dramatically when balancing pleural pressure relationships are disrupted. Tension pneumothorax in children decreases systemic venous return and cardiac output. Aerophagia and tachypnea result in gastric distention and less effective diaphragmatic function. Nasogastric intubation relieves gastric distention and may decrease risk of aspiration. Placement of a nasogastric tube is also helpful in recognizing left hemidiaphragmatic rupture with herniation of the stomach into the left chest. Deviation of the intraesophageal tube to the right in the presence of a widened mediastinum suggests aortic rupture. The deviation is due to esophageal displacement resulting from periaortic hematoma. In rare cases, perforation of the upper digestive tract leads to massive pneumoperitoneum, which may require needle decompression as a lifesaving maneuver.[58]

When thoracotomy is required in children, consideration of future development is important. Asymmetric growth of a child's thorax owing to injury or surgical change results in scoliosis and the associated cosmetic and physiologic derangement. In young females, incisions placed too anteriorly may alter subsequent breast development. Great care should be taken to preserve nerves emanating from the axilla. Significant deformity can be prevented if careful technique spares the long thoracic and thoracodorsal nerves.[11]

INITIAL MANAGEMENT

It is helpful to group thoracic injuries into two categories: immediately life threatening and potentially life threatening. Seven immediately life-threatening injuries are airway obstruction, open pneumothorax, tension pneumothorax, flail chest, massive hemothorax, pericardial tamponade, and air embolism. The potentially life-threatening injuries are tracheobronchial rupture, pulmonary contusion, diaphragmatic rupture, esophageal perforation, myocardial contusion, and injury to the great vessels.[2,53]

After the child's airway is secure, adequacy of ventilation is assured. Chest examination and auscultation provide information about adequacy and symmetry of ventilation, neck vein status, and heart tones. If breathing remains inadequate after endotracheal intubation with assisted ventilation and there is asymmetry of breath sounds, needle thoracentesis may demonstrate pneumothorax. The definitive treatment is placement of a thoracostomy tube. When open pneumothorax occurs and the chest wall defect has a greater cross-sectional area than the trachea, air will preferentially enter the defect and ventilation will be ineffective. Positive pressure ventilation obviates this problem, but in spontaneously breathing victims, coverage of the defect with an impermeable dressing and placement of a remote thoracostomy tube is proper treatment. Endotracheal intubation and positive pressure ventilation is also the definitive therapy for flail chest segments that compromise ventilation. Assisted ventilation is often necessary in cases of flail chest to deal with the hypoxia that results from the inevitable parenchymal lung injury.

After intravenous access is secure, treatment of shock ensues. If volume resuscitation with crystalloid and blood fails to restore adequate perfusion in the child with chest injury, and other sources of blood loss seem less likely, consider pericardial tamponade as an etiology. Pericardiocentesis can be lifesaving pending definitive surgical intervention. Physical examination may reveal evidence of a massive hemothorax, or it may be seen in an emergency chest x-ray. Treatment of the hemothorax is essential, but sudden drainage of a massive hemothorax will alter pleural pressure relationships, permit further bleeding, and lead to cardiovascular collapse. It is important to have adequate intravenous (IV) access and, if available, an autotransfusion device. After the immediately life-threatening injuries are treated, the potentially life-threatening injuries are considered. Careful physical examination and ancillary radiographic studies are imperative to avoid oversight of these injuries. Emergency chest radiography is an essential part of the evaluation of chest injury after reversal of immediately life-threatening trauma. The radiograph provides invaluable information about air or blood in pleural spaces. The thorax is an area where significant occult blood loss can occur that defies detection by physical examination alone.

Emergency department thoracotomy is the most dramatic resuscitative effort and offers the only hope for survival in selected children. The outcome of children who require emergency department resuscitative thoracotomy is poor and is similar to that in adults.[44] When vital signs are absent in the blunt trauma victim, the chance for salvage is negligible. A more liberal use in victims of penetrating thoracic injury is justified, and this modality is occasionally useful in the blunt trauma victim with detectable vital signs who deteriorates in spite of resuscitative efforts.[6,44] Emergency department thoracotomy is most effective in penetrating chest injury with pericardial tamponade unrelieved by needle aspiration and with intrathoracic sources of bleeding, and with massive air leak from bronchial injury that is readily controlled. Application of a vascular clamp to the hilum of the lung helps to control air embolism or pulmonary vascular injury.[53]

CHEST WALL INJURY

Chest wall injuries usually result from blunt trauma, although the majority of penetrating thoracic injuries involve some degree of thoracic wall disruption. Rib fracture occurred in 1.6% of all children admitted to CNMC with blunt injury. In children admitted with thoracic injury, 32% had rib fractures.[16] Single rib fractures did not indicate severe injury; there were no deaths and only one multisystem injury—a mild concussion—among children with single rib fractures. As the number of rib fractures increase, there is a pattern of increasing severity of injury noted: 70% of children with two or more rib fractures sustained multisystem injury. Thirty-three of 2080 children in this study sustained rib fractures; 14 of these 33 children died, a mortality rate of 42%. The association with head injury is devastating. Children with multiple rib fractures and severe head injury had a 100% increase in mortality over those with thoracic injury alone. The highest mortality groups were children injured in motor vehicle crashes and those who were abused. Among CNMC children, there was no correlation between location or level of rib fracture and associated great vessel injury.[16] First rib fracture has been associated with major vascular injury in a small group of patients. Physical examination findings were uniformly abnormal in children with vascular injury associated with first rib fracture.[23]

Clinicians caring for injured children probably do not appreciate the frequency of rib fracture in children with chest wall trauma. Because frequency is commonly related to only a select group of children and not to the entire population at risk for injury, the frequency is up 30% to 50%.[33,36,45,48] In older children, traffic-related injury is the most common cause. In children younger than age 3, 63% of all rib fractures are caused by abuse.[16]

Rib fractures may not be seen on initial radiographs, and "rib series" are rarely helpful. It is the pleuritic and somatic pain with the resultant splinting and respiratory compromise that complicate rib fracture. Relief of pain and restoration of pulmonary function is the objective of treatment. Underlying pulmonary contusion adds to the deterioration in function. Pneumothorax and hemopneumothorax are additional sequelae of rib fracture. Bleeding from intercostal artery laceration is the most common reason that thoracotomy is required for hemorrhage. If life-threatening injury does not intervene, treatment is aimed at alleviation of pain and at restoration of adequate breathing mechanics. Analgesic medication, intercostal nerve block, and epidural analgesia are helpful adjuncts. Sternal and scapular fractures are rare in children; these fractures are indicators of significant energy absorption.

FLAIL CHEST

Flail chest is a rare form of thoracic injury in children. When multiple fracture of adjacent ribs occurs, the flail segment exhibits paradoxical movement with spontaneous respiratory efforts. The loss of coordinated chest wall function inhibits effective respiration. Chest wall hemorrhage and severe pulmonary contusion complicate the picture. The child's mediastinum is more mobile, and the sudden shifts, owing to the altered pleural pressure relationships, interfere with normal systemic venous return. Arterial blood gas determination allows assessment of adequacy of gas exchange. If spontaneous ventilation is insufficient, endotracheal intubation with mechanical support, oxygenation, and treatment of pulmonary contusion are essential. Careful attention to analgesia is very important in treatment of these severe injuries.

LUNG CONTUSION AND LACERATION

Pulmonary contusion occurs when sufficient force is applied to lung parenchyma, causing hemorrhage and edema.[54] Loss of alveolar capillary integrity results in immediate intrapulmonary shunt. Subsequent transudation of fluid may worsen the pulmonary condition as the contusion evolves, exacerbating ventilation-perfusion abnormalities and hypoxemia. Pulmonary contusion consistently tops the list of most frequently observed chest injuries in children.[36,41,48]

Injury of lung parenchyma may be missed in examination of initial chest radiographs. The computed tomography (CT) scan is a more sensitive tool for detection of pulmonary contusion (see Fig. 40-1; see also Chapter 22). Occult or early pulmonary contusion is frequently seen on CT scans performed to evaluate blunt abdominal trauma in children.[47] CT also permits identification of pneumothorax not seen on plain films.[55]

Mild contusion requires observation and supportive care. More severe forms of injury cause respiratory insufficiency and require endotracheal intubation and mechanical ventilation with positive end-expiratory pressure (PEEP). The injured lung loses compliance and, as increasing ventilatory pressures are required to maintain oxygenation, the detrimental effect on the residual normal lung is significant. Pulmonary artery pressure is helpful to guide fluid administration and monitor inotropic therapy. Avoiding hydrostatic pulmonary edema is

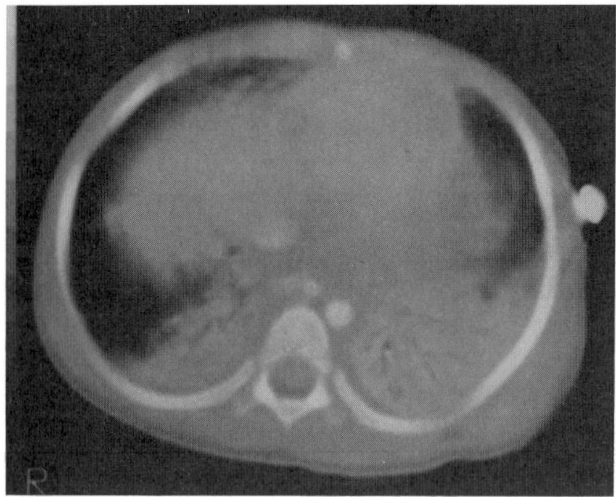

Figure 40–1 Pulmonary contusion seen on a CT scan of the lower chest.

accomplished by maintenance of euvolemia. In larger children with fulminant respiratory failure resulting from unilateral pulmonary contusion, simultaneous independent lung ventilation during the stage of maximal compliance and function derangement is possible.[14] This treatment requires placement of a double lumen endotracheal-endobronchial tube and two ventilators. Vigorous chest physiotherapy and clearance of secretions is essential. Prevention of secondary pneumonitis is ideal, but despite maximal efforts, it often occurs in the intubated child. Surveillance cultures of endotracheal aspirates help to guide initial antibiotic therapy.

Pulmonary laceration occurs frequently in cases of penetrating trauma but rarely in blunt injury. Significant blunt force is required to produce lung laceration, and this type of injury is often associated with rib fracture.[20] Rib fracture fragments may directly puncture the lung. This injury usually presents as pneumothorax or hemothorax, but with a large laceration hemoptysis may be noted. Most bleeding in the thorax emanates from chest wall sources.

A serious complication of lung laceration is air embolism. This diagnosis should be suspected in children with chest injury and focal neurologic findings in the absence of head injury, or in children who suddenly deteriorate after endotracheal intubation and positive pressure ventilation. Positive pressure ventilation of an injured lung, with open air passages and disruption of pulmonary vessels, is present with air embolism. The normally low pulmonary vascular pressure is lower during hypovolemia; this provides little resistance to passage of air into the pulmonary veins. When frothy blood is withdrawn from an arterial puncture, it signifies massive and usually fatal embolism.[20,53] Emergency thoracotomy and occlusion of the hilar structures on the injured side may be lifesaving while attempts to clear the coronary arteries proceed. Induction of high systemic blood pressure with vasopressors may help to speed the transit of bubbles through the coronary vessels. Air accumulation in the left ventricle is best treated by aspiration by direct apical puncture. None of these maneuvers are very successful if performed after cardiac arrest occurs.

Fortunately, the majority of lung lacerations require nothing more than tube thoracostomy placement for treatment of hemopneumothorax. More extensive procedures are required to treat ongoing hemorrhage, major air leak, clotted hemothorax, or air embolism.[20] Simple lacerations require suture or staple closure. Larger lung parenchymal destruction and major vascular injury often require lobectomy and, rarely, pneumonectomy.

INTRAPLEURAL INJURY

At CNMC, approximately 40% of children with thoracic injury had an intrapleural injury. Pneumothorax occurred in 12.5%, hemopneumothorax in 14.4%, and hemothorax in 13.5% of cases.[48] Additional studies of chest injury in children report similar incidence.[36] In contrast to the similar incidence of these injuries is the marked disparity in mortality. Pneumothorax was associated with a mortality of 15.4%. Hemothorax signifies severe injury in children; the mortality rate for children with this injury was 57%. The finding of intrapleural blood correlates with a prolonged hospital stay.[48]

PNEUMOTHORAX

The clinical presentations of children with pneumothorax range from no symptoms to severe distress. Careful inspection of the thorax reveals abrasion, crepitus, respiratory pattern change, and, occasionally, tracheal shift. Breath sounds may be diminished or absent. Tachypnea and labored respiration are early signs of respiratory compromise. Cyanosis is a late finding, seen in the child in extremis. Chest radiography reveals pleural space air with collapse of the ipsilateral lung. Severe shock with distended neck veins and tracheal shift signify pneumothorax under tension, one of the true immediately life-threatening injuries.

A small pneumothorax in the asymptomatic child (less than 15%), may not require treatment other than observation. It is a common pitfall to underestimate the size of a pneumothorax in observing the two-dimensional chest film. A 1 cm rim of intrapleural air is often called a 10% pneumothorax

when, in fact, cross-sectional examination reveals that this degree of whole lung collapse is closer to 50%, and what is often seen as a 50% pneumothorax on a plain film actually compromises 90% of lung tissue.[7] All children with symptomatic pneumothorax and those subject to positive pressure ventilation require treatment with tube thoracostomy. For most children, a 20 to 24 Fr thoracostomy tube is adequate; infants need only a 12 Fr tube.

Tension pneumothorax is common in children, occurring in up to 23% of all cases.[36] The compromise of functional lung tissue is severe and deterioration ensues when the mobile mediastinum of the child shifts and systemic venous return falls. Rapid treatment by needle thoracentesis in the second intercostal space at the midclavicular line is essential and must be followed by accurate placement of a thoracostomy tube. Suspect tension pneumothorax in any child with chest trauma who deteriorates suddenly, especially a child receiving assisted ventilation. If an intraabdominal operation is under way when deterioration occurs, quick inspection of the inferior diaphragmatic surfaces reveals evidence of tension that can be relieved by incision of the bulging diaphragm; diaphragm repair and tube thoracostomy through a separate incision follow. Preexisting lung disease, which compromises parenchymal compliance, places a child at increased risk of tension pneumothorax during positive pressure ventilation.

When lung rupture occurs on pleural surfaces that face the mediastinum, air dissection along the peribronchial and tracheal spaces will result in pneumomediastinum and subcutaneous emphysema of the neck and face. In spontaneously breathing children with these findings, injury of the lung tissue is the usual cause, but tracheobronchial disruption is an additional cause of massive subcutaneous emphysema. In major airway injury, acute exacerbation of emphysema occurs with institution of positive pressure ventilation.[7] Any child with a chest injury and evidence of a large air leak from one or more thoracostomy tubes requires bronchoscopy to rule out major airway injury.

Open pneumothorax and a sucking chest wound are less common variants of this class of injury. In the spontaneously breathing child, these injuries are catastrophic. The normal pleural and intrathoracic pressure relationships are upset; if the open chest defect exceeds the cross-sectional area of the upper airway, air will preferentially enter the chest wall defect and severely compromise respiration. Treatment consists of restoration of chest wall integrity by an occlusive dressing and placement of an intrapleural thoracostomy tube. Antibiotic coverage is recommended for these frequently contaminated wounds.

HEMOTHORAX

The thorax is one of the few areas where occult bleeding may result in severe shock. The emergency department anteroposterior chest x-ray provides invaluable information about hemothorax and pneumothorax. Major injury to the vascular structures of the mediastinum and lung hila that decompress into the thoracic spaces is usually fatal. The usual cause of hemothorax is injury to systemic vessels, such as an intercostal artery or an internal mammary artery. Approximately 5% to 10% of cases are due to pulmonary vascular bleeding from an injured lung.[7] The pulmonary vascular mean pressures are low and drop even further following hemorrhage. With lung expansion there is effective tamponade of most pulmonary sources of hemorrhage.

Tube thoracostomy is the treatment for hemothorax; however, there are several caveats. Rapid evacuation of a large hemothorax may acutely lower pleural pressure and eliminate any tamponade of bleeding. Serious recurrent or ongoing hemorrhage will ensue and may result in cardiovascular collapse. Large-caliber intravenous access is important in children with massive hemothorax; most will sustain profound shock. Autotransfusion devices are particularly applicable in this situation. Overtly unstable children require urgent thoracotomy and, occasionally, emergency department thoracotomy for control of hemorrhage. In most cases intrapleural hemorrhage will be less dramatic. The stable child is carefully observed, and a precise record of thoracostomy drainage is established. Hemorrhage that continues at a rate greater than 1 to 2 ml/kg of body weight per hour requires thoracotomy for control of bleeding.[11]

Complete evacuation of a hemothorax is essential. Unfortunately, failure to drain the hemothorax with one large chest tube usually indicates intrapleural adhesions or a clotted hemothorax.[7] Occasionally, a second tube will drain the residual blood, but thoracotomy is necessary if complete drainage is not possible. The sequelae of clotted hemothorax in children are often severe. Fibrothorax may impede pulmonary function and alter symmetry of thoracic growth; scoliosis is the end result of this complication. Infection of a residual hemothorax results in empyema, requiring prolonged hospitalization and thoracotomy. Small amounts of noninfected residual blood or clot warrant observation and will be absorbed over several weeks.[50]

CHYLOTHORAX

As the thoracic duct ascends from the cisterna chyli into the chest, it lies to the right of the aorta. At the midesophageal level the duct crosses to the left side on its way to join the venous system at the confluence of the left internal jugular and subclavian veins.[43] Injury to the thoracic duct resulting from trauma is rare, but may result either from blunt or penetrating forces. Blunt injury to the duct is most often caused by torso hyperextension, with or without concomitant thoracic spine fracture. This type of traction injury during birth is responsible for cases of congenital chylothorax.[43] Iatrogenic injury occurs during operations for tracheoesophageal fistula, esophageal resection, gastroesophageal reflux, and cardiovascular anomaly such as patent ductus arteriosus.

Once injury to the thoracic duct occurs, drainage of chyle into the mediastinum and pleural space follows.[42] The thoracic duct transit volume is dependent on the diet of the child, as to both quantity and content. Symptoms appear when the chylous accumulation is large enough to cause respiratory embarrassment. This may not occur until a large collection forms. Fortunately, infection is rare, owing to the bacteriostatic nature of chyle. The diagnosis is made when cloudy white fluid with high fat and lymphocyte content is aspirated from the pleural space.

Treatment is individualized, based on the amount and trend of the drainage pattern.[42] Initial management consists of thoracostomy drainage and dietary manipulation. Complete expansion of the lung promotes pleural symphysis and obliterates the pleuromediastinal spaces, increasing resistance to the flow of chyle. A fat-free diet with medium chain triglyceride (MCT) supplements is an excellent initial food. MCTs are absorbed directly into portal blood and do not directly stimulate chyle flow. Total parenteral nutrition is successful in selected cases. Before the first report of successful ligation of the thoracic duct, the mortality associated with this process exceeded 50%.[30] The timing of surgery is best individualized. With persistent thoracostomy output despite maximal therapy, recommendations for operative intervention range from 5 days to 4 weeks postinjury.[11,30,42] The operative approach entails exploration of the involved side or, in the case of bilateral effusion, exploration of the right side first. Several maneuvers aid in localization of the duct injury, such as intragastric instillation of cream, olive oil, or consumption of a preoperative high-fat meal. Methylene or Evans blue dye is cleared in the lymphatics and when it is injected in the thigh preoperatively, the duct may be visualized. There are times when none of these measures is effective. Careful mass ligation of all tissues between the azygos vein and aorta above the diaphragm via right thoracotomy is indicated if direct visualization of the leak is impossible.[39]

Persistent loss of chylous fluid results in hypoproteinemia, lymphocytopenia, and, ultimately, death from inanition and immune deficiency. Cell-mediated immunity is compromised and opportunistic infections, especially fungal sepsis, ensue.

TRACHEOBRONCHIAL INJURY

Tracheobronchial injury is rare in children. The true incidence in all ages is unknown inasmuch as many victims with this injury die before they reach a hospital.[12,19] Tracheobronchial injury may be due to penetrating trauma, but this is exceedingly rare. The majority of such injuries in children are due to blunt trauma. Severe crush injury and rapid deceleration with impact, as in a motor vehicle crash, may result in this type of trauma.[36,48] Tracheobronchial disruption must be suspected when a dyspneic child has sustained a massive air leak from a thoracostomy placed to treat a common or tension pneumothorax. Findings of hemoptysis, subcutaneous emphysema, and pneumomediastinum on a chest radiograph are additional clues to this diagnosis. Massive atelectasis that fails to improve with chest tube placement raises suspicion of a bronchial injury. Dyspnea is an almost universal finding, and subcutaneous emphysema occurs in 85% to 100% of patients.[5,27,28]

Sudden chest impact or crush drastically decreases the antero-posterior diameter of the thoracic cage. This measurement is less in children regardless of external forces. As the transverse diameter widens, the lungs are distracted laterally and abnormal forces are applied to the main bronchi and carina. If the glottis is closed and the tracheobronchial structures are crushed between the sternum and the vertebral column, a tremendous rise in intrabronchial pressure may lead to rupture. The membranous posterior portion is prone to this injury. Shearing injuries tend to occur at points of maximal fixation, namely the cricoid and carinal regions.[29]

Bronchoscopy must be performed expeditiously in all children with suspected tracheobronchial injury. The best diagnostic yield is achieved with rigid bronchoscopy performed by an experienced surgeon.[19] Flexible fiber-optic bronchoscopy is useful if the child has an endotracheal tube already in place. The endoscopic appearance of these injuries may underestimate the actual damage. Once the injury is identified, prompt treatment is essen-tial. The vast majority of children who have sustained tracheobronchial trauma have multisystem injury which may dictate the surgical approach. Direct surgical repair at the earliest possible time yields the best results. Delay in diagnosis is associated with intrathoracic infection, persistent pulmonary dysfunction, and progression to multiple-system organ failure.[19]

High tracheal injuries are approached through a cervical collar incision. Standard posterolateral thoracotomy is utilized for unilateral bronchial injury; right-sided bronchial injuries predominate.[19,29] Median sternotomy is satisfactory for anterior tracheal injury. Selective endobronchial intubation, if practicable, makes repair with absorbable suture easier and ventilation safer. If possible, the repair should be buttressed with a vascularized segment of tissue such as a pleural flap. Major parenchymal resection is done only as a last resort; extensive injury may require cardiopulmonary bypass for repair. Thoracostomy drainage and perioperative antibiotic coverage are important aspects of surgical care in children with these injuries. Long-term follow-up of survivors is important because late stenosis of the airway is a known sequelae of this type of injury.[5]

TRAUMATIC ASPHYXIA

Traumatic asphyxia is a clinical syndrome characterized by subconjunctival and petechial upper-body cutaneous hemorrhages, cyanosis, facial edema, and variable degrees of pulmonary and central nervous system dysfunction. It is caused by severe and sudden compression of the chest and upper abdomen.[17,21] In anticipation of impending injury, the response of the child is maximal inspiration, tensing of thoracoabdominal muscles, and closure of the glottis. Glottic closure or tracheobronchial obstruction appears to be prerequisite for this injury.[56] Clinical pictures similar to traumatic asphyxia have been reported in association with asthma, seizures, violent vomiting, whooping cough, and difficult obstetric deliveries.[17,56] Blast injuries, close-range shotgun wounds, and positive pressure ventilation following cardiac surgery are other reported causes.[21]

As positive pressure is transmitted to the mediastinum, blood is forced out of the right atrium into the valveless large veins of the chest and neck. This rapid retrograde pressure propagation dilates venules and capillaries, producing the characteristic petechial hemorrhages. The subconjunctival vessels are most profoundly affected because of the paucity of supporting tissue. Desaturation of blood produces the cyanotic hue. It is interesting that these discolorations blanch with digital pressure, indicating that the blood is still intravascular. Skin beneath pressure points such as hat bands or collars is frequently spared the typical changes; presumably, these areas are protected by the counterpressure.[17]

The external appearance of a child with traumatic asphyxia is quite dramatic. There is marked disparity between the cutaneous manifestations of the head and neck and the lower body. Pulmonary contusion and intraabdominal injury, especially hepatic trauma, are associated with this phenomenon. Cardiac injury is very rare.[17] In spite of the alarming physical appearance, the prognosis is good. The most severe injuries cause immediate death, and most victims who survive the first several hours will recover.[56] Central nervous system injury appears to be most closely related to degree of hypoxemia, and not to cerebral hemorrhage. It is postulated that the rigid cranium provides counterpressure protection and limits intracranial hemorrhage. The prognosis for return of normal cognitive function in children is excellent.[17]

AORTIC AND GREAT VESSEL INJURY

Traumatic rupture of the thoracic aorta is an uncommon injury of childhood. The mortality rate (75%) for children with injury to the heart and great vessels was the highest of any injury type in the CNMC study of thoracic injury in childhood.[40] Although young age is generally considered to be a favorable predictor of survival in this injury, the mortality rate associated with aortic rupture resulting from blunt trauma was found to be greater in children than in adults in one epidemiologic study.[10] In this study, only 2.1% of 551 accidental deaths in children were due to traumatic rupture of the aorta. The incidence of adult deaths resulting from this injury is higher. Aortic rupture in children is usually associated with a motor vehicle crash; the injured child may be either a passenger or a pedestrian. The use of car restraints for children virtually eliminates the impact and deceleration required for this injury.[10]

The site of aortic injury caused by blunt trauma, the ligamentum arteriosum, seems to be consistent across all age groups.[10] There is a frequent association with multisystem injury, and most victims do not live to reach the hospital. For a child with blunt injury, especially central chest impact, who exhibits a widened mediastinum on a chest radiograph or a hematoma on a CT scan, urgent aortography must be performed to determine whether great vessel injury is present. CT scan alone is not the diagnostic test of choice for this lesion.[35] An arteriographic finding of a ductus diverticulum, particularly in children, may be confused with aortic injury. A ductus diverticulum is smooth walled and limited to the inferior, medial aspect of the aorta; intimal irregularity seen in acute injury is absent.[7] The location and level of associated thoracic skeletal injury, such as first rib fracture, does not correlate well with aortic injury in children.[40] When first rib fracture occurs in association with major vascular injury in children, the findings in vascular examination are invariably abnormal as well.[23]

Prompt surgical repair of aortic injury in all surviving children is mandatory to prevent death resulting from subsequent rupture and exsanguination. Left posterolateral thoracotomy is the incision used to expose and repair this injury. There is controversy concerning the use of bypass techniques in aortic repair. Treatment must be individualized and includes factors such as the effects of systemic anticoagulation on associated injuries. Coexistent intraabdominal injury frequently exists, and repair precedes the aortic reconstruction. This approach presupposes hemodynamic stability and temporary containment of the aortic injury. Direct suture repair is optimum; in some cases an interposition graft may be required to make up for significant tissue loss.[52] The additional time required for placement of an interposition graft necessitates some form of bypass.

Blunt or deceleration injury may damage any of the other great vessels of the chest. Penetrating injury is increasingly common in many urban centers and is associated with high mortality. Left subclavian artery injury is treated through a left posterolateral thoracotomy. Median sternotomy gives the best exposure of the other vessels and can be extended into either side of the neck. Addition of a "trap-door" incision in the left third interspace allows visualization of the left subclavian vessels from the median sternotomy.[53]

CARDIAC INJURY

Cardiac injury in children may result from blunt or penetrating trauma, but is extremely rare. Blunt cardiac injury spans a relatively large spectrum of disorders—from contusion to rupture. The majority of these injuries are due to motor vehicle-related trauma. Penetrating injuries of the heart are equally dramatic, but the frequent lack of association with multi-system injury makes survival more likely than in severe blunt cardiac injury. Iatrogenic penetrating injury during cardiac catheterization is more frequent in young children than in adults. More recent reports indicate that the rates are equal.[15]

Among the most physiologically devastating sequelae of cardiac injury is pericardial tamponade. Tamponade may occur in children when either blood from intrapericardial injury, or air from airway barotrauma, accumulates in the pericardial space. Sudden distention of the pericardial space is poorly tolerated. Both systemic and pulmonary venous return decrease and cardiac output falls. The diagnosis of cardiac tamponade is difficult in small children. With blunt injury, there is frequently a concomitant head injury which alters examination findings. A child's pericardial sac has a smaller volume, and tamponade will occur with smaller accumulations of air or fluid. It is also more likely for a child to harbor an occult congenital heart defect, which may alter diagnosis.[15] Persistent hypotension in spite of maximal fluid resuscitation, neck vein distention, shock, and elevated central venous pressures all suggest a diagnosis of tamponade. The classic pulsus paradoxus is difficult to measure in the injured child, and Beck's triad (rising venous pressure, falling arterial pressure, and a small, quiet heart) is not often evident.[15] Salient signs on chest radiographs are rare and electrocardiogram findings are not reliable.

In the unstable child, especially one with penetrating injury and signs of tamponade, emergency thoracotomy may be required. Pericardiocentesis is useful for diagnosis and temporizing therapy; aspiration of blood or air may result in dramatic improvement. If pericardiocentesis is unsatisfactory or if more definitive information is needed and immediate thoracotomy is not planned, creation of a subxiphoid pericardial window may be diagnostic.[8,34] This may be performed independently, as a diagnostic test, or created during laparotomy if suspicion of cardiac injury arises.

Cardiac laceration caused by a knife, gun, or other penetrating object is best repaired by direct suturing.[38] Knife wounds or injuries such as those caused by shards of broken glass present the fewest obstacles to repair. Blunt myocardial rupture is usually fatal, and few victims survive transport to a hospital.[24] Thoracotomy for repair of cardiac injuries is best performed in a fully equipped operating room. Anterolateral thoracotomy extended across the sternum for additional exposure or median sternotomy is the incision of choice. Pericardial incision is performed, avoiding injury to the phrenic nerves, and tamponade is relieved. Digital pressure is an effective means of occluding most small holes and lacerations. Atrial injuries can be temporarily controlled by a curved vascular clamp while repair is performed. Use of pledget sutures helps to prevent extension of lacerations; pledgets are especially useful during repair of atrial and right ventricular injuries.[24] Unfortunately, the mortality

rate for children with heart and great vessel injury is 75%.[41]

Myocardial contusion is not a commonly reported injury of childhood. Its true incidence is probably not known. Cardiac contusion is an injury related to blunt trauma. Although most childhood injuries involve blunt mechanisms, the lack of central chest deceleration injury, seen with steering-wheel impact in adult drivers, probably accounts for the lower incidence of cardiac contusion. Motor vehicle-pedestrian crashes are the mechanisms most likely to cause cardiac contusion in children.[31,51] The child's chest is capable of significant anterior-posterior deformation during impact, allowing compression of the heart between the sternum and spine.

The diagnosis of myocardial contusion is made clinically and supported by a variety of investigations. Electrocardiographic changes are variable and range from mild S-T abnormality to conduction abnormality. Measurement of creatine phosphokinase MB levels may be helpful, but false positives in trauma patients limit the sensitivity.[51] Echocardiography, radionuclide angiography, and MUGA scanning are all helpful in diagnosis by defining abnormalities in ejection fraction or regional wall motion.[25,31,51] Children with suspected cardiac contusion are continuously monitored for dysrhythmia. The incidence of dysrhythmia is lower in children with cardiac contusion than in adults, and, barring serious myocardial dysfunction, children with contusion tolerate general anesthesia well.[25] Serious sequelae of myocardial contusion are related to infarction, delayed rupture, rupture of papillary muscles or the ventricular septum, and valvular dysfunction. These are rare in children. Echocardiography appears to be the best test for acute diagnosis, and for evaluation of these delayed complications.[51]

DIAPHRAGMATIC INJURY

Sudden forceful impact of the lower chest or upper abdomen is the most common cause of diaphragmatic rupture or laceration in children.[1] The hemidiaphragm most commonly injured in blunt trauma is the left. Motor vehicle crashes are, again, the most common mechanisms. This injury may be associated with use of a lap-belt type of restraint. The injured child with diaphragmatic rupture frequently has a truly scaphoid abdomen and respiratory distress. An emergency chest radiograph examination is very helpful in establishing the diagnosis. Early nasogastric tube placement helps in diagnosis if displacement of the stomach into the chest is seen on x-ray. Abdominal organs, including the spleen, may be injured during thoracostomy tube placement. Diaphragmatic hernia is best approached via laparotomy for repair of the diaphragm and evaluation of concomitant abdominal injury. In penetrating injury, careful diaphragmatic exploration is mandatory to avoid overlooking even small injuries. Small diaphragmatic rents enlarge with time, allowing herniation of abdominal contents into the chest.

BURN INJURY

Thermal injury alters thoracic function in several ways. Burn wounds of the chest and neck interfere with the mechanics of ventilation, and gas exchange suffers from inhalation of smoke and heated products of combustion. Burns are the second leading cause of death in childhood. The majority of burns in children requiring admission are scald injuries; these rarely have inhalation components. The highest mortality results from flame injury. Pulmonary complications resulting from flame burns are the most common cause of death.[41] Upper airway injury with rapid progression of edema may result in airway obstruction. Early intubation is prudent if there is any doubt about the security of the upper airway. Endotracheal intubation alone will be insufficient treatment if cervical eschar is adding to the problem. Escharotomy in conjunction with intubation is essential.[49] Chest burns with unyielding eschar inhibit respiratory excursions and must be treated by thoracic escharotomy.

Children burned in closed-space fires sustain direct tracheobronchial injury from smoke inhalation[32]; thermal injury and chemical tracheobronchitis often coexist. Several phases of response to pulmonary injury are identified. The earliest component of the spectrum is an acute respiratory distress phase characterized by bronchospasm, laryngeal edema, and lung consolidation. This is followed by variable degrees of pulmonary edema and, finally, by bronchopneumonia. The pneumonia usually occurs beyond postburn day 3 and is universally present in all survivors.[49] Early in the course of inhalational injury, chest x-rays and bronchoscopy may underestimate the severity of injury. Treatment is centered on scrupulous pulmonary care and treatment of bronchospasm. Assisted ventilation and PEEP are often necessary for prolonged periods. Surveillance sputum cultures will help to guide antibiotic therapy of the inevitable lung infection. Significant fluid requirements and shifts are the rule during the acute-phase response of these critically ill children. Pulmonary artery catheterization helps to optimize fluid administration and monitors cardiopulmonary function at a time when pulmonary edema is problematic and must not be exacerbated.

ESOPHAGEAL INJURY

Esophageal injury is rare in children. Penetrating trauma accounts for the majority of esophageal injuries, and among these iatrogenic perforation is most common. Esophageal perforation may occur during endoscopic instrumentation or with traumatic passage of tubes. Caustic ingestion is an additional source of esophageal injury that is predominantly seen in children.

Injury to the esophagus during instrumentation characteristically occurs at areas of physiologic narrowing: the cricopharyngeus-inferior constrictor, the region of the aortic arch, or the diaphragmatic hiatus.[26] Direct penetrating injuries resulting from thoracic gunshot wounds are extremely uncommon in children.[4] Postemetic rupture of the esophagus is quite unusual in children, but distal esophageal rupture may occur during major chest compression. Accidental insufflation of high-pressure air into the esophagus can cause rupture.[50] This injury has been described in a child who bit an inner tube of a tire that had been inflated under pressure.[9]

Esophageal perforation may be difficult to detect and mandates a disciplined diagnostic approach. Delay in recognition and treatment of this injury turns a simple problem into a very complicated one. Clinical signs that suggest perforation are subcutaneous emphysema, pneumothorax or pneumomediastinum, pleural effusion, shock, and mediastinal "crunch" observed upon auscultation. Pain response depends on the segment of the esophagus that is injured. Torticollis and resistance to motion result from cervical injury, and midchest pain from thoracic injury. Perforation of the intraabdominal esophagus usually causes tenderness and rigidity.[50] Progression of the injury pattern may be insidious. Small rents in the intrathoracic esophagus are subject to negative intrathoracic pressures, which provide a favorable gradient for leakage into the mediastinum.[37] In the patient who does not need immediate exploration, the esophagus is studied with contrast esophagography and esophagoscopy. These studies should be considered as complementary. Combining the two lessens the chance of misdiagnosis of esophageal injury.

Prompt treatment is essential to success. Initial measures include suspension of all oral intake, nasogastric suction, fluid resuscitation, and administration of broad-spectrum antibiotics.[50] Cervical injury is repaired via a modified collar incision or one that parallels the anterior border of the sternocleidomastoid muscle. Upper- and midthoracic esophageal wounds are repaired through a right posterolateral thoracotomy, and lower esophageal injury through left posterolateral incision. It is important to make repairs in viable tissue, and it is wise to buttress the suture line with vascularized flaps of parietal pleura or muscle.[50] Complicated injury necessitates proximal cervical diversion with occlusion of the distal esophagus and delayed repair after resolution of mediastinal sepsis. In all cases of esophageal repair, adequate external drainage of the adjacent tissues is mandatory.

Caustic esophageal injury requires prompt esophagoscopy to the most proximal level of the burn. Significant injury is treated with antibiotic therapy and meticulous nutritional support. Gastrostomy or parenteral nutrition is required when voluntary intake is insufficient. Careful follow-up is necessary after initial healing. There are numerous options for short segment stricture. Long segment stricture that fails to dilate is resected and replaced with a gastric tube or colon interposition.

NEONATAL THORACIC INJURY

One of the results of advanced neonatal therapy is the survival of preterm infants who require prolonged intensive care and mechanical ventilatory support. These small infants are at increased risk for barotrauma resulting from high airway pressures and injury during endotracheal suctioning or placement of vascular lines and thoracostomy tubes.[11] High airway pressure and use of PEEP predispose to tension pneumothorax, which occurs in up to 25% of cases.[18] Initial improvement follows needle thoracentesis. Chest tube placement must be done with great care; lung injury occurs as often as 25% of the time in these sick neonates.[57]

Bronchial perforation and pneumothorax may follow suctioning of endotracheal tubes if precautions are not taken to limit length and force of insertion. This injury should be suspected in any infant who suddenly deteriorates after suctioning, has a new onset of bloody tracheal aspirate, or has a persistent air leak.[3] Thoracotomy may provide the only means to control an air leak that persists despite adequate drainage. Nonoperative treatment of these infants is often doomed to failure, resulting from progressive pulmonary insufficiency, and death.[3,18]

Vigorous insertion of transoral or nasogastric tubes may result in neonatal esophageal perforation. This usually occurs at the junction of the hypopharynx and the cervical esophagus, and the radiographic appearance may mimic proximal esophageal atresia.[11] After removal of the tube, antibiotic therapy is started and oral feedings are suspended for 1 week. Contrast swallow is performed to confirm healing, at which time feeding is resumed. The need for cervical drainage depends on the clinical response. Intrathoracic perforation of the esophagus may be caused by instrumentation

or may occur spontaneously in the newborn.[22] In contrast to spontaneous esophageal rupture in adults, neonatal rupture occurs most frequently into the right chest. Although selective nonoperative treatment of contained thoracic esophageal perforation is possible, early repair, pedicle flap buttressing, and excellent drainage provide the best opportunity for successful outcome.

REFERENCES

1. Adeymi SD, Stephens CA: Traumatic diaphragmatic hernia in children, *Can J Surg* 24:355-359, 1981.
2. American College of Surgeons: *Advanced trauma life support manual,* 1989.
3. Anderson KD, Chandra R: Pneumothorax secondary to perforation of sequential bronchi by suction catheters, *J Pediatr Surg* 11:687-693, 1976.
4. Barlow B, Niemirska M, Gandhi RP: Ten years' experience with pediatric gunshot wounds, *J Pediatr Surg* 17:927-932, 1982.
5. Baumgartner F, Sheppard B, de Virgilio C et al: Tracheal and main bronchial disruptions after blunt chest trauma: presentation and management, *Ann Thorac Surg* 50:569-574, 1990.
6. Beaver BL, Colombani PM, Buck JR et al: Efficacy of emergency room thoracotomy in pediatric trauma, *J Pediatr Surg* 22:19-23, 1987.
7. Blaisdell FW: Pneumothorax and hemothorax. In Blaisdell FW, Trunkey DD, editors: *Cervicothoracic trauma.* New York, 1986, Thieme.
8. Brewster SA, Thirlby RC, Snyder WH III: Subxiphoid pericardial window and penetrating cardiac trauma, *Arch Surg* 123:937-941, 1988.
9. Cole DS, Burcher SK: Accidental pneumatic rupture of the esophagus and stomach, *Lancet* 1:24, 1961.
10. Eddy AC, Rusch VW, Fligner CL et al: The epidemiology of traumatic rupture of the thoracic aorta in children: a 13-year review, *J Trauma* 30:989-992, 1990.
11. Eichelberger MR, Anderson KD: Sequelae of thoracic injury in children. In Eichelberger MR, Pratsch GL, editors: *Pediatric trauma care,* Rockville, Md, 1988, Aspen, pp 59-68.
12. Eichelberger MR, Randolph JG: Thoracic trauma in children, *Surg Clin North Am* 61:1181-1197, 1981.
13. Eichelberger MR, Mangubat EA, Sacco WS et al: Comparative outcomes of children and adults suffering blunt trauma, *J Trauma* 28:430-434, 1988.
14. Frame SB, Marshall WJ, Clifford TG: Synchronized independent lung ventilation in the management of pediatric unilateral pulmonary contusion: case report, *J Trauma* 29:395-397, 1989.
15. Galladay ES, Donahoo JS, Haller JA: Special problems of cardiac injuries in infants and children, *J Trauma* 19:526-531, 1979.
16. Garcia VF et al: Rib fractures in children: a marker of severe trauma, *J Trauma* 30:695-700, 1990.
17. Gorenstein L, Blair GR, Shandling B: The prognosis of traumatic asphyxia in childhood, *J Pediatr Surg* 21:753-756, 1986.
18. Grosfeld JL, Lemans JL, Ballantine TN et al: Emergency thoracotomy for acquired bronchopleural fistulae in the premature infant with respiratory distress, *J Pediatr Surg* 15:416, 1980.
19. Grover FJ, Ellested C, Arom KU: Diagnosis and management of major tracheobronchial injuries, *Ann Thorac Surg* 28:384-391, 1979.

20. Guernsey JM, Blaisdell FW: Pulmonary injury. In Blaisdell FW, Trunkey DD, editors: *Cervicothoracic trauma,* New York, 1986, Thieme.
21. Haller JA, Donahoo JS: Traumatic asphyxia in children: pathophysiology and management, *J Trauma* 11:453-457, 1971.
22. Harrell GS, Friedland GW, Daily WJ et al: Neonatal Boerhaave's syndrome, *Radiology* 95:665-668, 1970.
23. Harris GJ, Soper RT: Pediatric first rib fractures, *J Trauma* 30:343-345, 1990.
24. Hurley EJ, Mayfield W: Cardiac injuries. In Blaisdell FW, Trunkey DD, editors: *Cervicothoracic trauma,* New York, 1986, Thieme.
25. Ildstad ST, Tollerud DJ, Weiss RG et al: Cardiac contusion in pediatric patients with blunt thoracic trauma, *J Pediatr Surg* 25:287-289, 1990.
26. Jones KW: Thoracic trauma, *Surg Clin North Am* 50:957-965, 1980.
27. Jones WS, Mavroudis C, Richardson JD et al: Management of tracheobronchial disruption resulting from blunt trauma, *Surgery* 95:319-322, 1984.
28. Kaiser LR, Cooper JD: Tracheobronchial injuries. In Turney SZ, Rodriguez A, Cowley RA, editors: *Management of cardiothoracic trauma,* Baltimore, 1990, Williams & Wilkens.
29. Kirsh MM, Orringer MB, Behrendt DM et al: Management of tracheobronchial disruption secondary to nonpenetrating trauma, *Ann Thorac Surg* 22:93-101, 1976.
30. Lampson RS: Traumatic chylothorax: a review of the literature and report of a case treated by mediastinal ligation of the thoracic duct, *J Thorac Surg* 17:778, 1948.
31. Langer JC, Winthrop AL, Wesson DE et al: Diagnosis and incidence of cardiac injury in children with blunt thoracic trauma, *J Pediatr Surg* 24:1091-1094, 1989.
32. Maylan JA: Smoke inhalation and burn injury, *Surg Clin North Am* 60:1533-1540, 1980.
33. Meller JL, Little AG, Shermeta DW: Thoracic trauma in children, *Pediatrics* 74:813-819, 1984.
34. Miller FB, Bond SJ, Shumate CR et al: Diagnostic pericardial window: a safe alternative to exploratory thoracotomy for suspected heart injuries, *Arch Surg* 122:605-609, 1987.
35. Miller FB, Richardson JD, Thomas HA et al: Role of CT in diagnosis of major arterial injury after blunt thoracic trauma, *Surgery* 106:596-603, 1989.
36. Nakayama DK, Ramenofsky ML, Rowe MI: Chest injuries in childhood, *Ann Surg* 210:770-775, 1989.
37. O'Neil MB: Pharyngoesophageal injury. In Blaisdell FW, Trunkey DD, editors: *Cervicothoracic trauma,* New York, 1986, Thieme.
38. Ordog GJ, Wasserberger J, Schatz I et al: Gunshot wounds in children under 10 years of age: a new epidemic, *Am J Dis Child* 142:618-622, 1988.
39. Patterson GA, Todd TRJ, Delarue NC et al: Supradiaphragmatic ligation of the thoracic duct in intractable chylous fistula, *Ann Thorac Surg* 32:44, 1981.
40. Peclet MH, Newman KD, Eichelberger MR et al: Patterns of injury in children, *J Pediatr Surg* 25:85-91, 1990.
41. Peclet MH, Newman KD, Eichelberger MR et al: *Thoracic trauma in children: an indicator of increased mortality, J Pediatr Surg* 25:961-966, 1990.
42. Ramzy A, Rodriguez A, Cowley RA: Pitfalls in the management of chylothorax, *J Trauma* 22:513-515, 1982.
43. Randolph JR, Gross R: Congenital chylothorax, *Arch Surg* 74:405, 1957.
44. Rothenberg SS, Moore EE, Moore FA et al: Emergency department thoracotomy in children: a critical analysis, *J Trauma* 29:1322-1325, 1989.
45. Schweich P, Fleisher G: Rib fractures in children, *Pediatr Emerg Care* 1:187-189, 1985.
46. Shorr RM, Crittenden M, Indeck M et al: Blunt thoracic trauma: analysis of 515 patients, *Ann Surg* 206:200-205, 1987.
47. Sivit CJ, Taylor GA, Eichelberger MR: Chest injury in children with blunt abdominal trauma: evaluation with CT, *Radiology* 171:815-818, 1989.
48. Smyth BT: Chest trauma in children, *J Pediatr Surg* 14:41-47, 1979.
49. Stone HH: Pulmonary burns in children, *J Pediatr Surg* 14:48-52, 1979.
50. Symbas PN: Cardiothoracic trauma. *Curr Probl Surg* 28:742-797, 1991.
51. Tellelz DW, Harden WD, Takehaski M et al: Blunt cardiac injury in children, *J Pediatr Surg* 22:1123-1128, 1987.
52. Townsend RN, Colella JJ, Diamond DL: Traumatic rupture of the aorta, *J Trauma* 30:1169-1174, 1990.
53. Trunkey DD: Thoracic trauma. In Trunkey DD, Lewis FR, editors: *Current therapy of trauma 1985.* Philadelphia, BC Decker, 1984.
54. Wagner RB, Crawford WO Jr, Schimpf PP: Classification of parenchymal injuries of the lung, *Radiology* 167:77-82, 1988.
55. Wall SD, Federle MP, Brett CM: CT diagnosis of unsuspected pneumothorax after blunt abdominal trauma, *AJR* 141:919-921, 1983.
56. Williams JS, Minken SL, Adams JT: Traumatic asphyxia reappraised, *Ann Surg* 167:384-392, 1968.
57. Wilson AJ, Kraus HF: Lung perforation during chest tube placement in the stiff-lung syndrome, *J Pediatr Surg* 9:213, 1974.
58. Young GM, Eichelberger MR: Initial resuscitation of the child with multiple injuries. In Grossman M, Dickmann RA, editors: *Pediatric emergency medicine: a clinician's reference,* Philadelphia, 1990, JB Lippincott.

PART TEN

Abdominal Injury

41 Patterns of Injury

W. Raleigh Thompson

Although isolated abdominal trauma occurs in children, it is usually encountered within the context of the multiply injured patient. In a series of 600 children admitted to a pediatric trauma center with blunt abdominal trauma, 30% were found to have significant intraabdominal injury. Mortality in that group was 4%, primarily reflecting the seriousness of associated injury.[6] Although blunt trauma remains the most frequent source of abdominal injury in the pediatric population, physicians who care for children must be increasingly aware of the proper management of penetrating injuries. This chapter reviews diagnostic methods and accepted therapy in the management of suspected abdominal trauma in children.

MECHANISM OF INJURY

Most abdominal trauma in children occurs as the result of motor vehicle, pedestrian, and bicycle accidents. Falls, sports injuries, and child abuse also account for a significant number of these injuries. All of these mechanisms are similar in that they result in blunt trauma. In blunt trauma, kinetic energy is transferred to intraabdominal organs through the abdominal wall. Solid organ injury predominates, and there is an approximately equal incidence of liver and spleen injuries. Subcapsular hematoma and parenchymal fracture result in hemorrhage, but bleeding often stops spontaneously, allowing for nonoperative management in the majority of cases. Despite the frequency of self-limited solid organ injury in children, it is critical to remember that massive hemorrhage, hollow viscus perforation, bladder rupture, and other life-threatening injuries do occur. Nonoperative management requires accurate diagnosis, vigilant resuscitation, and careful monitoring in an intensive care environment with the rapid availability of expert surgical care. Figure 41-1 is an algorithm for the management of blunt abdominal trauma.

Penetrating trauma, particularly that resulting from gunshot wounds, is more often associated with injuries incompatible with nonoperative therapy. Bowel perforation, ureter or bladder laceration, and large vessel injury occur with greater frequency and require repair to prevent peritonitis or massive bleeding. Unlike blunt trauma, penetration of the peritoneal cavity usually requires laparotomy. Kinetic energy, and therefore injury potential, is related to the mass and velocity of the penetrating object, as illustrated in the formula

$$KE = mv^2$$

whereas gunshot wounds are associated with significant and unpredictable collateral injury, stab wounds have much lower injury potential because of the relatively low velocity. These characteristics have led to different management schemes for the various types of penetrating injury. Stab wounds may be amenable to nonoperative therapy, given the application of the same criteria for accurate diagnosis and careful monitoring required in blunt trauma management. Gunshot wounds in which peritoneal penetration is proven, or even suspected, are best managed by laparotomy and direct inspection of all intraabdominal organs.[3] Figure 41-2 is an algorithm for management of penetrating abdominal trauma.

RESUSCITATION AND DIAGNOSIS
Initial management and assessment

Adequate respiratory and fluid resuscitation must be the initial focus in the treatment of any injured child. After management of the airway and correction of shock, the central issue becomes identification of injury. This may be difficult because of a child's fear or altered consciousness, or the severity of concomitant injuries. History and physical examination, including a digital rectal examination, are part of the initial assessment of the injured child. Adequate venous access, nasogastric tube decompression of the stomach, and bladder catheterization are integral to resuscitation.

The mechanisms of injury correlate with the incidence of severe abdominal injury and mortality. In a recent study, victims of assault or abuse were found to have abdominal injuries in nearly 40% of cases, and a mortality of 12.5%. Bicycle and motor vehicle crashes involved a high incidence of injury, but mortality was much lower, less than 5%.

Physical findings of gross hematuria and abdominal tenderness and trauma scores <12 are partic-

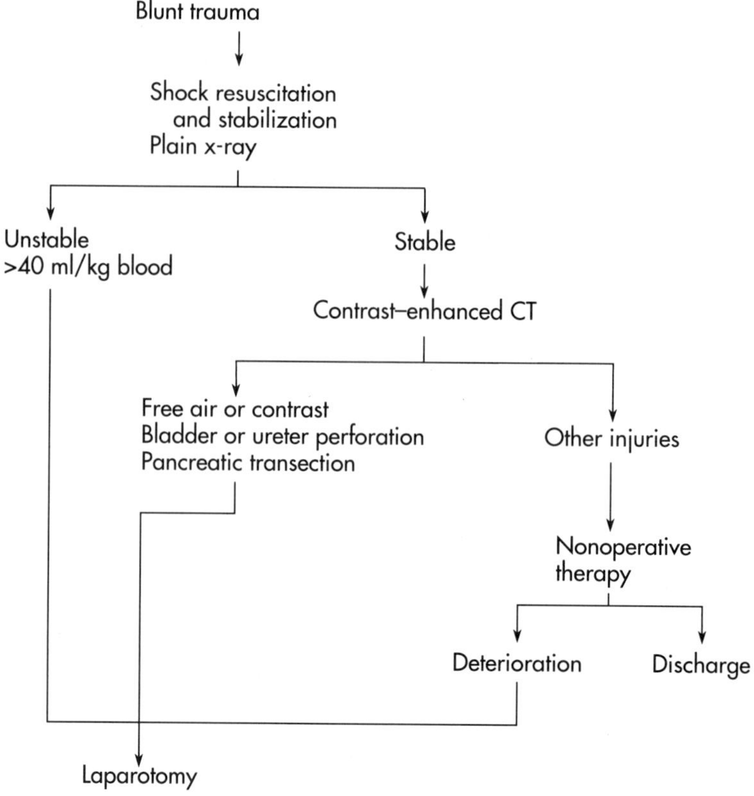

Figure 41–1 Algorithm for management of blunt abdominal trauma.

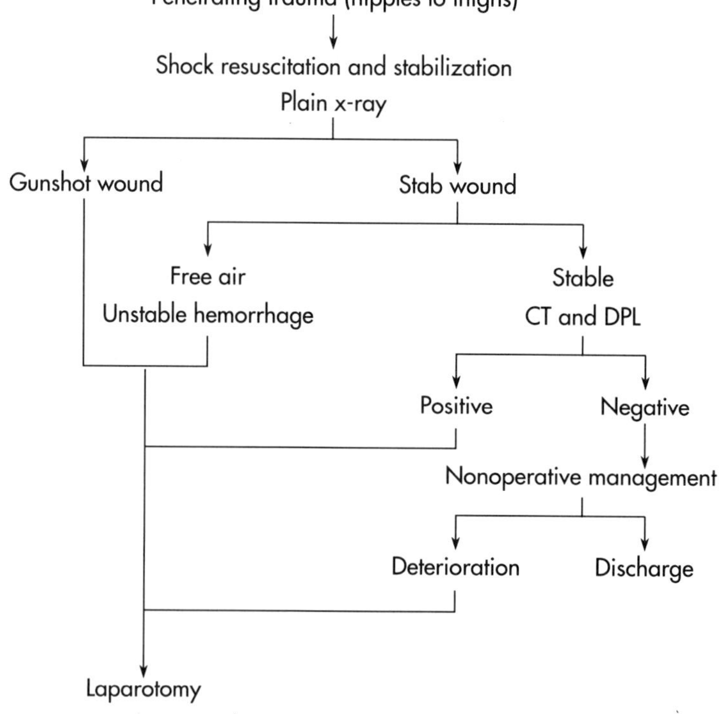

Figure 41–2 Algorithm for management of penetrating abdominal trauma.

ularly reliable predictors of serious injury. Interestingly, isolated neurologic deficit and dipstick or microscopic hematuria are not associated with an increased incidence of intraabdominal injury.[1] Plain radiographs of the chest, abdomen, and pelvis may show free intraperitoneal air, an indication for laparotomy. More often, they demonstrate lesions that should increase the physician's level of suspicion for intraabdominal injury.

A recent study of the association of pelvic fracture with intraabdominal trauma revealed abdominal injury in less than 1% of pelvic remus fractures, 15% of iliac or sacral fractures, and 60% of multiple pelvic ring fractures.[5] Rib fractures have also been shown to be markers for serious injury.

Table 41-1 lists the most important indicators for abdominal injury available on initial assessment of the injured child.

Assessment of extent of injury

A parallel goal to diagnosis is the determination of the extent of injury, in order to guide therapy and prevent unnecessary intervention. In addition to history and physical examination, a number of tools aid in the recognition and management of intraabdominal injury.

Computed tomography and ultrasound. The most useful diagnostic procedure in the treatment of children is the abdominal computed tomography scan, (CT), with both intraluminal and intravenous contrast. Numerous reports document the accuracy of this study in identifying and quantifying abdominal injury. Enhanced CT scan allows examination of the solid organs, of the anatomy and function of the urinary tract, and of the hollow viscera. Intraperitoneal air and blood are easily identified as well. This wealth of information has allowed for safe, nonoperative treatment in 81% of children with blunt trauma and proven intraabdominal injury. Only 15% of children with hemoperitoneum required laparotomy for repair of injury or control of bleeding. CT is a rapidly available, noninvasive test and has largely replaced ultrasound and liver-spleen scan in the evaluation of the trauma patient. Although ultrasound is enjoying some renewed interest, neither of these modalities provides the quantitative information available through CT.

Diagnostic peritoneal lavage. Diagnostic peritoneal lavage (DPL) is a surgical procedure used to detect the presence of blood bacteria, bile, or other visceral contents within the peritoneal cavity. It requires introduction of a plastic catheter into the peritoneal cavity, followed by infusion of 10 ml/kg normal saline. The infusate is then allowed to drain from the abdomen and is sent for cell count and amylase and microscopic analysis. Criteria for positive lavage are listed in Table 41-2. Although

Table 41–1 Indicators for serious abdominal injury (SAI)

Three or more clinical signs
Gross hematuria (52% SAI)
Abdominal tenderness (22% SAI)
Hematocrit <25%
Lap-belt injury
Assault or abuse as mechanism
Trauma score <12

Table 41–2 Criteria for positive diagnostic peritoneal lavage

10 ml gross blood upon catheter insertion
>100,000 red blood cells/mm^3
>500 white blood cells/mm^3
Bile or amylase >175IU/dl
Bacteria or vegetable matter upon microscopic examination

DPL has become the standard diagnostic procedure in adults, it has limited utility in children for several reasons. The most important drawback in DPL is that it provides little useful information. In contrast to enhanced CT, DPL only confirms the presence or absence of blood or bowel contents in the peritoneal fluid. Although its accuracy is well demonstrated (over 95% in most studies) it may miss significant injuries such as retroperitoneal hematoma and subcapsular liver or spleen injury. More important, exploration for positive DPL in children leads to unnecessary or even harmful laparotomies.[6] Early surgery for renal and splenic injury probably increases the incidence of splenectomy and nephrectomy. Transfusion of packed red blood cells is required in fewer than half of the children managed nonoperatively to maintain adequate blood volume and hematocrit of >20%. There is no evidence that early laparotomy reduces the necessity for transfusion. Other problems are that DPL is painful and potentially dangerous in the uncooperative patient. Incisional pain may interfere with follow-up examination, a factor especially important in safe nonoperative management.

Despite its limitations, DPL is quite useful in selected clinical settings in which CT is unavailable or has been proven less than adequate (Table 41-3). Stab wounds, particularly to the flank or lower chest, where peritoneal penetration is difficult to determine, can often be managed without laparotomy in the stable child. A negative lavage, with or without CT data, has proven valuable in reducing nontherapeutic laparotomy. Lap-belt injuries, a clear subgroup of blunt abdominal trauma, are associated with a much higher incidence of occult

Table 41–3 Indications for diagnostic peritoneal lavage

Stable patient, for whom nonoperative management is preferred, with:
Lap belt injury and normal enhanced CT
Stab wound to abdomen or flank with fascial penetration, but no other indication for laparotomy
CT not available and injury suspected

Table 41–4 Indications for laparotomy

Acute deterioration during resuscitation
Peritoneal penetration by gunshot
Gastrointestinal perforation
Persistent hemorrhage (40 ml/kg)
Hypotension or peritoneal signs during nonoperative management
Positive diagnostic peritoneal lavage

hollow viscus injury.[4] Such injury may be identified by DPL in patients with stigmata of the "lap-belt complex" whose abdominal CT scans reveal no abnormality. A third setting in which DPL has proven helpful is in evaluating the patient unavailable for CT because of prolonged or emergent orthopedic or neurosurgic procedures.

Assessment of penetrating trauma

Penetrating trauma may be further classified by mechanism of injury. Organ damage is directly proportional to the kinetic energy transferred to surrounding tissue by a penetrating object. Stab wounds are low-energy injuries, and gunshot wounds high-energy injuries. It is clear from the formula previously discussed that both mass and velocity of the penetrating object are important determinants of tissue injury. Practically speaking, most civilian gunshot injuries are low-velocity (but still high-energy) wounds caused by handguns. Rifle projectiles are much faster and cause even more tissue destruction. Shock waves can cause tissue damage several centimeters from the path of the projectile. Both of these high-energy injuries must be examined at laparotomy if penetration of the peritoneal cavity is proven or even strongly suspected (Table 41-4). A bullet may change course inside the body, making accurate prediction of its path impossible. For this reason, the general rule is that wounds between the nipples and the upper thigh must be presumed to penetrate the peritoneum.

Although knife wounds and other low-energy penetrating injuries often cause bowel perforation or other intraabdominal injuries when peritoneal penetration occurs, exploration of the abdomen (using the criteria outlined for gunshot wounds) results in as many as 80% nontherapeutic laparotomies. The mobility of the intestine within the peritoneal cavity may prevent perforation. Even deep flank wounds often fail to penetrate the peritoneal cavity. These conditions allow opportunities for selective nonoperative management. Contrast-enhanced CT combined with peritoneal lavage has been shown to provide accurate diagnostic information. Criteria for positive DPL are the same as those used in cases of blunt trauma, with the exception of lower chest wounds. Because of the frequency of occult diaphragmatic laceration, a lower RBC count (5000 to $10,000/mm^3$) should suggest the need for laparotomy in this setting. These studies, combined with close follow-up, should allow safe management and render nontherapeutic laparotomy less likely.

CONCLUSION

Abdominal trauma remains a significant cause of morbidity and mortality in the injured child. Shock resuscitation must be the initial priority in treatment of all children, but after resuscitation, the management strategies for blunt trauma and penetrating trauma are quite different. If hemodynamic stability can be achieved and accurate diagnosis established, most patients with blunt trauma can be treated safely without laparotomy. Enhanced CT and diagnostic peritoneal lavage have become useful tools in directing therapy, but it must be emphasized that the physiologic condition of the patient is the primary determinant of therapy. Nonoperative therapy has obvious advantages: postoperative pain, anesthetic complications, wound problems, and expense are all prevented. Nonoperative treatment may also prevent removal of damaged but salvageable spleens and kidneys. (Specific techniques of trauma laparotomy and organ repair are discussed in other chapters.) Regardless of the therapy chosen, abdominal trauma requires intensive monitoring and frequent reevaluation by experienced surgeons, because urgent intervention may be required at any time after the patient arrives in the emergency room.

REFERENCES

1. Bond SJ, Gotschall CS, Eichelberger MR: Predictors of abdominal injury in children with pelvic fractures, *J Trauma* 31:1169-1173, 1991.
2. Davis JW, Hoyt DB, Mackerskie RC: Complications in evaluating abdominal trauma: diagnostic peritoneal lavage versus computed axial tomography, *J Trauma* 30:1506-1509, 1990.

3. Eichelberger MR, Randolph JG. Abdominal trauma. In Welch KG, Randolph JG, Ravitch M et al, editors: *Pediatric surgery*, Chicago, 1986, Year Book Medical Publishers, pp 154-174.
4. Taylor GA, Eggli KD: Lap belt injuries of the lumbar spine in children: a pitfall in CT diagnosis, *AJR* 150:1355-1358, 1988.
5. Taylor GA, Eichelberger MR: Abdominal CT in children with neurologic impairment following blunt trauma, *Ann Surg* 210:229-233, 1989.
6. Taylor GA, Eichelberger MR, ODonnell R et al: Indications for computed tomography in children with blunt abdominal trauma, *Ann Surg* 213:212-218, 1991.
7. Taylor GA, Fallot ME, Potter BM et al: The role of computed tomography in blunt abdominal trauma in children, *J Trauma* 28:1660-1664, 1988.

42 Splenic Trauma

Ronald J. Scorpio and *David E. Wesson*

The spleen is one of the most commonly injured organs in blunt abdominal trauma. Recent advances in understanding of splenic function, splenic wound healing, and surgical technique have revolutionized the treatment of splenic injuries. Surgeons have played a major part in this process; pediatric surgeons in particular have championed selective nonoperative management of splenic injuries, the single most radical change in splenic surgery in the past 25 years.

Galen called the spleen "an organ filled with mystery." Ignorance of the physiologic role of the spleen colored the management of splenic injuries well into the twentieth century. Treatment, according to Roger Sherman, was based on four misconceptions[13]:

1. The spleen is not necessary for the maintenance of life.
2. The spleen cannot heal spontaneously.
3. Delayed rupture of the spleen is a true entity.
4. The number of complications following methods to conserve splenic function is greater than the number of complications following splenectomy.

In this chapter we present information about the anatomy, physiology, and pathophysiology of the spleen, as well as clinical data on the management of splenic injuries that will correct these misconceptions. We also outline a practical approach to the diagnosis and treatment of splenic injury.

ANATOMY

The spleen is located in the left hypochondrium. In adolescents and adults, it is protected by the rib cage, which covers the spleen in its entirety. However, in infants and small children the rib cage does not extend down far enough to provide adequate protection. Moreover, because the rib cage in children is much more pliable, it does not provide the same degree of protection as the more ossified adult rib cage. The spleen of children and adolescents is more susceptible to disease that can make it larger and more friable, thereby increasing the chances of injury.

The spleen is an intraperitoneal structure in close proximity to the diaphragm, stomach, tail of the pancreas, and left kidney. The tail of the pancreas lies close to the splenic hilum. The spleen is held in place by four ligaments, three avascular (splenophrenic, splenorenal, and splenocolic) and one vascular (gastrosplenic, containing the short gastric arteries).

The spleen is a conduit between the systemic and portal circulations. The arterial supply is dual, including the splenic artery (a branch of the celiac trunk) and the short gastric arteries (branches of the gastroepiploic artery). The splenic artery traverses the posterosuperior margin of the pancreas. Its proximity to the pancreas can present problems during application of a clamp to the artery in an attempt to control hemorrhage. The venous drainage that does not overlap the arterial segments occurs via the splenic vein. The splenic vein joins the superior and inferior mesenteric veins to form the portal vein. The architecture of the spleen is arranged in transverse segments with a separate blood supply to each segment. This favors segmental resection (Figure 42-1).[15]

PHYSIOLOGY

The spleen has three main functions: clearance and phagocytosis of particulate matter from the blood, antibody formation, and hematopoiesis. It performs these functions through a combination of specific microanatomy and a high rate of blood flow; 6% of resting cardiac output is directed to the spleen. The parenchyma is composed of red and white pulp. The red pulp serves as the site of phagocytosis, the removal of old red cells, and, in the infant, red cell production. The white pulp comprises the germinal centers, which produce IgM antibody and opsonizing proteins. The high rate of blood flow attests to the physiologic importance of the spleen and explains the risk of exsanguination in splenic trauma.

IMMUNOLOGY

The spleen is an important immunologic organ that plays a major role in combating infection. In addition to IgM, the spleen produces tuftsin and properdin, proteins that aid the phagocytosis of encapsulated bacteria, specifically pneumococcus, *H.*

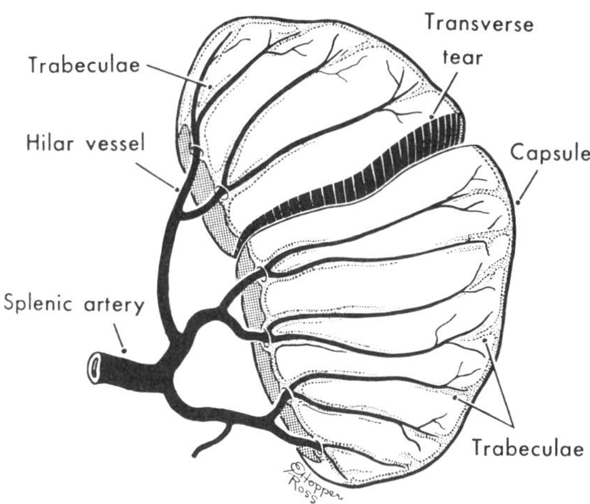

Figure 42–1 Segmental blood supply of spleen. (From Upadhyaya P, Simpson JS, in *Surg Gynecol Obstet*, April 1968. By permission of Surgery, Gynecology, & Obstetrics.)

influenzae, and meningococcus. The opsonizing proteins act on neutrophils to enhance the phagocytosis of these bacteria. In 1919 Morris and Bullock provided a scientific model reflecting the importance of the spleen in preventing infection.[8] This report was ignored until 1952, when King and Schumacker[6] reported the development of overwhelming infection in 5 asplenic infants, 2 of whom died. King reported an additional 15 patients, of whom 6 developed serious infections and 3 died. This report generated concern and controversy about splenectomy in children and raised several questions:

- Is the spleen important in preventing or fighting bloodstream infection?
- Is age an important factor?
- Is underlying disease a factor?
- Is the length of time from splenectomy significant?
- Is the patient at a higher risk for infection in general?

Numerous reports have now established that splenectomy increases the incidence of serious and perhaps fatal infection. Robinson and Sturgeon, reporting on 110 patients who underwent splenectomy, found 13 cases of infection.[11] However, in 63 cases of splenectomy for nonhematologic disease, only one patient developed a severe infection. Lucas and Krivit reported an infection rate of 4.1% in a series of 74 patients under 16 years of age.[7] Of the 18 trauma patients, none developed a severe infection. Erickson and colleagues,[5] in a review of 1467 patients, reported a serious infection rate of 2.8%. For children over 1 year of age, the rate was 1.1%. These authors also reported that 94% of patients developed their infections within 30 months of surgery. Diamond, in summarizing these data, coined the term "overwhelming postsplenectomy sepsis" (OPSI).[3] Eraklis and Filler, in a review of 1413 cases of splenectomy in children less than 16 years of age, found only 3 cases of infection in 342 trauma patients (0.9%).[4] Singer reviewed 2795 patients, including 388 children whose spleens were removed for trauma,[14] and found that only 4 trauma patients died from OPSI (mortality rate 0.58%). Even though this incidence is low, it is still 58 times greater than that in the general population. Wählby and Dömellof[17] reported that only 2.4% of 413 children whose spleens were removed because of trauma developed OPSI and that the mortality rate was 1.2%.

In summary, splenectomy predisposes patients to OPSI, especially children less than 1 year of age and those undergoing splenectomy for hematologic disorders. This predisposition persists for life.

EPIDEMIOLOGY

Splenic injury is three times more common in boys than in girls. The main causes are motor vehicle collisions, falls, bicycling accidents, and sports injuries, in that order. Penetrating injuries are rare. Motor vehicle–occupant injuries predominate among adolescents, whereas pedestrian injuries are more common among schoolchildren and domestic falls among preschoolers.

BIOMECHANICS

In children, the spleen is not well protected by the ribs and the parenchyma is friable. The forces of injury are usually transmitted through the abdominal wall directly to the spleen. The amount of parenchymal disruption depends on the force. Accelerating or decelerating forces may also injure the splenic hilum.

DIAGNOSIS

Diagnosis depends on the history of the injury, the symptoms and signs, and appropriate imaging. The latter confirms the clinical diagnosis and documents the degree of injury. In a child with multiple injuries, exclusion of splenic injury is important.

The force required to injure the spleen need not be excessive; a seemingly trivial blow can result in a splenic laceration. The diseased spleen is even more susceptible to injury. A history of a blow to the abdomen, left flank, or lower left chest should alert physicians to the possibility of a splenic injury.

Symptoms and signs of splenic injury are varied and usually nonspecific (Table 42-1). Symptoms include generalized or localized left upper quadrant abdominal or left flank pain. Other symptoms in-

Table 42–1 Symptoms and signs of splenic injury

Symptoms
Generalized abdominal pain
Localized abdominal pain
Nausea and vomiting
Left shoulder pain (Kehr's sign)
Dyspnea

Physical signs
Diffuse abdominal tenderness
Abdominal distention
Localized tenderness in left upper quadrant or flank
Peritoneal irritation
Rigidity
Muscle guarding
Rebound tenderness
Dullness in left upper quadrant
Ecchymosis in the left flank (Gray-Turner's sign)
Ecchymosis in the umbilical region (Cullen's sign)
Bruising in the left upper quadrant
Unexplained hypotension

Table 42–2 X-ray findings suggestive of splenic injury

Chest x-ray findings
Lower left rib fractures
Elevation of the left hemidiaphragm
Pleural effusion

Abdominal x-ray findings
Raised left hemidiaphragm
Stomach dilatation or medial displacement
Opacification of the left hypochondrium
Downward displacement of the transverse colon
Fluid between coils of intestines

clude pain referred to the left shoulder (Kehr's sign), dyspnea, nausea, and vomiting. Physical signs are reported to be present in only two thirds of cases of splenic injury. They include distention and tenderness, which may be localized or diffuse. The tenderness may be associated with signs of peritoneal irritation, including rigidity, muscle guarding, and rebound tenderness. Dullness of the left upper quadrant or shifting dullness may be present. A mass may be palpable in the left upper quadrant. Ecchymosis in the flank (Turner's sign) or in the umbilical region (Cullen's sign) may be present. Ecchymosis in the left upper quadrant or left flank strongly suggests an underlying injury. Unexplained hypotension is a nonspecific but worrisome indicator of intraabdominal bleeding, which may be of splenic origin.

Plain radiography is usually unhelpful; however, chest x-ray examination may suggest a splenic injury (Table 42-2).

Abdominal films can also be suggestive of splenic injury (Table 42-2). The important signs are elevation of the left hemidiaphragm, dilatation or medial displacement of the stomach, opacification of the left hypochondrium, downward displacement of the transverse colon, and fluid between loops of small intestine. Plain radiography will not confirm the diagnosis of splenic injury but will provide evidence to support the clinical signs and symptoms. It is important to remember that in ad-

olescents and children, even more than in adults, left lower rib fractures are highly suggestive of underlying organ injuries. However, rib fractures are uncommon in children and infants, and their absence does not exclude the presence of splenic injury.

More objective methods for diagnosis of splenic injury include diagnostic peritoneal lavage (DPL), nuclear medicine scintigraphy (NMS), ultrasonography (US), and computed tomography (CT).

To some extent, the method of treatment dictates the method of diagnosis. If nonoperative management of splenic injury is to be used, some type of diagnostic imaging (NMS, US, or CT) is necessary. DPL is not indicated in children who are to be managed nonoperatively; it is most useful in assessing the unstable child who is hypotensive and not responding to fluid resuscitation or the child who requires emergency surgery for extraabdominal injuries. DPL is very sensitive for the diagnosis of hemoperitoneum, which is almost always present in splenic trauma. In the stable child, however, hemoperitoneum is not an indication for surgery. Therefore DPL is not usually indicated in cases of suspected splenic injury because it does not alter treatment. The true value of DPL may lie in assessing injuries to other intraabdominal organs such as the small bowel.

CT is the diagnostic test of choice in hemodynamically stable children with suspected splenic injury. It can confirm a clinical diagnosis of splenic injury and quantify the severity of the injury. The advantages of CT include the availability of the scanning equipment, the speed at which the scan is completed, the specific detail of organ injury provided, and the ability to scan other areas at the same time, specifically the head and chest and other intraabdominal organs. A proper CT scan for trauma requires intravenous and gastrointestinal contrast. A qualified radiologist is also needed to interpret the results.

NMS is a simple, reliable method to establish the diagnosis of splenic injury. However, the child must be hemodynamically stable, and the suspected injury should be confined to the spleen or liver. The test uses the reticuloendothelial function of the liver and spleen, which take up a radiopharmaceutical from the blood. The scan requires about 30 minutes. Liver-spleen scans are more sensitive than CT in detecting splenic injury,[1] although injuries missed by a CT scan are unlikely to be clinically significant. A liver-spleen scan by NMS is easier to perform because the child need not be completely immobilized. However, small congenital abnormalities such as lobulation may mimic an injury on a liver-spleen scan, giving a false-positive result.

A newer but less reliable method for the diagnosis of splenic injury is US. Its advantages include its availability and noninvasive nature. However, difficulty is sometimes experienced in obtaining adequate images in the presence of a dressing, tube, or wound, in positioning the patient, and from interference of bowel gas. Ultrasound provides information on the presence of free peritoneal fluid and increased or decreased echogenicity of the spleen, and is most useful in following up documented splenic injuries.

Arteriography has no primary role in the diagnosis of splenic injury unless it is being performed for another indication.

In summary, most children with massive intraabdominal bleeding from splenic trauma who require urgent laparotomy are recognized on clinical grounds alone. In the unstable child without obvious signs of intraabdominal bleeding, the preferred diagnostic test is DPL; it can be done expeditiously and the results made available within minutes. In all cases of suspected splenic injury in hemodynamically stable children, the diagnosis should be confirmed by diagnostic imaging. The test of choice is usually CT, although NMS scan is acceptable.

CLASSIFICATION

CT demonstrates the quantity of hemoperitoneum and the exact type of splenic injury, which can be graded as shown in Table 42-3.

Radiographic classification has proven to be of some value in deciding whether or not operation is required in adults with splenic injuries (Figure 42-2). Its use as a guide to treatment of children has not been confirmed.

An operative grading system for splenic trauma has been developed by Shackford,[12] as follows: grade 1 injury is a nonbleeding capsular tear that

Table 42–3 CT classification of splenic injury severity

Grade	Description
1	Capsular avulsion, superficial laceration, or subcapsular hematoma
2	Parenchymal laceration 1-3 cm deep and/or central/subcapsular hematoma <3 cm
3	Laceration >3 cm deep, and/or central/subcapsular hematoma >3 cm
4	Fragmentation of three or more sections, devascularization of splenic parenchyma

requires no treatment; grade 2 injury is a capsular or parenchymal injury requiring only pressure for hemostasis; grade 3 injury is a parenchymal injury requiring suture ligation or suture approximation of splenic tissue or partial splenectomy; and grade 4 injury requires splenectomy. This system has not been applied to the treatment of children. Radiologic and operative grading systems are more useful for documentation and research than for the management of individual patients.

TREATMENT

Treatment is aimed at preserving the spleen by either operative or nonoperative means (Table 42-4). In most cases it can be preserved by selective nonoperative management.

All injured children require resuscitation as described in the guidelines set forth by the American College of Surgeons in the Advanced Trauma Life Support Course. Children who manifest persistent hypotension, expansion of abdominal girth, or a low or falling hematocrit level (<30%) in spite of adequate resuscitation (including transfusion of up to 20 ml/kg of packed red blood cells) require prompt operation.

Upadhyaya and Simpson[15] reported the first series of children with splenic injuries who were treated nonoperatively. The 12 children included had symptoms and signs that strongly indicated splenic rupture. They were all treated nonoperatively and did well. However, none of these injuries was confirmed by either radiographic or operative findings.

Since that time numerous reports have confirmed the value of selective nonoperative management of splenic injury. During the 15-year period from 1972 to 1986, 203 children with splenic injuries were treated at the Hospital for Sick Children in Toronto. Of these, 47 (23%) were treated operatively and 156 (77%) were treated nonoperatively.

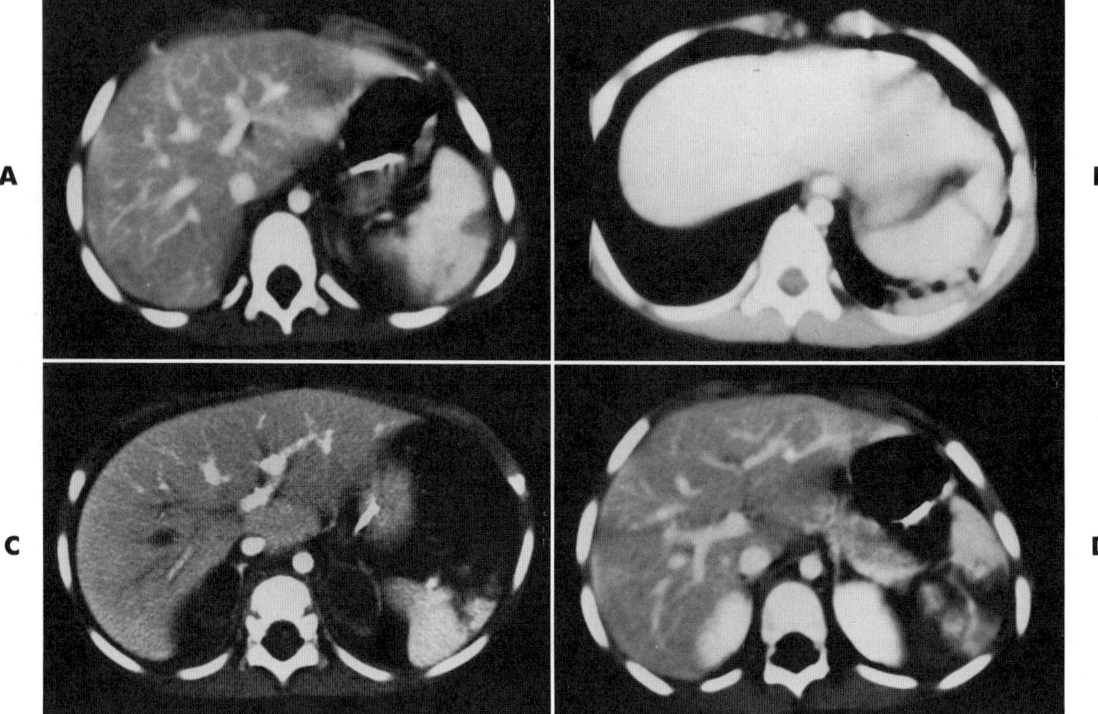

Figure 42–2 A, Splenic hematoma. **B,** Parenchymal laceration. **C,** Laceration and hematoma >3 cm. **D,** Fragmentation (this injury healed completely).

Table 42–4 Treatment of splenic injury

  I. Nonoperative
 II. Operative
    A. Splenorrhaphy
       1. Coagulation devices
       2. Hemostatic agents
       3. Direct suturing of bleeding points
       4. Mattress suturing of parenchyma:
          a. Without pledgets
          b. With pledgets
       5. Partial splenectomy
       6. Splenic artery ligation
    B. Splenectomy

The decision to operate should be based on the clinical course, not the presence of hemoperitoneum or the appearance of the CT scan. Nonoperative treatment is indicated in all hemodynamically stable children. It is also indicated in children who stabilize after initial resuscitation with crystalloid and/or blood (<20 ml/kg packed red blood cells or the equivalent). The clinical diagnosis of splenic injury must be confirmed by either a liver-spleen scan or a CT scan.

Once the diagnosis is confirmed, there are several prerequisites for nonoperative treatment:
1. The child must be monitored closely for at least 48 hours; vital signs must be measured frequently and hemoglobin and hematocrit levels determined at least daily.
2. The surgical team must be available to follow the child closely. The team must be in-house and prepared to operate at any time if necessary.
3. Adequate support from anesthesiology staff and the blood bank must be available.

If any of these conditions is not met, it is safer to operate and repair or remove the damaged spleen.

When treating a child nonoperatively, check the vital signs frequently, maintain venous access for 48 hours, and obtain serial hematocrit levels. Keep the child on strict bed rest and under close observation until he has been stable and has not required any blood for >48 hours. At this point the child may be allowed to ambulate, and may leave the hospital after 5 to 7 days. After discharge, the child may return to school but should refrain from sports and any other activities that might result in further bleeding or injury to the spleen for at least 8 weeks.

Operative care involves two methods of treatment: splenectomy and splenorrhaphy. Both require an adequate incision. In small children and infants, a transverse incision above the umbilicus is preferred. In adolescents, a midline incision provides better exposure. Regardless of age, in life-threatening cases the surgeon should use the incision that will allow access to the peritoneal cavity in the shortest amount of time. In most urgent cases, a midline incision is best.

Upon entering the abdomen, pack the four quadrants as needed and then assess the bleeding sites in a systematic fashion. When a splenic injury is detected, mobilize the spleen completely and deliver it out of the abdomen into the operative field. Mobilization proceeds by incision of the splenophrenic, splenocolic, and splenorenal ligaments and division of the short gastric vessels. Temporary hemostasis is possible if the first assistant occludes the blood supply to the spleen by compressing the splenic artery and vein between the index and middle fingers. Once the spleen is delivered into the operative field, an accurate assessment of the injury and the degree of splenic damage is possible. If the injury is severe, for example, a massive parenchymal injury or an injury extending into the hilum, perform splenectomy. Theoretically, reimplantation of splenic tissue is of value; however, no data are available on the clinical effectiveness of this therapy in humans. Thus there is no indication for autotransplantation of splenic tissue. If the child is stable and without multiple severe injuries, and the spleen is not beyond repair, attempt splenic salvage either by nonmechanical methods or splenorraphy.

Nonmechanical methods of hemostasis include simple pressure or the use of hemostatic agents such as fibrin glue or Avitene, or an absorbable mesh. Fibrin glue or Avitene applied to the splenic parenchyma with pressure, using gauze packs, may stop the bleeding. Another option is to compress and tamponade the spleen with an absorbable mesh. Coagulation is useful in stopping parenchymal, but not arterial, bleeding. Other nonmechanical methods of coagulation include either an argon beam or a carbon dioxide laser. However, we have found that nonmechanical methods are time-consuming and often ineffective; by the time they have been set up, the bleeding will have stopped in most cases.

Splenorrhaphy involves suturing the spleen. The procedure can range from partial splenectomy and direct suture of the splenic parenchyma and capsule with mattress sutures, to simple suture ligation of individual vessels. Recent reports have also described the use of stapling devices. It may be necessary to support the splenic sutures with pledgets

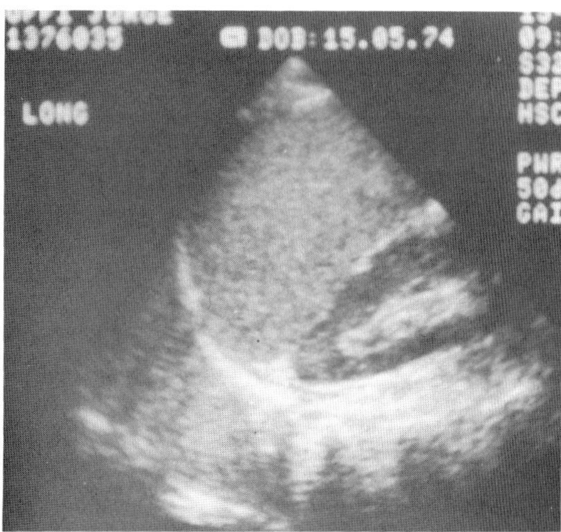

Figure 42–3 Follow-up ultrasound.

to prevent them from tearing through the spleen. The closeness of the splenic artery to the pancreas can result in injuries to the pancreas with disastrous complications. We have found that partial splenectomy, leaving at least one third of the spleen with its arterial blood supply intact, or suture ligation of individual bleeding points is the best way to achieve hemostasis. Splenic artery ligation with preservation of the short gastric arteries should be used only as a last resort.

AFTERCARE

The aftercare of the child with splenic injury depends on the treatment. Avoid respiratory complications such as atelectasis and pneumonia by encouraging the child to sit upright and to walk around.

After discharge, prohibit vigorous physical activity for 8 weeks for any child treated nonoperatively to allow maximum wound healing. Follow-up ultrasound examinations should be performed to document healing (Figure 42-3).

Following laparotomy, allow the child to walk as soon as possible. Monitor vital signs and urine production closely. Leave a nasogastric tube in place until the postoperative ileus has resolved.

The child who undergoes splenorrhaphy runs little risk of OPSI but could suffer from bowel obstruction.

Most aftercare guidelines deal specifically with the small percentage of children who undergo splenectomy. Unlike children treated nonoperatively or by splenic repair, these children are at risk of OPSI and must be protected from infection by two means: vaccination and administration of prophylactic antibiotics.

Vaccines are available against the three main bacteria involved in OPSI. Pneumovax 23 consists of a mixture of purified capsular polysaccharides derived from 23 pneumococcal subtypes. Bolan[2] has shown that the new 23-valent vaccine is 85% effective in asplenic patients over the age of 15 for at least 2 years. More detailed information on younger children is not available.

The most common adverse reactions to pneumococcal vaccines are fever, localized edema, pain, and swelling. Severe local and systemic reactions are more common in adults than in children and are much more common after a second injection or a booster dose of the vaccine. These reactions include weakness, myalgia, headache, photophobia, chills, nausea, and fever. The severe reactions are thought to result from antigen-antibody interaction. Consequently, booster injections should not be given within 5 years of the initial dose. Perkins[10] demonstrated that the antibody level achieved in asplenic patients is less than 50% of that achieved in patients with intact spleens. Nevertheless, he suggests that in most cases the antibody levels still provide protection. Vella and colleagues[16] found that adults had a 50% decline in the pneumococcal antibody titer at 3 years, whereas children showed a similar decline after only 21 months.

The second vaccine available is the *H. influenzae* type B (HIB) vaccine. Type B strain is responsible for virtually all invasive HIB disease. Most children of 24 months or more develop protective antibody levels following vaccination with the HIB polysaccharide antigen.[9] Fewer than half of children between the ages of 12 and 17 months respond well. The earliest age at which adequate antibody titers can be induced with the HIB vaccine is 18 months. If the vaccine is used earlier, then a booster dose is recommended after the child's second birthday.

Of the seven types of *Neisseria* meningitis that have been identified, only five groups (A, B, C, Y, W) are important causes of human disease. At present, a tetravalent meningococcal vaccine is available. This vaccine offers protection against groups A, C, Y, and W. Vaccination for group B meningococcal infection has been much more difficult to achieve. Among children under 2 years of age, vaccination against group A infection is the only one considered effective. There are no available reports of the vaccine's efficacy in the asplenic patient of any age. We do not routinely vaccinate children against meningococci after splenectomy in cases of trauma.

Because data concerning vaccine efficacy are difficult to obtain and because failure of any component is regarded as failure of the whole product, it is recommended that penicillin prophylaxis be used in addition to the vaccine to protect against the wider range of pneumococcal serotypes. Penicillin prophylaxis should be continued until the child reaches adolescence. Some authors have recommended amoxicillin instead of penicillin because it is effective against HIB. Erythromycin is an alternative in treatment of children who have penicillin allergy.

Patient compliance with antibiotic prophylaxis is poor. Moreover, infections can still occur despite antibiotic prophylaxis and vaccination. There are numerous reports of prophylactic antibiotics failing to prevent infection. Singer[14] has pointed out that half of the septic episodes in asplenic patients are due to organisms not sensitive to penicillin. Parents should therefore be taught to recognize signs of infection, warned to look for them, and advised, at the first sign, to begin antibiotic treatment and seek medical attention promptly.

In summary, the use of pneumococcal and HIB vaccines is strongly recommended following splenectomy in cases of trauma. However, vaccines are not a panacea because they only provide limited protection. Because of the unreliability of the vaccines, antibiotic prophylaxis is recommended, especially in infants and young children. Parental education is one of the most important factors in detecting and preventing infection.

COMPLICATIONS

Complications of nonoperative treatment of splenic trauma are mostly associated with rebleeding. After a diagnosis of splenic injury, the child should be advised to refrain from vigorous physical activity. However, the risk of delayed rupture of the spleen has been greatly exaggerated. Delayed splenic rupture has little, if any, clinical significance.

The time period during which the child should refrain from physical activity is not well defined. Based on our knowledge of wound repair, we recommend 8 weeks; this provides ample opportunity for splenic healing.

Complications of operative treatment are essentially the same, with the exception that the child who undergoes splenectomy is at risk of developing OPSI, whereas the patient who undergoes splenorrhaphy is not. The complication rates of splenic surgery in children are not well defined; however, rebleeding may occur following splenorrhaphy, with the result that a splenectomy must be performed.

Respiratory complications may follow any splenic operation. These include atelectasis, pleural effusion, and pneumonia; atelectasis is the most common and pleural effusion the least common.

Subphrenic abscess may also occur. However, the incidence of this complication is decreasing as the use of drains decreases.

Injury to the pancreas occurs in 2% to 3% of patients and results either in a pancreatic fistula caused by damage to the tail of the pancreas, or in pancreatitis.

Thrombocytosis is another complication of splenectomy, with platelet counts reaching their maximum value (~ 1 million) within 2 weeks of splenectomy. The most severe complication associated with thrombocytosis is mesenteric or portal vein thrombosis. In spite of this, there are no data to support the use of anticoagulants.

Although the complication rate among children is unknown, complications among adults and children generally have been reported to range anywhere from 6% to 61%, and among trauma patients specifically in the range of 30%.

SUMMARY

Splenic injury usually results from a direct blow to the abdomen. The physical signs vary from the typical mild local tenderness with little if any alteration in pulse or blood pressure, to frank peritonitis with profound shock resulting from massive intraabdominal bleeding. In the stable child with a suspected splenic injury, a CT scan should be performed to confirm the diagnosis. Most of these injuries can be treated nonoperatively because they will heal spontaneously. Massive bleeding requires immediate operation and the performance of splenorrhaphy, if possible, or splenectomy to stop the bleeding. In general, splenic salvage rates approach 90% in most case series. After splenectomy, there is a low but definite risk of OPSI, about which the child and parents must be advised. Pneumococcal and HIB vaccines should be given to reduce this risk. Systemic antibiotics are also indicated at the first sign of sepsis in the asplenic child.

REFERENCES

1. Bass DH, Mann MD, Cremin BJ et al: A comparison between scintigraphy and computed abdominal tomography in blunt liver and spleen injuries in children, *Pediatr Surg Int* 5:443-445, 1990.
2. Bolan G, Broome CV, Facklam RR et al: Pneumococcal vaccine efficacy in selected populations in the United States, *Ann Int Med* 104:1-6, 1986.
3. Diamond LK: Splenectomy in childhood and the hazard of overwhelming infection, *Pediatrics* 43:886-889, 1969.
4. Eraklis AJ, Filler RM: Splenectomy in childhood: a review of 1413 cases, *J Pediatr Surg* 7:382-388, 1972.
5. Erickson WD, Burgert EO Jr, Lynn HB: The hazard of infection following splenectomy in children, *Am J Dis Child* 116:1-12, 1968.
6. King H, Shumacker HB Jr: Spleen studies. I. Susceptibility to infection after splenectomy performed in infancy, *Ann Surg* 136:239-242, 1952.
7. Lucas RV Jr, Krivit W: Overwhelming infection in children following splenectomy, *J Pediatr* 57:185-191, 1960.
8. Morris DH, Bullock FD: The importance of the spleen in resistance to infection, *Ann Surg* 70:513-521, 1919.
9. Peltola H, Küyhty H, Virtanen M et al: Prevention of *Hemophilus influenzae* type B bacteremic infections with the capsular polysaccharide vaccine, *New Engl J Med* 310:1561-1566, 1984.
10. Perkins AC, Joshua DG, Gibson J et al: Fulminant postsplenectomy sepsis, *Med J Aust* 148:44-6, 1988.
11. Robinson TW, Sturgeon P: Post-splenectomy infection in infants and children, *Pediatrics* 25:941-951, 1960.
12. Shackford SR, Sise MJ, Virgilio RW et al: Evaluation of splenorrhaphy: a grading system for splenic trauma, *J Trauma* 21:538 542, 1981.
13. Sherman R: Management of trauma to the spleen, *Adv Surg* 17:37-71, 1984.
14. Singer DB: Postsplenectomy sepsis, *Perspect Pediatr Pathol* 1:285-311, 1973.
15. Upadhyaya P, Simpson JS: Splenic trauma in children, *Surg Gynecol Obstet* 126:781-790, 1968.
16. Vella PP, McLean AA, Woodhour AF et al: Persistence of pneumococcal antibiotics in human subjects following vaccination, *Proc Soc Exp Biol Med* 164:435-438, 1980.
17. Wählby L, Dömellof L: Splenectomy after blunt abdominal trauma: a retrospective study of 413 children, *Acta Chir Scand* 147:131-135, 1981.

43 Hepatobiliary Trauma

Ascension M. Torres and Victor F. Garcia

Emergency surgery for traumatic liver injury had its foundation in Germany.[47] In 1870 Bruns reported one of the earliest achievements of success in management of a gunshot wound to the liver, which he treated with resection of the injured area.[2] The early 1900s witnessed the development of many of the operative techniques currently employed for hepatic injury: the use of blunt needles, overlapping mattress sutures, mass ligation, thermocautery, and intrahepatic packing. In 1902 Beck emphasized the importance of meticulous hemostasis and discouraged the use of drains during hepatic surgery.[2] In 1908 J. Hogarth Pringle was the first to demonstrate that manual occlusion of the porta hepatis in humans was nonfatal.[49] The "Pringle maneuver" remains a valuable adjunct for hepatic hemorrhage control.

In 1954 Sparkman and Fogelman[57] described the complications of transfusion-associated coagulopathy and the pitfalls of superficial closure of deep hepatic laceration. They emphasized that the empiric use of systemic antibiotics did not prevent abscess formation and was not a substitute for hemostasis, debridement, and adequate drainage. In addition, they demonstrated that although hepatic wounds can be closed without drainage, the high incidence of associated complications subjects the patient to needless risk. In their experience with 100 civilian liver injuries, the principle determinants of outcome were the amount of blood loss, the number and type of associated injuries, and the extent of hepatic damage. Although hemorrhage was the greatest immediate threat to life, complications related to infection, liver necrosis, and inadequate drainage contributed to a 10% mortality rate.

By 1955 Madding's recommendations to explore all liver wounds, to perform resectional debridement of damaged tissue, to suture lacerations, and to establish external drainage were generally accepted by the surgical community.[30]

The 1960s ushered in a trend toward major hepatic resection as a primary treatment modality.[4,33,48] In 1963 Merendino and associates suggested T-tube insertion into the common duct or cholecystostomy in major hepatic injury to prevent biliary fistula.[34] This was vigorously impugned by Lucas in 1971.[28]

E. Truman Mays's contributions to the management of major hepatic injury prevailed in the 1970s and, to a large degree, are still valid today. He emphasized the importance of meticulous hepatic hemostasis and advocated hepatic artery ligation as a safe and effective method to control hemorrhage from the injured liver.[32]

A renewed appreciation of the importance of surgical exposure prompted the use of median sternotomy for exposure and vascular control in liver surgery, as reported by Miller in 1972.[36]

By the late 1970s and early 1980s, surgeons adopted a more conservative approach to hepatic injury. Debridement of only devitalized tissue and selective use of biliary drainage were promulgated.[59]

In the mid-1980s most centers of pediatric surgery recognized and advocated the safety and efficacy of treating selected blunt hepatic injuries nonoperatively.[9,21,26,41]

Because of the great strides made over the past century—the advances in general anesthesia, use of aseptic techniques, discovery of antibiotics, and the availability of blood banking technology, blood warmers, and rapid infusion equipment, as well as better-trained personnel caring for the injured patient not only in the prehospital phase but also during the acute phase—more and more patients survived injuries that were once considered lethal.

The overall mortality resulting from traumatic liver injury has decreased from 66% during World War I to a low of 9% during the Vietnam War. Today, the overall mortality of all liver injuries, blunt and penetrating, varies from 10% to 31%.[1,7,13,19]

EPIDEMIOLOGY

Not surprisingly, the etiology of liver injury parallels the leading causes of trauma-related death among children.[6,22] Each year in the United States, 20,000 to 25,000 children between birth and 19 years of age die of injuries: trauma remains the leading cause of childhood death. Motor vehicles were involved in 47% of injury-related deaths of

Table 43–1 Number, rate, and percentage of fatal injuries in children from birth to 19 years of age caused by motor vehicle accidents and falls in the United States, 1986

Causes of injury	Number	Annual rate/ 100,000	Percentage
Motor vehicle			47%
Occupant	7,412	10.5	33%
Pedestrian	1,787	2.5	8%
Other	1,336	1.9	6%
Falls	322	0.5	1.4%

From Childhood injuries in the United States: report to Congress. *Am J Dis Child* 144:627-646, 1990.

children in 1986 (Table 43-1). The patterns of injury are age related. From birth to 19 years of age, injuries to motor vehicle occupants are the major causes of death in the United States. Motor vehicle occupant injuries have the third highest hospitalization and emergency department visitation rates.

Pedestrian injuries are the fifth leading cause of injury-related deaths in children. Among children aged 5 to 9 years, pedestrian injuries account for more deaths than any other cause of injury. Childhood falls cause few deaths but have the highest rate for hospitalization and emergency department visits of all causes of injury.

The prevalence of penetrating injury in children is low, so it is not surprising that the overwhelming majority of hepatic injuries in children are the result of blunt trauma related to motor vehicle accidents. Completing the list of causative mechanisms are falls, handlebar injuries, and child abuse.

Because most hepatic injuries in childhood are the result of blunt trauma, multiple organ involvement is common, most notably of the head, musculoskeletal system, and chest.

Penetrating trauma, especially in areas of our country plagued by drug and gang wars, is usually the result of intentional injury. Interestingly, the liver is the organ most frequently injured in penetrating intraabdominal trauma.[31]

The most severe liver injuries are usually fatal early in their course, and exsanguination is the most common cause of death. Mortality associated with blunt liver injury stems from associated injuries and correlates with the number of organs injured. The shearing forces resulting from sudden deceleration and, consequently, the pattern of injury in the liver parenchyma, varies widely, and trauma is apt to be diffuse and associated with other organ injuries. Right lobe injury is four times more common than left lobe injury, and the posterior segment of the right lobe is involved in more than half of

all cases.[64] Fortunately, the majority of right-sided injuries are superficial and simple. In contrast, left-sided injuries tend to be deeper and more complex, because the usual direction of force is to the epigastrium.[58] Statistically, right hepatic vein injuries are most common, with right hepatic vein disruption occurring where the vein exits the liver parenchyma to join the inferior vena cava.[37]

The severity, extent, and nature of penetrating hepatic injuries depend on the trajectory, caliber, and the blast effect of the missile. The kinetic energy delivered by a projectile to the tissues depends on the projectile mass and the square of the velocity.

HISTORY AND PHYSICAL EXAMINATION

Historical information about an injury may prove very beneficial. When obtaining a history, the clinician should specifically inquire about the speed of the car, whether the child was restrained or unrestrained, how far from the point of impact the child was found, the need for extrication, and the condition of the child and of the vehicle at the scene. In cases of penetrating injury, queries should explore the type of assaulting weapon, caliber of the bullet, and the distance from which the weapon was fired.

The priorities of the primary examination are airway, breathing, and circulation. External signs of trauma, such as abrasions, ecchymosis, seat-belt markings, and entrance or exit wounds, especially to the right hemithorax and right upper quadrant, should be noted. Hypotension and abdominal distension with or without tenderness should also be recorded. Associated injuries to the head, long bones, ribs, and pelvic girdle should raise the level of suspicion for concomitant significant intraabdominal injury. Findings upon initial physical examination may correlate poorly with the presence of intraabdominal injury, especially if the child's sensorium is altered, whether by drugs or neurologic injury. Trauma scoring schemes may not offer the sensitivity once suggested. Saladino and colleagues confirmed that neither initial clinical findings nor a pediatric trauma score reliably predicts liver or spleen injury in children with focal abdominal injury.[50]

LABORATORY AND RADIOLOGIC EVALUATION

Initial laboratory studies include a cell blood count, urinalysis, and serum glutamic oxaloacetic transaminase (SGOT), serum glutamic pyruvic transaminase (SGPT), and amylase studies. It has been noted that elevations in SGOT and SGPT correlate with the presence of hepatic injury. When upon admission SGOT was greater than 200 IU and

SGPT greater than 100 IU, the probability of image-demonstrable hepatic injury was 62%.[40] Therefore, levels of SGOT greater than 200 IU and SGPT greater than 100 IU serve as useful guidelines for computerized axial tomography (CAT) imaging of the upper abdomen. Surprisingly, the degree of liver enzyme elevation above this threshold does not correlate with the severity or type of hepatic injury, nor does it predict a child's clinical course.[9,21,26]

Plain radiographs of the abdomen are of limited value. They may reveal displacement of the hepatic flexure or a mass effect in the right upper quadrant with hepatic injury, but overall they are not sensitive or specific and, if negative, do not rule out the presence of significant intraabdominal injury. In the event of penetrating intraabdominal trauma, plain films may delineate the trajectory of the missile and the organs that are at risk of injury.

Diagnostic peritoneal lavage (DPL) has limited use in the child with blunt trauma. DPL is not organ specific, and with the prevalent use and demonstrated efficacy of nonoperative management of the majority of pediatric hepatic injuries, a positive lavage rarely influences the decision to operate. Nevertheless, peritoneal lavage is used extensively in the diganosis of intraabdominal injuries in adults after blunt trauma.[44,45] A positive peritoneal lavage includes a red cell count greater than 100,000/mm^3, a white cell count greater than 500 per mm^3, the presence of bile or fecal material, and an elevated amylase.

After plain radiographs, the preferred radiographic modality in hemodynamically stable children is abdominal computed tomography (CT) with double contrast. No other single study or combination of studies defines the detail and extent of injury produced by abdominal CT.[25,60,62] Indicators for abdominal CT include a history or physical examination suggestive of specific injury to the liver, spleen, or kidneys; SGOT greater than 200 IU and SGPT greater than 100 IU upon admission; gross or microscopic hematuria; equivocal physical examination; head injury, altered sensorium or planned general anesthesia, which make serial abdominal examinations unreliable or unavailable (Table 43–2).[40] Children with unstable vital signs or progressive intracranial injury are not suitable candidates for a CT scan. In this event, peritoneal lavage is indicated as an adjunctive diagnostic measure.[11]

Some pediatric centers employ hepatic sonography in their diagnostic armamentaria.[21] Although sonography is noninvasive, portable, and readily available, its sensitivity is technician and radiologist dependent and its resolution is adversely altered by obesity and overlying bowel gas. It is,

Table 43–2 Indications for CT imaging in blunt abdominal trauma at Cincinnati Children's Hospital Medical Center

History or physical examination suggestive of liver, spleen, or renal injury
Admission SGOT > 200 IU and SGPT > 100 IU
Gross or microscopic hematuria
Unreliable physical examination owing to head injury, drugs, or general anesthesia

however, very useful in assessing the rate and completeness of healing in a hepatic injury.

Scintigraphy has also been used routinely in some centers in the initial evaluation of liver injury.[10] The limited availability of 24-hour in-house personnel trained in nuclear medicine limits the usefulness of this technique in the acute trauma setting.

There are few indications for the use of arteriography as a diagnostic modality in the acute setting. Typically, it is used in the evaluation of post-traumatic children who develop complications. When combined with embolization, it serves as a diagnostic, as well as therapeutic, tool in the treatment of selected hepatic injuries.

CLASSIFICATION OF LIVER INJURIES

Liver injuries can be classified according to the grading of the Organ Injury Scaling Committee of the American Association of Surgery of Trauma (Table 43-3).[38] This classification, which considers the location and the extent of the injury, fundamentally lists anatomic descriptions scaled from I to VI, representing the least to the most severe injury. It is, however, based on adult liver injuries, and its usefulness in treatment of children has not been evaluated. Except for those that invalue hypovolemic shock and hemodynamic instability, most hepatic injuries in children can be managed nonoperatively.

NONOPERATIVE MANAGEMENT

The safety and efficacy of nonoperative treatment of the hemodynamically stable child with blunt hepatic injury is well established.[9,10,21,26] Once diagnosis is made and the liver injury identified, resuscitation and serial evaluation is of utmost importance in nonoperative management. Operating room personnel, anesthesiology, and other ancillary critical care facilities must be available and able to respond immediately, 24 hours a day, for safe and successful nonoperative treatment of the injured child.

The child with a hepatic injury is kept at strict

Table 43–3 Grading of liver injuries

Grade*		Injury description†
I.	Hematoma	Subcapsular, nonexpanding < 10% surface area
	Laceration	Capsular tear, nonbleeding, with < 1 cm deep parenchymal disruption
II.	Hematoma	Subcapsular, nonexpanding, hematoma 10% to 50%; Intraparenchymal nonexpanding < 2 cm in diameter.
	Laceration	< 3 cm parenchymal depth < 10 cm in length
III.	Hematoma	Subcapsular, > 50% of surface area or expanding; ruptured subcapsular hematoma with active bleeding; intraparenchymal hematoma > 2 cm
	Laceration	> 3 cm parenchymal depth
IV.	Hematoma	Ruptured central hematoma
	Laceration	Parenchymal destruction involving 25% to 75% of hepatic lobe
V.	Laceration	Parenchymal destruction > 75% of hepatic lobe
	Vascular	Juxtahepatic venous injuries
VI.	Vascular	Hepatic avulsion

*Advance one grade for multiple injuries.
†Based on most accurate assessment at autopsy, laparotomy, or radiology study.
From Organ Injury Scaling Committee: *J Trauma* 29:1664-1666, 1989.

bed rest and closely monitored, usually in an intensive care setting. As suggested by the severity of the injury, the child requires nasogastric decompression until intestinal ileus resolves. An indwelling bladder catheter can be used to assess urine output accurately. Abdominal examinations are serially performed by a single experienced surgeon. Serial hematocrit levels assessed every 4 hours or more often, depending on the clinical course, are helpful. If hemodynamically stable and not in need of a transfusion, the child continues strict bed rest, and serial hematocrit determinations are made every 12 hours. Upon normalization of liver transaminase, the child is allowed to ambulate. Activity is restricted until complete healing of the liver injury is documented by ultrasound.

Karp and colleagues described four healing stages of nonoperatively managed blunt hepatic injury.[25] Stage 1 occurs over the first 2 weeks following injury and involves resorption of intraperitoneal and intrahepatic hematoma and injured tissue. Stage 2 involves coalescence of stellate lacerations until one large cavity of lesser density is found. Stage 3 shows an increased density and decreased size of the area of injury, at approximately 1 month postinjury. Stage 4 reveals a reduction in size to a point where parenchymal homogenicity is restored, at about 3 to 4 months postinjury. Follow-up CT or ultrasound examination of the liver is reserved for those children with documented grade III or greater liver injuries.

OPERATIVE MANAGEMENT

The need for exploratory celiotomy is evident by refractory hemodynamic instability, transfusion re-

quirements of greater than 50% of child's blood volume (40 cc/kg day) within a 24-hour-period, pneumoperitoneum or associated intraabdominal injuries themselves requiring surgical exploration, for example, renal vascular injury, ureteral transection, bladder rupture.

Liver injury

Priorities in the surgical management of hepatic injuries are control of hemorrhage, mobilization and identification of the liver injury, definitive control of hepatic bleeding, debridement of devitalized tissue, and establishment of adequate drainage.

A midline incision is preferred for rapid access and for exposure. Occasionally, in the younger child in whom the maximum transverse dimension of the abdomen is greater than the cephalad-caudad dimension, an upper transverse or chevron type of incision with a vertical limb (inverted T) is acceptable (Figure 43-1). In the child with refractory hypovolemic shock, occlusion of the descending thoracic aorta prior to celiotomy is advocated. Large-diameter, short intravenous cannulas (Cordis introducer, nasogastric tubes) combined with commercially available rapid infusion pumps are invaluable in this setting.

If O-negative blood is used, the empiric use of blood components should be considered. To avoid preventable delays, a simultaneous order of fresh frozen plasma, platelets, and cryoprecipitate is reasonable.

At least two large suction catheters should be available in the operative field. Once the abdomen is opened, however, blood is most expeditiously evacuated by manually scooping out the large clots.

After blood clot removal, pack all four quadrants tightly with large laparotomy tapes. Properly and deliberately performed, this maneuver can effectively tamponade abdominal bleeding and allow the anesthesia team to replenish the intravascular volume before mobilization and identification of the hepatic injury.

The injured liver is mobilized by dividing the falciform ligament between clamps. The right and left triangular and coronary ligaments are divided with scissors or electrocautery (Figure 43-2). After a diligent search, hepatic bleeding is controlled by packing and a plan formulated with the anesthesia team to time repair and anticipate blood loss. Good communication between surgical and anesthesia teams is essential.

An adjunctive maneuver to control hepatic bleeding is the Pringle maneuver (occlusion of the portal vein, common bile duct, and hepatic artery at the hepaticoduodenal ligament), which can be quickly performed and is usually tolerated up to 1 hour[14,42,43,49] (Figure 43-3). Persistent inflow bleeding can be seen despite the Pringle maneuver in children with an aberrant right or left hepatic artery. Ongoing massive bleeding, even with use of the Pringle maneuver, may be due to injury to a hepatic vein or retrohepatic cava.

Portal vein injury is usually the result of penetrating trauma. The best results are achieved with primary lateral venorrhaphy or end-to-end anastomosis. If there is extensive tissue destruction, then portal vein ligation, interposition grafts between portal vein segments, a portocaval shunt or splenic vein to superior mesentery vein bypass are other options, less desirable because of associated increased mortality.[20]

A simple, yet practical, method for immediate control of intrahepatic venous hemorrhage is to compress the liver against itself (Figure 43-4). The use of hepatotomy (finger fracture technique) with selective vascular ligation for deep laceration and debridement of devitalized tissue are more direct maneuvers to control deep parenchymal bleeding. An omental patch or use of hemostatic agents such as Surgicel, Avitene, thrombin-soaked gelfoam, or fibrin glue provides other useful adjunctive options.

A Penrose drain can be placed circumferentially around the liver and used as a tourniquet to control hemorrhage from the lateral aspect of the right or left lobe of the liver (Figure 43-5).

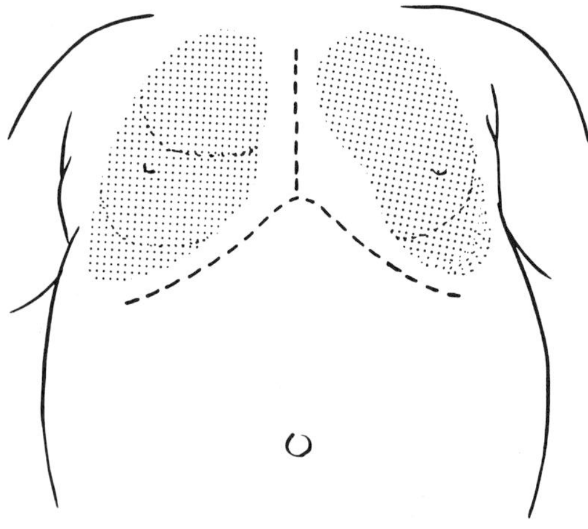

Figure 43–1 A chevron type of incision, with or without an upward vertical extension, is an alternative option in treatment of the young child undergoing laparotomy for trauma.

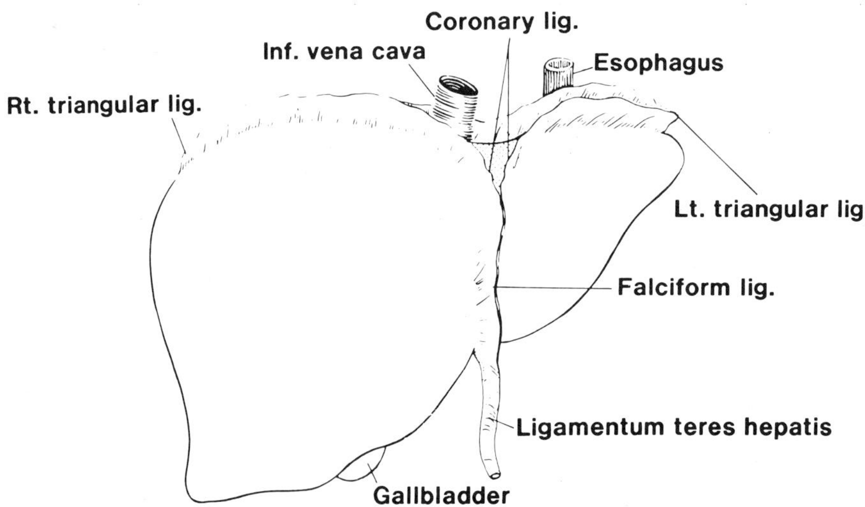

Figure 43–2 Anterior view of the liver. Note the relationship between the falciform ligament, ligamentum teres hepatis, coronary and triangular ligaments.

Sequential occlusion to achieve hepatic vascular isolation is poorly tolerated by the hypovolemic injured child. It entails occlusion of the supraceliac aorta, of the hepatoduodenal ligament, and of the suprahepatic and infrahepatic inferior vena cava

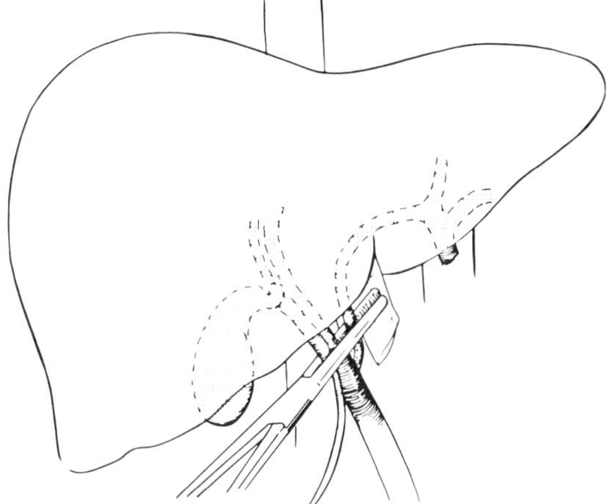

Figure 43–3 The Pringle maneuver.

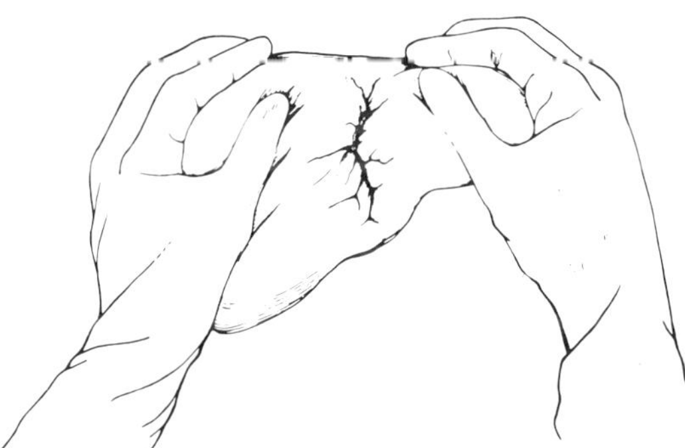

Figure 43–4 Manual compression of the liver is helpful in controlling intrahepatic venous hemorrhage.

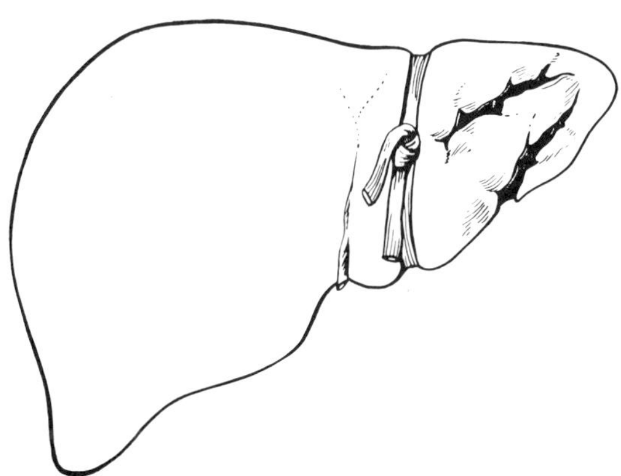

Figure 43–5 Penrose tourniquet technique.

(Figure 43-6). In the hypovolemic child this maneuver is frequently associated with cardiac arrhythmia or arrest, secondary to poor venous return.[27,61]

The right or left hepatic artery can be ligated when the bleeding is arterial but the distal site cannot be identified. If the right hepatic artery is ligated, cholecystectomy should be performed.[5,52,61] Major anatomical resections are required in only 2% to 4% of all hepatic injuries and carry a 20% to 45% mortality.[14,19]

Disruptions of the posterior aspect of the liver are often difficult to identify. When a retrocaval or hepatic vein injury is suspected, hepatic vascular isolation should be performed with minimal delay. A variety of techniques have been described.

An atriocaval shunt may be inserted via the atrium, infrarenal vena cava, or saphenofemoral junction.[27,46,54] The latter approach, developed by Moore and Pilcher,[46] may be the least practical in the child with small distal vessels (Figure 43-7). Atriocaval shunting via the right atrial appendage is the most commonly recommended approach (Figure 43-8).

The abdominal incision is extended cephalad as a median sternotomy. In the adolescent, the standard shunt is a no. 36 argyle chest tube with an extra hole cut approximately 20 cm above the most proximal hole in the distal tube for venous return. In smaller children, estimate the size of the inferior vena cava and choose a chest tube of appropriate caliber. The surgeon must quickly measure the dis-

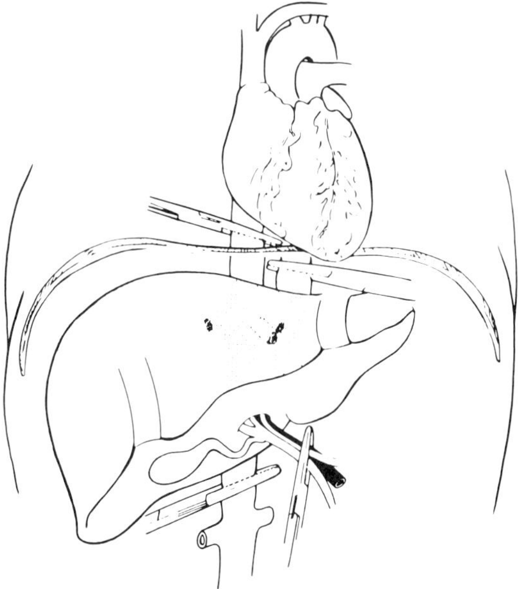

Figure 43–6 Sequential clamping technique for complete vascular isolation.

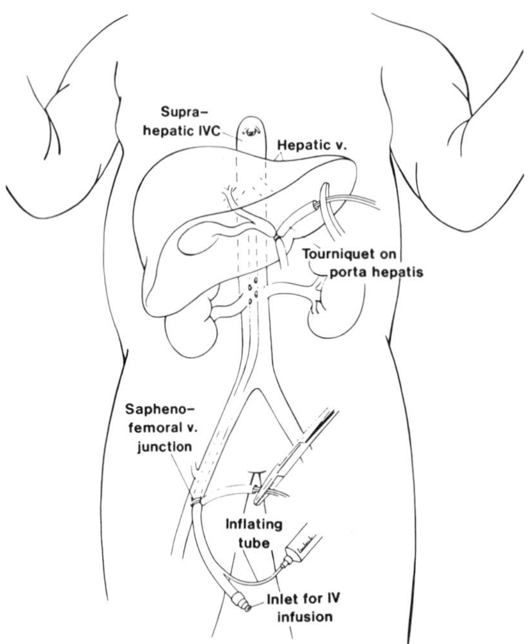

Figure 43–7 Saphenofemoral atriocaval shunt.

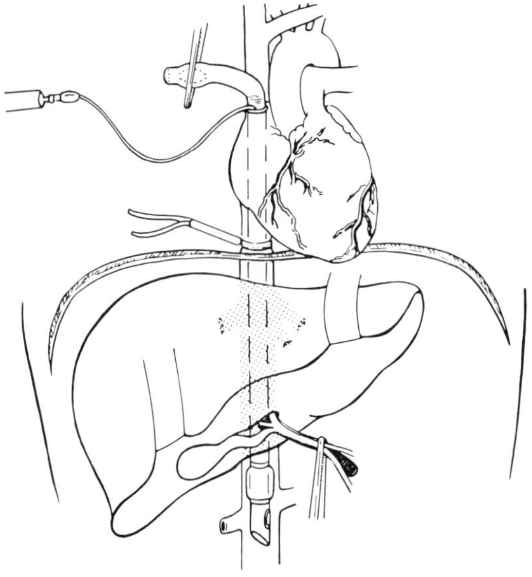

Figure 43–8 Atriocaval shunt.

tance from the renal veins to the right atrium in order to place a side hole accurately in the atrium. Intrapericardial suprahepatic caval and suprarenal caval tourniquets are placed, but not secured, prior to shunt insertion. A Satinsky vascular clamp is placed over the right atrial appendage, followed by a purse-string suture of 2-0 or 3-0 nonabsorbable suture material in the atrial appendage. A small opening is made inside the purse-string and, with a clamp just below the extra hole, the shunt is passed down to the inferior vena cava to the level of the renal veins. Once the shunt is filled with blood, the clamp is moved toward the end of the tube and the extra hole in the shunt is advanced so as to lie inside the right atrium. (These steps will lessen the chance of air embolus.) The suprahepatic caval and the suprarenal caval tourniquets are then tightened. Porta hepatis occlusion is required to complete vascular isolation.

An indwelling bladder catheter or cuffed endotracheal tube has also been employed as an atriocaval shunt. A saline-inflated balloon eliminates the need of one of the caval tourniquets. The end of the bladder, chest tube, or endotracheal tube catheter can be used as a site for rapid fluid infusion if there is need for additional volume replacement.[5,20,27,43,52,54,61]

Retrohepatic venocaval injury is the most lethal of hepatic vascular injuries. Mortality results from exsanguination or from transfusion-related disseminated intravascular coagulopathy (DIC), renal insufficiency, or pulmonary failure.

In children whose bleeding cannot be controlled, application of dressing packs into the abdomen with large laparotomy tapes and closure of the incision with staples or towel clips is a viable option.[8,15,16,18,24] A "second look" operation is performed 24 hours later, after hypothermia and coagulopathy are corrected.

Biliary injury

Extrahepatic biliary trauma is rare in the pediatric population.[3,12,23,55,56] Perforation of the gallbladder, usually as the result of penetrating trauma, is managed by simple cholecystectomy. In contrast to earlier reports in which falls, kicks, or blows were the most common factors causing blunt gallbladder injury, motor vehicle crashes are now the leading cause of such injury. The spectrum of gallbladder injuries includes contusion, avulsion, and perforation.[55] Cholecystectomy is the operation of choice for traumatic gallbladder rupture, but there have been several reports of successful treatment of such injuries in children by simple closure of the perforations, cholecystostomy, or both.[3,12,56] An intraoperative cholangiogram is necessary to rule out or delineate the extent of biliary ductal injury.

Disruption of the biliary ductal system by blunt abdominal trauma is also rare. The most common causes are motor vehicle accidents and falls. The most common site of injury of the duct is the superior border of the pancreas.[35]

Presentation varies, depending on the interval of time between injury and diagnosis. Early diagnosis is usually made at the time of laparotomy for other

Table 43-4 Review of 19 patients with hepatic injury

Patient	Age/race/sex	Mechanism	Abdominal examination	SGOT SGPT	Assoc injuries	
#1	21 mo WM	Fall	Normal	a) 297 b) 143	None	
#2	8 yr WM	Occupant	Tender	a) 1346 b) 817	Renal pedicle	Right lobe
#3	8 yr WM	Crush	Distended	a) 691 b) 403	Ribs, renal, and spleen	Right lobe
#4	11 mo WM	Blow	Tender	a) 2049 b) 1163	Spleen and renal	Right and left lobes
#5	15 yr WF	Occupant	Tender	a) 123 b) 98	None	Right lobe
#6	7 yr WF	Occupant	Tender	a) 582 b) 369	Renal lac	Right lobe
#7	22 mo WM	Fall	Normal	a) 1458 b) 853	None	Left lobe
#8	3 yr WM	Blow	Tender	a) 1932 b) 776	None	Right lobe
#9	7 yr WM	Pedestrian	Tender	a) 779 b) 363	Lung and ribs	Right lobe
#10	10 yr WM	Gunshot	Tender	a) 33 b) 17	None	Right lobe
#11	12 yr WF	Fall	Tender	a) 340 b) 228	None	Left lobe
#12	6 yr WM	Pedestrian	Tender	a) 381 b) 173	None	Left lobe
#13	2 yr WM	Occupant	Distended	a) 952 b) 417	Lung, renal, tib/fib	Right lobe
#14	9 yr WM	Fall	Tender	a) 527 b) 298	None	Right lobe
#15	3 yr WM	Pedestrian	Tender	a) 752 b) 330	Lung	Right lobe
#16	3 yr WF	Fall	Tender	a) 839 b) 433	None	Right lobe
#17	7 yr BF	Fall	Tender	a) 272 b) 252	None	Not done
#18	3 yr WF	Child abuse	Tender	a) 6582 b) 3009	Spleen	Right lobe
#19	9 yr BF	Penetrating	Tender	a) 88 b) 55	Kidney	Right lobe

injuries. Signs of delayed diagnosis include anorexia, vomiting, abdominal distension, and jaundice. Laboratory studies are of little use; abdominal paracentesis may be diagnostic. Radionuclide scans may demonstrate the leak with extravasation of radionuclide into the peritoneal cavity.

Common bile duct injury may be repaired over a stent. Primary end-to-end anastomosis may be technically more difficult in the small child with a normal size common duct. In these instances a preferable technique is a duct-to-enteric anastomosis, usually as a Roux-en-Y. A tension-free anastomosis with mucosa-to-mucosa apposition is essential. In a child with hepatic injury but intact extrahepatic biliary tree, routine T-tube common bile duct drainage results in increased morbidity and mortality and is not recommended.[28]

COMPLICATIONS

Exsanguination, secondary to uncontrolled bleeding, is the most frequent cause of death in children with hepatic and biliary injuries. Persistent uncontrolled hemorrhage, either from the actual injury itself or from a disseminated coagulopathy owing to massive blood transfusions, hypothermia, or metabolic acidosis secondary to inadequate resuscitation, is usually noted in children dying within 24 to 48 hours after injury. Because of hemodynamic instability at the time of presentation, these are the children usually treated with immediate surgical exploration. Not surprisingly, they are the same children who are at an increased risk for subsequent morbidity. Intraabdominal sepsis, respiratory failure, pyrexia, biliary leaks, and hemobilia complete the list of the more common complications encountered in the patient with a severe liver injury.

In the absence of sepsis, fever is attributed to resorption of the injured tissue. However, atelectasis is also common and may contribute to pyrexia in patients with trauma to the upper abdomen. The cause of fever that persists or recurs after the first 5 days postinjury requires diligent investigation; treatable intraabdominal sepsis is the leading cause of late morbidity. The incidence is higher in children with concomitant colon injury and in children in whom a Penrose drain, rather than closed suction drainage, is employed.[1,39,51,66]

Hemobilia is evidenced by painless upper gastrointestinal bleeding or colicky right upper quadrant pain and tenderness, associated with jaundice and fever. This is due to rupture of an intrahepatic pseudoaneurysm. The biliary system becomes obstructed with blood or blood clots, and there is subsequent elevation of serum bilirubin, alkaline phosphatase, and SGOT. Upper endoscopy usually reveals blood from the ampulla of Vater. This finding rules out other causes of gastrointestinal hemorrhage. Selective angiography may be diagnostic and therapeutic, demonstrating the pseudoaneurysm and providing a road map for angiographic embolization, the treatment of choice.[29,66]

A biliary leak, secondary to traumatic disruption of an intraparenchymal hepatic duct, leads to bile peritonitis or biliary fistula. Typically, such leaks are seen as perihepatic fluid collection, which is generally evident on ultrasound. Aspiration usually reveals the biloma.[17,35,53] Technetium-99–labeled scintigraphy can aid in the diagnosis of biliary leaks.[63] Most leaks will resolve with adequate external drainage and do not require surgical intervention, as reported in the experience of many pediatric trauma centers.

Nineteen patients with hepatic injury admitted to the Cincinnati Children's Hospital Medical Center from January to December 1990 were reviewed (Table 43-4). Their ages ranged from 11 months to 15 years. There were 12 male and 7 female children; 17 were white and 2 were black. The mechanism of injury was blunt in 17 children and penetrating in 2. Of the 17 children with blunt abdominal trauma, 41% had injuries resulting from motor vehicle crashes (4 occupants and 3 pedestrians). Other mechanisms included 6 falls, 3 intentional blows, and one instance of child abuse. SGOT and SGPT levels upon admission were greater than 200 IU and 100 IU, respectively, in all but one child who underwent a CT scan to evaluate abdominal tenderness noted at the time of admission. The right lobe of the liver was involved in 14 of the 19 cases. Sixteen children (84%) were treated nonoperatively. Three children underwent abdominal exploration, two with penetrating trauma and one child with blunt trauma who had an associated renal pedicle injury. In all children surgically explored, the liver laceration had stopped bleeding and drains were not used. Nine children had associated injuries. No significant morbidity resulted from liver injury in any of the children, and there were no deaths over this 12-month period. Nonoperative management was successful in all children in whom it was employed.

Nonoperative management of the hemodynamically stable child with liver injury is now well established. The complication rate varies between 4% and 8%, and most deaths occur as a consequence of an associated injury. In the hemodynamically unstable child, hemorrhage remains a major cause of morbidity and mortality, and surgeons continue the search for improvement in the expeditious vascular isolation of the injured liver. The role of veno-venous bypass and orthotopic liver transplantation for those children who have sustained isolated massive hepatic injury is currently in evolution.[65]

REFERENCES

1. Aldrete JS, Halpern NB, Ward S et al: Factors determining the mortality and morbidity in hepatic injuries: analysis of 108 cases, *Ann Surg* 189:466-474, 1979.
2. Beck C: Surgery of the liver, *JAMA* 38:1063-1068, 1902.
3. Benson CD, Prust FW: Traumatic injuries of the liver, gallbladder, and biliary tract in the infant and child, *Surg Clin Am* 33:1187-1191, 1953.
4. Byrd WM, McAfeem DK: Emergency hepatic lobectomy in massive injury of the liver, *Surg Gynecol Obstet* 113:103-105, 1961.
5. Canizaro PC, Pessa ME: Management of massive hemorrhage associated with abdominal trauma, *Surg Clin N Am* 70:621-634, 1990.
6. Childhood injuries in the United States: Report to Congress, *Am J Dis Child* 144:627-646, 1990.
7. Cox EF, Flancbaum L, Dauterive AH et al: Blunt trauma to liver: analysis of management and mortality in 323 consecutive patients, *Ann Surg* 207:126-134, 1988.
8. Cue JI, Cryer HG, Miller FB et al: Packing and planned re-exploration for hepatic and retroperitoneal hemorrhage: critical refinements of a useful technique, *J Trauma* 30:1007-1013, 1990.
9. Cywes S, Rode H, Millar AJW: Blunt liver trauma in children: nonoperative management, *J Pediatr Surg* 20:14-18, 1985.

10. Cywes S, Bass DH, Rode H et al: Blunt abdominal trauma in children, *Pediatr Surg Int* 5:350-354, 1990.
11. Drew R, Perry JF Jr, Fisher RP: The expediency of peritoneal lavage for blunt trauma in children, *Surg Gynecol Obstet* 145:885-888, 1977.
12. Evans JP: Traumatic rupture of the gallbladder in a 3-year-old boy, *J Pediatr Surg* 11:1033-1034, 1976.
13. Fabian TC, Croce MA, Stanford GG et al: Factors affecting morbidity following hepatic trauma: a prospective analysis of 482 injuries, *Ann Surg* 213:540-548, 1991.
14. Feliciano DV: Surgery for liver trauma, *Surg Clin N Am* 69:273-284, 1989.
15. Feliciano DV, Pachter HL: Hepatic trauma revisited, *Curr Probl Surg* 26:453-524, 1989.
16. Feliciano DV, Mattox KL, Jordan GL Jr: Intraabdominal packing for control of hepatic hemorrhage: a reappraisal, *J Trauma* 21:285-290, 1981.
17. Feliciano DV, Bitondo CG, Burch JM et al: Management of traumatic injuries to the extrahepatic biliary ducts, *Am J Surg* 150:705-709, 1985.
18. Feliciano DV, Mattox KL, Burch JM et al: Packing for control of hepatic hemorrhage, *J Trauma* 26:738-743, 1986.
19. Feliciano DV, Mattox KL, Jordan GL et al: Management of 1000 consecutive cases of hepatic trauma (1979-1984), *Ann Surg* 204:438-445, 1986.
20. Firsh JC: Reconstruction of the portal vein, *Am Surg* 32:472-478, 1966.
21. Grisoni ER, Gauderer MWL, Ferron J et al: Nonoperative management of liver injuries following blunt abdominal trauma in children, *J Pediatr Surg* 19:515-518, 1984.
22. Haller IA: Emergency medical services for children: what is the pediatric surgeon's role, *Pediatrics* 79:576-579, 1987.
23. Hartman SW, Greaney EM: Traumatic injuries to the biliary system in children, *Am J Surg* 108:150-156, 1964.
24. Ivatury RR, Nallathambi M, Gunduz Y et al: Liver packing for uncontrolled hemorrhage: a reappraisal, *J Trauma* 26:744-753, 1986.
25. Karp MP, Cooney DR, Berger PE et al: The role of computed tomography in the evaluation of blunt abdominal trauma in children, *J Pediatr Surg* 16:316-323, 1981.
26. Karp MP, Cooney DR, Pros GA et al: The nonoperative management of pediatric hepatic trauma, *J Pediatr Surg* 18:512-518, 1983.
27. Kudsk KA, Sheldon GF, Lim LC: Atrial caval shunting after trauma, *J Trauma* 22:81-85, 1982.
28. Lucas CE, Watt AJ: Analysis of randomized biliary drainage for liver trauma in 189 patients, *J Trauma* 12:925-930, 1972.
29. MacGillivray DC, Valentine RJ: Nonoperative management of blunt pediatric liver injury-late complications: case report, *J Trauma* 29:251-254, 1989.
30. Madding GF: Injuries of the liver, *Arch Surg* 70:748-756, 1955.
31. Marx JA: Abdominal traumatic injuries. Vol 1. In Rosen P, editor, *Emergency medicine*, ed 2, St Louis, 1988, Mosby pp 515, 526.
32. Mays ET: Hepatic trauma, *Curr Probl Surg* 13:5, 1976.
33. McClelland R, Shires T, Poulos E: Hepatic resection for massive trauma, *J Trauma* 4:282-291, 1964.
34. Merendino KA, Dillard DH, Cammock EE: The concept of surgical biliary decompression in the management of liver trauma, *Surg Gynecol Obstet* 117:285-293, 1963.
35. Michelassi F, Ranson JH: Bile duct disruption by blunt trauma, *J Trauma* 25:454-457, 1985.
36. Miller DR: Median stenotomy extension of abdominal incision for hepatic lobectomy, *Ann Surg* 175:193-196, 1972.
37. Moore EE, Eiseman B, Dunn E: Current management of hepatic trauma, *J Contemp Surg* 15:91-114, 1979.
38. Moore EE, Shackford SR, Pachter HL et al: Organ injury scaling: spleen, liver and kidney, *J Trauma* 29:1664-1666, 1989.
39. Noyes LD, Doyle DJ, McSwain NE: Septic complications associated with the use of peritoneal drains and liver trauma, *J Trauma* 28:337-346, 1988.
40. Oldham KT, Guice KS, Kaufman RA et al: Blunt hepatic injury and elevated hepatic enzymes: a clinical correlation in children, *J Pediatr Surg* 19:457-461, 1984.
41. Oldham KT, Guice KS, Ryckman F et al: Blunt liver injury in childhood: evolution of therapy and current perspective, *Surgery* 100:542-549, 1986.
42. Pachter HL, Spencer FC: Recent concepts in the treatment of hepatic trauma: facts and fallacies, *Ann Surg* 190:423-429, 1979.
43. Pachter HL, Spencer FC, Hofstetter SR et al: Experience with the finger fracture technique to achieve intrahepatic hemostasis in 75 patients with severe injuries of the liver, *Ann Surg* 197:771-778, 1983.
44. Perry JF Jr, Strate RG: Diagnostic peritoneal lavage in blunt abdominal trauma: indications and results, *Surgery* 71:898-901, 1972.
45. Perry JF Jr, DeMueles JE, Root HD: Diagnostic peritoneal lavage in blunt abdominal trauma, *Surg Gynecol Obstet* 131:742-744, 1970.
46. Pilcher DB, Harman PK, Moore EE: Retrohepatic vena cava balloon shunt introduced via the saphenofemoral junction, *J Trauma* 17:837-841, 1977.
47. Ponfick VA: Surgery of the liver, *Lancet* 1:881, 1890.
48. Poulos E: Hepatic resection for massive liver injuries, *Ann Surg* 157:525-531, 1963.
49. Pringle JH: Notes on the arrest of hepatic hemorrhage due to trauma, *Ann Surg* 48:541-548, 1908.
50. Saladino R, Lund D, Fleisher G: The spectrum of liver and spleen injuries in children: failure of the pediatric trauma score and clinical signs to predict isolated injuries, *Ann Emerg Med* 20:636-640, 1991.
51. Scott CM, Grasberger RC, Huran TF: Intraabdominal sepsis after hepatic trauma, *Am J Surg* 155:284-288, 1988.
52. Sheldon GJ, Rutledge R: Hepatic trauma, *Adv Surg* 22:179-194, 1989.
53. Sheldon GF, Lim RC, Yee ES et al: Management of injuries to the porta hepatis, *Ann Surg* 202:539-545, 1985.
54. Shrock T, Blaisdell W, Mathewson C: Management of blunt trauma to the liver and hepatic veins, *Arch Surg* 96:698-704, 1968.
55. Sonderstrom CA, Malkawa K, Dupriest RQ et al: Gallbladder injuries resulting from blunt abdominal trauma, *Ann Surg* 193:60-66, 1981.
56. Songsanand P, Gruff DB: Treatment of gallbladder rupture in an infant, *Am Surg* 38:335-337, 1972.
57. Sparkman RS, Fogelman MJ: Wounds of the liver: review of 100 cases, *Ann Surg* 139:690-719, 1954.
58. Stalker HP, Kaufman RA, Towbin R: Patterns of liver injury in childhood: CT analysis, *Am J Radiol* 147:1199-1205, 1986.
59. Stone HH, Ansley JD: Management of liver trauma in children, *J Pediatr Surg* 12:3-10, 1977.
60. Taylor GA, Eichelberger MR, O'Donnell R et al: Indications for computed tomography in children with blunt abdominal trauma, *Ann Surg* 213:212-218, 1991.
61. Trunkey D, Blaisdell FW: Trauma management, vol 1, *Abdominal trauma,* New York, 1982, Thieme Stratton.
62. Vock P, Kehrer B, Tschappeler H: Blunt liver trauma in children: the role of computed tomography in diagnosis and treatment, *J Pediatr Surg* 21:413-418, 1986.

63. Weissman HS, Chun KJ, Frank M et al: Demonstration of traumatic bile leakage with cholescintigraphy and ultrasound, *Am J Radiol* 133:843-847, 1979.
64. Welch KJ: Abdominal injuries. In Ravitch MM, Welch KJ, Benson CD, editors: *Pediatric surgery Chicago year book,* 1979, pp 125-140.
65. West JC, Kelley SE, Squiers EC: Future directions in hepatic injury, *Trauma Quarterly* 7:118-123, 1991.
66. Yoshida J, Donahue PE, Nyhus LM: Hemobilia: review of a recent experience with a worldwide problem, *Am J Gastroenterol* 82:448-453, 1987.

44 Gastric and Intestinal Injury

Kurt D. Newman

Historically, injuries of the stomach and small intestine in children are rare. In recent years, however, the incidence of gastric and intestinal injuries has been increasing. This trend relates to improved recognition of these injuries and to societal influences. The growth of urban violence and child abuse has resulted in an increase in abdominal injuries with potential for hollow viscus trauma. Moreover, the widespread availability of guns has led to an increase of penetrating injuries in children. For example, the incidence of such injury to patients less than 19 years of age increased threefold in the last 3 years in the Washington, D.C., metropolitan area. In addition, higher speed limits and greater compliance with seat-belt laws has heightened the potential for abdominal injury in children. Fortunately, today's improved prehospital care increases the likelihood of survival for children with abdominal injury.

In a study of 2300 consecutive admissions for traumatic injury at Children's National Medical Center, a regional pediatric trauma center, approximately 2.3% of children required operation for gastric or intestinal injury.[14] For children with abdominal injury caused by a blunt mechanism of trauma, damage to the stomach or intestine ranks third in frequency, just below injury to the liver or spleen. In penetrating trauma, the small intestine is the most frequently injured abdominal organ, largely because it occupies so much of the abdominal cavity.

Several factors put children at an increased risk for gastric or intestinal injury. The unique behavior patterns and natural curiosity of children establishes the possibility for injuries such as caustic ingestion or foreign-body aspiration. The lack of motor vehicle restraints specifically for children creates potential for injury when a lap belt is not positioned properly.[9] In addition, a child's propensity for air swallowing leads to gastric perforation. Thus the distinctive anatomic and behavioral characteristics of children must be considered when one is caring for victims of abdominal trauma.

MECHANISMS OF INJURY

The mechanisms of abdominal injury are traditionally classified as penetrating and blunt. Penetrating injury is usually the result of a stab or gunshot wound. Unusual mechanisms, however, such as a dog bite or a wooden splinter can cause penetrating injury. Stabbing generally produces a sharp, clean wound, which may involve the stomach or small bowel in one or more locations; these wounds are typically simple to repair. Because the intestines often slide away from a penetrating object of low velocity, there may be no bowel injury or there may be damage distant from the wound tract.

Most civilian gunshot wounds are of relatively low velocity. They produce variable patterns of tissue destruction owing to blast effects and to unpredictability of the bullet's course. The path of a bullet is variable and cannot be deduced from entrance and exit wounds because of ricochet and deflection of the missile. Gunshot wounds to the stomach and intestine may involve large areas of tissue destruction and require wide debridement. The current use of assault weapons and more powerful handguns has exacerbated the trend toward more extensive injury.

Blunt injury results most frequently from a direct blow to the abdomen, as happens to a subject of child abuse or a victim in a motor vehicle crash. The force is transferred directly to the abdominal organs and produces a burst mechanism, a shear effect, or a crush injury.[19] A burst injury is produced in a fluid-filled stomach or in a bowel loop that is stretched to bursting by an increase in intraabdominal pressure. A recent review of patients with gastric injury found that 60% had a history of a recent meal ingestion, which predisposed them to burst injury.[17] A common example of burst injury is that which results from insertion of an endotracheal tube into the esophagus during resuscitation. Forceful ventilation causes distention and perforation of the stomach and intestine. Shear injuries result from a deceleration force by which the stomach or bowel is torn at a fixed point, such as at the ligament of Treitz. Crush injuries derive from a

475

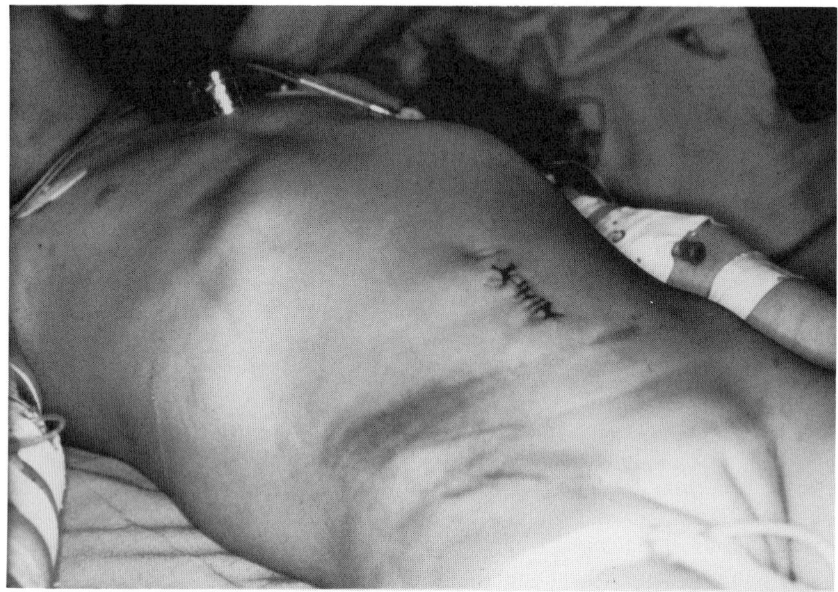

Figure 44–1 Photograph of child with lap-belt ecchymosis. Note the characteristic location across the lower abdomen. Diagnostic peritoneal lavage has been performed to assess the possibility of intestinal injury.

force that compresses the stomach or bowel against a stationary object, such as between a lap belt and the spine. Bicycle handlebars are notorious for producing duodenal injuries in this manner.

The "lap-belt complex" refers to a distinctive pattern of injury increasingly recognized in children who were restrained by lap belts.[13] The constellation of injuries involves a lap-belt ecchymosis associated with intestinal injury and/or spine injury (Figure 44-1). The complex results from sudden flexion of the child's torso around a fixed belt, which leads to visceral and spine compression. Children are at increased risk because they are more likely to be passengers in rear seats where only lap belts are available. Because the belts are designed for adults, they tend to ride up over the abdomen of the child instead of resting at the recommended across-the-hips position.

In a series of 61 children with lap-belt ecchymosis at the Children's National Medical Center, 21% had a lumbar spine injury, 23% had a hollow viscus injury, and 8% had both (Figure 44-2).[18] Several intestinal injuries were missed when computed tomography (CT) scanning alone was used for diagnosis. Free air was present in only one quarter of the children with bowel injuries and the intestinal tear frequently occurred on the mesenteric side of the bowel (Figure 44-3). For children with a lap-belt mark, diagnostic peritoneal lavage and early laparotomy are indicated. In addition, evaluation of the lumbar spine should include a lateral radiograph. A heightened level of suspicion for intestinal injury is required in this high-risk subgroup of children with blunt abdominal injury.

Intestinal stricture may be a late finding after a lap-belt injury.[16] Localized ischemia produces scarring and fibrosis, leading to compromise of the intestinal lumen. Children with such sequelae are seen several weeks after the injury to have bowel obstruction. Resection of the involved segment is curative.[5]

RESUSCITATION

As in treatment of all injured children, the fundamental priority in initial treatment of children with intestinal or gastric injury is stabilization of the airway, followed by cardiopulmonary resuscitation. In a hollow viscus injury, abdominal distention caused by a perforation that results in pneumoperitoneum may hinder ventilation by impingement of the diaphragm. Children are prone to gastric distention resulting from aerophagia or from bag-valve-mask ventilation. Occasionally, a nasogastric tube does not decompress the stomach. In that event, needle decompression of the stomach or pneumoperitoneum is lifesaving. Careful attention to volume resuscitation is essential, because abdominal trauma, particularly penetrating trauma, frequently produces hemorrhage and hypotension. Specifically, injuries to the stomach can cause sufficient hemorrhage to produce hypotension because of the rich four-vessel blood supply.

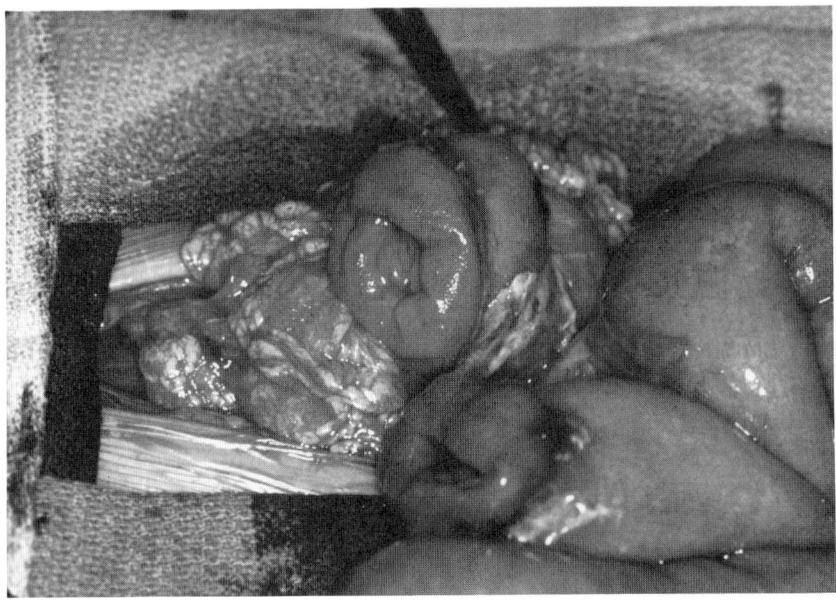

Figure 44–2 Operative photograph of a lap-belt intestinal injury suffered by a teenager, showing complete transection of the jejunum. This child also had an associated lumbar spine injury.

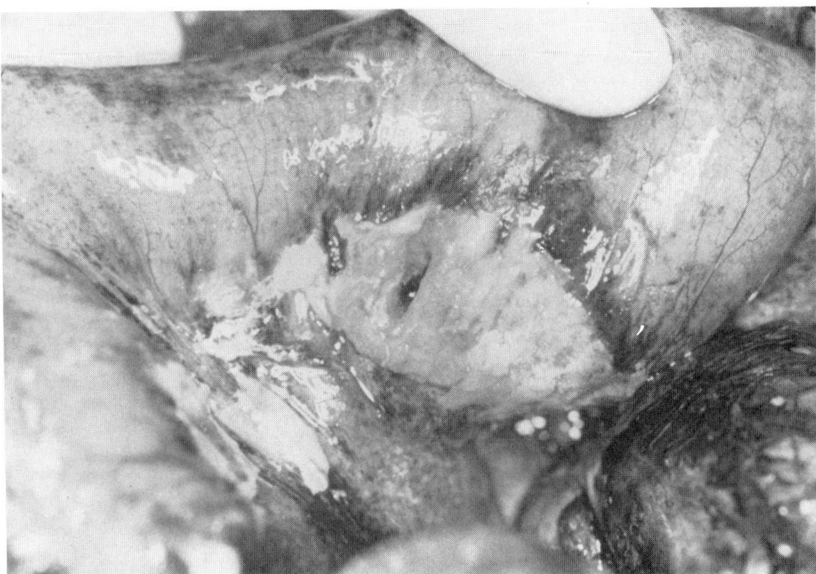

Figure 44–3 Lap-belt complex. Note small bowel perforation located on the mesenteric side. Treatment required segmental resection and anastomosis.

DIAGNOSIS

The keys to management of gastric and intestinal injury are a high level of suspicion and an expeditious, systematic scheme for diagnosis. The diagnostic approach to penetrating injuries is simple: the determination is made with surgical exploration. A safe policy is to explore virtually all penetrating injuries of the abdomen. Only when a stab wound conclusively fails to enter the peritoneal cavity is operation avoided. Explore all gunshot wound injuries to the abdomen; there is no latitude for speculative management. The presence of blood in the nasogastric tube is suggestive of injury; however, the experience at Parkland Hospital, revealed that blood was present in only 45% of gunshot wounds and 37% of stab wounds.[7] Free air is present radiographically in up to 60% of gastric injuries, and therefore is also not a reliable guide for exploration.[2]

The diagnosis of gastric or intestinal injury from blunt force is more problematic. A child who is experiencing pain or alteration of consciousness is especially difficult to examine. Therefore, rely on objective signs of injury. Physical examination is useful if peritoneal signs are present or if there is a lap-belt ecchymosis, tire track, or handlebar mark suggestive of injury; suspect hollow viscus injury with these signs. Following the secondary survey, the usual initial diagnostic approach for hemodynamically stable children with abdominal blunt injury is a CT scan. Although perforation may be demonstrated on a CT scan, free air may not be seen, nor is it specific for perforation. Pneumomediastinum, bladder rupture, or previous peritoneal lavage may confuse the diagnosis of pneumoperitoneum on a CT scan.[3]

Unexplained free intraabdominal fluid without evidence of injury to the liver or spleen on a CT scan is suggestive of bowel injury, particularly in children with a lap-belt complex. Diagnostic peritoneal lavage (15 cc/kg) is useful in children when the diagnosis is uncertain, when the child is unstable or unconscious, or when urgent operation is required for other injuries. The presence of bile, bacteria, or a high amylase content is indicative of intestinal injury. Follow children with blunt injury closely, reexamine them frequently, and if signs of peritonitis develop, use a low threshold for exploration. Employ upper gastrointestinal contrast series and contrast CT scans to evaluate injuries to the duodenum. Ultrasound is useful in evaluation of concomitant pancreatic injury.

GASTRIC INJURY

Explore the abdomen with a generous midline incision for suspected gastric or intestinal injury. Once hemorrhage is identified and controlled, mobilize the stomach and duodenum completely and examine the front and back for injury. The most common sites for missed injury are the gastroesophageal junction, the greater curvature of the stomach within the omentum, the lesser curvature, and the posterior wall. Always examine for an entrance and an exit site; suspect concomitant diaphragmatic injury if penetration is the mechanism of injury. Most stomach injuries are easily debrided and simply closed with two layers of sutures: an inner mucosal running layer of absorbable suture and a seromuscular interrupted layer of nonabsorbable suture. Burst injuries of the stomach may require more extensive debridement and closure;

nevertheless, avoid compromise of the gastric lumen. Irrigate the abdomen copiously to remove gastric contents. Gastrectomy and drainage of gastric injuries is rarely necessary. A nasogastric tube helps decompress the stomach until gastric peristalsis returns.

The chief complication of gastric injury is infection. Its incidence is low, however, because the acidic environment of the stomach retards bacterial colonization.[11] Following meals, acidity is neutralized and bacterial contamination is higher, accounting for a greater incidence of infection. Perioperative antibiotics aid in lessening the chances of infection. When a postoperative abscess does result, CT-assisted percutaneous drainage is an important adjunct. For combined gastric and diaphragmatic injury, wide drainage of the pleural space by thoracostomy tube is essential to avoid empyema. Despite the abundant blood supply of the stomach, postoperative bleeding is rare, particularly following careful hemostatic closure of the injury.

DUODENAL INJURY

The management of duodenal injury creates frequent dilemmas. A thorough and careful approach is essential because of the high mortality associated with such injury. The location of the duodenum in the retroperitoneum and its close anatomic relationship to the pancreas create the potential for occult injury and catastrophic complications. Blunt injury carries a higher risk of mortality than penetrating injury. This increase is probably due to the great amount of force required to injure the duodenum in its posterior location and the concomitant injury to other organs.

An isolated intramural hematoma of the duodenum is treated nonoperatively if the child does not manifest a perforation or peritonitis.[20,23] Common mechanisms of injury are kicks, blows from a fist, and direct handlebar compression. An upper gastrointestinal contrast examination shows a "coiled spring" and duodenal obstruction (Figure 44-4). CT scan or ultrasound also demonstrates the intramural hematoma. Associated pancreatic injury is present in 25% of cases. Nevertheless, treatment with total parenteral nutrition and with nasogastric suction is usually effective. Allow 2 or 3 weeks for resolution, but if obstruction persists, evacuate the hematoma surgically.[22] If a simple duodenal hematoma is encountered at the time of surgical exploration for abdominal trauma, incise the serosa and remove the offending clot, with care to avoid entry into the lumen.

Approach more complex duodenal injuries cautiously. Primary closure is suitable for many injuries, especially those that are limited, linear, and

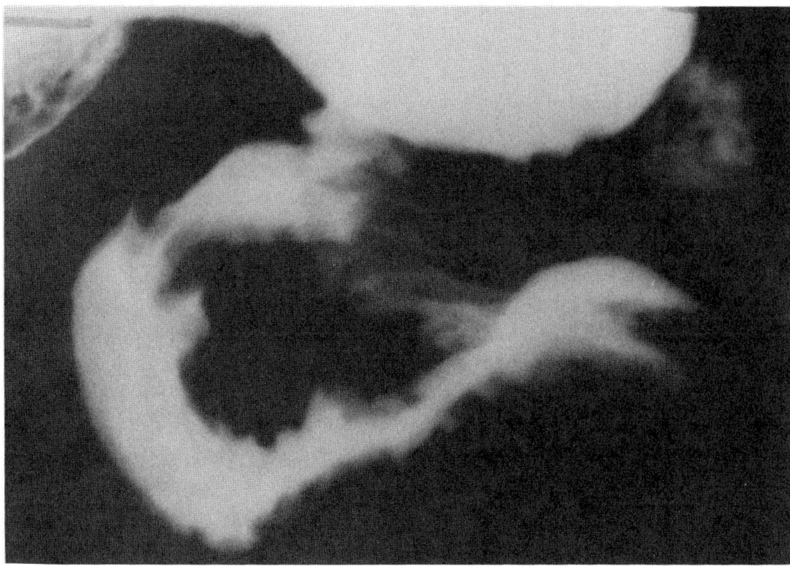

Figure 44–4 Upper GI contrast radiograph in a child kicked in the midabdomen by a horse. Note the complete obstruction of the duodenum (third to fourth portion), which resolved without operation.

lateral.[4] Mobilize the duodenum extensively, including the third and fourth portions. Exclude associated pancreatic or bile duct injury by careful inspection and intraoperative cholangiography. Be careful not to compromise the duodenal lumen with the closure; conversion of a longitudinal wound to a transverse closure (Heinecke-Mickulicz) is useful.

Selection of the ideal surgical management of a duodenal injury is best individualized according to the nature of the injury and the condition of the child.[15] Simple closure and adequate drainage are required for most injuries. For more extensive injuries, such as those with pancreatic involvement or major devitilization of tissue, consider anastomosis of the jejunum to the duodenal wound, with or without tube decompression.[8] Occasionally, temporary diversion through a pyloric exclusion procedure is required.[1] Oversew the pylorus with an absorbable suture, perform a gastrostomy, and create a gastrojejunostomy, thus bypassing the injured duodenum. Close the duodenal wound primarily, or with a jejunal patch, and drain extensively. Begin feeding and remove the drains after contrast studies show patency of the closure without leakage.

The major complication of duodenal wounds is fistula formation.[21] A fistula that is well drained usually closes spontaneously. Nutritional support, histamine-receptor blockade, and control of infection are integral components of management. Somatostatin and its analogues are helpful in decreasing pancreatic and intestinal secretions. Failure of a fistula to close after 6 to 8 weeks of medical treatment is an indication for surgical exploration.

SMALL BOWEL INJURY

Injuries to the small intestine are usually simple to repair. Primary closure following debridement of devitalized tissue suffices in most instances, particularly for penetrating injury. Resection with anastomosis may be required for multiple holes in a segment of intestine or for burst injuries where major necrosis is identified. Examine the entire length of the intestine; the mesenteric surface of the bowel is a common site for missed injuries. Search assiduously for an even number of holes. Diversion with a stoma is rarely required for children with small bowel injuries.

The most frequent complication of small bowel injury is wound infection. Perioperative antibiotic administration, wound irrigation and delayed primary closure are useful in the prevention of infection. Anastomotic leaks are rare, but, if present, intestinal diversion and local drainage can be used to help control sepsis. Confirm suspicion of postoperative abscess with ultrasound and CT. Percutaneous drainage is effective in the management of an infected intraabdominal collection.

MESENTERIC HEMATOMA

Treatment of a hematoma of the mesentery that is at the base or is expanding is a major priority during abdominal exploration for trauma (Figure 44-5).[10] First, be certain that the child has received appropriate volume resuscitation. Obtain proximal and

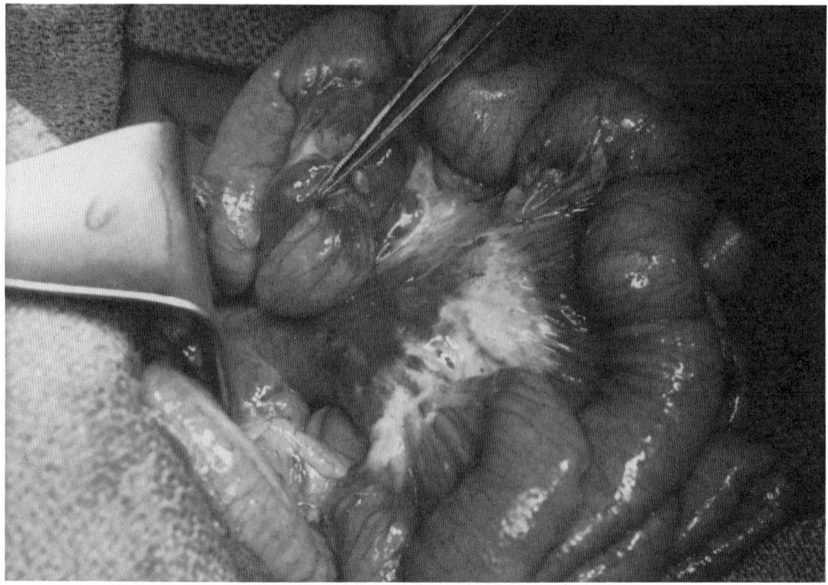

Figure 44–5 Operative photograph of expanding hematoma in the mesentery due to disruption of the superior mesenteric artery. Also noted is a perforation on the mesenteric side of the bowel.

distal control of the mesenteric vessels by extensive exposure of the aorta and vena cava.[12] If technically possible, repair the superior mesenteric artery; if not, use ligation, which children generally tolerate well. Venous injuries may be repaired with lateral venorrhaphy but often require ligation.

TRANSLOCATION AND ULCERATION

In recent years the role of bacterial translocation via the gastrointestinal tract has received much attention. Desai and Herndon identified the gut as a major source of sepsis and morbidity in a series of children with extensive burns.[6] The incidence of stress ulcers and Curling's ulceration is well documented in children. Use antacids and histamine-receptor blockade prophylactically to prevent these complications in children with major trauma or burns.

ACID INGESTION

The ingestion of acid substances causes extensive injury to the stomach and intestine, whereas the esophagus is often spared—in contradistinction to alkaline injury. To treat a child who has ingested an acid substance, urgently evacuate the stomach contents with a nasogastric tube, and administer antacids to neutralize the acid. Evaluate with endoscopy; however, if peritonitis supervenes, explore the abdomen. Gastric resection is occasionally required owing to the coagulative necrosis produced by strong acids.

FOREIGN BODY INGESTION

Foreign body ingestion is a potential source of gastric or intestinal injury in children. Most foreign bodies will pass spontaneously. The pylorus, ileocecal valve, and anomalous congenital narrowing are common sites of holdup. Failure of the object to move or pass for 6 weeks, as determined on an x-ray, suggests the need to remove the object surgically or endoscopically.

CONCLUSION

Although incidence is increasing, the morbidity and mortality of gastric and intestinal injury in children are low. Key components of a treatment plan are a high level of suspicion for injury and a low threshold for surgical exploration. Careful attention to the mechanism of injury allows for a streamlined and expeditious approach to diagnosis and therapy.

REFERENCES

1. Berne CJ, Donovan AJ, White EJ et al: Duodenal "diverticularization" for duodenal and pancreatic injury, *Am J Surg* 127:503-507, 1974.
2. Brunstig LA, Morton JH: Gastric rupture from blunt abdominal trauma, *J Trauma* 27:887-891, 1987.
3. Bulas DI, Taylor GA, Eichelberger MR: The value of CT in detecting bowel perforation in children after blunt abdominal trauma, *AJR* 153:561-564, 1989.
4. Cogbill TH, Moore EE, Feliciano DV et al: Conservative management of duodenal trauma: a multicenter perspective, *J Trauma* 30:1469-1475, 1990.
5. Czyrko C, Weltz C, Markowitz R et al: Blunt abdominal trauma resulting in intestinal obstruction: when to operate? *J Trauma* 30:1567-1570, 1990.

6. Desai MH, Herndon DN, Rutan RL et al: Ischemic intestinal complications in patients with burns, *Surg Gynecol Obstet* 172:257-261, 1991.
7. Durham R: Management of gastric injuries, *Surg Clin N Am* 70:517-527, 1990.
8. Feliciano DB, Martin TD, Cruse PA et al: Management of combined pancreatoduodenal injuries, *Ann Surg* 205:673-680, 1987.
9. Hoffman MA, Spence LJ, Wesson DE et al: The pediatric passenger: trends and seat belt use in injury patterns, *J Trauma* 27:974-976, 1987.
10. Lucas AE, Richardson JD, Flint LM et al: Traumatic injury of the proximal superior mesenteric artery, *Ann Surg* 193:30-34, 1981.
11. McNulty CM, Wise R: Gastric microflora, *Br Med J* 291:367-368, 1985.
12. Mattox KL, McCollum WB, Jordan GL et al: Management of upper abdominal vascular trauma, *Am J Surg* 120:823-828, 1974.
13. Newman KD, Bowman LM, Eichelberger MR et al: The lap belt complex: intestinal and lumbar spine injury in children, *J Trauma* 30:1133-1140, 1990.
14. Peclet MH, Newman KD, Eichelberger MR et al: Patterns of injuries in children, *J Ped Surg* 25:85-91, 1990.
15. Pokorny WJ, Brandt ML, Harberg FJ: Major duodenal injuries in children: diagnosis and operative management, *J Ped Surg* 21:613-616, 1986.
16. Shalaby-Rana E, Eichelberger MR, Kerzner B et al: Intestinal stricture due to lap belt injury, *J Radiol* 1991 (in press).
17. Siemens RA, Fulton RL: Gastric rupture as a result of blunt trauma, *Am Surg* 43:229, 1977.
18. Sivit CJ, Taylor GA, Newman KD et al: Safety belt injuries in children with lap belt ecchymosis: CT findings in 61 patients, *AJR* 157:111-114, 1991.
19. Stevens SC, Maull KI: Small bowel injuries, *Surg Clin N Am* 70:541-560, 1990.
20. Touloukian RJ: Protocol for the non-operative treatment of obstructing intramural duodenal hematoma during childhood, *Ann J Surg* 145:330-334, 1983.
21. Weigelt JA: Duodenal injuries, *Surg Clin N Am* 70:529-539, 1990.
22. Winthrop AL, Wesson DE, Filler RM: Traumatic duodenal hematoma in the pediatric patient, *J Ped Surg* 21:757-760, 1986.
23. Wooley MM, Mahour JH, Sloan T: Duodenal hematoma in infancy and childhood, *Am J Surg* 136:8-14, 1978.

45 Colonic, Rectal, and Perineal Injury

Thomas M. Rouse

Injuries of the colon, rectum, and perineum are uncommon in children. Most penetrating trauma results from wounds to the abdomen by gunshot, stabs, or falls onto sharp objects. Blunt trauma is most often due to motor vehicle–related injuries, abuse, or assault.

Penetrating injury of the rectum may also be due to domestic violence but is less common than penetrating injury of the colon. Perforation caused by thermometer probe or biopsy forceps is fortunately a rare event. Major impalement may cause extensive perineal, rectal, and intraabdominal injury. Blunt rectal and perineal trauma is seen with some frequency at pediatric trauma centers. Usually it is due to a straddle injury in which a child, at play or while being bathed, falls a short distance onto a flat surface, striking the perineum. Minor lacerations of the perineal body, vagina, or anus require suture closure after careful examination with the child under anesthesia. Extensive soft tissue disruption may follow falls from heights or forceful abduction of the hip or crush injury in motor vehicle–pedestrian crashes or automobile-motorcycle collisions. Anorectal and vaginal injury in children should raise a suspicion of child abuse. Black reported in 1982 that 24% of patients seen in a large urban trauma center because of sexual abuse were less than 16 years of age. One third of this group alleged anal trauma, in two-thirds of the patients the anorectal trauma was caused by sexual abuse, and more than two-thirds of this group were boys. Ages ranged from 3 months to 14 years.[1] It is important to obtain the details of the injury from the child as well as from the parent or guardian to establish the true nature of the injury. Consultation with social workers and Department of Human Resource personnel is often necessary.

PENETRATING COLON INJURY

The management of colon injuries has evolved over the last several decades. During World War I, Cuthbert Wallace reported primary closure of penetrating colon wounds in two thirds of 155 patients.[12] Following experience in North Africa during World War II, all colon injuries, even suspected ones, were treated by creation of a colostomy.

In 1951 Woodhall and Ochsner advocated that most civilian colon injuries be treated with primary repair, and they reported a lower morbidity and mortality in their patients.[13] Since then many authors advocate selective management of penetrating colon injury. A prospective randomized study by Chappius shows comparable outcomes in patients with penetrating colon injury treated by primary colon repair versus staged treatment with a colostomy.[2]

Penetrating injury in the colon is commonly the result of gunshot or stab wounds. Colon injuries are present in up to 20% of abdominal gunshot wounds but are less common in stab wounds (5%). Occasionally, a swallowed foreign body or endoscopic manipulation perforates the colon. Falls onto sharp objects with penetration through the abdominal wall or into the flank or back may also cause colon injury.

All gunshot wounds that penetrate the peritoneal cavity necessitate exploration of the abdominal cavity. A low-velocity injury from a BB gun or air rifle does not require exploration if a cross-table radiograph demonstrates the pellet to be superficial to the peritoneum.

A stab wound permits selective management. An isolated stab injury that does not penetrate the peritoneal cavity requires local wound care and discharge from the emergency room. A child with a stab wound that causes signs of hemodynamic instability such as tachycardia, decreased pulse pressure, or hypotension, or signs of peritoneal irritation, should proceed to exploratory laparotomy following appropriate resuscitation. Any child who manifests gross or hemoccult positive blood upon rectal examination following a penetrating wound usually has an associated injury to the colon or rectum.

The specific diagnosis of penetrating colon injury is usually made at laparotomy. Small perforations may produce only minor physical signs early after injury, but most children with such injuries manifest some abdominal pain and tenderness. Muscular guarding and rebound tenderness are common and should prompt early laparotomy.

Injury to the colon requires operative management. The first step is to stabilize the child's cardiorespiratory system. In the hemodynamically unstable child, fluid and, if necessary, blood transfusion are administered. Administration of a broad-spectrum antibiotic also precedes exploratory laparotomy. Because of the high bacterial colony count in the colon, the best combination of drugs is clindamycin, an aminoglycoside, and ampicillin.

A midline laparotomy incision permits rapid control of the sites of hemorrhage. It is uncommon for a colon injury to cause massive hemorrhage unless laceration of a large mesenteric vessel occurs. Following hemostasis, the management of contamination of intraluminal bowel contents is best achieved by approximation of the injury with either an Allis or a Babcock clamp. If colon transection occurs, minimize spillage by application of a Kocher clamp across each end.

A thorough abdominal exploration includes inspection of the colon from the cecum to the peritoneal reflection, with special concern for the integrity of the vascular supply of the colon. Open the lesser sac to examine the posterior surface of the transverse colon. Routine mobilization of the ascending and descending colon is unnecessary unless a missile has tracked close to these areas. A small retroperitoneal hematoma in the retrocolic region is a sign of colon injury; appropriate evaluation includes incision of the pericolic peritoneal fold and direct inspection of the retroperitoneal colon. In the absence of a suspicious missile track, however, careful inspection of the colon, mesentery, and retroperitoneum is sufficient.

After thorough exploration, several options for repair of a colon injury exist. Increasingly, primary suture repair without colostomy or a segmented resection and an anastomosis are being used for treatment of intra-abdominal colon injury. Clean stab wounds and low-velocity gunshot wounds permit wound debridement and closure in two layers: join adjacent wounds to facilitate a single closure.

Closure of a luminal perforation is best in the transverse plane to avoid narrowing of the colon. Minimal serosal defects do not require suture repair; however, management of an extensive partial-thickness injury includes approximation by suture. Chappius reports a randomized trial of penetrating colon injury in adults that shows no difference in outcome or complications between a group with primary repair and a group with colostomy diversion.[2] It is interesting to note that success in the treatment of right or left colon injury by either suture repair or resection and anastomosis was the same. The majority of the patients, however, had only one colon injury, and only two sustained injuries of the colon mesentery; most were treated

within 2 hours. Extensive wounds of the right colon were managed by right colon resection and ileocolostomy.[2]

Despite the encouraging reports of the primary repair of unselected colon injury, it is prudent to treat certain colon injuries in a less definitive manner. Children who are in shock preoperatively require expeditious treatment by primary repair if possible. Treatment of children whose diagnosis has been delayed and who have extensive fecal contamination of the peritoneal cavity requires injury resection and performance of a colostomy at the proximal margin.

Colon wounds with extensive injury to the kidney, liver, or pancreas require colostomy for fecal diversion. Management of injury in the distal colon is best by the creation of a mucous fistula or, if low in the sigmoid colon, by a Hartman's procedure.

Severe infections of the missile tract occur following transcolonic gunshot wounds.[4] Seven patients with such injuries developed infections of either bone, soft tissue, retroperitoneum, or a vascular structure. Diagnosis of infection is difficult; two of seven patients died as a direct result of missile tract infection. Aggressive debridement of a transcolonic missile tract, removal of all accessible missiles and foreign debris, and administration of adjuvant antibiotic therapy can reduce the infection rate.

Voyles and Flint reviewed the incidence of wound infection following primary skin closure of laparotomy in patients with colon injury. They identified an infection rate of 56% in wounds with primary closure, as compared with 19% in those with delayed primary closure or with closure by secondary intention.[11] Infection in open wounds was associated with an intraperitoneal abscess in 73% of their patients. The best management of a laparotomy wound is delayed primary closure or secondary healing by granulation. If a wound infection develops, evaluate the child for intraperitoneal abscess.

BLUNT COLON INJURY

Colon injury due to blunt trauma is uncommon. In adult studies less than 5% of patients who undergo laparotomy for injuries caused by blunt forces are found to have colon injury. Injuries range from small subserosal hematomas and partial-thickness lacerations to total disruption of the bowel or avulsion of the mesentery. Motor vehicle trauma is the primary cause of blunt colon injury in children. Lap-belt injury occurs less frequently to the colon than to the small intestine. However, the child who shows the characteristic lap-belt mark on his lower abdomen may also have an intraabdominal hollow viscus injury, which can include the cecum or sigmoid colon. Blunt injury to the colon is rarely isolated; it is often found with multiorgan system injury.

Three mechanisms of blunt injury are possible. The most common is a crushing force that compresses the colon between the vertebrae and the impacting object; the transverse and sigmoid colon are often injured in this way. Vertebral and pelvic fractures, as well as pancreatic disruption, may be associated injuries. Howell and associates identified 4 of 19 patients with simultaneous blunt pancreatic and colon injury.[5]

Another mechanism is a shear force that affects those areas of the colon that are relatively fixed in location by the peritoneum. Sudden deceleration can tear or avulse the more mobile intraperitoneal colon from its adjacent retroperitoneal component. Injuries of the cecum, hepatic and splenic flexures, and distal sigmoid colon are likely to occur through this mechanism. Finally, sudden decompression or burst injury due to an abrupt increase in intraluminal pressure rarely occurs within the colon lumen.

Blunt injury to the bowel wall that results in perforation or extensive disruption is usually manifested early with signs and symptoms of peritonitis. Mesenteric injury that causes ischemia may show perforation several hours to days following injury, or stricture formation even weeks after the traumatic event. There are reports of total colon disruption seen several days after blunt injury with signs of sepsis and bowel obstruction.[5]

Many children with blunt colon injury have multisystem trauma, including head injury, which makes evaluation for intraabdominal injury particularly difficult. The evaluation of these children mandates a stepwise approach to minimize delays in diagnosis. Physical examination of the abdomen is essential after resuscitation from life-threatening injuries. The abdominal wall, flank, and back may manifest abrasion, contusion, or penetrating wounds. Lap-belt contusion, a handlebar mark, or a tire track imprint should increase suspicion of serious intraabdominal injury. These areas are usually tender, which makes it difficult to differentiate between abdominal wall tenderness and peritonitis. A tear in the abdominal wall musculature caused by the force of the injury negates the reliability of the physical examination. Children thus injured often have significant head trauma that further diminishes the reliability of the physical examination. The finding of gross or occult blood upon rectal examination increases the likelihood of colorectal injury.

Many children with multisystem injury undergo a computed tomography (CT) scan of the abdomen to aid in diagnosis of a solid organ injury. This technique is highly sensitive to injuries to the liver, spleen, or kidneys. However, it is not a reliable means of detecting bowel injury. Pneumoperitoneum was present in only 39% of children with intestinal injury. However, peritoneal fluid in the absence of solid organ disruption or pelvic fracture is a helpful sign of a bowel injury.[8] Treatment of a child with an abdominal wall contusion or abrasion, particularly from a lap belt, requires peritoneal lavage or early exploratory laparotomy.

Any child with abdominal wall abrasion following blunt injury who does not have exploratory laparotomy requires close serial observation for signs of bowel injury. Frequent physical examinations by the same physician aid in the early identification of peritonitis. Worsening abdominal pain, persistent ileus, signs of sepsis or peritonitis, including hypovolemia and oliguria, are indications for abdominal exploration.

When there is a strong suspicion of colon injury, an urgent laparotomy is imperative, following adequate fluid resuscitation with lactated Ringer's solution and administration of intravenous antibiotics (ampicillin, gentamicin, and clindamycin). Proceed with laparotomy through a midline abdominal incision, and control active bleeding and contamination by intestinal content prior to thorough exploration.

Blunt colon injury varies from minor subserosal contusion or hematoma to partial-thickness tear, perforation, or complete transection of the bowel. A seromuscular tear is reapproximated with 3-0 silk sutures. Unroof and evacuate the blood from a small subserosal hematoma, inspect the bowel and, if it is intact, close the defect with seromuscular sutures of 3-0 silk. In contrast, a large intramural hematoma requires management with extreme caution; delayed ischemia causes perforation or stricture formation. If there is any uncertainty of the integrity of the vascular supply, perform a resection of the involved area and fashion a colostomy at the proximal margin. Anastomosis of the colon in this setting is inappropriate since ischemia at the resection margins may develop because of the crushing injury, even though the ends appear to be grossly uninvolved at the time of laparotomy. Blunt injury that results in perforation or necrosis requires resection, construction of a proximal colostomy, and the creation of a mucous fistula. Right hemicolectomy and ileotransverse colon anastomosis is the best treatment for a severe right colon injury if one is confident that the blood supply is adequate for the anastomosis, fecal contamination is minimal, and associated intraabdominal injury is not significant.

Hematoma of the colon mesentery is a potentially treacherous injury that requires thoughtful consideration. This injury causes ischemia and delayed perforation of the colon and implies significant morbidity and the potential for mortality. Hemorrhage is controlled by complete mobilization of the right and left colon from the retroperitoneal attachments and division of the gastrocolic ligament. Digital pressure on each side of the bowel mesentery will control bleeding and allow identification of the specific site of hemorrhage. Precise suture ligation permits preservation of the collateral mesenteric blood supply; even small vessels may be the only source of blood to that section of the colon if the collateral blood supply is inadequate. The splenic flexure and the rectosigmoid colon are notorious for their susceptibility to ischemia, and disruption of the marginal artery may make these points particularly vulnerable to ischemia and perforation. It is essential to be fully confident of the adequacy of the collateral blood supply to the colon following ligation of mesenteric vessels. Doppler ultrasound and intravenous fluorescein may be helpful, but surgical judgment remains paramount. If there is any question of vascular integrity, resect the involved area of the colon and form a colostomy.

Pericolic hematoma signals injury to the retroperitoneal right or left colon; open the hematoma and carefully inspect the bowel wall. If a bowel wall injury is present or if the integrity of the bowel is in question, resect the injury site and create a colostomy and mucous fistula.

Postoperative care requires careful attention to a child's hemodynamic status, particularly when diagnosis has been delayed and peritonitis is present. This may complicate the treatment of children with multisystem organ injuries. If necessary, a central venous catheter or Swan-Ganz catheter helps to guide fluid administration. Continue antibiotics for at least 24 hours for those children whose injuries were identified and treated early. Injuries identified with established peritonitis are treated with antibiotics for at least 7 to 10 days; regular monitoring of aminoglycoside levels helps in prevention of toxicity.

Once bowel function resumes, remove the nasogastric tube and begin enteral nutrition. Closure of the colostomy is possible 6 to 12 weeks following injury; the incidence of complications increases when closure is performed beyond this period.[9] A barium study of the distal colon and rectum is essential prior to colostomy closure.

PENETRATING RECTAL INJURY

Rectal injuries, uncommon in children, are caused by either blunt or penetrating trauma. Penetrating injury can occur following minor impalement with a thermometer or an enema tip; more extensive injury can result from a fall onto an object such as a picket fence, post, household tool, or other sharp object. Gunshot injury, the most common cause of rectal trauma in adults, is also seen in children. A gunshot wound in which the missile trajectory is between the upper thigh and the pelvic rim and which crosses the midline frequently results in rectal injury. Likewise, the presence of blood upon rectal examination, hematuria, blood in the vagina, or wounds of the buttocks, perineum, or anus raises the suspicion of rectal injury.

The extent of preoperative evaluation for rectal injury depends on the hemodynamic stability of the child. A hypotensive child with a gunshot wound to the pelvis who does not respond to fluid resuscitation requires prompt laparotomy to control hemorrhage; there is often a major pelvic vascular injury that is difficult to control. Transection of the iliac artery and vein frequently occurs with gunshot injuries of the rectum.[3]

Hematoma within the pelvis resulting from a penetrating wound compels vascular control and exploration. Injury to the genitourinary tract can occur with this mechanism and requires thorough evaluation. Hematoma below the retroperitoneal reflection strongly suggests rectal injury; nonexpanding hematoma does not require exploration. Rather, assume a rectal injury and create a diverting colostomy.

The stable child with a penetrating injury due to domestic violence or accidental impalement can undergo a more thorough preoperative assessment. A rectal examination is mandatory in all children with such injuries. The finding of blood within the rectal vault is presumptive evidence of rectal injury, and, occasionally, palpation of a defect in the wall of the rectum is possible. In addition, hematuria should be evaluated with a voiding cystourethrogram. Children infrequently tolerate proctoscopy in the resuscitation area; therefore, examination is best when a child is under general anesthesia.

Except for minor injury distal to the mucocutaneous junction of the rectum and anal canal, treatment of rectal injury requires total fecal diversion with a colostomy, rectal irrigation, and presacral drainage (Fig. 45-1). There is some controversy as to whether an extraperitoneal rectal injury needs repair, but Tuggle and Huber report that it is not required for safe treatment.[10]

Once all pelvic and abdominal injuries are evident, there are several ways to divert the fecal stream; however, a loop colostomy with a stapled distal limb is the most expeditious means of complete fecal diversion (Fig. 45-2). Rectal irrigation is especially beneficial when a large amount of stool is present in the rectum. After closure of the

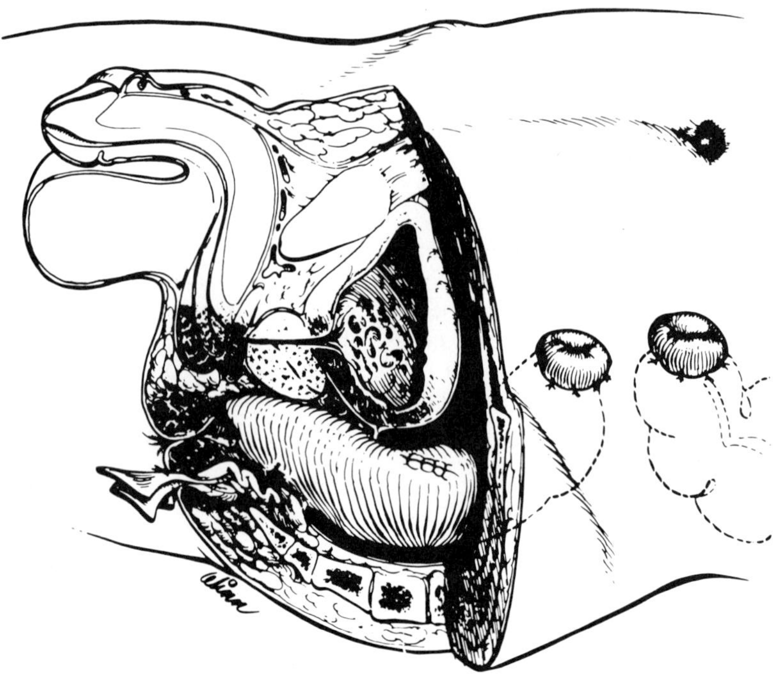

Figure 45–1 The essentials of rectal trauma management, i.e., a diverting colostomy and retrorectal drain. Closure of an intraperitoneal wound and an open extraperitoneal wound. (From Trunkey D et al. Management of rectal trauma, *J Trauma* 13:411-415, 1973.)

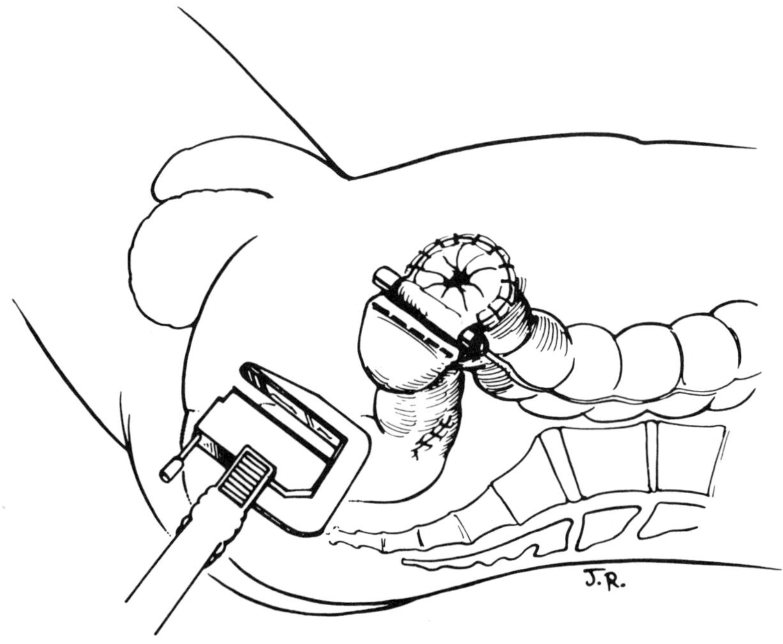

Figure 45–2 Loop colostomy with closure of distal limb, using a stapler. The distal limb can also be closed with a suture. (From Burch JM et al: Colostomy and drainage for civilian rectal injuries: is that all? *Ann Surg* 209:600-611, 1989.)

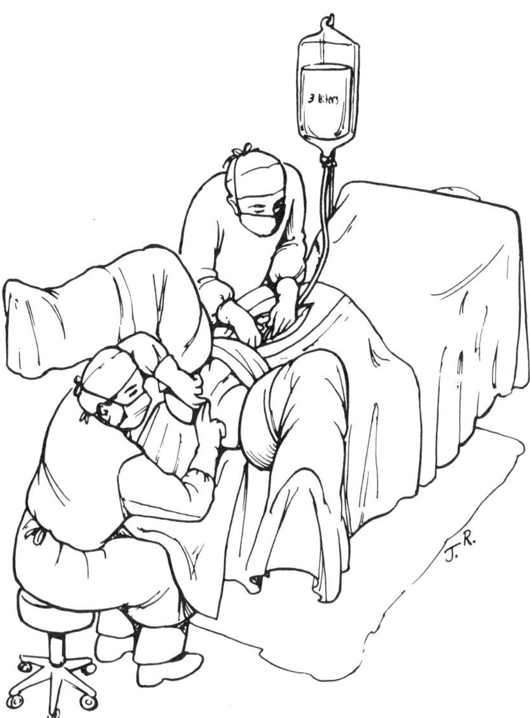

Figure 45–3 Setup for rectal irrigation. The anus should be held open while the irrigant is running. (From Burch JM et al: Colostomy and drainage for civilian rectal injuries: is that all? *Ann Surg* 209:600-611, 1989.)

abdominal fascia, place a purse-string suture at the distal colostomy site and insert a large-bore rubber catheter within the purse-string. Instillation of normal saline through the catheter clears the distal rectum while an assistant dilates the anus. Continue irrigation until the effluent from the anus is free of solid stool (Fig. 45-3).

Presacral drainage is an essential part of the management of rectal injury. A curvilinear incision is made between the tip of the coccyx and the posterior margin of the anus; extension through the endopelvic fascia by blunt dissection with a finger, or by blunt clamp into the presacral space, is imperative. Placement of a Penrose drain up to the level of the injury assures appropriate dependent drainage (Fig. 45-4). Drains are left in place for at least 5 days and slowly withdrawn thereafter.

Very rarely, extensive injuries of the rectum and pelvis result in extensive loss of the intraabdominal rectum; resection of the injured area via a Hartman's procedure is appropriate treatment. Even less common is an injury that disrupts both the rectal wall and the anal sphincter mechanism. Proximal diversion and distal mucous fistula permits isolation of the injury and subsequent effective debridement and hemorrhage control.

BLUNT PERINEAL INJURY

Blunt trauma to the perineum in children causes injury to the genitourinary system, the anus, and the rectum. Such injury usually follows a minor fall, for example, from straddling a bedpost, edge of bathtub or swimming pool, or a handlebar. Falls from playground apparatus are another common mechanism for this injury. A significant number of rectal and perineal injuries in children occur secondary to sexual abuse.[1] These injuries vary in severity from perianal erythema and pain to anal fissures or extensive vaginal laceration that disrupts the anal sphincter. Young children occasionally manifest extensive anorectal laceration and perineal injury that extends into the perineal cavity.[1]

Injury that results in deep perineal laceration may be associated with extensive disruption of the pelvic vasculature and soft tissues, often with massive, life-threatening hemorrhage. This type of injury often follows an extensively forceful trauma caused by a fall from a significant height or a motor vehicle–pedestrian collision that results in extreme abduction of the hip or a crushing injury to the pelvis. Mortality may be extremely high, ranging from 42% to 59%.[6,7] Essential management requires hemorrhage control, debridement of devi-

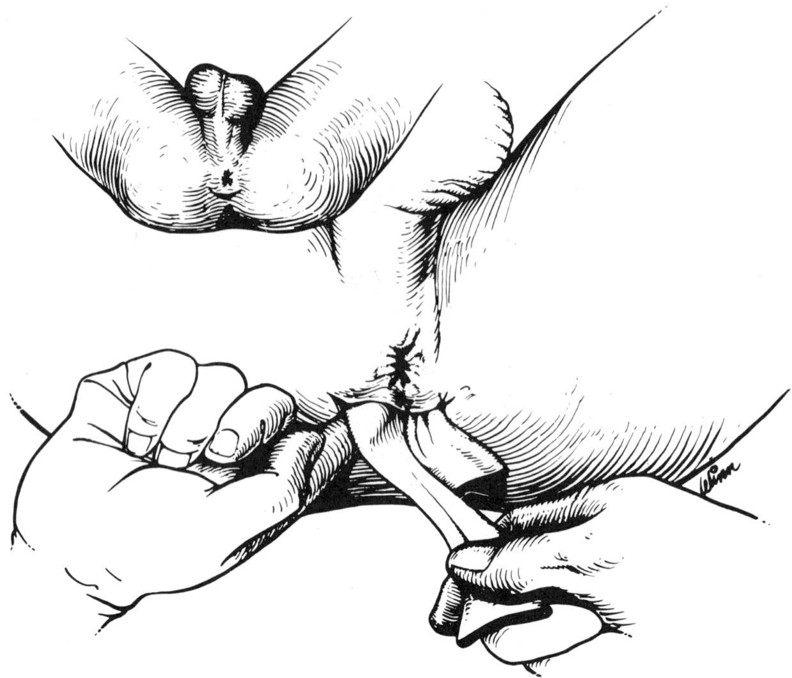

Figure 45–4 A curvilinear incision is made over the posterior anal area. By blunt dissection, the rectal area is entered and Penrose drains are inserted. (From Trunkey D et al: Management of rectal trauma, *J Trauma* 13:411-415, 1973.)

talized tissue, total fecal diversion, and presacral drainage; frequent operative debridement enhances wound healing. Without careful management, uncontrolled sepsis and death occur.

A thorough physical examination following blunt injury is important. Radiographic assessment helps to identify fracture of the pelvis. A high-riding prostate discovered in a rectal examination or the presence of a perineal hematoma necessitate a cystourethrogram to identify urethral injury.

Physical examination of the perineum in an alert child is difficult. The child is usually apprehensive and becomes more frightened and anxious when attempts are made to examine the perineum by abduction of the hips. Active bleeding obscures the extent of injury. It is best to examine the child while he or she is under anesthesia, rather than risk an incomplete evaluation of the injury. In examination of girls, placement of a urethral catheter prevents obstruction if there is edema adjacent to the urethra. In many cases laceration of the perineal body occurs. Determination of the depth of injury is essential for proper management because it can extend anteriorly and involve the posterior vagina; occasionally avulsion of the distal floor of the vagina occurs. Vaginal lacerations can bleed extensively, and hemostasis of the larger vessels is best achieved by ligature. Mucosal approximation with a running 3-0 chromic suture permits a secure closure. Careful reapproximation of the posterior mucosa to the perineal body minimizes the risk of stenosis.

Occasionally a perineal injury involves the vagina, perineal body, and anorectum. When the laceration extends up to the dentate line, suture approximation to the level of the anal canal permits closure by secondary intention. Frequent sitz baths and close observation of the wound for infection are necessary. When the laceration extends proximal to the mucocutaneous junction and involves full thickness of the rectum, it is safest to divert the fecal stream to minimize the risk of pelvic sepsis and rectovaginal fistula. Occasionally, an injury causes extensive disruption of the anal sphincter, and it is best, if possible, to approximate these anatomically at the time of repair of the laceration. Performance of a diverting colostomy, irrigation of the rectum, and presacral drainage constitute the best treatment. At 6 weeks, colostomy closure is possible after a barium enema demonstrates an intact rectal wall with no evidence of rectovaginal communication.

SUMMARY

Colon, rectal, and perineal injuries occur infrequently in children. Many penetrating colon wounds are safely treated with primary closure, and blunt colon injury is best managed with resection of the involved segment and proximal colostomy.

The standard of treatment for rectal injury includes total fecal diversion, rectal irrigation, and presacral drainage. Surgeons should be aware that a significant number of perineal and rectal injuries in children and adolescents are due to intentional abuse and require investigation. Proper management results in salvage of rectal continence and avoidance of pelvic sepsis.

REFERENCES

1. Black CT, Pokorny WI et al: Ano-rectal trauma in children, *J Ped Surg* 17:501-504, 1982.
2. Chappuis CW, Frey DJ et al: Management of penetrating colon injuries, *Ann Surg* 213:492-498, 1991.
3. Duncan AO, Phillips TF et al: Management of transpelvic gunshot wounds, *J Trauma* 29:1335-1340, 1989.
4. Flint LW, Voyles CR et al: Missile tract infections after transcolonic gunshot wounds, *Arch Surg* 113:727-728, 1978.
5. Howell HS, Bartizal JF et al: Blunt trauma involving the colon and rectum, *J Trauma* 16:624-632, 1976.
6. Kusminsky RE, Shbeeb I: Blunt pelviperineal injuries: an expanded role for the diverting colostomy, *Dis Col and Rect* 25:1787-1790, 1982.
7. Maull KI, Sachatello CR et al: The deep perineal laceration—an injury frequently associated with open pelvic fractures: a need for aggressive surgical management, *J Trauma* 17:685-696, 1977.
8. Sivit CJ, Taylor GA et al: Blunt trauma in children: significance of peritoneal fluid, *Radiology* 178:185-188, 1991.
9. Thal ER, Yeary EC: Morbidity of colostomy closure following colon trauma, *J Trauma* 20:287-291, 1980.
10. Tuggle D, Huber PJ: Management of rectal trauma, *Am J Surg* 148:806-808, 1984.
11. Voyles CR, Flint LM: Wound management after trauma to the colon, *South Med J* 70:1067-1069, 1977.
12. Wallace C: A study of 1200 cases of gunshot wounds of the abdomen, *Br J Surg* 4:679, 1917.
13. Woodhall J, Ochsner A: The management of perforating injuries of the colon and rectum in civilian practice, *Surgery* 29:305, 1951.

46 Pancreatic Injury

Frederick J. Rescorla and Jay L. Grosfeld

Trauma to the pancreas is a relatively uncommon injury among pediatric patients. Unfortunately, because of the retroperitoneal location of the pancreas, recognition of the injury is often delayed. Children with complete glandular fracture and ductal disruption may have relatively few symptoms initially, as the pancreatic secretions are contained within the retroperitoneum. Diagnosis of pancreatic injury is sometimes difficult, and the management of the patient at times controversial. Several of these observations are supported by the following case presentations.

Case report

A 6-year-old boy sustained a blunt abdominal injury when he struck the handlebars in a fall from his bicycle. Initial evaluation at a local community hospital demonstrated abdominal tenderness without peritoneal irritation. Results of the laboratory evaluation were normal, although a serum amylase level was not obtained. A computed tomography (CT) scan of the abdomen was interpreted as normal, and the child was observed for 24 hours and subsequently released as the pain subsided. The child returned to the emergency room 18 days later with abdominal pain and vomiting. At this time the serum amylase level was 1524 IU/L, and an abdominal CT scan demonstrated a pseudocyst occupying the lesser sac over the body and tail of the pancreas (Fig. 46-1). The child was transferred to the J.W. Riley Hospital for Children, Indianapolis, Indiana, and underwent placement of an ultrasound-guided percutaneous catheter into the pseudocyst and removal of fluid with an amylase level of 324,000 IU/L. The child's condition improved with resolution of his obstructive symptoms and return of his serum amylase level to normal. He was kept without oral intake and was maintained on total parenteral nutrition (TPN). The volume of drainage from the catheter gradually decreased and then stopped after 9 days. Unfortunately, the child's serum amylase level began to increase, and a second pseudocyst was noted in abdominal ultrasound examination. A major ductal injury was suspected, and endoscopic retrograde cholangiopancreatography (ERCP) demonstrated an abrupt cutoff of the pancreatic duct at the level of the spinal column (Fig. 46-2). Because of the ductal disruption, the child underwent laparotomy, at which time a complete pancreatic transection was noted. The distal pancreas was resected with splenic salvage. The proximal pancreatic duct could not be identified with certainty, and an autostapling device (Linear Stapler, 60 mm, Ethicon,

Somerville, New Jersey) was used to close the proximal pancreas and two closed-suction drains (Jackson Pratt, American V. Mueller, Chicago, Illinois) were placed near the pancreatic closure. The child recovered uneventfully; he was released 10 days after operation and allowed a full diet. He has been asymptomatic for 28 months.

This case illustrates the delay in diagnosis of pancreatic injury that is occasionally inevitable. Initial CT scan was normal, and the child improved and did well for a short period before presenting with pancreatitis and a pseudocyst. In assessing this child, some clinicians have recommended initial observation of the pseudocyst with later internal drainage; however, as noted in the following sections of the chapter, percutaneous external drainage alone may be effective in children with pancreatic trauma.

ETIOLOGY

Injury to the pancreas is a relatively uncommon occurrence following either blunt or penetrating abdominal trauma in children. Approximately 88% of cases of abdominal trauma in children are due to blunt injuries.[26] The mechanism of blunt injury to the pancreas is related to compression of the relatively fixed body of the pancreas against the spinal column. Common causes include falling from a bicycle with injury caused by the handlebar, pedestrian traffic accident, motor vehicle crash, and, unfortunately, child abuse. Most patients are between 2 and 13 years of age; bicycle injury constitutes up to 40% of cases of pancreatic trauma.[2,11,24,29]

DIAGNOSIS

An injured child who is hemodynamically stable upon arrival at the emergency room or becomes stable after initial resuscitation is evaluated on the basis of mechanism of injury, history, and complete physical examination. In cases of isolated pancreatic injury, evaluation of the abdomen can often be difficult and abdominal tenderness frequently absent. The retroperitoneal location of the pancreas may delay the lack of pancreatic enzymes into the peritoneal cavity. Consequently, the abdominal ex-

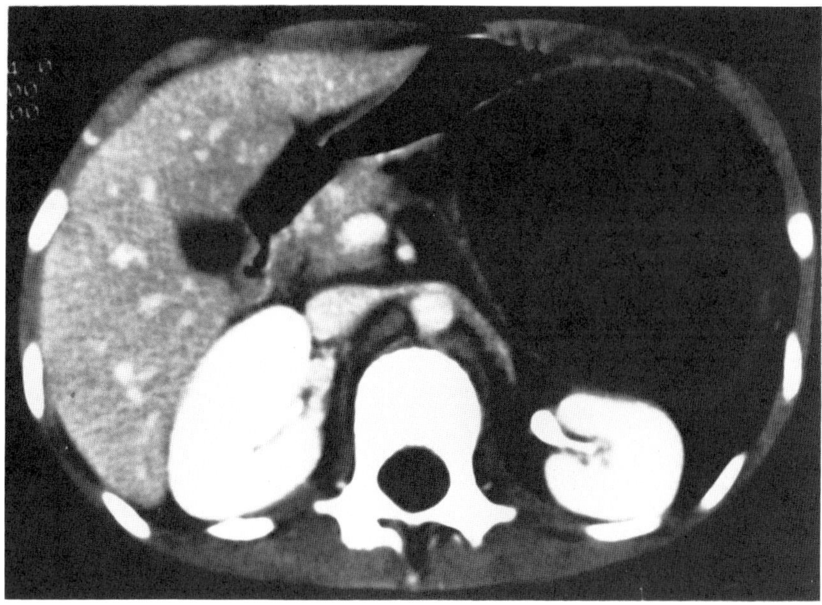

Figure 46–1 CT scan demonstrating a large pancreatic pseudocyst.

amination of a child with a significant injury to the pancreas may show no abnormalities except for superficial abdominal wall tenderness. Typically, the pain occurs in the midepigastrium; however, it may become diffuse with leak of pancreatic enzymes into the lesser sac or peritoneal cavity. Nausea and vomiting are often noted, and the abdominal pain may radiate to the back or left flank.

Serum amylase level remains one of the most useful indicators in detecting pancreatic injury. Unfortunately, hyperamylasemia also occurs with bowel perforation, appendicitis, intestinal obstruction, mesenteric thrombosis, injury with intracranial hemorrhage, and salivary gland trauma.[21,25] Amylase is produced by several organs, the major two of which are the pancreas and salivary glands. The assessment of amylase isoenzymes by the use of electrophoresis, isoelectric focusing, or chromatography has been reported to increase the specificity of an elevated serum amylase level by excluding salivary hyperamylasemia in cases of associated facial trauma.[5,12,25] Unfortunately, the data are conflicting in the evaluation of trauma patients. Some clinicians have noted an increase in the nonpancreatic fraction of amylase in facial trauma.[12] Others have reported patients with major pancreatic injuries to have normal amylase and isoamylase levels, although the pancreatic isoamylase level was elevated in several patients without evidence of pancreatic injury.[5] In addition, it has been noted that patients with intracranial hemorrhage have marked elevations of total serum am-

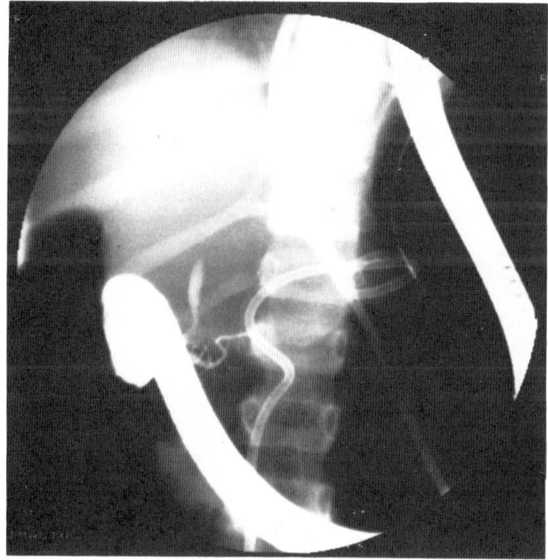

Figure 46–2 ERCP shows an abrupt cutoff of main pancreatic duct at the level of the spinal column.

ylase, which, upon fractionation, have been attributable to pancreatic and nonpancreatic sources.[4] Thus, the determination of pancreatitis in a child with head injury is difficult, even with the use of isoenzymes. As important as the elevation of serum amylase is the trend of amylase determinations. Although a single isolated serum amylase level is not a reliable indicator of a major pancreatic injury,

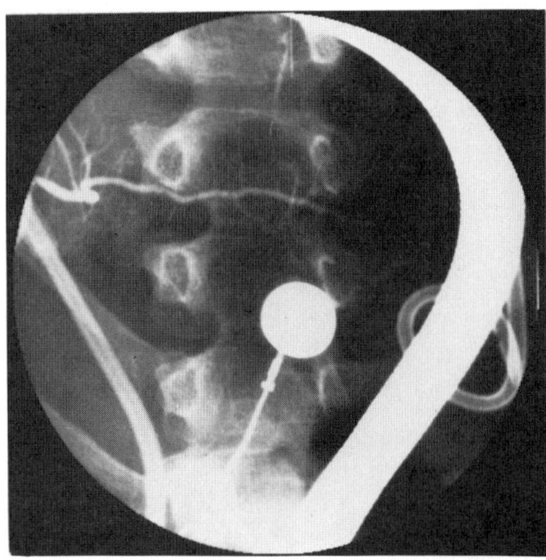

Figure 46–3 ERCP demonstrates cutoff in distal pancreatic duct. Distal pancreatectomy was performed for complete glandular and ductal disruption.

a trend of increasing serum amylase levels is indicative of a significant pancreatic injury, and an initially high level followed by subsequent decreasing levels may indicate a contusion of the gland without ductal injury. In many of such cases, evaluations of serum lipase level may complement serum amylase determinations as a diagnostic test. Lipase is primarily of pancreatic origin and as such should be a more sensitive and specific indicator of pancreatic injury than an increased amylase level. In clinical trials, however, it has not been proven superior to serum amylase as an indicator. When the two levels are used together, however, diagnostic accuracy is improved.[22]

The initial evaluation of a seriously injured child includes radiographic examination of the chest, abdomen, and pelvis, primarily to assess for associated injuries. A child with significant abdominal pain or suspected abdominal injuries who is hemodynamically stable upon arrival in the emergency room or after initial resuscitation is evaluated with an abdominal CT scan. Both intravenous and oral contrast and, in selective cases, rectal contrast, are administered. Abdominal CT scan documents associated splenic, hepatic, renal, and duodenal injuries extremely well.[18] Unfortunately, CT examination has not been as accurate in the diagnosis of acute pancreatic injury. The evaluation of the pancreas is difficult immediately after the injury and can lead to a false-negative ("normal") CT scan in the presence of transection of the pancreatic duct. If abdominal pain persists or the serum amylase level remains elevated or increases, a repeat CT scan to focus on the pancreas enhances the

likelihood of documentation of edema fluid within the lesser sac.

The use of endoscopic retrograde cholangiopancreatography (ERCP) has recently been reported in adults with acute traumatic pancreatic injury, and can be used to clearly identify ductal disruption.[1,14] Although ERCP should not be used routinely in acute cases of pancreatic trauma, it may be of occasional use if exploration is required for pain or rising serum amylase levels. The finding of a normal proximal pancreatic duct on ERCP allows the surgeon to perform a distal resection without the need to visualize the proximal ductal anatomy intraoperatively. In addition, normal results of an ERCP study may allow nonoperative management of a child with an intact pancreatic duct even in the presence of increasing pain or a rising serum amylase level. It should be emphasized that the use of ERCP in the presence of pancreatitis may be hazardous, and this technique should be employed selectively in acute cases when the surgeon is anticipating the need for a surgical procedure. ERCP is quite useful in cases that fail nonoperative management and are no longer in the acute phase of injury, providing the surgeon an accurate evaluation of the ductal anatomy (Fig. 46-3).

Ultrasound examination has a limited role in early management of pancreatic injury. It is, however, a very useful method of following the course of pancreatic pseudocysts and is also effective in guiding aspiration of cysts by placement of percutaneous external drainage catheters.

In the present era, diagnostic peritoneal lavage (DPL) is rarely employed in children with blunt traumatic injuries, and we would not recommend this technique for evaluation of pancreatic injury. DPL may result in a false-negative tap because of the retroperitoneal location of the gland.

CLASSIFICATION

Classification of pancreatic injury is based primarily on the presence of injury to the gland, major ductal system, or duodenum.[7,17,23,28] Because the location of the injury in the duct (proximal or distal) is important in determining the type of operative procedure, the classification listed in Table 46-1 is preferable.[17,23]

MANAGEMENT

Initial resuscitation of the injured child requires specific attention to the airway, breathing, and circulation. An isolated injury to the pancreas rarely requires emergent laparotomy, except in instances of penetrating abdominal trauma. Occasionally, a child with blunt trauma requires an emergent operation for exsanguinating a splenic or hepatic injury or bowel perforation. Following control of

Table 46–1 Classification of pancreatic injury

Type	Pancreatic injury
1	Contusion and laceration without ductal injury
2	Distal transection or parenchymal injury with ductal injury
3	Proximal transection or parenchymal injury with probable ductal injury
4	Combined pancreatic and duodenal injury

bleeding, visualization of the pancreas by dividing the gastrocolic ligament to enter the lesser sac is important. In addition, the presence of a hematoma around the pancreas, or bile stain around the duodenum and head of the pancreas, suggests a duodenal injury, biliary ductal disruption, or pancreatic injury. If the associated injury is severe and the child is unstable, the most expeditious management of the pancreatic injury may be simple external drainage, with the realization that a pancreatic fistula likely will result. In some cases, the fistula closes spontaneously; however, distal resection of the tail of the pancreas or internal drainage of the pseudocyst is sometimes necessary. If a child with an associated injury is stable, immediate treatment of the injured pancreas is indicated as described in "Operative Management" later in this chapter.

Children with abdominal pain, with an elevated serum amylase level and a normal CT scan, or with an abnormal CT scan due to injury involving other organs (spleen, liver, kidney) not requiring exploration, are treated with intravenous fluids and bed rest and maintained without oral intake. Insertion of a nasogastric tube prevents gastric distention and gastric stimulation of the exocrine pancreas and decreases the acid stimulation of the duodenum, thus preventing secretin release. In addition, cimetidine can block acid stimulation of the pancreas. Although these steps in patient care are physiologically sound, there have been no studies that clearly demonstrate the effectiveness of gastric decompression in adults or children with pancreatitis.[9,20] Occasionally, a child can have severe, unrelenting abdominal pain with evidence of peritoneal irritation and subsequently require laparotomy. Small bowel perforation is a more common finding than pancreatic disruption; however, the pancreas requires careful examination during the course of exploration.

If CT scan of the pancreas demonstrates ductal disruption, pancreatic edema, or lesser sac fluid collection, the options for treatment include observation, percutaneous drainage, and/or exploration. The method of treatment of a child with a suspected or documented pancreatic injury is controversial. Some authors have recommended urgent exploration because many such children eventually require an operation for gland disruption, pseudocyst, or fistula (if percutaneous drainage is used). Smith and colleagues, in a review of 22 children with pancreatic injury, noted a much shorter hospital stay for those children treated with prompt laparotomy.[29] There is no question that early operation allows confirmation of the diagnosis and prompt definitive treatment. The disadvantage is that many children with contusions and small lacerations who may not require surgery or may be treated successfully by other methods (observation or percutaneous drainage) are all subjected to laparotomy.

Our current preference is initial observation, even if the serum amylase level increases. If a lesser sac fluid collection occurs and the child has a rising amylase level or increasing abdominal pain, place a percutaneous external drainage catheter under CT or ultrasound guidance. The following report illustrates a recent case of pancreatic injury managed in this fashion.

Case report

A 10-year-old boy developed a sudden onset of intense periumbilical pain 2 days after a fall from a minibike. The fall produced numerous extremity abrasions; however, the child denied injuring his abdomen and was asymptomatic for 48 hours after the incident. The serum amylase level was 1450 IU/L, and the serum lipase level was 19,000 IU/L. An abdominal CT scan demonstrated fluid within the pelvis and left upper quadrant and edema of the tail of the pancreas (Fig. 46-4). Upon admission to the hospital 3 days after the injury, examination revealed diffuse abdominal tenderness and a serum amylase level of 2113 IU/L and lipase level of 12,936 IU/L. The child was kept without oral intake and supported with intravenous fluids. Percutaneous aspiration of the fluid, performed under ultrasound guidance, demonstrated straw-colored fluid with an amylase level of 8100 IU/L. A catheter was placed for continued drainage. Twelve hours following percutaneous drainage, abdominal pain began to abate and a repeat determination of serum amylase level was 1076 IU/L. The child was treated with octreotide acetate (Sandostatin) 50 µg subcutaneously b.i.d. The serum amylase level fell to normal within 72 hours. The amylase level in the drain fell below the serum level by the fifth day and the child's diet was resumed. He remained asymptomatic, the catheter was removed, and he was released 12 days after the injury.

In this case the ductal anatomy was never ascertained because the patient improved clinically. Although a catheter was left in place, it may in fact have been unnecessary in this situation of traumatic pancreatitis. The child described in the pre-

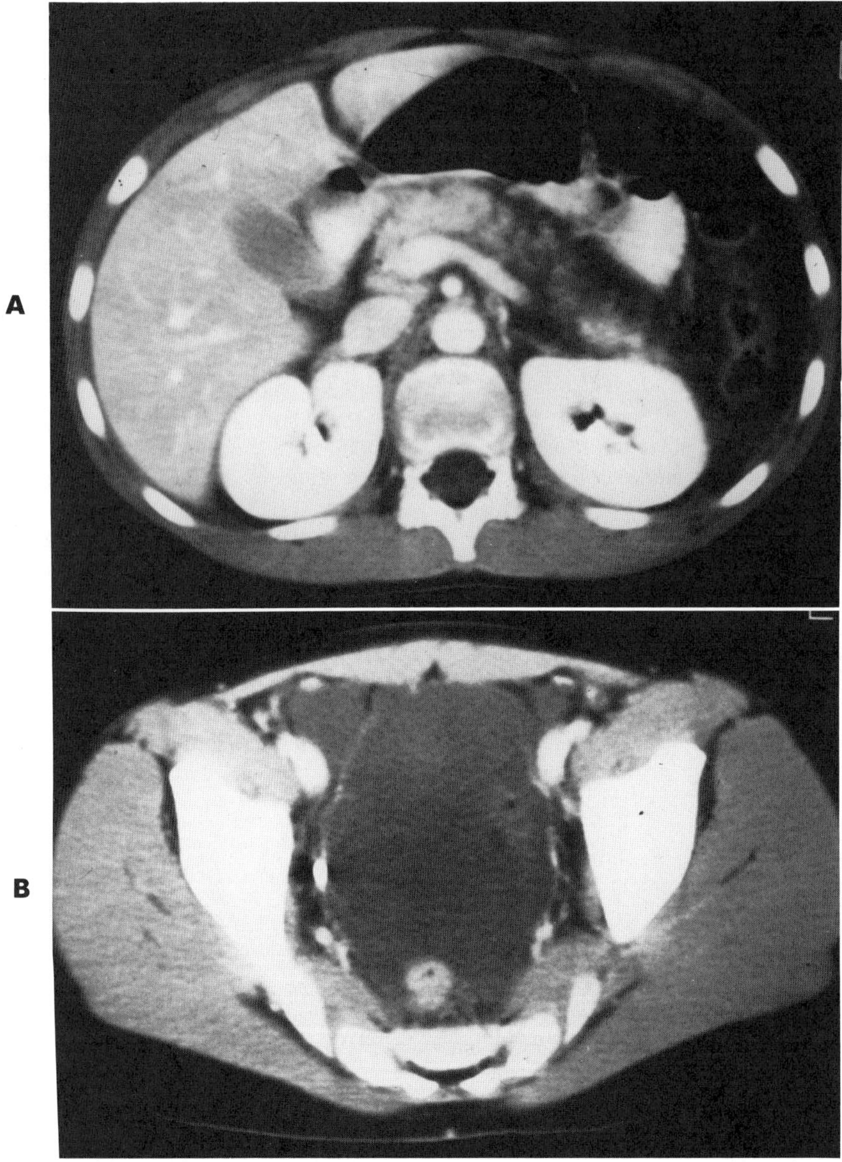

Figure 46–4 CT scans demonstrate (**A**) edema of the distal pancreas and (**B**) free fluid within the pelvis.

vious case was also treated with octreotide acetate (Sandostatin) in an attempt to decrease the pancreatic exocrine secretions. Octreotide acetate and somatostatin both act by suppressing secretion of gastrin, vasoactive intestinal polypeptide, insulin, glucagon, secretin, motilin, and pancreatic polypeptide.[13] The advantages of octreotide acetate are a longer half-life (90 to 113 minutes) and longer duration of action (8 to 12 hours) than somatostatin (half-life, 1 to 3 minutes). It can also be admin-

istered subcutaneously, whereas somatostatin must be administered by continuous intravenous infusion owing to its shorter half-life.

The role of ERCP in pediatric pancreatic trauma is unclear. ERCP is very useful in delineating the pancreatic ductal anatomy prior to surgical exploration in cases with delayed presentation or in those that have failed percutaneous drainage. If a major ductal injury is observed on ERCP, laparotomy is indicated to treat the injury, although some authors

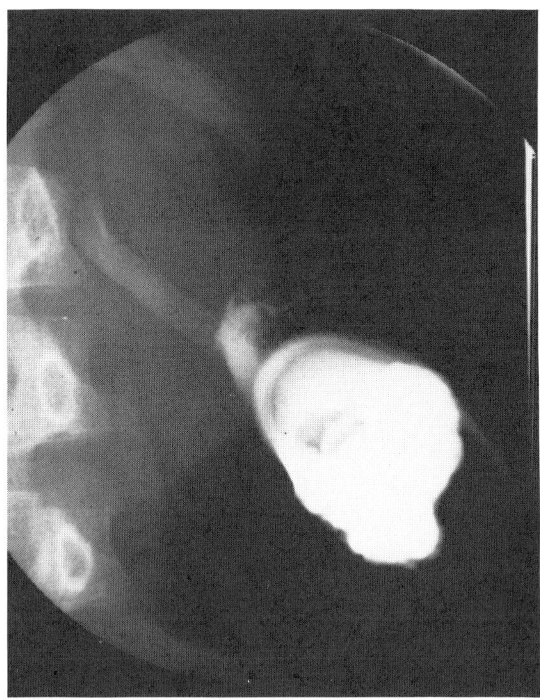

Figure 46–5 Cyst injection demonstrates filling of distal pancreatic duct without proximal drainage in a child with prolonged drainage from a percutaneously placed catheter. Complete glandular and ductal disruption was noted at operation.

have noted resolution of pancreatitis with conservative nonoperative management, even in the presence of ductal disruption.[24]

The role of percutaneous drainage of the lesser sac or free peritoneal cavity is controversial. Advantages are that drainage removes the enzyme-containing fluid from the abdomen and frequently results in resolution of the pain caused by peritoneal irritation. The disadvantages of percutaneous drainage are the prolonged period of drainage and the need for hospitalization, as well as for treatment with TPN. Percutaneous treatment of a severe ductal disruption may have little chance of success. Injection of the cyst through the drainage catheter or ERCP, however, is helpful if percutaneous drainage is unsuccessful within 2 weeks (Fig. 46-5). If ductal disruption is noted in association with prolonged drainage or pancreatitis, laparotomy with distal resection of the pancreas is appropriate treatment. This is a controversial point and some clinicians would argue for continued percutaneous catheter drainage. Jaffe and colleagues, in a report concerning seven children in whom percutaneous treatment was successful, noted drainage for as long as 66 days.[16]

A stable child for whom initial abdominal CT examination showed no abnormality, and who subsequently has continued abdominal pain, elevated amylase, or an upper abdominal mass should be examined by ultrasound or CT for a possible pseudocyst, lesser sac fluid collection, or pancreatic edema. As noted previously, several children with initially normal CT scans have been found later to have major pancreatic injuries missed by the initial study.

OPERATIVE MANAGEMENT

If a child has an associated extrapancreatic intraabdominal injury requiring exploration, the surgeon should repair the injury and evaluate the status of the pancreas. The most common conditions requiring emergent exploration are injuries to the spleen, liver, and small bowel. Many of these injuries are related to a significant force applied to the abdomen, which increases the possibility of a pancreatic injury. Visualization of the pancreas is important. The lesser sac is entered by dividing the greater omentum just above the colon, allowing visualization of the body and tail of the pancreas. If injury to the head of the pancreas is suspected, or if air or bile is noted in the retroperitoneum, a Kocher maneuver permits complete visualization of the head of the pancreas and duodenum and, thus, evaluation of the injury. For further visualization of the pancreas, the spleen may be mobilized from the left upper quadrant and then, along with the pancreas, mobilized medially. This allows visualization of the posterior surface of the pancreas to the level of the superior mesenteric vessels.

Operative strategy is based on the presence of parenchymal, ductal, or duodenal injury. The overall goals of the operative procedure are to control hemorrhage, to debride or resect devitalized pancreatic tissue, to preserve adequate pancreatic tissue (20% to 40%), and to provide appropriate internal and external drainage.

If a pancreatic contusion or laceration without ductal injury (type I) is noted, simple external drainage is adequate therapy. Placement of two closed suction catheters permits quantification of drainage volume and prevention of skin excoriation. Drains are left in place until they no longer drain or until the amylase level in the drain effluent is less than the serum amylase level. During the perioperative period, TNP is indicated for nutritional support of the child. When postoperative ileus resolves, the regimen may be advanced to a low-fat diet as long as drain output does not increase with advancement of feedings. Several authors have recommended needle-catheter jejunostomy at the time of initial exploration for most pancreatic injuries, to allow early enteral feeding of an elemental diet.[7,17] If a low-output pancreatic fistula remains, the child can be managed on an outpatient basis, as most fistulas will close with time.

Case report

A 15-month-old boy sustained a blunt abdominal injury when he was run over by the rear wheels of a pickup truck. The child was initially stable and was treated in a community hospital with only intravenous fluids. Sixteen hours after the injury he developed increasing abdominal distention and hypotension and underwent emergent laparotomy. Operative findings included a nearly complete transection of his small bowel 2 cm past the ligament of Treitz. This injury was repaired with a primary bowel anastomosis. Over the next 48 hours the child developed tachypnea, increased inspired oxygen requirement, abdominal distention, and a rising serum amylase level. He was transferred to our institution and shortly after admission required endotracheal intubation for progressive hypoxemia. An abdominal CT scan demonstrated edema of the pancreas with significant fluid within the lesser sac. Because of the child's deteriorating condition, he was taken to the operating room for exploratory laparotomy. During surgery, a laceration was noted on the ventral surface of the pancreas. Owing to the extensive inflammation and edema, the injury was treated with external drainage, rather than resection, with the use of two closed suction drains. The child's condition improved dramatically, and he was extubated 24 hours after the procedure. He was supported with TPN for 2 weeks. One drainage catheter was removed; however, the other continued to drain 25 cc of fluid per day while the amylase level was over 5000 IU/L. The drainage amount was unaffected by dietary intake, and the child was therefore discharged and allowed a regular diet. The fistula gradually closed, and the drain was removed during a follow-up office visit 6 weeks after the operation. At 8 months following the injury, the child remained asymptomatic.

This report again illustrates the delay in diagnosis frequently seen in cases of blunt pancreatic injury. It also demonstrates that external drainage may be adequate treatment even for rather major pancreatic injuries in children with otherwise normal pancreatic ducts. If the lesser sac had been explored at the initial operation, the injury might have been noted and either drainage or resection performed.

If a laceration of the pancreas is centrally located and close to the duct, or drains a large amount of pancreatic fluid, an operative pancreatogram may be useful in assessing ductal integrity and excluding a type II injury. An operative pancreatogram can be performed by opening the duodenum, inserting a small catheter into the ampulla of Vater, and filling the common bile and pancreatic duct with contrast. It is also possible to amputate the tail of the pancreas and perform a retrograde study; however, we would not recommend this procedure in children. Some authors have assessed ductal anatomy in penetrating trauma in adult patients with intraoperative ERCP.[19] We have no personal experience with this technique. Two alternatives to an operative pancreatogram are simple external drainage of the injury, and resection of the distal pancreas with splenic preservation. If a major ductal injury seems likely, we do not perform a pancreatogram (with the risks of duodenal closure) but instead perform a distal resection. If the inflammation is severe and if a resection appears hazardous, external drainage is the procedure of choice. In the foregoing case a ductal injury healed with simple external drainage. Long-term follow-up is needed to assess the course of such injuries, particularly regarding growth and scarring of the pancreatic duct. We have seen one child treated with external drainage who developed a symptomatic high-grade stricture of the pancreatic duct 3 years later, requiring a distal pancreatectomy.

If a complete distal transection of the pancreas or parenchymal injury with ductal injury (type II) is noted, a distal pancreatectomy with splenic salvage is the procedure of choice. The inferior border of the pancreas is mobilized, and the pancreas is then separated from the splenic artery and vein with care to ligate the many small vessels penetrating the pancreas. The proximal pancreas is managed by one of two methods. The proximal duct can be ligated with a nonabsorbable suture, and the remainder of the pancreas closed with mattress sutures placed in a full-thickness fashion. An alternative method (which we prefer in children) is to use one of the readily available autostapling devices to seal the end of the gland. This may be easier in children because the gland is smaller and softer and the proximal ductal anatomy is almost always normal. Ligation of the pancreatic duct is preferred but may not be necessary with the stapling technique. The suture line is externally drained with one or two closed, soft silastic suction catheters. Some authors have suggested that an omental patch be placed over the suture line; however, we have not routinely used this technique. If there is concern regarding the integrity of the proximal pancreatic duct, a pancreatogram can be performed through the open duct prior to closure. Although a small fistula may result in the end of the transected pancreas, it will usually close with time.

In cases in which the proximal pancreas is injured (type III) it is necessary to identify the pancreatic ductal anatomy with a pancreatogram or intraoperative ERCP. If the major pancreatic duct is intact, simple external drainage is the treatment of choice. If the duct is disrupted, a distal pancreatectomy is recommended, as long as the head of the pancreas is preserved. We have generally performed distal pancreatectomy for injuries occurring directly over the superior mesenteric vessels. If the injury is proximal to this level, the proximal pancreas can be closed and a Roux-en-Y pancreaticojejunostomy constructed to drain the distal pancreas in order to preserve endocrine and exocrine function. Although it has been described in adult series, we have never performed this procedure in a child with a pancreatic injury.

Combined pancreaticoduodenal (type IV) injuries in children are rare, usually occurring with penetrating trauma. Careful assessment of the pancreatic duct and common bile duct is necessary in these cases. If the duodenum is open and the ampulla can be visualized, a retrograde cholangiogram can be performed. If the common bile duct is intact, the duodenum can be closed and the pancreatic injury treated according to the status of the duct (as in a type III injury). Occasionally, in severe injuries to the duodenum it may be useful to divert gastric and biliary contents away from the duodenum by performing a duodenal "diverticularization" procedure described by Berne and colleagues.[3] This procedure includes a vagotomy, antrectomy with end-to-side gastrojejunostomy (Billroth II), duodenal closure, T-tube drainage of the common bile duct, and tube duodenostomy. In children, tube cholecystostomy may be preferable to T-tube drainage because of the small size of the common bile duct. An alternative operation for severe duodenal injury is the "pyloric exclusion" procedure described by Vaughan and colleagues.[31] In this procedure the pylorus is closed with an absorbable purse-string suture through a gastrotomy and a loop gastrojejunostomy constructed. This temporarily diverts gastric juices from the duodenum. Eventually, the pylorus opens and the gastrojejunostomy becomes nonfunctional. The trend in treatment of adult trauma over the past few years has been away from radical resections for combined injuries, and toward the use of duodenal closure and pancreatic resection or drainage as primary therapy.[8] If a ductal injury is missed and results in a high-output fistula, distal resection may be performed safely at a later date.

Occasionally, a pancreaticoduodenectomy (Whipple) or pylorus-preserving Traverso-Longmire procedure may be required in a case of extensive devitalization of the head of the pancreas, ductal disruption of the pancreatic head in association with a duodenal or common bile duct injury, injury to the ampulla of Vater or uncontrollable bleeding from the pancreatic head.[30] This is rarely required in children, and we have performed a pancreaticoduodenectomy on only one occasion for pediatric pancreatic trauma in the past 19 years.

PSEUDOCYSTS AND LESSER SAC FLUID COLLECTIONS

There are several therapeutic options available for treatment of children with pancreatic pseudocysts. If there are no signs or symptoms (other than a mass), we advocate simple observation of the child, as a significant number of pseudocysts (perhaps 44% to 60%) spontaneously resolve with time.[2,11,24] In patients with signs and symptoms such as pain, obstruction, anorexia, or pancreatitis, several interventional options are available (Table 46-2). If the pseudocyst has been present for a significant period of time (more than 6 weeks), the treatment is usually internal drainage by a Roux-en-Y cystjejunostomy. Cystgastrostomy is useful if the cyst is adherent to the posterior wall of the stomach. Cystduodenostomy is not recommended. Distal resection is advised if the pseudocyst is located in the tail of the pancreas. In children in whom a pseudocyst is noted soon after injury, treatment options include observation, operative external drainage, or percutaneous external drainage. Resection of the pseudocyst is rarely an option.

For a child in whom a mass is the only finding, observation of the child on an outpatient basis is possible. Symptomatic children with pain, obstruction, or pancreatitis who are being treated conservatively by observation require withholding of oral intake, TPN, and, in cases of obstruction, nasogastric decompression. If the pseudocyst persists, internal drainage is the treatment of choice. External operative drainage is rarely required, and we have not used this technique in the past 15 years because of prolonged drainage and the reported recurrence rate of approximately 8%.[6]

Percutaneous external drainage of pseudocysts and lesser sac fluid collections has been reported by several authors with varying degrees of success.[2,15] This procedure offers several advantages in that it relieves the obstructive symptoms, alleviates the associated pancreatitis, allows drainage

Table 46–2 Pseudocysts: management options

Observation
External drainage
Percutaneous External drainage
Internal drainage
Cystgastrostomy
Cystduodenostomy
Cystjejunostomy
Resection

of a thin-walled cyst that may not be amenable to internal drainage, and may provide definitive therapy. We have recently reported four children with pseudocysts treated with percutaneous drainage, three of whom eventually required resection for continued drainage or a persistent cyst. In each case, ERCP or cyst injection demonstrated unsuspected ductal disruption.[27] Other authors have reported much higher success rates following percutaneous drainage by allowing a longer duration of drainage or placement of additional catheters.[15] Percutaneous transgastric drainage and percutaneous pancreatic cystgastrostomy have also been reported.[10]

COMPLICATIONS

Complications associated with the care of pancreatic injuries in children are, fortunately, quite rare. Pseudocysts may be noted after nonoperative treatment, and presenting symptoms generally include a mass, fever, abdominal pain, vomiting, or pancreatitis.

A pancreatic fistula may complicate an operative procedure or percutaneous external drainage. Most fistulas will close with time, particularly if the proximal pancreatic duct is normal. A high-output fistula may indicate ductal obstruction or disruption and warrant evaluation by drain or catheter injection or by ERCP.

Although pancreatic insufficiency has been observed in adults following pancreatic resection, children tolerate resection well and rarely require exogenous pancreatic enzymes.

SUMMARY

The contemporary methods of management of pancreatic injuries in children has evolved over the past decade. The availability of imaging modalities such as CT, ERCP, and ultrasound have provided the surgeon with improved methods of evaluating these injuries. In an increasing number of cases, close observation and percutaneous external drainage have obviated the need for laparotomy in many children. Despite the success achieved by these newer treatment modalities, the surgeon must carefully follow the patient's course and be prepared to explore the child and perform appropriate operative procedures, including pancreatic resection, if the child does not respond to nonoperative measures.

REFERENCES

1. Barkin JS, Ferstenberg RM, Panullo W et al: Endoscopic retrograde cholangiopancreatography in pancreatic trauma, *Gastroenterol Endosc* 34:102-105, 1988.
2. Bass J, Lorenzo MD, Desjardins JG et al: Blunt pancreatic injuries in children: the role of percutaneous external drainage in the treatment of pancreatic pseudocysts, *J Pediatr Surg* 23:721-724, 1988.
3. Berne CJ, Donovan AJ, White EJ: Duodenal "diverticulization" for duodenal and pancreatic injury, *Am J Surg* 127:503-507, 1974.
4. Bouwman DL, Altshuler J, Weaver DW: Hyperamylasemia: a result of intracranial bleeding, *Surgery* 94:318-323, 1983.
5. Bouwman DL, Weaver DW, Walt AJ: Serum amylase and its isoenzymes: clarification of their implications in trauma, *J Trauma* 24:573-578, 1984.
6. Cooney DR, Grosfeld JL: Operative management of pancreatic pseudocysts in infants and children: a review of 75 cases, *Ann Surg* 182:590-596, 1975.
7. Feliciano P, Lowe DK: Pancreatic trauma. In Maull KI, editor: *Advances in trauma*, Chicago, Ill, 1990, Mosby–Year Book, pp 101-102.
8. Flynn WJ Jr, Cryer HG, Richardson JD: Reappraisal of pancreatic and duodenal injury management based on injury severity, *Arch Surg* 125:1539-1541, 1990.
9. Fuller RK, Loveland JP, Frankel MH: An evaluation of the efficacy of nasogastric suction treatment in alcoholic pancreatitis, *Am J Gastroenterol* 75:349-353, 1981.
10. Gandini G, Jullani E, Grasso M et al: Nonsurgical treatment of 68 pancreatic pseudocysts including percutaneous pseudocystogastrostomy. Paper presented at the meeting of the Radiological Society of North America, Chicago, November 1988.
11. Gorenstein A, O'Halpin D, Wesson DE et al: Blunt injury to the pancreas in children: selective management based on ultrasound, *J Pediatr Surg* 22:1110-1116, 1987.
12. Greenlee T, Murphy K, Ram MD: Amylase isoenzymes in the evaluation of trauma patients, *Am Surg* 50:637-640, 1984.
13. Grosman I, Simon D: Potential gastrointestinal uses of somatostatin and its synthetic analogue octreotide, *Am J Gastroenterol* 85:1061-72, 1990.
14. Hayward SR, Lucas CE, Sugawa C et al: Emergent endoscopic retrograde cholangiopancreatography, *Arch Surg* 124:745-746, 1989.
15. Hendrickson M, Matlak ME, Jaffe RB et al: Treatment of traumatic pancreatic pseudocysts in children: the role of percutaneous drainage, *Pediatr Surg Intl* 5:347-349, 1990.
16. Jaffe RB, Arata JA Jr, Matlak ME: Percutaneous drainage of traumatic pancreatic pseudocysts in children, *AJR* 152:591-595, 1989.
17. Jurkovich GJ, Carrico CJ: Pancreatic trauma, *Surg Clin N Am* 70:575-593, 1990.
18. Karp MP, Cooney DR, Berger PE et al: The role of computed tomography in the evaluation of blunt abdominal trauma in children, *J Pediatr Surg* 16:316-323, 1981.
19. Laraja RD, Lobbato VJ, Cassaro S et al: Intraoperative ERCP in penetrating trauma of the pancreas, *J Trauma* 26:1146-1147, 1986.
20. Levant JA, Secrist DM, Resin H et al: Nasogastric suction in the treatment of alcoholic pancreatitis, *JAMA* 229:51-52, 1974.
21. Levitt MD: Clinical use of amylase clearance and isoamylase measurements, *Mayo Clin Proc* 54:428-431, 1979.
22. Lifton LJ, Slickers KA, Pragay DA et al: Pancreatitis and lipase: a reevaluation with a five minute turbidimetric lipase determination, *JAMA* 229:47-50, 1974.
23. Lucas CE: Diagnosis and treatment of pancreatic and duodenal injury, *Surg Clin N Am* 57:49-65, 1977.
24. Millar AJW, Rode H, Stunden RJ et al: Management of pancreatic pseudocysts in children, *J Pediatr Surg* 23:122-127, 1988.
25. Moosa AR: Diagnostic tests and procedures in acute pancreatitis, *N Engl J Med* 311:639-643, 1984.
26. Ramenofsky ML: Pediatric abdominal trauma, *Pediatr Ann* 16:318-326, 1987.
27. Rescorla FJ, Cory D, Vane DW et al: Failure of percuta-

neous drainage in children with traumatic pancreatic pseudocysts, *J Pediatr Surg* 25:1038-1042, 1990.

28. Smego DR, Richardson JD, Flint LM: Determinants of outcome in pancreatic trauma, *J Trauma* 25:771-776, 1985.

29. Smith SD, Nakayama DK, Gantt N et al: Pancreatic injuries in childhood due to blunt trauma, *J Pediatr Surg* 23:610-614, 1988.

30. Traverso LW, Longmire WP Jr: Preservation of the pylorus during pancreaticoduodenectomy, *Surg Gynecol Obstet* 146:959-962, 1978.

31. Vaughan GD III, Frazier OH, Graham DY et al: The use of pyloric exclusion in the management of severe duodenal injuries, *Am J Surg* 134:785-790, 1977.

PART ELEVEN

Genitourinary Injury

47 Genitourinary Injury*

Michael J. Allshouse and *James M. Betts*

Injury is the leading cause of mortality in children between the ages of 1 and 15, surpassing the next four leading causes of death combined. The majority of deaths resulting from trauma are related to severe head or truncal injuries or a combination of both. Genitourinary injury is rarely a cause of trauma-related accidental death but occurs frequently enough to warrant careful consideration during the secondary survey and treatment phase of trauma care. Significant morbidity may be attributable to genitourinary injury. Sequelae may have delayed manifestations, as well as life-long implications.

Estimates compiled from pediatric trauma data suggest that 5% of all injured children have involvement of the genitourinary tract.[16] Most of these injuries are due to blunt trauma, either intentional or unintentional. Approximately 80% of genitourinary injuries result from blunt trauma, and the remaining 20% from penetrating trauma.[20] The ratio of blunt to penetrating genitourinary trauma varies, depending on the location of the reporting institution. Urban trauma centers tend to treat a greater number of penetrating injuries because of patterns of urban crime and violence. It is likely that genitourinary injury is underreported in injured children for several reasons. First, more life-threatening central nervous system, thoracic, abdominal, or musculoskeletal injuries are present in 40% to 50% of children with renal injuries.[20] Additionally, many of the isolated genitourinary injuries may not necessitate admission to an inpatient unit. A review of 3587 admissions to the Children's National Medical Center (CNMC) in Washington, D.C., for blunt and penetrating trauma revealed only 58 children (1.6%) with genitourinary injury. There were 27 documented injuries in 2020 admissions (1.3%) to the trauma service at Children's Hospital, Oakland, California.

There are anatomic and developmental differences between children and adults that influence the patterns of genitourinary trauma. A peculiarity of urinary tract trauma in children is the frequent association of the injury with the initial presentation of a preexisting disease or anomaly. The coexistence of childhood genitourinary anomaly with renal or urinary tract injury occurs in up to 23% of cases.[16] Hydronephrosis, renal and ureteral ectopia, and tumors all predispose various portions of the genitourinary tract to injury. Hematuria after trivial or minor trauma in school-aged children is often the first sign of hydronephrosis.[9] In younger children, hematuria after minor trauma may be the initial finding with unrecognized Wilms' tumor or other renal or adrenal neoplasm.

The goal of evaluation and treatment in genitourinary injury is the same as in other areas of trauma care. Every attempt should be made to preserve life, maintain tissue functioning, and ensure the eventual ability to return the child to home life and family as expeditiously as possible.

KIDNEY INJURY

In both the adult and pediatric populations, injury to the kidney is the most common form of genitourinary injury, accounting for 34% to 68% of all genitourinary tract trauma.[16] The most common source of urinary tract injury is blunt trauma. Blunt trauma causes proportionately more injuries in children than in adults, most of which result from motor vehicle crashes. Children suffer a significant number of kidney injuries after seemingly minor trauma. Certain anatomic and developmental characteristics of the child's kidney, as compared with the adult's, increase vulnerability to injury from blunt trauma[11]:

1. The kidney is larger in proportion to the abdomen.
2. Underdevelopment of abdominal wall musculature and a lack of extensive perirenal fat provide less protection for the kidney.
3. The lower ribs do not afford the same degree of renal protection.
4. The persistence of fetal lobulations may provide cleavage planes that are less resistant to blunt forces.
5. The presence of multiple renal arteries acts in concert with fetal lobulation to increase

---

503

the risk of segmental separation or laceration of the child's kidney resulting from blunt trauma.[22] These same anatomic findings may ultimately result in the preservation of function in these injured segments.

Mechanism of injury

Renal injury caused by blunt trauma generally falls into one of two categories. The kidney absorbs energy from direct compression via an external force or it experiences deceleration injury. Direct forces often result in a crush of the kidney against adjacent viscera, ribs, spinal column, or abdominal wall; deceleration injury primarily causes contusion and laceration. The most potentially devastating effect of significant deceleration force is injury of the renal artery; stretch of the renal vascular pedicle results in intimal disruption and subsequent thrombosis. Occasionally, laceration of the renal vein occurs, predominantly on the left side, and is associated with other major retroperitoneal vascular injury.[9]

Children with congenital renal abnormality are more vulnerable to injury from blunt trauma than other children. The hydronephrotic, ectopic, or diseased kidney (e.g., if tumor is present) is prone to injury resulting from even trivial trauma. Hematuria following minor trauma is often the presenting symptom of hydronephrosis in school-aged boys.[9] The incidence of renal injury in children who have a preexisting anomaly or disease is between 5% and 21%.[9,11]

Penetrating trauma is a rare cause of renal injury in children; only 7% of kidney injuries are due to a penetrating mechanism.[19] Stab and firearm wounds certainly cause renal injury, although today iatrogenic sources predominate as the cause of penetrating renal injury. Percutaneous invasive procedures, including amniocentesis, are responsible for penetrating renal injury in the fetus, infant, and child.

Indirect renal injury often occurs as a result of sequelae of major trauma. Electrical, crush, and ischemia-reperfusion injuries, which cause tissue necrosis and myoglobin release, can initiate tubular injury of the renal parenchyma. Thrombosis of the renal artery can also occur following high-voltage electrical injury.[20] The association of acute renal injury with low perfusion states is well established. This association is seen less frequently in children who have unique responses to major trauma. Children have a lower overall incidence of the syndrome of multiple organ system failure as a delayed response to major injury.

Initial evaluation and diagnosis

The mechanism of renal injury is evident during the initial evaluation of an injured child. In the case of penetrating trauma, the proximity of a wound to genitourinary structures prompts thorough investigation. The child who has sustained blunt trauma may be asymptomatic or complain of abdominal or flank pain. The spectrum of signs ranges from none to shock with a large flank hematoma. Hematuria, the laboratory hallmark of renal injury, occurs in up to 90% of cases.[10] Unfortunately, there is no correlation between the magnitude of injury and the degree of hematuria; devastating injury such as renal artery occlusion or collecting system destruction may occur in the absence of hematuria.[20] Frequently, hematuria in the hypovolemic child will manifest only after volume replacement.

Initial assessment and resuscitation, which take highest priority in the treatment of any injured child, influence the choice of diagnostic modality for evaluation of the renal system. A low threshold is important in evaluation of the upper urinary tract when the history is suspicious or a penetrating injury of the chest or abdomen is in proximity to the kidney.

A plain abdominal or KUB film can provide clues which suggest renal trauma. Obliteration of the renal or psoas shadow suggests the presence of hematoma or of urinoma. Lumbar scoliosis and fracture of the body or of the transverse processes of the spine indicate significant injury transmission to the retroperitoneal region of the kidney. Unfortunately, up to 85% of plain abdominal radiographs are normal in spite of proven kidney injury.[20] The excretory urogram (IVP) is the standard for diagnosis of renal injury. The selective application of the IVP is useful for evaluation of urinary tract trauma. In cases of penetrating trauma, the emergency IVP provides valuable information about the location, function, and number of kidneys. The standard dosage is 1 ml of iodinated contrast per pound of body weight administered after establishment of a functional intravenous line. Hypotension with low perfusion or vigorous intravenous fluid resuscitation, however, causes poor upper urinary tract visualization and makes the IVP a limited imaging technique.[10]

Ultrasonography is portable and prevents ionizing radiation, but its application in the evaluation of injured children is limited. A renal ultrasound examination can locate a kidney if it is not visualized with an IVP. It is also useful as a serial examination technique to follow the course of perinephric hematoma or of a urinoma. Doppler-enhanced ultrasound may provide information on renal perfusion and verify the integrity of the vascular pedicle of the kidney. Ultrasonography gives no information on function, however, and does not visualize intrarenal pathology as well as other techniques do.[20] Trauma centers in Europe have championed the application of ultrasound in

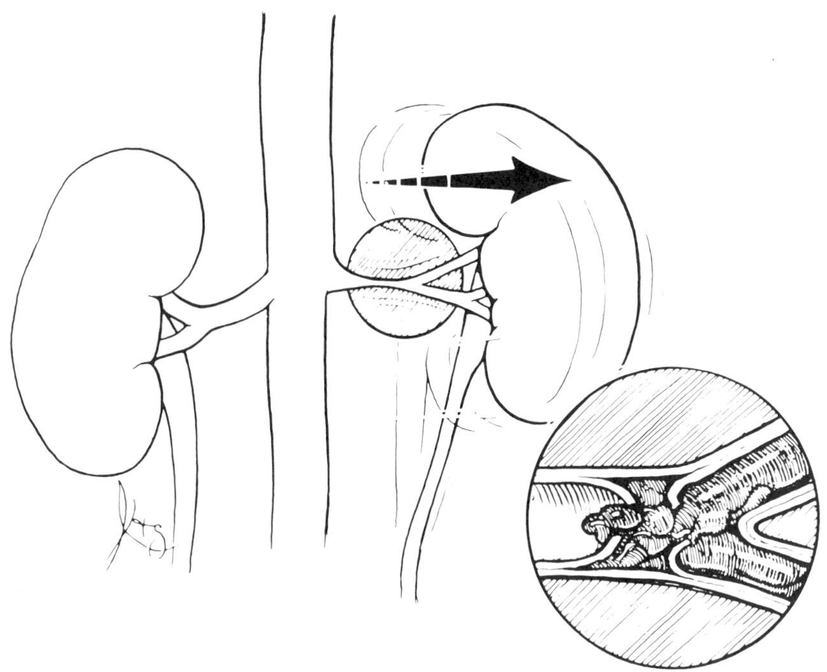

Figure 47–1 Mechanism of deceleration renal pedicle injury. Forces transmitted to the kidney result in stretch of the vascular pedicle. The intima disrupts, and subintimal dissection with thrombosis occurs. This commonly occurs in the middle third of the artery. (From Guerriero WG: *Management of acute and chronic urologic injury,* Englewood Cliffs, NJ, 1984, Prentice-Hall.)

the evaluation of the abdomen of the trauma patient.

Computed tomography (CT) is the standard imaging study for acute renal trauma in children. Its main advantages over other imaging techniques are as follows[9,10,16,20]:

1. More accurate demonstration of renal injury.
2. Visualization of nonvascularized areas of renal tissue.
3. Greater accuracy in definition of criteria for surgical intervention.
4. Simultaneous visualization of associated intraabdominal injuries.

The widespread availability of the CT scanning device enhances the preference of this imaging modality for evaluation of renal trauma in children.

The CT scan makes arteriography less important during the acute evaluation of renal trauma. Arteriography is time-consuming and more technically difficult in small children as compared with adults. In certain instances, such as in cases of horseshoe kidney, arteriographic information may be essential in planning surgical treatment.[10] The findings in arteriography can confirm acute arterial obstruction, such as traumatic occlusion of the renal artery which characteristically occurs in the middle third of the vessel and is more common on the left side.[18,20] It is frequently impossible to differentiate spasm, partial or complete laceration, and external compression on standard arteriographic images (Fig. 47-1).

A radionuclide renal scan provides useful information related to function, perfusion, and urinary extravasation. It is applicable for following renal perfusion and injuries resulting in extravasation of urine. The technique is also useful in very young children who have an allergy to contrast material.[9,10,16]

The future holds promise for additional imaging techniques to aid the surgeon in evaluation of the child with acute renal trauma. It is conceivable that refinements in magnetic resonance imaging (MRI) angiography will soon replace conventional contrast arteriography in the evaluation of renal trauma and its sequelae.

Classification

There is no standard classification of renal injury. Nevertheless, it is useful to categorize renal injuries based on their clinical severity (Fig. 47-2)[16,20]:

1. Minor—simple contusion and laceration within an intact capsule, in a child with stable clinical signs
2. Major—more extensive laceration with or without extravasation, in a child with stable clinical signs

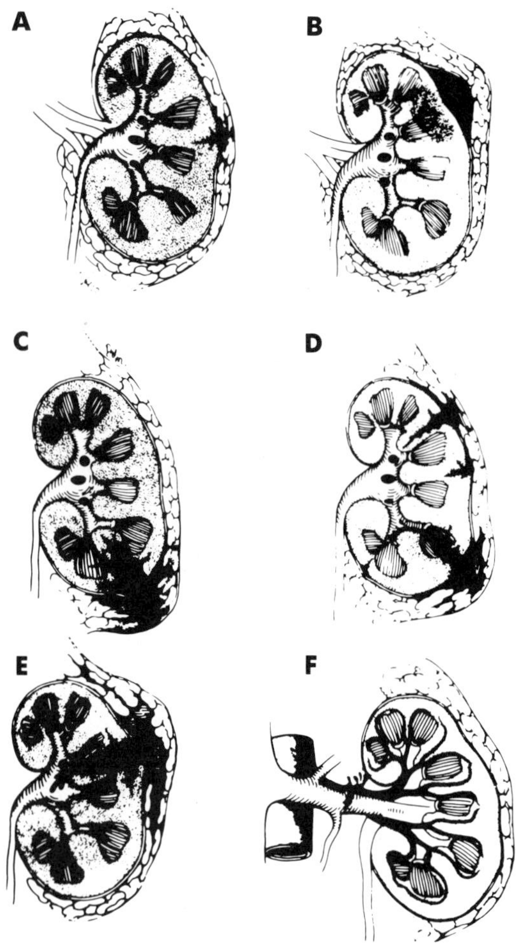

Figure 47–2 Classification of renal injuries. **A, B,** These represent minor injuries such as superficial laceration, hematoma, and contusion. **C, D, E,** Major parenchymal injury extending into the deep medulla with or without extravasation. **F,** Vascular pedicle injury which, along with "shattered kidney," represents critical renal injury. (From Nicolaisen GS, McAninch JW: Evaluation and management of traumatic renal injuries; *AUA Update Series*, lesson 37, vol 4, 1985.)

3. Critical—major vascular injury, shattered kidney, uncontrollable hemorrhage, in a child with unstable clinical signs

Management

There are often other injuries associated with renal trauma that are life threatening. In the absence of exsanguinating renal hemorrhage, the associated injuries frequently take precedence for resuscitation by the pediatric trauma team. For the most part, evaluation of renal injury proceeds simultaneously with evaluation of abdominal injury after a child is stable. The severity of renal injury, status

of the other kidney, and overall condition of the child are important factors that affect treatment options.

There is less controversy concerning management of penetrating trauma than there is about management of blunt renal trauma. Most penetrating renal injuries require surgical exploration during laparotomy for associated intraabdominal injury. A minor renal stab wound without associated intraabdominal injury may be observed in a child with stable vital signs and with radiographic evidence of parenchymal function. In contrast, all gunshot wounds generally require exploration.[16] It is crucial to have vascular control of the pedicle prior to renal exploration, and improved renal salvage rates are possible if excellent vascular control is secured prior to exploration and repair.[14]

The management of blunt kidney injury in children is dependent on the stability of the child and the extent of the injury. Up to 85% of such injuries are minor injuries that require only observation.[11,12,13,16] Treatment consists of bed rest until gross hematuria resolves. A decreased level of activity is recommended until microscopic hematuria clears. If results of initial radiographic studies were abnormal, a repeat CT, renal scan, or Doppler ultrasound exam is necessary at 6 to 8 weeks postinjury to document injury resolution. A 1-year postinjury renal scan will verify long-term renal function[10]; biannual documentation of blood pressure is essential to assess the presence of occult hypertension secondary to renal compromise.

There is controversy regarding operative versus nonoperative treatment of renal injury in children with major renal trauma. Currently, there is no evidence that early surgery reduces long-term complications such as hypertension or loss of renal function. Advocates of early surgery believe that this approach reduces blood loss, lowers the risk of abscess, sepsis, and ileus, and shortens a child's hospital stay.[10] There is a subset of children with severe injury who are categorized as critical. For these children, surgical exploration is lifesaving; transabdominal exploration and rapid control of the renal vascular pedicle are essential. The opening of Gerota's fascia prior to securing vascular control may result in hemorrhage that leads to nephrectomy (Fig. 47-3).[16,19] With adequate control of the vascular pedicle, Gerota's fascia is entered and debridement and repair may begin. Topical microfibrillar collagen is helpful in controlling small vessel bleeding following debridement, and fibrin glue can help in repair of major renal laceration.[4] The proximity of the pancreas, duodenum, and colon to the kidneys accounts for associated injury to these structures. Interposition of peritoneal or omental tissue between repair of these structures

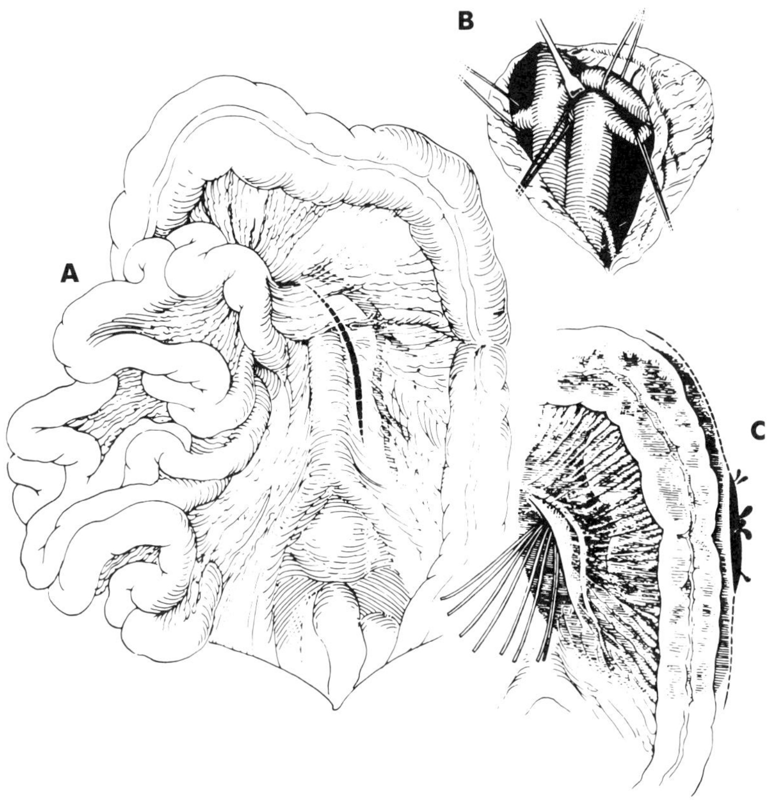

Figure 47–3 Operative exposure of renal vessels. **A,** The bowel is retracted superiorly, and the retroperitoneal tissue overlying the aorta and medial to the inferior mesenteric vein is opened. **B,** Exposure and control of the renal vessels is obtained. **C,** After vascular control is secured, the colon is mobilized and reflected from lateral peritoneal attachments in order to permit visualization of the kidney. (From McAninch JW, Carroll PR: Renal trauma: kidney preservation through improved vascular control—a refined approach, *J Trauma* 22:285, 1982.)

is prudent. Establish adequate drainage in the perinephric retroperitoneum. The use of antibiotics for injuries that involve extravasation is controversial.

If surgical intervention is necessary for urinary extravasation alone, delay of treatment for 3 or 4 days after the injury is appropriate. A large amount of extravasated urine may diminish with time and obviate the need for surgical exploration. Also, active hemorrhage will be less of a problem after stabilization of the injury, allowing drainage of the urinoma through a flank incision or by percutaneous catheter aspiration.[10]

Injury to the renal vascular pedicle is a formidable surgical challenge even under the best of circumstances. In most cases of blunt trauma involving the renal pedicle, nephrectomy is preferable to renal artery reconstruction and renorrhaphy when there is massive parenchymal disruption. Vascular repair, however, is more appropriate for vascular pedicle disruption due to penetrating injury. Restoration of arterial inflow is crucial to suc-

cessful repair. Ligation of the left renal vein is possible because of collateral drainage via gonadal and adrenal veins, but the right renal vein requires repair.[20]

Traumatic renal artery thrombosis is largely a disease of young men.[18] Diagnosis is difficult because signs and symptoms are few and association with other severe injuries is frequent. Unfortunately, the end result of arterial injury and thrombosis is most often irreversible infarction. Diagnosis is usually delayed, made long after there is salvageable renal function. Bilateral infarction has a dismal prognosis for native renal functional return, but there are scattered reports of return of function after bilateral renal artery thrombosis. A few of these patients appear to develop renal hypertension regardless of functional status. There is some benefit in retention of native kidneys with respect to intrinsic calcium metabolism and hematopoiesis; therefore, routine bilateral nephrectomy is not essential in every case.[18] Successful treatment of renal artery thrombosis requires a high level of suspicion regarding the presence of the injury and the earliest possible repair.

Long-term follow-up of renal injury is important because hypertension is occult and frequently associated with vascular trauma. The arterial injury responsible for posttraumatic hypertension can be at either the main or the segmental renal artery level. Occasionally, arteriovenous fistula occurs after blunt or penetrating trauma. However, the most common cause is iatrogenic injury following percutaneous renal biopsy.[9] The ability to perform selective renal vein sampling may guide any subsequent elective surgery for posttraumatic hypertension.[9] Children with major renal injury require follow-up renal radionuclide scans at 6 weeks and at 1 year, as a minimum, to evaluate function. Biannual blood pressure determination is also a helpful adjunct.[10] Posttraumatic renal hypertension usually develops several months after injury but can occur as early as 1 month and as late as 14 years after injury.[18]

URETERAL INJURY

Traumatic injury of the ureter in children is an uncommon upper genitourinary tract injury. Penetrating injury from low-velocity firearm or stab wounding usually causes simple laceration. Extensive tissue loss from high-velocity firearm wounding is common. High-velocity gunshot wounds can damage the ureter several centimeters from the path of the projectile and produce delayed necrosis of the ureteral wall.[6] In contrast, ureteropelvic junction avulsion of the ureter is the most common blunt injury to the ureter seen in children. Hypermobility of the child's spine permits excessive truncal flexion and extension, with transfer of energy to the ureteropelvic transition zone, during trauma (Fig. 47-4).[17] Lower ureteral injury rarely occurs in children with blunt trauma, but is seen in association with pelvic fracture.[16] Because of its smaller caliber, a child's ureter is more prone to injury resulting from endoscopic manipulation, yet fewer iatrogenic ureteral injuries occur in children during open procedures. A paucity of retroperitoneal fat often makes the identification of the ureter much easier in children than in adults.[9,16,20] An unrecognized congenital ureteral anomaly, such as a megaureter or duplication, increases the overall risk for injury.[20]

Initial evaluation and diagnosis

Isolated ureteral injury is rare and often occurs as a part of a multisystem event. Consequently, diagnosis may be delayed until the appearance of complications such as extravasation, obstruction, or infection provide clues to ureteral injury. Un-

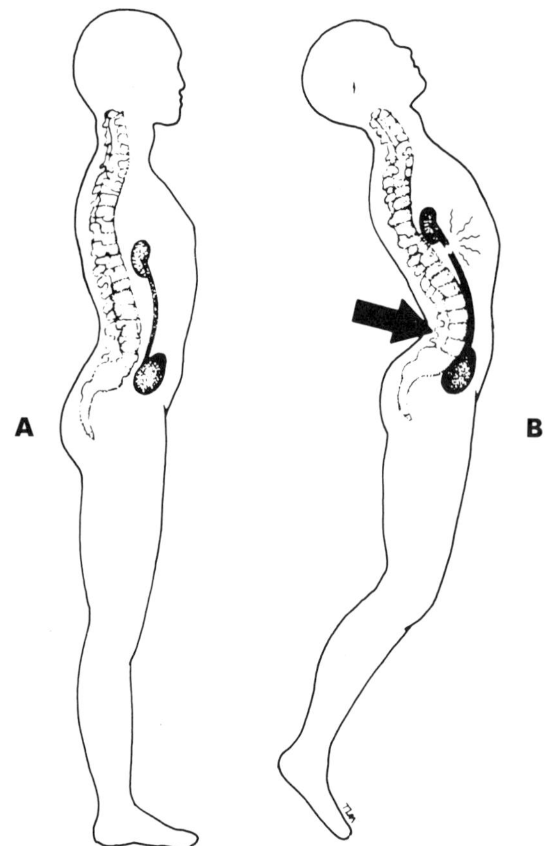

Figure 47–4 Ureteropelvic injury in children. **A,** Demonstration of the normal anatomic relations of the spine and urinary tract in the child. **B,** The sudden application of blunt force in the anterioposterior plane causes exaggerated spinal extension and results in ureteropelvic junction disruption. (From Gillenwater JY, Grayhack JT, Howards SS et al, editors: *Adult and pediatric urology,* ed 2, St Louis, 1991, Mosby–Year Book, p 492.)

fortunately, hematuria is frequently absent.[16] Recognition depends on a high level of suspicion and careful exploration during laparotomy for abdominal trauma. Reliance on CT scan evaluation of the hemodynamically stable child with blunt abdominal trauma enhances simultaneous demonstration of the anatomy and function of an injured ureter.

Management

For blunt ureteropelvic avulsion injury, the ureteropyelostomy is the repair of choice. Midureteral injury requires careful debridement and spatulated end-to-end anastomosis over a stent (Fig. 47-5). Mobilization of the kidney helps reduce the tension at the anastomosis. Ideal management of distal ureteral injury with only a short-gap tissue loss is by ureteroneocystostomy. Reconstruction of a long ureteral segment injury requires special techniques,

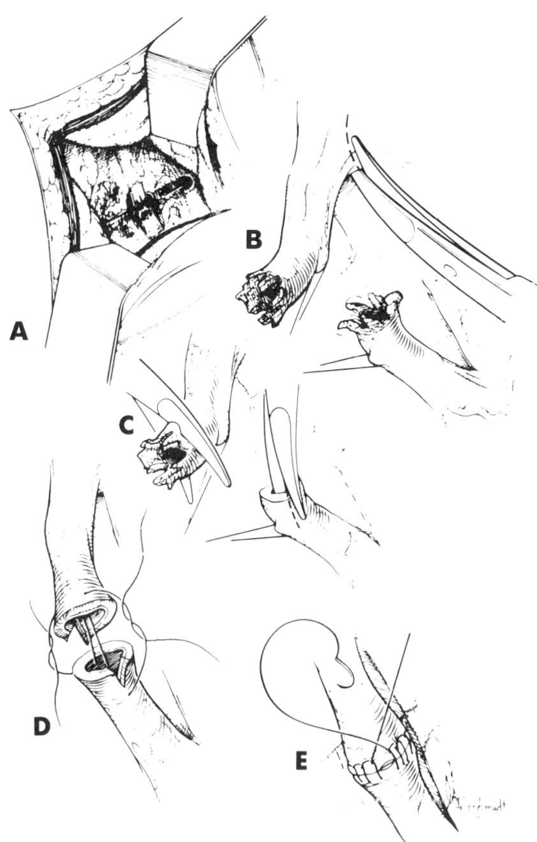

Figure 47–5 Technique of ureteral repair following traumatic disruption. The steps emphasize important principles: **A,** Adequate exposure; **B,** mobilization to allow tension-free anastomosis; **C,** debridement of devitalized tissue; **D,** spatulation of ureteral ends prior to anastomosis; **E,** watertight closure. (From Guerriero WG: Management of acute and chronic urologic injury, Englewood Cliffs, NJ, 1984, Prentice-Hall.)

including a bladder-psoas hitch, with or without a bladder (Boari-Ockerblad) flap for ureteroneocystostomy, transureteroureterostomy, or renal autotransplantation (Figs. 47-6 and 47-7). Transureteroureterostomy is best avoided because of the risk of cross contamination or damage to the contralateral system.[9] If ureteral injury is suspected during exploratory laparotomy, injection of 5 ml of indigo carmine followed by a loop diuretic (Lasix) aids localization of the defect through dye extravasation or staining of the injured urothelium. Adequate external drainage following repair is customary. In most cases, use of a stent for ureteral repair is advisable.

The short-term complications of ureteral injury are persistent extravasation, infection, and fistula formation. Treatment of a pelvic or retroperitoneal urinoma is possible by retrograde decompression, percutaneous aspiration, or operative drainage. Long-term complications such as stricture, urinary tract infection, hydronephrosis, and calculus formation require further treatment; consequently, long-term follow-up through radiographic imaging is important.[20]

BLADDER INJURY

The characteristics of bladder injury in children are closely linked to the anatomic and developmental differences that distinguish the injured child from the adult. The child's bladder is predominantly an intraabdominal organ. When it is full, it rises further out of the pelvis, increasing its vulnerability. Blunt trauma is the mechanism in 80% of all bladder injuries. Seventy percent of all children with bladder injury also have a pelvic fracture.[20] Estimates of the incidence of bladder injury among all pelvic fractures range from 5% to 20%.[16,20] A recent review of 2248 injured children, admitted consecutively to CNMC with blunt trauma over a 48-month period, identified a subset of 54 with pelvic fracture. Only two of those children (4%) had bladder injuries, both of which were intraperitoneal ruptures.[3]

Bladder rupture resulting from blunt trauma is the most common major bladder injury. This may occur as an extraperitoneal or intraperitoneal event (Fig. 47-8). The mechanism of injury and the urine volume of the bladder at time of impact influence the type of injury. Over 80% of bladder ruptures are of the extraperitoneal type seen with pelvic fracture. Multiple fracture sites increase risk for rupture of the bladder and for injury to other intraabdominal organs.[3] The mechanism of injury often involves laceration of the bladder by bone fragments, usually near the bladder neck.[16] The full bladder exposes the expanded and vulnerable dome. The dome is located above the pelvis, which permits intraperitoneal rupture following abdominopelvic impact and increase of the intraabdominal pressure (Fig. 47-9).[20] Intraperitoneal bladder rupture also occurs infrequently as part of the complex of injuries seen in children who are restrained by lap belts during motor vehicle crashes.[16a]

Penetrating trauma to the bladder from stab or gunshot wounds creates a variety of injuries that require a customized management scheme. Unfortunately, iatrogenic injury of the bladder during hernia repair and umbilical artery catheterization in neonates is possible.[9,16]

Initial evaluation and diagnosis

The strong association of bladder injury with blunt abdominal trauma and concomitant pelvic fracture must heighten suspicion, especially during evaluation of the multiply injured child. Simple bladder

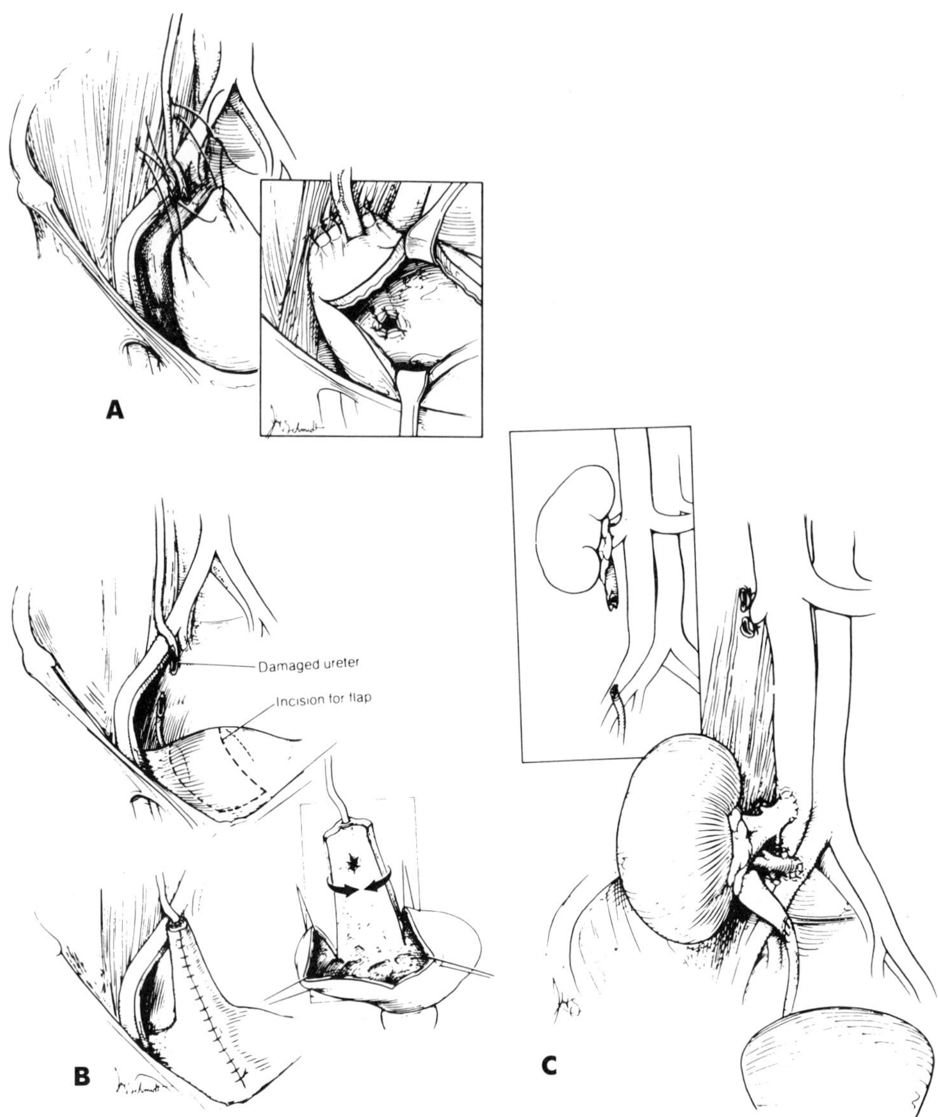

Figure 47–6 Techniques for repair of lower ureteral injury with a long gap tissue deficit. **A,** Vesico-psoas hitch with ureteroneocystostomy; **B,** vesical flap (Boari-Ockerblad flap); **C,** for extensive ureteral loss not amenable to above techniques, renal autotransplantation is required. (From Guer-riero WG: *Management of acute and chronic urologic injury,* Englewood Cliffs, NJ, 1984, Prentice-Hall.)

contusion can manifest impressive hematuria, in-travesicle clot, and retention of urine, whereas a more severe bladder injury, including rupture, may be asymptomatic.[20] Extraperitoneal rupture may initially appear much like an uncomplicated pelvic fracture.[8] The disparity between the severity of an injury and its symptoms requires a disciplined ap-proach to prevent diagnostic errors in management of bladder trauma.

The child with bladder injury complains of su-prapubic tenderness, pelvic pain, dysuria, or in-ability to void. Gross hematuria is the hallmark laboratory finding that compels evaluation by cys-tography. A complete cystographic examination with anteroposterior and oblique views is important to obtain following a CT scan that demonstrates extravasation. In most cases, and especially in the presence of pelvic fracture in the male, retrograde

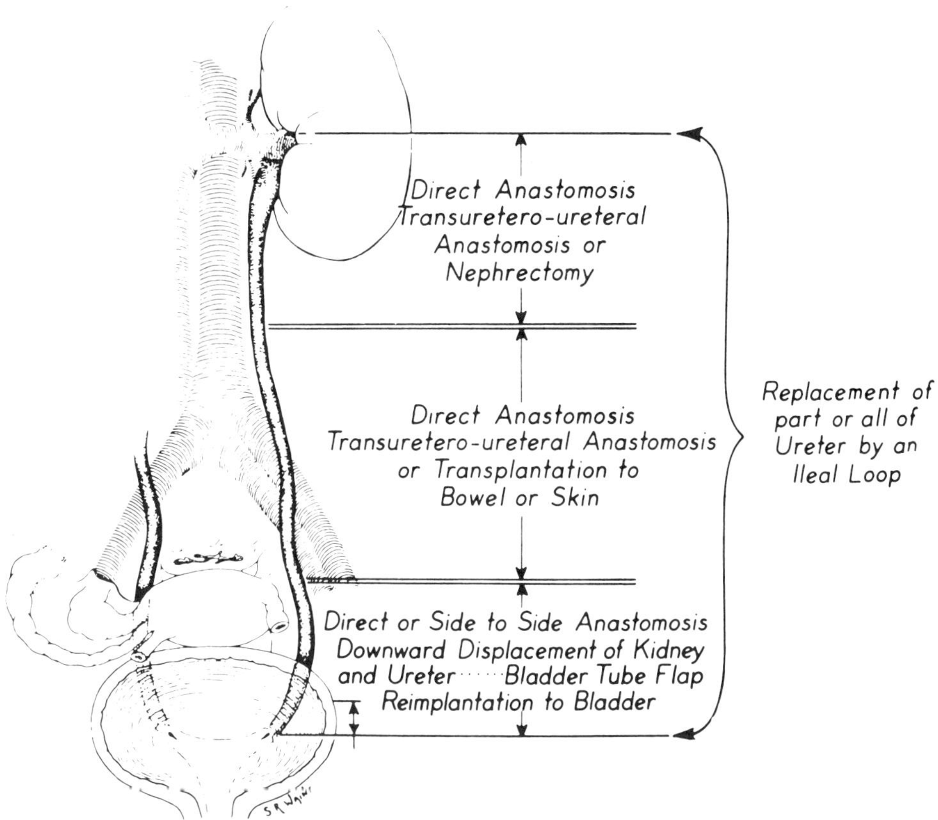

Figure 47–7 Summary of treatment options for ureteral injuries. (From Walsh PC, Gittes RT, Perlmutter AD et al, editors: *Campbell's urology,* ed 5, Philadelphia, 1986, WB Saunders, p 1212.)

urethrogram evaluation precedes the cystographic study. Gravity infusion of the bladder with contrast dye until the child experiences discomfort, or use of the predicted bladder capacity appropriate for age, is the best method for diagnosis[20]:

Bladder capacity in ounces = Age in years + 2

Following drainage of the contrast material, a second set of views greatly reduces the risk of overlooking a small amount of extravasation that was obscured by the contrast-filled bladder. IVP examination or evaluation of the upper genitourinary tract by CT scan is important. Unfortunately, only 10% to 15% of children with a bladder injury have findings confirmed by a standard IVP.[5] The combination of upper and lower tract and bladder studies must be obtained to ensure timely diagnosis of these injuries.

Management

Treatment of extraperitoneal bladder rupture is best accomplished through a selective approach. The extent of the injury and the sex of the child are important considerations when formulating a treatment plan. With the exception of large or complicated extraperitoneal ruptures, bladder catheter drainage permits complete healing in most cases. This approach is advantageous because it does not convert a closed pelvic fracture to an open one. If the suspected injury is due to penetrating bone fragments, surgical exploration to remove or reduce the bone fragment is preferable to prevent persistent leakage and sepsis.[20] Surgical repair and suprapubic drainage is the best treatment for a small male child or infant. This prevents the morbidity of prolonged transurethral catheterization (Fig. 47-10).

Intraperitoneal rupture usually requires surgical repair, although there are reports of successful nonoperative treatment.[16,20] Continued intraperitoneal spillage of urine leads to metabolic derangements such as azotemia and acid-base disorders which potentially lead to death of the child.

The principles of bladder repair are quite standard: adequate debridement of devitalized tissue and water-tight closure with absorbable suture. Ad-

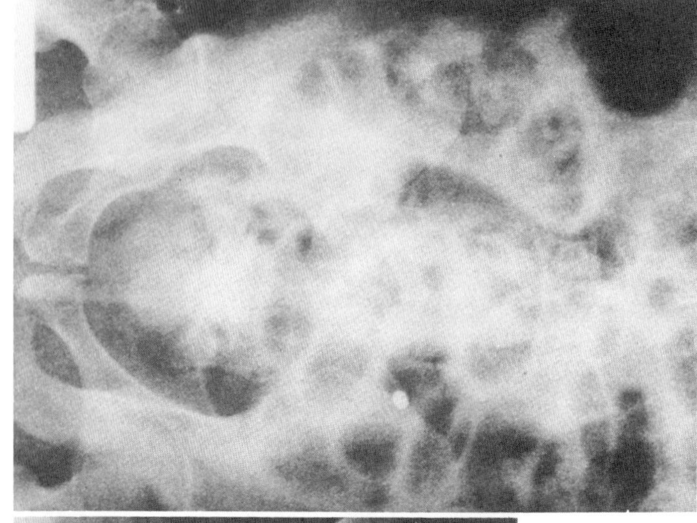

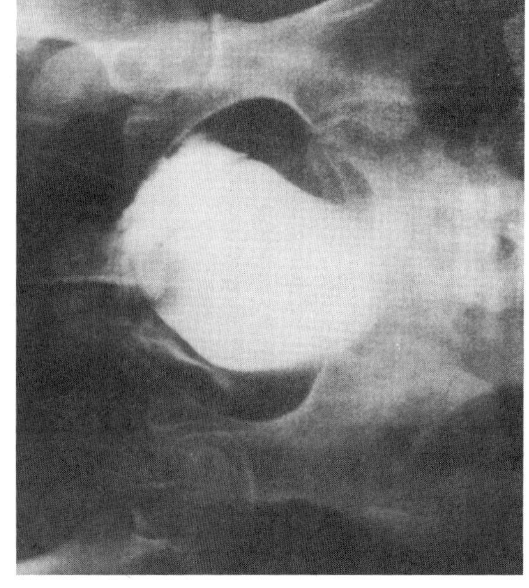

Figure 47–8 A, Intraperitoneal bladder rupture due to blunt abdominal trauma; **B,** extraperitoneal bladder rupture associated with pelvic fracture. (From Gillenwater JY, Grayhack JT, Howard SS et al, editors: *Adult and pediatric urology,* ed 2, St Louis, 1991, Mosby–Year Book, p 492.)

equate drainage of the repair site and proper bladder decompression are essential. In certain instances, it is useful to open the bladder in an uninjured area and suture the laceration from within. This technique permits visualization of trigone structures and avoids the distorted tissue planes associated with the primary injury.[10] To recognize concomitant rectal or vaginal injury that can be missed during abdominal exploration, perform endoscopic examination with the child under anesthesia.[20] Prior to removal of drainage catheters, contrast cystography, performed approximately 10 days after injury repair or institution of drainage, confirms the adequacy of repair and healing.

Mortality in bladder injury is very low. Children with bladder injury who die almost always do so because of associated serious injury. Fortunately, long-term morbidity is also uncommon. Posttraumatic vesicovaginal or vesicorectal fistulae usually occur in association with penetrating trauma. Urinary tract infection in combination with a foreign body or blood clot may result in the development of the occasional posttraumatic bladder stone.[20] Periodic follow-up and symptom-oriented evaluation will help in detecting these problems.

URETHRAL INJURY

Urethral injury in children occurs in two distinct patterns, each associated with a classic mechanism of injury. Anterior urethral injury occurs distal to

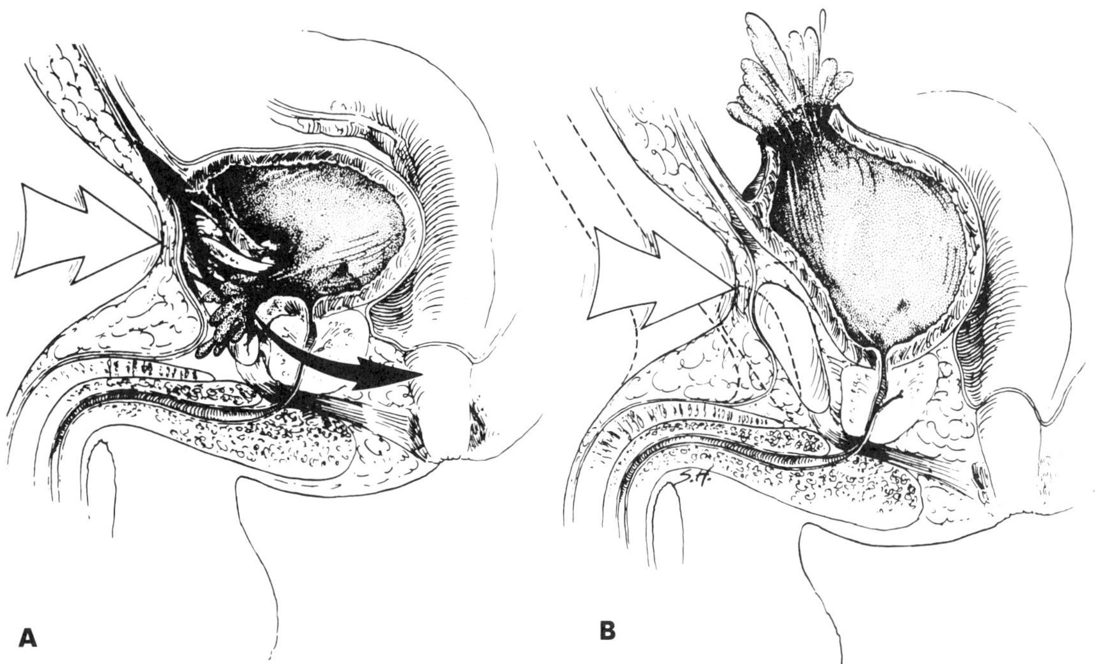

Figure 47–9 Mechanism of bladder injury from blunt trauma. **A,** Pelvic fracture of pubic rami results in laceration by bone fragments. **B,** Blunt force applied to lower abdomen of child with full bladder results in rupture of the bladder at its most vulnerable point, the dome. (From Walsh PC, Gittes RT, Perlmutter AD et al, editors: *Campbell's urology,* ed 5, Philadelphia, 1986, WB Saunders, p 1212.)

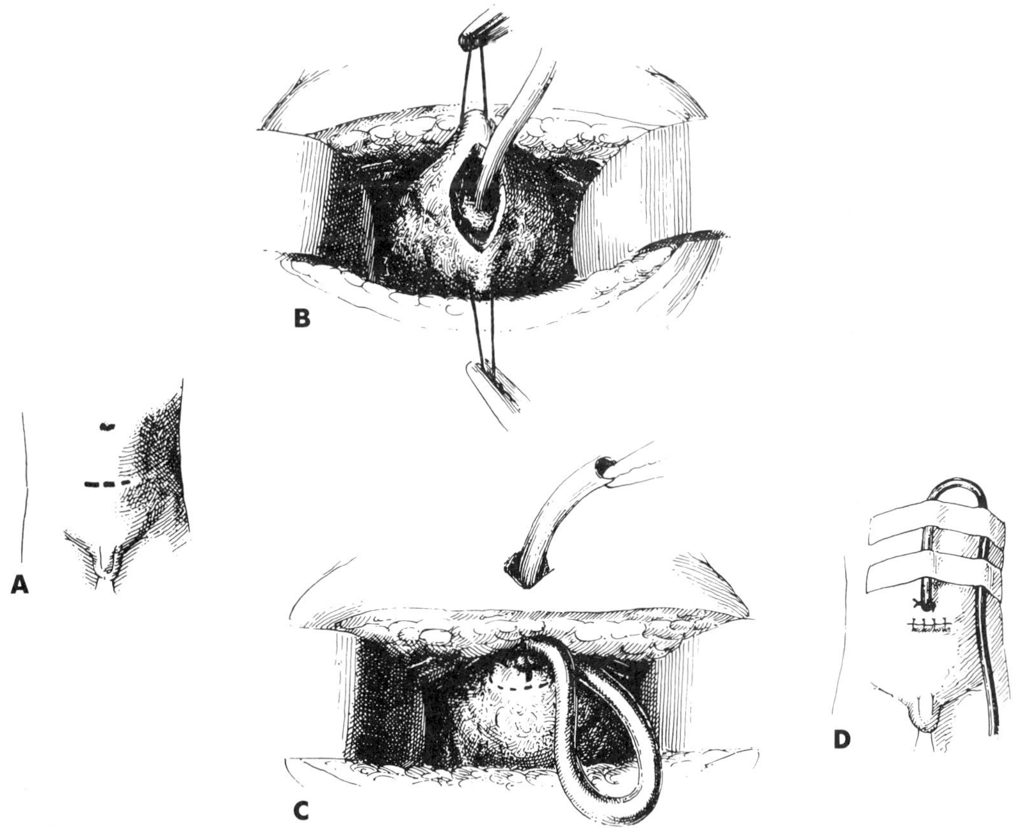

Figure 47–10 Technique of suprapubic cystostomy in the child. (From Kelalis PP, King LR, Belman AB, editors: *Clinical pediatric urology,* ed 2, Philadelphia, 1985, WB Saunders, p 588.)

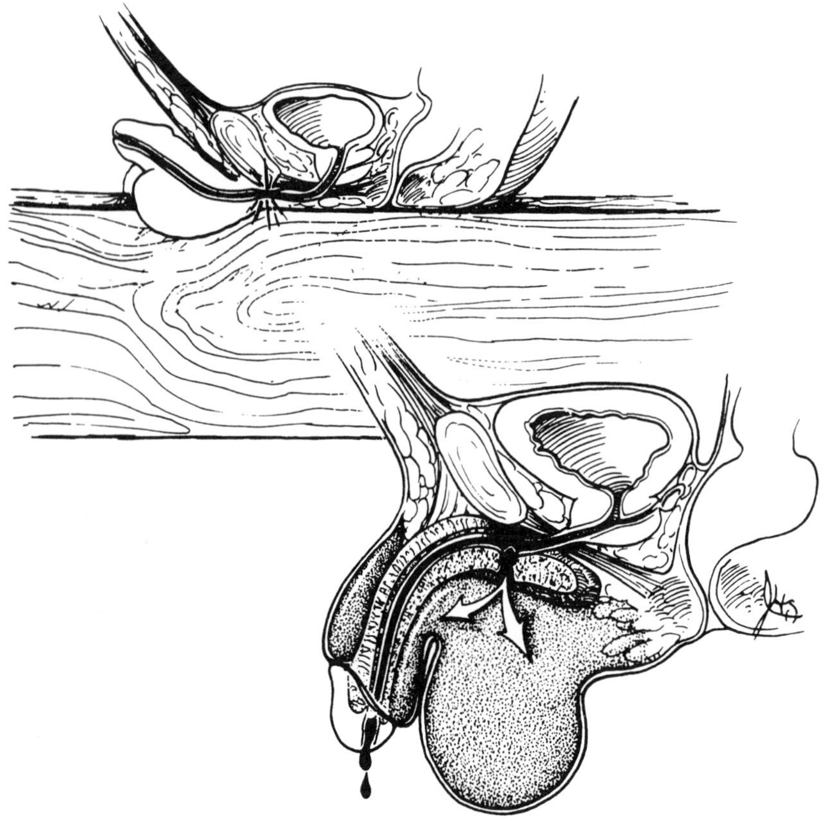

Figure 47-11 Mechanism of anterior urethral straddle injury. The urethra is crushed against the inferior aspect of the pubis. (Guerriero WG: *Management of acute and chronic urologic injury,* Englewood Cliffs, NJ, 1984, Prentice-Hall.)

the urogenital diaphragm and involves either the pendulous or bulbous urethral division. Posterior urethral injury is more common and involves the divisions of the urethra which are proximal to the urogenital diaphragm: the membranous and prostatic portions.[16,20]

Mechanism of injury

The etiology of most anterior urethral injuries involves blunt trauma in the form of a straddle injury. This is often an isolated injury, occurring when a straddle blow to the perineum causes a direct crush of the anterior urethra against the undersurface of the symphysis pubis (Fig. 47-11).[20] The spectrum of injury extends from small, simple contusion to complete disruption. A shearing force or pressure necrosis associated with an excessively large instrument, foreign body, or catheter is occasionally responsible for anterior urethral injury.

Approximately 90% of posterior urethral injuries in children are associated with fracture of the pelvis, yet only 10% of all pelvic fractures in children are associated with urethral injury.[20] However, the risk of urethral injury increases to 40% in cases of multiple pelvic fracture sites and the "butterfly" fracture of the bilateral superior and inferior pubic rami.[9] In general, urethral injury in children is actually quite rare.[3] The impact of blunt trauma sufficient to cause pelvic fracture may impart shearing forces to the posterior urethra at a point where it is firmly fixed by the urogenital diaphragm and puboprostatic ligaments. These forces may induce injury ranging from contusion to complete avulsion.[16] In children, iatrogenic injury of the posterior urethra is less common than injury of the anterior portion; this type of injury is commonly associated with surgical ablation of posterior urethral valves in young boys.

Initial evaluation and diagnosis

A detailed and complete history of the traumatic incident is important. Common signs of urethral injury include blood at the meatus, perineal or penoscrotal hematoma, presence of pelvic fracture, and abnormal rectal examination results manifested by fullness, tenderness, or mobility of the prostate.

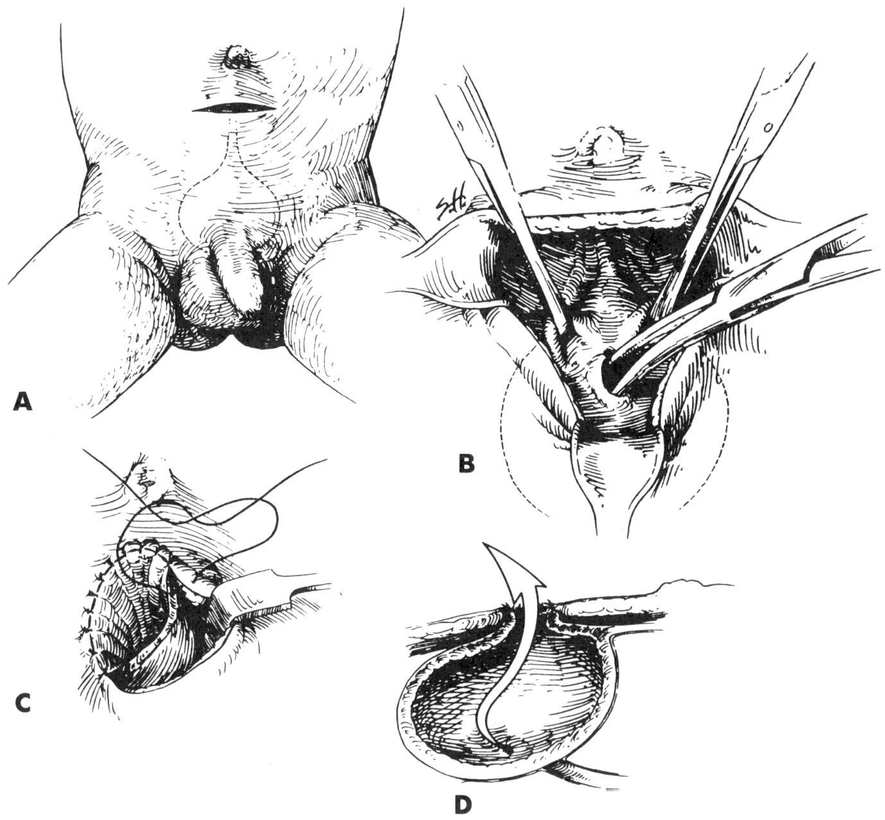

Figure 47–12 Technique of cutaneous vesicostomy. **A,** Transverse incision 2 cm below the umbilicus; **B,** bladder entry; **C,** vesicocutaneous stoma fashioned; **D,** final pathway of urine flow. (From Walsh PC, Gittes RT, Perlmutter AD et al, editors: *Campbell's urology,* ed 5, Philadelphia, 1986, WB Saunders, p 1225.)

It is difficult to feel evidence of prostatic displacement in a child.[20] The only symptom may be dysuria or an inability to void.

In the presence of a suspicious mechanism of injury and signs or symptoms of urethral injury, a retrograde urethrogram completed prior to any instrumentation of the urethra is essential. If an indwelling catheter is in place, perform the retrograde urethrogram examination by inserting a smaller tube alongside the urethral catheter. A sterile lubricant with a topical anesthetic, such as lidocaine, often makes this maneuver easier for the young child to tolerate; examination with the child under anesthesia may be necessary. Extravasation of contrast material confirms at least partial disruption of the urethra. Significant contusion can occur without extravasation and can result in delayed stricture formation.[16] A more deliberate injection is sometimes necessary to overcome external sphincter spasm and delineate posterior urethral injury. When the urogenital diaphragm tissues are intact, extravasation usually remains confined within the pelvis. Disruption of the urogenital diaphragm allows ex-

travasation of contrast downward into the perineum.[20]

Management

Treatment of incomplete and minor anterior urethral disruption is possible by either temporary suprapubic urinary diversion or the gentle transurethral passage of a small Silastic catheter.[16,20] More extensive damage of the anterior urethra is rare in boys, but if it does occur, the approach to treatment is individualized. Significant anterior urethral injury requires diversion and staged urethroplasty. In very small boys it is advantageous to perform temporary vesicostomy and delay urethroplasty until the child is older (Fig. 47-12).[9] The most common complication of this type of injury is stricture formation. The initial manifestation of voiding difficulty or infection in boys is often due to a short anterior urethral stricture. In the vast majority of cases the etiology is an old injury, long since forgotten, that caused an incomplete urethral injury.

Posterior urethral injury is associated with pelvic fracture and is more challenging to manage. Chil-

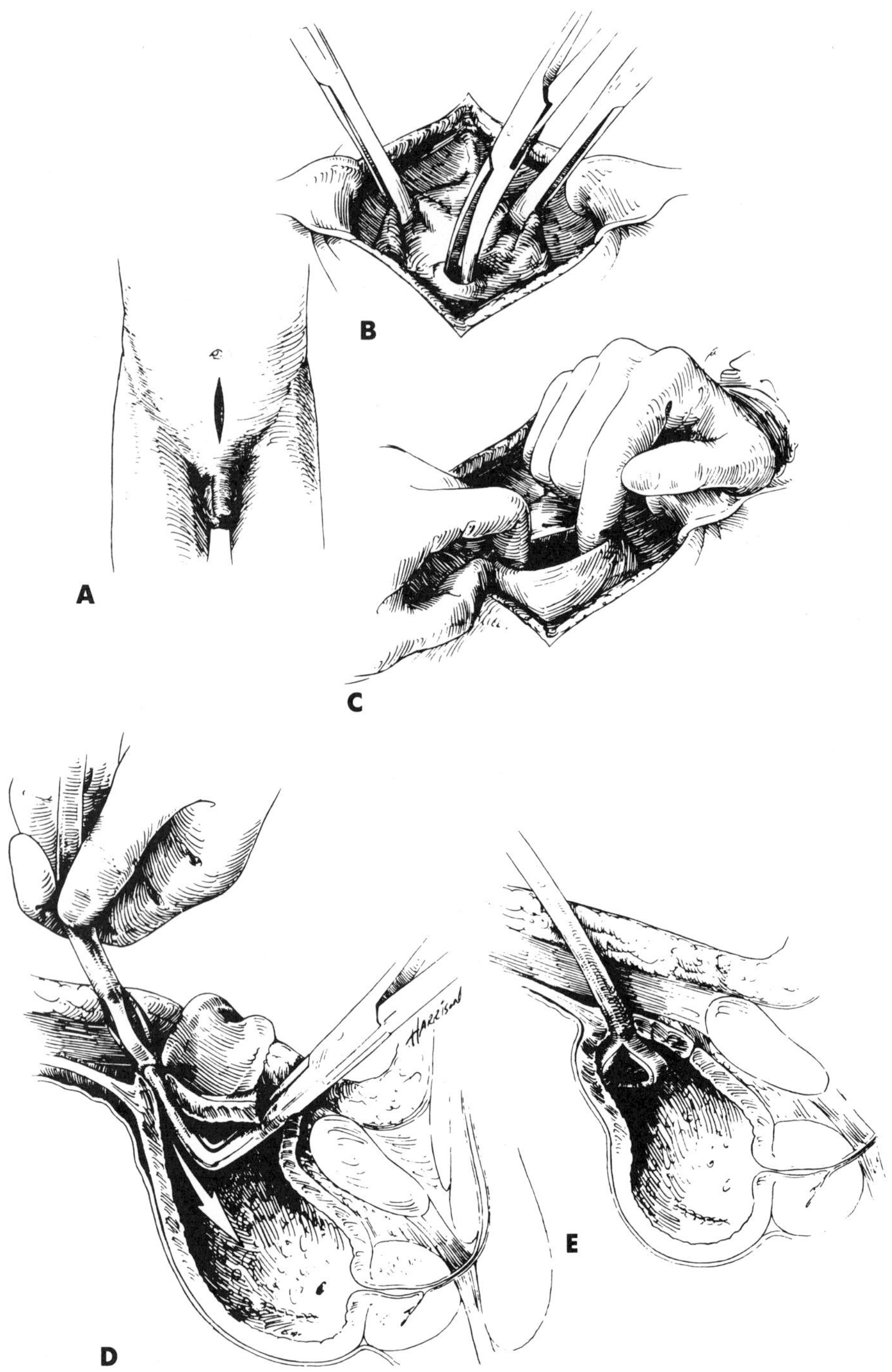

Figure 47-13 Technique of suprapubic cystostomy. **A,** Midline incision depicted here allows liberal extension cephalad if needed. If abdominal exploration is not required, a transverse incision is acceptable. **B,** The bladder is grasped between Allis forceps and a tonsil forceps is quickly inserted. Failure to use quick, sustained motion results in submucosal dissection. Electrocautery is helpful. **C,** Blunt enlargement of opening minimizes bleeding. **D,** Malecot catheter is inserted obliquely through the bladder and abdominal wall, with care to avoid intraperitoneal structures. **E,** Cystostomy tube in place. (From Walsh PC, Gittes RT, Perlmutter AD et al, editors: *Campbell's urology,* ed 5, Philadelphia, 1986, WB Saunders, p 1216.)

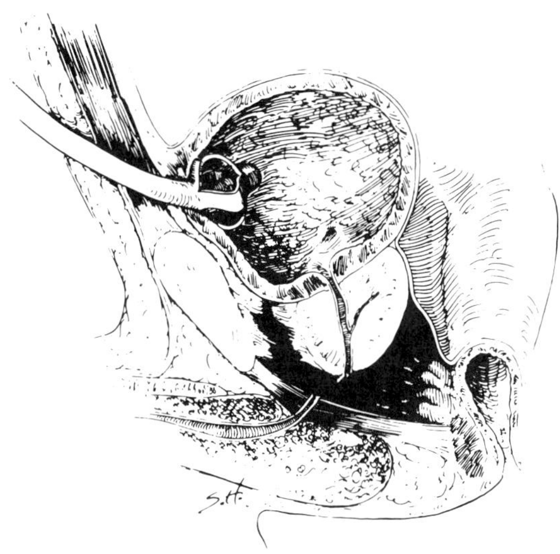

Figure 47–14 Initial placement of suprapubic cystostomy for treatment of urethral injury. This approach avoids pelvic dissection and perivesical drainage. (From Walsh PC, Gittes RT, Perlmutter AD et al, editors: *Campbell's urology*, ed 5, Philadelphia, 1986, WB Saunders, p 1224.)

dren with this injury will have more severe and multisystem trauma. There is little disagreement that a partial posterior urethral tear requires suprapubic diversion and delay of treatment of any resultant stricture. This approach is preferable for a complete urethral tear, although some clinicians favor early operative intervention with primary realignment and anastomosis. In general, suprapubic diversion and treatment delay is best, because complications such as stricture, incontinence, and impotence are infrequent.[15] If an unstable child requires immediate surgery for other injuries and urethral injury is suspected, proceed with suprapubic cystostomy at the time of surgery and delay urethrography until the child is stable (Figs. 47-13 and 47-14).[10]

Urethral injury is much less common in girls. Although the frequency of pelvic fracture and urethral injury is rare in all children, pelvic fracture remains the most common etiology of urethral disruption in both boys and girls. Examination while the child is under anesthesia is often necessary to evaluate the extent of such injuries. There is the distinct possibility of an associated vaginal injury.[9] Early surgical repair of these complete and complex vesicovaginal injuries is important for optimal functional results. Treatment of a partial tear is best accomplished by suprapubic or transurethral catheter drainage.[12,16,20] If the anus or rectum is also involved, primary repair may be performed, with concomitant proximal colostomy diversion based on the degree and complexity of the injury.

In the absence of associated pelvic fracture, the presence of complex urethral and vaginal wounds in a female child raises the suspicion of possible sexual abuse, especially in the absence of a straddle mechanism of injury.

TESTICULAR INJURY

As is true of most other types of genitourinary injury, the common element in trauma to the testis and scrotum is a blunt mechanism of injury. Penetrating injury of the scrotum and testis is less common in children than adults.[2] In general, penoscrotal injury in the child is rare, probably a consequence of the small size and the mobility of the prepubertal testis.[9] Blunt or penetrating injury causes rapid swelling, which distorts the normal anatomy and makes the determination of testicular rupture impossible. In this instance, ultrasonography is helpful in determining the integrity of the tunica albuginea.[20] If there is any doubt concerning rupture of the testis, proceed with surgical exploration, evacuation of the hematoma, and testis repair (Fig. 47-15).[9,16,20] Extensive loss of scrotal skin is uncommon in boys but may present the surgeon with a management dilemma. Testicular relocation in subcutaneous thigh pouches is possible but results in an unacceptably high rate of testicular atrophy or tissue loss. The scrotum has an impressive propensity to heal, and the testis survives for extended periods with moist saline dressings until delayed closure or grafting is possible.[2]

Torsion of the spermatic cord related to trauma occurs in as many as 5% to 12% of cases.[7] Testicular swelling and cremaster spasm may initiate the torsion.[16] If torsion of the cord is the suspected diagnosis, surgical exploration is required for definitive assessment. Seemingly trivial trauma to the testis that results in significant swelling and hematoma should alert the examiner to the possibility of an occult testis tumor, which will influence the choice of operative approach. All of the testicular problems of childhood are rare, and differentiation on clinical grounds alone is difficult. Additional information gained from nuclear scan and ultrasound examinations is helpful; nevertheless, if there is any doubt regarding the integrity of the testis or spermatic cord, the appropriate approach is surgical exploration (Table 47-1).

SUMMARY

Genitourinary injury is uncommon, occurring in less than 5% of all injured children, but the incidence is often underestimated because of the paucity of signs and symptoms in the injured child. Children with even severe genitourinary trauma can be strikingly asymptomatic. A thorough and dis-

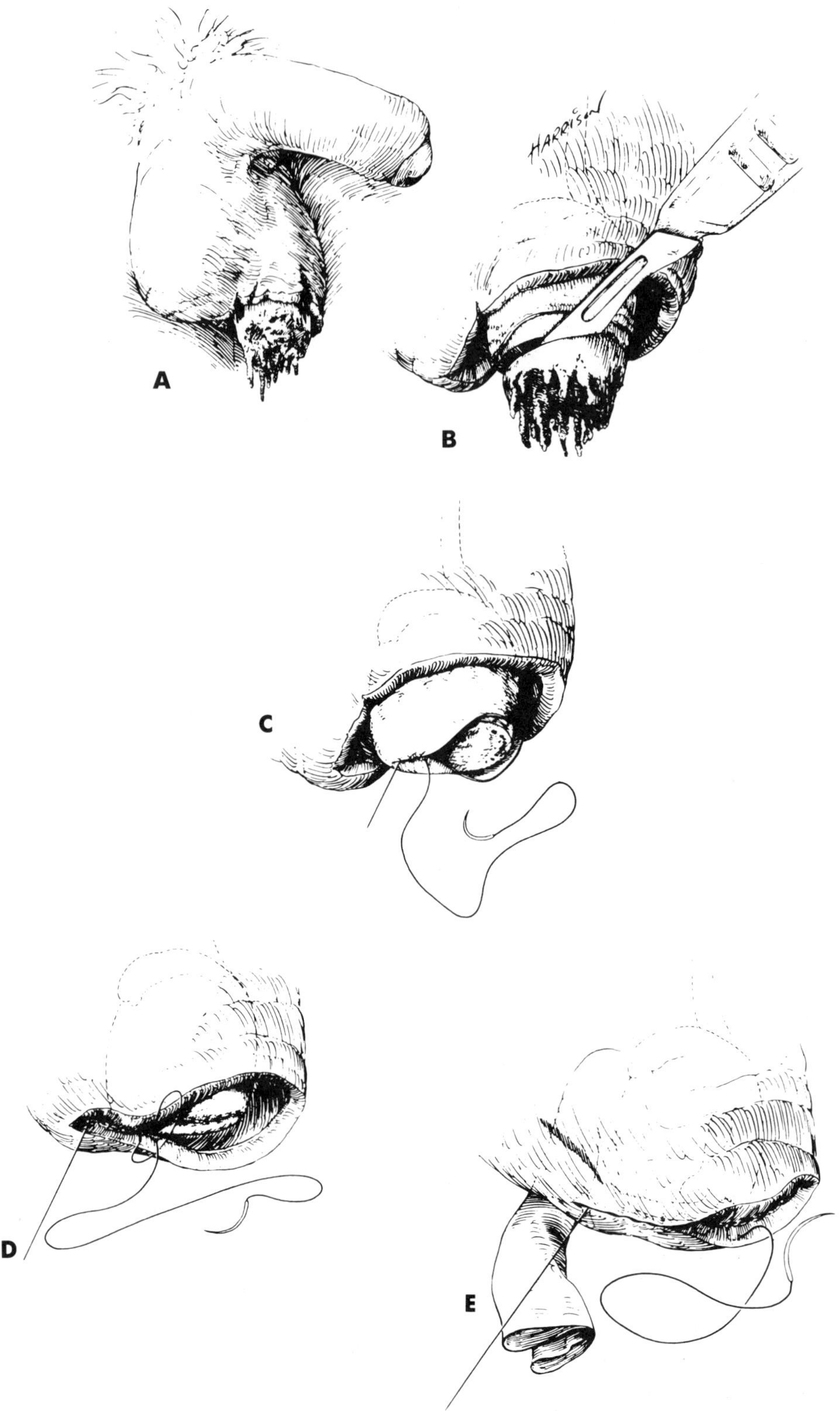

Figure 47–15 Closure of traumatic testicular and scrotal defect. **A,** Initial appearance; **B,** sharp debridement of devitalized tissue and seminiferous tubules; **C,** tunica albuginea closure. **D** and **E,** Dartos layer and skin closure for hemostasis and optional drainage. (From Walsh PC, Gittes RT, Perlmutter AD et al, editors: *Campbell's urology,* ed 5, Philadelphia, 1986, WB Saunders, p 1241.)

Table 47–1 Differential diagnosis of testicular trauma, torsion, tumor, and epididymitis

	Torsion	Trauma	Tumor	Epididymitis
Urine	Normal	Normal	Normal	Pyuria Bacteriuria
Palpation	1. Pain	1. Pain and swelling	1. Painless unless hemorrhage	1. Discrete epididymis
	2. Indefinable structures 3. Horizontal lie	2. Related to nature of injury	2. Diffuse or local testicular swelling	2. Soft testis (early)
Onset	1. Sudden 2. Previous episodes 3. During sleep or vehicle ride	Sudden	Gradual unless hemorrhagic	1. Gradual 2. Groin pain 3. Previous funiculitis
Scan (Stage et al, 1981)	Decreased activity	Depends on injury	Normal	Increased activity
Small parts sonography	↑ Size	Rupture seen	Complex pattern	Enlarged epididymis
Doppler (Thompson et al, 1975)	Flow	Depends on injury	Normal	Normal

From Walsh, et al, editors: *Campbell's urology*, ed 5, Philadelphia, 1986, WB Saunders, p 1242.

ciplined approach to the pediatric trauma patient is essential to avoid errors and delays in the diagnosis of these injuries. Trivial trauma often results in genitourinary injury, and minor injury frequently leads to identification of occult genitourinary anomaly or malignancy.

The management of genitourinary injury is primarily nonoperative and is aimed at prevention of complications and maintenance of function. Fortunately, the outcome in genitourinary injury is usually excellent. Careful immediate treatment and comprehensive long-term follow-up result in the return to normal activity for the majority of children.

REFERENCES

1. Belman AB, Kaplan GW: Trauma. In Belman AB, Kaplan GW, editors: *Genitourinary problems in pediatrics*, Philadelphia, 1981, WB Saunders.
2. Bertini JE, Corriere JN: The etiology and management of genital injuries, *J Trauma* 28:1278-1281, 1988.
3. Bond SJ, Gotschall CS, Eichelberger MR: Predictors of abdominal injury in children with pelvic fractures, *J Trauma* 31:1169-1173, 1991.
4. Brands W, Haselberger J, Mennicken C et al: Treatment of ruptured kidney by gluing with highly concentrated human fibrinogen, *J Ped Surg* 18:611-613, 1983.
5. Brosman S, Faye R: Diagnosis and management of bladder trauma, *J Urol* 113:687, 1973.
6. Cass AS: Ureteral contusion with gunshot wounds, *J Trauma* 24:59-60, 1984.
7. Elsaharty S, Pranikoff K, Magess IV et al: Traumatic torsion of the testis, *J Urol* 132:1155-1156, 1984.
8. Flarety JJ, Kelley R, Burnett B et al: Relationship of pelvic bone fracture patterns to injuries of urethra and bladder, *J Urol* 99:297, 1968.
9. Gonzales ET Jr, Guerriero WG: Genitourinary trauma in children. In Kelalis PP, King LR, Belman AB, editors: *Clinical Pediatric Urology*, Philadelphia, 1985, WB Saunders.
10. Kass EJ: Genitourinary injury. In Eichelberger MR, Pratsch GL, editors: *Pediatric trauma care*, Rockville, Md, 1988, Aspen Publications.
11. Kuzmarov IW, Morehouse DD, Gibson S: Blunt renal trauma in a pediatric population: a retrospective study, *J Urol* 126:648, 1981.
12. Livne PM, Gonzales ET: Genitourinary trauma in children, *Urol Clin N Am* 12:53-65, 1985.
13. Mandour WA, Lai MK, Lincke CA et al: Blunt renal trauma in pediatric patients, *J Ped Surg* 16:669-676, 1981.
14. McAninch JW, Carroll PR: Renal trauma: kidney preservation through improved vascular control—a refined approach, *J Trauma* 22:285-290, 1982.
15. Morehouse DD, MacKinnon KJ: Posterior urethral injury: etiology diagnosis, initial management, *Urol Clin N Am* 41:69, 1977.
16. Murphy JP: Genitourinary trauma. In Ashcraft KW, editor: *Pediatric urology*, Philadelphia, 1990, WB Saunders.
16a. Newman KD, Bowman LM, Eichelberger MR, et al: The lap belt complex: intestinal and lumbar spine injury in children. *J Trauma* 30:1133-1140, 1990.
17. Palmer JM, Drago JR: Ureteral avulsion from nonpenetrating trauma, *J Urol* 125:108-111, 1981.
18. Peterson NE: Review article: traumatic bilateral renal infarction, *J Trauma* 29(2):158-167, 1989.
19. Scott R Jr, Carlton CE, Goldman M: Penetrating injuries

of the kidney: an analysis of 181 patients, *J Urol* 115:229, 1976.

20. Snyder HMcC III, Caldamone AA: Genitourinary injuries. In Welch KJ, Randolph JG, Ravitch MM et al, editors: *Pediatric Surgery,* ed 4, Chicago, 1986, Mosby–Year Book.

21. Taylor GA, Eichelberger MR, Potter BM: Hematuria: a marker of abdominal injury in children after blunt trauma, *Ann Surg* 208:688-693, 1988.

22. Yamazaki J, Nakao N, Inmoto K et al: Traumatic laceration of the kidney in children with supernumerary renal arteries, *Urol Radiol* 2:245, 1981.

PART TWELVE

Pelvic and Retroperitoneal Trauma

48 Pelvic Fracture and Retroperitoneal Hematoma

Sheldon J. Bond

Pelvic fracture is an uncommon injury in injured children. When treating children who have sustained such injury, a team approach is absolutely essential. Effective communication among specialties, such as urology and orthopedic surgery, can provide these children the best possible care and long-term outcome free from disability.

The essential function of the pelvis is transmission of weight from the trunk to the lower supportive skeleton. The stability of the pelvis depends on the integrity of the entire posterior weight-bearing sacroiliac complex from the major sacroiliac, sacrotuberous, and sacrospinous ligaments. In addition to its function as a weight-bearing element, the pelvis has a major role as a point of origin and insertion for a wide variety of muscles. These muscles set the position of the pelvis relative to the trunk, and of the femurs relative to the pelvis. In general, in anterior pelvic fractures, the muscle forces and the contents of the pelvis restore normal anatomy, whereas in posterior pelvis injuries they further distort the normal anatomy.[12] The pelvis is important also because vessels and nerves essential to the function of the lower extremities and intrapelvic organs are closely approximated to the pelvis; thus bony injuries may produce hemorrhage or neurologic deficits. These complications are much more common in posterior pelvic fractures than in anterior pelvic fractures.[12]

The pelvis is a ring structure. If the ring is broken in one area and the fragments displaced, there is also a fracture or dislocation in another portion of the ring. There are three general subsets of forces that result in pelvic fracture. These are the anterior, lateral, and shearing mechanisms.[12,16] The anterior mechanism denotes a force to the pubic symphysis in which one, two, or all four of the pubic rami are broken. This is also referred to as a straddle or external rotational injury, because the extremity is externally rotated relative to the pelvis. Although not life-threatening in terms of hemorrhage or disabling owing to neurologic sequelae, this fracture can result in significant disability resulting from associated injury to the genitourinary system. The urethra, which exits inferior to the pubic symphysis, is especially at risk.

Lateral compression, also known as internal rotation, may be caused by a direct blow on the outer aspect of the iliac crest or indirect force through the femoral head. This produces compression fractures of the posterior elements and of the rami anteriorly. The injury can, through compression of a full bladder, result in intraperitoneal bladder rupture. The possibility of life-threatening hemorrhage resulting from fracture of this type is not as great as that caused by a shearing mechanism. Lateral compressions can result, however, in significant disability because the acetabulum may be involved if the femoral head is driven through the hip joint. This has significant potential for long-term arthritic changes.

A shear injury is the most life-threatening because of its potential for hemorrhage. The forces are applied parallel to the sacroiliac joint, producing disruption of the sacroiliac segments and sacrotuberous ligaments posteriorly. This results in contusion or laceration of nerve roots as they exit the sacral foramina; significant retroperitoneal bleeding can occur. There is generally no end point to damage by this force, and even traumatic hemipelvectomy may result.[16] The clinician must always be attentive to the inadequacies of routine radiography to reveal posterior element disruption. It is generally agreed that computed tomographic (CT) scans are indicated when there is clinical suspicion of a disruption of posterior elements of the pelvis and when there is a displaced fracture of the pubic rami anteriorly (see Chapter 22).

PELVIC FRACTURE
Initial stabilization: management of hemorrhage

The appropriate management of hemorrhage from pelvic fracture is the subject of controversy and of much effort by trauma surgeons for well over 30 years. In 1978 Rothenberger, in a series of 604 patients, noted a 12% mortality with 60% of the deaths related to hemorrhage or pelvic sepsis.[14] He correlated a greater risk of hemorrhage and increased mortality with posterior element disruption. Postmortem injection studies disclose that most pelvic fracture hemorrhage results from lacerations of large venous channels and smaller moderate arterial vessels near the sacroiliac joints, rather than from major arterial injury.[5] However, disruption of major branches of the internal iliac system does occur.

The management of hemorrhage from pelvic fractures has evolved over time. Initial efforts were directed at surgical exposure of the retroperitoneal hematoma with hypogastric artery ligation or tamponade by pressure with sponges. These efforts were futile because of the loss of tamponade effect caused by opening the hematoma and by subsequent infectious complications. Dissatisfaction with these operative approaches led to attempts to control pelvic fracture hemorrhage by nonoperative means. In adults, this was first attempted with pneumatic pressure trousers.[6] Pneumatic trousers have two potential advantages in the treatment of such fractures. First, they allow for compression of the pelvic area, which may tamponade hemorrhage. Second, they immobilize the fracture so that no further disruption of vessels may occur. Protocol requires that the extremity compartments be inflated to 50 mm Hg and the abdominal compartments to 40 mm Hg. In addition, tracheal intubation of patients is necessary for ventilation because of abdominal pressure and elevation of the diaphragm, regardless of respiratory status.[6] Failure of pneumatic pressure therapy necessitated arteriography for study of the major pelvic vessels and embolization to stop hemorrhage. This approach has reduced the mortality of pelvic fracture hemorrhage.

Additional refinements in the treatment of adult pelvic fracture have involved the use of external fixation devices. External fixation prevents the risk of compartment syndrome and ischemic necrosis that can be associated with the use of pneumatic pressure trousers. In general, fixation of fractures within the first 48 hours reduces the risk of subsequent multiple organ failure.[15] Currently, the most comprehensive treatment of pelvic fracture hemorrhage includes the immediate application of pneumatic pressure trousers in the field or in the emergency room. Patients who continue to bleed despite external compression require application of an external fixation device, which provides better hemorrhage control through fracture-fragment apposition. Failure of these two forms of therapy indicates a need for arteriographic evaluation and embolization. The large majority of arteriographically demonstrated bleeding originates from the hypogastric artery and its branches. Occlusion of these

vessels through embolization is successful in most cases.[9]

Inherent in this discussion is the appropriate evaluation for additional bleeding sites other than the pelvis. The thorax and abdomen are frequent locations for occult blood loss. Exclusion of bleeding in the chest is possible by a combination of physical examination, chest x-ray examination, and tube thoracostomy. In cases of severe hypotension unresponsive to fluid and blood resuscitation, the abdomen is best evaluated by diagnostic peritoneal lavage or laparotomy. However, the combination of pelvic fracture and diagnostic peritoneal lavage may produce false-positive examination results from two sources; one, directly entering the anterior extension of the pelvic hematoma, and two, diapedesis of red cells across an intact retroperitoneum. Avoid the first risk by attention to placing the lavage incision above the umbilicus in the patient with a concomitant pelvic fracture. Reduction of the second risk of false-positive lavage is possible by early performance of the diagnostic peritoneal lavage before diapedesis occurs; unfortunately, even with these precautions there is still a significant incidence of false-positive exams.[4]

Experience with patients who have concomitant pelvic fracture and abdominal injury reveals that if a patient cannot undergo CT, a diagnostic peritoneal lavage is performed in the operating room. If the lavage yields grossly positive, laparotomy is performed first. If hypotension persists, an external fixator is applied. Patients who do not have grossly positive lavage but are positive by RBC count alone (greater than 100,000), require external fixation and arterial embolization first. Abdominal CT or laparotomy enhances evaluation of intraabdominal injury once the patient is hemodynamically stable.[2,4]

The majority of cases of abdominal trauma in children permit evaluation by CT scan. However, in the event a child is hemodynamically unstable, the clinician must know whether there is concomitant intraabdominal injury that needs immediate laparotomy. Peritoneal lavage is helpful for differentiation.

Initial evaluation: associated injuries

The determination of all associated injuries in the abdomen, genitourinary system, and lower extremities are critical in deciding the next stage of management. First, determine whether the pelvic fracture is open or closed; is there communication via a break in the skin to the fracture site? The presence of an open pelvic fracture increases morbidity and mortality substantially, secondary to infection in the region of the fracture site.[13] A good examination of the perineum and the rectum is essential. Identification of blood in the rectum suggests a rectal laceration. These patients require proctoscopic examination in the operating room. If a major rectal laceration is present, diverting colostomy and irrigation of the distal rectum is therapeutic.[7] Additional treatment of the soft tissue injuries includes debridement, irrigation, and appropriate dressings. The wound is left open, not closed, and the patient receives broad-spectrum parenteral antibiotics. Laceration of the vagina occurs in females, and treatment depends on recognition. Debridement of devitalized vaginal tissue and copious irrigation of the vagina are usually adequate. A CT scan of the abdomen is best to delineate injury; however, diagnostic peritoneal lavage is useful for the assessment of the unstable patient. All males with anterior fracture of the pelvis, because of the possibilities of urethral injury, require a urethrogram examination. The technique is simple and is possible by placement of a syringe in the urethral meatus and injection of 15 to 20 ml of contrast material, followed by immediate x-ray examination. If the urethra is intact, placement of an indwelling catheter to obtain a cystogram is indicated. If urethral dye extravasation occurs, avoid insertion of a catheter.

Careful attention to detail in performing cystography is also crucial. The two major pitfalls in this procedure are failure to fill the bladder adequately, so that a leak is not detected, and failure to obtain post-emptying films to disclose posterior bladder extravasation that may not be visible with the bladder completely filled with contrast material. The treatment of intraperitoneal bladder rupture is, generally, exploration, debridement, and multiple layer closure with urinary bladder decompression. The treatment of extraperitoneal bladder rupture can be limited to urinary bladder decompression. Be extremely attentive in assessment of patients with such injuries, because the smallest laceration can result in pelvic sepsis and death.

As in the evaluation of any patient who has sustained trauma, neurovascular supply to the lower extremity should be examined. Unique to the patient with pelvic fracture is the possibility of pelvic nerve damage. This is best assessed by examination of rectal tone and by evaluation of the bulbocavernosus and cremasteric reflexes; defects are usually evident.

Pelvic fractures: complications

Following initial assessment, resuscitation, and treatment of injuries, the two greatest threats to the patient are multiple-system organ failure and intercurrent infection. Supportive therapy is all that can be done for multiple-system failure. Yet, as previously mentioned, there is evidence that early fixation of fractures and patient mobilization result in better pulmonary toilet and reduced incidence of the symptom complex.[15] With careful attention to details in supportive management, the period of multiple-system dysfunction can be overcome.

Often perplexing is the patient who has persistent fever despite negative cultures of sputum, urine, and blood. If the patient exhibits signs of sepsis, one must exclude the possibility of an infected retroperitoneal hematoma. This occurs most frequently with an open pelvic fracture; however, it can occur because of hematogenous infection. Needle aspiration guided by CT scan is useful in obtaining material from the hematoma for culture and sensitivity and for directing the appropriate antibiotic therapy. A hematoma may drain through an open fracture site or, if necessary, through surgical evacuation of a contaminated clot—an infrequent requirement. Nevertheless, life-threatening infection occurs with genitourinary or rectal injury when bacterial contamination happens at the time of injury.

Fracture management and outcome

The treatment of pelvic fracture depends on the type of fracture.[16] Various methods available for fixation include traction, external fixation, open reduction, and combinations of these. Simple fractures that are stable and do not involve the posterior elements are treated with bed rest and active mobilization when the patient can tolerate weight-bearing devices such as crutches. These include isolated fractures of the pubic rami and chip fractures of the iliac wing.

Fractures that involve distraction or instability of the pelvic ring often require traction as their initial treatment, unless hemorrhagic complications require early application of an external fixation device. Traction alone is effective in children to achieve and maintain reduction. Unfortunately, this requires long-term immobilization, but does not increase complications such as pulmonary embolism as it does in adults.

Studies show that an external bone fixator, regardless of the configuration, cannot immobilize a posterior disruption in an unstable pelvic injury. Consequently, application is used for approximation of anterior disruption; internal fixation is best for posterior segments. There is a reluctance on the part of many surgeons to employ the techniques of external internal fixation in children, partly because of a false sense of security in the expectation that children's bones will always heal and "remodel" their injury; unfortunately, this is not the case.[10] Candidates for external fixation devices include patients with extensive associated soft tissue

Table 48–1 Associated injury by location of pelvic fracture

Fracture site	N	%	Abdominal injury		Genitourinary injury	
Pubic ramus	32	59.3	2	6	0	
Ilium or pelvic rim	9	16.7	3	33	0	
Sacrum	3	5.6	0	0	0	
Multiple	10	18.5	6	60	4	40.0
Total	54		11	20	4	7.4

injury, epiphyseal, diaphyseal, and joint injuries, polytrauma, and unstable pelvic fractures. There are certainly complications with external fixators, including pin sepsis and erosion, that are more likely to occur in the smaller pelvis of the child. However, the balance of treatment seems to be shifting toward the use of external fixation devices.

The sources of long-term disability include genitourinary injuries, especially injury to the urethra, which is devastating if not treated appropriately. Fractures involving articular cartilage and growth centers resulting in leg-length discrepancy and arthritic change are additional sources of long-term morbidity.

Pediatric experience

Most information concerning the management of pelvic fractures evolved from treatment of adult patients. To date, only four studies[1,8,11,17] deal with the specific entity of pelvic fracture in children. Our own study[17] reviewed a 48-month period ending September 1989. During that time 2248 children with blunt trauma were admitted to Children's National Medical Center in Washington, D.C. Evaluation of these children included routine radiographic examinations. CT examinations of the abdomen and pelvis were selectively performed, based on physical examination and clinical signs. The location of pelvic fracture, transfusion requirements within the first 48 hours after injury, associated injuries, and patient outcomes were recorded.

Fifty-four (2.4%) of the 2248 children with blunt trauma, in consecutive admissions, had sustained pelvic fractures. The mean age of the injured children was 8.6 years. Eighty-nine percent of the pelvic fractures related to motor vehicle crashes (59% pedestrian, 30% vehicle occupant). The motor vehicle continues to pose the greatest risk to the child. Children with pelvic fracture tended to be severely injured, representing a mean Injury Severity Score (ISS) of 18.9 and a mean trauma score of 13. The pelvic fractures were classified as pubic rami fractures, ileum or pelvic rim fractures, sacral fractures, and multiple fractures of the pelvis (Table 48-1).

Ten children (18.5%) had multiple fracture sites in the pelvis, primarily the Malgaigne or open-book type. Eleven children had concomitant abdominal injury (20.3%), and there were four injuries to the genitourinary system (7.4%). Contingency table analysis revealed differences between children with isolated versus multiple pelvic fractures. Type of fracture was strongly associated with the probability of intraabdominal injury. Eighty percent of children with multiple pelvic fractures had concomitant abdominal or genitourinary injury, as compared with 33% of children with fracture of the ileum or pelvic rim and 6% with isolated pubic rami fracture. When the frequencies of abdominal and genitourinary injury were compared for children with isolated versus multiple pelvic fracture, these differences were statistically significant (p = less than 0.001 for abdominal injury; p = less than 0.002 for genitourinary injury).

Six children died as a result of their injuries, representing a mortality rate of 11.1% (Table 48-2). Five deaths were attributed to irreversible neurologic injury. The other fatality occurred with intraperitoneal rupture of a retroperitoneal hematoma with uncontrollable bleeding. Nine children (17%) required infusion of packed red cells; the median volume of transfusion was 11.5 cc/kg. Fracture type was not significantly associated with mortality or the need for transfusion.

The incidence of associated injuries to the abdomen and genitourinary tract in this study is similar to that in other pediatric institutions (Table 48-3). This is also consistent with experience in treatment of adults, except that genitourinary injury has a slightly lower frequency in the pediatric population; urethral injury appears to be especially uncommon in children. The most consistent predictor of abdominal or genitourinary injury in children is the presence of multiple sites of fracture within the pelvic circle. The increased incidence of abdominal and genitourinary injury with multiple fracture sites was also evident in Toronto.[16] Therefore, children

Table 48–2 Fracture site versus transfusion requirements and mortality

Fracture site	N	Transfusion		Deaths	
		N	%	N	%
Pubic ramus	32	3	9	3	9
Ilium/pelvic rim	9	3	33	0	0
Sacrum	3	0	0	0	0
Multiple	10	3	30	3	30
Total	54	9	17	6	11

Table 48–3 Comparative studies of pelvic fracture in children

	Location			
	Washington	Baltimore*	Houston†	Toronto‡
Population:				
Time period (yr)	4	17	5	10
Patients	54	120	57	141
Patients/year	13.5	7.1	11.4	14.1
Injury mechanism				
Motor vehicle (%)	87	92	98	83
Auto vs pedestrian (%)	59	67	61	78
Associated injuries				
Abdominal (%)	20.3	12	21	18.4
Genitourinary (%)	7.4	10	5.2	13.4
Deaths				
Mortality rate (%)	11.1	1.4	14	8
Head injury (%)	83.3	50.0	100	72.7

*Reichard, 1980.[11]
†Musemeche, 1987.[8]
‡Torode, 1985.[17]

with multiple pelvic fractures require early identification, radiologic assessment, and appropriate treatment of intraabdominal injury. The association between fracture type and intraabdominal injury also occurs in adult patients.[4,6]

Pediatric pelvic fracture does differ in one important clinical respect from pelvic fracture in adults. In adults, the two major conditions leading to death from severe pelvic fracture are hemorrhage and infection of intrapelvic hematoma. In contrast, death in children with pelvic fractures is usually caused by associated head injury. Consolidation of data from the studies listed in Table 48-3 reveals that 21 of 27 pediatric deaths (77%) were due to head injury. Despite having anatomic fracture sites similar to those in adults, only 5 of the 372 children, (1.3%) listed in Table 48-3 died as a result of hemorrhage. These findings are different from those in adult patients, of whom at least 10% die of pelvic fracture hemorrhage or subsequent infection.[3,4,6] Plausible explanations for this difference include the more vasoreactive vessels in children, which reduce hemorrhage, or the more densely adherent periosteal envelope, which limits bleeding.

Summary

Pelvic fracture is an uncommon injury in children, occurring in only 2.4% of all blunt trauma admissions to the Children's National Medical Center (mean age 8.6 years), with a mortality of 11.1%. Initial resuscitation and stabilization are followed by screening for associated injuries. Genitourinary injuries occur in 5% to 10% of children with pelvic fracture, and abdominal injuries were noted in 10% to 20%. The likelihood of finding such an associated abdominal or genitourinary injury increases when there are multiple fracture sites in the pelvis. Unlike adults, however, children are not prone to life-threatening hemorrhage and death in association with multiple fracture sites in the pelvis. In children, the primary determinant of mortality is associated head injury.

Close communication between trauma surgeons and their urologic and orthopedic colleagues will continue to give the best care for children with pelvic trauma. The primary mechanism of such injury continues to be related to motor vehicles (90%). Further efforts at preventing pediatric pedestrian injury and enforcing motor vehicle restraint laws will certainly reduce the incidence and, perhaps, the severity of pelvic fracture in children.

RETROPERITONEAL HEMATOMA

The surgeon is often confronted with the decision of whether to explore or to conservatively manage a collection of blood discovered in the retroperitoneum intraoperatively or on CT scan. Attention to both the mechanism of injury and the location of the hematoma permits the most judicious decision on whether to explore or to open these collections. The retroperitoneum is defined by the mesothelial plain covering the distal esophagus, duodenum, aorta, inferior vena cava, kidneys, adrenal glands, lateral gutters and posterior surfaces of the ascending and descending colon, and the pelvis. There are many classifications of retroperitoneal hematoma,[3] which recognize the upper midline, paraduodenal, perirenal, pericolonic, pelvic, portal, and retrohepatic spaces. In delineation of pelvic hematoma and perirenal hematoma, however, there is some confusion.

In cases of blunt trauma, pelvic hematoma is most likely to emanate from bleeding edges of a pelvic fracture. If the patient with a pelvic hematoma is stable, without evidence of injury to the urethra or bladder, and there are arterial pulsations in both lower extremities and rate of expansion is slow, the hematoma is left undisturbed. In this situation much of the bleeding is venous in origin and is not amenable to direct suture repair or hypogastric artery ligation. Injudicious manipulation or rupture of the hematoma frequently requires tamponade of bleeding by packing the pelvis. Pelvic hematomas resulting from penetrating injury differ from those associated with pelvic fractures. Pelvic hematoma resulting from penetrating injury requires exploration after adequate proximal and distal vascular control, because bleeding may be arterial.

Management of perirenal hematoma depends on radiologic demonstration of an intact, functioning kidney. In the instance of blunt trauma, it is usually a CT scan that demonstrates arterial inflow. If a preoperative CT scan does not afford visualization, an arteriogram investigation of the renal pedicle is essential. If at operation a renal hematoma is found without preoperative radiologic analysis, the procedure is as follows: if the hematoma is not expanding, is not pulsatile, or is not freely ruptured, intraoperative intravenous pyelogram is helpful. If this produces a nephrogram showing good excretion, the renovascular pedicle is intact and the hematoma is not disturbed. Otherwise, exploration is the proper treatment.

Perirenal hematoma secondary to penetrating trauma requires exploration, unless preoperative staging by CT shows a limited renal injury. Before exploration, radiologic evaluation of the contralateral kidney for function is imperative. Proximal and distal control of the renal vascular pedicle is best prior to opening the hematoma, to lower the necessity for nephrectomy and to enhance the possibility of renal salvage.

Upper midline hematoma requires exploration. This injury is best approached with aortic control at the hiatus. Opening the chest and taking down the diaphragm may be necessary prior to opening the hematoma. This provides adequate exposure for the upper aorta, celiac trunk, superior mesenteric artery, and left renal artery. A hematoma overlying the pancreas and duodenum should be explored. Perform a proper Kocher maneuver and inspect for signs of crepitus or bile staining in the retroperitoneum. Pericolonic retroperitoneal hematoma requires exploration to rule out any colonic injury; this is always necessary in cases of penetrating trauma. There are some cases, however, in which a pelvic fracture results in pelvic hematoma dissecting into the lateral gutters. In these cases the retroperitoneal hematoma, although it is pericolonic, emanates from the pelvis and does not require exploration.

A hematoma surrounding the porta hepatis requires exploration for assessment of injury to the common duct, portal vein, and hepatic artery. If there is any question, an intraoperative cholangiogram evaluation helps to demonstrate patency of the biliary ductal system. Retrohepatic injury in both blunt and penetrating trauma is best let alone if no overt, active hemorrhage occurs once the overlying hepatic injury is treated. If the retrohepatic hematoma is associated with moderate bleeding, however, one may elect either to pack the area, if a severe coagulopathy with hypothermia is present, or to proceed with an atrial-caval shunt to isolate the liver.

In summary, most retroperitoneal hematomas are explored, with the exception of pelvic hematoma associated with pelvic fracture and uncomplicated perirenal hematoma. The surgical approach to these injuries depends on the mechanism and location of injury and the clinical status of the patient.

REFERENCES

1. Bond SJ, Gotschall CS, Eichelberger MR: Predictors of abdominal injury in children with pelvic fracture, *J Trauma* 31(8):1169-1173, 1991.
2. Evers BM, Cryer HM, Miller FB: Pelvic fracture hemorrhage: priorities in management, *Arch Surg* 422-424, 1989.
3. Feliciano DV: Management of traumatic retroperitoneal hematoma, *Ann Surg* 109-123, 1990.
4. Flint L, Babikian G, Anders M et al: Definitive control of mortality from severe pelvic fracture, *Ann Surg* 703-707, 1990.
5. Flint LM, Brown A, Richardson JD et al: Definitive control of bleeding from severe pelvic fractures, *Ann Surg* 709-716, 1979.
6. Huittinen V, Slatis P: Postmortem angiography and dissection of the hypogastric artery in pelvic fractures, *Surgery* 454, 1973.
7. Maull KI, Sachatello CR, Ernst CB: The deep perineal laceration—an injury frequently associated with open pelvic fractures: a need for aggressive surgical management, *J Trauma* 685-696, 1977.
8. Musemeche CA, Fischer RP et al: Selective management of pediatric pelvic fractures: a conservative approach, *J Pediatr Surg* 538-540, 1987.
9. Panetta T, Sclafani S, Goldstein A et al: Percutaneous transcatheter embolization for massive bleeding from pelvic fractures, *J Trauma* 1021-1029, 1985.
10. Reff RB: The use of external fixation devices in the management of severe lower-extremity trauma and pelvic injuries in children, *Clin Ortho Rel Res* 21-33, 1984.
11. Reichard SA, Helikson MA, Shorter N et al: Pelvic fractures in children: review of 120 patients with a new look at general management, *J Pediatr Surg* 727-734, 1980.
12. Richardson JD, Polk HC, Flint LM: *Trauma: clinical care and pathophysiology,* Chicago, 1987, Mosby–Year Book, pp 421-432.
13. Richardson JD, Harty J, Amin M et al: Open pelvic fractures, *J Trauma* 533-538, 1982.
14. Rothenberger DA, Fischer RP, Strate RG et al: The mortality associated with pelvic fractures, *Surgery* 356-361, 1978.
15. Seibel R, LaDuca J, Hassett J et al: Blunt multiple trauma (ISS 36), femur traction and the pulmonary failure-septic state, *Ann Surg* 283-289, 1985.
16. Tile M: Pelvic ring fractures: should they be fixed? *J Bone Joint Surg (Br)* 1-12, 1988.
17. Torode I, Zieg D: Pelvic fractures in children, *J Pediatr Ortho* 76-84, 1985.

PART THIRTEEN

Skeletal Injury

49 Musculoskeletal Injury

Michael D. Thomas

Skeletal injury occurs in approximately 20% of all trauma sustained by children. In 1980 the National Center for Health Statistics, National Health Interview Survey, reported 21.7 million nonfatal pediatric injuries.[9] This total number of injuries represents some 4 million children of all ages who sustained fractures requiring treatment in that year.

At birth, skull and clavicle fractures are the most common, although fractures of nearly every bone have been reported. Fractures are rare during the first year of life. During the first 2 years of life, fractures may be the first indications of skeletal dysplasia, metabolic bone disease, or the battered child syndrome. Most fractures caused by intentional trauma occur during the first 2 years of a child's life. Identification and evaluation of victims of child abuse are discussed in Chapter 52.

In children from age 2 through adolescence, fractures of the upper extremity outnumber fractures of the lower extremity 7:1; fracture of the radius is the most common. From 2 to 5 years of age, a toddler's fracture of the distal tibia is common. Clavicle fractures are common at all ages. The automobile is mainly responsible for producing blunt trauma, the primary mechanism of injury to children in the United States, who suffer both as passengers and as pedestrians. Other mechanisms of injury include falls and occasional penetration by knives, bullets, and other sharp objects.

Fractures are more common in children than adults and are more likely to occur following seemingly minimal trauma. Complications are different and the different methods of fracture treatment receive different emphasis.

DIFFERENCES IN BONE OF CHILDREN AND ADULTS

Children differ from adults in their response to injury for psychological and physical reasons. The major differences between fractures in adults and those in growing children involve anatomic, physiologic, and biomechanical differences in their bones.

The most important part of a child's bone is the radiolucent growth plate. The growth plate and the variably radiolucent chondro-osseus epiphyses of long bones in a child may make diagnosis by radiographic examination uncertain.

The biomechanical properties of the immature skeleton differ because a child's bone is more porous. The effect of porosity is realized in incomplete fractures unique to the immature skeleton. The physiologic characteristics specific to children's bones allow rapid healing and useful remodeling after fracture, which can result in progressive deformity.

PATHOPHYSIOLOGY OF FRACTURES

Fractures occur when a bone sustains a deforming load that exceeds its elastic limits or its ability to dissipate the applied force to adjacent structures. The load limit varies from bone to bone and regionally within a bone, depending on its density and shape, and is rate dependent. Fracture occurs as a result of compression, tension, or rotatory forces. The magnitude and direction of force determines the type of fracture sustained. High-energy trauma, most commonly the result of motor vehicle crashes, may also be seen in falls from substantial heights. High-energy trauma usually results directly in fractures at the site of load application. Dissipation of energy occurs locally, at the significant expense of soft tissues surrounding the fractured bone. Fractures secondary to high-energy trauma are frequently associated with severe concomitant injury to other body systems. Even when present as isolated fractures, these are more commonly open fractures and are complicated by greater muscle, nerve, and vascular injury and periosteal stripping than are fractures resulting from low-energy trauma. Such extensive injury results in less predictable, slower healing with greater risk of complications. Low-energy trauma is typical of household and playground falls, falls from bicycles, collisions in contact sports, or injury caused by truncheons and most civilian handguns. Fracture owing to low-energy trauma usually results in less injury to surrounding structures and, therefore, the likelihood of healing with fewer complications. These fractures, however, may be open and contaminated, or include nerve or vascular injuries, resulting in problems of management equal to those of high-energy fractures.

Pain, usually sharp and severe but of a variable degree, is the common denominator among children with acute fractures. Fracture pain is primarily caused by injury to the periosteum, surrounding soft tissues, and the cancellous portion of the bone. Local biochemical and metabolic changes initiate an inflammatory response that includes the sensitization of nociceptors. Concomitant primary nerve or vascular injury may cause additional pain. Hemorrhage, which occurs to a variable degree with nearly all fractures, leads to local swelling. Moderate to severe hemorrhage into a closed compartment of one of the extremities may result in the development of a compartment syndrome, which produces ischemic muscular pain. The pain of muscle ischemia is constant and increases in intensity until the ischemia progresses sufficiently to obliterate afferent nerve impulses.

Extrinsic arterial compression after fracture may also result in ischemic pain. Reflex muscle spasm in the same and adjacent spinal cord segments often occurs in response to painful stimuli from the fracture. Suprasegmental responses to pain result in neuroendocrine and metabolic responses that stimulate ventilation and circulation and selective metabolites, which leads to a catabolic state and negative nitrogen balance. Cortical responses result in the perception of pain as an unpleasant sensation and the initiation of anxiety, apprehension, and fear.

The causes of pain in response to trauma are additive and may create a vicious circle wherein local pain produces muscle spasm, which produces more local pain, both resulting in suprasegmental and cortical responses. These normal responses to pain are intended to maintain homeostasis but may become abnormal and increase morbidity and mortality. Under these circumstances interruption of the cycle of pain is necessary to promote homeostasis.

INJURIES: GENERAL TYPES
Incomplete fractures

The unique qualities of children's bones account for three patterns of incomplete fracture (Fig. 49-1):

1. Torus or buckle fracture. Results from failure of the bone in compression. Generally occurs in the metaphyseal region of long bones and resembles the raised band at the base of an architectural column (torus).
2. Traumatic bowing. Results from plastic deformation in a bone bent beyond its elastic limits; most commonly seen in the radius,

ulna, and fibula. No evidence of microscopic fractures that occur is seen on radiograph, and remodeling is incomplete.

3. Greenstick fracture. Occurs when bending of an immature bone results in a fracture of that half of the cortex on the convex (tension) side of the bowed bone; the concave (compression) side remains intact. Greenstick fractures may result in impressive deformity, especially those of the radius and ulna.

Complete fractures

Complete fracture patterns are described below (Fig. 49-2):

4. Transverse fracture. The line fracture passes at a right angle to the long axis of the bone and results in two fragments caused by direct trauma.
5. Comminuted fracture. The bone is broken into three or more fragments.
6. Oblique and spiral fractures. These terms describe the appearance of the bone fragment at the fractured edge and indicate the mechanism of injury. Oblique = axial loading. Spiral = rotary force.
7. Closed fracture. One in which the skin barrier overlying the fracture is intact.
8. Open fracture. One in which the skin barrier overlying the fracture is broken, and thus the fracture is considered to be contaminated.

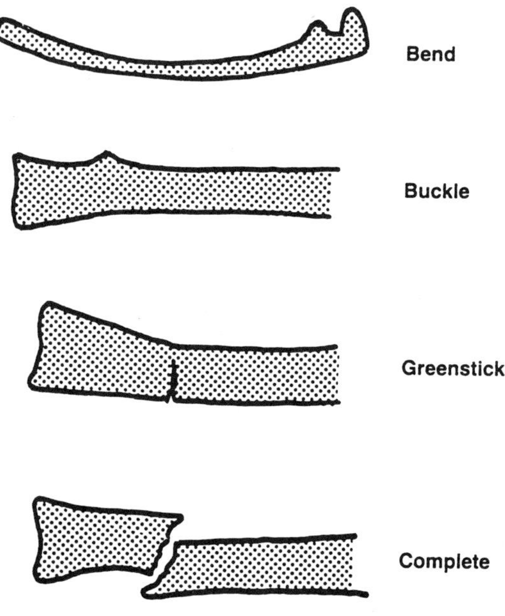

Figure 49–1 Fracture types in children. (From Rang M: *Children's fractures,* ed 2, Philadelphia, 1983, JB Lippincott.)

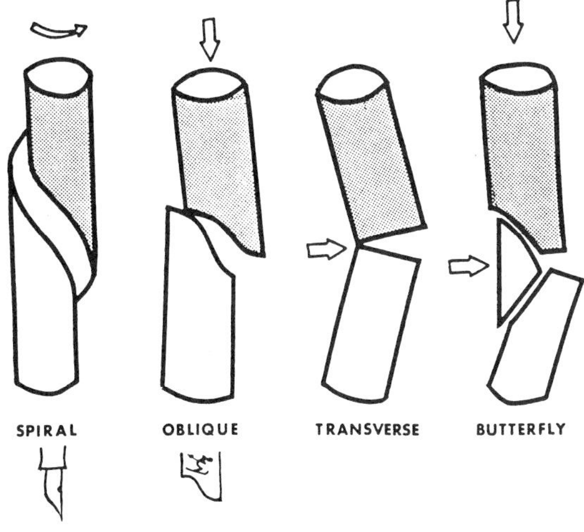

Figure 49–2 Shape of the fracture tells how it was produced. Spiral fractures are shaped like a pen nib. Oblique fractures are like a ski jump. (From Rang M: *Children's fractures,* ed 2, Philadephia, 1983, JB Lippincott.)

Growth plate injuries

The growth plate (physis plate) is a cartilaginous disc located between the epiphysis and metaphysis at the ends of long bones in the immature skeletal. Three zones within the physis have been identified (Fig. 49-3). Injury to the zone of growth by any means, including avascular necrosis, infection, or fracture, may result in disturbances of growth that may be manifested in acceleration, deceleration, or arrest of longitudinal growth, or progressive angular deformity. Most fractures of the growth plate pass through the zone of cartilage transformation and hence do not disturb growth.

The Salter-Harris classification of epiphyseal fractures published in 1965 assists in determining the mechanism of injury, appropriate treatment, and prognosis of such fractures (Fig. 49-4). Their classification of epiphyseal fractures is as follows:

Type I. Complete separation of the epiphysis from the metaphysis through the zone of cartilage transformation. Results from a shearing

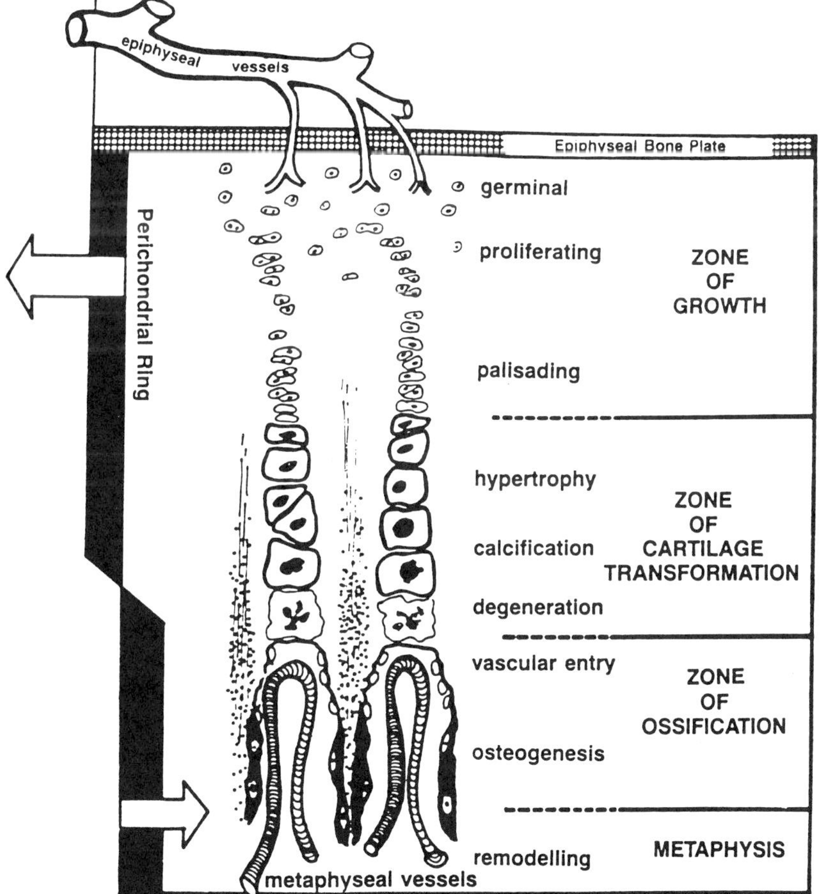

Figure 49–3 A schematic representation of the growth plate. Separation of the growth plate invariably occurs through the zone of cartilage transformation. (From Siffert RS, Gilbert MD: Anatomy and physiology of the growth plate. In Rang M, editor: *The growth plate and its disorders,* Baltimore, 1969, Williams & Wilkins.)

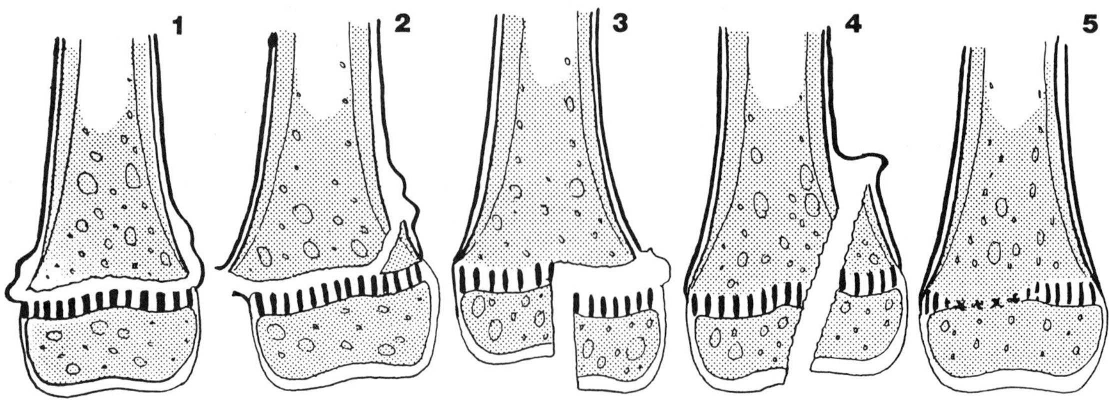

Figure 49–4 The types of growth plate injury as classified by Salter and Harris. (From Salter RB, Harris WR; Injuries involving the epiphyseal plate, *J Bone Joint Surg* 45A:587, 1963.)

(side-to-side) force. Displacement is variable and risk of growth disturbance is generally low.

Type II. Results in a fracture fragment, consisting of the epiphysis and a triangular portion of the metaphysis, caused by shearing and bending forces. Displacement is variable and risk of growth disturbance is generally low.

Type III. An uncommon injury seen when the growth plates are partially closed. The fracture line passes through a portion of the open growth plate, then through the epiphysis, becoming intraarticular. Accurate fracture reduction, frequently open and with internal fixation, is indicated to restore joint incongruity and minimize risk of growth disturbance. Most common site of occurrence is the distal end of the tibia.

Type IV. The fracture line in this injury passes from the articular surface across the epiphysis and the growth plate, and exits through the metaphusis. Open reduction and internal fixation are frequently indicated to obtain accurate reduction; otherwise, nonunion, growth disturbance, and joint incongruity are very likely.

Type V. Implies a crush injury of the growth plate. This may be primary, or occur secondary to uncontrolled motion of the flail limb or manipulation for fracture reduction. This injury is rare and diagnosis is commonly made in retrospect.

Growth disturbances after an epiphyseal fracture may not become apparent in the time required for the fracture to heal. Therefore, all fractures involving the growth plate require prolonged follow-up, some even through skeletal maturity.

Epiphyseal fracture may also occur without injury to the growth plate. Three fracture patterns are recognized as follows:

1. Avulsion fractures. These occur at the site of ligament attachment to bone.
2. Compression fracture. This is a rare fracture in children.
3. Osteochondral fracture. Shearing or avulsing forces result in the detachment of a fragment of the boney epiphysis and its articular cartilage, creating a defect of the articular surface. Large defects should be repaired by replacement and pinning of the fragment; small fragments are better removed. The distal femoral condyles, patella, and radial head are the most common sites of this injury.

Apophyseal fractures

Avulsion fractures also occur at accessory growth centers known as apophyses. These centers serve as origins or insertions of muscle-tendon units such as the anterior superior and inferior iliac spines of the ilium (respective origins of the sartorius and rectus femoris muscles) and the anterior tibial tubercle (insertion of the patellar tendon). Sudden acceleration or deceleration muscle contractions may result in avulsion of bone at the site of muscle attachment.

Sprains

A sprain is a joint injury in which fibers of a supporting ligament are ruptured, resulting in proportionate symptoms, instability, and dysfunction. Sprains are graded I through IV, according to severity. A grade I sprain implies minimal fiber disruption, which results in mild pain, no instability, and minimal dysfunction. A grade II sprain results in immediate joint instability, pain, and dysfunction attributable to moderate fiber disruption. A grade III injury manifests complete fiber disruption within its substance and gross joint instability. A grade IV injury implies rupture of the ligament from the bone, with or without a fragment of bone attachment to the avulsed part.

Dislocation and fracture dislocation

A dislocation is a joint injury in which there is a complete disruption of a joint so that the articular surfaces are no longer in contact. A fracture dislocation is a joint injury of dislocation combined with concomitant fracture of one or more of the displaced bones.

Dislocations and fracture dislocations can result in severe joint injuries and neurovascular compromise. Dislocations and fracture dislocations of the major joints—shoulder, elbow, wrist, hip, knee, and ankle—are orthopedic emergencies.

TREATMENT
Initial resuscitation

The timing of fracture treatment depends on the general condition of the child. Emergency measures are necessary to combat pain, hemorrhage, and shock and to ensure adequacy of airway, breathing, and circulation; attention may then be directed to skeletal injuries. Although fractures are rarely fatal injuries, their contribution to morbidity owing to hemorrhage must not be underestimated. The goals of first aid for fracture are the prevention of further injury and relief of pain. The successive steps of first aid (pain control, reduction, immobilization, cold packs, and elevation) are encoded in the mnemonic PRICE. These measures will reduce suffering and pain and elicit gratitude.

Pain control

Pain control is accomplished by (1) immobilizing proven or suspected fractures, and (2) administering analgesics in adequate doses: potent narcotic analgesics, ketamine, local or regional anesthesia, inhalational analgesics, or adjuvant drugs.

Reduction

Most fractured extremities need not be reduced acutely but are better splinted in the position found, to reduce pain and risk of further injury. If gross displacement of a fracture or dislocation results in circulatory compromise (pulselessness distal to the injury), however, reduction and immobilization are indicated. A splint is prepared while the analgesics take effect. The proximal fragment is then steadied by an assistant while application of gentle, firm, steady manual longitudinal traction and if necessary rotation is applied to the distal fragment until anatomic alignment is approximated. Evaluation of distal pulses will determine the best position for

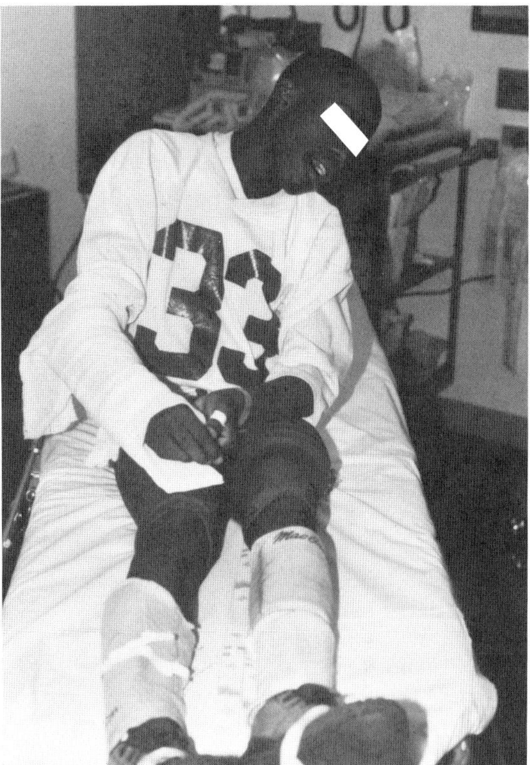

Figure 49–5 This athlete was guarding his dislocated right elbow with his left hand at his right wrist, upon presentation. He continued to support his elbow in this manner because the arm board provided no immobilization of the elbow.

the extremity to be splinted. Dislocated joints may require flexion or extension in addition to traction. Avoid reduction if circulation is not compromised, because injudicious manipulation of a fracture may create unnecessary risk for the child.

Immobilization

Immobilization alone provides remarkable relief from pain and suffering and reduces hemorrhage and risk of further injury. To be effective, a splint must immobilize the joint just proximal and distal to the fractured bone. Longer splints are more effective; for example, the splint for a radius and ulna fracture should extend as far as the axilla above the elbow and stop just proximal to the metacarpophalangeal joints to immobilize the elbow and wrist most effectively. Splints for dislocations should extend at least to the joints immediately proximal and distal to the dislocated joint. Effective splints relieve the child of the need to guard an injury actively (Fig. 49-5). A plaster splint molded on the spot is preferable to an ill-fitting commercial splint. The use of circumferential bandages, especially elasticized ones, should be avoided to prevent circulatory compromise.

Cold packs

Ice packs generously applied to the site of injury reduce hemorrhage, swelling, and pain. The metabolic demands of the muscle are reduced, thereby increasing its resistance to ischemia.

Elevation

Dependent swelling impedes healing. Unless there is a coexisting compartment syndrome, an injured extremity should be elevated to reduce swelling and promote circulation. Once stabilized, the child is ready for transport from the field or within the hospital.

General assessment

A history, as complete as possible, is obtained and followed by a head-to-toe physical examination of the patient with multiple trauma. The examination is appropriately scaled down according to the condition of the patient with lesser injuries. Physical examination should proceed in a logical sequence, in a search for signs suggestive of injury including:

Swelling
Open wounds, with or without exposed bone
Deformity of an extremity
Abnormal color of skin (ecchymosis, cyanosis, pallor)
Local hypothermia
Absence of pulse
Diminished capillary refill
Loss of asymmetry of voluntary motion
Pain or tenderness

Systematic palpation of the cervical spine, thorax, and upper extremities is followed by palpation of the pelvis and lower extremities. All joints are examined and put through active and passive range of motion series. Abnormal posturing and muscle tone implies potentially serious neurologic injury. Swelling or instability of major joints is an indication of a possible joint dislocation. Even in the absence of significant swelling, considerable displacement after epiphyseal fracture or dislocation may have occurred. Considerable fracture or joint displacement, especially about the elbow and knee, may result in injury to the adjacent neurovascular structures. Any loss of pulse or reduced capillary refill in the extremity distal to the swollen traumatized joint should raise the level of suspicion for vascular injury. If it is suspected, a vascular surgeon should be alerted to assist in evaluation for vascular injury.

Once the physical examination is documented, radiographic examination is necessary to confirm and define the extent and nature of skeletal injuries.

The spine and all extremities with proven or suspected skeletal injury must be splinted prior to transportation of the child to the radiology department. Radiologic technicians must be instructed not to disturb or alter the splints to obtain radiographs.

Open injuries

A review of the literature on open fractures shows that 30% of children with open fractures sustain multiple injuries; that the severity of associated soft tissue injury is of prognostic significance; that the majority of open fractures, open dislocations, and deep wounds are colonized by bacteria at the time of admission; and that open fractures require emergency treatment. Gustilo has classified open fractures based on the amount of coexistent soft tissue injury as follows[21]:

Type I. Small wounds of 1 cm or less caused by low-velocity trauma, such as the protrusion of a fragment of bone, out from within, or by a low-velocity bullet passing in from without with minimal damage to soft tissue.

Type II. Wounds extensive in length and width but with little or no avascular or devitalized soft tissue and relatively little foreign material.

Type III. Wounds of moderate or massive size with considerable devitalized soft tissue, foreign material, or both, or traumatic amputation.

With the exception of fractures of the tuft of the distal phalanges, open skeletal injury is a surgical emergency.

In the emergency room a culture is taken of the wound, which is then covered with sterile dressings until the child is in the operating room. Documentation of the dimensions of the wound with a sketch is helpful. Tetanus prophylaxis is indicated for all open fractures, following the guidelines in Table 49-1. Appropriate and adequate antibiotic therapy is started in the emergency room. Gustilo recommends a first-generation cephalosporin in an initial dose of 2 g intravenously, then 1 to 2 g every 4 to 6 hours for 3 days. For wounds contaminated by soil, add 10 to 20 million units of penicillin daily. An aminoglycoside, 3 to 5 mg/kg of body weight is added for patients with type II and type III wounds.[2]

Once the child is in the operating room, the skin about the wound is surgically prepared. The wound is then irrigated with large volumes (5 liters or more) of normal saline, lactated Ringer's solution, or sterile water and debrided of dead and devitalized tissues. A culture of the wound is taken after the debridement. The fracture must then be stabilized. The wound is left open, and an external fixator or other methods that facilitate frequent

Table 49–1 Tetanus prophylaxis in open fractures

Immunization data	Action to be taken
Immunization completed previously; last booster within 1 year	None.
Immunization completed within the previous 10 years; no subsequent booster dose	0.5 ml of tetanus and diphtheria toxoid, adult type (Td).
Immunization completed more than 10 years previously; last booster within the previous 10 years	0.5 ml of Td.
Immunization completed more than 10 years previously; no booster within the previous 10 years; wound minor and relatively clean, treated promptly and adequately	0.5 ml of Td.
Immunization completed more than 10 years previously; no booster within the previous 5 years; wound other than minor and clean and/or not minor and clean and/or not treated promptly	0.5 ml of Td and 250 to 500 units of human tetanus immune globulin (TIG[H]); 500 units if wound is clostridia prone, otherwise 250 units; give Td and TIG(H) by separate syringes and needles at separate sites.
No history or record of immunization; wound minor and clean; wound surgery prompt and adequate	Begin immunization program with 0.5 ml of Td; schedule further immunization.
No record of immunization; wound other than clean and/or treated promptly and adequately	250 units of human tetanus immune globulin (TIG[H]); begin immunization with 0.5 ml of Td. Give 500 units of TIG(H) if wound is prone to *Clostridium;* otherwise give 250 units; give Td and TIG(H) by separate syringes and needles at separate sites.

From Gustilo RB, editor: Orthopaedic infection: diagnosis and treatment, Philadelphia, 1989, WB Saunders.

wound examinations and dressing changes are employed for fracture stabilization. Repeated surgical debridement is often indicated. Antibiotics are adjusted, as indicated by cultures, and discontinued after 3 days if cultures are negative. Delayed primary wound closure is performed when feasible. Open fractures should be left open until the wounds are surgically clean.

SPECIFIC FRACTURES BY ANATOMIC REGION[4]

The treatment of traumatic skeletal injury, including fracture and associated injury, is herewith presented by anatomic region. The discussion emphasizes presenting symptoms and signs of the skeletal injury, acute complications, and the principles of initial management of common injuries. Definitive care is discussed briefly to provide those who administer first aid for fractures some information to allay the concern of children and their parents.

Definitive treatment of fractures and other skeletal injuries in children consists primarily of nonoperative treatment, unlike the care of adult fracture which commonly involves operative treatment. Some fractures in children, however, are indications for operative treatment. This category includes open fracture, displaced intraarticular fracture, long bone fracture in a comatose child with a head injury or with multiple trauma, unstable fracture dislocations, and fractures including many supracondylar fractures of the humerus, which require extreme positions to maintain a closed reduction. Children generally heal rapidly and nonunions are rare. Rehabilitation needs following the treatment of fracture in children are generally minimal and best determined case by case. Allowing a child to resume normal activity and providing instructions for home exercises to improve range of motion are usually sufficient to restore normal function.

Clavicle, scapula, and shoulder

The clavicle is the most frequently fractured bone in children. Fractures may be complete or incomplete and result from direct or indirect trauma. Presenting signs include swelling, variable deformity, and guarding.

An infant may have pseudoparalysis of the upper extremity; the differential diagnosis includes clavicle or proximal humerus fracture, brachial plexus palsy and septic arthritis. Diagnosis is confirmed on a standard anterior-posterior or 40° apical lordotic view radiograph. Because the periosteum remains partially intact, healing is usually rapid. Malunion is frequent, but remodeling is usually complete. Complications are rare in spite of the proximity of the subclavian neurovascular structures. Closed treatment is the method of choice. Infants are best treated by immobilization of the ipsilateral upper extremity to the trunk for 1 week. Older children usually heal within 3 weeks, and a figure-eight clavicle strap can provide comfort during this period.

Posteriorly displaced epiphyseal fractures of the medial clavicle may mimic posterior sternoclavicular dislocation. Both are uncommon in children, and both constitute indications for reduction if symptomatic tracheal compression occurs. Injuries of the acromioclavicular region, usually attributable to direct trauma, result in fractures or sprains with variable prominence of the medial fragment. Nonoperative treatment, usually a figure-eight strap applied for comfort, is generally sufficient.

Fractures of the scapula, which are rare, are the result of violent trauma. Associated injuries must be sought out. Except for intrathoracic dislocation, closed treatment with a sling and swathe is sufficient.

Proximal humerus

Fractures of the proximal humeral epiphysis are common; Salter-Harris type I and type II fractures predominate. The mechanism of injury is usually a backward fall onto the outstretched hand. The proximal end of the distal fragment may create an abrupt projection visible beneath the coracoid. Muscular attachments to the fragments determine the degree of angulation. Displacement is usually not severe. Radiographs may be difficult to interpret because of the radiolucent physis; orthogonal and comparison views of the uninjured shoulder are helpful. Substantial angulation will remodel, so precise anatomic reduction is unnecessary. Closed treatment, consisting of immobilization with a Velpeau sling and swathe or a shoulder spica splint or cast, is usually effective. If the position of stable reduction is in extreme abduction, brachial plexus injury may result. In that case, placement of a percutaneous pin allows the use of a sling and swathe. Three weeks of immobilization, followed by 3 weeks of protected, progressive mobilization and strengthening are prescribed prior to resumption of normal activities. Neurovascular complications are rare. Injudicious manipulation can cause an arrest in the growth of this physis, which is responsible for 80% of the longitudinal growth of the humerus.

Shaft of humerus

Fractures of the shaft of the humerus are more common in adults than in children. Most are attributable to direct trauma causing a transverse fracture to or rotatory forces that result in a spiral

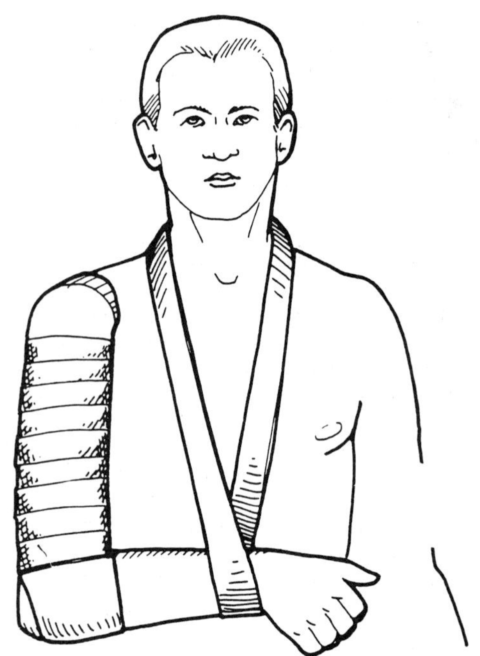

Figure 49–6 A sugar-tongs arm splint has been used to immobilize a humeral fracture, and a sling is used to support the arm. (From Wu KK: *Techniques in surgical casting and splinting,* Philadelphia, 1987, Lea & Febiger. Reproduced with permission.)

fracture pattern. Falling on the outstretched hand may produce a buckle fracture in the metaphyseal region. Infants with incomplete fractures may be presented because of a caregiver's concern about a firm swelling that represents a healing callus of a recent fracture. Acute fractures result in swelling, pain, and guarding of the extremity. The radial nerve wraps around the humerus and is especially vulnerable in fractures of the junction of the middle and distal thirds of the humerus.

Neurovascular function must be documented prior to splint application to the extremity for radiographic examination. Standard anteroposterior and lateral views including the shoulder and elbow are obtained so that an associated but less apparent injury becomes apparent.

A sling and swathe incorporating a plaster splint, or a long arm hanging cast, is the usual means of fracture immobilization (Fig. 49-6). Complications are rare. Serial examinations of the radial nerve are indicated; a change of status may affect the management of the fracture.

Elbow

Among the commonly occurring fractures in children, none poses more difficulties in diagnosis and treatment or threat of complications than a displaced supracondylar fracture of the distal humerus. Other common elbow injuries, medial and lateral humeral condyle fractures, displaced fracture of the medical epicondyle, the Monteggia lesion (a fracture of the proximal ulna with dislocation of the radial head), and elbow dislocations may also result in severe complications.

The usual mechanism of injury is a fall onto the outstretched hand or extended elbow. The elbow should be immobilized in the position in which it is found, to reduce the risk of further injury. Applying a splint to the elbow in flexion invites vascular complications and must be avoided. Careful serial assessment and documentation of median (grasp and finger abduction), radial (thumb extension), and anterior interosseous (flexion of distal interphalangeal joint of the thumb) nerve motor function, sensation (in each digit and dorsal thumb web space), and circulation (pulses, capillary refill) is mandatory.

Diagnosis requires radiographs in the anteroposterior and lateral projections to define the fracture pattern and degree of displacement.

Early reduction of the displaced fracture or dislocation is the most important step in eliminating complications, which include deep volar compartment syndrome (which can lead to Volkmann's ischemic contracture), brachial artery injury, radial nerve paralysis, median nerve paralysis, and malunion causing cubitus varus ("gunstock" deformity).

A displaced supracondylar fracture requires management by a skilled orthopedist. Definitive treatment is best rendered under general anesthesia and may include manipulation, skeletal traction, closed percutaneous pinning, or open reduction and internal fixation.

Radius and ulna

Fractures of the radius and ulna are common in children and usually result from falls on an outstretched hand. Fractures of the shaft of the radius and ulna, Salter-Harris types I and II fractures of the distal radius, and torus fractures are the most common. Pain and swelling are proportionate to the extent of the injury. A long-arm or forearm sugar tong splint can protect the child during transport and exposure to radiography.

Radiographs in the anteroposterior and lateral planes which include the elbow and wrist can reveal the primary fracture and the occasional Monteggia's lesion and Galeazzi's lesion (fracture of the radius with dislocation of the distal radioulnar joint).

The majority of radius and ulna fractures in children are best managed by closed treatment methods; however, open reduction and internal fixation

is sometimes necessary for optimal restoration of function, principally in children nearing skeletal maturity.

Complications are infrequent and can be minimized by the avoidance of circular bandages or casts during the initial fracture treatment and by close follow-up for maintenance of reduction.

Hand and fingers

The hand and fingers are subject to injuries caused by either accidental or intentional exposure to a variety of hazards. Fractures, open and closed, stable and unstable, as well as dislocations, may result. Initial management with analgesics, ice packs, elevation, and splint application in the position found can ease pain while standard radiographs in the anteroposterior and lateral projections are obtained.

Stable fractures are usually managed by nonoperative methods. Open fractures, excluding those of the tuft of the distal phalanx and human bite wounds (resulting from an intentional bite or from striking the tooth during a round of fisticuffs), are treated as a surgical emergency. Swelling and deformity localized to the metacarpophalangeal joints (MCP) or to the proximal (PIP) or distal interphalangeal joints (DIP) occur after dislocation of these joints. Dislocations usually result from hyperextension injury. The temptation to reduce an unwitnessed dislocation prior to radiographic assessment should be avoided. Following radiographic examination, the reduction of a confirmed dorsal dislocation by applying longitudinal traction to the digit with one hand, while applying pressure to the volar side of the deformity with the other, is recommended. Failing in a single attempt, this manipulation should not be repeated, because the deformity may not be reducible by nonoperative means and continued reduction attempts may be harmful. Injuries that result in significant swelling should be dressed with a pressure dressing consisting of fluffed gauze squares placed between the fingers and in the palm. Apply the splint in the "safe position" with MCP joints in 60° to 70° of flexion and the PIP joints flexed 15° to 20°. This is preferable to the "position of function" when possible (Fig. 49-7). Definitive treatment may include simple splintage, closed or open reduction, a percutaneous pin, or external or internal fixation. Secure splints are necessary to protect the injured part from further injury by usually active children.

SPINE

Traumatic injury of the spine and spinal cord is relatively uncommon in the pediatric population. Trauma to the spine may result in spinal cord injury

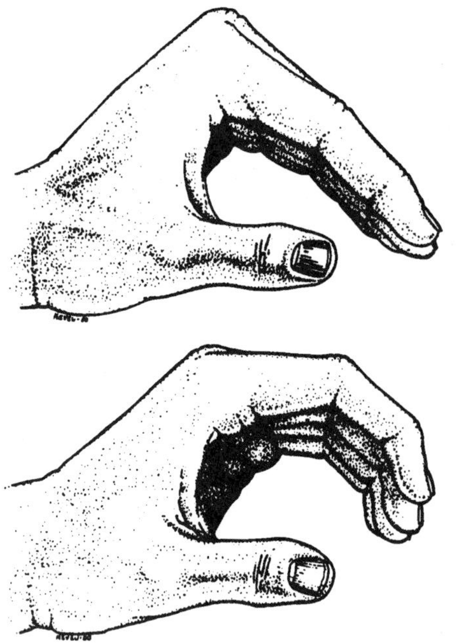

Figure 49–7 The safe position *(top)* and standard "position of function" *(bottom)*. (From O'Brien ET: Fractures of the hand. In Green DP, editor: *Operative hand surgery,* ed 2, New York, 1988, Churchill Livingstone, p 745.)

with or without fracture or dislocation, or fracture or dislocation alone. Skeletal injuries of the spinal column include compression fractures, burst fractures, seat-belt injuries, and fracture dislocations. Growth plate injuries and dislocations without radiographic evidence of fractures also occur. The goals in management of injury of the spinal column are (1) immobilization of the spine to prevent further injury, (2) immediate decompression of the spinal cord in cases of incomplete spinal cord lesions, and (3) realignment of the spine to prevent deformity.

Definitive management of bony, cartilagenous, and ligamentous injuries depends on the location, nature, extent of injury, and, especially, the presence and extent of spinal cord injury. Good results are usually obtained through nonoperative treatment, but operative treatment is indicated in perhaps 20% of children. The reader is referred to Chapter 33 for a detailed discussion of acute and chronic spine and spinal cord injury management.

Pelvis

Fracture of the pelvic ring is usually the result of motor vehicular trauma. Concomitant injuries to the head, chest, and abdomen are frequent and result in significant mortality and morbidity. Recognition of the potential complications in injuries to the major nerves and vessels of the pelvis, abdominal viscera, urethra, and bladder is crucial to resuscitation. Severe pelvic hemorrhage may result.

Fractures of the pelvis may be classified as (1) avulsion fractures of apophyses, (2) fractures involving the pelvic ring, and (3) fractures involving the acetabulum. Palpation of the pelvis and neurovascular examination are mandatory for every child struck by an automobile. Manual compression of the iliac wings toward the midline and of the symphysis pubis is used to elicit tenderness of a fracture. Examination of the vagina and rectum or the presence of hematuria may reveal genitourinary or rectal injury and indicate the need for a urethrogram in addition to standard radiographs. Rapid hemorrhage may respond to the application of pneumatic antishock trousers or manual compression of the iliac wings toward the midline in the field or in the emergency room. Angiography and selective embolization, the application of an external fixator, or laparotomy may be required to control hemorrhage while adequate blood replacement occurs.

Avulsion fractures of the iliac crest, anterosuperior iliac spine, and ischial tuberosity are usually the result of vigorous muscle contraction during running or jumping and are common in adolescents. Closed treatment usually results in restoration of function. Definitive management of pelvic ring and acetabular fractures usually involves closed treatment, including bed rest and traction, but may require external or internal fixation. Pelvic and retroperitoneal trauma are discussed in detail in Chapter 48.

Hip

Skeletal injuries about the hip include fractures of the femoral head and neck, intertrochanteric fracture, and dislocation. These injuries place the child at risk for avascular necrosis of the femoral head, which may lead to disturbance of growth or traumatic arthritis. Displaced proximal femoral fractures and anterior dislocations result in a foreshortened, extended, adducted, externally rotated thigh, whereas posterior dislocations result in a flexed, adducted, internally rotated thigh. Sciatic nerve injury may result, thus careful motor and sensory examination and documentation are required.

Adequate immobilization of the hip is usually possible with strategic placement of pillow bolsters. Dislocations require emergency reduction, but not before radiographs are obtained, as a fracture dislocation may complicate hip reduction. Radiographs of the hip should include the pelvis and the entire ipsilateral femur in anteroposterior and lateral views. Definitive treatment of hip dislocation requires early reduction to minimize the risk of avascular necrosis and to relieve pain. Adequate muscle relaxation is the key to a gentle reduction,

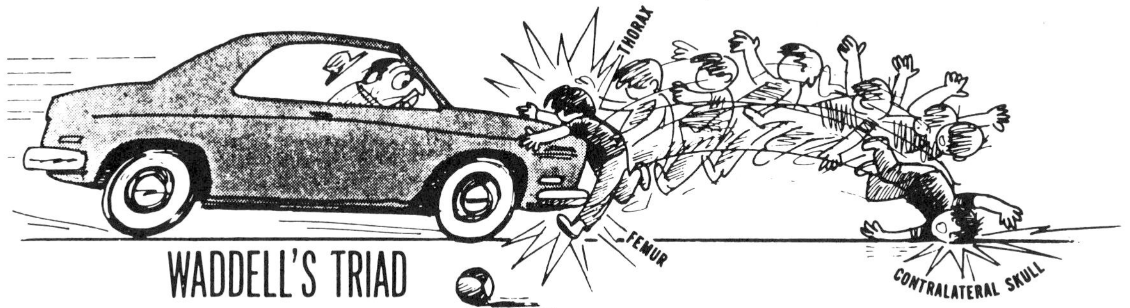

Figure 49–8 Waddel's triad of injuries in children. (From Rang M: *Children's fractures,* ed 2, Philadelphia, 1983, JB Lippincott.)

which may be accomplished in the emergency room or, with greater ease, with the child under a general anesthetic in the operating room. Fractures of the proximal femur may be treated by closed techniques with cast immoblization or by manipulation and percutaneous or open internal fixation methods, followed by cast immobilization or limited weight bearing.

Femoral shaft

Fracture of the femoral shaft is frequently the result of trauma caused by a motor vehicle. Concomitant injuries to the head and chest (Waddell's triad, Fig. 49-8) are common and should be sought. Hemorrhage owing to femoral shaft fracture in a child is usually less severe than in an adult and may contribute to but not cause shock. A child in shock is presumed to have other injuries (e.g. splenic rupture) until proven otherwise. Concomitant injuries of the ipsilateral hip or knee that may occur are sometimes difficult to document by physical examination because of the presence of the fractured femoral shaft. Therefore, radiographs must include the entire femur, hip and knee joints to avoid missing injuries about the joints.

Immobilization of the femur with a hairpin traction splint or Buck's traction can provide more comfort and reduction of hemorrhage than most splints. Definitive treatment commonly consists of immediate spica cast application, traction and delayed cast application, or closed intramedullary rodding. The choice of treatment is dependent on several factors, including the child's age, severity of injury, and the child's general condition. Close follow-up and allowances for the potential of femoral overgrowth results in minimal complications from treatment.

Knee

Skeletal injury about the knee includes supracondylar and Salter-Harris types I through V epiphyseal fractures of the distal femur, fractures of the proximal tibia, avulsion fractures of the tibial spine, patella, and anterior tibial tubercle, and dislocations of the knee. Ligamentous injuries are rare in the young child, but become more frequent as skeletal maturity occurs. The degrees of pain, swelling, and deformity experienced vary in proportion to the severity of the injury to the knee. Most knee injuries are due to direct trauma; motor vehicle crashes are the prime cause of high-energy trauma to the knee.

Injuries that result in displacement of the femur from the tibia, as in similar injuries about the elbow, can lead to severe complications, including compartment syndrome, tibial and peroneal nerve injury, and posterior tibial artery injury. Vigorous quadriceps contraction during the course of running, jumping, or kicking may cause avulsion fractures of the patella and anterior tibial tubercle, which results in a marked hemarthrosis and loss of ability to fully extend the knee. Hyperextension knee injury may result in avulsion fracture of the tibial spine. Injury of the knee generally results in swelling, or swelling and deformity, which may be marked; however, severe injury may occur without hemarthrosis because of a rupture of the knee joint capsule. When present, aspiration of a hemarthrosis may reveal fat globules within the aspirate, indicating the presence of an intraarticular fracture. Aspiration provides significant pain relief if the hemarthrosis is tense.

Very rapid swelling suggests the possibility of an arterial injury. If an arterial injury is suspected, a vascular surgery team is alerted immediately to minimize delay should arterial repair be needed. A careful examination for the location of tenderness indicates likely areas of pathology. Reserve manipulation of the knee until after review of radiographs. Immobilization of the knee, in the position found, with a long leg splint, application of ice packs, elevation of the extremity, and provision of appropriate analgesic can provide pain relief and prevent injury during transport and radiography.

Standard anteroposterior and lateral radiographs are essential initial views. Oblique views aid in the identification of nondisplaced fractures that might otherwise be missed. If no fractures are present, the stability of the knee is assessed by manual examination.

Early management involves close monitoring and documentation of the neurovascular status of the lower extremity, as indicated by the severity of injury and risk of complications. Reduction of a dislocation can often be accomplished in the emergency room because of a significant loss of ligamentous integrity. Muscle relaxation is key to reduction; therefore, reduction is often best accomplished with the child under general anesthesia. Epiphyseal fractures should be reduced under a local anesthetic with sedation, or preferably, a general anesthetic. Residual instability may be treated by nonoperative or operative means. Loss of reduction is common in epiphyseal fractures of the distal femur unless the child is placed in a hip spica cast or the fracture is stabilized with a percutaneous pin and a long leg cast. Therefore, general anesthesia increases treatment options. Definitive treatment of the variety of skeletal injury patterns that may affect the knee includes nonoperative and operative methods to obtain optional results.

Tibia and fibula

Fractures of the tibia and fibula are the most common injuries of the lower extremity in children. Fracture patterns vary relative to the child's age, the mechanism of injury, and the anatomic location of the injury. Physical findings of swelling and deformity are variable, depending on the degree of trauma and whether one or both bones are fractured. Indirect trauma caused by rotary forces, commonly the result of falls, produces oblique or spiral fractures. Direct trauma is a less common mechanism of injury and is usually associated with a transverse fracture pattern. Falls and motor vehicle crashes account for the majority of tibia and fibula fractures. Older children are at greater risk for fractures of this type caused by motor vehicle accidents because of the correlation of leg height with the height of a car bumper; whereas younger, shorter children are more likely to sustain a femur fracture. Because the tibia is subcutaneous throughout much of its length, open tibia fractures are common. Fractures of the tibia and fibula may be complete or incomplete and may involve one or both bones.

Signs and symptoms depend on the severity and mechanism of the injury. Young children may be seen to limp or to refuse to bear weight on the extremity, even with minimal to no history of trauma. Swelling can be so slight as to go unde-

tected. At the other extreme, swelling alone or swelling with deformity may leave no doubt about diagnosis. Nerve and vascular injuries and compartment syndromes may complicate tibia and fibula fractures. Complications of fracture healing may result in malunion, angular deformity, premature closure of the upper tibial physis, and leg-length discrepancy. Nonunion is rare and most likely associated with operative treatment.

Initial treatment should include a history of the injury, which indicates the potential for injuries to other body parts and the severity of the local injury. The neurovascular status of the lower extremity distal to the injury must be documented in the initial examination and, based on the risk of complications, in subsequent serial examinations. Pain out of proportion to the injury, tenderness over the muscles greater than the tenderness at the fracture site, and muscles that are hard on palpation suggest the existence of a compartment syndrome. It is important to document the presence and volume of the pulses, sensation, active motor function, and pain response to passive stretch of the muscles of the compartment in question. The anterior compartment is traversed by the common peroneal nerve and contains the anterior tibial, extensor hallucis longus, and extensor digitorum longus muscles. When untreated, the results are paralysis and contracture of the muscles and loss of sensation over the dorsum of the foot proximal to the web space between the great and second toes. The deep posterior compartment syndrome involves the posterior tibial nerve, which supplies the intrinsic muscles of the foot (except the extensor digitorum brevis, the flexor hallucis and flexor digitorum longus), the posterior tibial muscles, and the posterior tibial nerve and artery. The autonomous zone of sensation of the posterior tibial nerve is the plantar surface of the sole of the foot and the toes, excepting the instep.

First aid for fracture should include careful reduction of gross fracture displacement. Steady longitudinal traction applied to the leg through the ankle can improve alignment prior to application of a long leg splint. Care must be taken to avoid laceration of the skin on the sharp bone fragments. Avoid the use of constrictive bandages that increase the risk of compartment syndrome. Should arterial injury occur, the vascular surgery team performs immediate repair if indicated.

Standard radiographs in the anteroposterior and lateral projections should be obtained and supplemented with oblique views as needed to define nondisplaced fractures that might otherwise be missed.

Children with nondisplaced and torus fractures require application of a short or long leg cast, depending on the fracture pattern. The knee should be in the flexed position to prevent early weight bearing. Displaced tibia fractures require immobilization of the knee and ankle in a long leg splint. Parents must be instructed on how to perform a basic neurovascular examination (testing capillary refill, sensation, active motion, and pain response to passive motion of the toes) and a plan established for response to any abnormality. The application of ice packs for 48 hours and near-continuous elevation of the affected extremity above the level of the heart constitute treatment until the child is seen for the first orthopedic follow-up examination. Children who are at more than a minor risk for developing a compartment syndrome, including all with displaced tibia fractures, require admission to the hospital for observation and care overnight. Likewise, concerns over the adequacy of home monitoring justifies admission for 24 hours even in children deemed to have low risk for compartment syndrome. Definitive care of closed tibia and fibula fractures in children usually consists of nonoperative treatment; however, for open fractures, external fixation devices have an important role.

Ankle

Injury to the ankle is uncommon in young children, but increases in frequency with age. The incidence is highest in adolescents regularly involved in running sports. Injuries of the ankle are usually the result of indirect trauma that overloads the joint, exceeding the limits of the normal ranges of motion. Sprain is the most common injury, followed by fractures involving the growth plate. After growth plate closure (at 14 to 15 years of age), adult injury patterns emerge. Salter-Harris type I fractures of the distal fibula, followed by type II fractures of the distal tibia, are most common, whereas types III through V injuries are relatively less frequent. Growth arrest of the distal tibia or fibular physis may result in limb length discrepancy or angular deformity. Intraarticular fractures of the tibia (type III or IV) or talus may result in traumatic arthritis. Dislocation of the tibiotalar articulation may result in circulatory compromise, vascular injury, or nerve injury.

Children can have variable degrees of pain, swelling, deformity, and dysfunction, depending on the severity of trauma and the location of injury. Sprains result in swelling and tenderness that is greatest over the ligament, whereas fracture tenderness is greatest over the involved bone. A child in whom radiographic examination reveals no apparent abnormality, whose point of maximal tenderness is over the lateral malleolus rather than the anterior talofibular ligament, is more likely to have a nondisplaced type I fracture of the distal fibula epiphysis than a sprain. A careful physical exam-

ination of the lower extremity from the knee to the toes is indicated as more proximal injury may exist, such as the Maisonneuve lesion: proximal fibula fracture associated with medial ankle instability.

The neurovascular status of the extremities must be documented upon initial examination and prior to any manipulation of the ankle. If circulatory compromise exists in the instance of significant ankle deformity, immediate reduction of the deformity may restore circulation, thereby preventing serious complications. Reduction of the deformity with longitudinal traction applied to the foot should be maintained with a short leg splint.

Standard radiographic views for the assessment of ankle injuries consist of anteroposterior, lateral, and mortise (15° to 20° internal rotation) views of the ankle on a film long enough to include the knee joint on the anteroposterior and lateral views. Other oblique views of the ankle may be necessary to define the presence and extent of bony injuries.

Application of ice for 48 hours and near continuous elevation of the ankle, along with analgesic medication, are important elements in the control of acute pain. Treatment of grades I and II sprains may involve early motion, with or without selective immobilization, or a period of complete immobilization followed by motion therapy. Grades III and IV sprains frequently require surgery. Therefore, grading a sprain at the initial encounter is important; otherwise, the inevitable delay between initial and first follow-up examination can compromise the potential to obtain a good surgical treatment result. The treatment of fractures consists primarily of nonoperative methods. Operative treatment is primarily used for the management of displaced intraarticular fractures.

Foot

Fractures of the foot in children are caused by direct or indirect trauma; more complications are likely to result from high-energy injuries to the soft tissues and swelling than from fractures themselves. Displaced fractures of the talus carry a high risk of avascular necrosis; fortunately, most talus fractures are nondisplaced and heal well when placed in a cast. Fractures of the os calcis are infrequent in children and may be missed without an axial radiographic view. Midtarsal injury includes fracture and dislocation, usually resulting from high-energy rotational forces. Fracture of the metatarsals, however, commonly results from low energy trauma and may be a single or multiple.

Multiple metatarsal fractures and stress fractures produce varying degrees of forefoot tenderness and swelling. Radiographic examination of the entire foot and ankle is imperative, as traumatic metatarsal fractures may coexist with tarsal-metatarsal fractures; these injuries to the phalanges generally heal well if the toes are protected from further injury. However, intraarticular fractures of the great toe metatarsal phalangeal joint and epiphyseal fractures of the nail fold require adequate reduction and wound care, including open reduction to restore articular congruity when necessary.

Initial management requires observation for signs of injury and documentation of neurovascular status. Anteroposterior and lateral radiographs are obtained to define fractures, and additional views are taken as necessary. A bulky compressive dressing of pound cotton about the foot, fluffed cotton gauze squares between the toes, and elevation of the foot can retard swelling. A history of a severe injury or massive swelling is cause for admission to ensure adequate management of soft tissue injury and early detection of neurovascular problems. Treatment of foot fractures by closed techniques usually results in satisfactory healing. Displaced tarsal fracture, dislocation involving the tarsal bones, and intraarticular fracture, however, frequently require manipulation, or manipulation and fixation by percutaneous or open pinning.

Tennis shoes, the footwear of choice for children and adolescents, commonly harbor *Pseudomonas* species bacteria. Puncture wounds of the foot may result in *Pseudomonas* cellulitis, osteomyelitis, or septic arthritis of the foot. In cases of puncture wounds of the foot, take a culture, assure adequate tetanus immunization, and begin treatment with gentamicin. Should an established infection be present, more aggressive treatment may be indicated. If the bone changes to osteomyelitis, which takes 3 to 4 weeks to appear, operative irrigation and debridement are necessary.

SPECIAL CONSIDERATIONS
Obvious fracture trap

Avoid focusing on the obvious fracture. Such selective attention can lead to a failure to diagnose and to treat less obvious injuries and is a trap to be avoided. The discovery of a missed fracture or other skeletal injury after treatment of acute skeletal trauma results in prolonged suffering and expense for the child and parents, accusation and recrimination among the treatment team, and possible litigation. Late discovery of skeletal injuries is most often the result of an incomplete initial physical or radiographic examination of the child. Physical examination serves as a guide to appropriate radiographic examination. This is especially important in treatment of a child with multiple injury and of a child whose ability to communicate is limited in any way. Radiographs of the extremities must include the joints just proximal and distal to the bone of interest. The clinician should examine the radiograph in a systematic fashion, looking for subtle abnormalities of soft tissue and of

apparently intact bone before giving attention to any obvious injury. Only by complete and careful examination can a reduction in late diagnosis and complications occur.

Compartment syndrome

Compartment syndrome is defined as a symptom complex caused by elevated pressure of tissue in a closed osseofascial compartment of a limb that interferes with the circulation to the muscles and nerves of that compartment. Since 1881, when Richard von Volkmann first described a contracture involving the injured muscles and nerves of the forearm, correlations have been made between fractures, arterial injuries, embolus, postischemic edema, and external compression, with the occurrence of Volkmann's ischemic contracture.[7] The incidence of compartment syndrome varies from 1% to 30% in closed fractures, open fractures, venous injuries, and arterial injuries, in ascending order. Supracondylar fracture of the humerus, fracture of the radius and ulna, fracture of the femur treated with skin traction, and fracture of the tibia are the most common injuries associated with compartment syndrome and Volkmann's ischemic contracture.

The normal tissue fluid pressure within a compartment of an extremity is 3 or 4 torr. Normal perfusion pressure of muscles is 30 torr. Compartment pressure may rise in response to intrinsic or extrinsic causes. Any condition that increases the content of the compartment (intrinsic) or decreases the compartment volume (extrinsic) will raise compartment pressure and possibly lead to the development of a compartment syndrome.

Compartment content may be increased by hemorrhage following severe soft tissue injuries or fractures, by increased capillary permeability following burns, and by temporary periods of ischemia following arterial injuries. Compartment syndrome associated with arterial injury usually develops after arterial flow is restored. Ischemic injury of the muscle that occurs between the time of arterial injury and its repair leads to an increase in capillary permeability. Therefore, once arterial flow is reestablished, renewed blood flow increases fluid transudation across the capillary, which causes interstitial fluid pressure to rise. When the end-closing pressure of the muscle arterioles is exceeded, blood will cease to enter the muscle compartment and shunting will occur. A rise in pressure sufficient to cause complete muscle ischemia need not be great enough to occlude major arteries traversing the compartment. Therefore, *pulses are present* in an acute compartment syndrome and pulselessness is a late finding of this disorder.

Ischemia of muscles and nerves may result in tissue injury or destruction, depending on the completeness and duration of the ischemic event. Permanent loss of nerve function and muscle integrity occurs after 8 to 12 hours of complete ischemia. The results are contracture of the muscles of the compartment and sensory loss in the distribution of the nerves that traverse the compartment. If relief from ischemia occurs in less than 6 hours, muscle and nerve injury is completely reversible.

The diagnosis of compartment syndrome is often difficult, and delay in diagnosis, which is all too common, risks disaster. The single most important symptom is pain out of proportion to the injury. Fracture immobilization usually provides instant reduction in pain. Persistence of pain after fracture reduction and immobilization can be attributed to ischemia, until proven otherwise. Children who need frequent administration of analgesia or who complain loudly about pain require careful examination for signs of a compartment syndrome. The pain is constant and unrelieved by elevating the limb or splitting the cast. The most reliable clinical signs of compartment syndrome include severe pain on passive motion of the involved compartment, pain on palpation of the involved compartment, and sensory deficit in the distribution of any nerves traversing the compartment. A careful sensory examination is essential. Young children are apt to respond that they "can feel" sensation discriminately if they are allowed to see the area of skin being tested. Response to pain and sensation depend on an alert and conscious child. A child with a long bone fracture, who is unconscious or has a head injury, and an alert child with equivocal signs must undergo invasive compartment pressure measurement by a needle manometer, wick catheter, or slit catheter technique.

The differential elements in diagnosis of compartment syndrome in a child include arterial injury, peripheral nerve injury, and a complaining, uncooperative child. The former two must be ruled out before the latter circumstance is credited. In the absence of arterial injury, pulses and even adequate capillary refill are usually present in an acute compartment syndrome. Treatment of an acute compartment syndrome by clinical diagnosis or by compartment manometry (compartment pressure 30 to 35 torr, or 10 to 30 torr < diastolic pressure) must be via an appropriate fasciotomy of the involved compartment. There is no role for operative management in established cases.

CONCLUSION

The presenting symptoms of child trauma victims are pain and some degree of anxiety and apprehension, which is shared by their parents. Although management of the child's physical injuries is of first priority, attention must be given to the psychological response to pain and the loss of sense of control experienced by the child and parents. Physical pain will respond substantially to analgesia and local measures. Psychological stress diminishes gradually when there is an understanding of the extent of the injury and requirements for proper treatment. Clear communication, concise, simple, and understandable, begins the care of the child. Complications such as growth plate injury, and especially, neurovascular injury must be documented and, time permitting, explained to parents prior to therapeutic intervention. This sequence minimizes the possibility that liability for any posttraumatic deformity or dysfunction will be attributed to the treatment rendered. Accurate documentation is the best protection against litigation.

Once acute care is complete, follow-up care proceeds. A child with a fracture should be seen in 24 to 72 hours; occasionally, within 1 week, depending on the location and nature of the injury. Children with adequate immobilization of a fracture quickly resume a level of activity that approaches the premorbid level. Slower progress may result from failure to elevate the extremity, to apply ice appropriately, and to remove the cast or splint. Communication with the child and parent, including home care instruction, and the provision of sturdy splints, helps to childproof the gains of initial management until the first follow-up visit. Fracture care commonly results in a relatively long child and parent relationship with the physician. Although some fractures heal well with nothing more than first aid measures, early and close follow-up care by an orthopedic surgeon is important to ensure that the concerns of the child and parents receive proper attention, especially in achievement of the goals of definitive fracture management, relief of pain, prevention of deformity, and restoration of optimal function.

REFERENCES

1. Bonica J. *The management of pain* ed 2, Philadelphia, 1990, Lea & Febiger.
2. Gustilo RB, editor: *Orthopaedic infection: diagnosis and treatment*, Philadelphia, 1989, WB Saunders.
3. NCHS: Current estimates from the national health interview survey. United States, 1980, DHS Publication No. (PHS) 82-1567. Hyattsville, MD, National Center for Health Statistics 1981.
4. Rang M: *Children's fractures* ed 2, Philadelphia, 1983, JB Lippincott.
5. Rockwood CA Jr, Wilklins KE, King RE: *Fractures in children*, Philadelphia, 1991, JB Lippincott.
6. Salter RB, Harris WR: Injuries involving the epiphyseal plate, *J Bone Joint Surg* 45A(3):587-622, 1963.
7. von Volkmann R: Die ischaemischen muskelahmungen and kontrakturen, *Zentralbl Chir* 8:801, 1881.
8. Willis RB, Rorabeck CH: Treatment of compartment syndrome in children, *Orth Clin N Am* 21(2):401-412, 1990.
9. Wu KK: *Techniques in surgical casting and splinting*, Philadelphia, 1987, Lea & Febiger.

  Crush Injury and Compartment Syndrome

William W. Robertson, Jr.

In a 1964 article for the *American Journal of Public Health*, J.E. Press noted that there were 100,000 accidents per year involving washing machine wringers and children under 15 years of age.[5] At that time most crush injuries of an extremity were caused in accidents with this common household appliance. Although the etiology of this entity was readily apparent and its treatment well described, the pathophysiology was not well understood. In his paper, Press does not mention anatomical compartments nor tissue pressures.

Another well-described entity, Volkmann's ischemic contracture, has been the bane of physicians who treat elbow fractures in children. Vascular compromise and constrictive dressings were known to lead to muscle necrosis, scarring, and contractures.

In the 1970s the common mechanism of these and numerous other problems was found to be increased intracompartmental pressure. A compartment syndrome results from increased pressure within a closed anatomic area, which causes compromise of the circulation and function of the tissues within that space.[1]

Compartment syndromes can occur in any anatomic site in which fascia tightly binds muscle groups. The most familiar regions for the occurrence of compartment syndrome are the four compartments of the lower leg (Fig. 50-1). However, the process can occur in many other sites, including the buttocks and the intrinsic muscles of the hand.

There are no major differences between children and adults in the presentation or treatment of compartment syndromes. In spite of the child's increased tolerance of injury, the most significant determinant of the outcome of compartment syndrome treatment in children is the duration of symptoms prior to decompression of the compartment.[2] Prompt recognition of the potential for development of ischemia from increased pressure can lead to timely decompression prophylaxis and treatment of the potentially maiming condition.

ETIOLOGY

An increase in the tissue pressures in a compartment can be produced by "exogenous" sources, resulting in a decrease in the size of the compartment, or by "endogenous" problems, which result in an increase in the contents of the compartment.

A decrease in the volume of a compartment can result from constricting dressings or casts. Localized external pressure resulting from the "old-fashioned" wringer injury or the "new-fashioned" compression caused by lying on an arm following a drug overdose also leads to increased compartmental pressure owing to a decrease in volume. Surgical repair of a fascial defect can also lessen the size of a compartment.

The volume of the contents of a compartment can increase as a result of intracompartmental bleeding. This can be due to laceration of vessels, bleeding from fractured bone, surgical bleeding, anticoagulation therapy, or hemorrhagic dyscrasia. Interstitial edema can also increase intracompartmental volume. Edema can result any time vascular permeability is increased, such as during muscular ischemia, exercise, or trauma, or with burns, snake bites, intraarterial infusions, or surgical manipulation of tissue. Elevated intracapillary pressure and subsequent edema may result from venous obstruction. Muscular hypertrophy can increase the intracompartmental pressures and lead to a chronic elevated pressure syndrome. An additional cause of increased intracompartmental volume is intravenous infusion infiltration.

Compartmental tamponade, no matter what the cause, gives rise to arteriolar spasm. This effect may be aggravated by shock and extremity elevation. The resulting decrease in arteriolar pressure diminishes tissue perfusion and leads to closure of the arterioles. Tissue necrosis begins if the process is not reversed within 4 hours. Low tissue perfusion causes increased capillary permeability, increasing interstitial leakage, and increasing compartment content. The vicious circle continues, causing irreversible muscle death.

DIAGNOSIS

The clinical diagnosis of a compartment syndrome is not very accurate. Because intracompartmental pressures of 30 to 60 mm Hg can begin the process, they are not sufficient to obliterate the arterial pulse

548

pressures that traverse the involved compartment. That is, a full-blown compartment syndrome may occur with distal pulses remaining intact. For the same reason, skin color is a poor indicator of compartment compromise. Nerve function may be a more sensitive test inasmuch as hypesthesia and paresthesia may occur within 30 minutes of the onset of intracompartmental ischemia. Pain upon passive stretching of the muscles of the involved compartment is the most sensitive clinical test for compartment ischemia. However, this test is of little use in the unresponsive patient or in the patient whose extremity is insensate.

Because the development of a compartment syndrome is time related, sequential reexamination is mandatory for the child who is at high risk for compartment compromise.

The earliest indicator of incipient compartment problems is increased interstitial fluid pressure, which may be directly measured by needles introduced into the affected compartment and into other surrounding compartments for comparison.[4] Arterial pressures are measured concurrently to determine the perfusion gradient within the compartment. Gradients of less than 30 mm Hg suggest the need for decompression fasciotomy.

TREATMENT

In children who are suspected of developing a compartment syndrome, the first step in treatment of the compression is to relieve any constricting bandages and remove any casts from the extremity. It is interesting to note that the compression caused by pneumatic antishock trousers has been implicated in the development of compartment syndromes in some severely injured children.

Infrequently, diuretics may be employed in the early stages of the syndrome if this treatment is not otherwise medically contraindicated.

Surgical fasciotomy is required early in the course of the problem. The fasciotomy must relieve the pressures throughout the compartment involved and must be performed on all involved compartments. The schematic approach to a two-incision, four-compartment fasciotomy of the leg is illustrated in Fig. 50-2. Of course, the fascia and skin are not closed at the time of a fasciotomy. Further wound care may involve debridement of necrotic

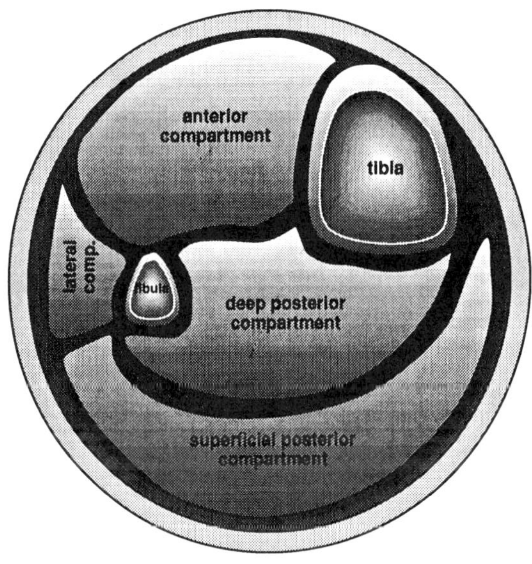

Figure 50–1 The four compartments of the lower leg.

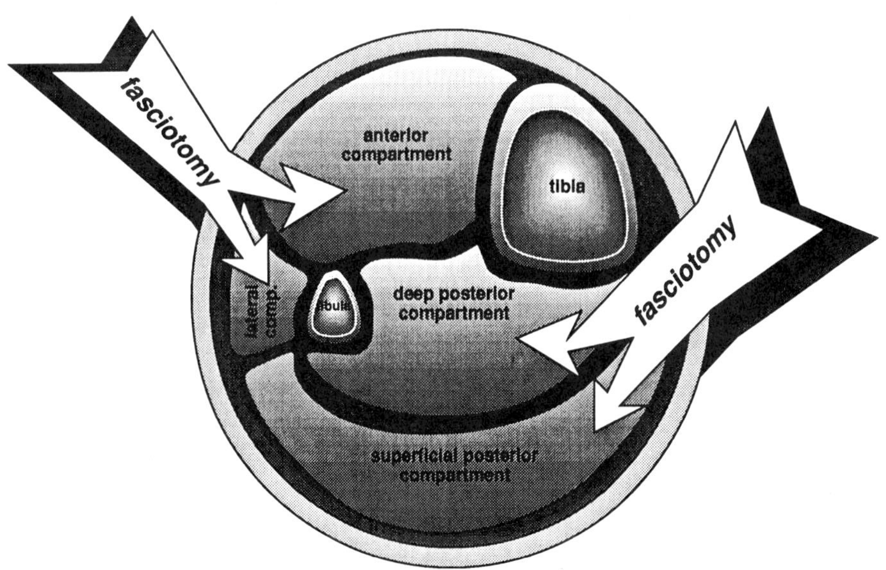

Figure 50–2 The schematic approach to a two-incision, four-compartment fasciotomy of the leg.

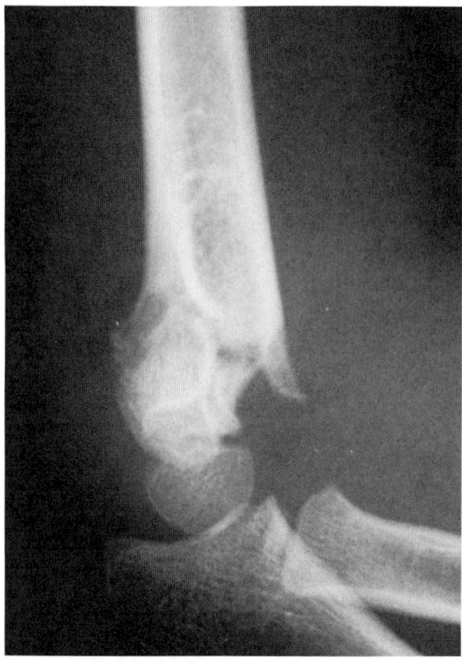

Figure 50–3 A displaced supracondylar fracture of the distal humerus in a child.

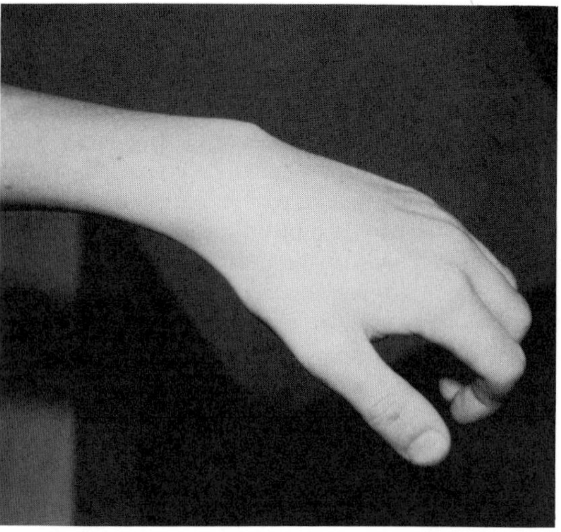

Figure 50–4 The hand of a child following a Volkmann's ischemia.

muscle and delayed skin closure or application of skin grafts.

The use of splints and physical or occupational therapy is necessary for restoration of function following fasciotomy. Internal or external fixation of fractures may aid wound care and speed rehabilitation.

PROPHYLAXIS

Because the greatest determinant of the outcome of a compartment syndrome is the time of ischemia, prevention of increased pressure is the best treatment. Careful handling of tissue, in both traumatic wounds and fresh surgical incisions, will diminish edema after surgery. In sites that are known to have a high risk of subsequent compartment compromise, such as the leg and forearm, internal or external skeletal fixation and splint application are preferable to constrictive dressings and casts.

Prophylactic fasciotomy should be performed in cases where limb ischemia time from vascular injury or occlusion is greater than 4 hours. Extremities with shorter ischemic times require close observation. When prophylactic fasciotomy is performed for significant ischemia, all compartments distal to the occlusion should be opened; these include the intrinsic compartments of the hands and feet. Prophylactic fasciotomy for a localized crush injury requires decompression of only the involved compartments.

In the case of crush injuries with concomitant amputation, a compartment that is transected by the amputation does not need fasciotomy. However, all the muscles of the compartment will swell into the open amputation site when a significant crush or ischemia occurs. As in fasciotomy, the fascia and skin layers of these wounds should not be closed.

COMPLICATIONS

The most significant complication of an incompletely treated or unrecognized compartment syndrome is ischemic contracture. The classic example is Volkmann's ischemic contracture following a displaced supracondylar fracture of the distal humerus in a child (such as the fracture pictured in Fig. 50-3). The spike of anterior humeral cortex of the proximal fragment may injure the brachial artery at the elbow. That injury, followed by constricting casting, has been known to lead to a compartment syndrome of the deep and superficial compartments of the forearm. The dead muscle contracts and heals into fibrous scar tissue. Function is limited not only by the degree to which nerve function returns, but also by the physical contractures of the soft tissues. Figure 50-4 shows the hand of a child following such a Volkmann's ischemia. Occasionally, tendon transfers and releases may make the extremity more functional.

Another aspect of the spectrum of crush injuries is the development of a "crush syndrome."[3] Crush syndrome is the end-stage systemic manifestation of muscle necrosis. If compartment pressure is not relieved and the involved muscle dies, the muscle releases myoglobin as it degrades. The myoglobin circulates to the kidney, where it causes renal failure. Also in muscle degradation, there is an increasing third-space fluid loss leading to shock, increasing acidosis, and hyperkalemia, which can precipitate cardiac arrhythmia. Treatment of this syndrome consists of resuscitation of the child from hypovolemic shock with intravenous fluids. Because the development of a crush syndrome is time related, early surgical fasciotomy will prevent its appearance.

Another complication of a compartment syndrome is the loss of the involved extremity. Amputation may be required if secondary infection makes the distal extremity nonviable or if nerve loss is permanent, leaving an insensate foot.

REFERENCES

1. Matsen FA: Compartmental syndrome: a unified concept, *Clin Orthop* 113:3-14, 1975.
2. Matsen FA, Veith G: Compartmental syndromes in children, *J Pediatr Orthop* 1:33-41, 1981.
3. Mubarak SJ, Owen CA: Compartmental syndrome and its relation to the crush syndrome: a spectrum of disease, *Clin Orthop* 113:81-89, 1975.
4. Mubarak SJ, Rorabeck CH: Treatment of compartment syndromes. In Dudley H, Carter DC, Russell RCG, editors: *Rob and Smith's Operative Surgery*, ed 4, London, 1989, Butterworth and Co, pp 585-594.
5. Press JE: Wringer washing machine injuries, *Am J Public Health* 54:812, 1964.

51 Amputation

William W. Robertson, Jr.

The indications for amputation in cases of extremity trauma have been widely discussed.[2,8,12,13] At times early amputation is considered to be the "conservative" approach to massive injury.[12] When weighed against the time, energy, and emotional upheaval involved in the salvage of an extremely compromised extremity, the immediate mobilization and rehabilitation possible with amputation may become the deciding factors.

The frequently mentioned indications for amputation—crush injury (or irreparable soft tissue damage); vascular compromise (including failure of revascularization); irreparable neurologic loss; complex fractures; wound sepsis; and burns—have been refined through the use of various injury scores[7,9,10] as predictive indicators of outcome. Although these indices have not found universal acceptance, their use has facilitated decision making in treatment of the severely injured patient and can be applied to such problems as possible replantation of amputated extremities.[8]

Even in cases of severe trauma, the extremity salvage rate in children may be higher than reported in the literature on adults. Type III-C fractures of the tibia (open fractures with concomitant arterial injury requiring repair) commonly lead to amputation in adults.[4] Buckley[3] reports the salvage of two lower extremities with type III-C fractures of the tibia in children.

Although the indications for early amputation must be individualized, the Mangled Extremity Severity Score (MESS) of Johansen[10] is a useful tool in the evaluation of children (Table 51-1). This scale uses a combination of points related to four categories: skeletal and soft tissue injury, limb ischemia, shock, and age. The last category is not relevant in children because no "points" are added for any patient's age under 30 years. The most heavily weighted criterion is ischemia, the points for which double after 6 hours from the time of injury. A MESS score of 7 or more predicts a nonsalvageable extremity.

TECHNIQUES: CHILD VERSUS ADULT

The techniques of amputation in the child vary from those recommended for adults primarily in the level of amputation.[1] In a child, every effort must be made to preserve length of the involved extremity. A longer remaining limb provides better proprioception, energy efficiency when walking, self-image, and weight distribution in the prosthetic socket. Modern bone lengthening (Ilizarov) technology[5] can be employed to lengthen a short amputation stump, but only after growth has ceased. This technique is also limited by the soft tissue over the transected bone.

The weight-bearing end of the stump should be full thickness, mobile, and preferably sensate skin. The traditional anterior- and posterior-based flaps of equal length can be altered significantly in a child as long as the skin has adequate circulation. Neurovascular pedicle flaps (such as the latissimus

Table 51–1 Mangled Extremity Severity Score variables*

	Points
Skeletal/soft tissue injury	
Low energy (stab, simple fracture, "civilian" gunshot wound)	1
Medium injury (open or multiple fractures, dislocation)	2
High energy (close-range shotgun or "military" gunshot wound)	3
Very high energy (above + gross contamination, soft tissue avulsion)	4
Limb ischemia	
Pulse reduced or absent but perfusion normal	1
Pulseless, paresthesia, diminished capillary refill	2
Cool, paralyzed, insensate, numb	3
Points are doubled for ischemia >6 hours.	
Shock	
Systolic pressure >90 mm Hg	0
Hypotensive transiently	1
Persistent hypotension	2

*Modified for children—no age variable

dorsi flap in the upper extremity of the lateral prox-imal gastrocnemius flap in the lower extremity) and the technique of tissue expansion improve distal skin coverage. Rotation of sensate flaps from non–weight-bearing portions of the stump to the weight-bearing surface may allow preservation of addi-tional length. Closure of the non–weight-bearing donor site is possible with full- or split-thickness skin grafts. Free neurovascular pedicle grafts are not so desirable for the weight-bearing end of the extremity because of variable sensory return. They are, however, preferable to full- or split-thickness grafts that contact the distal prosthetic socket.

Another imperative in amputation technique for children is to preserve all epiphyses possible. There are two reasons for this principle, both related to growth problems. The first is that although the stump will remain constant in length in adults, it will become relatively shorter in children with growth plate injury. Meanwhile, intact physes will allow growth of the remaining extremity. The sec-ond growth problem with children's amputations occurs with through-bone amputations. When a distal epiphysis is not present, overgrowth of the bone in the stump occurs in 12% to 20% of chil-dren. This may take the form of bony spurs, which can penetrate the end of a stump and therefore require revision of the amputation. Preservation of the distal physis prevents this problem. For this reason through-joint amputations in children are preferred to amputations through bone proximal to the physis.[6]

There is a caveat to this principle. In spite of the emphasis on maintenance of a distal physis, the importance of a motored, functional knee joint in a prosthetic gait is paramount. Given a choice between a short below-knee amputation and one at a through-knee level, one should always choose the lower level if the knee joint is normal.

PROSTHETICS AND REHABILITATION

The fitting of prostheses following amputation in children may be done as soon as the wound is closed. In clean lower extremity amputations, this can happen at the time of surgery with the use of an "instant-fit" prosthesis. The instant-fit prosthesis has a plaster socket that is molded to the stump on the operating room table. The socket is then at-tached to a pylon and a prosthetic foot. Weight bearing can begin as soon as the child's general condition warrants. Formal gait training with phys-ical therapy does not have to wait for the "tem-porary" prosthesis, which will follow once the stump has reached its residual size and shape. Fig-ure 51-1 shows a boy in his temporary prosthesis, following a below-knee injury. External knee hinges substitute for injured knee ligaments.

If the fitting of a prosthesis is delayed for any reason (because of the stump wound, other injuries, or the child's general condition), physical therapy should begin as soon as possible after injury to prepare the child for ambulation when other factors permit.

For children, acceptance of a lower extremity prosthesis and rehabilitation to independent am-bulation occur rapidly. Growth is a problem in the lower-extremity amputee as the volume of the stump increases with growth. Changes in length of the legs are easily handled with lengthening of the prosthesis. Newer technology has provided the means to fabricate "sports" prostheses that more nearly mimic normal joint motion, weigh less, and allow energy "storage" in the prosthetic mechanism for activities such as jumping.

There is greater acceptance of a prosthesis in the upper extremity if it is fitted before the child is 2 years of age. Because of the fine motor control required in the hand, the artificial hand is at best a useful tool to assist the normal extremity. My-oelectric prostheses remain expensive in terms of financial outlay and "down time" required for re-pairs and maintenance.

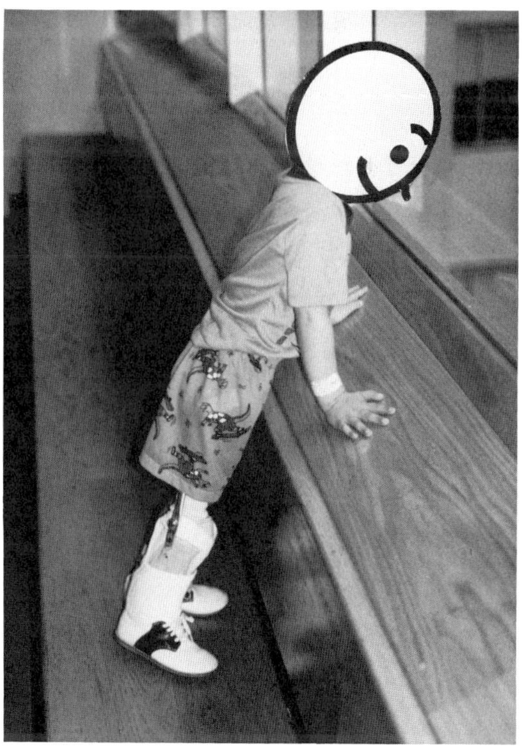

Figure 51–1 Boy in a temporary prosthesis following a below-knee injury.

REFERENCES

1. Aitken GT. Surgical amputation in children, *J Bone Joint Surg* 45A:1735-1741, 1963.
2. Bondurant FJ, Cotler HB, Buckle R et al: The medical and economic impact of severely injured lower extremities, *J Trauma* 28:1270-1273, 1988.
3. Buckley SL, Smith G, Sponseller PD et al: Open fractures of the tibia in children, *J Bone Joint Surg* 72A:1462-1469, 1990.
4. Caudle RJ, Stern PJ: Severe open fractures of the tibia, *J Bone Joint Surg* 69A:801-807, 1987.
5. Eldridge JC, Armstrong PF, Krajbich JI: Amputation stump lengthening with the Ilizarov technique, *Clin Orthop* 256:76-79, 1990.
6. Gillespie R: Principles of amputation surgery in children with longitudinal deficiencies of the femur, *Clin Orthop* 256:29-38, 1990.
7. Gregory RT, Gould RJ, Peclet M et al: The mangled extremity syndrome (M.E.S.): a severity grading system for multisystem injury of the extremity, *J Trauma* 25:1147-1150, 1985.
8. Hervé C, Gaillard M, Andrivet P et al: Treatment of serious lower limb injuries: amputation versus preservation, *Injury* 18:21-23, 1987.
9. Howe HR, Poole GV, Hansen KJ et al: Salvage of lower extremities following combined orthopedic and vascular trauma, *Am Surg* 53:205-208, 1987.
10. Johansen K, Daines M, Howey T et al: Objective criteria accurately predict amputation following lower extremity trauma, *J Trauma* 30:568-573, 1990.
11. Pozo JL, Powell B, Andrews BG et al: The timing of amputation for lower limb trauma, *J Bone Joint Surg* 72B:288-292, 1990.
12. Seiler JG, Richardson JD: Amputation after extremity injury, *Am J Surg* 152:260-264, 1986.
13. Weaver FA, Rosenthal RE, Waterhouse G et al: Combined skeletal and vascular injuries of the lower extremities, *Am Surg* 50:189-197, 1984.
14. Zong-Wei C, Meyer V, Kleinert HE et al: Present indications and contraindications for replantation as reflected by long term functional results, *Orthop Clin N Am* 12:849-870, 1981.

Environmental Injuries

52 Intentional Injury: Abuse

Mireille B. Kanda, Lavdena A. Orr, Sheryl Brissett-Chapman and Tobey S. Lawson

An oft-asked question in a trauma center is, "How did this happen?" The answer may be routine, obvious, or unimportant, or the answer—the real truth—may be fraught with significance if it involves *intentional* injury. Sometimes intentionality is obvious in the presenting symptoms of a child. At other times suspicion is triggered by identification of one of a number of patterns of injury commonly associated with maltreatment of children. Questions may also be raised by repeated requests for care of a chronic illness coupled with previous noncompliance with a prescribed regimen.

Although child victimization by parents and other caregivers has come into recognition by both professionals and the general public during the past decade, it remains a poorly identified, inadequately understood, and greatly understated phenomenon. Most adults experience tremendous inner resistance to even visualizing sexual or physical exploitation of the "innocent, defenseless" young. Traditional rhetoric about the family—let alone the concurrent debates about the economic and political meaning of valuing and supporting the family—also makes it almost unthinkable to many adults (including medical professionals) that parents may be maltreating their own child. Unexamined and unsupported assumptions about the socioeconomic privilege of some parents may make such incidents even more incomprehensible to the physician or nurse.

In 1961, however, Dr. C. Henry Kempe described the battered child syndrome and thus led the way for the medical community—assisted by the contributions of several allied disciplines—to establish scientifically based diagnoses of child abuse and neglect. Since then, the number of identified victims has continued to increase relentlessly. Part of this increase has been due to new legal mandates for reporting child maltreatment, which are now in effect in all 50 states and the District of Columbia.

Yet there is another set of causes for the rise in reported numbers of child victims. Social phenomena such as increased poverty, substance abuse by parents, domestic violence, and community violence have assuredly contributed to the multiplication of cases of abuse and neglect. When 2.5 million cases of suspected maltreatment are reported every year—with the rate of occurrence doubtless much higher—it is inevitable that every single facility offering pediatric care will encounter maltreated children.

The spectrum of child victimization has been classified into four broad categories: physical abuse, sexual abuse, emotional abuse, and child neglect. These kinds of maltreatment are typically defined in terms of parental accountability and include acts of commission or omission on the part of parents and substitute caregivers. The systematic study of child maltreatment is relatively new, and the definition of *intentionality* is approached gingerly and more as a means of separating unintentional injuries from those caused directly by a caregiver or allowed to occur as a result of inadequate parental performance. In many cases of child abuse or neglect, even those resulting in death, it is difficult to ascertain and to conclude that a parent premeditated the harmful behavior. For the purpose of this discussion, the term intentional abuse will be used as a general equivalent of the four areas outlined above.

Because of the complexities of assessing and of intervening in cases of child maltreatment, the suspicion or disclosure of childhood victimization warrants a multidisciplinary, multiagency approach that can respond to the medical, mental health, and legal issues of the situation. Despite the current inability to predict precisely the actual long-term effects of child maltreatment, it is generally acknowledged that the disclosure or discovery of abuse and the subsequent intervention by various professionals typically precipitate a psychosocial crisis for both the child victim and the family. A competent professional response is necessarily a team approach, one that is both specialized and comprehensive.

The three major dimensions of the professional response, discussed in following sections, are medical intervention, psychosocial intervention, and legal issues.

MEDICAL INTERVENTION

In addition to its primary diagnostic and therapeutic goals, medical evaluation of traumatic injuries in children serves to establish a reasonable basis for suspicion of abuse and neglect, and to differentiate intentional injuries from events that may have been beyond the control of a child's caregiver. Gathering data for a complete medical history is extremely important, a process requiring organization, thoroughness, and patience. Historical data may be obtained from a variety of sources including eyewitnesses, emergency transport personnel, and emergency room staff. Because most injuries occur to young children in the home or under the supervision of primary caregivers, the participation of parents or caregivers is crucial to an understanding of the course of events leading to a child's injuries. Regardless of initial suspicions, parents or caregivers should be approached in a courteous, nonjudgmental, and nonthreatening manner, and the history gathered objectively. Historical information must include the circumstances of the injury, the past medical history, the developmental history of the child, and, finally, an assessment of family dynamics. Table 52-1 lists the areas to be explored during the interview.

Age and abuse

It is crucial to determine the developmental status of a child in order to assess the veracity of the explanation for injury offered by a caregiver. A detailed discussion of developmental milestones is beyond the scope of this chapter but is readily available in standard pediatric texts. Suffice it to say that motor development is determined by age and that even the most precocious child cannot attain milestones sometimes claimed or expected by parents.

Conversely, the particular age of children may predispose them to certain injuries that can be inflicted by others. For example, most shake-impact injuries resulting in closed head trauma occur in infants and children below age 2. Some behaviors prevalent at this age (persistent crying and lack of control over elimination) may be particularly annoying to caregivers, resulting in frustration expressed by shaking, hitting, or immersing the child in hot water. In older children, however, injuries are more likely to be related to neglect or to inappropriate techniques of discipline.

Explanation of injury

An explanation given by a parent or caregiver to describe trauma sustained by a child may be inconsistent or even implausible when compared with the developmental stage of the child or with the unique features of the injuries—specifically, type,

Table 52–1 Historical information pertinent in the evaluation of intentional injury

Circumstances that led to injury

Exact time and place
Location of injury
Child's symptoms at the time of injury
Child's condition prior to acute injury
Development of symptoms over time
Chronology of events between onset of symptoms and seeking of medical intervention
Eyewitnesses accounts

Past medical history

Previous trauma
Prior hospitalizations
Other illnesses
Immunization status
Routine health care supervision
Medication history
Brief review of systems

Developmental history

Milestones
Delays
Unusual or unexpected behaviors
Child's personality traits

Family psychosocial profile (Social worker, nurse, or other team member can gather this data.)

Household configuration and composition
Siblings or other children in the home
Primary caregiver or multiple caregivers
Child care arrangements
Other environmental factors: poverty, poor housing, family losses, alcohol use, substance abuse, domestic violence, physical or psychiatric impairment of parent(s)

age, severity, and multiplicity. Table 52-2 presents a list of factors that should raise the practitioner's level of suspicion.

The child must be interviewed apart from the accompanying adult, if at all possible. This gives the examiner a chance to establish rapport with the child, to ask questions freely, and to provide an opportunity for the child to impart information that might not be offered spontaneously in the presence of the parent. The examiner should be careful not to suggest any explanation to the child but, rather, in age-appropriate language, should ask open-ended questions and convey clearly a desire to help the child. Promises to protect the child from any harm should not be made, however, because failure to carry out impossible promises may further increase the child's sense of betrayal and powerlessness.

Table 52–2 Factors suggestive of intentional injury

Lack of explanation
Discrepancy between history and physical presentation
  Injury pattern
  Child's development
Changing stories
  Unexplained or inappropriate
Delay in seeking care
Assignation of blame to another
  Patient
  Sibling
  Pet

Table 52–3 Age estimation of bruises

Age of bruise	Discoloration
<24 hours	Red to blue or purple
1 to 5 days	Blue to purple
5 to 7 days	Green
10 to 14 days	Yellow to brown
2 to 4 weeks	Resolution

Adapted from Wilson EF: Estimation of the age of cutaneous contusions in child abuse, *Pediatrics* 60:750, 1977.

Additional, and sometimes invaluable, information may be obtained from emergency transport personnel, who may be able to report specifics about the condition of the site where injury occurred (e.g., hot or cold water in the tub, no food in house, evidence of alcohol or drug abuse), the condition of other siblings, the behavior of the child in the field, and the caregiver's initial behavior and explanation.

Issues specific to sexual abuse

Acute care facilities are currently encountering an increasing number of children who present with expressed suspicion (an allegation by an accompanying adult), or disclosure by the child, of sexual abuse. There are yet other children who raise the suspicions of acute-care professionals because presenting symptoms (e.g., abdominal pain, genital trauma, evidence of sexually transmitted disease) strongly suggest the possibility of sexual victimization.

The general principles of history gathering apply to these children and their families, but there are important differences. Although the physical trauma exhibited may not be as dramatic, particularly in young children, the dynamics of the abusive situation may often be more complex and the possibility of denial on the part of both the family and the professionals involved may be even greater. The examiner should guard carefully against underestimating or trivializing the significance or consequences to the child in sexually abusive situations.

Physical examination

The physical examination of a battered, sexually abused, or neglected child must be complete and thorough. The careful, caring examiner can sometimes discover physical injuries not revealed in the history, and the time spent with the child can pro-vide an opportunity to obtain further information. During the physical examination, the physician may inspect the injuries and inquire about the way the child was hurt.

Objective documentation of pertinent physical findings, as well as lack of physical findings, is necessary. The absence of external injury never rules out abuse. Children with severe cranial or intraabdominal trauma may have no visible, external trauma. The tools necessary for examination include a good light source, measuring tape, and anatomic diagrams for labeling the size, color, location, and shape of injuries. Any photographs taken by medical personnel must be labeled with patient name, date, name of photographer, and a brief legend. If indicated, appropriate written consent should be obtained from the parent prior to photographic documentation. Photographs and diagrams must be secured with the medical record.

Sites of intentional injury

Signs and symptoms of maltreatment may be limited to one organ system (e.g., bruises) or may affect multiple organ systems (e.g., burns that destroy soft tissue, resulting in overwhelming secondary infection, cardiovascular compromise, and respiratory distress). Abuse-related trauma may range from no physical morbidity (e.g., healed rib fracture) to extensive sequelae (e.g., neurologic impairment from closed head trauma).

The skin and soft tissues are the most common sites of manifestations of intentional injury. Bruises, abrasions, contusions, lacerations, and burns represent a substantial proportion of abusive injuries. Bruises in particular may be in various stages of healing, may be evident at multiple body sites, and often have distinctive patterns characteristic of the instrument of abuse (handprints, loop marks, slap marks, bite marks, grab marks). Typical sites for intentional injury include the face, trunk, buttocks, earlobe, neck, and frenulum of the tongue. The age of a bruise may be estimated by its color, as described in Table 52-3.

Bite marks may suggest intentional injury, depending on location, size, shape, and configuration.

Burns of the extremities are suspicious if both sides are involved in a symmetrical and circumferential pattern. Isolated circular lesions with deep ulcerated centers on the palms or soles may represent cigarette burns.

Extraocular and intraocular damage may result from intentional injury. Periorbital soft tissue ecchymosis and hyphema may result from blunt trauma, from a punch or from a belt buckle injury. Dislocated lens, detached retina, and retinal hemorrhage may result from traumatic head injury. Retinal hemorrhage may be a further clue to intracerebral damage, particularly subdural and subarachnoid hematoma in infants and children who have otherwise unexplained central nervous system symptoms. Retinal hemorrhages may last from 3 to 21 days. An intraocular examination by an ophthalmologist can be helpful in confirming such findings in the eye of an acutely ill child. The association of retinal hemorrhage and cardiopulmonary resuscitation is uncommon but has been documented by some investigators.[4,7,8] Retinal hemorrhage should not be dismissed as secondary to resuscitative efforts, but warrants a thorough evaluation for trauma after other medical conditions have been excluded.

Intentional trauma to the head can cause traumatic alopecia, subgaleal hematoma, scalp contusion, subdural and subarachnoid hemorrhage, and cerebral edema. Guthkelch[5] and Caffey[2] were among the first to describe the shaken baby syndrome and its classic triad of intracranial injury, retinal hemorrhage, and long-bone fractures in young infants. More recent studies by Duhaime and colleagues[3] demonstrated that a direct blow to the head probably contributes to the severity of injury in this syndrome. Helfer[6] and Billmire[1] have documented the finding that severe head injury is unlikely to be caused by falls from a height of less than 3 feet (i.e., from a crib or bed). Examination of the chest and abdomen of a child can be supplemented by appropriate radiologic procedures to exclude internal injury. Blunt trauma to the abdomen in particular may leave no visible bruises or marks, and the presenting symptoms may easily be attributed to more benign causes, such as gastroenteritis. Abdominal injury is the most lethal form of physical abuse, because the internal injury may remain undetected. The most common such injuries include duodenal hematoma, pancreatic injury, renal injury, intestinal perforation, and rupture of the spleen or liver.

A complete physical examination includes inspection and palpation of the extremities to detect ecchymoses, abrasions, or the presence of fractures. Healed skeletal injury may not manifest as gross deformity and is often detectable only with use of radiologic procedures. The age, type, location, and number of fractures may be helpful in distinguishing accidental from nonaccidental trauma.

A variety of skeletal injuries occur in abused children. Injuries highly specific for abuse-related trauma are metaphyseal "corner" or "bucket handle" fractures and fractures to bones such as the posterior ribs, scapulae, sternum, and spinous processes of the vertebrae. Spiral fractures are suggestive of twisting injury and should raise concern if found in children who are not yet walking independently.

Genital trauma can also result from intentional injury. Again, historical information is extremely important in establishing the etiology of such an injury. In both boys and girls, the external genitalia should be palpated for tenderness and inspected for swelling, laceration, redness, abrasion, blisters, and ulcers. In girls, in addition, the diameter of the vaginal orifice should be measured, the condition of the hymen assessed, and evidence of trauma to the vulva and perineum described. If there is evidence of a foreign body in the vagina of a prepubertal child, or extensive genital injury, an examination under anesthesia is necessary, and surgical intervention may be indicated in some cases. The timing of this intervention should, of course, be based on the acuteness of the symptoms.

The anus and rectum should be inspected and palpated as indicated. Instrumentation of the rectum should be performed only when absolutely necessary, as it may be perceived by the child as an added violation. Any bruises, lesions, or laxity of the anal sphincter should be noted.

Table 52-4 categorizes injuries by type or site and lists features that are helpful in differentiating unintentional versus intentional injury.

Injury resulting from neglect

Many childhood injuries can be prevented. A substantial number of injuries occur because of neglectful or uninformed behavior of a parent or caregiver. Contact burns from irons, curlers, or other household appliances, for example, can be the result of inadequate safety precautions. Lack of adult supervision has contributed to the drowning of many children and to their falling out of open windows in the summertime. Physical injury of children can also be the direct result of violence between adults in the home, the children receiving blows which, although not meant for them, can be lethal nonetheless. In recent years children have been suffering gunshot wounds resulting from the

Table 52–4 Characteristics: intentional versus unintentional injury

Type of injury	Intentional	Unintentional
Bites	Ovoid, elliptical shaped intercanine distance Usually greater than 3 cm May involve neck, ear lobes May have reddened area in the center Crushing, bruising injuries	Sharp punctures, lacerations Usually involve extremities Tearing injuries
Bruises	Different colors (age) Multiple May have a specific pattern Inner thigh, back, buttocks, upper arm	Single color Single to few Rounded Prominent bony surfaces
Contact burns	Distinct patterns, margins Uniform depth Partial to full thickness	Blurred margin Uneven depth Superficial to partial thickness
Splatter burns	Irregular margins Usually anterior chest, arms	Irregular margins Multiple areas
Immersion burns	Symmetric Distinct margins Usually no splash marks Stocking or glove pattern Spare flexure points	Asymmetric Blurred margins Splash marks Random distribution
Alopecia	Multiple sites Patchy Tender, red	Isolated Defined borders May be associated with braids, fungus
Skull fractures	Unilateral or bilateral One site or multiple Linear, complex, depressed May be associated with cerebral injury or hemorrhage	Unilateral One site Linear Usually no cerebral injury
Extremity fractures	Single or multiple Spiral or transverse Associated with occult metaphyseal fractures	Single Consistent with explanation
Eye trauma	Bilateral or unilateral Intraocular, i.e., retinal hemorrhage	Usually unilateral, but can be bilateral Rare intraocular hemorrhages may be associated with medical conditions
Head trauma	Bilateral or unilateral Submeningeal blood May have no external sign of injury	Soft tissue injury Unilateral meningeal
Abdominal trauma	Delay in seeking medical treatment May have no external signs of injury Duodenal hematoma most common	Immediate medical intervention
Genitalia	Lacerations asymmetrical Foreign bodies May be associated with sexually transmitted disease	Straddle injury May have symmetrical soft tissue injuries Lacerations infrequent

crossfire of street violence or from the failure of parents to secure firearms properly. Lack of adequate parental supervision can place a child in great danger if harmful household chemicals, over-the-counter medications, prescription medications, alcohol, and illegal substances are not out of reach of the child.

Occasionally a child may be seen in an advanced state of starvation or dehydration because of parental ignorance or impairment (owing to mental illness or substance abuse). Most cases of neglect, however, are less dramatic, and children are often seen suffering from a chronic failure to thrive.

Diagnostic tests

Laboratory tests and radiologic procedures are essential elements in the provision of good clinical care, often enabling diagnosis or validation of a suspicion of intentional injury. An appropriate diagnostic evaluation can be helpful in establishing the extent of injury, confirming that an injury is secondary to another medical condition, or ruling out the possibility of a medical illness as the etiology of the injury. Table 52-5 summarizes studies that are most commonly useful in evaluating intentional injury to children. Additional tests useful when there is suspicion of sexual abuse are listed in Table 52-6.

A medical assessment of trauma etiology in children provides data that may play a decisive role in the outcome of cases of suspected child maltreatment. Public agencies involved in the investigation and prosecution of these cases rely greatly upon medical information and opinion to separate organic conditions and unintentional events from intentional injuries.

Establishing the time of occurrence of head trauma, estimating the age of a bruise, or recognizing the severity of an injury as inconsistent with a child's developmental ability can help investigators clarify a pattern of events and may even inculpate or exculpate a possible suspect.

Maximizing the medical evaluation

The value of an evaluation is strengthened by the use of established protocols, chain-of-possession forms, medicolegal forms, and sex offense kits. Protocols ensure that suspected child abuse evaluations are thorough, well organized, and reliable. The use of a standard protocol decreases lapses in procedure and increases effective collaboration of all professionals involved.

Chain-of-possession forms document the passage of specimens through the hands of the many individuals who must work with them. This procedure minimizes subsequent legal challenges, and is essential in processing toxicology tests and forensic materials for suspected sexual abuse cases.

Medicolegal forms, which are usually provided by law enforcement agencies, enable examining physicians to provide medical information in a uniform and consistent manner. The forms must be completed fully and legibly with terminology that clearly documents historical data, carefully describes injuries, and appropriately states the results of diagnostic studies and professional consultations. Sex offense kits are used for a comprehensive

Table 52–5 Intentional injury evaluation: laboratory and radiographic studies

Test	Comments
CBC with platelet count	Clarifies allegations of "easy bruising"; leukemia, pancytopenias
Coagulation profile	Identifies intracranial hemorrhage, disseminated intravascular coagulopathy (DIC) or sepsis-related coagulopathy, inherited coagulopathy
Urinalysis, urine toxicology	Detects renal trauma, exposure to drugs or illegal substances
Electrolytes, glucose, amylase	Detects abdominal trauma
Skeletal survey	Child under 2 years: full survey
	Ages 2–5: as indicated by clinical examination
	Older than 5 years: usually not positive
Bone scan	Detects occult fractures to spine, ribs, and metaphyses; not helpful with skull fractures
CT scan	Determines suspected head or viseral trauma
MRI	Provides differential delineation of intracranial fluid collections

and organized collection of forensic evidence. They are most useful if the suspected sexual contact has occurred less than 72 hours prior to the examination. Beyond that time, yield does not usually justify their use.

Medical conditions that mimic child abuse

The challenge in determining whether a child's injuries were caused by abuse or neglect is further complicated by the very similar presentation of certain medical conditions. These conditions may represent normal variants or may result from diseases or other processes that do not represent abusive or neglectful behavior of caregivers. Table 52-7 outlines the most commonly seen conditions that may be confused with intentional injuries.

Table 52–6 Sexual abuse: forensic tests

Site/specimen	Test
Vagina/cervix	*Gram stain (sperm identification)
	*Swabs for seminal fluid (acid phosphatase, semen glycoprotein (P30), mouse antihuman sperm-5 (MHS-5) monoclonal antibody, DNA fingerprinting)
	†/‡ Gonorrhea culture
	†/‡ Chlamydia culture
	†/‡ Routine vaginal culture
	‡ Wet mount (sexually transmitted disease [STD] and motile sperm)
Rectum	‡ Wet mount (STD and motile sperm)
	*Swabs for seminal fluid (as above)
	†/‡ Gonorrhea culture
	†/‡ Chlamydia culture
	‡ Wet mount (STD)
Oropharynx	†/‡ Gonorrhea culture
	‡ Wet mount or Gram stain (sperm)
	*Saliva
	*Swabs for seminal fluid (as above)
Blood	†/‡ Serology test for syphilis, herpes,§ HIV antibody,§ hepatitis§
	*Typing
Urine	†/‡ Urinalysis
	†/‡ Urine culture
	†/‡ Pregnancy in postpubertal girls (repeat in 2 weeks)
Other	*Clothing and debris collection
	*Fingernail scrapings
	*Hair samples

* = part of sex offense kit—use only if alleged abuse occurred less than 72 hours before examination; †/ baseline evaluation for sexually transmitted diseases and pregnancy; ‡ = deliver to hospital laboratory; § = as indicated.

PSYCHOSOCIAL INTERVENTION

To be most effective in the child's behalf, the pediatrician or nurse practitioner who deals with the family in a situation of suspected child abuse should fully understand the need for comprehensive psychosocial intervention for both child victim and family. This intervention is best provided by a trained medical health professional—clinical social worker, psychologist, or clinical nurse specialist—trained and experienced in the subspeciality of child maltreatment.

At the time of initial medical evaluation, the mental health professional should be introduced to the case for three main purposes: (1) to interview and observe the child and family for mental health or clinical difficulties that may be suggestive of child maltreatment, (2) to ascertain with the medical professional the need for reporting to a child protective service or law enforcement authorities, and (3) to respond to the emotional needs of the child and family at the time of initial suspicion or disclosure.

Common indicators of maltreatment—sexual, physical, and emotional—are described in Table 52-8.

The mental health professional should assess not only the status of the child, but also the parent-child relationship. The parent or other adult who accompanies the child to the hospital is usually an important resource in the initial assessment of the situation in which the child's maltreatment has occurred. Is the abuse condoned because it serves a reportedly higher principle (teaching obedience or teaching about sexuality from one who "loves the child")? Does the parent minimize or deny the incident or have a selective memory? Does the parent blame the child or shift the blame to others? Are parents derogatory in their attitude or inadequately attached to the child? Do they use verbal insults and put-downs in speaking to the child? What is the level of support provided by the parent and the family? by the extended family and community?

During the initial face-to-face contact with the family, the mental health professional tries to gain information to build an accurate history of the abusive event, to assess the child's present mental health needs, and to allow preliminary determination of the appropriate treatment (of both child and family) to follow.

The clinician's goals for the child and family in the initial hospital encounter are as follows:

1. Cognitive understanding of what has hap-

Table 52–7 Medical conditions that mimic child abuse

Organ system	Differential diagnosis
Integument	Impetigo
	Mongolian spots
	Cao Gao (coining)
	Staphylococcal scalded skin syndrome
	Cupping
	Moxibustion
	Healed chickenpox marks
	Multiple nevi and cafe-au-lait spots
	Phytophotodermatitis
	Dermatorrhexis
	Ehlers-Danlos syndrome (type I)
	Idiophathic thrombocytopenia purpura
	Hemophilia
	von Willebrand disease
	Henoch-Schönlein purpura
	Vasculitis
	Erythema multiforme
Skeletal system	Osteogenesis imperfecta
	Congenital syphilis
	Leukemia
	Osteomyelitis
	Vitamin A intoxication
	Caffey's disease
	Rickets
	Scurvy
	Osteopenia secondary to chronic illness
Ocular system	Coagulopathies
	Neoplasm
	Hypertension
	Infection
	Arteriovenous malformation
Gastrointestinal system	Peritonitis
	Meckel's diverticulum
	Renal stone
	Torsion of spermatic cord
	Ovarian cyst
Central nervous system	Mollera caida (fallen fontanelle)
	Infection (meningitis)
	Neoplasm
	Metabolic abnormalities

pened and of the actual or potential consequences within the family

2. Reinforcement and encouragement of positive or adoptive responses and functioning
3. Perception of the clinician and the hospital team as a resource

4. Knowledge of at least the basics of the legally mandated responses to maltreatment and any other public/systemic ramifications
5. Understanding of the rationale and logistics of plans for follow-up and treatment—both medical and mental health—for child and family

The approach of the entire team, especially of the mental health professional, should be carefully balanced between providing nonjudgmental support and probing for relevant psychosocial information. Establishing positive rapport is crucial in this aspect of intervention and requires professional maturity, including the ability to monitor one's own emotional responses to various forms of child maltreatment (anger, repulsion, denial, disbelief, grief, and avoidance). The mental health professional must pace the intervention and actively assess the concerns and capacities of all those involved. This wide-angle focus may sometimes have to include professional colleagues, for example, in cases of brutal sexual abuse of young children or severe physical injuries resulting in permanent disfigurement or death.

Another function of psychosocial intervention is to assess not only the parental relationship with the child, but also how the suspicion or disclosure evolved. How are the child and family experiencing the crisis of disclosure? Sometimes families do not appear to be traumatized when, in fact, they are.

Finally, the mental health professional should address the level of risk for the child in the current situation. A structured risk-assessment instrument may be used by the mental health professional to help objectify the estimation of the child's safety or the family's ability to ensure the child's protection. Is the parent supportive or overwhelmed? Do the adults in the child's life have a clear understanding of what constitutes abuse and of its implications for the child? Are family members suffering from psychiatric problems or drug addiction? What resources—human and financial—are available for the family? What has been the family's experience with the authorities and with "helping" professionals?

In many cases, there is need for additional mental health services for the family as well as for the child. Typically, these are families who need assistance in rebuilding their coping mechanisms or who need to integrate the child's victimization experience in such a way that future vulnerability of the child victim (and siblings) is reduced. Mental health resources for these families include parenting education, psychotherapy, and supportive counseling. The mental health professional makes the appropriate referral of children and families to

Table 52–8 Behavioral indicators of child maltreatment

Sexually related behavior

Sexual victimization of younger children
Overt sexual acting out toward adults
Excessive masturbation
Sex play with others
Knowledge of sexual matters or details of adult sexual activity inappropriate for age or developmental level
Hinting about sexual activity
Promiscuity

Violence in behavior

Combination of violence and sexuality in artwork, written school work, language, or play
Violence against younger children
Fire setting

Aberrant behavior

Acting-out behavior
Overcompliant behavior
Pseudomature behavior
Repulsion or extreme fear when touched by an adult
Fear of being alone with adults
Excessive bathing
Fear of bathrooms and showers
Sleep disturbances
Encopresis, enuresis
Regressive behavior
Clinical depression
Dissociative disorders
Self-mutilation

Other indicators and associated factors

Suicidal ideation or attempts
Psychosomatic complaints
Drug or alcohol abuse
Poor peer relationships
Change in school performance
Problems in concentrating in school
Refusal to dress for gym at school
Avoidance of physical or recreational activities
Running away
Delinquency
Developmental delay
Chronic illness
Eating problems

Parental behaviors associated with risk

Inappropriate expectations for child, including toilet training
Psychiatric impairment
Substance abuse
Domestic violence

services beyond the emergency room, working in concert with the public child welfare system, which is legally responsible for the protection and care of vulnerable children.

LEGAL ISSUES

Although child maltreatment is a relatively new arena for the law, all states have child protection statutes. Professionals working in a pediatric setting are legally required to report any knowledge or suspicion that a child has been abused. *Abused child* has a legal definition: the term generally means *a child whose parent, guardian, or custodian has inflicted—or failed to prevent—physical injury to the child, including excessive corporal punishment or acts of sexual abuse or exploitation.*

Many statutes also require health care professionals to report any suspicion that a child has been injured because of exposure to drug-related activity (e.g., drug ingestion or inhalations). It is important to note that the term *custodian* now includes not only one who is acting *in loco parentis* (in the place of a parent), but out-of-home day-care providers as well.

In deciding whether to report, professionals must bear in mind that the law requires them to have a "good faith" suspicion, that is, a reasonable belief that a child has been abused. To report a child for any other reason may subject the reporter, as well as the pediatric institution, to civil or criminal liability. With the intent of ensuring appropriate reporting of all suspected cases, child protection laws generally stipulate that any person who is required to make a report but who willfully fails to do so may be subject to civil or criminal sanctions. Moreover, failure to identify, to establish the diagnosis, or to report suspected child victimization that results in physical injury or death may very well subject the professional to further liability for damages caused by the oversight.

To meet their legal responsibilities, professionals must report cases of child abuse to the Department of Human (Social) Services (or, in some instances, the police department) located within the jurisdiction in which the abuse occurs. Legal responsibility for investigating reports of suspected abuse and for making decisions about custody and placement rests with the Department, not with the professional who makes the report. Only the Department—again, not the professional—can ask the local prosecutor's office to file a petition in family court and/or criminal court. Thus, there are legal limits to what a health care professional can do in advocacy for children.

If the family court becomes involved in a reported case of suspected abuse, the court's paramount concern is the best interests (safety, health, welfare) of the child. Because child protection laws are written to be entirely consistent with the constitutionally protected right of family integrity, the court tries to arrange the "least restrictive" placement of a child. Consequently, a child might remain at home under court supervision or be placed under the supervision of a relative or family friend. In other cases, custody may be temporarily transferred from parents to the Department of Human Services.

Contrary to popular belief, parental rights are not terminated when a child is placed in the custody of the Department. The ultimate goal is reunification of the family. In actuality, parental rights are retained until a parent voluntarily relinquishes them or, more typically, until a legal proceeding results in a court order terminating parental rights. Once parental rights have been severed, a child becomes available for adoption. Because child protection laws are designed to keep families intact, the road to termination of parental rights is a very long one.

In addition to child protection laws, each state has criminal statutes that provide for the prosecution of parents, guardians, and custodians, as well as non-caregivers who abuse children. The focus of criminal proceedings is essentially twofold: to determine whether the accused is guilty and, if so, what punishment is appropriate. Thus the criminal court, unlike the family court, cannot protect a child victim of abuse except in the limited instance when the accused is ordered by the court to stay away from the child.

Because professionals working in a pediatric setting are legally mandated to report suspected child abuse, they are likely to receive subpoenas to appear in family court or in criminal court to testify. Although a court appearance may cause disruption in the delivery of services to other patients, the professional's advocacy for an abused child necessarily extends to the courtroom once a report has been made. A subpoena should never be disregarded, and legal counsel (for example, general counsel for the pediatric center) should be sought before responding to the subpoena and testifying.

A witness may be called upon to give either factual or expert testimony. If a professional makes a court appearance as a factual witness, only testimony regarding his or her personal observations will be elicited. In the prosecution of a child abuse case, however, the trier of fact often needs a witness with specialized knowledge to assist the judge or jury in better understanding the evidence or in determining a fact at issue. Thus, the professional may be qualified as an expert witness by providing testimony about his or her educational and expe-

riential background. The witness can then testify in the form of an opinion on matters that are beyond the common knowledge or skills of the trier of fact (judge or jury).

The professional should be adequately prepared for testifying in court. This can best be accomplished by arranging a conference, prior to the court hearing, with the attorney who issues the subpoena. The professional will then be provided an opportunity to learn more about the facts of the case, to discuss the nature of the testimony to be elicited, and to educate the attorney regarding his or her area of expertise.

Because professionals working in a pediatric setting are likely to become witnesses in child abuse cases, their medical records may be subpoenaed and disclosed to a prosecutor, defense attorney, guardian *ad litem,* and/or a judge. Therefore, complete and accurate record documentation is crucial. Again, legal counsel should be sought before responding to a subpoena and releasing information.

Oral requests are frequently made for the release of information from the professional who reports suspected child abuse. Whether information may be released depends on local child protection laws, as well as laws governing confidentiality. As a general rule, professionals are required to maintain the confidentiality of medical records and the information contained therein. Information may be released only with the written consent of the parent, legal guardian, or the child. Failure to obtain appropriate consent prior to releasing records or information could expose the professional to civil or criminal liability.

Child protection laws and laws governing confidentiality are (and no doubt will continue to be) controversial. Although such laws are admittedly imperfect, they cannot and must not be ignored. If the spirit of these laws is fulfilled, they will serve to protect not only children—who are the intended beneficiaries—but also the professionals and the institutions who serve the children.

CONCLUSION

The role of the trauma specialist is vital to successful intervention in situations of abuse and neglect. As gatekeepers, emergency room specialists can make a difference—literally between life and death—for countless wounded and vulnerable children. Trauma specialists cannot and should not shoulder this burden alone: their commitment and efforts must proceed in tandem with the expertise of colleagues in mental health, social work, and law, as hospital professionals work together in assessment, treatment, and advocacy in their shared mission to heal and protect children.

REFERENCES

1. Billmire EM, Myers PA: Serious head injury in infants: accident or abuse? *Pediatrics* 75:340, 1985.
2. Caffey J: On the theory and practice of shaking infants, *Am J Dis Child* 124:161, 1972.
3. Duhaime AC, Gennarellia TA et al: The shaken baby syndrome: a clinical, pathological and biomechanical study, *J Neurosurg* 66:409, 1987.
4. Goetting M: Retinal hemorrhage after cardiopulmonary resuscitation in children: an etiologic re-evaluation, *Pediatrics* 85:585, 1990.
5. Guthkelch AN: Infantile subdural hematoma and its relationship to whiplash injuries, *Br Med J* 2:430, 1971.
6. Helfer RE, Slovis TL, Black M: Injuries resulting when small children fall out of bed, *Pediatrics* 60:533, 1977.
7. Kanter RK: Retinal hemorrhage after cardiopulmonary resuscitation or child abuse, *J Pediatr* 180:430, 1986.
8. Levin AV: Retinal hemorrhages after cardiopulmonary resuscitation: literature review and commentary, *Pediatr Emerg Care* 2:269, 1986.
9. Newberger E, editor: *Child abuse*, Boston, 1982, Little Brown.
10. Wilson EF: Estimation of the age of cutaneous contusions in child abuse, *Pediatrics* 60:750, 1977.

53 Management of Burn Injuries

David N. Herndon, Randi L. Rutan, William E. Alison, Jr., and Charles S. Cox, Jr.

Even the most routine hospitalization can be a traumatic and terrifying experience for a child. Hospitalization for a severe burn injury can produce an even greater psychological impact. The child has undergone a frightening and painful experience at the time of injury and is then hurried away from his family and placed into an environment full of ominous noisy machines and strangers. The child experiences multiple painful procedures such as debridement, dressing changes, blood tests, and surgery, frequently with inadequate or inappropriate preparation. It is often necessary for the child to remain immobilized in an uncomfortable position and to be required to perform exercises of the injured areas when every movement is exquisitely painful. This sudden traumatic change, for which most children have no coping skills, may elicit responses such as regression, anger, fear, depression, and anxiety.

The demands placed on acute-care providers frequently allow the unique situation of the pediatric patient to be forgotten. Children are not, however, "little adults," and special consideration of their needs should commence at the time of injury. Children may be unable, or unwilling, to express their needs or wishes, and the staff must be sensitive to their feelings and requirements.

INCIDENCE AND ETIOLOGY

Each year in the United States more than 2.5 million people seek medical attention for burn injuries, about 100,000 require hospitalization, and 12,000 die. Fire and burns are the leading cause of accidental death in the home for children under the age of 14 years. One half of all burned children will require up to a month's hospitalization, 25% will require up to 2 months, and 25% will require 3 months or more. As many as 50% will need additional reconstructive surgery to correct cosmetic or functional defects following recovery from acute injury.

The home is the most common site of burn injuries in children; the kitchen is the room most often involved. Infants and toddlers are frequently victims of scalding, and medical staff should be familiar with the characteristic patterns of intentionally inflicted scald injuries. Older children are more frequently injured by burning substances. Ignition of clothing significantly increases the size and depth of injury.

Burn survival in pediatric cases is primarily a function of burn size and concomitant injuries. Overall, pediatric burn victims of all ages survive well. Over the past decade, the size of a survivable injury has increased from 70% total body surface area to an injury of more than 95% total body surface area in children under the age of 15. The decrease in mortality can be attributed to advances in surgical techniques, infection control, and nutritional support. The postburn morbidity associated with scar contracture has been significantly reduced by improved surgical techniques, the near universal use of pressure garments, advanced splinting techniques, and aggressive attention to physical and occupational therapy.

INITIAL MANAGEMENT

The initial treatment of thermal injury begins at the scene of the accident. The most immediate concern is to *stop the burning* without injury to the rescuers. Should the incident be in progress, emphasize "Stop, drop, and roll" or use a blanket to smother the flames. As with all traumatic injuries, airway patency is of utmost priority. Oxygen should be administered by face mask in all cases in which inhalation of smoke or carbonaceous material may have occurred. At the slightest indication of impending obstruction, prophylactic intubation should be performed. If a cutaneous chemical injury is suspected, copious lavage with water should be performed. Care should be taken to rinse the affected areas away from the uninjured ones. Never immerse a chemically contaminated person, but instead use a hose or shower to rinse and simultaneously dilute the chemical agent. All burn injuries should be covered with a clean, dry sheet. Cold wet compresses may be applied to small injuries, but only briefly to large injuries, as prolonged exposure may induce hypothermia. As with all trauma patients, stabilization of fractures and control of frank hemorrhage may be necessary prior to transporting the burn victim to the nearest health

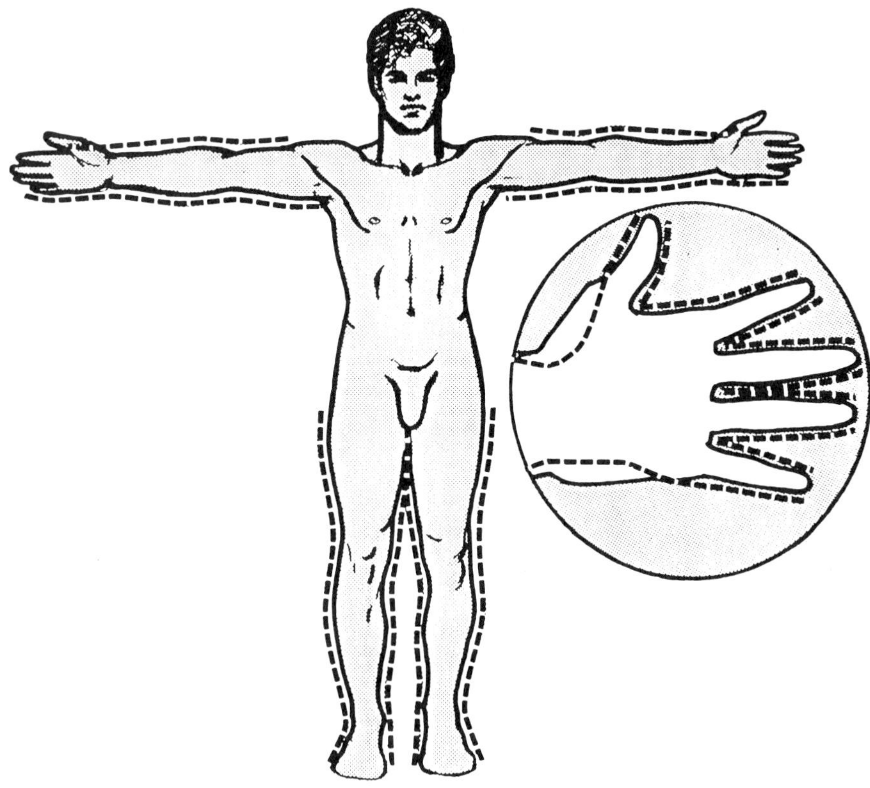

Figure 53–1 Placement of escharotomies. Midaxial escharotomies should be performed if vascular compromise occurs. Incisions should be performed through the dermal tissue to allow maximal expansion of the underlying fascia.

care facility. Upon arrival at the hospital, the patient's cardiopulmonary system should be carefully evaluated. For those children with burn injuries of more than 15% total body surface area, two large-bore intravenous catheters should be placed, in addition to a nasogastric tube and an indwelling urinary bladder catheter.

A rapid initial examination of the burn wounds should be performed, including assessment of distal pulses. This is of particular importance in areas distal to circumferential burns. Full-thickness injury produces a constricting eschar that will increase tissue pressure and impede circulation. Pulses may be absent at the time of admission or may diminish or disappear as tissue edema develops in an affected extremity. The extremity may appear cyanotic and have an abnormal capillary refill time. Should hypoperfusion continue, obstruction of the arterial network will occur, leading to deep tissue death. Midaxial escharotomies should be performed when decreased capillary circulation is obvious (Figs. 53-1 and 53-2). The total absence of arterial pulses may indicate a prolonged occlusion, and even escharotomies may not release

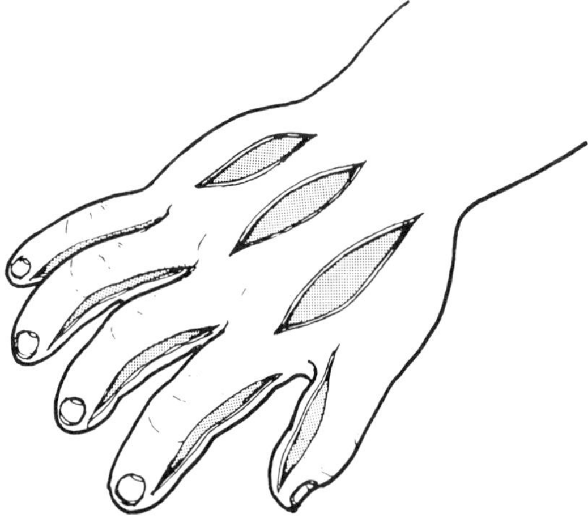

Figure 53–2 Hand and digital escharotomy. Medial and lateral digital escharotomies performed to preserve the distal phalanges when digits are circumferentially burned. Dorsal intermetacarpal escharotomies are used with circumferentially burned hands.

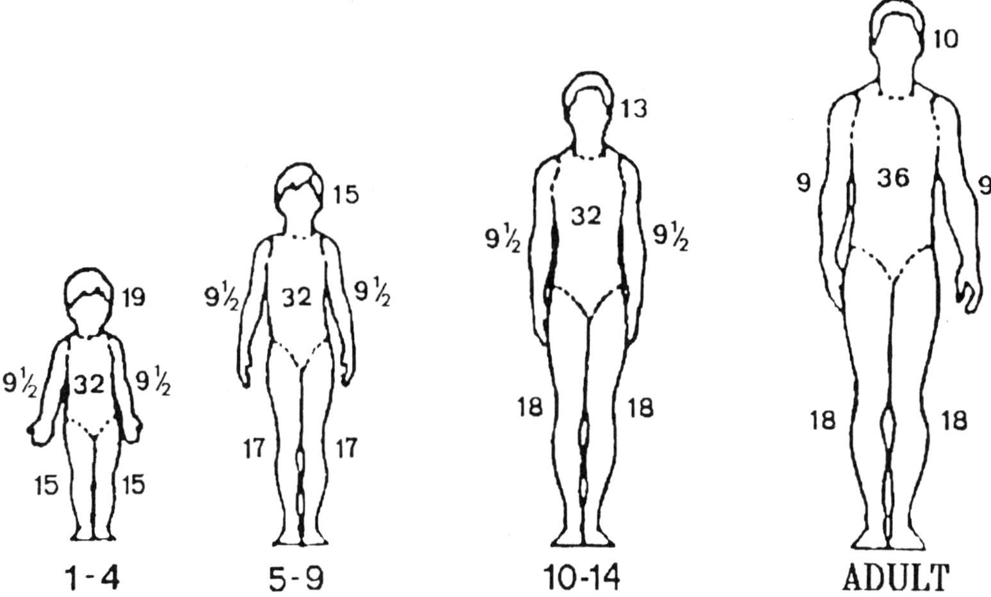

Figure 53–3 Modified "Rule of Nines" to include the pediatric anthropomorphic differences.

the tissue pressure. If vascular compromise has been prolonged, the return of circulation permitted by escharotomy will cause a reactive hyperemia, similar to reperfusion injuries, and lead to gross edema formation. In these cases, fasciotomies may be required to release the pressures within muscle compartments.

Tetanus toxoid as prophylaxis should be given to all patients who have not received tetanus toxoid within the past 6 months, and human tetanus hyperimmune globulin should be administered to children who have never received tetanus toxoid or who have not received it within the past 10 years.

An accurate estimation of the area burned and the depth of burn is essential, the former being the most important at this point. The commonly used "Rule of Nines" does not accurately reflect the surface area of children less than 15 years of age (Fig. 53-3). Infants have a larger cranial surface area in proportion to the extremities than do adults. An inexperienced physician may overestimate the surface area burned and administer excessive fluid volumes. The most accurate method of determining surface area burned is by mapping the injured areas on a Lund and Browder–like body chart (Fig. 53-4) and then calculating the burned area from body surface area nomograms (Fig. 53-5).

All children with burn injuries of greater than 10% to 15% of body surface area (BSA) involving the hands, face, feet, perineum, or joint surfaces, or with electrical injuries in which deep tissue in-volvement is suspected, should be hospitalized. Infants with a greater than 10% body surface area injury and older children with a greater than 15% injury require immediate institution of fluid resuscitation. Hypovolemic shock can appear quickly in these patients, and even in those with smaller burns, if they are full-thickness burns or occur in children of less than 1 year of age. Even small burn injuries can produce severe hypovolemia in infants, whose circulating volume is proportionally less than that of adults, but volume losses are similar cm² to cm² surface area. Children frequently receive insufficient fluid because they refuse to take fluids orally or because intravenous access is difficult to obtain. However, *replacement fluid must be administered.* It is imperative that intravenous fluid be given if oral resuscitation cannot be accomplished. Children can maintain a normal blood pressure, with tachycardia, for a period of time, but then quickly decompensate into severe hypotension and hypoxia. Unlike adults, in children this decompensation occurs rapidly and with little warning. Impending decompensation may be signaled by increasing irritability and restlessness.

FLUID RESUSCITATION

Initial fluid resuscitation should begin with the administration of the isotonic electrolyte solution, lactated Ringer's, at a rate of 400 to 500 ml/m² body surface area, titrated to maintain urine output at 0.25 ml/kg/15 minutes. This will administer

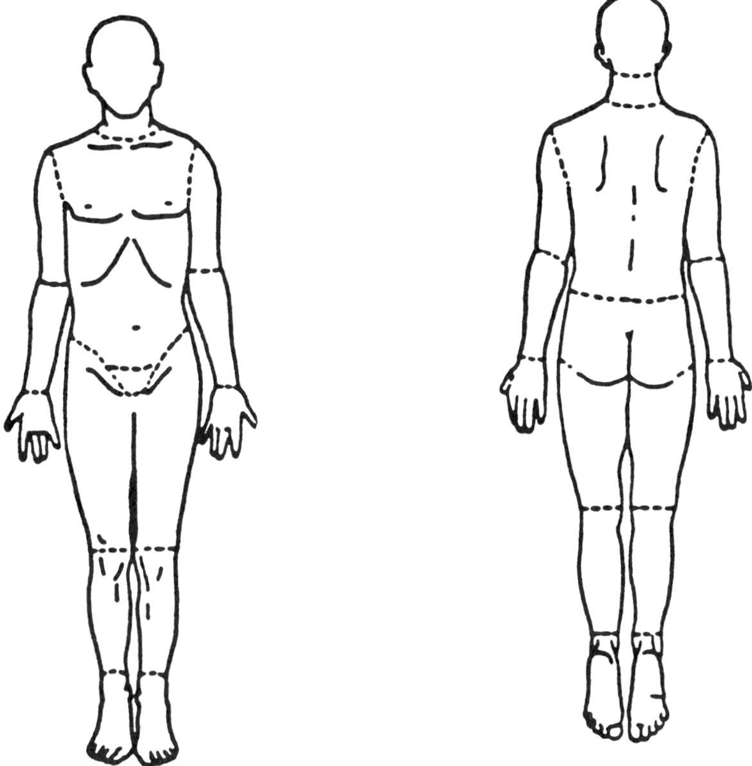

	Age (yr)					
	0	1	5	10	15	Adult
Head	19	17	13	11	9	7
Neck	2	2	2	2	2	2
Ant. trunk	13	13	13	13	13	13
Post. trunk	13	13	13	13	13	13
Buttock	2.5	2.5	2.5	2.5	2.5	2.5
Genitalia	1	1	1	1	1	1
Upper arm	2.5	2.5	2.5	2.5	2.5	2.5
Lower arm	3	3	3	3	3	3
Hand	2.5	2.5	2.5	2.5	2.5	2.5
Thigh	5.5	6.5	8	8.5	9	9.5
Leg	5	5	5.5	6	6.5	7
Foot	3.5	3.5	3.5	3.5	3.5	3.5

Figure 53–4 The Lund and Browder type form yields a more precise estimate of the area of burn injury than the Rule of Nines.

sufficient volume to allow time for more precise calculation of fluid needs. At this time, to ensure accurate mapping of the burned area, the wounds should be carefully cleaned and debrided, and more accurate calculations of fluid requirements performed. Great caution must be exercised in the use of opiates (see "Pain Management" later in this chapter) and the corporeal cooling of children prior to the restoration of plasma volume. Body temperature must be maintained above 37° C at all

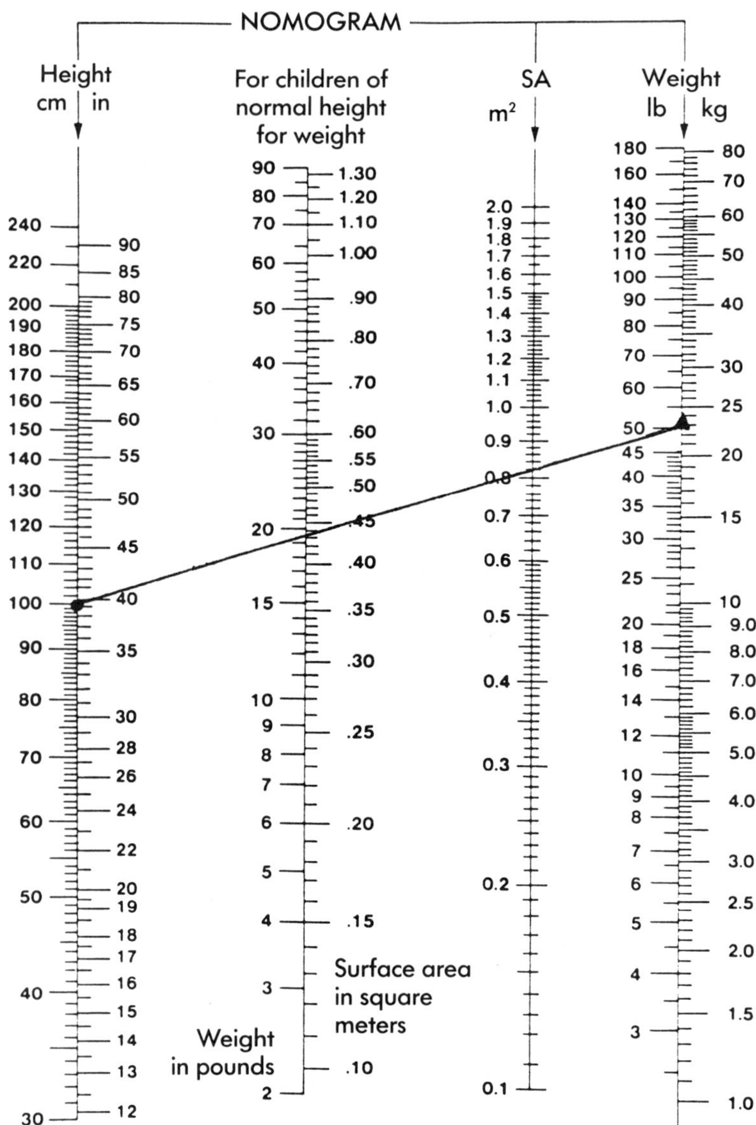

Figure 53–5 Standard surface area nomogram which converts height and weight into body surface area measurements, used to calculate fluid and nutritional requirements. For example, a child of 100 cm in height and 23 kg in weight, would have a body surface area of 0.82 m².

times with the use of environmental heating, overbed warmers, and blankets.

Several formulas have been proposed for resuscitation in children, most based on the weight of the patient, as in adults. However, a difficulty in appropriately employing these formulas in pediatric patients is that surface area and weight relationships are not linear in growing children. Children have a greater body surface area in relation to their weight, and formulas developed for use in treatment of adults do not address the additional fluid losses accrued through the higher ratio of exposed surface area. Weight-based formulas underresuscitate small injuries in small children, sometimes even providing less than maintenance fluid requirements, and grossly overresuscitate large injuries in older children.

Owing to these inconsistencies, a more appropriate means of calculating fluid resuscitation requirements is based on body surface area burned, with additional fluids administered to meet maintenance requirements. Such a formula has been developed and calls for the administration of 5000 ml/m² BSA burn plus 2000 ml/m² total BSA for maintenance, given over the first 24 hours, with one half of the volume infused during the first 8 hours postinjury. Albumin should be added after the first 6 hours postinjury in amounts needed to prevent hypoalbuminemia (<2.0 g/dl).

Resuscitation fluids should be administered, as needed, to maintain acceptable clinical parameters; however, great care should be taken to avoid fluid overload, particularly in the pediatric patient. Children are more prone to edema formation than adults, and of particular concern is the development of cerebral or pulmonary edema.

Regardless of the formula used to calculate fluid requirements, it should be remembered that these formulas are *guides* for fluid administration (Fig. 53-6). Fluid requirements for individual patients will vary, and the adequacy of resuscitation should be assessed through other clinical parameters. Urine output should be maintained at a rate of more than 0.5 to 2 ml/kg/hr, and serum electrolytes, osmolality, and albumin should be normal. Sensorium should be unclouded, pulse rate and pulse pressure should be within normal parameters for age, and adequate capillary refill should be observed in the distal extremities. In only very complicated or severe cases, for example, preexisting disease states such as juvenile diabetes or cystic fibrosis, should arterial, central venous, or pulmonary artery pressure monitoring be necessary.

After the first 24 hours, when vascular integrity is restored, fluid requirements decrease to a constant which remains as long as the burn wound is open. During this period, the fluid requirements are a reflection of the transcutaneous evaporative losses, and fluid should be administered in amounts calculated by a second surface area–based formula: 3750 ml/m² BSA burn plus 1500 ml/m² total BSA/ 24 hr. The primary solution administered should be 5% dextrose with varying sodium concentrations, the goal being to maintain normal serum sodium concentrations. Sudden shifts in sodium concentration can cause convulsions in children, which, although not lethal themselves, may cause other complications such as aspiration pneumonia and postictal traumatic injuries. Sodium requirements are usually quite low after the first 24 hours, and 5% dextrose plus 0.33% normal saline is generally sufficient to replace urinary and cutaneous sodium losses. Children under 1 year of age require slightly larger amounts of sodium replacement because of their different renal function. Additional amounts of potassium are often required. Potassium replacement should be administered as potassium phosphate rather than potassium chloride, as hypophosphatemia is frequently observed.

Variations of the resuscitation fluid itself have been proposed, such as the use of hypertonic lactated saline. The advocates of this fluid regime believe that intravascular volume can be obtained by osmotically pulling fluid from the interstitial space rather than adding additional exogenous fluid. This regimen is also purported to decrease the amount of edema formation incurred through the vascular permeability following thermal injury.[24] However, potential hypernatremia, hyperosmolarity, and intracellular dehydration are severe drawbacks to the use of this resuscitation method, particularly in children. This form of fluid replacement can be dangerous except in very expert hands and is not recommended for use by any other than the most experienced practitioners.

There is further controversy as to whether, and when, colloid should be added to resuscitation fluids. The vascular permeability following thermal injury allows the leakage of fluid, solutes, and protein into the interstitial spaces, decreasing the colloid oncotic pressure of the circulating plasma. The most marked loss occurs in the first 6 to 8 hours postinjury, and vascular integrity is restored by 24 hours postinjury. The most commonly used colloid is albumin, although some institutions use fresh frozen plasma which has the advantage of possessing clotting factors. However, in this era of serotransmitted diseases, the risk of viral transmission may outweigh the advantages of fresh plasma over processed albumin. Whole blood or packed red blood cells should not be incorporated into the resuscitation regimen unless necessary to normalize a rapidly falling hemoglobin or hematocrit level.

Colloid administration can commence after the first 6 hours postinjury. Salt-poor albumin can be added to the established crystalloid fluids (to make a 5% solution) or may be infused in a "piggyback" fashion. Either way, sufficient albumin should be given to maintain stable intravascular albumin levels at 2 to 3 mg/dl. The administration of colloid early in the postburn course may decrease peripheral edema formation through the maintenance of normal serum oncotic pressures, although this has not been specifically demonstrated.

Albumin losses following burn injury are in the form of wound exudate and so will continue until the wounds are closed. In burns of less than 20% total BSA, these losses do not normally produce a significant hypoalbuminemia. However, in a larger injury the protein extravasation can be extreme. Bacterial colonization of the wound will increase the exudate formation and proportionally increase protein losses. In addition, the synthesis of plasma proteins by the liver, particularly albumin, may be impaired, and losses from the gastrointestinal or urinary tracts may magnify protein deficiencies. In the absence of septicemia, administration of 100

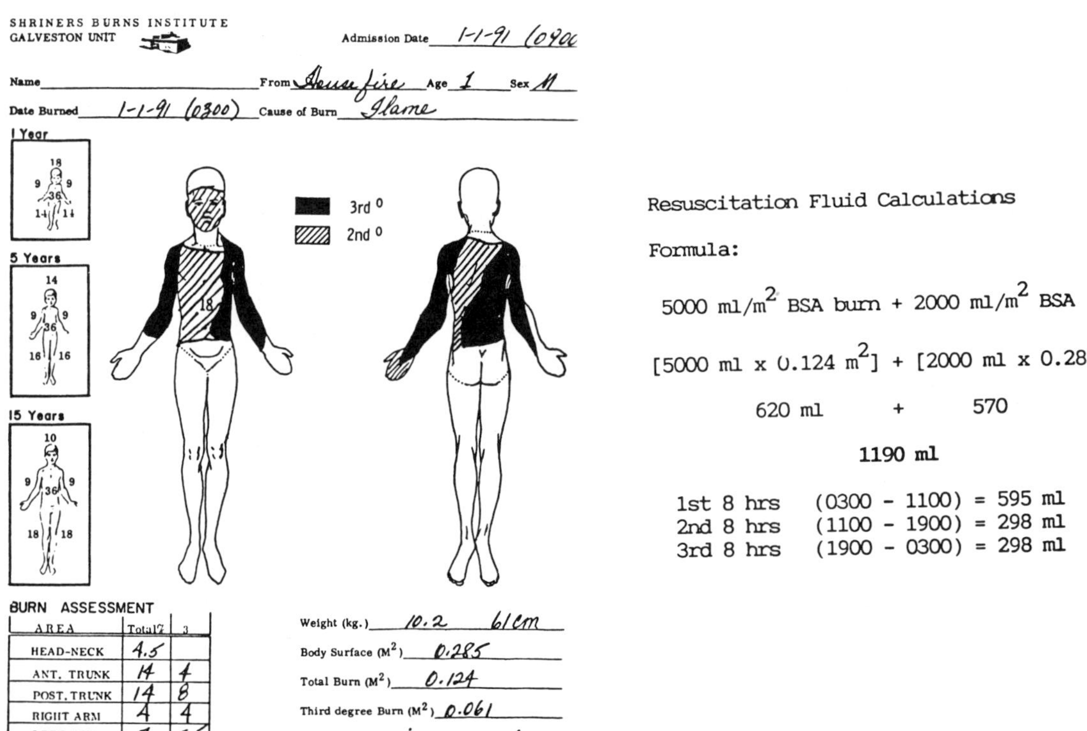

SHRINERS BURNS INSTITUTE
GALVESTON UNIT

Admission Date **1-1-91 (0900)**

Name ________________ From *House fire* Age *1* Sex *M*

Date Burned **1-1-91 (0300)** Cause of Burn *Flame*

BURN ASSESSMENT

AREA	Total 2	3
HEAD-NECK	4.5	
ANT. TRUNK	14	4
POST. TRUNK	14	8
RIGHT ARM	4	4
LEFT ARM	7	5.5
RIGHT LEG		
LEFT LEG		
TOTAL	43.5	21.5

Weight (kg.) *10.2   61 cm*

Body Surface (M^2) *0.285*

Total Burn (M^2) *0.124*

Third degree Burn (M^2) *0.061*

REMARKS *no inhalation by bronchoscopy*

Resuscitation Fluid Calculations

Formula:

$$5000 \text{ ml/m}^2 \text{ BSA burn} + 2000 \text{ ml/m}^2 \text{ BSA}$$

$$[5000 \text{ ml} \times 0.124 \text{ m}^2] + [2000 \text{ ml} \times 0.285]$$

$$620 \text{ ml} \quad + \quad 570$$

$$\textbf{1190 ml}$$

1st 8 hrs	(0300 − 1100)	= 595 ml
2nd 8 hrs	(1100 − 1900)	= 298 ml
3rd 8 hrs	(1900 − 0300)	= 298 ml

Flow Sheet — Physiologic Data

Hourly Time	Peripheral Pulses	BP 00	BP 15	BP 30	BP 45	HR 00	HR 15	HR 30	HR 45	Resp 00	Resp 15	Resp 30	Resp 45	Temp 00	Temp 30
08															
09	✓✓		90/50	82/50	82/54		130	128	130		22		24		36.9
10	✓✓	96/56	96/60	95/58	96/60	132	130	131	130	24		24		37.2	37.4
11	✓✓	98/62	96/60	96/60	94/58	132	132	134	134	22		22		37.6	
12	✓✓	100/40	90/56	82/60	94/60	140	136	132	130	22		24		37.7	
13	✓✓	94/60	94/58	94/62	94/60	132		130		22				37.8	
14	✓✓	95/60	94/58	94/60	94/58	130		131		23				37.9	
15	✓✓	94/60		94/58		130		132		22				38	
16	✓✓	98/60		94/60		130		132		23				38	
17	✓✓	94/58		94/60		128		128		22				38.1	
18	✓✓	96/60		94/60		130		131		23				38	
19															
20															
21															
22															
23															

DATE **1-1-91**   Signature/Title ________ RN

Flow Sheet — Intake / Output

Hourly Time	LR + 25gm SPA 00	15	30	45	LR + 25gm SPA 00	15	30	45	FEEDING Milk	Hourly TOTALS	Cumulative Total Intake	Cumulative Total Output	Out 00	Out 15	Out 30	Out 45
08										04-09	500	26				
09		↑	5	5		↑	5	5		20	520	6			3	3
10	5	4	5	3	5	4	3	3		30	550	16	3	3	2	2
11	3	3	3	3	3	3	3	3	5	29	579	24	2	2	2	2
12	2	10	2	2	2	2	2	2	10	34	613	34	2	2	3	3
13	2	2	1	1	2	2	1	1	15	27	640	45	3	3	3	2
14	1	1	1	1	1	1	1	1	20	28	668	53	2	2	2	2
15	2				2				25	29	697	61	2	2	2	2
8 Hr. Total										197		61				
16	2				2				30	34	731	7	2		5	
17	1				1				35	37	768	14	4		3	
18	1				DC				40	41	809	20	3		3	
19																
20																
21																
22																
23																
16 Hr. Total																

Figure 53–6 J.D., a 1-year-old male, sustained a 43.5% total body surface area burn in a house fire. J.D.'s burn injury has been mapped on the burn diagram, and total body surface area calculated *(upper left)*. Fluid requirements *(upper right)* and infusion rates have been calculated, based on total body surface area and BSA burn. The flow sheet *(lower)* demonstrates the clinical evaluations performed and the titration of administered fluid to maintain urine output. Note the hypotensive episode at 1200, the fluid bolus given, and the subsequent urine output and return of baseline blood pressure. Enteral feeding was initiated at 1100 hours, approximately 8 hours postinjury, and gradually increased. Calculation of J.D.'s caloric requirements are depicted in Table 53-1.

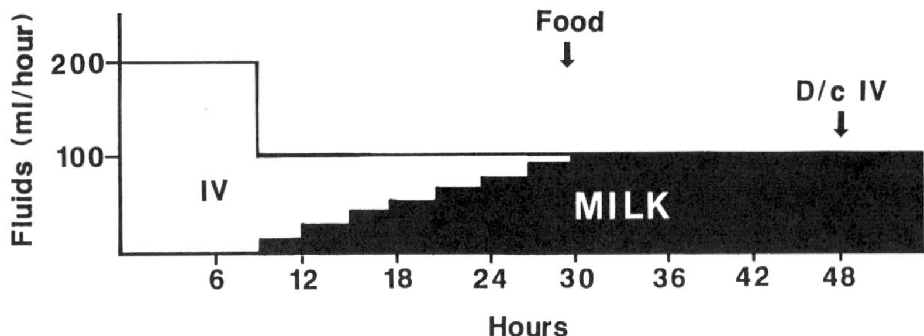

Figure 53–7 Intravenous resuscitation fluid can be tapered as enteral nutrition is increased. By 48 hours postinjury, all fluid and nutritional requirements can be met enterally.

gm/m² BSA burn of albumin or an equivalent amount of plasma, each week in three divided doses, will usually maintain normal serum albumin levels and colloid oncotic pressures >15 mm Hg. This is best administered as a 5% solution in 5% dextrose and ⅓ normal saline over a 6- to 12-hour period.

Any blood loss incurred as a direct result of injury or complication should be replaced on the second to fifth day postinjury. As much as 10% of the circulating red blood cell volume may be destroyed or trapped in the burned areas. The time of administration is dependent upon the severity of the trauma and the actual amount of loss. The usual amount of blood replacement in a 24-hour period is 10 ml/kg body weight infused over a 3- to 4-hour period. Unless there is active blood loss, no more than 15 ml/kg should be given over any 24-hour period, as larger quantities will frequently result in cardiopulmonary congestion or severe hypertension.

Volumes of enteral feedings should be included in the calculation of total fluids administered. As the volume of enteral feedings is increased, the volume of intravenous fluid should be decreased (Fig. 53-7). Continuous enteral infusion of milk or other liquid feedings may be started as early as 6 hours postinjury and slowly increased over the subsequent 12 hours. By 24 hours postinjury, all but the most severely burn-injured patients may be receiving all their fluid needs as enteral feedings.

MEETING ENERGY DEMANDS

Hypermetabolism, increased glucose flow, and severe protein and fat wasting are characteristic of the response to major trauma and infection. No other disease state produces as great an effect on these responses as thermal injury. Patients with multiple fractures experience a 5% to 25% increase in metabolic rate, whereas patients who are ventilator dependent and who have sustained multiple trauma may exhibit elevations of 30% to 75%

Resting Metabolic Expenditure (RME): Early Convalescence from Injury

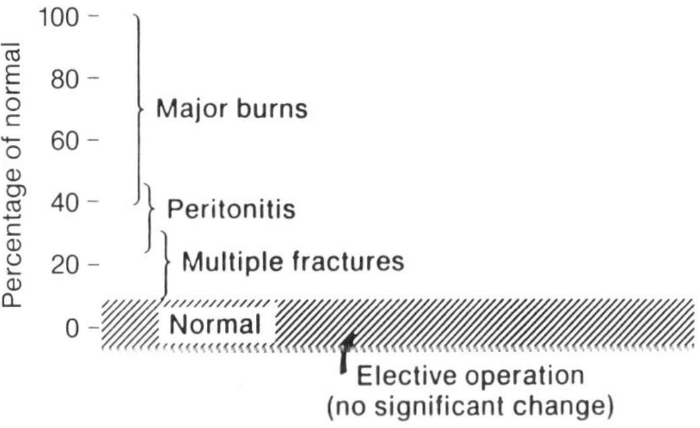

Figure 53–8 Major burns result in a 40% to 100% increase in resting energy expenditure. Other surgical populations experience significantly lower metabolic responses than burn patients.

above normal. Patients with greater than a 40% BSA burn may experience elevations in metabolic rate of up to twice normal (Fig. 53-8). As much as 30 grams of nitrogen each day can be liberated by catabolic activity following severe thermal injury. Without exogenous nutritional support, this catabolism will exhaust essential protein stores within 3 to 4 weeks postinjury in the adult. In a child with limited stores, caloric support is even more essential. Resting energy expenditure increases in a curvilinear fashion with increasing burn size, ranging from near normal with burns of less than 10% BSA to a 50% increase with injuries of greater than 25% and a maximum of twice normal for injuries of greater than 40% BSA.

The 14 interleukins, tumor necrosis factor, prostaglandins, glucagon, corticosteroids, and catecholamines have been implicated as the primary mediators of the hypermetabolic response following thermal injury. Elevations in urinary catecholamine excretion in proportion to increases in metabolic rate have been demonstrated, and the hypermetabolic response may be at least partially blocked with combined alpha- and beta-adrenergic blockade. Elevated prostaglandin levels have been found in burn wound exudate, in wound lymph drainage, and in serum of acutely burned or septic patients.[1] Increased catecholamine output stimulates increased glucagon secretion. Cortisol levels are elevated. These hormones promote hepatic gluconeogenesis and ureagenesis when increased relative to insulin levels. During the resuscitative phase, insulin levels are low but return to normal in the uncomplicated, fed patient. Insulin appears to regulate skeletal muscle uptake and release of amino acids, with relatively low levels increasing release. Catecholamines and glucagon stimulate both amino acid and lactic acid efflux from muscle and lipolysis. Support with glucose and insulin does not ablate hypermetabolism, but does preserve body weight, decrease nitrogen losses, and increase body fat. Levels of human growth hormone and IGF-1 initially ebb following thermal injury. Exogenous support, recently with recombinant human growth hormone, has been demonstrated to encourage positive nitrogen balance, preserve lean muscle mass, and increase the rate of wound healing.[15,20,29]

The hypermetabolic response is temperature sensitive, but not temperature dependent. Increased metabolic rate can be minimized but not abolished by environmental heating. Owing to a central temperature reset, thought to originate in the hypothalamus, patients with large thermal injuries strive for core and skin temperatures of 1° to 2° C above normal. The ambient temperature must be maintained at 28° to 33° C to minimize metabolic expenditure for maintenance of core temperature and to maximize comfort. Patients allowed to select their own environmental temperatures will choose temperatures within this range. In addition, the increased ambient temperature decreases evaporative water losses, which can be as high as 22 ml/cm^2 of open wound.

Almost all routine events of burn care increase metabolic rate and catecholamine release through increasing pain and anxiety. Rational use of narcotic sedatives and supportive psychological interventions help reduce these effects. Caution in the use of narcotics is advised because preservation of gastrointestinal motility is of critical importance. In addition, the critical need for uninterrupted sleep intervals should not be overlooked.

Nutritional support

Increased oxygen consumption, metabolic rate, urinary nitrogen excretion, lipolysis, and a steady erosion of lean body mass are directly related to burn size and gradually return toward normal as the wound heals or is physiologically closed. Children with a greater than 40% BSA burn have been demonstrated to lose as much as 25% of their preburn weight by 3 weeks postinjury. It has only recently been possible, through vigorous enteral and parenteral hyperalimentation, to deliver sufficient exogenous calories to prevent massive postburn weight loss.

The precise energy requirements needed to reach weight and nitrogen balance have been calculated from linear regression analysis of weight change versus predicted dietary intake in large burns in adults, producing the Curreri formula, which calls for 25 kcal/kg plus 40 kcal/% BSA burn per day. Like resuscitation requirements, caloric requirements vary with age, and Curreri has recently developed a formula for use in children.[4] However, as previously stated, weight and surface area are disproportionate in children. Moreover, relative percentages of burn area are not accurate reflections of the surface area injured and its subsequent heat, fluid, and protein losses.

A formula based on body surface area is a more accurate means of calculating caloric requirements in children. Recent evidence has suggested that the historic formulas for nutrition supplementation overestimated caloric requirements. A new formula, developed at the Shriners Burns Institute in Galveston, calls for 1800 kcal/m^2 BSA plus 2200 kcal/m^2 BSA burn per day (Table 53-1).

Calories should be provided through the enteral route if at all possible. Most children will tolerate enteral feedings as early as 3 to 6 hours postburn, if not immediately. Several studies have demonstrated that the implementation of early alimentation is safe and may help to maintain the integrity of the intestinal mucosa, sustaining normal and efficient digestion and absorption. A frequent argument against the use of early enteral alimentation has been the incidence of paralytic ileus during the initial postburn period. However, it should be recognized that postburn ileus and dilatation affect the stomach, and not the small intestine, so successful enteral feeding can be accomplished with the use of small bowel feeding tubes. In addition, some studies indicate that early enteral feeding can decrease the degree of postburn hypermetabolism and subsequent catabolism.[8]

With hourly enteral administration of milk, one third of severely burned children can gain weight, one third maintain a stable weight, and the remaining third lose less than 10% of their preadmission weight. Milk, at 0.6 kcal/ml, is the least expensive and best tolerated of all feedings. In addition, it is palatable and easily recognized by children when they are able to tolerate oral feed-

Table 53–1 Nutritional requirement calculation

JD is a 1-year-old male who has sustained a 43.5% burn injury. He weighs 10.2 kg and is 61 cm tall. Using a nomogram (Fig. 53-5) to calculate his body surface area, it was determined that JD has a body surface area of 0.285 m^2 and a burn surface area of 0.124 m^2. His caloric requirements would therefore be

$$1800 \text{ kcal}/m^2 \text{ body surface area} + 2200 \text{ kcal}/m^2 \text{ body surface area burn}$$
$$(1800 \text{ kcal} \times 0.285 \text{ m}^2) + (2200 \text{ kcal} \times 0.124 \text{ m}^2)$$
$$513 + 273$$
$$= 786 \text{ kcal}/\text{day}$$

To calculate actual volume requirements, the caloric value of the feeding must be known. JD will receive milk, which contains 0.66 kcal/ml.

$$\frac{786 \text{ kcal}}{0.66 \text{ kcal}/\text{ml}} = 1191 \text{ ml}/\text{day} = 50 \text{ ml}/\text{hr}$$

ings. However, because of the low sodium content of cow's milk, sodium supplementation is frequently required. The administration of enteral feeding can commence as early as 6 hours postinjury. As the rate of enteral feeding increases, intravenous fluid support should be decreased, to avoid fluid overload. In some cases, intravenous support can be discontinued within 12 hours postinjury and replaced by enteral feedings (see Fig. 53-7). The feedings can be given continuously via a bedside pump or can be administered as hourly boluses, although consensus leans toward continuous feeding. Various commercially prepared formulas may be used, particularly if the volume of feeding required to meet caloric demands grossly exceeds fluid requirements. Hyperosmolar feedings, however, can cause diarrhea.

Diarrhea is the most common complication of enteral nutrition. In infants less than 1 year of age, this may be due to the continuing development of the gastrointestinal tract. Moreover, many drugs, such as H_2 antagonists, antacids, and antibiotics, predispose patients to diarrhea. Recently, the incidence of diarrhea has been linked to the administration of formula with high fat content and limited vitamin A uptake. The introduction of dietary fiber, administration of bulk-forming agents such as bran, maintenance of fat content to less than 20% of caloric intake, and a balanced approach to antacid therapy can reduce the incidence of this complication. Continuous infusion of milk into the stomach will usually provide a sufficient buffer and obviate the need of antacids. Constipation should also be aggressively treated with serial enemas. When such large volumes are administered enterally, a single day of constipation can cause serious problems.

All patients should additionally receive increased amounts of ascorbic acid (vitamin C), ret-

Table 53–2 Amounts of vitamins and elements necessary for reparative processes

Vitamin or element	Daily amount
Ascorbic acid	1-6 g in 3 divided doses
Zinc	110-220 mg
Vitamin A	5000-20,000 IU
Multivitamin	1 tablet
Ferrous sulfate	300-1000 mg
Folate	0.1-1 mg

inol (vitamin A), vitamin E and zinc. Iron and folate supplementation should also be considered, particularly in infants and adolescent females. Daily intake of a balanced multivitamin plus additional amounts of the above named elements is essential to provide the patient with sufficient nutritional substances for reparative processes to occur (Table 53-2).

Parenteral hyperalimentation should be avoided. It has been demonstrated that the early administration of parenteral hyperalimentation has detrimental effects on immune function and survival, despite the fact that the use of this method enabled the administration of significantly more calories.[16,18] However, if weight loss occurs despite maximal enteral feeding, or if the patient was malnourished prior to injury, parenteral alimentation may be necessary. Peripheral parenteral nutrition (PPN), with its lower carbohydrate load, carries fewer risks than total parenteral nutrition (TPN) and is preferable to TPN. Should central venous access be required for TPN administration, absolute aseptic technique in the insertion and maintenance of the catheter, as well as the rotation of insertion sites every 3 days, is essential in preventing septic thrombophlebitis in these surface-contaminated patients. Insulin supplementation may be required when sufficient calories are administered, and as much as 1 IU/kg/day may be necessary to normalize serum glucose levels. During parenteral hyperalimentation, serial liver function tests to monitor possible fatty liver degeneration, as well as frequent serum and urine glucose determinations, are obligatory. Potassium supplementation may also be necessary. All hyperalimentation fluids, in addition to containing amino acids and glucose load, should contain vitamins and trace elements. Intravenous fat emulsions may be administered, with as much as 20% to 25% of the required calories given in this form.

Failure to meet the caloric loads required for weight maintenance, nitrogen balance, and energy equilibrium results in delayed and abnormal wound healing with defects in fibroblast and white cell metabolic rates. Red blood cell active transport is reversibly inhibited in patients with a negative energy balance, and decreases in leukocyte chemotaxis and phagocytosis have also been noted.

WOUND MANAGEMENT

Immediately after the burn injury, wound care is not of the highest priority; however, ultimate survival of the patient depends on the success of wound management. Many authors have presented various methods of wound care, ranging from fairly conservative to highly aggressive. A thorough understanding of the pathophysiology of burn wounds is required to make clinical decisions as to the most appropriate approach to wound management in any particular patient.

In general, the pathophysiology of burn wounds is no different in the pediatric population than in the adult. The end product of the application of heat to tissue is the denaturization of proteins, destruction of cellular parts, and the abolition of cellular metabolic processes. The extent of the injury, in both size and depth, is determined by the intensity of the applied heat source, the duration of the exposure, and the thickness of the exposed skin. Children have relatively thin skin, so grease and chemical burns are more frequently full-thickness injuries, whereas water scalds are commonly partial-thickness injuries.

Control of infection

A major function of viable skin is the prevention of bacterial invasion. Burn wound surfaces provide a warm, moist, protein-rich growth media for microorganisms. Colonization of the wound with bacteria and fungi presents a constant potential reservoir of microbes and their by-products. It is unrealistic to keep the burn wound sterile through environmental techniques, as the patient serves as his own pool of potential microbial contaminants, by either normal surface or endogenous intestinal flora. However, control of the wound's microbial flora can be achieved with the application of prophylactic topical agents.

Wound cultures. It is essential to realize that no single topical agent is effective against all burn wound microbial contaminants. For this reason, constant surveillance through qualitative and quantitative wound cultures should be used to guide appropriate topical treatment. One to two samples should be collected for every 18% of body surface area burned, three times a week. Gross classification of the contaminating organism can be made 24 hours after wound culture. Specific identification and antibiotic sensitivities can be available at 48 hours after sampling. Rapid identification is possible with a Gram stain and rapid histologic biopsy; this method is useful when clinical suspicion of burn wound sepsis is high, and the rapidity of treatment implementation may be an important factor in the ultimate survival of the patient.

There are clinical implications to the results of quantitative cultures. The goal in use of topical antimicrobial agents is to maintain bacterial quantities at less than 10^3 organisms/g of tissue. Should quantities rise above this level, a change in the antimicrobial agent is indicated. Bacterial quantities of greater than 10^5 indicate a progressive wound infection, which should be systemically treated with antibiotics selected according to the particular sensitivity of the infecting organism(s). Bacterial invasion of viable tissue is indicated should bacterial counts rise above 10^7. Invasive infections must be treated with systemic antibiotics and wound excision.[9]

Topical agents. Through the years, many agents have been used for topical treatment of burn wounds. These include 0.5% silver nitrate solution, mafenide acetate, nitrofurazone, povidone iodine, silver sulfadiazine, gentamicin, and nystatin. However, povidone iodine ointment, nitrofurazone cream, and 0.5% silver nitrate fail to inhibit bacterial growth in agar diffusion assays. The effectiveness of mafenide acetate, silver sulfadiazine, and nitrofurazone ointment against organisms commonly colonizing a burn wound has been noted. All these agents increase metabolic rate upon application and decrease the rate of wound healing.[14]

Silver sulfadiazine is the most widely used topical agent. This white cream is easy to apply and painless to the patient. It has a broad spectrum efficacy, although it does not penetrate eschar. The most common adverse reaction to silver sulfadiazine is a transient leukopenia. For this reason, serial white blood cell counts should be monitored.

The agent should be replaced if the counts fall below 3000 cells/mm^3, but may be reinstituted after they return to normal ranges. The leukopenia observed is usually a reflection of granulocyte margination rather than an allergic response. A small number of patients demonstrate a true allergy to this agent by exhibiting a leukopenia or skin rash upon reapplication, and in such cases it should be permanently replaced by another agent.

Mafenide acetate may be used on areas of full-thickness injury or contaminated wounds. This is the only agent, other than sodium hypochlorite, demonstrated to penetrate the eschar to the necrotic-viable tissue interface, and it does so within 3 hours of application. It is also easy to apply, but may be transiently painful to the patient. Some patients may develop a rash around the site of application; however, this is usually transient. If the rash persists or worsens, the agent should be discontinued.

Mafenide acetate is also a potent carbonic anhydrase inhibitor, increasing the potential for metabolic acidosis. Should this occur, hyperventilation initially compensates for the increased carbon dioxide levels. The amount of acid-base change and the renal and pulmonary complications of its use are related to the surface area treated. Intravenous or oral administration of sodium bicarbonate usually corrects the imbalance. When no more than 20% of the body surface area is treated with this agent at any one time, there are usually minimal effects on the acid-base balance or pulmonary function. An effective regimen is to rotate application sites every 2 to 4 hours, replacing the mafenide acetate with a second topical agent. A rotation schedule is established so that all burn areas are treated with the agent twice each day. This is commonly referred to as "pulse therapy." Wound colony counts of over 10^5/g of tissue have been reduced to less than 10^2/g of tissue with a 2- to 9-day pulse therapy treatment period.[11]

Nystatin ointment has generally been reserved for use on wounds with documented *Candida* infection. However, the combination of nystatin and silver sulfadiazine, or bacitracin (mixed 1:1, that is, gram for gram) has significantly reduced the incidence of *Candida* superinfection in our population. Nystatin cannot be mixed with mafenide acetate because they inactivate each other, but instead should be alternated every 12 hours. In addition, 5 to 15 ml doses of oral nystatin, given three times daily, has decreased the incidence of thrush. In combination, topical nystatin and enteral nystatin have reduced the occurrence of *Candida* septicemia in our population to virtually nil.

In general, dressings should be changed at least every 8 to 24 hours and wounds should be cleansed and gently debrided with each dressing change. Topical agents can be maintained in intimate contact with the wound by applying a layer of fine mesh gauze over the agent and securing it with bulky dressings and elastic wraps. The use of closed dressings is more comfortable for the patient than open techniques of wound care. Dressing changes should be conducted under aseptic conditions and wound cleansing performed with a antimicrobial soap or a dilute (1:240) hypochlorite solution. Maintaining wounds at low contamination levels reduces the number and duration of septic episodes caused by wound flora and decreases the incidence of cross-contamination within the burn unit. Decreasing septic episodes, in turn, decreases the caloric and fluid demands of the patient. Skin graft survival is increased in wounds with fewer than 10^2 organisms per g of tissue, and scarring as a result of graft loss is decreased. Fifty percent of grafts applied to wounds with more than 10^5 bacteria/g of tissue are lost.[25]

Systemic antibiotics. Systemic antibiotics are generally reserved for use in cases of documented infection. Children should be examined daily for signs of sepsis, and the presence of any three of the following signs or symptoms should stimulate prophylactic administration of systemic antimicrobials. The child should be monitored for obtundation or changed sensorium, hyperventilation, hyperglycemia, thrombocytopenia, hypothermia or hyperthermia, and leukocytopenia or leukocytosis. When these signs are present and colony counts in the wound exceed 10^5 organisms per g of tissue, systemic antimicrobial therapy should be instituted specifically for the organism cultured. However, if the wound appears clean, other sources of sepsis such as the lungs, genitourinary tract, or thrombophlebitis, should be suspected. Routine cultures of sputum and urine should be performed two to three times each week. If no specific bacteriologic data are available and rapid assessment techniques are unrevealing, empiric therapy should be instituted, based on epidemiologic data available from the health care facility. This presumptive therapy should provide antimicrobial coverage for the predominant organisms endogenous to each specific burn unit; in our institution, vancomycin and amikacin are given. All children should receive broad-spectrum perioperative antibiotics, with the first dose administered just prior to surgical excision and subsequent doses continued for 48 hours postoperatively. As the bacteremia rate following excision is quite high and bacterial seeding following wound manipulation may occur, it is prudent to attempt to protect the patient from a systemic bacteremia.

Topical antimicrobial agents present a mechanical obstruction to epithelial migration and so inhibit the rate of wound healing. Some of these agents can cause electrolyte abnormalities, can disturb the acid-base equilibrium, and may increase metabolic rate. For these reasons, there has been a major effort to develop biologic dressings capable of physiologically closing the wound without impeding wound healing.

Biologic dressings

Biologic dressings such as porcine heterograft (also known as xenograft), human cadaveric allograft (also known as homograft), and amnion have been demonstrated to adhere to the wound surface, reduce wound bacterial colony counts, limit fluid and protein loss, reduce pain, and increase the rate of epithelialization over topical antimicrobial agents. Current uses of biologic dressings include (1) immediate (within 16 hours) closure of superficial, fully debrided, partial-thickness injuries; (2) coverage of an excised, granulating wound awaiting autografting; (3) as test grafts prior to autografting; and (4) debridement of patchy necrotic areas still adherent on granulating wounds.

Application of porcine heterograft or such synthetic skin substitutes as Biobrane, OpSite, or Omniderm to fresh, clean partial-thickness injuries provides a physiologic environment for reepithelialization. Partial-thickness injuries treated in this fashion heal at a faster rate than those treated with mafenide acetate or silver sulfadiazine. Success of this technique is dependent on the adherence of the heterograft or synthetic material to the wound. Any remaining necrotic tissue or accumulation of serum produces a closed loculation, which may become infected and destroy remaining epidermal components. Application of heterografts or synthetics should be carried out with the same diligence as an autograft procedure. The graft areas should be protected from shearing and frequently inspected for developing infection. The adherent heterograft or skin substitute will detach as keratinization occurs, leaving a normal epidermal covering.

Long-term wound coverage with heterograft is not recommended. Cadaveric allograft is a more suitable cover for wounds awaiting autograft. If homograft is unavailable, xenograft can be used but must be changed every 3 to 4 days to prevent suppuration. When homograft is used, the readiness of the granulating wound can be assessed by the degree of "take" of the allograft. The successful adherence and vascularization of homograft demonstrates the readiness of the wound to accept an autograft.

Although debridement of granulating wounds with adherent, patchy necrotic tissue can be accomplished with serial applications of biologic dressings, this seems to be somewhat wasteful of a valuable resource. The use of closed dressings for debridement results in high wound colony counts which must subsequently be reduced prior to autograft application, and the bacteria-laden wounds serve a reservoir of bacterial contaminants for an entire burn unit. Coarse mesh gauze, when frequently changed, has been demonstrated to effectively debride granulating wounds better than biologic dressings.

Artificial skin has been used successfully in limited clinical trials. The results of a multicenter trial using artificial skin demonstrated its efficacy in closing full-thickness wounds.[10] However, the use of artificial skin requires two surgical procedures separated by a 2-week interval: the first is the application of the substance to a debrided wound, and the second is placement of epithelial grafts over the vascularized substance.

Surgical intervention

The ultimate solution to the derangements associated with thermal injury in children is closure of the burn wound. Controversy exists, however, as to who, when, and how to appropriately intervene and surgically close the wounds. Excision of all deep components of the burn wound, whether deep partial-thickness or full-thickness wounds, becomes the treatment of choice if the patient can withstand the rigors of the procedure.

It is at this point that the determination of the depth of burn injury becomes a priority. A variety of techniques have been used for estimating the depth of burn injury, but none has proven to be reliable and reproducible. Superficial injuries, which will spontaneously heal within 3 weeks, can be recognized accurately on a clinical basis. The similarities of the physiologic and functional sequelae of a deep partial-thickness injury and a full-thickness injury make their distinction somewhat moot. A deep partial-thickness injury allowed to close through epithelial migration and wound contracture will cause the same deformity as a full-thickness injury going through the usual time of eschar separation and subsequent grafting.

Traditionally, burn wounds have been allowed to separate spontaneously through bacterial action over 3 to 5 weeks, the proliferation of granulation tissue encouraged and grafting performed on the neovascularized granulated bed. Although this method allows the wound to fully demarcate, it also prolongs the period in which the patient is at risk for infection, fluid and electrolyte imbalances, and malnutrition.

The more conservative technique may be complicated by a high incidence of burn wound infection in spite of the use of topical antimicrobial

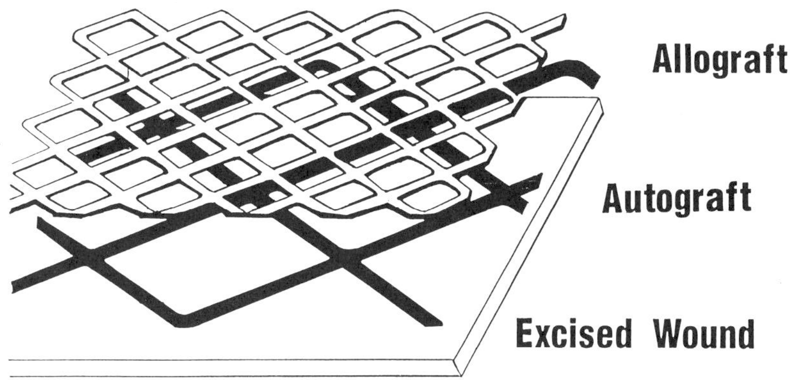

Figure 53–9 Widely meshed autograft continues to allow fluid and protein fluxes until interstices are completely epithelialized. Physiologic closure of grafted wounds can be obtained by overlaying widely meshed autograft with 2:1 meshed allograft.

agents. Organisms may invade viable tissue, resulting in bacteremia, which may eventually cause multiorgan failure. However, this approach has been used for years and is the basis for our current methods of treatment. Children treated with aggressive surgical excision of all eschar during the early postburn period have been noted to have shorter hospital stays, as well as fewer and shorter surgical procedures. However, a comparison of the techniques has demonstrated no differences in mortality.

Operative excision of as much of the burn wound as possible should, therefore, be performed as early in the burn course, as soon as the child is hemodynamically stable. The first surgical procedure can be safely performed within the first 48 hours postburn, and the risks of the surgical procedure will not increase mortality. This decision, however, should be tempered by such considerations as concomitant trauma (such as an inhalation injury), age (younger than 1 year), or premorbid medical conditions (e.g., juvenile diabetes, cystic fibrosis), all of which would significantly increase the surgical risk factors. In addition, early excision (fewer than 3 days postburn) of scald burns appears to increase blood loss without shortening hospital stay. The surgeon must weigh all of these factors against the risk of burn wound infection and sepsis, which generally occurs no earlier than 5 days postinjury. The optimal time for the surgical excision of most burns is, therefore, within the first 72 hours postinjury.

Tangential excision, a method of sequentially removing thin layers of burned tissue to viable punctate bleeding, is generally accepted as the method of choice for burn wound excision since its introduction by Janzekovic 20 years ago. However, its very nature requires the availability of blood for replacement. If the technique is used on burns of larger surface area, blood loss may approach two to three times the circulating volume. Blood loss of 0.4 ml/cm^2 of tissue excised should be expected if the excision is performed within the first 24 hours postinjury. The amount lost between 48 hours and 14 days postinjury during tangential excision is 0.75 ml/cm^2 of tissue excised.

Fascial excision of burn wounds is reserved for large full-thickness injuries (over 60% BSA burn) in which the risks of infection, blood loss, and skin slough may lead to higher mortality. Expanded meshed autografts are used to cover the excised beds. Expansion ratios of split-thickness skin grafts should not exceed 1:4, as higher ratios produce a suboptimal result with contracture and friable skin. Although meshed autograft has been used to cover open wound beds, wounds covered with meshed skin continue to leak protein and fluids. Complete closure can be obtained by placing 2:1 meshed cadaveric homograft over the meshed autograft (Fig. 53-9), as described by Alexander.

The amount excised at each procedure is dependent on the stability of the child, the rapidity at which the surgeon can perform the debridement, the adequacy of anesthesia, the availability of autograft or substitute, and the blood loss incurred during the procedure. Injuries of less than 40% BSA burn can usually be completely excised in a single procedure. Sufficient donor sites are available to graft the excised bed despite the fact that about 30% BSA is unavailable for donation (i.e., face, neck, hands, and feet). However, donor site availability is limited in children with greater than 40% BSA burn. The first donor-site harvest usually provides the best graft tissue, so early consideration should be given to the closure of articulating surfaces, particularly the hand. Excision of the entire burn wound in the first procedure allows for the complete removal of all necrotic tissue. When there is insufficient autograft to close all excised beds, fresh cadaveric homograft is the dressing of choice, although antimicrobial agent–impregnated fine mesh gauze, Biobrane, and other biologic dressings have been used.

There are several methods for the surgical management of burn wounds. One of the earliest methods employed involves treatment with topical antimicrobial agents while performing blunt debridement of the nonadherent eschar in daily bathing procedures. The wounds are grafted as granulating surfaces appear. A somewhat more radical approach involves the surgical excision of eschar as soon as the child is hemodynamically stable.

Although it may seem that early definitive closure of a burn wound would eliminate or reduce the hypermetabolic responses following thermal injury, this has not been demonstrated. Preliminary data demonstrated no significant differences in resting energy expenditure, oxygen consumption, or carbon dioxide production when the two treatment methods were compared. Moreover, it has not yet been determined exactly when, in the postburn course, metabolic rates return to normal.

Most burn wounds (less than 30% BSA burn), whether of deep partial or full thickness, can and should be excised and grafted within the early postburn period. Larger burns in hemodynamically stable patients who are physiologically good surgical risks should undergo massive excision with autograft placement and cadaveric allograft coverage of those excised beds in which sufficient autograft is unavailable. Current research efforts are directed toward the development of tissue culture epithelium and artificial dermis.

Intraoperative management

Early excision of massive burn wounds requires the coordination of the entire burn team. The total support of the anesthesiologists is essential, as they are responsible for continuing resuscitation and maintaining volume during the procedure. Preoperatively, sufficient venous access should be obtained to ensure a timely response to adverse events. If the procedure will be lengthy, arterial cannulation and pressure monitoring for enhanced physiologic surveillance is indicated. Nasogastric intubation and urinary bladder catheterization are also necessary. Ketamine is the anesthetic agent of choice for pediatric patients, even in the excision of massive injuries. Nasotracheal intubation is infrequently needed, although supplemental oxygen should be provided by face mask.

Blood losses associated with early burn wound excision are predictable. A series of equations have been developed to predict blood loss (Table 53-3).[7] Blood loss can be decreased with the use of tour-

Table 53–3 Blood losses related to excision

Time of excision	Burn area excised	Formula
First 24 hours postinjury	>30% BSA burn	0.35 ml/cm² excised
Postburn days 2 to 16	>30% BSA burn	0.6 ml/cm² excised
Anytime postburn	<30% BSA burn	0.68 ml/cm² excised

niquets during extremity excisions, with the application of topical and local pressure. Epinephrine solutions can be used to control bleeding but must be employed judiciously. Pediatric patients are particularly sensitive to topical epinephrine, and paroxysmal tachycardia may occur, particularly in infants or children with small (<30% BSA burn) injuries.

WOUNDS REQUIRING SPECIAL CONSIDERATION
Head

Burn injuries to the head present many different problems. Cutaneous facial burns are usually treated conservatively, allowing demarcation and spontaneous eschar separation over 14 to 21 days. Bacitracin/polymyxin B is the antimicrobial agent of choice, and rarely are gauze dressings necessary. Ointments may be applied by a gloved hand as frequently as necessary. Following the first 2 to 3 weeks, careful tangential excision may be performed. A dermabrader is occasionally useful, as maximal tissue conservation is essential. Facial wounds are usually closed with sheet grafts donated from the scalp, upper chest, or upper arm for the best color match. Coverage should be performed in "cosmetic units," with sheet graft seams falling into the normal folds of the face. Full-thickness grafts and flap reconstruction may be performed in specific instances, usually in small injuries or nose reconstruction. Occasional releases of contractures may be needed for severe ectropion or microstomia, particularly when mucosal surfaces are continuously exposed.

Evaluation of the eyes is of utmost importance, and if any injury is suspected, an ophthalmologist should be consulted. Initial eye care includes copious irrigation with a balanced saline solution. Burn injuries to the eyelid or canthi may necessitate application of additional lubricative gels or antibiotic ointments to prevent corneal dessication or infection. Surgical tarsorraphy should be avoided, and early eyelid release is rarely indicated unless ectropion is severe.

Partial-thickness or full-thickness injuries to the pinna of the ear should be treated conservatively. Because of the limited vascularity of this cartilaginous tissue, mafenide acetate is the topical agent of choice. The eschar is allowed to spontaneously separate prior to grafting which frequently requires several attempts before final closure. Reconstructive surgery is usually required and is undertaken only after the scar tissue has matured.

Scalp burns are treated as any other cutaneous injury. Small areas may be primarily closed, owing to the great elasticity of the scalp. Grafts can also be placed directly over exposed periosteum. Should the injury be sufficiently deep to injure the periosteum, however, the outer table of the cranium can be removed and allowed to granulate prior to grafting.

Hands

One of the involuntary actions during a burn injury is clenching of the fists. Palmar burns are therefore rare, although the dorsal aspects of the hands are frequently injured. Early tangential excision of deep partial-thickness or full-thickness injuries that do not involve the tendon sheaths is the treatment of choice. The early closure of these injuries allows for a rapid remobilization and preservation of function. Split-thickness skin grafts should be expanded no more than 2:1, and optimal results are obtained if the dorsum is closed with sheet grafts. Early splinting and progressive range of motion exercises promote the best functional results. If the injury is sufficiently severe to imperil phalanges or involves the tendon sheaths, the wounds should be allowed 14 to 21 days to demarcate. By allowing a full declaration of the injury, the phalanges can be maximally preserved.

Severe palmar injuries are rare and portend a poor prognosis for the entire hand. These injuries should be allowed to heal primarily. Full-thickness injuries to the palm cause severe contracture of all phalanges which, despite aggressive exercise and splinting, rarely regain full range of motion.

Feet

Severe burn injury to the soles of the feet is infrequent. Like the palmar aspect of the hands, they are usually protected from the causative agent. Early tangential excision of deep partial-thickness or full-thickness injuries and closure with no more than a 2:1 meshed autograft allows for early mobilization and ambulation. The single exception is a scald injury, the depth of which is difficult to assess accurately in the early postburn period. Like hand injuries, those injuries sufficiently severe to involve the tendon sheaths should be treated conservatively.

Perineum, genitalia, and buttocks

In its protected location, the perineum is rarely injured other than with large surface area burns or intentional burning. This area heals primarily by contracture rather than epithelialization. If the total injury is sufficiently small, early debridement and closure is optimal. However, with large surface area burns, the perineum is frequently allowed to heal by secondary intention. Should the buttocks or anal area be severely burned, the patient may be maintained prone until closure is obtained or, alternately, placed in an air-suspension bed. It is essential that the patient be kept clean of fecal material, as wound contamination with enteric bacteria is possible, if not probable. This is particularly difficult in treatment of the infant and small child. Diverting colostomies should be avoided, as the anus and rectum are prone to the development of strictures.

Burns to the penis are usually treated conservatively, although early debridement with split-thickness skin grafts is acceptable. Complete loss of the scrotal epidermis is infrequent because the deep rugae protect islands of intact tissue, which slowly coalesce into total coverage. Should skin grafting be necessary, split-thickness grafts may be applied, but further surgical reconstructive procedures are frequently needed.

Breast

Burn injury to the anterior chest often involves the nipple-areolar complex (NAC), and severe injuries may result in a partial or total loss of the NAC. Despite this, female breast development does not appear to be affected, as the prepubescent breast bud receives minimal injury. However, aggressive fascial excision of the chest could damage the breast bud and subsequent glandular development, leading to significant breast deformities later in life. Tangential excision with 2:1 split-thickness skin grafting provides the optimal cosmetic result, although larger expansion ratios can provide acceptable coverage. The majority of prepubescent females will require breast releases because the scar tissue will restrict development. In those injuries that result in the loss of the NAC, acceptable reconstruction can be performed.

INHALATION INJURY

The presence or absence of an inhalation injury is the major determinant of mortality. Pulmonary pathology accounts for 20% to 84% of burn mortalities.[17] About 5% of burn-injured children below the age of 4 and 7% of those between 5 and 14 years sustain an inhalation injury. The mortality rate of children with isolated cutaneous injuries is 1% to 2%, but increases to about 40% if the injury is complicated with a concomitant inhalation injury, irrespective of total surface area burn.

The pathophysiology of inhalation injury is complex and of multifactorial etiology. The mechanisms of upper-airway injury are markedly different from those of injury to the lower airways and pulmonary parenchyma. Oropharyngeal and supracarinal airway injuries are related to direct thermal injury and subsequent edema formation. Direct thermal injury to the lower airways occurs only with steam inhalation.

In inhalation injury, the injured mucosa is shed and combines with fibrinous exudate and polymorphonuclear leukocytes to create pseudomembranous casts. These casts cause airway obstruction and atelectasis, predisposing the lung to pneumonia and infection. Lower airway and parenchymal damage is mediated by the polymorphonuclear leukocytes and their proteolytic enzymes. The release of these enzymes and oxygen-free radicals are most probably the causative agents of the progressive permeability changes observed following inhalation injury. The changes in microvascular permeability make the lung extremely sensitive to the deleterious effects of volume overload and sepsis.

In addition, it appears that surfactant is deactivated with inhalation injury. Many investigators have demonstrated an immediate decrease in thoracic compliance in children suffering from smoke inhalation. The loss of surfactant function also increases the work of breathing, which increases the metabolic demands placed on the child.

Inhalation injury is suspected if the injury occurred to the child in an enclosed space and if the child exhibits carbonaceous sputum, wheezing, or bronchorrhea. Abnormal carboxyhemoglobin levels are of significant value if the measurement is made soon after injury. Carbon monoxide levels over 30% may cause headaches, nausea, and behavioral disturbances, the characteristic cherry-red skin discoloration occurring at levels over 40%. By itself, however, an elevated carboxyhemoglobin level is a poor predictor of later complications. Likewise, standard chest radiographs are insensitive to inhalation injury. Bronchoscopy is the most frequent method used for determination of an inhalation injury. The direct visualization of airway edema, mucosal hyperemia, tissue sloughing, and carbonaceous matter in the airways confirms these classic signs of inhalation injury. Various other methods, such as xenon[133] scans, evaluation of extravascular lung water, and assessment of pulmonary mechanics, may be used to evaluate the presence of inhalation injury in the parenchymal tissue, but as yet there is no method for the quantitation of inhalation injury.

Patients with inhalation injury pass through a fairly predictable clinical course of three distinct stages: pulmonary insufficiency, pulmonary edema, and bronchopneumonia. The first stage appears up to 72 hours postinjury. During the burning process, the fire consumes the available oxygen, and carbon monoxide poisoning may contribute to the development of hypoxia. In addition, the toxic products of combustion irritate the tracheobronchial lining and produce bronchospasm, which decreases airway compliance. Treatment must begin immediately upon the suspicion of inhalation injury. Oxygen should be administered by face mask at the scene of the injury. One hundred percent oxygen will reduce carboxyhemoglobin levels by one half in 1 hour. Hyperbaric oxygen therapy will also hasten the removal of carbon monoxide from the blood, although this therapy is not universally available. Endotracheal intubation should be performed with the earliest indication of impending airway collapse, or may be necessary to preserve the airway when the patient has sustained full-thickness nasolabial or circumferential neck burns. We do not prophylactically intubate pediatric patients solely with the diagnosis of inhalation injury. In field situations or during transport, however, it may be prudent to ensure an uncompromised airway. Serial bronchoscopy and pulmonary lavage may help to remove carbonaceous debris and airway casts. Aggressive chest physiotherapy may also be of assistance.

Positive end-expiratory pressure (PEEP) is essential to the intubated patient to prevent atelectasis, consolidation, and subsequent pneumonia. The normal regulatory mechanism of epiglottic closure is ablated with endotracheal intubation, and the injury has inactivated the pulmonary surfactant. Although the microvascular permeability exhibited following inhalation injury promotes fluid sequestration in the parenchymal tissue, resuscitation fluids should not be restricted. Patients with inhalation injury and concomitant cutaneous burns will require additional resuscitation fluid, and administered volumes should be guided by urine output, blood pressure, and distal vascular response. Should insufficient fluid be administered, it appears to increase the severity of pulmonary injury by allowing a greater sequestration of polymorphonuclearcytes in the pulmonary tissue.

As pulmonary edema develops, increased levels of oxygen and PEEP may be required to maintain acceptable gas exchange. Both underhydration and volume overload should be prevented. The former predisposes the patient to other systemic insults, such as renal failure, and the latter promotes the development of hydrostatic pulmonary edema. Antibiotics should be administered only in cases of documented infection.

Should clinical symptomatology indicate the development of pneumonia, sputum cultures should be obtained and empiric antibiotics initiated. Early pneumonias (earlier than 7 days postinjury) are usually the result of staphylococcal organisms, whereas later pneumonias are generally caused by gram-negative organisms, such as *Pseudomonas*. Serial sputum cultures should guide antibiotic changes. Aggressive pulmonary toilet and early mobilization are useful care modalities. Although there have been anecdotal reports of the therapeutic effects of hyperbaric oxygen, we do not routinely employ this technique. Corticosteroids have also been examined as supportive agents but they have demonstrated no clear clinical benefit and they may, in fact, predispose the patient to bronchopneumonia.

ELECTRICAL INJURY

Although extensive electrical injuries are uncommon in children, about 3% to 5% of all admitted burn patients have sustained injury as a result of electrical contact. Of these, about one third are under the age of 15 and 90% are male. One of the most common injuries, injury to the oral commissure, is caused by biting an electrical cord, although this injury is caused more by heat than by electrical conduction.

Electrical current produces an injury unlike other burns in that the visible areas of tissue necrosis represent only a small portion of the destroyed tissue. Deep tissue destruction is produced by the heat generated from the electrical resistance of the tissues. Tissues surrounding long bones usually sustain the most extensive damage, as bone is the least able to conduct electricity. Periosseous muscle is the most significantly damaged, and progressive destruction occurs as a result of microvascular thrombosis. The most significant injury, therefore, is within the deep tissue, and subsequent edema formation can cause vascular compromise to any area distal to the injury. Fascial compartment pressures may quickly rise, and fasciotomy is frequently necessary to prevent the loss of the distal areas. Serial muscle compartment explorations are usually required to sequentially debride nonviable tissue. Should the muscle compartment be extensively injured, amputation may be necessary.

Resuscitation fluid should be given to maintain urine output of more than 1 ml/kg/hr. Because of the relative smallness of the visible injury, it is easy to underestimate fluid requirements. Should insufficient fluid be administered, the tissue detritus produced will lodge in the renal glomeruli or tubules and will compromise renal function. Systemic alkalinization with sodium bicarbonate can prevent the myoglobin deposition in the renal tubules; however, care should be taken to monitor serum sodium levels and prevent hypernatremia.

Myocardial damage and arrhythmias, including asystole, may occur with high-voltage electrical injuries. The most serious derangements occur in the first 24 hours postinjury. Any significant ECG abnormalities should be treated appropriately.

Only a sustained, high-voltage injury will produce long-term neurologic deficits, although approximately two thirds of patients exhibit neurologic symptoms immediately following such injury. Most patients experience a transient loss of consciousness without any ill effects. Peripheral neuropathies and myelopathies occur less frequently. Serial neurologic evaluations should be performed as part of the routine monitoring of these patients.

CHEMICAL INJURY

Chemical injuries are not as common as thermal injuries. Most commonly, they are sustained by children who come in contact with household chemicals, such as various cleaning agents and other household products. Parents should be forewarned of this danger and admonished to maintain these products in secure areas. In particular, these products should not be kept in the lower cabinets of the kitchen, where especially young children can gain access to them. The local Poison Information Center telephone numbers should be provided to new parents, and first-aid products, such as syrup of ipecac, should be kept in all households with children.

The chemical burn is unique in that tissue destruction will continue until the agent is completely removed or, if ingested, sufficiently diluted. Strong acids and strong alkalis cause the most severe chemical burns. Dilution is the key to all chemical burn treatment. Neutralization is not generally chosen over dilution as a treatment because the heat produced in the neutralization reaction may exacerbate the injury. Early excision should always be considered.

Alkali burns are usually full-thickness injuries. The wounds require continuous and copious irrigation for 24 hours. This process must begin within 1 hour postburn to be effective. The repair process cannot begin until the irritant has been removed. Uncleared residue that remains in the eschar increases the depth of the burn wound. Intravenous fluid resuscitation is similar to that for thermal burns.

Acid burns also require copious lavage with water or saline, and some unique acid burns require additional therapy. Hydrofluoric acid burns are additionally treated with subcutaneous 10% calcium gluconate injections around and under the burned area. We reserve the subcutaneous injections for acid burns with acid concentrations of greater than 10%. A calcium gluconate gel (2.5%) may be topically applied to help inactivate the fluoride ion and decrease the severity of the injury. Complications of hydrofluoric acid burns include hypocalcemia and possible pulmonary edema if the fumes are inhaled. To prevent hypocalcemia in this setting, we routinely add 20 ml of 10% calcium gluconate to the first liter of resuscitation fluid.

Phosphorous burns are seen primarily in battlefield situations. Exposure is characterized by gray discoloration of the skin. Early death may occur as a result of a reversal of the calcium-phosphorus ratio, leading to malignant cardiac arrhythmias. Treatment centers on removing the phosphorous from the burn wound and keeping the wound moist with damp bandages. In summary, a chemical burn can have a deceptively benign appearance on initial examination, progressing over time to a severe full-thickness injury. The cornerstone of treatment is early copious lavage with tap water or isotonic saline.

PREVENTION

Even young children can be taught the fundamentals of self-preservation during a fire. Emphasis should be placed on the drill of "Stop, drop, and roll" in the event that clothing catches fire, and the use of blankets to smother flame. Fire drills should be conducted in homes, day-care facilities, and schools for preschool and school-aged children. These drills should include not only the children's orderly exit from classrooms or homes to the outdoors, but other procedures such as low-crawling to decrease exposure to smoke, closing doors behind them, feeling doors prior to opening them, and not opening hot doors. Emergency first-aid techniques, such as application of cold (not icy) water to burn injuries and avoidance of oral fluids, and instructions on how to contact emergency personnel (e.g., 911) should also be emphasized.

Rescue fundamentals should be taught to parents and older children. Wooden or rubber objects should be used to dislodge a person in contact with a high-voltage electrical source. Caustic chemicals should be properly stored out of reach of children, and the local Poison Information Center telephone number should be readily available.

Burn prevention should continue at home. Water heaters should be set at no more than 140° F. This temperature is more than sufficient for dishwashers. There is a direct, linear relationship between water temperature and length of exposure to the resulting burn injury. By decreasing the water temperature from 140° F to 120° F, the risk of an accidental burn is greatly decreased by increasing the length of exposure time necessary to produce a significant burn injury.[23] In addition, gas water heaters should be installed at least 18 inches above the floor, to reduce the risk of explosion in the presence of volatile substances. Petroleum-based products, such as turpentine, paint, and kerosene, should be used and stored in an isolated location, away from any natural gas–fueled appliance.

Mortality associated with thermal injury has been drastically reduced because of extensive lobbying by burn "preventionists" in legislative agencies on such issues as the use of flame-resistant fabric in children's nightwear.

REHABILITATION

Successful attainment of rehabilitation goals is dependent on the active participation of the child (or the primary caregiver in the case of infants) in the process. Children, in general, respond well to an organized, consistent routine. Care should be scheduled so that medical, rehabilitation, and play or relaxation periods occur at consistently regular intervals. The rehabilitation process should be carefully explained in language appropriate to the age and developmental level of the child. Major efforts should be expended in preparing a child well in advance of any change in the treatment plan or surgical procedure.

During the acute postburn period, a large portion of rehabilitation is positioning. It is common for a child to be restricted to bed rest after grafting procedures or during periods of acute illness. Proper positioning provides joint alignment, decreases contracture formation, and prevents undue pressure on peripheral nerve plexes. Appropriate positioning should be implemented upon admission and continued throughout the child's hospital stay.

Splinting is used to immobilize a specific body part. Most commonly used for splints are thermoplastic materials. These substances can be molded directly to the patient when they are warm and retain their molded shape when cool. It is especially important to employ splinting techniques early in infants and toddlers because they rarely comply with positioning regimens. Splints should be used to maintain immobility of a newly grafted wound and to maintain position of function and prevent contracture of a burned hand, foot, or other injured joint. Specially created splints can be used to prevent microstomia, which is particularly common with burns of the oronasal area or injuries of the oral commissure incurred by biting electrical cords. Serial splinting can be used to increase gradually the range of motion of a contracted joint.

Skeletal suspension has been used to facilitate skin grafting and to preserve position of function during the correction of burn-acquired deformities. This technique is safe and effective, having only a 4.4% incidence of complications, of which 90% are local cutaneous pin-site infections that resolve with pin removal and local antibiotic treatment. With this low rate of complications, skeletal suspension should be considered a useful adjunct in the care of severely burned children.

Hypertrophic scarring is a common result of deep thermal injuries. Usually, hypertrophic scar formation is a function of the time required for initial burn wound closure. The earlier closure is accomplished, the less likely hypertrophic scarring will occur. A large number of injuries that are closed after 21 days postinjury will produce hypertrophic scars, whereas those closed in less than 14 days have a lower incidence of such scarring.

The effectiveness of controlled constant pressure on suppressing hypertrophic scar formation has been demonstrated, and custom-fitted elastic garments are commercially available. However, elastic wraps or tubular elastic bandages can be used to accomplish the same goal. Constant pressure should be applied 24 hours a day until scars mature, usually 6 to 18 months following injury. Children, in general, are more prone to hypertrophic scar formation than adults, probably because of the rapid cell mitosis associated with growth. The use of pressure to reduce the occurrence of hypertrophic scarring is essential to achieve an optimal cosmetic and functional result.

Positioning, splinting, and elastic garments should be used in conjunction with a specifically tailored exercise program. Exercises should be designed to encompass activities of daily living, and children often respond more enthusiastically if the program is presented in terms of play. Written guidelines for the exercise program, which can be given to the patient or family at the time of discharge, will help them continue the program at home. Family members should be involved early in the course of treatment, so that they are familiar with the regime and feel comfortable in implementing it with little or no supervision.

A growth delay in burned children has been described.[26] This delay was noted in children sustaining a greater than 40% BSA burn and continued for as long as 3 years postinjury. No "catch up" growth spurt was experienced by these children, although they resumed age-normal growth rates within a 3-year period following injury. This phenomenon has both physical and psychosocial implications, and the children and their families should be advised that it may occur.

Reconstructive procedures should be planned well in advance, and should not be implemented prior to scar maturation. However, if such procedures are necessary to provide sufficient motion for activities of daily living, they should be performed with the full knowledge that revisions may be necessary. In designing a reconstructive plan, the child should be involved in the decisions, because the child's reconstructive priorities may not coincide with those of the medical staff.

PSYCHOSOCIAL ISSUES

Research into the effect of hospitalization on children has extensively documented the emotional responses of separation anxiety, regression, anger, fear, and depression. The behavior patterns of burned children are similar to those observed in other hospitalized children, but appear to be more extreme. The trauma of the injury, the removal from a familiar environment, and the disruption of daily routines can leave a child bewildered and emotionally drained.

Responses to hospitalization are related to the developmental stage of the child. Infants and toddlers exhibit acute separation anxiety, manifested as agitation, fear, and social withdrawal during parental absence. School-aged children are more frequently upset by activity restrictions and become agitated, angry, and manipulative. Adolescents are affected most by the loss of environmental and personal control and frequently become demanding, manipulative, and angry. In addition, school-aged and adolescent patients are deeply aware of body image and concerned about peer acceptance. They are likely to become depressed and withdrawn, particularly as the time of discharge nears.

Each child is a member of a functioning familial environment, and the child and his family should be treated as a single unit. Many of the emotions exhibited by the child are echoed among family members, and all require emotional support throughout the hospital stay. Guilt, felt by both the child and family members, is a major source of emotional stress. The child and his family should be encouraged to express their feelings about this issue.

Information alleviates many of the stresses experienced during hospitalization. Clear, rational explanations of the procedures, the expected results, and the potential complications should be given in small doses. These explanations will have to be repeated several times before the child and family members can accept and incorporate the information.

Parents should be allowed to participate actively in the care of their child. In the early stages, their involvement may be only peripheral, but even then infants can be held and rocked and toddlers and school-aged children can be read to or told stories. Some burn units have even initiated "rooming-in" or unlimited visiting hours with success. In later stages, parents can assist with feeding and dressing

Table 53–4 Pain medications useful in pediatric patients

Drug	Dose	Indication	Outcome
Chloral hydrate	250-500 mg q8h	Preop; sleep	Amnesia
Diazepam	1-2 mg q3-4h	Preop; anxiety	Disassociation
Demerol	1-2 mg/kg q2-3h	Acute pain	Analgesia/amnesia
Ketamine	0.2-0.5 mg/kg	OR; debridement	Analgesia/amnesia
Morphine sulfate	0.2-0.5 mg/kg q2-3h	Acute pain	Analgesia/amnesia
Midozalam	0.5 mg/kg q3-4h	Acute pain	Analgesia/amnesia
Pedi Cocktail*	0.1 ml/kg q3-4h	Acute pain	Analgesia/amnesia

*Pedi Cocktail contains meperidine 25 mg/ml, promethazine 6.25 mg/ml, and chlorpromazine 6.25 mg/ml.

changes and thus provide the child with some sense of normalcy.

Few long-term studies have been conducted on burned children, and evaluations of the psychosocial impact of burn injury are sparse in the literature. In a group of 12 children who had survived a greater than 80% BSA burn, static measurements of range of motion and hearing demonstrated severe disabilities. However, all the children were functioning at age-appropriate levels with nearly all attending age-appropriate school programs and participating in extracurricular activities. In a second group of 38 children at least 2 years postburn, a battery of psychological tests including the Minnesota Multiphasic Personality Scale, Family Environment Scale, and Suicide Probability Scale demonstrated that all patients fell within normal limits for psychological adjustment. No correlations could be found with any demographic or burn-related variables. The few patients noted to have some psychological disturbances perceived their families as less cohesive, less independent, less self-sufficient and less likely to make their own decisions. The implications of this study are that professionals working with burn victims should stress the importance of a familial support system and encourage the values of autonomy and self-sufficiency.

PAIN MANAGEMENT

Pain and its control are major issues in burn care. Medical personnel who work with burn patients consistently underestimate the amount of pain associated with the injury as compared with the patient's reported level of pain. Burned children tend to exhibit extreme pain during treatment procedures but seem able to recover more quickly than adolescents or adults.

Although no one can describe how preverbal neonates and infants experience pain, it is unrealistic to assume that they do not feel pain. However, burned children are more likely than adults to receive no pain medication. Morphine and its derivatives are the most frequently used analgesic, alone or in combination with mood-altering drugs. Hypnosis has been proven efficacious in relieving pain for pediatric patients, although less successful than in adults. Other interventions such as relaxation therapy or guided imagery have also been employed, with success, in the pediatric population. Children are more amenable to guided imagery therapy than adults, and this is thought to be due to a more active fantasy life and less fear associated with loss of control.

Effective pain control techniques need not compromise the recovery of the patient. Selective use of analgesics or amnesics, in combination with other mood-altering drugs, makes the required medical care more tolerable (Table 53-4). Relaxation techniques and guided imagery methods can be taught to nursing and paraprofessional staff and do not require the full-time presence of a professional psychologist to be effective. Hypnotherapy does require the initial intervention of a trained professional, but the techniques can be used by other staff members after the process is mastered by the patient.

CHILD ABUSE BY BURNING

Many deliberately inflicted burn injuries can pass as accidents unless practicing physicians are cognizant of the characteristics of the burn-abused child. Legal mandates require the reporting of suspected child abuse cases. Reported incidences of inflicted burn injury range from 4% to 10% of all acute burn admissions; however, as many as one out of every four children hospitalized for scald injuries has been deliberately burned.

Although the burned child may have a history of frequent medical treatment for bruises, fractures, or hematomas, this is not always the case. The abused child may also display evidence of physical neglect and malnutrition. There are, in addition, other clues that should elicit a high degree of suspicion of inflicted injury: there has been an inexplicable delay between the time of injury and the first attempt to gain medical attention; the burns appear older than they would had they happened on the alleged day of the incident; the parent's account of the incident is inconsistent with the injury present; there are no witnesses to the incident; the injury is reported to have been inflicted by a sibling or a person other than the parent present with the injured child.

Abused children may be excessively withdrawn, unresponsive, or submissive. They rarely cry during painful procedures. Their burns are most frequently symmetrical in nature (e.g., "stocking" burns) and are full-thickness injuries. Splash marks, which would indicate an attempt by a child to get out of a bath of hot water, are absent. Symmetrical injuries and isolated burns to the buttocks are almost impossible to produce accidentally.

SUMMARY

The pediatric burn patient requires a carefully tailored treatment plan from the time of admission through the entire hospitalization. Children present a unique combination of physiologic and psychological factors that affect all postinjury care regimens. Each member of the treatment team must be aware of and prepared to compensate for the physiologic and psychological impact of a burn injury on the pediatric patient.

Successful resuscitation of the burned child can be addressed through specifically designed formulas for fluid replacement and nutritional support. Precise fluid management in the pediatric patient is more crucial than in the adult, especially in infants and toddlers. Careful and frequent monitoring of clinical signs of impending decompensation is essential. Nutritional supplementation beginning with the initial postburn period is of prime importance in the child, who is undergoing not only reparative processes, but also growth and development.

Early surgical intervention, with removal of necrotic tissue and graft application, is desirable in all pediatric burns other than scald injuries. Positioning and splinting should be incorporated into the care plan for each child upon admission, followed by constant, continuous pressure application after healing is accomplished.

Psychosocial support should be provided to burned children and their families, and all effort should be made to provide adequate information about the care plan to the entire family unit. Depression, anger, withdrawal, regression, and manipulation are emotional reactions to be expected, and appropriate interventions should be in-corporated into the treatment plan. Pain control can be achieved with judicious use of analgesics, psychotropics, and other measures such as hypnosis, relaxation therapy, and guided imagery.

REFERENCES

1. Arturson G: Prostaglandins in human burn wound secretions, *Burns* 3:112, 1977.
2. Artz CP, Moncrief JA, Pruitt BA Jr, editors: *Burns: a team approach*, Philadelphia, 1979, WB Saunders.
3. Boswick JA, editor: *The art and science of burn care*, Rockville, 1987, Aspen Publications.
4. Curreri PW: Assessing nutritional need for the burned patient, *J Trauma* 30(suppl 12):S20, 1990.
5. Davies JWL: *The pathophysiology of burning*, London, 1979, Ballier & Tindall.
6. Demling RH, LaLonde C: *Burn trauma*, New York, 1989, Thieme Medical Publishers.
7. Desai MH, Herndon DN, Broemeling LD et al: Early burn wound excision significantly reduces blood loss, *Ann Surg* 211(6):753, 1990.
8. Enzi G, Casadei A, Sergi G et al: Metabolic and hormonal effects of early nutritional supplementation after surgery in burn patients, *Crit Care Med* 18(7):719, 1990.
9. Heggers JP, Robson MC: Infection control in burn patients. In Ruberg RL, editor: Clinics in plastic surgery, Philadelphia, 1986, WB Saunders.
10. Heimbach D, Luterman A, Burke J et al: Artificial dermis for major burns: a multicenter randomized clinical trial, *Ann Surg* 208(3):313, 1988.
11. Herndon DN, Kraft ER: Temporary reduction of burn wound quantitative bacterial counts to $<10^2$ with subsequent 95% overall autograft survival, *Surg Forum* 33:61, 1982.
12. Herndon DN, Traber DL: Inhalation injury: pathophysiology, diagnosis and treatment. In Sarro M, editor: *Multiple organ failure*, New York, 1990, Thieme Medical Publishers.
13. Herndon DN, Thompson PB, Desai MH et al: Treatment of burns in children. In Lamsback WJ, editor: *Pediatric clinics of North America*, Philadelphia, 1985, WB Saunders, p 1131.
14. Herndon DN, Wilmore DW, Mason AD Jr et al: Increases in postburn hypermetabolism caused by application of topical ointments, *Surg Forum* 29:49, 1978.
15. Herndon DN, Barrow RE, Kunkel KR et al: Effects of recombinant human growth hormone on donor site healing in severely burned children, *Surgery* 212(4):424, 1990.
16. Herndon DN, Barrow RE, Stein MD et al: Increased mortality with intravenous supplemental feeding in severely burned patients, *J Burn Care Rehabil* 10(4):309, 1989.
17. Herndon DN, Curreri PW, Abston S et al: Treatment of burns. In Ravitch MM, editor: *Current problems in surgery*, vol 24, Chicago, Mosby–Year Book, p 341.
18. Herndon DN, Stein MD, Rutan TC et al: Failure of TPN supplementation to improve liver function, immunity and mortality in thermally injured patients, *J Trauma* 27:195, 1987.
19. Jacoby FG: *Nursing care of the patient with burns*, St Louis, 1976, Mosby–Year Book.
20. Liljedahl S, Gemzell C, Plantin L et al: Effect of human growth hormone in patients with severe burns, *Acta Chir Scand* 122:1, 1961.
21. Larson DL, Abston S, Evans EB et al: Techniques for decreasing scar formation and contractures in the burned patient, *J Trauma* 11:807, 1971.

22. Moncrief JA: Topical antibacterial therapy of the burn wound, *Clin Plast Surg* 1(4):563, 1974.

23. Moritz AD, Henriques FC Jr: Studies of thermal injury. II. The relative importance of time and surface temperature in the causation of cutaneous burns, *Am J Pathol* 23:695, 1947.

24. Onarkein H, Lund T, Reed R: Thermal skin injury. II. Effects on edema formation and albumin extravasation of fluid resuscitation with lactated Ringer's, plasma and hypertonic saline (2,400 mosmol/l) in the rat, *Circ Shock* 27(1):25, 1989.

25. Robson MC, Krizek TS: Predicting skin graft survival, *J Trauma* 13(3):213, 1973.

26. Rutan RL, Herndon DN: Growth delay in postburn pediatric patients, *Arch Surg* 125(3):392, 1990.

27. Willis BS, Larson DL, Abston S: Positioning and splinting the burned patient, *Heart Lung* 2:696, 1973.

28. Wilmore DW, Long JM, Mason AD Jr et al: Catecholamines: mediator of the hypermetabolic response to thermal injury, *Ann Surg* 180:653, 1974.

29. Wilmore DW, Moylan JA, Bristow BF et al: Anabolic effects of human growth hormone and high calorie feedings following thermal injury, *Surg Gynecol Obstet* 138:875, 1974.

54 Nutritional Management of Children with Burns and Trauma

Orrawin Trocki

Nutritional support is an essential component in critical care of pediatric trauma patients. Although many children are healthy and well nourished before injury, their survival after initial stabilization still depends on effective nutritional support to preserve vital organ functions, prevent sepsis, and promote wound healing. Severe trauma induces several metabolic responses which are characterized by hypermetabolism and hypercatabolism resulting from hormonal derangement and stress mediators. If these responses are not treated by appropriate nutritional therapy, they may lead not only to malnutrition, but also to delayed wound healing, immunodeficiency, complications, prolonged recovery, and even death resulting from multiorgan failure.

Management of nutritional support can be more difficult in injured children than in injured adults. In injuries of similar types and extents, children are at greater risk for developing malnutrition than adults. Children normally have higher metabolic rates, smaller nutrient stores, and greater nutrient requirements per unit of body weight than adults. Moreover, the nutritional needs of injured children have been poorly studied. Current nutritional support of pediatric trauma patients is based on studies of animals and adult trauma patients. Nutritional therapy that is used successfully for adult trauma patients may not be as successful for children.

The keys to successful nutritional support are early assessment of nutritional requirements, timely implementation of the appropriate intervention, continuous monitoring of the children's progress, and modification of the nutritional regimens to meet their changing needs.

ASSESSMENT OF NUTRITIONAL STATUS

Every injured child should be screened for nutritional status. If a child is found to be at nutritional risk, a comprehensive nutritional assessment should be performed. There is no one simple method that can be used for defining the nutritional status of a child.

Nutritional assessment begins with obtaining a history that includes medical, surgical, social, and dietary data. Of particular interest are preexisting conditions, such as chronic diseases affecting nutrient utilization, surgical resections of the gut or accessory organs for digestion, food allergies, feeding intolerances, and vitamin and mineral deficiencies.

Height and weight should be determined upon admission, as many methods used to estimate energy and protein requirements are based on height and weight. Preinjury weight is also the best indicator of the existing nutrient store. If possible, weight should be ascertained before the injured child receives fluid resuscitation. Height and weight should be plotted on graphs and compared with reference standards prepared by the National Center for Health Statistics (NCHS).[37] This is a useful tool for identifying children whose size is small for their age and weight is low as compared with length or stature. Measurements of weight or height above the 95th or below the 5th percentile indicate nutritional excess or deficit, respectively. Other anthropometric measurements such as skinfold thickness and midarm circumference are useful to estimate current total body fat and to determine chronic undernutrition.

Biochemical asssessment provides objective data that can support dietary and anthropometric evaluation. Measurements of visceral proteins such as albumin, prealbumin, and transferrin upon admission will detect preexisting protein and calorie malnutrition and provide a baseline for evaluating the effectiveness of nutritional intervention.

ESTIMATION OF ENERGY REQUIREMENTS

The primary goal of nutritional support in critically injured children is to provide adequate calorie intake to maintain weight during the acute phase of injury and allow age-appropriate growth during convalescence. Both inadequate and excess provision of calories should be avoided. Underfeeding has detrimental effects on wound healing, immunocompetence, organ functions, and mortality.

Table 54–1 Recommended dietary allowance of energy and protein for children

	Age (years)	Reference weight (kg)	REE (kcal/kg)	Energy (kcal/kg)	Protein (g/kg)
Infants	0.0-0.5	6	53	108	2.2
	0.5-1	9	56	98	1.6
Children	1-3	13	57	102	1.2
	4-6	20	47	90	1.1
	7-10	28	40	70	1.0
Males	11-14	45	32	55	1.0
	15-18	66	27	45	0.9
Females	11-14	46	28	47	1.0
	15-18	55	25	40	0.8

Adapted from Food and Nutrition Board: *Recommended dietary allowances,* ed 10, Washington, DC, 1989, National Academy Press.

Overfeeding can cause complications such as hyperglycemia, liver abnormalities, and respiratory distress. Therefore, an accurate estimation of caloric needs is essential.

Energy requirements of injured children are highly individual. They vary widely with sex, age, activity, previous nutritional status, and hypermetabolic state resulting from injury.

The first step in estimating total energy requirements is to determine the basal metabolic requirements (BMR).

Resting energy expenditure (REE), which represents the energy expended by a person at rest and differs from BMR by less than 10%, may be used interchangeably with BMR. The type of injury, whether head, spinal, skeletal, or thermal, blunt, or penetrating, and its severity determine the magnitude and duration of postinjury increase in basal metabolic rate. Winthrop and colleagues studied the changes in energy expenditure resulting from blunt trauma in children and demonstrated that the initial increase in BMR varied directly with the injury, as reflected in the injury severity score (ISS).[73]

The most accurate way to estimate REE is to use indirect calorimetry. It has been demonstrated that REE can be measured safely in critically ill pediatric patients.[67] REE should be measured when the child is awake and 2 hours after meals. If the child is receiving continuous nutritional support, measurements can be taken while he or she is receiving nutrition. Measurements should not be taken immediately after physical therapy, dressing change, blood drawing, or other activities that agitate children.

If actual measurement by indirect calorimetry is not possible, BMR can be estimated from many available formulas that are based on weight or surface area. Boothby and colleagues[12] developed a monogram for the calculation of BMR for males and females aged 6 to 68 years based on surface area. Altman and Dittmer[4] provided a table for BMR prediction in infants and children less than 16 years old, based on body weight. These two methods are widely used among pediatric dietitians.

Recently, the World Health Organization (WHO) published equations for predicting REE in different age groups from body weight, based on a survey of indirect calorimetry studies.[74] The most recent U.S. Recommended Dietary Allowances (RDA) for energy used these WHO equations for the calculation of REE (Table 54-1.)[26]

The well-known Harris-Benedict equations for predicting resting metabolic requirements in adults should not be used for small children, especially infants. These equations were formulated from observations of adults, in which women were found to have lower basal caloric requirements than men. Therefore, this method is appropriate for use only in adolescents. The estimates of BMR or REE obtained through the methods described above are for normal children. The energy requirements then must be adjusted upward to account for the increased metabolic rate resulting from injury. Long and colleagues[50] proposed that BMR should be multiplied by the following injury factors: 1.2 for a minor operation, 1.35 for skeletal injury, 1.6 for major sepsis, and 2.1 for severe thermal burn. Sporadic data are available to validate these predictive formulas in injured children in some age groups.

Winthrop and colleagues reported that the BMR of children with blunt trauma increased by 14% when compared with baseline values.[73] Phillips and colleagues examined the metabolic responses in children and adolescents with severe head injury and found that the mean measured energy expenditure was 1.3 times the Harris-Benedict predicted values for energy expenditure.[63] In a review of patients aged 3 to 67 years with severe head trauma who required mechanical support, Moore and colleagues reported the percentage increase of the actual measured REE over the predicted REE derived from Harris-Benedict equations to be 160%.[60]

Tilden and colleagues measured the REE in mechanically ventilated critically ill children and found that the measured REE averaged 48% more than REE predicted from the Harris-Benedict equations.[67] Upon examining REE measurements obtained in burned children, Goran and colleagues suggested that REE could be estimated by multiplying Harris-Benedict predicted values by 1.29.[29]

Groner and colleagues measured REE in children aged 8 to 19 years before and after major selective operations and found no significant increase in REE.[34] They theorized that children might be able to convert energy expended on growth to energy spent on wound repair and healing, thus avoiding the overall increase in energy expenditure seen in adults.

Not every injury results in a hypermetabolic rate. Kolpek and colleagues compared measured energy expenditure in spinal cord injury and in nonsteroid-treated head trauma in adult patients.[49] During the first week following injury, the mean measured energy expenditure/predicted REE by the Harris-Benedict equations ratio was 0.56 for spinal injury and 1.4 for head trauma. There is no similar study in the pediatric trauma population.

Another determinant of total energy requirements is physical activity. For normal children, it represents the second largest component of total energy expenditure after resting energy expenditure. For injured children at bed rest, the energy requirements for activity are approximately 10% above basal needs.[71] Some children may be able to engage in light activity out of bed and thus their energy needs for activity increase to 30% above basal. Most authors recommend that the measured or calculated REE should be multiplied by 1.2 to 1.3 for activity factor.[50,34]

For most injured children, the total energy requirements estimated by multiplying BMR by injury and activity factors should be sufficient to meet energy expenditure and to maintain weight. However, there are situations in which energy requirements should be further adjusted. The presence of fever increases energy requirements by approximately 13% above the normal BMR per degree of temperature elevation.[47] Barbiturate therapy can decrease energy expenditure by eliminating postinjury hypermetabolism. Dempsy and colleagues reported that energy expenditure measurements performed in patients with severe acute trauma to the head during barbiturate therapy were 14% below those that would be predicted in nonstressed patients.[25]

Weight gain in underweight injured children or weight loss in obese children should be deferred until after the critical period has passed. Attempts to provide extra calories for catch-up growth in underweight children may lead to complications of overfeeding. It has been reported that in the early phase of severe injury, obese adult patients could not use their abundant fat fuel sources and had to depend on other fuel sources.[44] Traumatized obese patients mobilized relatively more protein and less fat, as compared with nonobese subjects.

ESTIMATION OF PROTEIN REQUIREMENTS

Following trauma, protein requirements for children are increased above the recommended allowances for normal children.[26] Additional quantities of protein are needed for synthesis of acute-phase proteins, for wound healing, and for replacing protein loss in skeletal muscle breakdown, drainage, or exudate. Just how much extra protein is needed is still unclear. Theoretically, it should be possible to determine protein requirements by estimating protein requirements by age for normal children and using an injury factor to correct for the degree of protein catabolism. To date, there is no consensus on what to use as correction factors for different types of injury.

Urinary nitrogen excretion reflects the protein catabolism in which amino acids are broken down to meet the increased demand for energy. The magnitude and the duration of increased nitrogen loss depend on the type and severity of injury.[6] Infection, fever, and surgery can all result in substantial nitrogen loss through the urine.[23] It is well known that bed rest and immobilization also cause increased nitrogen excretion. Although increased urinary nitrogen excretion after injury has been well documented in adults,[50] there is little information on children available. It is also very difficult to make comparisons among studies because of differences in ages, severity and types of injury, treatments, and calorie and nitrogen intake.

Ziegler and colleagues[75] conducted a study of nitrogen balance in normal children and reported the mean total urinary nitrogen to be 364 mg/kg/day for children 12 to 18 months old, 390 mg/kg/day for children 18 to 36 months old, 374 mg/kg/day for those 3 to 6 years old, and 339 mg/kg/day for those 6 to 11 years old. Phillips and colleagues studied nitrogen excretion in adolescents and children with severe head injury during 2 weeks after admission.[63] Their reported levels of urinary nitrogen excretion were lower than those reported by Ziegler and colleagues; mean urinary nitrogen excretion was 307 mg/kg/day for adolescents and 160 mg/kg/day for children between 2 and 5 years old. To the contrary, Cunningham and colleagues[21] reported much greater urinary nitrogen excretion in severely burned children under 3 years old: 3.1 g/day, with an additional nitrogen loss of 1.5 g from wound seepage.

Pharmacologic doses of steroids have been shown by Ford and colleagues to increase postinjury nitrogen excretion in children aged 4 to 14 years with closed head injury.[27] The steroid-treated group showed a significantly higher urinary excretion (mean 286 mg/kg/day) than the non–steroid-treated group (mean 149 mg/kg/day).

The most accurate means to estimate protein requirements is, then, to perform a nitrogen balance study. The nitrogen balance is calculated as the difference between daily nitrogen intake and output. Nitrogen output includes nitrogen losses in urine, feces, drainage fluids, gastric juices, and exudates. In clinical settings, it is practical only to determine urinary nitrogen loss. Under normal conditions, nitrogen losses via skin and feces are thought to be approximately 4 g of nitrogen per day in adults, but are unknown in children of different age groups. An estimate of total nitrogen output can be obtained by adding 4 g to the amount of nitrogen excreted in the urine. The course of protein catabolism over time differs among different types of injury, but it usually peaks at about the first week postinjury.

The goal of nutritional support is to provide adequate protein to maintain a positive nitrogen balance for anabolism. How high a positive nitrogen balance should be is unclear because the amount of protein needed for acute-phase protein production and tissue repairing is still unknown. Overzealous attempts to achieve a positive nitrogen balance may lead to the detrimental effects of overfeeding. It has been reported that there is an obligatory nitrogen loss due to paralysis in spinal cord–injured patients that prevents a positive nitrogen balance regardless of the calorie and protein intake.[65]

It is well recognized that urinary nitrogen excretion is influenced by the availability of total caloric intake. Therefore, protein requirements are tied to energy requirements. Long and colleagues suggested an alternate method for evaluating protein requirements in stressed adult patients; that is, by first determining the total daily caloric requirements and providing protein at a calorie:nitrogen (g) ratio of 150:1.[50] Cerra recommended a nonprotein calorie–nitrogen ratio ranging from 150:1 to 80:1 for adults, depending on the severity of injury.[16] These ratios seem rather low for small children, especially for infants who normally consume protein at approximate 250 to 300:1 ratio of nonprotein calories to nitrogen. Only in severely

burned children had these high levels of protein intake been studied. Alexander and colleagues demonstrated that a diet that provided approximately 20% to 25% of calories as protein, equivalent to a nonprotein calorie–nitrogen ratio of 80 to 100:1, had beneficial effects on outcome, as evidenced by improved survival, decreased incidence of infection, and better nitrogen balance.[2] More studies are needed to establish the efficacy of high protein intake in children with other types of injury.

CARBOHYDRATE AND FAT REQUIREMENTS

After protein requirements have been estimated, the nonprotein energy requirements can be met by carbohydrates and fats. Although there is no absolute dietary requirement for carbohydrate, the intake of the essential fatty acid linoleic acid must be at levels from 1% to 2% of total dietary calories to prevent essential fatty acid deficiency in humans.[41] The American Academy of Pediatrics has recommended that infants receive a minimum of 30% of total energy as fat, including 3% of total energy as the essential fatty acid linoleic.[5] After they are 6 months of age, there is no good reason to decrease fat intake in normal children and adolescents. However, many complications have been attributed to excessive fat intake during the acute phase following severe trauma. These include elevated plasma triglyceride levels, hepatomegaly, impaired clotting, and depressed reticuloendothelial system functions with resultant decreased resistance to infection.[38,69] Alexander and colleagues recommended diets containing between 5% and 15% of nonprotein calories as fat as optimal for nutritional support following burn injury.[3] Although low-fat diets have been used successfully in nutritional support of burned chidren,[32] similar diets have not been tried in children with other types of traumatic injury.

On the other hand, large quantities of carbohydrate may be detrimental to injured children. As part of the metabolic response to injury, most types of trauma result in an increase in glucose turnover rate.[66] Consequently, patients have a tendency to develop hyperglycemia and, occasionally, glycosuria. Trauma patients are also relatively resistant to insulin, and glucose tolerance is significantly reduced. Furthermore, Askanazi and colleagues have demonstrated in hypermetabolic adult patients that high glucose intake can increase carbon dioxide production and that the work load imposed by the high carbon dioxide production may precipitate respiratory distress in patients with compromised pulmonary function.[7] In such patients, fat is a better source of nonprotein calories and is associated with lower carbon dioxide production than isocaloric amounts of carbohydrate.

VITAMIN AND MINERAL REQUIREMENTS

The impact of trauma on vitamin and mineral requirements of injured children has not been studied adequately. Current practices in vitamin and mineral supplementation following trauma, for all but a few vitamins and minerals, represent the extrapolation of the requirements of normal children (Table 54-2) and are carried out empirically.

Because energy and protein requirements increase after trauma, the requirements for vitamins such as thiamine, riboflavin, niacin, and vitamin B_6, which are needed for energy and protein metabolism, must also increase proportionally to the increase in energy and protein requirements. Vitamin C is a cosubstrate in hydroxylation of proline, and lysine in the formation of collagen, which is necessary for wound healing. Vitamin C can also affect functions of leukocytes and macrophages and immune responses. Vitamin A is essential for cellular differentiation and proliferation and for the integrity of the immune system. Markedly depressed circulating vitamin K levels are found in patients with fractures, and the time needed for this level to return to normal appears to be influenced by the severity of the fracture.[10] Increased urinary output of carnitine after injury has been reported; the excretion of carnitine reflects the increased body protein catabolism.[42]

It is not surprising that many clinicians are prescribing multivitamin supplements during traumatic stress.[46] On the other hand, many clinicians do not provide vitamin supplementation because they feel that most available commercial enteral formulas have been designed to meet or exceed the RDAs when the caloric requirements are provided. The benefits of vitamin supplementation above the RDAs for critically injured children have not been demonstrated. Because of the possible dangers of toxicity resulting from megadoses, vitamin supplementation should be used cautiously.

Guidelines for vitamin supplementation have been established only for burned children,[31] but not for those with other types of traumatic injury. Children younger than 3 years with burns involving more than 10% of body surface area, and those older than 3 years with burns involving more than 20%, should be given multivitamin supplements daily. In addition to multivitamin supplements, children younger than 3 years with larger burns should be given 500 mg of vitamin C and 5000 IU of vitamin A, and children older than 3 years 1000 mg of vitamin C and 10,000 IU of vitamin A. Similar supplementations may be useful in treat-

ment of critically injured children for whom massive tissue repair is required. In general, vitamin supplementations more than twice the RDAs should not be given.[71]

To date, only fragments of information concerning mineral metabolism following trauma are available.

Severe trauma induces disturbances in phosphate metabolism. The immediate posttraumatic period is associated with a decrease in serum phosphate concentration and massive urinary phosphate concentration. Hypophosphatemia may lead to respiratory insufficiency, muscle weakness, anorexia, and neurologic symptoms. Severe hypophosphatemia may cause dysfunction of erythrocytes and gastrointestinal hemorrhage owing to platelet dysfunction. Loven and colleagues demonstrated that posttraumatic disturbances in erythrocyte phosphate metabolism may be prevented by the administration of phosphate.[51] Daily and colleagues suggested prophylactic administration of phosphate to prevent serum phosphate decrease.[24]

Hypocalcemia has been associated with decreased myocardial contractility, hypotension, congestive heart failure, and decreased cardiac output. Gauthier and colleagues evaluated calcium metabolism in critically ill children and adolescents and found that hypocalcemia occurs frequently and is associated with raised levels of calcitonin and parathyroid hormone.[28] In their study, mortality was significantly higher in hypocalcemic patients. After intravenous administration of calcium, hypotension was corrected and the cardiac output was improved.

During the early period following major trauma, there is a high incidence of hypomagnesemia. Among many factors that contribute to magnesium depletion are prolonged nasogastric suction, loss of fluids in wound seepage, hyperaldosteronism, and aminoglycoside therapy. Cunningham and colleagues examined the magnesium status of severely burned adolescents.[20] They concluded that magnesium requirement is increased during recovery from severe burn injury and that hypoglycemia can be prevented by magnesium supplementation.

Zinc deficiency may result in impaired wound healing, impaired immune function, diarrhea, and alterations in taste and smell and mental status. During the acute-phase response to injury, the serum zinc level can be depressed to less than half of the preinjury level.[61] McClain and colleagues reported strikingly reduced serum zinc concentrations early in the postinjury course of patients with head trauma, and elevated urinary losses that correlated with the severity of head injury.[53] Cunningham and colleagues reported that hypozincemia persisted in moderately to severely burned

Table 54–2 Recommended dietary allowances of vitamins and minerals for children

| Age (years) | Fat-soluble vitamins | | | | Water-soluble vitamins | | | | |
	Vitamin A (µg RE)*	Vitamin D (µg)†	Vitamin E (mg α-TE)‡	Vitamin K (µg)	Vitamin C (mg)	Thiamin (mg)	Riboflavin (mg)	Niacin (mg NE)§	Vitamin B₆ (mg)
Infants									
0.0-0.5	375	7.5	3	5	30	0.3	0.4	5	0.3
0.5-1	375	10.0	4	10	35	0.4	0.5	6	0.6
Children									
1-3	400	10.0	6	15	40	0.7	0.8	9	1.0
4-6	500	10.0	7	20	45	0.9	1.1	12	1.1
7-10	700	10.0	7	30	45	1.0	1.2	13	1.4
Males									
11-14	1000	10.0	10	45	50	1.3	1.5	17	1.7
15-18	1000	10.0	10	65	60	1.5	1.8	20	2.0
Females									
11-14	800	10.0	8	45	50	1.1	1.3	15	1.4
15-18	800	10.0	8	55	60	1.1	1.3	15	1.5

Adapted from Food and Nutrition Board: *Recommended dietary allowances,* ed 10, Washington, DC, 1989, National Academy Press, p 284.

*Retinol equivalents. I retinol equivalent = 1 µg retinol or 6 µg β-carotene.

†As cholecalciferol. 10 µg cholecalciferol = 400 IU of vitamin D.

‡α-Tocopherol equivalents. 1 mg d-α tocopherol = 1 α-TE.

§1 NE (niacin equivalent) is equal to 1 mg of niacin or 60 mg of dietary tryptophan.

children who received total parenteral nutrition supplemented with zinc at the recommended level for parenteral feeding.[22] In some burn centers, zinc supplementation is routinely given to burned patients.[70]

Copper deficiency is rare in humans. However, hypocupremia has been observed during parenteral nutrition in burned children.[22] Serum ceruloplasmin in burned patients was also depressed, and urinary excretion was elevated.[11] A deficiency of copper may lead to neutropenia, leukopenia, bone mineralization, or impaired immune function. Further studies are needed to determine whether copper supplementation following trauma is necessary.

INITIATION OF NUTRITIONAL SUPPORT

Traditionally nutritional support was not a major component of the early treatment of a child with acute traumatic injury. It was common for nutritional support to be delayed for several days, until gastrointestinal function returned. During this time patients might receive only intravenous glucose solution, which provided a minimal amount of calories and no protein sources. As a consequence, there was danger that a significant nutritional deficit could develop.

Despite the absence of specific injury to the gastrointestinal tract, gastric paralysis commonly occurs in traumatized patients. It may take 3 to 5 days

for the stomach to recover normal motility. On the other hand, the small bowel is more resistant to ileus and usually maintains normal motility and absorption. Therefore, it is possible to feed into the small bowel during the time of gastric ileus.

Recently, Alexander and colleagues advocated early enteral nutritional support in burned patients, starting immediately after admission.[56] They believe that early enteral feeding can blunt the postburn hypermetabolic response, decrease secretion of catabolic hormones, and prevent bacteria translocation resulting from atrophy of gut mucosal cells. Since then many studies have confirmed that immediate enteral feeding is safe and effective in patients with major burns.[18,54]

On the other hand, Herndon and colleagues reported that early administration of parenteral nutrition to patients with burns covering more than 50% of total body surface area for the first 10 days postinjury had no beneficial effects on immune function, liver function, or survival.[40] In a follow-up study, they reported that the group of patients receiving supplemental parenteral nutrition had twice the death rate of the group receiving enteral calories only.[39] They concluded that administration of intravenous supplementation decreases the amount of enteral calories that burned patients can tolerate. The use of intravenous supplemental nutrition in early postburn period should be discour-

Table 54–2 Recomomended dietary allowances of vitamins and minerals for children—cont'd

| | | Minerals | | | | | | |
Folate (µg)	Vitamin B_{12} (µg)	Calcium (mg)	Phosphorus (mg)	Magnesium (mg)	Iron (mg)	Zinc (mg)	Iodine (µg)	Selenium (µg)
25	0.3	400	300	40	6	5	40	10
35	0.5	600	500	60	10	5	50	15
50	0.7	800	800	80	10	10	70	20
75	1.0	800	800	120	10	10	90	20
100	1.4	800	800	170	10	10	120	30
150	2.0	1200	1200	270	12	15	150	40
200	2.0	1200	1200	400	12	15	150	50
150	2.0	1200	1200	280	15	12	150	45
180	2.0	1200	1200	300	15	12	150	50

aged and its use limited to only those patients with total enteral failure.

In a prospective randomized controlled clinical trial, Rapp and colleagues compared the effects of early parenteral nutrition and traditional delayed enteral nutrition on the outcome of patients with head injuries.[64] They reported that the patients receiving total parenteral nutrition had a more positive nitrogen balance, a higher serum albumin level, and higher total lymphocyte count than patients receiving enteral nutrition. However, the results of this study did not reflect the superiority of total parenteral nutrition over enteral nutrition, because parenterally fed patients were able to receive significantly higher amounts of calories than the enterally fed patients. Rather, the results reflected the effects of adequate nutrition versus undernutrition.

Later, Hadley and colleagues[36] compared the efficacy of total parenteral nutrition and enteral nutrition in patients with acute head trauma and found no significant differences between the two routes of nutritional support with respect to maintenance of serum albumin level, weight loss, incidence of infection, nitrogen balance, and final outcome.

Moore and colleagues[58,59] demonstrated the feasibility of immediate postoperative enteral feeding via needle catheter jejunostomy after major abdominal trauma. A needle catheter jejunostomy was placed just before abdominal closure, and infusion of an elemental diet was begun within 12 hours postoperatively. They reported that patients tolerated enteral feeding via needle catheter jejunostomy well. When compared with total parenteral nutrition, this early enteral nutrition was found to reduce septic complications in critically injured patients and to restore albumin, transferrin, and retinol-binding protein levels better than total parenteral nutrition.

Adams and colleagues conducted a similar study comparing the efficacy of total parenteral nutrition and enteral nutrition via jejunostomy following laparotomy in patients with multiple trauma.[1] In their study, patients in the enteral feeding group received a polymeric formula instead of an elemental formula. Their results confirmed that early postoperative jejunostomy feeding is a safe and efficacious choice for patients with multiple trauma undergoing laparotomy. They suggested that any patient undergoing a laparotomy who is likely to need nutritional support for more than 10 days postoperatively should be seriously considered for a feeding jejunostomy placement.

Most recently, Kirby and colleagues[48] demonstrated another approach for early enteral feeding of patients with severe brain injury by endoscopic placement at bedside of a percutaneous endogastrostomy (PEG) tube with a smaller feeding tube that had both gastric and intestinal ports. With this technique, the reduction in nitrogen loss appeared to be equal to or superior to either gastric feeding or total parenteral nutrition.

Although most of the previously mentioned studies were performed in adult trauma patients, it can be concluded that nutritional support should be provided to injured children as soon as possible, preferably within 24 hours of admission. If there is a functional gastrointestinal tract, the enteral route is preferred for nutritional support. Otherwise, the parenteral route should be used.

Increased understanding of posttrauma metabolism and the etiology of complications has increased the safety of both parenteral and enteral nutrition. The use of the parenteral route in nutritional support has recently increased significantly. At times it is abused, partly because parenteral nutrition appears to be easier and more convenient than enteral nutrition. Nevertheless, it carries high risks because the patient is exposed to the possible complications of parenteral nutrition. In addition, enteral nutrition continues to have a cost advantage over parenteral nutrition, which includes less expensive formulas and equipment and less preparation time.

Alert injured children are seldom able or willing to eat the foods necessary to meet their increased caloric and protein needs following trauma. Some children may be motivated to drink high protein, high calorie beverages to supplement oral intake. In most cases, to ensure adequate intake it is necessary to supplement oral intake with tube feeding. Continuous infusion is preferred if tube feeding is to provide all or most of the child's nutritional needs. Intrajejunal feeding should also be given by continuous infusion. Intermittent feedings, which are administered several times a day, and nocturnal feeding are more appropriate if tube feeding is to serve as a supplement to oral intake. During the acute posttrauma period, most children tolerate continuous infusion better than intermittent feeding.

In general, continuous tube feeding should begin with isotonic diets that provide 1 kcal/ml or infant formulas at full strength. More concentrated formulas should be diluted to 1 kcal/ml. The starting rate should be slow, at 1 ml/kg/hr. If tolerated, it should be increased by small increments as tolerated until the feeding goal is reached. If the gastrointestinal tract is functional, the feeding goal can be met within 48 hours.

Comatose children with severe traumatic injury need all their nutrient requirements to be administered via the enteral or parenteral route. Total parenteral nutrition can be implemented as soon as a catheter for nutritional support is inserted and its correct placement verified. Enteral feeding should be initiated and advanced as previously described. Parenteral nutrition may be used in conjunction with enteral nutrition while it is being advanced to the desired concentration and volume.

CONSIDERATIONS FOR SELECTING FORMULAS FOR NUTRITIONAL SUPPORT

Recent progress in understanding the physiology of the stress of critical illnesses has led to the development of a wide variety of commercially available specialized parenteral and enteral formulations for nutritional support. These products differ greatly in their sources and concentrations of proteins, carbohydrates, and fats. Consequently, they also differ in caloric density, calorie-nitrogen ratio, electrolytes, vitamin and mineral content, solubility, viscosity, and osmolality. Examples of commercially available enteral products are described in Table 54-3.

Some products are designed to meet the special nutritional needs of metabolically stressed adult patients but none are especially designed for stressed children. Infant, pediatric, and adult formulas must be modified to meet the increased protein and caloric requirements of severely injured children. Most commercial formulas are designed to meet the RDA requirements for vitamins and minerals when caloric requirements are met through consumption of a specified volume. If formula is diluted or volume is too low, intake of vitamins and minerals may be insufficient. Deficiencies can be corrected by the addition of liquid vitamin and mineral preparations. When ready-made formulations cannot be modified to meet the unique nutritional needs of an injured child, it is possible to design a special nutritionally complete formula for that child by using modular components. Currently, proteins, carbohydrates, fats, fiber, vitamins, and minerals are all commercially available in modular forms.

At present, the proteins in enteral feeding formulas are available in three forms: intact proteins, protein hydrolysates, and crystalline amino acids. Formulas with intact proteins are the products of choice for children with normal gastrointestinal tracts. It has been shown that formulas containing intact protein as their protein source are superior to formulas containing crystalline amino acids for postburn nutritional support, as evidenced by better nitrogen balance, higher visceral protein levels, and less postburn weight loss.[68] Only when the digestive or absorptive capability is impaired should children be given formulas containing proteins that have been prehydrolyzed into smaller peptides. It is now known that protein can be better absorbed

Table 54–3 Examples of commercially available enteral products

Product category	Product main characteristics	Examples of commercial products
Infant formulas		
Milk base	Intact macronutrients Contains lactose Provides 0.67 kcal/ml	Enfamil (Mead Johnson) Similac (Ross)
Soy base	Does not contain lactose	Prosobee (Mead Johnson) Isomil (Ross)
Premature	High-protein and high-calorie	Premature (Mead Johnson) Special Care (Ross)
Predigested protein	Contains hydrolyzed protein as nitrogen source	Pregestimil (Mead Johnson) Alimentum (Ross) Nutramigen (Mead Johnson)
Fat modified	Part of long-chain triglycerides replaced by MCT oil	Pregestimil (Mead Johnson) Portagen (Mead Johnson)
Pediatric formulas		
Standard formula	Especially designed for children 1-6 years old	Pediasure (Ross)
Adult formulas		
Standard	Intact macronutrients; isotonic; mimics composition of standard American diet; usually provides 1 kcal/ml and contains no lactose	Isocal (Mead Johnson) Osmolite (Ross) Isosource (Sandoz) Ensure (Ross)
High-calorie	Provides calories up to 2 kcal/ml	Isocal HCN (Mead Johnson) Magnacal (Mead Johnson)
High-protein	Provides high protein	Sustacal (Mead Johnson)
High-calorie, High-protein	Provides high amounts of calories and protein	Traumacal (Mead Johnson)
Predigested protein	Contains hydrolyzed protein as nitrogen source	Peptamen (Clintec) Reabilan (O'Brien) Vital HN (Ross)
Elemental	Contains free amino acids as nitrogen source	Tolerex (Norwich) Stresstein (Sandoz)
Low-fat	Contains only 1%-2% of calories as fat	Surgical Liquid Diet (Ross) Citrotein (Sandoz) Tolerex (Norwich)
High-fiber	Contains fiber from natural food sources or added soy polysaccharide	Enrich (Ross) Sustacal with Fiber (Mead Johnson)
Specialized formulas		
Metabolic stress	High amounts of protein and calories; some contain high branched-chain amino acids	Traumacal (Mead Johnson) Stressein (Sandoz) Impact (Sandoz)
Others	Nutrients are modified for certain disease states such as liver, renal, pulmonary, and so on	Pulmocare (Ross) Hepatic-aid II (Kendall) Nephro (Ross)

as dipeptides and tripeptides than as free crystalline amino acids.[52] Therefore the expensive elemental diets that contain free amino acids as protein sources should be reserved for use in jejunostomy feeding via a needle catheter, where polymeric diets may clog the needle. More recently, in a prospective randomized study, Meredith and colleagues found a lower incidence of diarrhea and better visceral protein levels in trauma patients fed peptide diets than in those fed whole proteins.[55] More studies showing the benefits of peptide diets over intact protein are needed before these diets can be recommended for all injured children.

Branched-chain amino-acid–enriched formulas have been proposed for use in nutritional support of severely stressed, traumatized, and septic patients.[13,17] It is believed that during stress branched-chain amino acids are used preferentially as an energy source; thereby they can reduce muscle protein breakdown, improve nitrogen retention, and stimulate protein synthesis. In addition, solutions with high percentages of branched amino acids have been shown to promote positive nitrogen balance and prevent hepatic encephalopathy in patients with chronic liver disease and liver failure.[57] However, not all studies found that enriched branched–amino-acid formulas are effective in improving nitrogen balance in traumatic injury.[57]

It has been demonstrated that there is an increase in gut consumption of glutamine in the catabolic state. Glutamine-supplemented total parenteral nutrition has been shown in animals to prevent bacterial translocation from gut and improve gut immune function.[15] Parenteral solutions supplemented with glutamine are not currently available, but elemental enteral formulas supplemented with glutamine are available. Glutamine is already abundant in intact protein, so supplementation of polymeric formulas is not necessary.

Arginine supplementation has been shown to reduce protein catabolism, reduce urinary excretion, and improve immune function in sepsis and trauma.[8] Enteral formulas rich in arginine are currently available. Arginine can also be added as crystalline amino acid to ready-made formulas to the desired levels.

Most commercially available polymeric enteral formulas are high in fat, providing approximately 30% to 50% of total energy as fat. Only a few elemental formulas have lower fat content. Most of the polymeric enteral products use vegetable oils that are rich in long-chain linoleic acid, an n-6 fatty acid, as fat sources. High levels of linoleic are associated with adverse effects such as alterations in immune function and thrombogenic and hyperlipidemic tendencies.[30] Since the detrimental effects of excessive intake of fats and n-6 fatty acids were reported, attempts have been made to lower the fat content in some enteral products and substitute part of the vegetable oils with fish oils. Fish oils that are low in linoleic and high in n-3 fatty acids do not have adverse effects on immunity. Another alternative to long-chain fatty acid is medium-chain triglyceride (MCT). The use of MCT is indicated in disorders of fat absorption and transportation.

Lactose intolerance due to lactase deficiency can occur postinjury or after gastrointestinal surgery. To prevent lactose-associated diarrhea, most enteral feeding formulas are lactose free, with carbohydrate provided as maltodextrin or hydrolyzed cornstarch.

Most enteral formulas contain little or no residue. Prolonged administration of low-residue formulas can cause constipation in some children. Soy polysaccharide, a dietary fiber, is currently added to some commercial formulas to help promote normal bowel function. However, the RDA requirement for fiber has not been established, and high fiber intake can cause adverse effects.

The potential beneficial effects of these specialized formulas can be realized only when they are chosen appropriately and when their use is based on nutritional needs, clinical situations, and gastrointestinal function.

MONITORING OF NUTRITIONAL SUPPORT

The safety, adequacy, and efficiency of nutritional therapy should be monitored continuously in order to identify potential complications and provide adjustments to meet children's changing needs.

Both parenteral and enteral nutrition are associated with several mechanical, metabolic, and gastrointestinal complications. These complications can be minimized through careful monitoring (Tables 54-4 and 54-5). All injured children receiving enteral or parenteral nutrition should be monitored according to the institution's established protocols for monitoring parenteral and enteral feedings.

Gastrointestinal complications of enteral feeding include nausea, vomiting, diarrhea, delayed gastric emptying, and abdominal distention. If there is a persistent large volume of gastric residuals, the formula concentration or the rate of administration should be reduced. If the gastric residuals exceed the volume infused during the preceding 2 hours, tube feeding should be stopped.

Diarrhea, which is the most often cited complication associated with tube feeding, may result from various causes: infection, antibiotic therapy, hypoalbuminemia, protein malnutrition, refeeding syndrome, zinc or vitamin A deficiency, or use of antacids, potassium, or phosphorus supplements.[14, 33, 35, 45] Therefore, the tube feeding formula may not be the cause of diarrhea and should not be automatically discontinued. The treatment for diarrhea depends on its etiology. A variety of antidiarrheal medications, such as agents that slow gastrointestinal motility, may be used to control diarrhea. If diarrhea continues, tube feeding should be stopped and the patient may need parenteral nutrition while waiting for diarrhea to subside.

The nutritional status of the injured child should be assessed continuously in order to determine the adequacy of nutritional support. This can be accomplished by using a combination of dietary, anthropometric, clinical, and biochemical data.

Daily intakes of calories and protein should be estimated from the daily food record kept at bedside. As oral intake increases or decreases, the

Table 54–4 Suggested laboratory monitoring of enteral nutrition in children

Parameter	First week and during critical illness	Later for stable patients
Electrolytes	Initially, twice weekly	Weekly
Calcium	Initially, weekly	Weekly
Phosphorus	Daily until stable	Weekly
Magnesium	Initially, weekly	Weekly
Zinc	Initially	Monthly
Blood urea nitrogen	Daily until stable	Weekly
Creatinine	Daily until stable	Weekly
Liver function tests	Initially, as needed	As needed
Glucose	Daily until stable	As needed
Albumin	Initially, weekly	Weekly
Prealbumin	Initially, weekly	Weekly
Transferrin	Initially, weekly	Weekly
Retinol-binding protein	Initially, weekly	Weekly
Nitrogen balance	Twice weekly	Weekly

Note: Monitor more frequently if any parameter is abnormal.

Table 54–5 Suggested laboratory monitoring of parenteral nutrition in children

Parameter	First week and during critical illness	Later for stable patients
Electrolytes	Daily until stable	Twice weekly
Calcium	Daily until stable	Weekly
Phosphorus	Daily until stable	Weekly
Magnesium	Initially, weekly	Weekly
Zinc	Initially, weekly	Monthly
Blood urea nitrogen	Daily until stable	Weekly
Creatinine	Daily until stable	Weekly
Liver function tests	Initially, weekly	Weekly
Serum osmolarity	Initially	Weekly
Glucose	Daily until stable	Weekly
Triglycerides	With every increase in fat	Twice weekly
Albumin	Initially, weekly	Weekly
Prealbumin	Initially, weekly	Weekly
Transferrin	Initially, weekly	Weekly
Retinol-binding protein	Initially, weekly	Weekly
Nitrogen balance	Daily until stable	Weekly

Note: Monitor more frequently if any parameter is abnormal.

supplemental enteral or parenteral nutrition should be adjusted accordingly. Weekly measurements of resting metabolic expenditure by indirect calorimetry should be used to confirm the adequacy of estimated caloric requirements or to make adjustments. Continual comparison of estimated caloric needs and calories consumed can prevent underfeeding or overfeeding.

Children should be weighed at least twice weekly. Serial anthropometric measurements, such as measurement of triceps skin-folds and arm muscle circumferences, may be useful in monitoring subcutaneous fat and muscle reserves in some long-hospitalized traumatized children. Nutritional support should at least be able to maintain preinjury weight and preserve lean body mass.

There is no one laboratory test, or group of tests, that is satisfactory for the assessment of protein-calorie status. Each test has its own applications and limitations, as recently reviewed by Benjamin.[9] Serial measurements of hepatically synthesized protein such as albumin, transferrin, prealbumin, and retinol-binding protein may be used to assess the adequacy of protein provision (Table 54–6). Reduction of these transport proteins is indicative of an impairment of hepatic protein synthesis, as well as depletion of visceral protein stores. Although low serum albumin levels are associated with increased morbidity and mortality,[19] serum albumin is not a sensitive indicator of acute or moderate degrees of protein-calorie malnutrition.

Transferrin and prealbumin are more sensitive indicators than albumin because of their shorter half-lives. Low transferrin levels have been associated with an increased incidence of bacteremia in burned patients.[62] The retinol-binding protein and prealbumin concentrations have been reported to change earlier than albumin and transferrin levels and to correlate better with nitrogen balance during nutritional therapy.[72]

One of the goals of nutritional support of injured children is to achieve a positive nitrogen balance. Although there are many determinants of nitrogen balance during recovery from trauma, nitrogen intake is the major determinant[43] and is the easiest to alter. A nitrogen balance study should be performed weekly to assess the adequacy of the current nitrogen intake. If a child is found to have a negative nitrogen balance, attempts should be made to increase protein intake. The accuracy of a nitrogen balance study depends on the completeness of urine collection, which is difficult to accomplish in infants and small children. Although nitrogen balance study is not practical in burned children because of difficulty in estimating nitrogen losses in burn wound exudates, it is useful in monitoring the adequacy of protein intake in children with other types of injury.

Table 54–6 Normal blood laboratory values (Children's National Medical Center)

Parameter	Normal range	Age
Sodium (mmol/L)	139-146	Newborn-2 yr
	138-145	2 yr-16 yr
	136-146	16 yr-18 yr
Potassium (mmol/L)	3.7-5.9	Newborn-2 wk
	4.1-5.3	2 wk-2 yr
	3.4-4.7	2 yr-16 yr
	3.5-5.1	16 yr-18 yr
Chloride (mmol/L)	95-100	Newborn-18 yr
Calcium (mg/dl)		
Total	8.0-10.5	Newborn-15 days
	9.0-11.0	15 days-18 yr
Ionized	4.2-5.9	Newborn-5 days
	4.7-5.1	5 days-18 yr
Phosphorus (mg/dl)	5.0-7.8	Newborn-15 days
	4.5-6.5	15 days-2 yr
	4.5-5.5	2 yr-16 yr
	2.7-4.5	16 yr-18 yr
Magnesium (mg/dl)	1.2-2.0	Newborn-15 days
	1.7-2.3	15 days-6 yr
	1.7-2.1	6 yr-12 yr
	1.6-2.2	16 yr-18 yr
Zinc (μg/dl)	68-94	Newborn-18 yr
Blood urea nitrogen (mg/dl)	4-18	Newborn-18 yr
Creatinine (mg/dl)	0.2-0.6	Newborn-2 yr
	0.3-0.7	2 yr-8 yr
	0.4-0.8	8 yr-11 yr
	0.4-0.9	11 yr-14 yr
	0.6-1.2	14 yr-18 yr
Albumin (g/dl)	2.4-4.8	Newborn-2 days
	3.0-5.1	2 days-7 days
	3.5-4.7	7 days-3 yr
	3.8-5.4	3 yr-16 yr
	3.8-5.2	16 yr-18 yr
Prealbumin (mg/dl)	10.9-27.3	Newborn-18 yr
Transferrin (mg/dl)	203-360	Newborn-18 yr
Ceruloplastin (mg/dl)	5-18	Newborn-3 mo
	33-43	3 mo-12 mo
	26-55	12 mo-3 yr
	27-56	3 yr-5 yr
	24-48	5 yr-7 yr
	18-48	7 yr-18 yr
Glucose (mg/dl)	40-60	Newborn-1 day
	50-80	1 day-1 wk
	60-100	1 wk-16 yr
	70-105	16 yr-18 yr
Total protein (g/dl)	4.6-7.0	Newborn-1 mo
	4.5-6.5	1 mo-6 mo
	5.4-7.5	6 mo-2 yr
	5.3-8.0	2 yr-16 yr
	6.0-8.0	16 yr-18 yr
Hemoglobin (g/dl)	14.5-22.5	Newborn-3 day
	13.5-21.5	3 day-1 wk
	12.5-20.5	1 wk-2 wk
	10.0-18.0	2 wk-1 mo
	9.0-14.0	1 mo-2 mo
	9.5-13.5	2 mo-6 mo

Table 54–6 Normal blood laboratory values (Children's National Medical Center)—cont'd

Parameter	Normal range	Age
Hemoglobin (g/dl)—cont'd	10.5-13.5	6 mo-2 yr
	11.5-13.5	2 yr-6 yr
	11.5-14.5	6 yr-12 yr
	13.0-16.0	12 yr-18 yr (male)
	12.0-16.0	12 yr-18 yr (female)
Hematocrit (%)	42-65	Newborn-3 day
	42-62	3 day-1 wk
	39-63	1 wk-2 wk
	31-55	2 wk-1 mo
	28-42	1 mo-2 mo
	29-41	2 mo-6 mo
	31-39	6 mo-2 yr
	34-40	2 yr-6 yr
	35-45	6 yr-18 yr
	37-49	12 yr-18 yr (male)
	36-46	12 yr-18 yr (female)

Wk = Week, mo = month, yr = year.

Thus the success of nutritional support depends on careful monitoring and ongoing assessment of safety, adequacy, and effectiveness of the therapy.

CONCLUSION

Severely injured children present a demanding and complicated challenge in nutritional support. Because nutrition plays an important role in the outcome of traumatic injury, each injured child deserves a thorough nutritional assessment, an individualized nutritional care plan, timely initiation of nutritional support, careful monitoring, and continuous tailoring of nutritional therapy to accomodate changing needs.

It is apparent that there is not sufficient information to make definite recommendations regarding optimal nutritional support of injured children. Further investigation is needed to settle many controversial issues and to provide guidance for nutritional treatment of seriously injured children.

REFERENCES

1. Adams S, Dellinger EP, Wertz MJ et al: Enteral versus parenteral nutritional support following laparotomy for trauma: a randomized prospective trial, *J Trauma* 26:882-891, 1986.
2. Alexander JW, MacMillan BG, Stinnett JW et al: Beneficial effects of aggressive protein feeding in severely burned children, *Ann Surg* 192:505-517, 1980.
3. Alexander JW, Saito H, Trocki O et al: The importance of lipid type in the diet after burn injury, *Ann Surg* 204:1-8, 1986.
4. Altman Pl, Dittmer DS, editors: *Metabolism*, Bethesda, Md, 1968, Federation of American Societies for Experimental Biology, p 344.
5. American Academy of Pediatrics, Committee on Nutrition, Commentary on breast feeding and infant formulas, including proposed standards for formulas, *Pediatrics* 57:278-285, 1976.
6. Andrassy RJ, Dubois T: Modified injury severity scale and concurrent steroid therapy: independent correlates of negative nitrogen balance in pediatric trauma, *J Pediat Surg* 20:799-802, 1985.
7. Askanazi J, Nordenstrom J, Rosenbaum SH et al: Nutrition for the patient with respiratory failure: glucose vs fat, *Anesthesiology* 54:373-377, 1981.
8. Barbul A, Sisto DA, Wasserkrug HL et al: Nitrogen sparing and immune mechanisms of arginine: differential dose-dependent responses during postinjury intravenous hyperalimentation, *Curr Surg* 40:114-116, 1983.
9. Benjamin DR: Laboratory tests and nutritional assessments, *Pediatr Clin N Am* 36:139-161, 1989.
10. Bitensky L, Hart JP, Catterall A et al: Circulating vitamin K levels in patients with fractures, *J Bone Joint Surg* 70:663-664, 1988.
11. Boosalis MG, McCall JT, Solem LD et al: Serum copper and ceruloplasmin levels and urinary copper excretion in thermal injury, *Am J Clin Nutr* 44:899-906, 1986.
12. Boothby WM, Berkson J, Dunn HL: Studies of the energy of metabolism of normal individuals: a standard for basal metabolism with a nomogram for clinical application, *Am J Physiol* 116:468-484, 1936.
13. Brennan MF, Cerra FB, Daly JM et al: Report of a research workshop: branched chain amino acids in stress and injury, *JPEN* 10:446-453, 1986.
14. Brinson RR, Kolts BE: Hypoalbuminemia as an indicator of diarrheal incidence in critically ill patients, *Crit Care Med* 15:506-509, 1987.
15. Burke DJ, Alverdy JC, Aoys E et al: Glutamine-supplemented total parenteral nutrition improves gut immune functions, *Arch Surg* 124:1396-1399, 1989.
16. Cerra FB: Branched chain amino acids. I. Stress nutrition, *Nutr Supp Serv* 5:8-40, 1985.
17. Cerra FB, Blackburn G, Hirsch J et al: The effect of stress level, amino acid formula, and nitrogen retention in traumatic and septic stress, *Ann Surg* 205:282-287, 1987.
18. Chiarelli A, Enzi G, Casadei A et al: Very early nutrition supplementation in burned patients, *Am J Clin Nutr* 51:1035-1039, 1990.
19. Ching N, Grossi CE, Angers J et al: The outcome of surgical treatment as related to the response of the serum albumin level to nutritional support, *Surg Gynecol Obstet* 151:200-205, 1980.

20. Cunningham JJ, Anbar RD, Crawford JD: Hypomagnesemia: a multifactorial complication of treatment of patients with severe burn trauma, *JPEN* 11:364-367, 1987.

21. Cunningham JJ, Lydon MK, Russell WE: Calorie and protein provision for recovery from severe burns in infants and young children, *Am J Clin Nutr* 51:553-557, 1990.

22. Cunningham JJ, Lydon MK, Briggs SE et al: Zinc and copper status of severely burned children during TPN, *J Am Coll Nutr* 10:57-62, 1991.

23. Cuthbertson DP: The metabolic response to injury and its nutritional implications: retrospect and prospect, *JPEN* 3:108-129, 1979.

24. Daily WH, Tonnesen AS, Allen SJ: Hypophosphatemia: incidence, etiology, and prevention in the trauma patient, *Crit Care Med* 18:1210-1214, 1990.

25. Dempsey DT, Guenter P, Mullen JL et al: Energy expenditure in acute trauma to the head with and without barbiturate therapy, *Surg Gynecol Obstet* 160:128-134, 1985.

26. Food and Nutrition Board: Recommended dietary allowances, Washington, DC, 1989, 10th National Academy Press, p 284.

27. Ford EG, Jennings LM, Andrassy RJ: Therapeutic steroid administration potentiates urinary nitrogen losses and may impair adequate nutritional support of the head injured child, *J Trauma* 26:674, 1986.

28. Gauthier B, Trachtman H, Carmine FD et al: Hypocalcemia and hypercalcitoninemia in critically ill children, *Crit Care Med* 18:1215-1219, 1990.

29. Goran MI, Broemeling L, Herndon DN et al: Estimating energy requirements in burned children: a new approach derived from measurements of resting energy expenditure, *Am J Clin Nutr* 54:35-40, 1991.

30. Gottschlich MM, Alexander JW: Fat kinetics and recommended dietary intake in burns, *JPEN* 80-85, 1987.

31. Gottschlich MM, Warden GD: Vitamin supplementation in the patient with burns, *J Burn Care Rehab* 11:275-279, 1990.

32. Gottschlich MM, Jenkins M, Warden GD et al: Differential effects of three enteral dietary regimens on selected outcome variables in burn patients. *JPEN* 14:225-236, 1990.

33. Gottschlich MM, Warden GD, Michel M et al: Diarrhea in tube-fed burn patients: incidence, etiology, nutritional impact, and prevention, *JPEN* 12:338-345, 1988.

34. Groner JI, Brown MK, Stallings et al: Resting energy expenditure in children following major operative procedures, *J Ped Surg* 24:825-828, 1989.

35. Guenter PA, Settle RG, Perlmutter S et al: Tube feeding–related diarrhea in acutely ill patients, *JPEN* 15:277-280, 1991.

36. Hadley MN, Grahm TW, Harrington T et al: Nutritional support and neurotrauma: a critical review of early nutrition in forty-five acute head injury patients, *Neurosurg* 19:367-373, 1986.

37. Hamill PV, Drizd TA, Johnson CL et al: Physical growth: National Center for Health Statistics percentiles, *Am J Clin Nutr* 32:607-629, 1979.

38. Harris RL, Frenkel RA, Cottam GL et al: Lipid mobilization and metabolism after thermal trauma, *J Trauma* 22:194-198, 1982.

39. Herndon DN, Barrow RE, Stein MD et al: Increased mortality with intravenous supplemental feeding in severely burned patients, *J Burn Care Rehab* 10:309-313, 1989.

40. Herndon DN, Stein MD, Rutan TC et al: Failure of TPN supplementation to improve liver function, immunity and mortality in thermally injured patients, *J Trauma* 27:195-204, 1987.

41. Holman RT: Biological activities of and requirements for polyunsaturated acids, *Prog Chem Fats Lipids* 9:607-682, 1970.

42. Iapichino G, Radrizzani D, Colombo A et al: Carnitine excretion: a catabolic index of injury, *JPEN* 12:35-36, 1988.

43. Iapichino G, Radrizzani D, Solca M et al: The main determinants of nitrogen balance during total parenteral nutrition in critically ill injured patients, *Inten Care Med* 10:251-254, 1984.

44. Jeevanandam M, Young DH, Schiller WR: Obesity and the metabolic response to severe multiple trauma in man, *J Clin Invest* 87:262-269, 1991.

45. Kelly TWJ, Patrick MR, Hillman KM: Study of diarrhea in critically ill patients, *Crit Care Med* 11:7-9, 1983.

46. King N, Goodwin CW: Use of vitamin supplements for burned patients: a national survey, *J Am Dietet Assoc* 84:923-925, 1984.

47. Kinney JM, Roe CF: Caloric equivalent of fever. I. Patterns of postoperative response, *Ann Surg* 156:610-622, 1962.

48. Kirby DF, Clifton GL, Turner H et al: Early enteral nutrition after brain injury by percutaneous endoscopic gastrojejunostomy, *JPEN* 15:298-302, 1991.

49. Kolpek JH, Ott LG, Record KE et al: Comparison of urinary urea nitrogen excretion and measured energy expenditure in spinal cord injury and nonsteroid-treated severe head trauma patients, *JPEN* 13:277-280, 1989.

50. Long CL, Shaffel N, Geiger JW et al: Metabolic response to injury and illness: estimation of energy and needs from indirect calorimetry and nitrogen balance, *JPEN* 3:452-456, 1979.

51. Loven L, Larsson L, Nordstrom H et al: Serum phosphate and 2,3 diphosphoglycerate in severely burned patients after phosphate supplementation, *J Trauma* 26:348-352, 1986.

52. Matthews DM, Adibi SA: Peptide absorption, *Gastroenterol* 71:151-161, 1976.

53. McClain CJ, Twyman DL, Ott LG et al: Serum and urine zinc response in head-injured patients, *J Neurosurg* 64:224-230, 1986.

54. McDonald WS, Sharp CW, Deitch EA: Immediate enteral feeding in burn patients is safe and effective, *Ann Surg* 213:177-183, 1991.

55. Meredith JW, Ditesheim JA, Zaloga GP: Visceral protein levels in trauma patients are greater with peptide diet than with intact protein diet, *J Trauma* 30:825-829, 1990.

56. Mochizuki H, Trocki O, Dominioni L et al: Mechanism of prevention of postburn hypermetabolism and catabolism by early enteral feeding, *Ann Surg* 200:297-310, 1984.

57. Mochizuki H, Trocki O, Dominioni L et al: Effect of a diet rich in branched chain amino acids in severely burned guinea pigs, *J Trauma* 26:1077-1085, 1986.

58. Moore EE, Todd NJ: Benefits of immediate jejunostomy feeding after major abdominal trauma: a prospective, randomized study, *J Trauma* 26:874-881, 1986.

59. Moore FA, Moore EE, Jones TN et al: TEN versus TPN following major abdominal trauma: reduced septic morbidity, *J Trauma* 29:916-923, 1989.

60. Moore R, Najarian MP, Konvolinka CW: Measured energy expenditure in severe head trauma, *J Trauma* 29:1633-1636, 1989.

61. Moser PB, Borel J, Majerus T et al: Serum zinc and urinary excretion of trauma patients, *Nutr Res* 5:253-261, 1985.

62. Ogle CK, Alexander JW, MacMillan BG: The relationship of bacteremia to levels of transferrin, albumin, and total serum protein in burn patients, *Burns* 8:32-38, 1981.

63. Phillips R, Ott L, Young B et al: Nutritional support and measured energy expenditure of the child and adolescent with head injury, *J Neurosurg* 67:846-851, 1987.

64. Rapp RP, Young B, Twyman D et al: The favorable effect of early parenteral feeding on survival in head-injured patients, *J Neurosurg* 58:906-912, 1983.

65. Rodriguez DJ, Clevenger FW, Osler TM et al: Obligatory

negative nitrogen balance following spinal cord injury, *JPEN* 15:319-322, 1991.

66. Shaw JHF, Wolfe RR: An integrated analysis of glucose, fat, and protein metabolism in severely traumatized patients, *Ann Surg* 209:63-72, 1989.

67. Tilden SJ, Watkins S, Tong TK et al: Measured energy expenditure in pediatric intensive care patients, *Am J Dis Child* 143:490-492, 1989.

68. Trocki O, Mochizuki H, Dominioni L et al: Intact protein versus free amino acids in the nutritional support of thermally injured animals, *JPEN* 10:139-145, 1985.

69. Wan JMF, Teo TC, Babayan VK et al: Invited comment: lipids and the development of immune dysfunction and infection, *JPEN* 12:43S-52S, 1988.

70. Williamson J: Actual burn nutrition care practices: a national survey, *J Burn Care Rehab* 10:185-194, 1990.

71. Wilmore DW: *The metabolic management of the critically ill*, New York, 1977, Plenum Medical Book, p 129.

72. Winkeler MF, Gerrior SA, Pomp A et al: Use of retinol binding protein and prealbumin as indicators of the response to nutrition therapy, *J Am Dietet Assoc* 89:684-687, 1989.

73. Winthrop Al, Wesson DE, Pencharz PB et al: Injury severity, whole body protein turnover, and energy expenditure in pediatric trauma, *J Pediatr Surg* 22:534-537, 1987.

74. World Health Organization: Energy and protein requirements. Report of Joint FAO/WHO/UNU Expert Consultation. Tech Rep Series 724. Geneva, 1985, World Health Organization, p 206.

75. Ziegler RE, O'Donnell AM, Stearns G et al: Nitrogen balances studies with normal children, *Am J Clin Nutr* 30:939-946, 1977.

55 Near-Drowning

Alan I. Fields

Near-drowning is a frequently preventable catastrophic event that still remains a significant source of morbidity and mortality in children.[5,6,8] New data on this hypoxic-ischemic insult has offered insight into the epidemiology of the problem, outcomes of pediatric resuscitations, and the effects of various treatment modalities on brain resuscitation. It is clear that education and efforts at prevention remain the most important means to effect a better outcome, as neurologic outcome may well be determined by the time the near-drowning victim arrives at the hospital.

DEFINITIONS

In the 1960s drowning had been defined simply as "a submersion incident leading to death." During the following decade, however, this definition became inadequate for describing all of the possible pathophysiologic events and sequelae associated with drowning, thus leading some authors to add multiple modifiers.[2] These definitions were cumbersome and only added confusion to the literature. Therefore, the definitions used in this chapter are that drowning is a submersion incident that leads to death within the first 24-hours, and near-drowning is a submersion incident in which there is survival for at least 24 hours, irrespective of eventual outcome.

EPIDEMIOLOGY AND POPULATION AT RISK

Drowning is the fourth leading cause of fatal injury in children between birth and 19 years of age (Table 55-1) and, in some states (e.g., Arizona) is the leading cause of fatal injury in children 4 years of age and younger. It is most common among children 4 years of age and younger and in males aged 15 to 19 years. Among the latter group, drownings occur in a wide variety of aquatic environments; alcohol use is associated with an estimated 40% to 50% of these events. Although preschool-aged children have the largest incidence, adolescents have the largest case fatality rate. A middle peak (8 to 12 years) involves boys almost exclusively and is often associated with disobedience or trespassing. In all states, up to 90% of drownings in this age group occur in residential pools, but the case fatality rate for victims is highest if drowning occurs in a lake or river. In addition, approximately 3000 children less than 5 years old are treated annually in hospital emergency rooms for submersion accidents; 80% are admitted for 1 or more days for treatment or observation.

In 1986 the U.S. Consumer Product Safety Commission studied drowning and near-drowning accidents that occurred in residential pools in children under 5 years of age.[8] Most of the victims were males aged 2 years or younger. Discussions with the parents of the victims revealed that 46% of the children were last seen in their home, 24% were in the yard, on the porch or patio, or at a neighbor's home, and 30% were in or around the pool itself. Most of the children were last seen playing alone (41%) or with others (32%).

Most accidents occurred between 3:00 and 7:00 PM, and a large number reported around noon and 6:00 PM—traditional mealtimes. Most children were being supervised by one or both parents at the time of the accident. Most parents were occupied with normal household chores at the time of the accident. The estimated time the child was noted to be missing was usually less than 5 minutes. Of additional interest, no caregiver ever reported hearing a splash (even when the caregiver was poolside) in the 142 incidents evaluated.

This study concluded that near-drownings in young children were due to momentary lapses in adult supervision. No matter what method was being used to safeguard the child, it was not sufficient: supervised children got into pools, complete barriers around pools were penetrated, or locked doors in houses were opened. These included locked sliding-glass doors that were opened for the first time by children less than 2 years old. In short, pools represented risks to toddlers in spite of optimal barriers.

Although swimming pools and natural bodies of water close to home present the greatest risk to young children and adolescents, two new risks have been reported and are worthy to mention. One previously unrecognized hazard is the home use of five-gallon industrial buckets, usually for mopping

Table 55–1 Number, percentage, and rate of fatal injuries for children ≤19 years of age, by leading cause of injury—United States, 1986

Cause of injury	No.	(%)	Rate per 100,000
Motor vehicle crash	10,535	(47.0)	14.9
Occupant	7,412	(33.0)	10.5
Pedestrian	1,787	(8.0)	2.5
Other	1,336	(6.0)	1.9
Homicide	2,877	(12.8)	4.1
Suicide	2,151	(9.6)	3.0
Drowning	2,062	(9.2)	2.9
Fire/burns	1,619	(7.2)	2.3
Other	3,167	(14.1)	4.5
All	22,411	(100.0)	31.7

Data from the Centers for Disease Control: Fatal injuries to children: United States, 1986, *MMWR* 39:442-451, 1990.

floors or containing leaks. The other newly identified risk is the use of solar pool blankets. These blankets have become an increasingly popular means of maintaining heat in private and public swimming pools. They can support reasonably heavy toys, thus tempting the toddler, and can obscure visualization of a submersed child, thereby delaying rescue efforts. Drowning can also occur on top of pool covers where water has collected from rain or melting snow.

Some 55,000 individuals each year are treated for nonsubmersion accidents in and around swimming pools, and another 13,000—most between 5 and 15 years of age—are injured when diving or using pool slides. At least 1600 more accidents involve spas. Injuries in these instances include

1. Neck and spinal injuries, including quadriplegia or paraplegia. There are approximately 700 to 800 diving injuries resulting in 300 spinal cord injuries each year. These tend to involve males aged 18 to 31. In almost 50% of cases, consumption of alcohol, usually beer, is involved. In most cases the diver is removed from the pool by friends who are unaware of the spinal injury and do not use a spine board. Children under 11 years of age are at considerably less risk of diving injuries as they are usually neither tall enough nor heavy enough to penetrate the water with sufficient velocity or force to cause a cervical spine injury if they touch the bottom of the pool.
2. Evisceration (resulting from suction caused by missing or broken drain covers on wading

pools), as well as chemical and electrical injuries, have also been reported.

Saltwater drowning and near-drowning

Among children, the "saltwater" accident rate is much lower than the "freshwater" accident rate. Although the surf involves special hazards (e.g., the undertow) to children, beaches are much safer than other types of swimming facilities because of the inaccessibility of the beach to toddlers (who generally will not be at a beach without an accompanying adult) and better surveillance of swimmers by lifeguards and other adults. Even in a "beach society," more children drown in inland lakes and canals than in the ocean. Although the saltwater drowning rate is increasing, fortunately the absolute risk of death remains small.

Boating and the use of surfboards currently account for a very small percentage of drowning deaths in children. Alcohol use is a prominent factor in many teen and adult drownings. Body surfing represents a larger threat for head and spinal injury.

Lakes and rivers

In states in which lakes and rivers are in abundance (Georgia, New Mexico, and Maryland), they are the most common sites for submersions and reported drownings, especially in the adolescent age group.[9] Submersion incidents are associated with (1) swimming in unofficial areas, (2) boating, (3) motor vehicle accidents, and (4) use of alcohol. The high mortality of adolescents involved in submersions at these sites is probably related to lack of supervision, difficulty of rescue, and the physiologic effect of alcohol. In addition, docks constitute risks for death for both toddlers and adolescents. Water depth and poor water clarity preclude rapid rescue and probably explain the large case fatality rate for these groups.

Hot tubs and spas

Another risk to the pediatric population is posed by hot tubs or spas. Associated entrapment injuries and deaths have been reported. Body part entrapment and hair entanglement in pool and spa drains with suction fittings are the most common causes of these accidents.

Bathtub drowning and near-drowning

Another primary source of submersion accidents involving infants and children is the bathtub. The child involved in a bathtub submersion accident usually is less than 1 year of age and is often left in the care of an older sibling, who is frequently of pre-school age. Bathtub drownings have also been reported as a form of child abuse. Children with epilepsy have a greater risk of drowning in

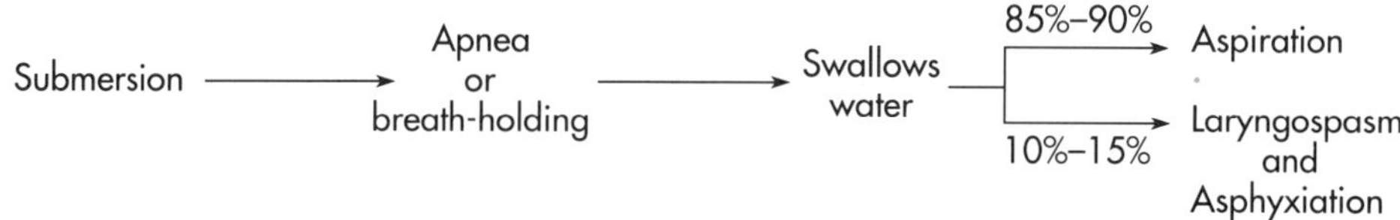

Figure 55–1 A plausible response to unexpected submersions. The victim will first aspirate or swallow small volumes of water. With increasing hypoxia and panic, the victim will then swallow water into the stomach. As the hypoxia increases, 85% to 90% of victims will lose airway reflexes and aspirate stomach contents. The other 10% to 15% will go into laryngospasm and asphyxiate ("dry drowning").

bathtubs than in pools or saltwater, because they often are inadequately supervised in bathtubs. For this reason it has been suggested that children with seizure disorders never bathe alone, although showering alone may be safe.

Children with seizure disorders have a four to five times increased risk of both drowning and near-drowning accidents than an equivalent population without seizures, but the absolute risk remains low. The American Academy of Pediatrics has stated that children with epilepsy should be allowed to swim (with increased vigilance), but not be allowed to engage in high diving or participate in competitive underwater swimming.

MECHANISM OF INJURY

Although there is no agreement on the exact sequence of events in a drowning episode, the description by Noble and Sharpe seems plausible (Fig. 55-1).[4] There is an initial period of panic, followed by violent struggling and automatic swimming movements. Apnea or breath-holding occurs, and the victim then swallows large amounts of water. Vomiting and gasping ensue, and water is aspirated. Once the child is unconscious, airway reflexes are lost and fluid is passively introduced into the airway. Cardiac arrest follows shortly thereafter. It should be noted that 10% to 15% of patients succumb to "dry" drowning from laryngospasm without significant aspiration.

PATHOPHYSIOLOGY
Aspiration

Animal studies have shown several physiologic and biochemical differences between saltwater drowning and freshwater drowning.[2] Based on these experimental data, a patient involved in drowning or near-drowning in fresh water was expected to show evidence of hemodilution, fluid overload, and hyperkalemia. Because the osmolality of seawater is approximately three to four times that of blood, patients involved in drowning or near-drowning in seawater were expected to show evidence of hemoconcentration, hypernatremia, hypovolemia, and pulmonary edema.

The differences in blood chemistry resulting from aspiration of fresh water and saltwater in these animal studies were contrary to the clinical data of various investigators. Several investigators[2,7] have shown that in both freshwater and saltwater near-drownings, adults and children who arrived alive at an emergency room rarely required correction of serum electrolytes initially. Furthermore, the presumed hypervolemia from freshwater aspiration has been noted to be clinically significant only occasionally, although hypovolemia resulting from saltwater aspiration often necessitated volume expansion to maintain circulatory volume.

The results of animal studies indicate that changes in serum electrolytes in near-drownings depend both on the tonicity of the fluid and on the volume of fluid aspirated, with abnormalities in electrolytes reported only in markedly hypertonic conditions such as found in the Dead Sea. It is presumed that patients who survive long enough to be transported to a hospital have aspirated less fluid (less than 22 ml of water per kg of body weight) into their lungs. The presence of chlorine in the water does not affect the pulmonary pathology or the outcome of drowning or near-drowning.

Hypoxemia

A review of experimental and clinical data shows clearly that the single most important consequence of near-drowning is hypoxemia. Acidosis is often associated with hypoxemia; hypoperfusion is associated less frequently. For the 10% to 15% of human drowning victims who die without aspiration, hypoxemia is due to laryngospasm with obstructive asphyxiation.

Results of animal studies suggest that there are many causes for the pulmonary insufficiency that occurs in near-drowning victims (Fig. 55-2). Hypoxemia from near-drowning in fresh water is predominantly due to inactivation of pulmonary surfactant, and thus causes atelectasis. Perfusion of the atelectatic areas can account for an increase in intrapulmonary shunting. In addition, loss of surface-active material and disruption of alveolar cells can cause the pulmonary capillaries to leak, which

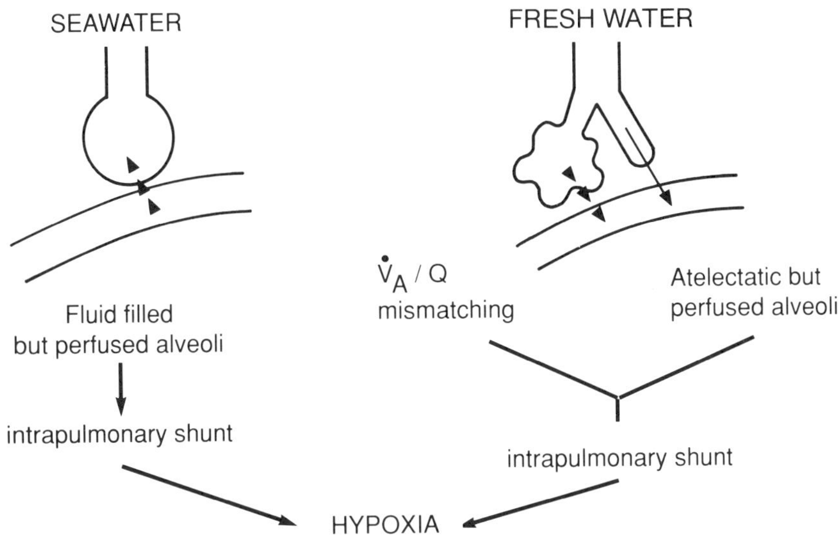

Figure 55–2 Near-drowning with aspiration. This represents the pulmonary pathophysiology seen in freshwater and saltwater submersions. Fresh water causes an inactivation of pulmonary surfactant and atelectasis. Saltwater causes pulmonary edema. Perfusion in both cases increases the intrapulmonary shunt.

leads to pulmonary edema. Therefore, freshwater near-drowning results in poorly compliant lungs, an increase in the intrapulmonary shunt, and ventilation-perfusion mismatch.[2,5]

The initial factor leading to hypoxemia associated with near-drowning in saltwater is hypothesized to be the establishment of an osmotic gradient across the alveolar-capillary membrane. This causes the protein-rich intravascular fluid to move into the alveoli that are already filled with fluid. The perfusion of these fluid-filled alveoli, with little or no ventilation or gas exchange possible, results in increased intrapulmonary shunt, ventilation-perfusion abnormalities, and, finally, hypoxemia. However, pulmonary edema is often found in both seawater and freshwater near-drownings.[5]

Other effects in the lung—so-called secondary drowning—may occur later. These effects may result from aspiration pneumonitis, superimposed bacterial pneumonia, or inhalation of foreign materials, and may appear as a delayed onset of lung pathology, including the adult respiratory distress syndrome (ARDS).

Other Organ Failures

Multisystem organ failure can occur as a result of a submersion injury. Ventricular fibrillation, previously thought to be secondary to electrolyte abnormalities and the most frequent cause of death in submersion victims, probably occurs in no more than 15% of cases.[2] Myocardial dysfunction, coagulation disorders (disseminated intravascular co-

agulopathy), renal failure (acute tubular necrosis), and central nervous system (CNS) dysfunction may result from hypoxia and the possible accompanying secondary problems such as acidosis, hypoperfusion, and hemolysis.

The common cause of injury to various organ systems in victims of near-drowning is the hypoxic-ischemic insult. However, there may be important physiologic differences between young children and adults that can affect their responses following submersion accidents.[5] First, young children can become hypothermic more rapidly than adults because they have a relatively larger surface area, proportionately smaller amounts of subcutaneous fat, and a tendency toward increased mobility when they are immersed. This hypothermia may be significant in view of documented cases of complete recovery of children who sustained prolonged submersion in cold water (in one case up to 66 minutes). Second, at least some investigators feel that the diving reflex may be important, as children may manifest this response. This reflex, which allows air-breathing mammals to submerge for prolonged periods, consists of bradycardia and redistribution of blood flow to the heart and brain, thereby affording greater protection against hypoxia. The reflex is triggered by submersion of the face while the individual is apneic, especially in water of less than 20° C. It has been thought to be most active in young children and potentiated by fear.

More recently, experimental studies have shown a decreased ability of children to hold their breath in cold water.[11] This has led some investigators to

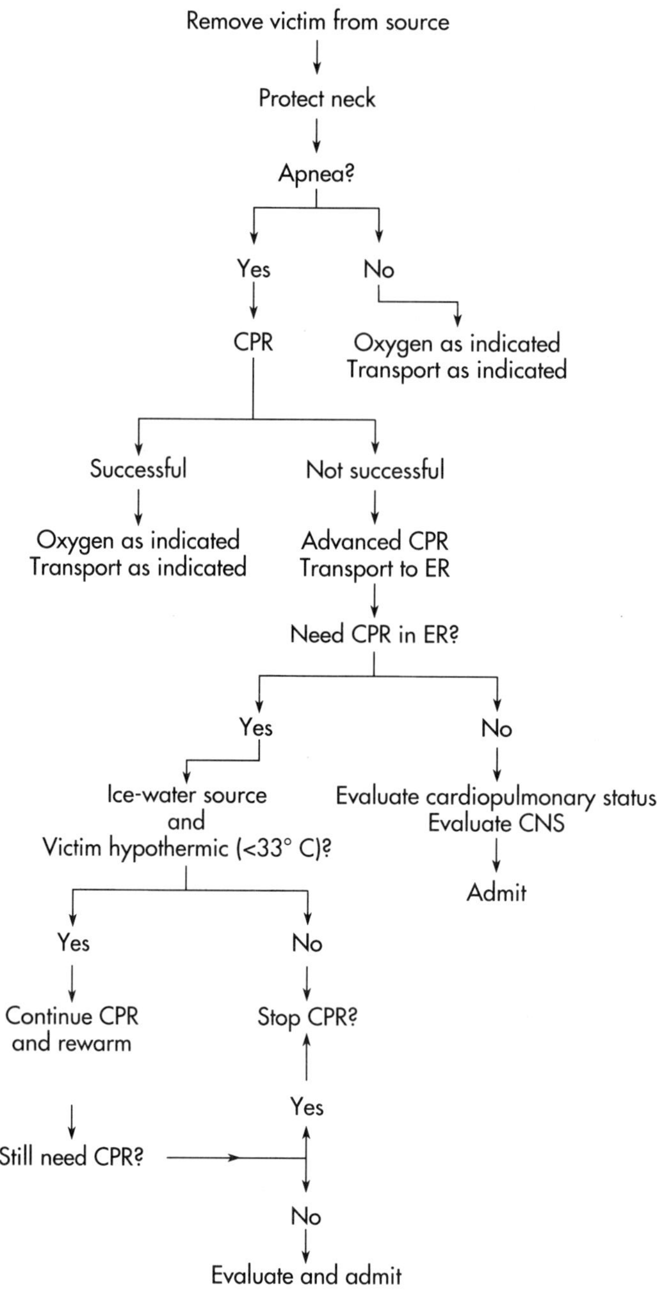

Figure 55–3 Resuscitation algorithm.

hypothesize that the better outcome of children in cold-water near-drownings is almost solely due to their ability to become hypothermic, and that the diving reflex plays but a small part in cerebral protection of this hypoxic-ischemic insult.

TREATMENT
Initial treatment at the scene

Most children who are pulled from the water and are unconscious will survive, and more than 90%

who survive will do so with minimal or no neurologic dysfunction.[10] Therefore, except for extremely long submersions or delayed discovery (see "Outcome and Prognosis" later in this chapter), all children should receive cardiopulmonary resuscitation (CPR) at the scene if needed (Fig. 55-3).

The most important treatment at the site of a near-drowning is immediate and effective CPR; this topic has been previously covered, but some points need emphasis:

1. Call for help, but do not delay the start or continuation of resuscitative efforts to do so.
2. Remove the child from the water as quickly as possible. If the child is apneic and the resuscitator is able, mouth-to-mouth resuscitation should be started before pulling the victim out of the water; it should not be delayed until the victim is on dry land if extrication will take more than a few seconds (often the case in lakes and rivers). If there is no pulse, closed chest cardiac massage should be started as soon as the child is in a boat or on land; external cardiac compressions cannot be effectively performed in water.
3. If a cervical spine or back injury is suspected, immobilize the child, if possible, before removal from the water. Turn the victim to the supine position, taking care to avoid bending the neck and torso. Support the neck and back until a board can be placed beneath the child and an immobilizing cervical collar applied. Great care must be taken not to increase the risk of aspiration.
4. Drainage procedures before resuscitation (such as pressure on the upper abdomen) waste valuable time, are ineffective, are likely to produce vomiting, and should not be attempted. It is very important that an unconscious but breathing near-drowned child be managed in the coma position (i.e., the semi-prone position while lying on the left side with the head down; see Fig. 55-4). If a head or neck injury is suspected, keep the head and neck supported and aligned with the body. Even without these procedures, more than half of all submersion victims vomit during resuscitation.
5. Assess the airway and clear it of any debris or vomitus. If the victim cannot be ventilated, obstructed airway maneuvers are indicated to clear the airway. The finger sweep maneuver is preferable, as the abdominal thrust (Heimlich) maneuver may induce further vomiting.
6. The risk of producing gastric distention with positive pressure at the airway is greater in children than in adults. Cricoid pressure during mouth-to-mouth or bag-valve-mask ventilation may decrease the risk of gastric aspiration by preventing regurgitation and reducing further abdominal distention during ventilation. Oxygen should be administered as soon as possible. If an artificial airway is needed, an endotracheal tube is indicated. An esophageal obturator should not be used. *Once the airway is protected*, a nasogastric tube can be placed for possible relief of gas-

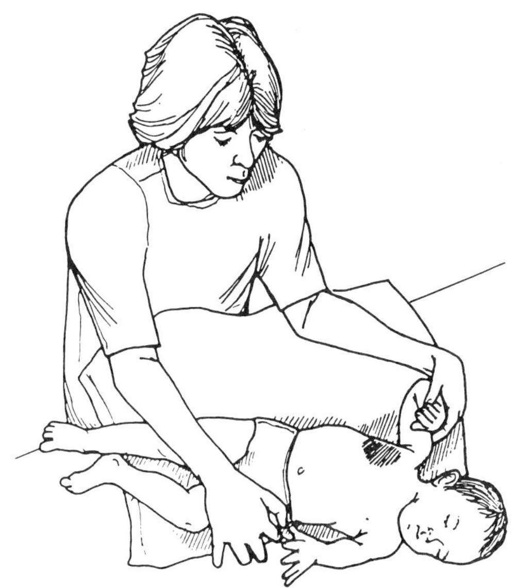

Figure 55-4 This represents the "coma position" for airway protection. In the older child, the neck should be protected for possible cervical spinal involvement. (From Levin D, Morriss F, Moore G. *Practical guide to pediatric intensive care,* ed 2, St Louis, 1984, Mosby–Year Book, p 559.)

tric distention. This is particularly important if distention is preventing adequate ventilation.

7. Keep the child warm and administer oxygen during transport. Resuscitative efforts (including ACLS) should continue until there is an adequate return of cardiac rhythm with adequate tissue perfusion or until arrival at the emergency room.

Resuscitation in the emergency room

Although one can strongly advocate the need to initiate and continue CPR in the field in most cases of pediatric near-drowning, the need to continue CPR or start advanced CPR in the emergency room becomes questionable (see "Outcome and Prognosis" later in this chapter). Continued resuscitation of the nonhypothermic victim (temperature >33° C) who arrives in the emergency room with an absence of vital signs, appears to be unwarranted, as the outcome is almost always either death or severe neurologic impairment.

In the emergency room, the presence or absence of spontaneous breathing, pulse, and blood pressure should be ascertained quickly. Because trauma is a possibility in all cases of near-drowning (especially in adolescent diving accidents), the neck should be stabilized until a cervical fracture is ruled out. Hypoxemia and acidosis are common complications of near-drowning and their possibility should be evaluated. If further resuscitation is indicated, the following interventions are suggested:

1. Administer 100% oxygen by face mask if the child is breathing spontaneously and can protect his or her own airway. If the child cannot, then intubate the trachea and administer oxygen (FiO_2 1.0). If oxygenation (either determined clinically or based on pulse oximetry) remains poor, add a 5 cm positive end-expiratory pressure (PEEP) valve while bagging by hand.
2. Place a nasogastric tube and empty the stomach to prevent further aspiration and help ventilation.
3. Insert an intravenous catheter to administer fluid and drugs. If the child is still in full cardiac arrest, the endotracheal or interosseous route for drug administration should be used. Most children who need CPR and who are still hypoperfused will need volume expansion in the emergency room. Colloid expansion during this phase is preferable. If volume expansion does not produce adequate perfusion, inotropic agents may be indicated.
4. Obtain a chest x-ray and cervical spine films as indicated.
5. Obtain arterial blood gas levels to evaluate acidosis, hypoxia, and the adequacy of ventilation.
6. After the child is resuscitated, a quick neurologic examination should be performed, as this may be prognostically important and dictate further therapy.

Ice-water immersions

The hypothermia of cold-water near-drownings may allow a more prolonged submersion time with good outcome. Although cold water is technically water with a temperature under 5° C, most of the "miraculous" saves have been rescues of victims submerged in ice water. In cases of cold-water near-drowning, body temperature should be assessed upon admission to the emergency room. This usually requires a glass thermometer, as many electronic thermometers may not register at these low temperatures.

Some clinicians believe strongly that all attempts at resuscitation of a hypothermic child who was involved in a submersion incident should be continued until the child's temperature is higher than 28° C, inasmuch as spontaneous cardiac activity or the ability to defibrillate the heart may be impossible below this temperature. Many disagree with this position and point out that successful resuscitation is the exception rather than the rule. Many children are hypothermic because they have

become poikilothermic after death.[5] Certainly, victims from a warm-water environment who are hypothermic would fit the latter description, and attempts at their resuscitation seem unwarranted.

Several methods of rewarming have been described, which include (1) surface warming, (2) administration of heated, humidified gases via an endotracheal tube, (3) peritoneal dialysis or gastric lavage with warmed solutions, and (4) extracorporeal rewarming. In rewarming, careful attention must be paid to cardiac rhythm, acid-base status, and electrolyte values. Arterial blood gases do not need to be temperature corrected in the presence of hypothermia.

ICU management

Monitoring. Near-drowning victims who are admitted to an intensive care unit (ICU) have varying degrees of organ system dysfunction, and their monitoring needs may differ. However, heart rate, ECG, systemic arterial blood pressure (frequently requiring an arterial line), and urine output should be monitored in all submersion victims for whom ICU admission is indicated. Central venous pressure or, preferably, pulmonary artery occlusion pressure, and cardiac output should be monitored if there is significant cardiac dysfunction (which frequently accompanies an hypoxic insult). Frequent neurologic assessments, including the Glasgow Coma Scale, should be made.

Respiratory management. Supplemental oxygen should be provided to relieve hypoxemia, and acidosis should be appropriately treated. If the airway is not protected naturally (e.g., if the child has a poor gag reflex or altered state of consciousness), an endotracheal tube should be inserted. Serial arterial blood gas determinations are required to monitor respiratory function, as chest x-ray films may not reflect functional abnormalities. Uneven ventilation should always alert the physician to the possibility of foreign-body aspiration.

Pulmonary insufficiency caused by near-drowning often produces ARDS and, in fact, is often used as the prototype of this syndrome. The treatment for near-drowning with ARDS is generally the same as for ARDS resulting from other causes. Briefly, it includes the use of PEEP or continuous positive airway pressure (CPAP) to decrease the intrapulmonary shunt, while maximizing oxygen delivery (the product of cardiac index and oxygen content), and decreasing the FiO_2 to less toxic levels (≤50%). To increase blood oxygen content at the expense of cardiac output is counterproductive.

There are no clear indications for the use of corticosteroids in near-drowning victims. General prophylactic use of antibiotics has not been shown to improve survival, but tends only to select ou more resistant and more aggressive organisms. However, the physician should consider antibiotic coverage if there is a possibility that water aspirated by the near-drowning victim is grossly contaminated. The child should be monitored continuously for signs of infection whether or not antibiotics are administered. An unexplained deterioration in pulmonary function after 48 to 72 hours could be due to a secondary bacterial infection. To evaluate the possibility of infection, a tracheal aspirate culture and Gram stain should be obtained. Appropriate antibiotic therapy should be instituted promptly at the first sign of infection, including fever, pulmonary infiltrates, or a white cell response in the tracheal aspirate. Bacteremia with shock occurring within the first 24 hours has been reported.

Cardiovascular management. The ventricular dysrhythmias and cardiac arrest that accompany drowning are probably secondary to combinations of hypoxia, acidosis, hypothermia, and, rarely, electrolyte disturbances. After the child undergoes resuscitation, persistent myocardial dysfunction is usually secondary to the hypoxic insult. Poor cardiac function may be manifested by poor perfusion (poor skin color, decreased urine output, and so forth), persistent or worsening metabolic acidosis, and hypotension. If there is evidence of cardiac dysfunction, objective measurement of cardiovascular hemodynamics and the adequacy of oxygenation is helpful. If the child has significant pulmonary involvement, the central venous pressure measurement often may not reflect the filling pressures in the left side of the heart. The technique of thermodilution cardiac outputs by a pulmonary artery catheter may be more reliable in these children. This will enable the physician to better assess cardiac function and oxygen delivery and to evaluate the effects of various therapies.

Central nervous system management. Studying pediatric victims of near-drownings has allowed evaluation of the effects of various treatment modalities on neurologic outcome after a hypoxic-ischemic event. Over a decade ago, "miraculous" outcomes were suggested after early and aggressive therapy to treat cerebral edema following near-drowning incidents. These therapies included evaluation and treatment of intracranial pressure and attempts at brain resuscitation using barbiturate coma and hypothermia. Ongoing analysis of this patient population as to the effectiveness of therapy can be summarized as follows[10]:

1. The use of intracranial pressure monitoring and attempts to treat elevations in intracranial pressure have failed to show conclusively any effects on outcome. Elevations in intracranial pressure, which frequently starts 24 hours after the insult, may at best be a predictor of poor outcome if present after 72 hours. Monitoring and treatment are no longer recommended in several intensive care units, including ours, that were previously involved in aggressive monitoring and treatment of this condition.

2. Barbiturate coma for cerebral salvage and protection does not increase the number of intact survivors and may, in fact, increase the number of survivors in a persistent vegetative state.

3. The use of induced hypothermia in the postresuscitation period has been unsuccessful in improving outcome. Induced hypothermia may result in increased morbidity resulting from sepsis.

4. The protective effects of hypothermia in icewater near-drownings apply only to the submersion incident and immediate postresuscitative period. Full recovery has been reported after prolonged submersion in ice water, and those who do well go on to recover fairly rapidly, as is the case in non-hypothermic arrests. Frequently, children who do well will have appropriate pain responses within 6 hours.[5] Children without appropriate pain responses and spontaneous eye opening, or who are unable to follow commands by 48 to 72 hours after resuscitation, usually have moderate to severe neurologic impairments if they survive.

Thus, present-day intensive care treatment is largely directed toward the respiratory and central nervous systems to minimize secondary neurologic damage from hypoxia, hypercapnia, hypotension, fluid overload, and uncontrolled seizure activity.[1] Such treatment may include elevation of the head of the bed, early paralysis (if indicated to treat respiratory failure), and treatment of seizures with anticonvulsants. Expectant treatment of cerebral edema with hyperosmolar agents does not affect outcome and, therefore, is not recommended.

In summary, near-drowning is a global hypoxic-ischemic insult that causes multisystem organ dysfunction, correlating in magnitude to the severity and time of hypoxia and ischemia. Although several organ dysfunctions can be treated in the ICU setting, neurologic outcome is usually predetermined by the time the child reaches the hospital. To significantly affect the associated morbidity and mortality, this catastrophe must be prevented.

OUTCOME AND PROGNOSIS

The primary determinant of the ultimate prognosis in drowning and near-drowning victims is the duration of the hypoxic-ischemic insult, which may be modified by hypothermia. Poor outcomes have been correlated with the length of time a child is missing, delayed arrival of emergency help, delay of CPR initiation while waiting for rescue personnel, and delay of CPR to telephone for help.[8] Nevertheless, large population studies have shown that the overall rate of survival is high for children who have lost consciousness in the water.

Several factors have been identified previously as predictive of poor outcome in children involved in near-drowning episodes:

1. Submersion time (increased morbidity and mortality starting at more than 5 minutes)
2. Serum pH below 7 at time of admission to the emergency room
3. The need for CPR in the emergency room
4. A delay before the first postresuscitation gasp
5. Poor initial neurologic evaluation upon resuscitation

However, recent data show that the ability of these predictors to determine outcome may be modified by early, aggressive advanced CPR in the prehospital setting[10] or hypothermia secondary to an ice-water near-drowning.[1] Only the need for CPR in the emergency room in the nonhypothermic individual has been consistently predictive of poor outcome.[3,10]

There are new data available concerning the effects of prehospital care and outcome for the near-drowning victim. A recent study has confirmed earlier studies showing that more than 90% of pediatric survivors of submersions have good outcomes.[10] An earlier study retrospectively evaluated 93 consecutive pediatric warm-water near-drownings.[3] The protocol and documentation of the need for CPR was often lacking, but 68% of the children who received only basic CPR survived intact. However, any child who needed cardiotonic drugs (including intravenous or endotracheal epinephrine or atropine, even when administered in the field) to establish a spontaneous cardiac rhythm with adequate tissue perfusion, either died or were left with severe neurologic impairment.

In a more recent study, outcome and predictors of outcome were evaluated for pediatric submersion victims receiving prehospital care in the state of Washington.[10] Emergency care was delivered by a tiered system of emergency medical technicians and paramedics. All children needing CPR were apneic, had no blood pressure, and were pulseless or bradycardic (pulse ≤40 beats per minute). This subgroup of children needing advanced CPR had a 32% survival rate, and two thirds of these survivors were unimpaired or only minimally impaired. The two risk factors for death or severe impairment were submersion time (≥10 minutes, 88% risk; ≥25 minutes, 100% risk) and CPR >25 minutes (100% risk). Thus, in agreement with the findings of others, the study found that submersion time is important in outcome, *but prompt prehospital advanced cardiac life support is the most effective means of medical intervention for the pediatric submersion victim.*

Recent data has supported earlier findings on outcome and the need for CPR in the emergency room, noting a uniformly poor outcome (either death or severe neurologic impairment) in all children who needed CPR in the emergency room after a warm-water near-drowning. These findings suggest that discontinuing CPR in the emergency room may be warranted.

The exception to the findings on the importance of CPR in the emergency room is cold-water near-drownings. Although cold water has been defined as a water temperature of 5° C or lower, most "miraculous" outcomes have been in children submerged in water covered with ice. This subject has been extensively reviewed by Orlowski.[5] In a recent review of a large series of children, the effects of hypothermia and cardiac arrest on outcome of near-drowning accidents in children were evaluated.[1] All children arriving in an emergency room with absent vital signs and body temperature of >33° C either died or survived in a persistent vegetative state. Of 14 children arriving in an emergency room with absent vital signs but with body temperature of <33° C, four survived intact. Thus, attempts at resuscitating a victim of an ice-water submersion who is hypothermic upon arrival in an emergency room with CPR in progress seem to be warranted.

As stated previously, neurologic improvement usually occurs within 48 to 72 hours if there is to be a good outcome. However, one may have to wait several months to determine the eventual neurologic outcome in children. In addition, a significant number of children who experience a submersion accident may have minimum cerebral dysfunction that may not become evident for years.

Those who treat a child victim of drowning or near-drowning should be aware of how devastating such an episode can be to the child's family. Separation and divorce may result, and accident-generated stresses within such families can persist for years; alcohol use and sleep disturbances are common. Siblings may also be affected. For these reasons the physician should continue to give support to parents and siblings. Tragically, parents of a child involved in a drowning or near-drowning episode often do not take effective measures to prevent such an accident from occurring again, and the child and siblings continue to remain at risk for additional submersion accidents.

PREVENTION

It is clear that the ability to treat victims of submersion accidents is limited and has not significantly changed the numbers of fatal outcomes; therefore, prevention is most important. Prevention takes generally two forms: (1) more effective barriers and (2) better supervision. The effectiveness of these two approaches has been shown in the literature.[6]

Because in almost half of all near-drownings the victim was last seen in the home, the U.S. Consumer Product Safety Commission (USCPSC) has recommended that pools be fenced in on all four sides. It is further recommended that the house should not serve as one side of this barrier (that is, the house should not directly access the pool). The fence should be at least 5 feet high with vertical spacing of no more than 4 inches. The gate should have a self-closing and self-latching lock that is properly maintained and easy enough to use that there is no temptation to circumvent the safety benefit. Pool covers and pool alarms have not been studied and cannot be considered to be effective alternatives.

There is substantial evidence that pool fencing is an effective drowning prevention measure; however, barrier requirements have to be legislated and often include only semipublic and public pools. Unfortunately, many such legislated actions are frequently unenforceable for residential pools, and the submersion frequency for this most important area of risk may not decrease if such regulations are not enforced.

Barriers would have prevented at most only 70% of submersion incidents in the USCPSC study, and, even when in place, several victims were able to overcome them. Experts agree that barriers can be effective and may frequently buy important time, but some fear that they may give the caregivers a false sense of security. *Barriers are no substitute for constant adult supervision,* which, when inadequate, is the most common factor associated with submersions.[6,8]

Statistics indicate that children and young adults can benefit most from water safety educational programs. Physicians, along with local government agencies, should share the responsibility for accident prevention and safety education. Pool owners should be required to be trained in adult and pediatric CPR. Most pool owners agree with voluntary CPR training, but resist its being mandated.

Infant swimming lessons and "drown-proofing" are undocumented methods that frequently lead parents to a false sense of security. Young children and infants are never "drown-proof" and swimming lessons (not recommended for children until age 3) cannot take the place of constant adult supervision. In addition, infants who swim frequently swallow water, and acute water intoxication with seizures has been reported.

Two other areas in which prevention strategies are important are adolescent activities around lakes and rivers, and submersions during bathing.[9] The dangers of alcohol consumption during recreational water activities should be publicized. Parents should be cautioned about leaving young children unattended in a bathtub and about the risk of leaving the supervision of an infant or toddler to another child who is less than 5 years of age. Children with seizures, even those older than 5 years, and their families should be warned of the risks of bathing unattended.

In spite of all the recommendations, children will continue to drown, as supervision cannot be mandated and lapses will continue to occur. Nevertheless, the incidence of drowning and near-drowning can be significantly decreased. It is the responsibility of all health care providers to generate and maintain awareness of this problem.

REFERENCES

1. Biggart MJ, Bohn DJ: Effect of hypothermia and cardiac arrest on outcome of near-drowning accidents in children, *J Pediatr* 117:179-183, 1990.
2. Modell JH: *The pathophysiology and treatment of drowning and near-drowning*, Springfield, Ill, 1971, Charles C Thomas.
3. Nichter MA, Everett PB: Childhood near-drowning: is cardiopulmonary resuscitation always indicated? *Crit Care Med* 17:993-995, 1989.
4. Noble CS, Sharpe N: Drowning: its mechanism and treatment, *Can Med Assoc J* 89:402-405, 1963.
5. Orlowski JP: Drowning, near-drowning, and ice-water submersions, *Ped Clin N Am* 34:75-92, 1987.
6. Pearn J, Nixon J: Swimming pool immersion accidents: an analysis from the Brisbane drowning study, *Med J Aust* 1:432-437, 1977.
7. Peterson B: Morbidity of childhood near-drowning, *Pediatrics* 59:364-370, 1977.
8. Present P: Child drowning study: a report on the epidemiology of drownings in residential pools to children under age five, Washington, DC, 1987, US Consumer Product Safety Commission.
9. Quan L, Gore EJ, Wentz K et al: Ten-year study of pediatric drownings and near-drownings in King County, Washington: lessons in injury prevention, *Pediatrics* 83:1035-1040, 1989.
10. Quan L, Wentz KR, Gore EJ et al: Outcome and predictors of outcome in pediatric submersion victims receiving prehospital care in King County, Washington, *Pediatrics* 86:586-593, 1990.
11. Ramey CA, Ramey DN, Hayward JS: Dive response of children in relation to cold-water near-drowning, *J Appl Physiol* 63(2):665-668, 1987.

56 Hand Injury

Michael J. Boyajian

Hand injuries represent one of the most common presentations to the emergency room or doctor's office, presumably because the hand is the organ of environment exploration. To carry out its function, the hand combines precision, mobility, power, and sensibility with unique intensity. Many hand injuries may be cared for by a primary physician; many others require referral to a specialist. The care rendered in the acute situation is the factor that most determines the final outcome.

As in other areas, the injured hand of a child differs in many aspects from the adult counterpart. The pattern of injury is different: whereas the adult commonly suffers occupational trauma, the child is often injured at play. Among the most frequent injuries are fingertip amputation or crush in a door, exercise equipment, folding chair, or stroller; contact burn; laceration from a fall; animal bite; and sports injury. Unfortunately, one might add self-inflicted teenage wrist injury to the list. Furthermore, for a given insult, periarticular ligament tear is less common, and epiphyseal fracture more common in children than in adults.

Evaluation of the injured hand of a child is difficult. The alarm the child feels, often compounded by the parents' anxiety and guilt, makes cooperation an unlikely possibility. A large measure of empathy and patience is required, and even then the examination may be limited. Lacerations that violate the dermis of the hand, especially on the volar aspect, require exploration in the operating room.

Postoperative management is a particular concern. The physician must accept minimal cooperation from the child. The dressing needs to be more extensive and secure, and plaster immobilization more sturdy. Physical rehabilitation of a child is both easier and harder: left alone, the child is quite active; in regimented therapy, he or she may be resistant.

The healing potential of the child is great. Good management is usually rewarded with a good functional result.

EVALUATION

All emergency visits are stressful for a child and family. Hand injuries are usually painful, and func-

tional evaluation involves further pain associated with motion. The first task of the physician is to comfort the child.

If a dressing is in place, obtain as much information as possible before removal. Careful observation before any contact is made with the injury will be of considerable value. For example, the posture of the digits (i.e., the positional "cascade") is a valuable indicator of the integrity of the underlying tendons. Detectable motion of the fingers will likewise rule out tendon laceration or motor nerve injury. Sensory examination is possible with the dressing in place.

Sensory examination in the child is difficult. Asking him if he feels light touch on even an anesthetic finger will most commonly elicit an affirmative answer. It is more productive to inquire whether the feeling is the same in a touch to an uninjured finger, perhaps on the opposite hand. The examiner must be familiar with the sensory territories of the three main nerves and test each. Detection of sweating on an injured finger, as compared with an uninjured finger, is a useful clue, because it depends on innervation. Immerse the hand in water for 15 minutes; the pattern of wrinkling will often reveal a nerve laceration, as this is a pseudomotor function. The motor function of the intrinsic muscles should be tested, if practical.

Ability to flex and extend each joint of both the fingers and wrist requires definition (Fig. 56-1). The deep and superficial flexors of each digit should be tested systematically. Although a partial tendon laceration can be present with normal motion, it may well be associated with pain upon motion against mild resistance. Tendon examination may be virtually impossible in the young child, and careful observation becomes critical.

The cardinal signs of bone fracture are swelling, tenderness, deformity, and loss of function. The latter two signs are the only constants, but they are nonspecific. Anteroposterior and lateral radiographs of the part suspected for fracture provide the basis of diagnosis. Analysis requires consideration of the chronology of secondary centers of ossification, which might suggest a chip fracture; otherwise, diagnosis of epiphyseal fracture is difficult.

Inspect the wound with respect to its nature and location. The significance of a particular site is based on the examiner's knowledge of hand anatomy. A small laceration can easily be associated with serious injury. All injuries that penetrate the dermis require exploration by the treating surgeon under operating room conditions. This is particularly important for injuries on the volar side of the hand. Conservative debridement of devitalized tissue is clearly indicated. In crush or avulsion injury, a delay in debridement and closure is commonly useful; a wet dressing will prevent desiccation for 24 hours.

SURGICAL TREATMENT

A thorough knowledge of hand anatomy, exploration under appropriate anesthesia and tourniquet control, adequate debridement and hemostasis, proper magnification, and primary repair whenever possible are the mainstays of good surgical care.

Hematomas assist discovery of injured structures. All injuries to bone, tendon, nerve, and vessel should be identified and tagged with fine sutures for subsequent retrieval. Only then is formulation of a systematic plan for repair possible. One common approach addresses the stronger structures before the more fragile: immobilize the fracture, repair the tendon, and follow these by microneurorrhaphy and microanastomosis. Many times this order is altered in the interest of exposure or urgent revascularization. Loop magnification is essential for optimum repair; however, the operating microscope is preferable for treating nerve or vessel injury.

Early primary repair is the rule whenever feasible. However, a delay of 24 to 48 hours does not worsen outcome. The longer the delay beyond that time, the more vessel thrombosis, muscle-tendon retraction, inflammation, edema, and scar formation will occur. Secondary repair, including nerve and tendon graft should be considered only when primary repair is hampered by extensive structural damage.

Fracture

In contrast to other parts of the skeleton, only minimal deformity is acceptable in the hand. However, a small amount of remodeling can take place in a child's hand if the angulation is in the plane of flexion-extension.

Fractures are designated as open or closed, intraarticular or extraarticular, and stable or unstable. In the hand, as elsewhere, open fracture requires debridement and closure; anatomic reduction of intraarticular fracture of any significant size (more than 30% of the articular surface) and stabilization of any fracture are imperative.

Treatment of an open fracture includes irrigation, debridement, and provision of systemic antibiotic and stabilization. If there is severe contamination, avoid wound closure. This is particularly important in the case of a human bite; delayed primary closure is a good option. An unstable fracture is one whose reduction is temporary and requires stabilization,

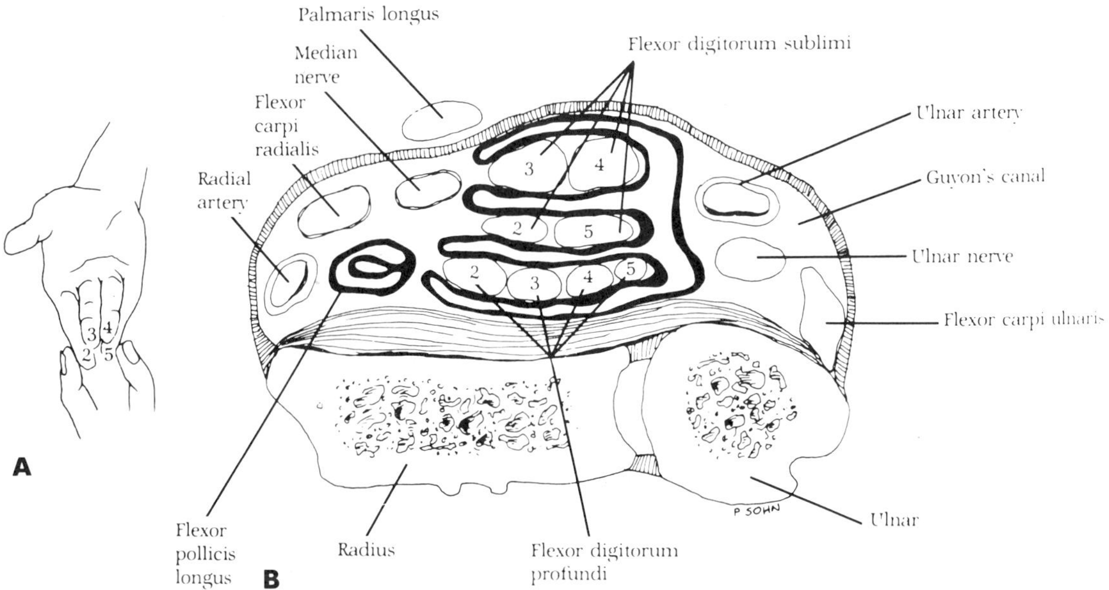

Figure 56–1 A, Relationship of superficialis tendons. **B,** Cross-sectional anatomy at the level of the wrist.

often by application of a cast or splint; otherwise internal fixation is indicated.

Metacarpal fracture is frequently unstable; evaluation of adequate reduction is best with the finger straight and in flexion to evaluate for rotational deformity. One very common metacarpal fracture is the "boxer's fracture": palmar angulation of the distal fifth metacarpal shaft, usually caused by striking the fist against a chin or wall. Reduction occurs by flexing the metacarpophalangeal (MCP) joint and by applying dorsal force to the proximal phalanx. An ulnar gutter splint then holds the reduction.

Avulsion fracture of the MCP joint where the collateral ligament attaches, and of the distal interphalangeal (DIP) joint where the extensor tendon inserts, are common manifestations of sports injury. Both usually require open reduction and pin fixation.

In general, fractures that are unstable even with plaster immobilization are treated by closed reduction and percutaneous Kirschner wire fixation, or open reduction and internal fixation with Kirschner wires or interosseous wires, to assure stabilization of rotation and angulation. Miniplates are of limited use in treatment of children.

Epiphyseal fractures are designated by the Salter-Harris classification:

Type I—slipped epiphysis

Type II—slipped epiphysis with metaphyseal fragment

Type III—isolated fracture of the epiphysis

Type IV—fracture through metaphysis, growth plate, and epiphysis

Type V—growth plate crush

Closed treatment usually suffices for types I, II, and III. Type IV commonly requires precise reduction and fixation to prevent premature fusion and subsequent growth deformity.

In summary, open treatment is indicated for:

1. Fractures that cannot be reduced
2. Fractures that are unstable after reduction
3. Intraarticular fractures involving over 30%
4. Type IV epiphyseal fractures

Flexor tendon injury

All lacerations that transgress the volar skin require exploration in the operating room to provide a clear assessment under tourniquet control. In general, repair both flexor tendons to each digit, even in "no man's land"; if the injury is too extensive, repair of the profundus tendon is important.

When exploring a tendon transection, it is helpful to remember that the position of the distal end is related to the posture of the digit at the time of laceration. If the fingers were flexed around the offending instrument, as in grasping a knife, the distal end will lie distal to the skin wound. If the fingers were straight, the distal tendon end and the skin laceration will be at the same level. The distal end may be exposed by extending the laceration with a Bruner incision; the proximal end may well be retracted. The retrieval of the tendon is aided by flexing all proximal joints and "milking" it distally. Explore the tendon sheath with a smooth-tipped clamp that permits gentle manipulation of the tendon. The tendon is drawn toward the distal tendon and transfixed with a needle. Every effort is made not to divide the pulleys.

Tendon repair is usually carried out after the technique of Bunnell or Kessler, using 4-0 nylon or polypropylene and finished with a running 6-0 epitendineum suture. The deep suture should not "collapse" the juncture, and the superficial suture should invert or enclose the raw tendon substance, thus providing a smooth surface to the sheath. Avoid manipulation of the tendon, and close the tendon sheath where feasible. There is evidence that partial tendon lacerations are better left unsutured if the injury is less than 25%. In this case, trim the frayed edges to prevent development of a trigger finger. Extensive partial lacerations require surgical reconstruction for best results.

After repair and closure are complete, the tendon junctures must be protected to prevent rupture. In the young child, the joints are immobilized just short of full flexion with a plaster splint for 3 to 4 weeks. The dressing is as important as the surgery; in this procedure, do not depend on the child's cooperation. The splint should be thick and should extend nearly to the axilla; be sure also to provide a secure external dressing. The significant problem with flexor tendon laceration is loss of excursion within the complex wound scar. Active motion is initiated after 3 to 4 weeks of immobilization, and passive motion after 6 weeks. A hand therapist familiar with the particular problems of this age group and an actively participating parent are essential for effective rehabilitation. Older children may be candidates for a program of dynamic splinting. In this system, active extension is allowed to the limits of a dorsal stop (wrist flexed 60, MVPs 20, IPs 0), and passive flexion is a result of rubber band traction applied to the fingertips.

Extensor tendon injury

In general, extensor tendons have less excursion than their flexor counterparts; the extensor muscles are weaker, and adhesive scar forms in injuries less frequently. Furthermore, lacerations to these structures are frequently incomplete. It is possible to repair the extensor tendon in the emergency room, depending upon the nature of the injury, adequacy of the visualization, and the child's willingness to cooperate. Nevertheless, most of these injuries require surgical repair in the operating room.

Mallet finger deformity is caused by division of the extensor mechanism over the middle phalanx with the DIP joint dropping into flexion. This is sometimes associated with a type II epiphyseal fracture; direct repair is best for open injury. Unfortunately, repair of a mallet finger requires placement of a pin and use of a splint for an extended period.

Injuries of the central slip may be open or closed. When this structure is functionally lost, the remaining extensor may drift in a volar direction to the midaxial line and cause a boutonnière deformity; this may not occur for some time. Therefore, suspect the deformity if forceful PIP flexion produces dorsal swelling of the joint or "jamming" of the digit; apply a splint to immobilize and reexamine frequently. Surgical repair is indicated if tendon rupture is present. Wounds over the MCP joint may be consistent with near-normal extension because the extensor mechanism injury is commonly incomplete, or because of connections between tendons. This simply underscores the necessity for exploration.

Laceration of the extensor tendon near its insertion is repaired with a horizontal mattress or a figure-eight nylon suture. Similar repair of a central slip laceration is possible, or repair with a Bunnell or Kessler suture. Partial lacerations may be treated with a running fine nylon suture.

The surgical dressing incorporates a plaster splint in full extension. In the case of mallet finger surgery, a Kirschner wire is a useful adjunct. Immobilization is held for 6 weeks before initiation of active motion involving the strong flexors.

Nerve injury

Avoid application of a hemostatic clamp to a bleeding artery in a volar laceration in the emergency room. The associated nerve is usually superficial, similarly divided, and subject to crush injury. Direct pressure is almost always sufficient to stop the bleeding. Excellent results occur from neurorraphy in the pediatric age group. The younger the patient, the sharper the injury, and the more tension-free the nerve, the better the result.

The median and ulnar nerves at the wrist comprise mixed sensory and motor nerves. The common and proper digital nerves are purely sensory. In case of nerve transection, every effort is necessary to note any surface vascular marking, bundle pattern, or obliquity of the cut ends to achieve perfect fascicle alignment. Damaged nerve ends, as in a crush injury, should be cut back to normal nerve, using a nerve cutter or wooden tongue blade as support. Some mobilization of the ends is possible, but a primary or secondary nerve graft is preferable to a repair with tension.

The larger nerves are best approached with a grouped fascicular repair. Smaller nerve junctures are made with epineural repair. Dissection and neurorraphy is best undertaken with the operating microscope, using 9-0 and 10-0 nylon suture. Splint application will follow the requirements of any concurrent tendon work; flexion is useful to minimize any tension across the nerve juncture.

Fingertip amputation

In young children, amputation of the fingertip is among the most common of hand injuries. This is almost always a crush injury rather than a sharp amputation. The injury is defined by the level and angulation of amputation, the condition of the amputation stump, especially the nail bed, and the condition of the amputated part. Near-amputation of the fingertip is best treated by replacement of the part with few sutures. This is true even when the vascularity is marginal or questionable, because the blood flow often improves after untwisting the pedicle and resolution of vessel spasm.

Microvascular replantation is indicated for any amputation proximal to the arterial branching at the DIP level. For an amputation distal to the germinal matrix, debridement and replacement as a composite graft is at least occasionally successful in the toddler. All devitalized tissue is cut away sharply, and a few absorbable sutures placed. The part is immobilized with a conforming dressing including a plaster splint.

In cases in which the lost part is extensively damaged, salvage of a full-thickness skin graft from the distal tip is possible. A tie-over bolster technique secures the graft onto a dry base; complete hemostasis is required in either grafting situation. Even when the graft fails to vascularize, it mummifies and serves as a biologic dressing. When it separates, near-complete epithelialization of the proximal digit occurs.

In cases in which the amputated part is not available, small to moderate defects, with little or no bone exposed, will heal quite well by secondary intention, providing an excellent result, with good, sensate, pain-free padding. A split-thickness skin graft, using the hypothenar eminence or another donor site, is a reasonable alternative, but after graft contraction the result is not better than spontaneous epithelialization.

Transverse or dorsal oblique amputation with broad bone exposure is usually closed by a local advancement flap and minimal bone shortening; the simplest closure is usually the best. Direct closure is sometimes possible, but the volar V-Y advancement is a common and useful approach.

Closure of a volar oblique amputation with local flaps is difficult without unacceptable sacrificed bone. Skin graft and nonsurgical management do not work well. A cross-finger flap from the dorsum of the adjacent ulnar digit is a good choice. The flap is taken at the level of the extensor paratenon and turned like a page of a book to cover the defect. The donor site is covered with a full or split skin graft. The best coverage of the volar oblique amputation is the thenar flap. A distally or proximally based flap from the thenar eminence is raised, and the digit is flexed into position to accept the flap. The donor defect is closed directly.

Management of either flap requires reliable immobilization for about 12 to 14 days, after which the pedicle may be divided and the flap inset. The thenar flap provides excellent controur and sensibility, and the donor scar is almost always quite acceptable.

Digit amputation

Unless the part is severely damaged, microvascular replantation is best for single or multiple digit amputation in children, who experience a better result than adult patients.

Management of the amputated part requires prevention of contamination and a cool environment without direct contact with ice. The best technique is to wrap the part in gauze moistened in saline or Ringer's lactate solution and place on ice. Alternatively, the part may be placed in a plastic bag of saline or Ringer's solution, and the bag set in ice. The child should receive gram-positive antibiotic coverage, appropriate tetanus prophylaxis, and aspirin. X-rays are taken of both the amputated part and the proximal finger.

The operation is begun on the amputated part before initiation of anesthesia. Using the operating microscope with a magnification of 15 to 20 power, the distal arteries, dorsal veins, and nerves are identified and tagged.

Surgical sequencing is as follows:
1. Definition of vessels and nerves
2. Bone shortening and internal fixation
3. Tendon repair
4. Microanastomosis and neurorraphy
5. Loose skin closure
6. Regional nerve block

A nonconstrictive, conforming dressing and splint are applied to permit hand elevation. The exposed fingertip is monitored with use of a pulse oximeter or thermocouple in addition to vascular checks. The child is kept warm and quiet because the risk of spasm is real, the dressing is not changed and the child not stressed for at least a week.

Replantation of finger amputation is less successful in children than in adults for several reasons. The amputation is more commonly an avulsion or crush injury rather than a sharp amputation. The surgeon usually attempts to replant a more damaged digit in a child. Unfortunately, tiny vessels and vasospasm are more commonly encountered. In spite of these concerns, a success rate of at least 60% with excellent function is possible.

REFERENCES

1. Campbell RM Jr: Operative treatment of fractures and dislocations of the hand and wrist region in children, *Orthop Clin N Am* 21, 1990.
2. Almquist EE. Hand injuries in children, *Pediatr Clin N Am* 33, 1986.
3. Serafin D, Georgiade N: *Pediatric plastic surgery*, St Louis, 1984, Mosby–Year Book.

57 Animal, Human, and Insect Bites

Charles G. Howell, Jr. and Robyn M. Hatley

Childhood emergencies are extremely common and generally occur in or near the home. Of the nearly two million phone calls to our nation's poison control centers in 1990,[9] more than half involved children less than 6 years of age. The broad category "Bites and Envenomations" included more than 60,000 total bites, nearly half occurring in children. Only 25% of these bites were serious enough to result in treatment at a health care facility, only 0.2% were subsequently categorized as "major outcome" (see Table 57-1 for all outcome definitions), and only one death was reported. The magnitude of the problem, however, is impressive.

Children, especially boys, tend to be aggressive in regard to animals. They are more likely to sustain a dog or snake bite to the face while teasing or holding an animal. They may sustain a serious spider bite to the finger as they explore a hole in the side of an old building, or a significant sting or stings to the body while playing with a beehive or wasp's nest. The effect of the actual bite in the child is also different than in the adult. Because of the child's smaller size, envenomation equal to that in an adult will produce a more serious effect.

The most effective therapy in the treatment of childhood bites is prevention, and the central theme of prevention is education, both at home and at school. Prevention becomes even more important when one studies the systemic consequences of a bite, which may include rabies, tetanus, Lyme disease, or acquired immunodeficiency syndrome.

SNAKE BITES
Pit vipers: rattlesnake, water moccasin, and copperhead

In the 1990[9] report from the 72 participating poison control centers across the United States serving a population of 192 million people, 3726 snake bites were reported, involving all age groups. Of the 3726 bites, 979 were poisonous but only 62 (6%) produced a subsequent "major outcome." Table 57-2 includes a comparison of snake bites in children less than 6 years of age with those 6 to 17 years of age. The older age group suffered three times as many bites in general, and more than twice as many poisonous bites. Even more significant is the fact that only 13% of the total bites in children were poisonous. A significant number of the snakes were of the exotic variety, and more than 50% were classified as "unknown"—information that is extremely important in planning therapy.

In general, the prepubescent male, barefoot, playing in the neighborhood woods, seems to be a prime target. Wagner[13] recently reported on 29 crotalid bites in children in Arkansas. All bites occurred close to the home, in spring and summer, and more than half happened to barefoot children, whose average age was 7 years.

The majority of rattlesnake bites occur in the Southwest, moccasin bites (cottonmouth and copperhead) in the Southeast, and coral snake bites in the South. Rarely does one encounter bites from poisonous snakes in the New England states.

Pathophysiology. Distinct characteristics of the bite allow for identification, especially in the category of pit vipers (Crotalidae), which include the rattlesnake, copperhead, and the cottonmouth. The pit vipers are distinguished by a triangular head, vertical elliptical pupils, facial pits, and a single row of subcaudal scales. In addition, rattles at the end of the tail section are specific for the genus *Crotalus*. Furthermore, the pit vipers have two fangs through which they may inject their venom.

Table 57–1 American Association of Poison Control Centers medical outcome definitions

Minor outcome	Minimal signs or symptoms, rapid resolution, no treatment required, skin involvement only
Moderate outcome	More pronounced, prolonged, systemic manifestations of toxicity
Major outcome	Life-threatening symptoms or manifested residual disability; that is, children requiring intubation or mechanical ventilation, or having cardiac instability or coma

Table 57-2 1990 Comparison of snake bites reported to poison control centers in children of less than 6 years and in those 6 to 17 years of age

	<6 Years of age	6-17 Years of age	Total
Rattlesnake	32	57	89
Copperhead	22	65	87
Coral	0	3	3
Cottonmouth	1	14	15
Crotalidae (unknown)	1	2	3
Exotic, poisonous	7	9	16
Exotic, nonpoisonous	22	50	72
Nonpoisonous	126	417	543
Unknown snake	206	614	820
Total	417	1231	1648

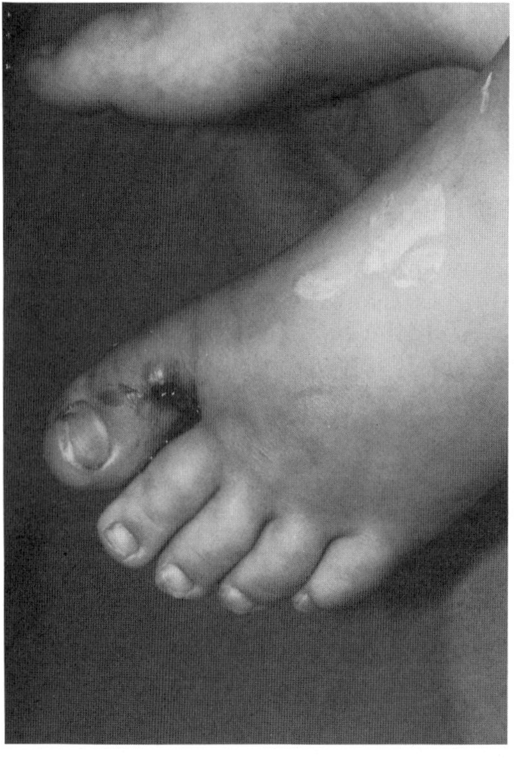

Figure 57-1 Six-year-old with crotalid envenomation of left great toe.

Specific identifying features of the genus *Agkistrodon* include the cottony appearance of the mouth in the cottonmouth moccasin and the lack of rattles.

The venom of pit vipers, a multiple poison, contains polypeptides that are used to first kill the victim and a multitude of enzymes, including phospholipase A, to aid in digestion. The polypeptides consist of cardiotoxins, neurotoxins, and hemorrhagins.

The symptoms following envenomation are those that occur in the area of the bite and those that occur systemically. Symptoms are dependent on the dose of venom the child has received, the location of the envenomation, whether it has been delivered subcutaneously or intravenously, and the size of the child.

In general, severe pain is followed by the development of edema of the extremity. Blebs or blisters may occur along with ecchymosis and subsequent local tissue necrosis (Fig. 57-1). Systemic symptoms of nausea, vomiting, weakness, diarrhea, and bleeding will follow in significant envenomations. Fasciculations and paresthesias, as well as neurologic deficits, may also occur. Depending on the site of the bite, the symptoms and signs will vary. Timber rattler envenomation is noted to cause a metallic taste in the mouth, whereas that of the Mojave rattlesnake may cause little local reaction but a significant neuromuscular blockade that can lead to respiratory arrest.

Diagnosis. The history of a bite in a child playing outdoors, along with the fang marks, may be the only information about a bite that is initially available. The snake may not have been identified. If no significant local or systemic reaction occurs within 4 hours, it is unlikely that a serious envenomation has occurred, but hospitalization is still required. Laboratory tests helpful in diagnosis include creatinine phosphokinase, prothrombin time, fibrinogen, fibrin split products, and platelet counts.

Initial resuscitation. First-aid treatment at the site of injury is important. This includes the placement of a loose tourniquet to retard lymphatic return, immobilization of the injured extremity, and elevation of the extremity just below the level of the heart. We believe that incision and suction (performed within minutes of the bite) should be avoided unless medical personnel are immediately

Table 57–3 Guidelines for initial dosage of antivenin

Envenomation	Signs	Dose of antivenin
None	No local or systemic signs	0 vials
Minimal	Local swelling, no systemic signs, normal laboratory data	2-4 vials
Moderate	Swelling beyond site of bite, one or more systemic signs, abnormal laboratory findings (drop in hematocrit or platelets)	5-9 vials
Severe	Marked local response, severe systemic signs, abnormal laboratory data	10-15+ vials

Data from Minton S: Venom diseases: snakebite. In Beeson P, McDermott W, editors: *Textbook of medicine*, Philadelphia, 1975, WB Saunders, pp 88-92; Russell F et al: Snake venom poisoning in the United States: experiences with 550 cases, *JAMA* 233:341, 1975; Russell F: Venomous bites and stings: poisonous snakes. In *The Merck Manual of Diagnosis and Therapy*, ed 14, 1982, pp 2450-2456; and Wingert W, Wainschel J: Diagnosis and management of envenomation by poisonous snakes, *South Med J* 68:1015, 1975.

available. The time required is better spent in transporting the victim to a medical facility. Furthermore, incision wounds inflicted by inexperienced individuals are often worse than the bite itself.

Noting the size of the snake is helpful in an estimation of potential venom dose. It is important to restrict activity in a child who has been bitten and to transport the child to an appropriate medical facility as soon as possible.

In-hospital care. Within minutes of arrival at a medical center, one should be able to establish a baseline status of the injured child. Determine whether the bite was from a venomous or nonvenomous snake, particularly because the overwhelming majority are of the nonvenomous variety. Question and examine the child or family members as to symptoms and signs relative to the bite; examine the bite and measure the area of local erythema and the size of the extremity. Also record the time of injury, initial treatment, and allergic status. Pertinent laboratory tests and data include CBC with platelet count, urinalysis, creatinine, electrolytes, creatinine phosphokinase, coagulation profile (protime, fibrinogen, fibrin-split products), blood type and cross-match. Administration of intravenous fluid such as Ringer's lactate with dextrose, NPO orders, monitoring of vital signs and urine output, administration of tetanus vaccine, and antibiotic administration are essential. Obviously, if the bite is considered poisonous and the use of antivenin is planned, test for hypersensitization to horse serum. The administration of antivenin is determined by the severity of envenomation and the type of snake that inflicted the bite. Some authors[3] believe that antivenin is almost never indicated, but others[15] believe that judicious use is prudent.

Despite the obvious controversy, guidelines[14] do exist and are useful in determining therapy. The envenomation from a rattlesnake bite is extremely serious and requires use of antivenin, whereas the bite of the less-dangerous water moccasin may be best treated by local wound care without the use of antivenin. Specifically, if a child sustains a crotalid envenomation with obvious fang marks and edema up to 12 inches from the site, begin with 5 vials of antivenin and titrate with additional antivenin based on response (Table 57-3). Larger doses of antivenin may be required when a small child is envenomated by a large rattlesnake.

An antivenin package insert outlines specific protocols for dosage, administration, and assessment of hypersensitivity to horse serum. A detailed plan of subsequent antivenin administration in the diluted form for use in the hypersensitive child is also available.

Wound care. Depending on the site of the original envenomation and the subsequent local reaction, the wound will require a minimum of immobilization, debridement, and local care. If a compartment syndrome requires a fasciotomy, leave the wound open for 7 to 10 days before secondary closure or split-thickness skin graft to the defect.

Aftercare. Subsequent care is dependent on whether a child has received antivenin. The development of serum sickness may occur as soon as 3 days after treatment or as late as 3 weeks. Symptoms include fever, urticaria, arthralgia, and evidence of lymphadenopathy. The subsequent treatment includes diphenhydramine hydrochloride and prednisone.

Outcome. Less than 1% of snakebite victims die from envenomation. Rattlesnakes continue to inflict the majority of snakebite envenomations associated with death, but the copperhead bite rarely results in fatality.

Coral snake

Coral snakes in the United States belong to the family Elapidae. The eastern coral snake ranges from Florida to Texas, and the western coral snake from Texas to Mexico. The coral snake is most often noted to be less than 2 feet in length, with smaller fangs than the rattlesnake, round instead of elliptical pupils, and a small mouth. One of the most important aspects of coral snake bites is accurate identification, because the coral snake has the same colors as the nonpoisonous king snake. The phrase "red on yellow, kill a fellow; red on black, won't kill Jack" is helpful in discerning the colored circles of the coral snake.

Our experience with bites from the coral snake suggests that the bite is not particularly painful, but soon thereafter leads to local hypesthesia, muscle weakness, fasciculations, and even paralysis. The size of the snake and the size of the fangs usually require that the bite be on a toe, finger, or fold of skin for envenomation to occur.

A clear strike mark with subsequent identification of the fang sites indicate a serious envenomation. The neurotoxicity of the venom usually leads to the slow progression of neurologic symptoms, with numbness or weakness developing in the involved extremity. Within hours there may be difficulty with speaking and excess salivation.

Other than the identification of the snake itself and the characteristic symptoms, there is no special clotting abnormality or local indicators to prove the diagnosis. The systemic effects of the venom may progress to paralysis of cranial nerves, with subsequent respiratory arrest within 4 to 6 hours of a significant envenomation. Treatment of the coral snake bite requires support of the circulation, tetanus immunization, antibiotic administration, and antivenin.

In addition, one must beware of the neurotoxic effect of the venom on respiration. Antivenin is available for bites of both the eastern and western coral snake (*Micrurus* species) and is made by Wyeth as a horse serum product.

ANIMAL BITES: DOG, CAT AND HUMAN

Mammalian bites, besides inflicting injury to the site of the bite, are also responsible for the transmission of diseases such as rabies, cat-scratch disease, and, possibly, acquired immunodeficiency syndrome. Bites of this nature are a common cause of emergency room visits and are difficult to manage. Litovitz[9] reported the experience of 72 of the nation's poison control center calls and noted some 3869 mammalian bites in 1990. More than half of all bites occurred in children less than 17 years of age, and 28% were dog-related. Overwhelmingly, the majority were categorized as "none" to "minor outcome," and no deaths were reported.

Dog bites

Sacks,[11] in a comprehensive review of dog bite–related fatalities over a 10-year period prior to 1989, reported 157 deaths (70% were in children aged less than 10). Pit bull breeds, German shepherds, huskies, and Doberman pinschers were the most common offenders, the pit bull being the most common. Of significant interest in this review was the fact that 110 of the 157 deaths were in children less than 9 years of age and, furthermore, that 16% of the deaths occurred in infants less than 1 year of age (9 patients were less than 1 month of age). The majority of the injuries are inflicted by a known animal in young boys, which suggests provocation as an etiologic factor. Older children are more often bitten on an extremity, whereas younger children are more likely to sustain bites to the head or neck.

The mechanism of injury in a dog bite is somewhat related to the breed involved. Pit bull breeds are especially ferocious in that they do not usually bite and run, but bite and hold while continuing to maul the victim. Significant laceration, puncture wounds, tears, and even fractures of bone with disruption of major nerves, tendons, and vessels can occur in attacks by large animals (Fig. 57-2).

Secondary injury from infection is common. Initial treatment is directed at the wound. Our expe-

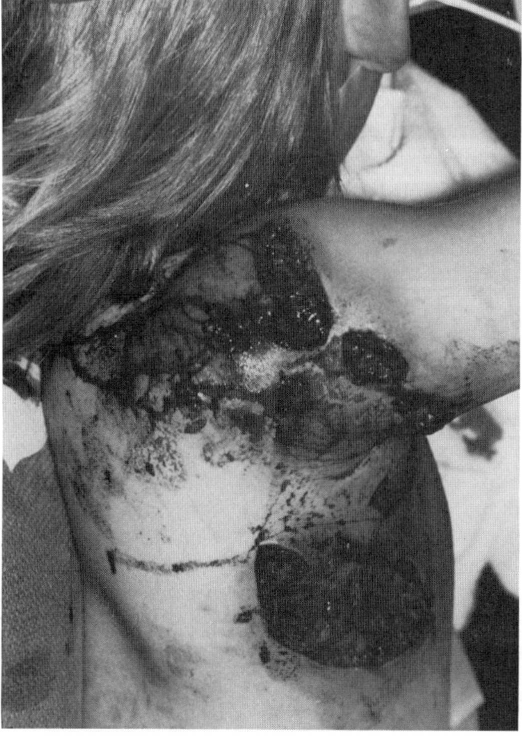

Figure 57–2 Four-year-old with severe dog bite–related injuries.

rience supports that of others,[12] that high pressure irrigation with a jet lavage of the wound (even the puncture wound), debridement of devitalized tissue, removal of foreign debris, and tetanus and rabies prophylaxis, when indicated, are the hallmarks of therapy. The majority of minor lacerations from dog bites do very well with primary closure and administration of antibiotics such as amoxicillin and clavulinic acid (Augmentin). Frequent examination of the wound for signs of infection is important; facial injuries are less likely to become infected than extremity injuries.

Major injury from a dog bite can require hospitalization, intravenous antibiotic administration, and primary repair or delayed reconstruction after extensive wound care. The site and age of the wound, age of the child, and the extent of the injury determine subsequent management. Treatment of avulsion injury is possible by replacement of the injured tissue after appropriate debridement, or by debridement with subsequent secondary reconstruction. Our experience with primary repair of avulsion injury has not been satisfactory, and we would not recommend this form of therapy.

Cat bites

Domestic cats as pets are as common as dogs, yet they account for few serious injuries. Marcy[10] has emphasized the infection potential of these injuries, which are predominantly puncture wounds. Basic wound management for cat bites is much the same as for dog bites, except that the wounds are generally left open and treated with frequent dressing change or irrigation, and antibiotic administration.

Of equal importance to the early wound infection induced by the cat's oral flora (*Pasturella multocida* is most common) is the subsequent development of cat-scratch disease.

Approximately 6000 cases of cat-scratch disease occur in the United States each year. The etiology of this illness is a bacterial organism that causes chills, fever, arthralgia, lymphadenopathy of the neck, axillae, or even the parasternal area, depending on the inoculation site. Recently, antibiotic regimens including ciprofloxacin[6] and trimethoprim and sulfamethoxazole[4] have been found useful in eradication of the sequelae of cat-scratch disease. Surgical excision of a lymphadenopathy is warranted for diagnosis when the history is atypical or when a draining sinus from an involved lymphadenitis fails to heal. The specimen reveals necrotizing granulomas in the enlarged node and the tiny organisms recently named *Afipia felis*.[2]

Human bites

Human bites in children are common occurrences. The data of Baker and Moore[1] suggest that bites occur most often in early adolescence, and that victims of human bites are notorious for delay in seeking treatment and for a high risk of infection. Successful treatment includes closure of lacerations of the face and treatment of all other wounds with delayed closure, debridement, daily wound care, and antibiotic administration, particularly in those with deep lacerations or punctures. Others,[12] however, recommend avoidance of primary closure of facial bites because of the high risk of infection.

Of particular interest is an injury over the metacarpophalangeal joint (caused by a blow of a closed fist to a tooth), as it may have penetrated the joint space and thus lead to a serious hand infection. If delay in presentation leads to a surrounding cellulitis of the area, hospitalization, culture of the depth of the wound site, and intravenous antibiotic administration are indicated. In general, gram-positive aerobic bacteria (*Staphylococcus* and *Streptococcus*) predominate, and thus a course of Augmentin is sufficient for early treatment and subsequent outpatient therapy. The transmission of other diseases, such as hepatitis B and acquired immunodeficiency syndrome, is also possible.

INSECT BITES

Insect bites and stings are among the most common envenomations that children sustain. In fact, of the 64,233 bites and envenomations reported to the American Association of Poison Control Centers in 1990,[9] 18,011 (29%) were in this group. Furthermore, 8831 (49%) of these bites occurred in children less than 17 years of age, but only 16 bites were categorized as "major outcome." No deaths were reported to the poison control centers; however, other studies have documented more deaths by hymenoptera stings than by any other group of venomous animals.[7]

Hymenoptera: bees, yellow jackets, wasps, and ants

Pathophysiology. Hymenoptera venom is not particularly toxic enough to produce fatality but can certainly lead to sensitization. After the development of sensitization, a subsequent sting may lead to an anaphylactic reaction and death. Specific hymenoptera such as ants, inflict bites that are characterized by the injection of irritants such as formic acid, and others, such as the fire ant, inject an alkaloid toxin that may cause severe pain with subsequent pustule formation. Wasps, on the other hand, can repeatedly inject venom-containing enzymes that can cause actual tissue destruction. A bee sting also delivers venom, and, except in the case of the bumblebee, the sting apparatus is left in the victim. The stinger must then be carefully removed. Much attention has been given to the African bees that travel in swarms and are particularly aggressive in their behavior. They may actually kill a victim by the overwhelming dose of venom delivered in swarm attacks.

The most serious problem with all hymenoptera stings is the development of anaphylaxis with subsequent stings following an initial sensitization. The systemic reaction that develops from this hypersensitivity may range from mild to severe anaphylaxis.

Diagnosis. The diagnosis of a hymenoptera sting is dependent on the identification of the particular insect involved. Clues to diagnosis range from development of pustules after fire ant bites to the presence of the barbed stinger and sac after a yellow jacket sting.

Treatment of sting. The treatment of hymenoptera stings consists of removal of the stinger apparatus, if still present, neutralization of ant bites with diluted ammonia or bicarbonate, and administration of antihistamine for wasp envenomation. Nonspecific means, such as application of ice at the time of the bite and calamine lotion for subsequent pruritis, may also be helpful. If cellulitis develops, oral antibiotics are appropriate. In children who have a prior history of allergic reactions, immediate transport to a medical facility is indicated.

Anaphylaxis treatment. Anyone who has already been sensitized to hymenoptera stings should be evaluated by an immunologist. Immunotherapy is very reliable in preventing a subsequent anaphylactic reaction. Preventive measures may also include avoidance of areas where one is at risk for stings. Kits containing epinephrine and antihistamine are available; however, they require special maintenance and periodic replacement. Medical alert bracelets are of the utmost importance for susceptible individuals. The treatment of an anaphylactic reaction consists of (1) airway management; (2) intravenous access with volume replacement; (3) subcutaneous epinephrine, 0.01 cc/kg (up to 0.3 cc total dose) repeated every 10 minutes; (4) aminophylline, 5 mg/kg (up to 500 mg total dose), intravenously over 15 to 20 minutes for bronchospasm; (5) corticosteroids; and (6) removal of the stinger, if still present.

SPIDER BITES

Nearly 18,000 phone calls were made to U.S. poison control centers[9] reporting probable spider bites in 1990. Of these calls, nearly one quarter were subsequently confirmed as either black widow or brown recluse spider bites. In children less than 17 years of age, there were nearly twice as many black widow spider bites (631) as brown recluse bites (364). Although the majority of spider bites are harmless, any spider with strong fangs may cause a local envenomation.

Black widow spider

The black widow spider, *Lactrodectus mactans,* is typically found under rocks, stones, boards, or logs throughout North America. The majority of bites occur in the rural areas of the South. The usual adult female (the male is harmless) is black with a red hourglass mark on the underside of the abdomen and two to three red marks along the midline.

The actual bite itself is rarely painful and may not be noticed by the child. Within the next hour however, the neurotoxic venom leads to muscle spasm, cramps, and toxicity. Characteristically, the child will develop abdominal rigidity without tenderness. Paresthesias, particularly in the soles of feet, vomiting, diaphoresis, and occasional facial (periorbital) edema and ptosis may occur. Hypertensive crises have been described, especially in cases of head and neck bites.[7] No specific laboratory data are available to aid in diagnosis.

The treatment of black widow spider bites in the majority of children is the use of simple analgesics such as aspirin. The younger the child, however, the more serious may be the envenomation and the less clear is the history. The search for a punctate bite with surrounding erythema in a child with periorbital edema, abdominal rigidity, and diaphoresis may yield clues to diagnosis.

Supportive care, of the utmost importance, includes attention to vital signs (particularly blood pressure), maintenance of airway, administration of intravenous fluids, and establishment of the correct diagnosis. Treatment of muscular rigidity may include intravenous calcium gluconate and a muscle relaxant such as Valium. Any agent that may depress respiration should be used only when airway management can be easily accomplished. In severe cases, antivenin has been used, with complications similar to those with horse serum antivenin used in snake bites. We advocate supportive care, antibiotic administration, analgesia, and Valium. If there is no relief, antivenin (Lyovac—Merck, Sharp and Dohme) may then be used (single vial diluted to 50 cc) as a slow intravenous infusion. Specific details for use of this antivenin are included in the package insert.

Brown recluse spider

The brown recluse spider, *Loxosceles reclusus,* is generally found in the South. It usually lives under stones, rocks, bark of dead trees, and in dry areas. Abandoned houses, shacks, attics, even playhouses, are common sites. The spiders bite children more often than adults, and the bite usually goes unnoticed.

The diagnosis of a brown recluse spider bite may be suspected with an accurate identification of the violin- or fiddle-shaped markings on the spider's thorax. Characteristic locations for bites include the extremities and the buttocks. Otherwise, diagnosis is suspected by the presence of a reddish blister surrounded by a blue-white halo. The involved area may subsequently be circumscribed by a spreading area of hemorrhage. The area of the bite may eventually become necrotic, with a central ulcer and surrounding cellulitis (cyanotic pustule). Systemic signs in children may include a scarlatiniform rash and fever. Treatment varies with the degree of envenomation, based on reaction in the individual child. In rare instances, a combination of DIC, fever, chills, hypotension, renal failure, and pulmonary edema develops. More commonly, treatment is centered on the actual site of the bite. Treatment is controversial, as some authors[7] recommend early excision of the bite focus and periodic secondary excisions as the induration and necrosis spread. Hollabaugh[5] recently reported an experience with 18 children who received simple curettage of the lesion; all wounds healed without necrosis. We have not used oral Dapsone[5] (which inhibits neutrophil function), and only rarely have had to perform a formal excision with subsequent skin grafting for complete healing. Tetanus prophylaxis and broad-spectrum antibiotics are also administered in addition to the usual daily wound management. Severe cases warrant hospitalization and steroid administration for treatment of systemic toxicity.

SUMMARY

Treatment for any bite requires rapid and accurate identification of the animal that inflicted the bite. Subsequent transport to an appropriate health care facility (or at least a phone call to the primary physician for assessment) is usually indicated. Local wound care, administration of antibiotics, tetanus prophylaxis, and consideration of the use of antivenin then follow. Depending on the circumstances, hospitalization (even in a pediatric intensive care unit), airway management, intravenous fluids, pharmacologic therapy, and surgical intervention may be necessary. Follow-up after the child leaves the hospital is important in treating the sequelae of the bite or of the therapy. Most childhood bites require little more than supportive care and time, but it is the responsibility of children's physicians to be prepared to care for the most serious of envenomations.

REFERENCES

1. Baker MD, Moore SE: Human bites in children, *AJDC* 141:1285-1290, 1987.
2. Brenner DJ, Hollis DG, Moss CW et al: Proposal of *Afipia* gen. nov. with *Afipia felis* sp. nov. (formerly the cat scratch bacillus), *Afipia clevelandensis* sp. nov. (formerly the Cleveland Clinic Foundation strain), *Afipia broomeae* sp. nov. and three unnamed gen species, *J Clin Micro* 29:2450-2460, 1991.
3. Burch JM, Agarwal R, Mattox KL: The treatment of crotalid envenomation without antivenin, *J Trauma* 28:35-43, 1988.
4. Collipp PJ: Cat-scratch disease therapy, *AJDC* 143:1261, 1989.
5. Hollabaugh RS, Fernandes ET: Management of the brown recluse spider bite, *J Pediatr Surg* 24:126-127, 1989.
6. Holley HP: Successful treatment of cat-scratch disease with ciprofloxacin, *JAMA* 265:1563-1565, 1991.
7. Johnson LA: Toxic bites and stings. In Schwartz GR et al, editors: *Principles and practice of emergency medicine*, vol 2, Philadelphia, 1986, WB Saunders, pp 1626-1638.
8. King LE, Rees RS: Dapsone treatment of a brown recluse spider bite, *JAMA* 250:648, 1983.
9. Litovitz TL, Bailey KM, Schmitz BF et al: 1990 annual report of the American Association of Poison Control Center National Data Collection System, *Am J Emerg Med* 9:461-509, 1991.
10. Marcy SM: Infections due to dog and cat bites, *Pediatr Inf Dis* 1:351-356, 1982.
11. Sacks JJ, Sattin RW, Bonzo SE: Dog bite-related fatalities from 1979 through 1988, *JAMA* 262:1489-1492, 1989.
12. Stucker J, Shaw GY, Boyd S et al: Management of animal and human bites on the head and neck, *Arch Otolaryngol Head Neck Surg* 116:789-793, 1990.
13. Wagner CW, Golladay ES, Crotalid envenomation in children: selective conservative management, *J Pediatr Surg* 24:128-131, 1989.
14. Watt C, Gennaro J: Pit viper bites in south Georgia and north Florida, *Tr South Surg Assoc* 77:378-386, 1966.
15. White RR, Weber RA: Poisonous snakebite in central Texas, *Ann Surg* 213:466-472, 1991.

PART FIFTEEN

Procedures

58 Procedures*

Martin R. Eichelberger

TUBE THORACOSTOMY

Insertion of a chest drain is indicated when there is a tension pneumothorax, hemothorax, or hydrothorax. In the presence of a hemothorax it is wise to establish an intravenous infusion before inserting the tube and evacuating large amounts of blood, as this can result in rapid decompensation of the cardiovascular system. If there is rapid decompression before venous access is established, it is advisable to clamp the tube until this is achieved. Decompression of the third space without volume resuscitation can result in irreversible shock and death.

Procedure

The skin is cleaned in the midaxillary line with an antiseptic solution such as Betadine (povidone-iodine) (Fig. 58-1, *A*). Local anesthesia is obtained by injecting 1% lignocaine (lidocaine) with adrenaline around the chosen rib and into the adjacent parietal pleura. The thoracostomy tube is usually inserted in the midaxillary line at the level of the nipple (fourth or fifth intercostal space). A skin incision is made two intercostal spaces below the intended thoracostomy site (Fig. 58-1, *B*). Blunt dissection with a curved hemostat is used to expose the muscle and fascia. The hemostat is then slid along the muscle layer to create a subcutaneous tunnel to the thoracostomy site. The tip of the hemostat is then turned over the superior border of the rib so that it penetrates the thorax. Opening the jaws of the hemostat enlarges the tunnel as the hemostat is withdrawn.

The thoracostomy tube is then grasped with a large hemostat and inserted into the chest (Fig. 58-1, *C*). Correct placement of the tube is confirmed by the appearance of condensation within the tube and by fluctuation in the water column when the tube is connected to an underwater sealed drain. It is also worth palpating the chest to ensure that the tube is indeed passing into the pleural cavity.

The thoracostomy tube is secured to the skin with heavy nylon sutures, dressed with a sterile ointment, and its base wrapped with petroleum gauze. It is then sprayed with a Holister spray or tincture of Benzoin and anchored with tape. A chest x-ray to confirm correct placement of the tube is obtained routinely.

Once the thoracostomy tube is in position (Fig. 58-1, *D*), the rate of efflux of blood from the chest is assessed. A rate of 1 to 2 ml/kg per hour suggests major vascular injury and is an indication for thoracotomy to obtain hemostasis.

VENOUS ACCESS

Venous access is essential for resuscitation. The upper extremity is preferred and two attempts can be made to gain access percutaneously. If these fail, distal saphenous vein cutdown should be attempted, followed by femoral vein cutdown if that is also unsuccessful. The saphenous vein is found one fingerbreadth below and lateral to the pubic tubercle; alternatively, the femoral artery can be palpated and the incision extended medially. Subclavian vein catheterization is used only as a last resort because of the high risk of subclavian artery laceration or hydrothorax from improper placement of the catheter.

Greater saphenous vein: cutdown technique

The great saphenous vein is constant in its location just anterior to the medial malleolus; it is the only structure of importance in this area. Cutdown is facilitated by the fact that the vein lies on a tough periosteum and has enough elasticity to permit traction through a small incision without the danger of avulsion.

Procedure. The foot is held in equinovarus (Fig. 58-2, *A*). The medial malleolus is palpated and the site of incision noted 1 cm anterior and 1 cm superior to the malleolus. The area is cleaned with an antiseptic solution and draped with sterile towels. The line of incision is marked by scratching the skin with a hypodermic needle before infiltrating the skin and subcutaneous tissue with 0.5 to

*This chapter has been modified and printed with permission from Eichelberger MR: Essential techniques in the resuscitation of paediatric trauma patients. I. In Dudley H, Carter D, Russell RCG, editors: *Rob and Smith operative surgery: trauma surgery,* ed. 4, Stoneham, Mass, 1989, Butterworth.

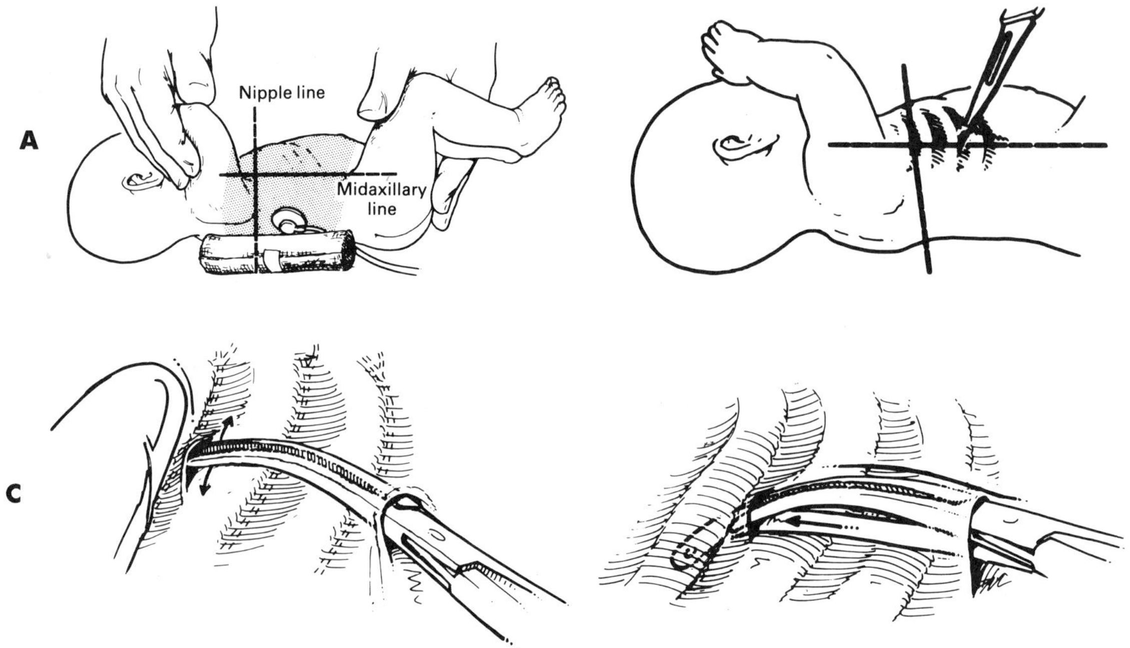

Figure 58–1 Procedure for tube thoracostomy. (From Eichelberger MR: Essential techniques in the resuscitation of paediatric trauma patients. I. In Dudley H, Carter D, Russell RCG, editors: *Rob and Smith operative surgery: trauma surgery*, ed 4, Stoneham, Mass, 1989, Butterworth.)

1.0 ml of lignocaine. A 1 cm transverse incision is then made through the skin, down to the superficial subcutaneous fat, avoiding transection of the superficial vein. A curved hemostat is introduced into the incision with its tip down.

Its blades are then spread parallel to the vein to dissect the tissues down to the periosteum until adequate visualization of the vein is achieved (Fig. 58-2, *B*).

The curved hemostat is then reintroduced as before and passed down to the periosteum (Fig. 58-2, *C*). Using a "scooping" motion, the tip of the hemostat is guided behind the vein, which is drawn into the incision.

The hemostat is opened carefully to spread the subcutaneous tissue, leaving the vein surface clean (Fig. 58-2, *D*). A 5-0 nylon suture is placed loosely around the vein and held in a hemostat to allow distal control of the vessel (Fig. 58-2, *E*). The ligature is not tied. The ligature and clamp are held in the left hand so that the ligature passes over the extended index finger, which is used to retract the vein upward and caudad (Fig. 58-2, *F*). A cannula/stylet is introduced into the vein at a 45° angle with its bevel pointing downwards. Once the vein has been entered, the cannula is angled to pass parallel to the vein. The cannula is advanced into the vein while withdrawing the inner needle stylet. A small volume of saline is infused to confirm that it lies within the lumen. The traction suture is now removed and the skin incision closed with one or two 5-0 nylon sutures. The cannula is attached to the infusion tubing and intravenous infusion is commenced.

Complications. Inadvertent infusion of local anesthetic into the artery or vein, damage to the vein as a result of too deep an initial incision, and infiltration of intravenous fluid into the body cavity are the commonest complications. The latter is usually the result of using too long a catheter. Indeed, such catheters should be avoided in neonates. When infusing an irritating or hypertonic solution, a central venous catheter should be used if at all possible.

ARTERIAL CANNULATION

Arterial cannulation is particularly useful for monitoring children with hypovolemic shock and associated head injury. Percutaneous cannulation of the radial artery is useful in children. Nevertheless, a cutdown technique is better for the infant because trauma to the artery precipitates vasospasm which makes cannulation of the small vessel difficult.

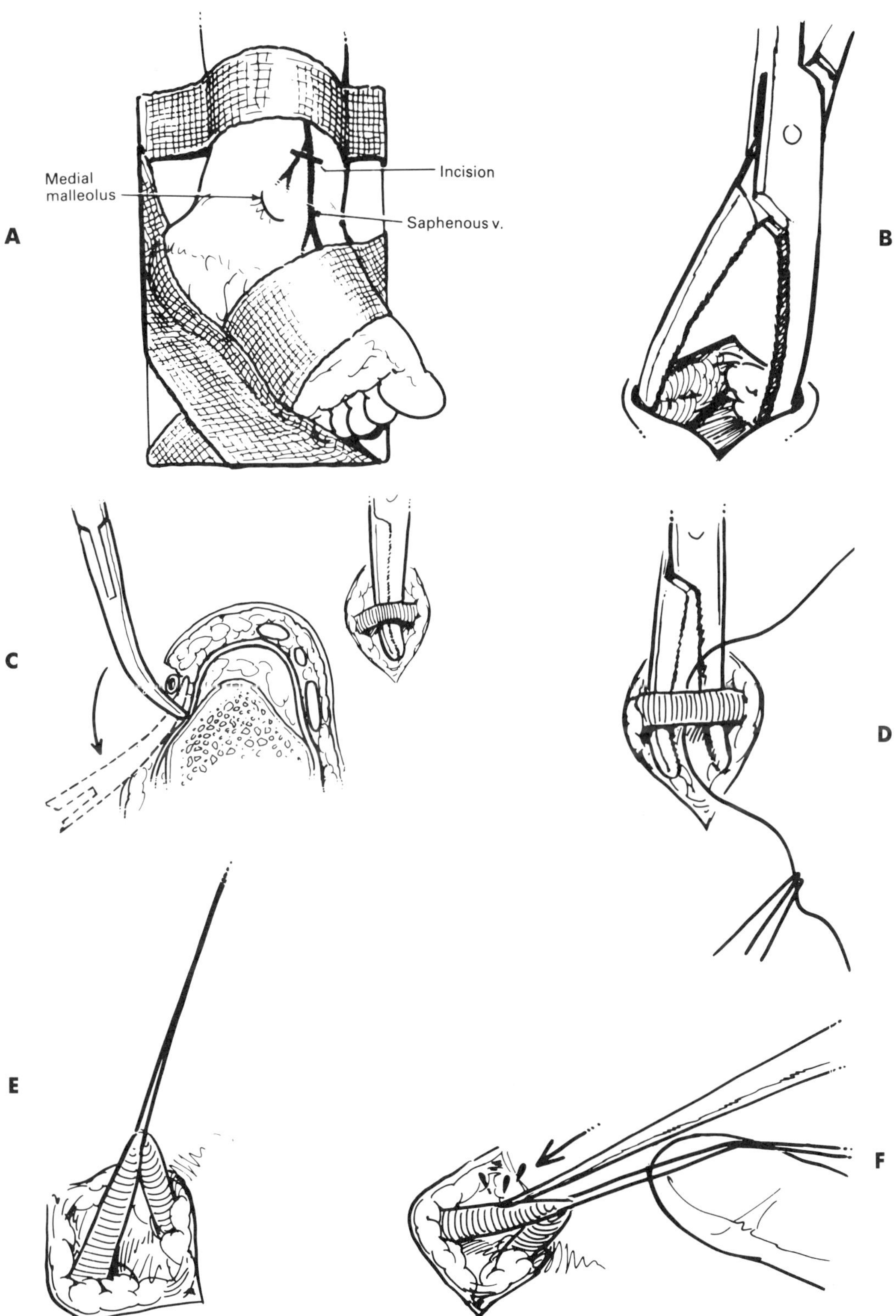

Figure 58–2 Procedure for cutdown of greater saphenous vein. (From Eichelberger MR: Essential techniques in the resuscitation of paediatric trauma patients. I. In Dudley H, Carter D, Russell RCG, editors: *Rob and Smith operative surgery: trauma surgery*, ed 4, Stoneham, Mass, 1989, Butterworth.)

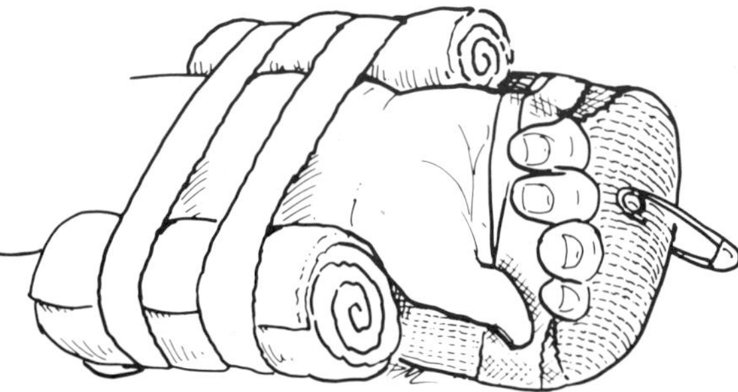

Figure 58–3 Procedure for percutaneous cannulation of the radial artery. (From Eichelberger MR: Essential techniques in the resuscitation of paediatric trauma patients. I. In Dudley H, Carter D, Russell RCG, editors: *Rob and Smith operative surgery: trauma surgery*, ed 4, Stoneham, Mass, 1989, Butterworth.)

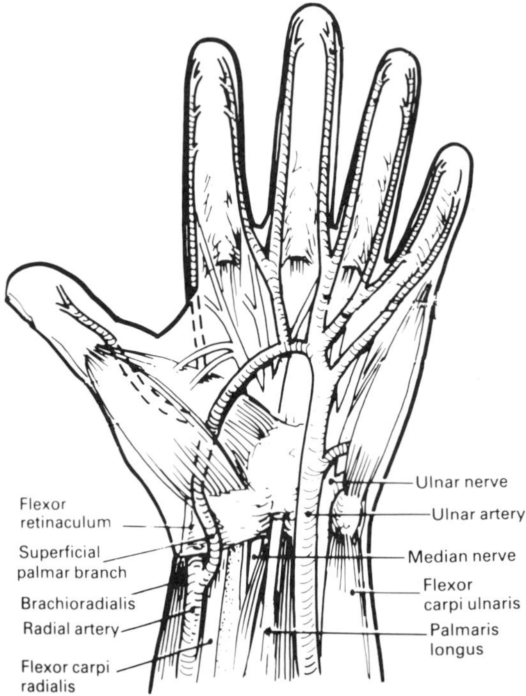

Figure 58–4 Diagram of the anatomy of the wrist. (From Eichelberger MR: Essential techniques in the resuscitation of paediatric trauma patients. I. In Dudley H, Carter D, Russell RCG, editors: *Rob and Smith operative surgery: trauma surgery*, ed 4, Stoneham, Mass, 1989, Butterworth.)

Cannulation of the radial artery

Percutaneous cannulation: procedure. Before commencing the procedure it is essential to assess the adequacy of ulnar collateral circulation by performing an Allen's test. The infant's forearm and hand are restrained with the wrist held in extension (Fig. 58-3).

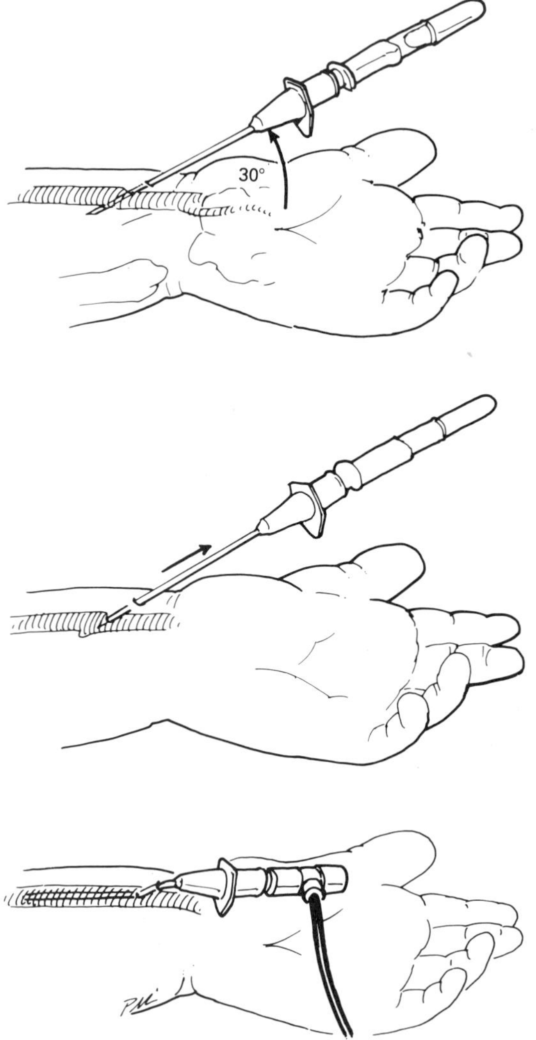

Figure 58–5 Alternative method of percutaneous cannulation of the radial artery. (From Eichelberger MR: Essential techniques in the resuscitation of paediatric trauma patients. I. In Dudley H, Carter D, Russell RCG, editors: *Rob and Smith operative surgery: trauma surgery*, ed 4, Stoneham, Mass, 1989, Butterworth.)

The artery is identified by palpation at the proximal wrist crease just lateral to the flexor carpi radialis (Fig. 58-4). Doppler ultrasound may help to identify the small vessel. Careful preparation of the skin and sterile technique are important if long-term complications from sepsis are to be avoided. A small puncture wound is made over the radial artery just distal to the proximal skin crease to ease passage of the cannula through the skin.

Using the needle with the bevel pointing downwards, the artery is punctured directly at an angle of 30 degrees. Blood should appear in the cannula before it is advanced into the artery.

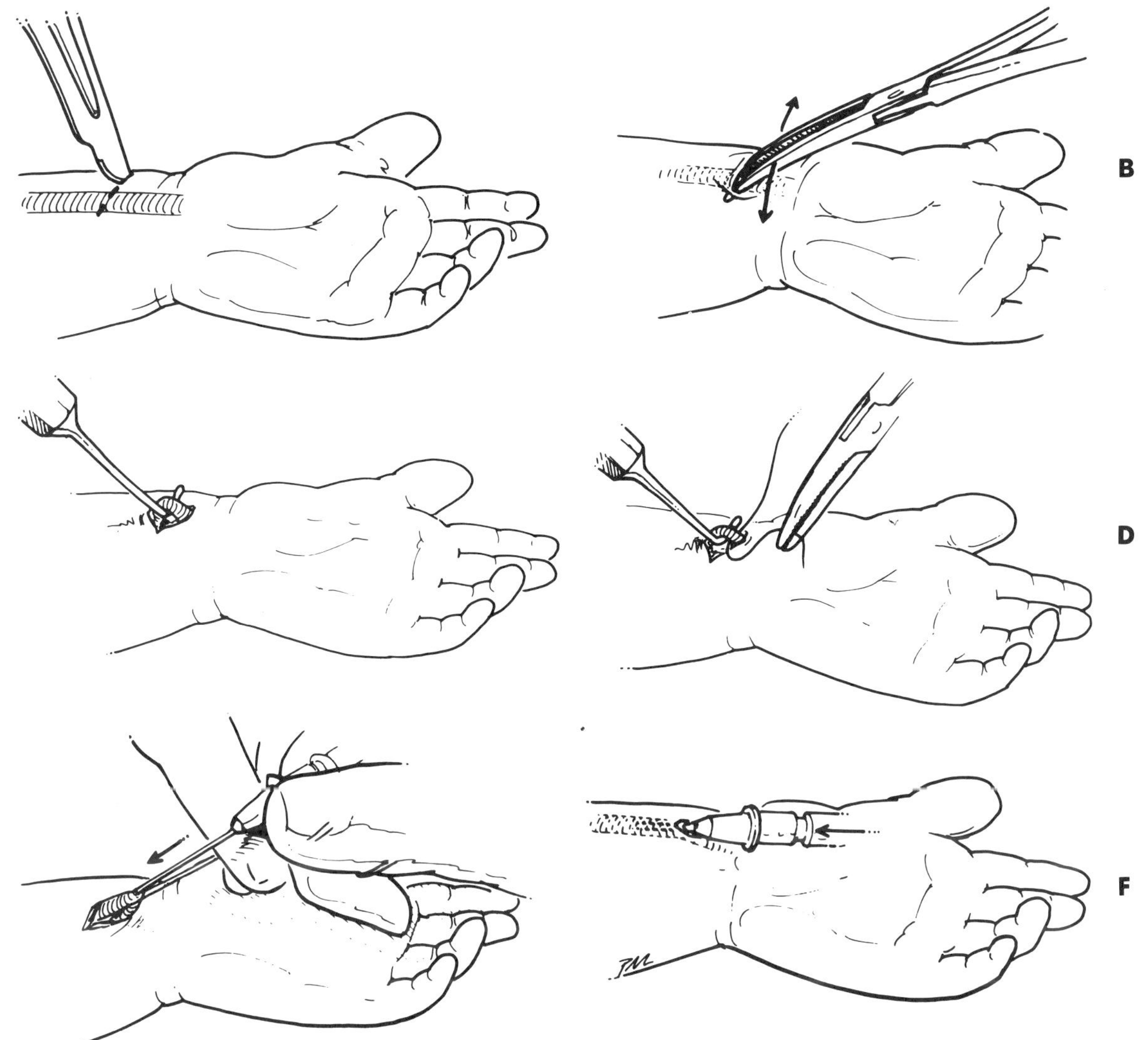

Figure 58–6 Procedure for cutdown cannulation of the radial artery. (From Eichelberger MR: Essential techniques in the resuscitation of paediatric trauma patients. I. In Dudley H, Carter D, Russell RCG, editors: *Rob and Smith operative surgery: trauma surgery*, ed 4, Stoneham, Mass, 1989, Butterworth.)

An alternative method is to pass the needle and cannula through the artery at a 30- to 40-degree angle to the skin (Fig. 58-5). The stylet is then removed and the cannula slowly withdrawn until arterial flow is established. The cannula is advanced into the artery once there is pulsatile flow through the catheter. Inability to insert the cannula into the lumen usually indicates failure to puncture the artery centrally; this often results in laceration of the artery with formation of a hematoma. The cannula is sutured to the skin with a 5-0 nylon suture and attached firmly to a T-connector for infusion with heparinized saline solution (1 ml/h). To reduce the risk of accidental decannulation and

facilitate sampling, a three-way stopcock may be inserted distal to the T-connector.

Cutdown cannulation: procedure. The skin and wrist are prepared as described for percutaneous insertion of the cannula. The site of incision is infiltrated with 0.5 to 1.0 ml of 1% lignocaine at the point of maximal pulsation just proximal to the distal wrist crease. A 0.5-cm transverse skin incision is made (Fig. 58-6, *A*) and deepened into the subcutaneous tissue by blunt longitudinal dissection with a curved mosquito hemostat (Fig. 58-6, *B*). The hemostat is then used to dissect the artery free, proceeding very gently to avoid arteriospasm. The artery is then lifted out of the wound

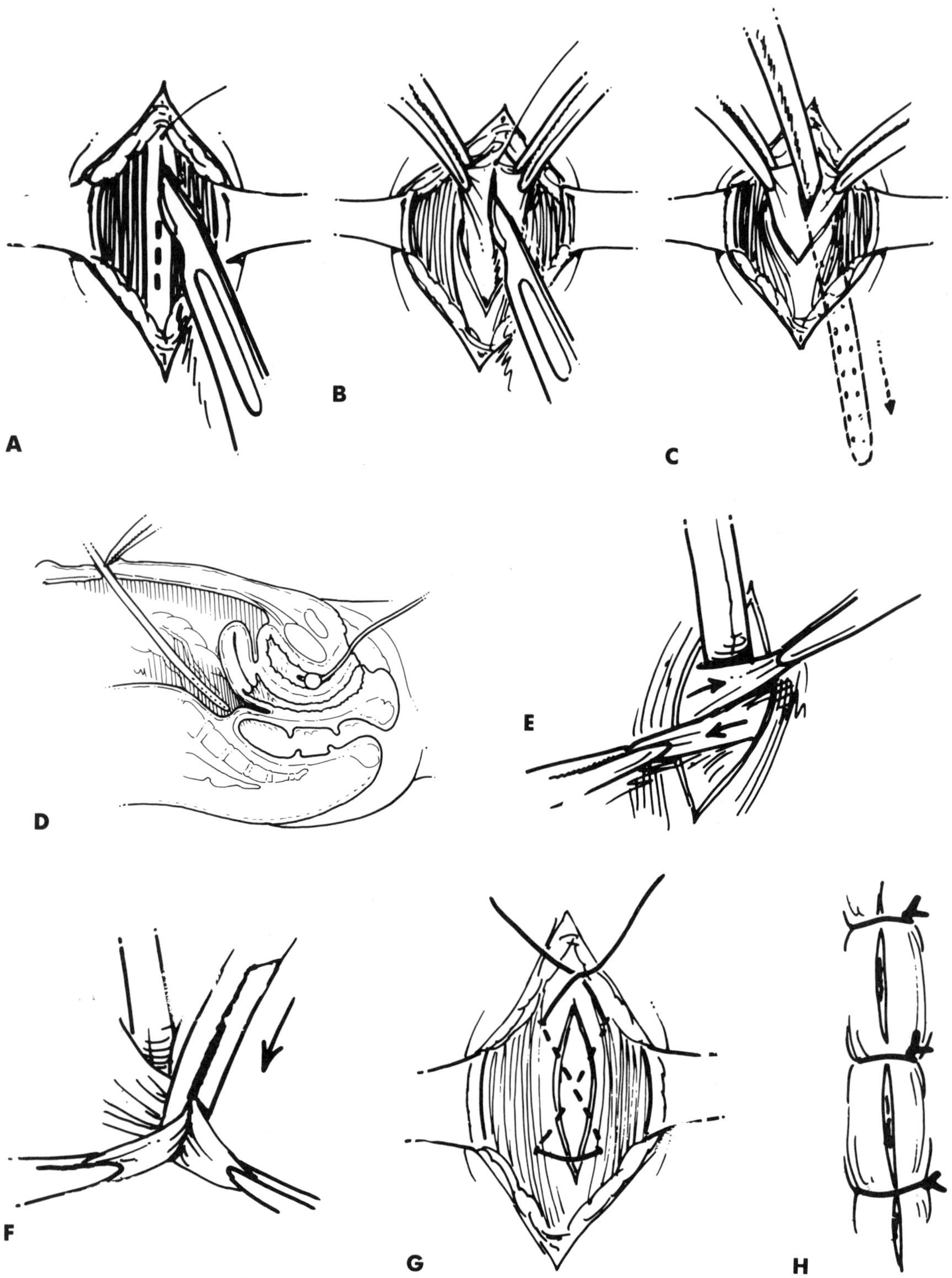

Figure 58–7 Procedure for peritoneal lavage. (From Eichelberger MR: Essential techniques in the resuscitation of paediatric trauma patients. I. In Dudley H, Carter D, Russell RCG, editors: *Rob and Smith operative surgery: trauma surgery*, ed 4, Stoneham, Mass, 1989, Butterworth.)

with a hemostat or nerve hook (Fig. 58-6, *C*) and a ligature (5-0 nylon) is looped around it for traction (Fig. 58-6, *D*). This ligature should not be tied. The cannula stylet is then advanced into the artery with the bevel pointing downward until the cannula is clearly within the vessel lumen (Fig. 58-6, *E*). The stylet is then removed and the cannula advanced to the hub (Fig. 58-6, *F*). Finally, the ligature is removed and the catheter fixed with a 5-0 nylon suture. The incision does not usually require a suture for closure.

PERITONEAL LAVAGE

Abdominal peritoneal lavage is rarely required in children and has been largely superseded by computed axial tomography (CT), which has a high resolution and is extremely reliable. Blood in the abdomen of a child does not demand exploratory laparotomy. The commonest cause of hemoperitoneum is injury to the liver, spleen, or mesentery of the small bowel. Pneumoperitoneum is also easily diagnosed by CT scanning. Peritoneal lavage is useful in children requiring immediate operative intervention for neurosurgical or orthopedic injuries. If the child is comatose and hypotensive, it is useful to perform peritoneal lavage in the operating room at the same time as the neurosurgical or orthopedic procedure. A positive tap should lead the surgeon to exploratory laparotomy in this rare instance.

Procedure

Minilaparotomy is preferred for abdominal peritoneal lavage since complications are rare and the procedure can be safely performed under direct vision. A urinary catheter is inserted to decompress the bladder, and a nasogastric tube passed into the stomach. A 3 to 4 cm midline vertical incision is made below the umbilicus. The skin is infiltrated with 1% lignocaine in adrenaline to minimize subcutaneous bleeding. A vertical incision along the linea alba permits proper access to the fascia (Fig. 58-7, *A*). A small peritoneal incision is then made between curved hemostats to allow access to the peritoneum (Fig. 58-7, *B*). A pediatric peritoneal catheter without a trocar is inserted into the pelvis and directed towards the left lower quadrant (Fig. 58-7, *C*).

The lavage catheter should lie in the depth of pelvis where most of the irrigant will collect (Fig. 58-7, *D*).

The hemostats holding the peritoneum are then crossed over to form a watertight seal (Fig. 58-7, *E*). A curved hemostat is used to approximate the peritoneum at the peritoneal lavage catheter (Fig. 58-7, *F*). Aspiration of 10 ml of blood is considered a positive tap. However, if less than this amount of blood is obtained, Ringer's lactate is infused at a rate of 15 ml/kg of body weight and a colorimetric analysis performed. On completion of the test, the catheter is removed and a single figure eight suture is used to close the fascia and peritoneum in one layer (Fig. 58-7, *G*). The skin closure is covered with a small dressing (Fig. 58-7, *H*).

PART SIXTEEN

Outcome Analysis

William J. Sacco, Wayne S. Copes and *Catherine S. Gotschall*

Physicians want to feel confident that they are providing the best possible care to children. But how can they be sure that they are? Scientific assessment of the care provided to injured children is possible only if accurate and reliable means of measuring both injury severity and resulting disability exist and are used. To this end, numerous scoring systems have been developed. These systems typically employ measures of physiologic or anatomic derangement to quantify the severity of injury. This chapter describes the construction, purposes, and practical application of several trauma scoring systems.

TYPES OF SEVERITY SCORES

Development of valid and useful methods for triage, quality assurance, comparison of trauma patient outcomes, and collection of basic epidemiologic trauma data are major trauma system needs. The most commonly used scores employ measures of the degree of a person's physiologic derangement, anatomic damage, or a combination of these two factors.

Physiologic scores

The body responds to injury with physiologic changes. Uncontrolled bleeding can cause hypotension, tachycardia, and shock; damage to the central nervous system can depress consciousness. These departures from normal physiology are reflected by changes in a child's vital signs. Consequently, many trauma scoring systems are based on assessments of blood pressure, pulse, respiratory rate, and level of consciousness. Because these scores have been shown to correlate strongly with mortality, they are used for patient triage, for assessing response to therapy, and for predicting patient outcome. Many such scores have been developed; those in greatest use or of historic importance are outlined in this chapter.

Glasgow Coma Scale. The Glasgow Coma Scale[44] (GCS) is a widely used assessment of level of consciousness. It is based on the sum of coded values for three behavioral responses: eye opening, best verbal response, and best motor response. Scores range from 3 to 15, with higher scores in-

dicating a higher level of consciousness (see Table 5-3 on p 47). The GCS is simple to use and has been correlated with mortality. The GCS is a component of the Trauma Score and the Revised Trauma Score, which are discussed later in this chapter.

Several coma scales have been proposed to compensate for perceived deficiencies in the GCS when used to assess preverbal children. Among the more widely used are the Pediatric Coma Scale,[38] the Children's Coma Scale,[37] and the Jacobi Scale.[23] Preliminary findings indicate differences in interobserver variability among the various coma scales currently used in pediatric practice.[47]

Triage index. The Triage Index[14] was developed using statistical techniques to select from 16 routinely collected biochemical and physiologic variables, those that best predicted mortality. Evaluation of the index on data from patients in both critical and general care environments showed that the index was easy to use, accurate in ranking patients according to the probability of death, and had high interrater and intrarater reliability. Although this score is no longer widely used, it is the predecessor of the Trauma Score.

Trauma score. The Trauma Score[12] (TS), a modification of the Triage Index, is based on the GCS and on assessments of cardiovascular status (capillary return and systolic blood pressure) and respiratory status (respiratory rate and respiratory expansion). Coded values assigned to the variables are added to obtain the TS, which ranges from 1 (worst prognosis) to 16 (best prognosis) (see Table 59-1). The TS was found to be a slightly poorer predictor of survival than the Triage Index[7,8] but more acceptable to the trauma community because of the addition of systolic blood pressure and respiratory rate.

Although originally developed for adults, the TS has been successfully applied to children. It has been widely used to characterize the physiologic status of injured children and adults. The TS has high interrater reliability[35] and is a good indicator of the need for pediatric triage.[20] In addition, the TS is a valuable tool for predicting survival among injured children.[18,21]

Table 59–1 Trauma Score

Attribute	Coded value
Respiratory rate	
10–24	4
25–35	3
>35	2
0–9	1
Respiratory effort	
Normal	1
Shallow, retractive	0
Systolic blood pressure	
>90	4
70–89	3
50–69	2
<50	1
Capillary refill	
Normal	2
Delayed	1
Absent	0
Glasgow Coma Scale	
14–15	5
11–13	4
8–10	3
5–7	2
3–4	1
Total Trauma Score:	__________

From Champion HR, Sacco WJ, Carnazzo AJ, et al: Trauma score, *Crit Care Med* 9:672, 1981.

Table 59–2 Revised Trauma Score

Attribute	Coded value
Respiratory rate	
10–29	4
>29	3
6–9	2
1–5	1
0	0
Systolic blood pressure	
>89	4
76–89	3
50–75	2
1–49	1
0	0
Glasgow Coma Scale	
13–15	4
9–12	3
6–8	2
4–5	1
3	0
Unweighted Revised Trauma Score:	__________

CRAMS scale. The Circulation, Respiration, Abdomen, Motor, Speech (CRAMS) Scale[24] resulted from an attempt to simplify the TS for field triage use. The CRAMS Scale eliminated assessments of eye opening and respiratory effort and added an assessment of thoracoabdominal trauma. Although neither interrater nor intrarater reliability for the abdominal and thoracic field assessments has been documented, the scale has been successfully applied in many areas.

Revised trauma score. Despite the high interrater reliability of the Trauma Score in prehospital and military settings, researchers have tried to simplify the score without sacrificing its accuracy or correlation with outcome.[31,34] Furthermore, field use of the TS revealed that capillary refill and respiratory expansion were difficult to assess at night and that "retractive" respiratory expansion is always difficult to observe. It was additionally noted that the TS underestimates the severity of injury for some patients with head injuries. For these reasons, the TS was revised.

The Revised Trauma Score[13] (RTS) is based on the Glasgow Coma Scale, systolic blood pressure, and respiratory rate. Variables are assigned coded values from 4 (normal) to 0 (see Table 59-2). For in-hospital outcome evaluation, coded values of the three variables are weighted and summed to yield the RTS, which takes values from 0 to 7.84. Higher values are associated with better prognoses. The RTS provides both more accurate predictions of outcome for patients with serious head injury and more reliable[27] outcome predictions for all patients.

The value of the RTS for triage has been demonstrated for both pediatric and adult populations. A lower than normal coded value for any RTS variable suggests the need for trauma center care.[10] For infants and toddlers, however, triage is not indicated if the sole RTS deduction is for increased respiratory rate.[20] The efficacy of the RTS for outcome evaluations of children has also been demonstrated.[18]

Anatomic scores

Several severity indices are based on assessments of a patient's anatomic injuries. These indices are designed to rate and compare injury severity by characterizing the anatomic damage associated with a patient's individual or collective injuries.

Abbreviated injury scale. The Abbreviated Injury Scale (AIS)[1] is a list of several hundred injuries, to each of which is assigned both a 5- or 6-digit descriptive code and a severity score from 1 (minor injuries) to 6 (nearly always fatal). The scale has undergone several revisions since its inception in 1969. The earliest versions coded only injuries resulting from blunt trauma; the 1985 revision (AIS-85) provided for the first time severity scores for penetrating injuries.

Table 59–3 Sample ISS for child with head, abdominal, and chest injuries

Body region	Injury	AIS-90 severity score
Head	Parietal skull fracture	3
	Subarachnoid hematoma	4
	Basal skull fracture	3
Abdomen	Ruptured spleen	2
Chest	Fractured ribs (3)	2
	Pulmonary contusion	3

The ISS is:

$$4^2 + 2^2 + 3^2 = 16 + 4 + 9 = 29$$

In the latest version, AIS-90, injuries are specified by naming anatomic structure, location (side, lobe), and internal measurements (some of which are age-dependent) of diameter, thickness, midline shift, and blood loss. There are moderate differences between AIS-85 and AIS-90 in terminology. Injury severity values for spinal, extremity, and external injuries are nearly unchanged in AIS-90. There are significant differences for head, thoracic, and abdominal injuries. Special consideration is given to the relatively greater severity to young children of wounds of a given size (e.g., 10 ml subdural hematoma) than to adults.

Injury severity score. The Injury Severity Score (ISS)[2,3] was devised to assess multiple injuries. The ISS ranges from 1 to 75, with higher scores indicating more severe injury. Any patient with an AIS 6 injury is assigned the maximum ISS value of 75. Otherwise, the ISS is the sum of squares of the highest AIS values for injuries to three different body regions (head and neck, face, thorax, abdomen and pelvic contents, extremities, and external). For example, the ISS for a child with multiple head injuries, a ruptured spleen, three fractured ribs, and a pulmonary contusion would be computed as shown in Table 59-3.

The ISS correlates with mortality both in children and in adults,[5,41] but has documented limitations[16]—it considers only the highest AIS value from any body region, and it considers injuries with equal AIS values to be of equal severity, regardless of body region. As a result, some ISS values can represent children with heterogeneous injury combinations who have substantially different survival prognoses. For example, if the child whose injuries are listed in Table 59-3 had sustained a fractured femur (AIS severity 3) instead of the two chest injuries, the ISS would not change. Despite these limitations, the ISS remains the most widely used summary measure of anatomic injury severity.

PODS. The Probability of Death Score (PODS)[42] is a logistic function that models probability of death based on the two greatest AIS values from 19 injury categories. These categories were refined from the six body regions used in AIS coding. The PODS has been shown to have a higher predictive value than the ISS for several sets of trauma patients.

Anatomic profile. The development of the Anatomic Profile (AP)[17] was motivated by increased demands for greater precision in quantifying injury severity and by the inherent limitations of the ISS. The AP classifies each injury into one of four categories, labeled *A* through *D*. The first three categories include serious injuries (injuries with AIS values of 3 or greater): *A*, injuries to the head-brain and spinal cord; *B*, injuries to the thorax and front of the neck; and *C*, all remaining serious injuries. Category *D* is a summary grouping of all nonserious injuries. These groupings were motivated by the observations of experienced trauma surgeons and research findings regarding the primacy of head injury and chest injury to mortality.[22]

An AP component value is the square root of the sum of squares of the AIS values for all injuries in a given category. For example, the *A* component for a patient with two AIS-5 injuries and one AIS-3 injury to the head is expressed as $A = \sqrt{(5^2 + 5^2 + 3^2)} = 7.68$. This method attributes a diminishing contribution to injuries other than the most severe in a body area. Component values account for multiple injuries and distinguish between body regions injured; for example, $B = 0$ if no serious thoracic injuries were sustained.

It is believed that the AP is a more precise description of anatomic injury, which will improve quality studies and effectively describe patient sets.

Other scores and systems

Trauma index. The Trauma Index[33] was an early attempt to assess injury severity using a combination of anatomic and physiologic data. The index is a numerical rating system based on the body region injured, injury type, and cardiovascular, central nervous system, and respiratory status. It is easy to use and predicts the need for hospitalization after injury. A field test of prehospital providers found consistent correlations between estimates of injury severity using a modified Trauma Index and actual hospitalization rates; however, the test also found that the index was less predictive of morbidity and mortality.[36]

Pediatric trauma score. The perceived need for an injury severity score designed expressly for children to led the development of the Pediatric Trauma

Table 59–4 Pediatric Trauma Score

Component	Category		
	+2	**+1**	**−1**
Size	>20 kg (40#)	10–20 kg	<10 kg
Airway	Normal	Maintainable	Unmaintainable
Systolic BP	>90 mm Hg	50–90 mm Hg	<50 mm Hg
CNS	Awake	Obtunded/LOC	Coma/decerebrate
Skeletal	None	Closed fracture	Open/multiple fractures
Cutaneous	None	Minor	Major/penetrating
			Sum _______

From Tepas JJ III, Ramenofsky ML, Mollitt DL et al: The pediatric trauma score as a predictor of injury severity: an objective assessment, *J Trauma* 28, 1988. © 1988 by Williams & Wilkins.

Score (PTS).[45] The PTS combines physiologic and anatomic measures to assess the severity of childhood injury (see Table 59-4). One of three severity assignments is made for each of the six component variables. The associated point values are summed to yield the PTS, the values of which range from −6 to 12.

It has been recommended that injured children with PTS ≤ 8 be considered for transfer to a Level I pediatric trauma unit.[20,32] Studies comparing the triage effectiveness of the PTS and the RTS concluded that the PTS offered no statistical advantage over the TS or the RTS.[20,32] In addition, it has been shown that the RTS can be applied to pediatric populations in evaluations of patient outcome.[18] Thus, although the PTS does correlate with injury severity as measured by the ISS and can accurately identify children needing triage to a trauma center, it offers no apparent advantage over either the TS or RTS.

TRISS methodology. TRISS methodology[4,10] comprises a series of techniques that can be used to assess the severity of a child's injury (as measured by probability of survival), to identify patients with unexpected survival or death outcomes, and to perform a severity controlled comparison of survival in a group of children with national norms identified in the Major Trauma Outcome Study (MTOS). TRISS gets its name from statistical techniques combining the *TR*auma Score and *I*njury *S*everity *S*core. The cornerstone of TRISS methodology is the estimation of children's survival probabilities. The probability of survival for an injured child is computed using the logistic model:

$$P_s = 1/(1+e^{-b}),$$
where:

P_s = probability of survival
e = 2.7183 (base of Napierian logarithms);

and:

$$b = b_0 + b_1 (RTS) + b_2 (ISS),*$$
where:

$b_0 = -1.2470$
$b_1p = 0.9544$
$b_2 = -0.0768$

RTS = Revised Trauma Score (on emergency department admission)
ISS = Injury Severity Score (as derived from final anatomic diagnoses)

By using estimated survival probabilities for all admitted children, an institution can compare its trauma outcomes to national norms derived from the MTOS.

PRE charts identify unexpected survivals and deaths.[10] These graphs display physiologic and anatomical severity information for each child and allow for the comparison of outcomes to national norms. Figure 59-1 illustrates a PRE chart, with an inverted RTS scale along the ordinate and the ISS along the abscissa; values for each child are plotted using separate symbols for survivals and deaths. The sloping line, identified as P_s50 isobar, represents combinations of RTS and ISS associated with a 0.50 probability of survival, based on MTOS data.

Survivors above the P_s50 isobar and deaths below this line represent statistically unexpected outcomes. Such survivors may represent therapeutic triumphs for the health care system. Unexpected deaths may reflect trauma system failures, misrepresentations by TRISS, or unavoidable compli-

---

*The b_is are weights derived by applying the Walker-Duncan regression algorithm to MTOS data. Outcomes for pediatric patients (age < 15 years) are evaluated using the adult blunt injury norms for 15- to 54-year-olds.

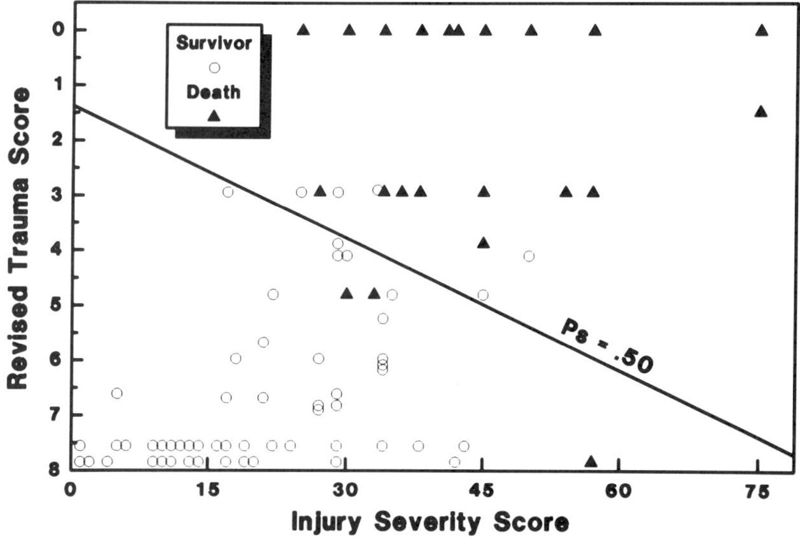

Figure 59–1 PRE chart.

cations. The cases of children with unexpected outcomes should be subjected to critical peer review.

The relationship between injury severity and survival also can be used to compare the performance of a hospital against a standard or norm. The z statistic is used to compare the actual number of survivors in an institution (A) with the number expected, based on current MTOS norms (E). The z value is the significance of differences between the actual (A) number of survivors among an institution's patients and the number expected (E) from outcome norms. z is defined as

$$z = \frac{(A - E)}{S},$$

where $E = \Sigma P_i$, and S is a scale factor that accounts for statistical variation $(S = \sqrt{\Sigma P_i(1 - P_i)})$. P_i is the TRISS survival probability for the ith patient. If z exceeds 1.96 (is less than $-$ 1.96), there are statistically significantly more (fewer) survivors than expected from MTOS–TRISS norms.

W is computed only when z is statistically significant. W measures the clinical significance of statistically significant differences between the actual (A) and expected (E) numbers of survivors in a patient group. The ability to detect such differences, called statistical power, increases with sample size.[43] Thus, for large samples, significant z values may indicate slight, but statistically significant, differences between A and E. W is defined as

$$W = \frac{(A - E)}{(N / 100)}$$

where A and E are as defined in z, and N is the number of children analyzed. A positive (negative) W is the number of survivors more (less) than would be expected per 100 children treated. W values based on small patient samples should be considered preliminary.

Computations of z and W are biased by the exclusion of patients with missing TRISS data. Patient exclusions are not uncommon, as some patients are intubated or under the influence of paralytic agents at emergency department admission, precluding assessments of respiratory and neurologic status needed for TRISS. Nonetheless, the range of possible survival probabilities (P_s) for such patients can be determined, enhancing both quality assessments and outcome evaluations. The highest possible value of P_s results when all missing values are assumed "normal." The lowest possible value of P_s results when the most pessimistic values are attributed to missing variables. "Truly" unexpected deaths and survivals are defined as children whose range of possible P_s values excludes 0.50.[26] "Possibly" unexpected survivors and nonsurvivors are patients whose range of P_s values includes 0.50.

An institution should include consecutive patients in the computation of z and W to avoid biased results. The degree of bias depends on injuries to excluded patients. The exclusion of deaths associated with extremely severe injuries and of survivors with minor severities ordinarily has little effect on z and W, but the exclusion of other patients can bias z and W substantially.

Because TRISS norms are based on adult data, the applicability of TRISS methodology to pediatric trauma has been questioned. Researchers using the adult, blunt trauma coefficients to estimate survival

Table 59–5 ASCOT "set-aside" data summary

	Blunt		Penetrating	
Set-aside	No.	% Survivors	No.	% Survivors
1. MAIS = 6, RTS = 0	48	0	22	0
2. MAIS < 6, RTS = 0	217	1.4	192	2.6
3. MAIS = 6, RTS > 0	35	22.9	9	22.2
4. MAIS = 1 or 2, RTS > 0	4262	99.8	1345	90.9

probabilities for children have shown that TRISS outcome predictions are highly reliable.[10,21,32] Recently, pediatric coefficients were derived using the MTOS data for children aged 14 and younger.[19] Comparisons of estimated survival probabilities using the adult and pediatric norms indicated that there were no statistically significant differences in the predicted and actual numbers of survivors using either norm. Given that both norms yielded equally good survival estimates, the authors recommended the continued use of the adult, blunt trauma norm, stressing the importance of a consistent system to evaluate trauma care.

ASCOT: a new severity characterization of trauma. Limitations of TRISS's component indices, TS and ISS, motivated the development of RTS and AP. ASCOT[11] combines emergency department admission values of the Glasgow Coma Scale, systolic blood pressure, and respiratory rate, as coded for RTS, with AP components and patient age. ASCOT values are related to patient survival probability (P_s) using the logistic function

$$P_s = 1/(1 + e^{-k}),$$

where:

$$k = k_0 + k_1GCS + k_2SBP + k_3RR + k_4A + k_5B + k_6C + k_7AGE$$

D, the summary score for all minor injuries, was found not significant in predicting P_s. For children, the AGE coefficient is 0.

Patients with very severe or very minor injuries are not evaluated by the ASCOT logistic model. These "set-aside" patient groups are defined, and their survival rates given, in Table 59-5.

The ability of TRISS and ASCOT to discriminate survivors from nonsurvivors and the reliability of their predictions, as measured by the Hosmer-Lemeshow statistic, were compared using MTOS patient data. ASCOT performance matched or exceeded TRISS's for large samples of patients with blunt injuries and for patients with penetrating injuries. The Hosmer-Lemeshow statistics indicate that ASCOT reliably predicts patient outcome for patients with penetrating injuries and nearly so for

patients with blunt injuries. Statistically reliable predictions were not achieved by TRISS for either set. When AIS-90 is implemented, new coefficients will be derived for ASCOT.

PARTITION—prehospital care evaluation. PARTITION, an extension of TRISS, is intended to estimate the contribution of prehospital care to a patient's "potential for survival" by separating its effects from those of hospital care.[39] The measure "potential for survival" is used here rather than "improved survival outcome," as the latter depends on both prehospital and hospital care. It is conceivable that superb prehospital care could be offset by poor hospital care, resulting in average or poor survival outcomes. Similarly, poor prehospital care could be overcome by superb hospital management, resulting in improved outcomes. Prehospital care personnel should not be penalized in examples of the first kind nor credited in examples of the second. PARTITION uses estimates of survival probabilities based on a patient's RTS (measured *both* at the scene of injury and upon hospital admission), ISS, and patient age.

The PARTITION score is the increase (decrease, if negative), per 100 patients, in the number of survivors above (below) the number expected to survive with MTOS baseline hospital and prehospital care.

USES OF SEVERITY SCORES

Trauma scoring systems have several related, but distinct, uses: field triage, assessment of the effectiveness of care, scientific comparison of patient populations, and epidemiologic research.

Triage

Triage, the classification of patients by medical need, is accomplished by assessing the severity of a patient's injuries and recommending appropriate care. For pediatric trauma, triage is usually performed by prehospital providers at the scene of injury or by physicians at non–trauma centers.

At the scene of injury, accurate determination of anatomic damage is difficult because of children's capacity to compensate for physiologic derangement resulting from injury and because of the inability of young children to articulate their injuries. Identifying patients at risk of dying may be aided by scores that have a quantified link with mortality.

Interhospital patient triage is appropriate for a child admitted to a hospital that cannot quickly provide the necessary care. The transfer decision may be prompted by deterioration of a child's condition or by physician diagnosis of injuries requiring trauma center care. Severity scores can assist in early identification of such patients.

Three scoring systems have been evaluated for the field triage of injured children: the TS, the unweighted RTS, and the PTS. Threshold values yielding the most accurate separation of severely injured patients have been shown to be a TS < 15, unweighted RTS < 12, and PTS < 9.[20] No significant differences have been found in the ability of these three scores to identify severely injured children as defined by ISS values of >15 or ≥20.

Quality assessment

Quality assessment is receiving increasing attention in medicine. The Joint Commission on the Accreditation of Healthcare Organizations requires hospitals to monitor and evaluate the quality and appropriateness of patient care.[29,30] In addition, trauma centers also must conduct ongoing quality assessment programs to meet criteria established by the American College of Surgeons.[15] Although both the Joint Commission and the College of Surgeons leave the means of conducting these programs to individual hospitals, appropriateness of care can be demonstrated by using injury scoring systems. TRISS and ASCOT methods can be used objectively to compare predicted and actual survival rates for children.

Comparison of trauma patients

Trauma severity scores provide the ability to compare the severity mix and outcomes of patients within and among institutions. It is only by using methodologies that incorporate such scores that the effectiveness of individual trauma centers or of regional trauma systems can be demonstrated. Given the labor- and capital-intensive resources required by trauma centers and systems, documentation of their efficacy and identification of nonproductive components is necessary.

Trauma centers have developed many methods for meeting quality assessment obligations, but there is no guarantee that their methods are valid. Many quality assessment methods focus on the process indicators of care, such as service utilization, and not on patient outcome. These methods are of limited value, however, since determinations of appropriate length of stay or type of procedures performed provide little indication of timeliness of care or appropriate outcome. Moreover, because injury severity can vary substantially among trauma patients with the same diagnosis, traditional quality assessment methods that do not account for injury severity are of little value in determining effectiveness of care.

Few published studies have demonstrated the trauma center's impact on outcome over time or its effect on children who survive their injuries. One such study by Wesson and colleagues found that a substantial proportion of children hospitalized with serious injuries had disabilities that limited their participation in normal activities 6 months after discharge.[46] A report from San Diego documented the impact of a regional trauma system on saving lives,[6] and a Washington, D.C., study showed a significant improvement in trauma patient outcome coinciding with a major institutional commitment to trauma care.[9] Both the San Diego and Washington studies used severity scales to control for case mix.

Regional quality assurance assessment

Ideally, a regional trauma system should be able to evaluate prehospital, hospital, and rehabilitative care for all trauma patients, whether managed in a trauma center or not. Such an evaluation would include patients who die before reaching a hospital. A method (partly futuristic) for continuum of care trauma outcome evaluation (from injury scene through rehabilitation) has been proposed.[40] This should be extended to such postdischarge outcomes as return to school or work, functional disabilities, and outpatient rehabilitative needs.

It is particularly important that regional trauma systems adopt effective and consistent quality assessment programs to identify areas where changes in care result in improved patient outcomes. This requires, at a minimum, the accurate characterization of the type and severity of patient injuries.

EPIDEMIOLOGIC NEEDS

A reliable system for gathering trauma data is necessary to address matters of trauma health care policy. To this end, the American College of Surgeons requires that all trauma centers maintain a data registry. Several organizations, including the Centers for Disease Control and the American Public Health Association, have specified "core" data elements for trauma registries. Basic data sets generally include information on injury types, causes, and severities; survival and death outcomes; complications; lengths of stay, costs of care; discharge disabilities; and methods of reimbursement. In addition to hospital-based trauma registries, many states and local jurisdictions collect similar information.

OTHER PATIENT OUTCOMES

Survival and death outcomes have been the thrust of most trauma management studies. Recently, researchers have reported studies of such other outcomes as lengths of hospital and intensive care unit (ICU) stays, serious complications, brain function, and functional dependencies. The Glasgow Outcome Scale,[28] measures brain function and has been used since the middle 1970s to characterize the outcomes of patients with head injuries. More recently, the Functional Independence Measure (FIM)[25] has been used to characterize patient disability. It includes 18 assessments of patient cognition and ability to perform activities of daily living. FIM is also used to assess the value of rehabilitation.

ASCOT-like and AP-like models may be more appropriate to predict outcomes other than survival. For example, to predict level of disability or resource requirements, one may be tempted to fashion a model that includes separate components for head, spinal, and orthopedic injuries.

Trauma registry

Many hospitals use trauma registries to store and analyze patient data including demographics; anatomic diagnoses; prehospital, emergency department and operating room clinical information; and outcomes (survival, lengths of stay, and disabilities).

Not all registry data need be collected on every patient. In-depth data collection can be productively limited to more severely injured patients requiring intensive care or surgery or hospitalization for at least 3 days. Such limitations lighten the data collection burden while fulfilling the trauma center needs for assessment of quality improvement, outcomes, and triage effectiveness.

Identification of trauma patients who can benefit from trauma care, together with documentation of benefits, is essential for future triage of trauma patients and for allocation of trauma research, training, and ever-dwindling fiscal resources. Such identification and documentation can be accomplished only through the use of trauma severity scores.

REFERENCES

1. American Association for Automotive Medicine: *The Abbreviated Injury Scale—1985 revision*, Des Plaines, Il, 1985, The American Association.
2. Baker SP, O'Neill B: The injury severity score: an update, *J Trauma* 16:822, 1976.
3. Baker SP, O'Neill B, Haddon W et al: The injury severity score: a method for describing patients with multiple injuries and evaluating emergency care, *J Trauma* 14:187, 1974.
4. Boyd CR, Tolson MA, Copes WS: Evaluating trauma care: the TRISS method, *J Trauma* 27:370-378, 1987.
5. Bull JP: The Injury Severity Score of road traffic casualties in relation to mortality, time of death, hospital treatment time and disability, *Accid Anal Prev.* 7:249-255, 1975.
6. Cales R: Trauma mortality in Orange County: the effect of implementation of a regional trauma system, *Ann Emerg Med* 13:1, 1984.
7. Champion HR: Field triage of the trauma patient, *Ann Emerg Med* 11:160, 1982.
8. Champion HR, Sacco WJ: The trauma score as applied to penetrating injury, *Ann Emerg Med* 13:6, 1984.
9. Champion HR, Sacco WJ, Copes WS: Improvement in outcome from trauma center care, *Arch Surg* 127:333-335, 1992.
10. Champion HR, Sacco WJ, Hunt TK: Trauma severity scoring to predict mortality, *World J Surg* 7:4-11, 1983.
11. Champion HR, Copes WS, Sacco WJ et al: A new characterization of injury severity. Paper presented at the fiftieth annual meeting of the American Association for the Surgery of Trauma. Submitted for publication.
12. Champion HR, Sacco WJ, Carnazzo AJ et al: Trauma score, *Crit Care Med* 9:672, 1981.
13. Champion HR, Sacco WJ, Copes WS et al: A revision of the Trauma Score, *J Trauma* 29:623-629, 1989.
14. Champion HR, Sacco WJ, Hannan DS et al: Assessment of injury severity: the triage index, *Crit Care Med* 8:201, 1980.
15. Committee on Trauma of the American College of Surgeons: hospital and prehospital resources for optimal care of the injured patient (and Appendices A through J), 1987.
16. Copes WS, Champion HR, Sacco WJ et al: The Injury Severity Score revisited, *J Trauma* 28:69-77, 1988.
17. Copes WS, Champion HR, Sacco WJ et al: Progress in characterizing anatomic injury. Proceedings of the thirty-third annual meeting of the Association for the Advancement of Automotive Medicine, Baltimore, Md, 1989.
18. Eichelberger MR, Bowman LM, Sacco WJ et al: Trauma Score versus Revised Trauma Score in TRISS to predict outcome in children with blunt trauma, *Ann Emerg Med* 18:939-942, 1989.
19. Eichelberger MR, Champion HR, Sacco WJ et al: Pediatric coefficients for TRISS analysis, *J Trauma* 1993 (in press).
20. Eichelberger MR, Gotschall CS, Sacco WJ et al: A comparison of the Trauma Score, the Revised Trauma Score, and the Pediatric Trauma Score, *Ann Emerg Med*, 18:1053-1058, 1989.
21. Eichelberger MR, Mangubat EA, Sacco WJ et al: Comparative outcomes of children and adults suffering blunt trauma, *J Trauma* 28:430-434, 1988.
22. Gennarelli TA, Champion HR, Sacco WJ et al: Mortality of patients with head injury and extracranial injury treated in trauma centers, *J Trauma* 29:1193-1202, 1989.
23. Gordon NS, Fois A, Jacobi G et al: Consensus statement: the management of the comatose child, *Neuropediatrics* 14:3-5, 1985.
24. Gormican SP: CRAMS scale: field triage of trauma victims, *Ann Emerg Med* 11:132, 1982.
25. Hamilton BB, Granger CV, Sherwin FS et al: *A uniform national data system for medical rehabilitation*. In Fuhrer MJ, editor: *Rehabilitation outcomes: analysis and measurement*, Baltimore, 1987, Paul H Brookes.
26. Harviel JD, Landsman I, Greenberg A et al: The effect of autopsy on injury severity and survival probability calculations, *J Trauma* 15:766-773, 1989.
27. Hosmer DW, Lemeshow S: Goodness of fit tests for the multiple logistic regression model, *Commun Statistics—Theor meth* A9(10):1043-1068, 1980.
28. Jennett B, Teasdale G, Braakman R et al: Predicting outcome in individual patients after severe head injury, *Lancet* 1:1031, 1976.

29. Joint Commission on the Accreditation of Healthcare Organizations: *Overview of the Joint Commission's Agenda for Change,* August 1987, The Commission.

30. Joint Commission on the Accreditation of Hospitals: Accreditation Manual for Hospitals. Chicago, 1985.

31. Kamers DR: *Trauma score simplified,* UAMES Annual Meeting, Kansas City, Mo, 1985 (abstract).

32. Kaufmann CR, Maier RV, Rivara FP et al: Evaluation of the pediatric trauma score, *JAMA* 263:69, 1990.

33. Kirkpatrick JR, Youmans RL: Trauma index: an aid in the evaluation of injury victims, *J Trauma* 11:711, 1971.

34. Koehler JJ, Meindertsma MS, Baer LJ: Prehospital index: a scoring system for field triage of trauma victims. UAMES Annual Meeting, Kansas City, Mo, 1985 (abstract).

35. Moreau M, Gainer P, Champion HR et al: Application of the trauma score in the prehospital setting, *Ann Emerg Med* 14:1049, 1985.

36. Ogawa M, Sugimoto T: Rating severity of the injured by ambulance attendants, *J Trauma* 14:934, 1974.

37. Raimondi AJ, Hirschauer J: Head injury in the infant and toddler: coma scoring and outcome scale, *Child's Brain* 11:12-35, 1984.

38. Reilly PL, Simpson DA, Sprod R et al: Assessing the conscious level in infants and young children: a paediatric version of the Glasgow Coma Scale. *Child Nerv Syst* 4:30-33, 1988.

39. Sacco WJ, Jameson JW, Copes WS et al: PARTITION: a quantitative method for evaluating prehospital services for trauma patients, *Comput Biol Med* 18:221-227, 1988.

40. Sacco WJ, Long WB, Copes WS et al: Continuum of care trauma outcome evaluations (submitted for publication).

41. Semmlow JL, Cone R: Application of the injury severity score: an independent correlation, *Health Serv,* Spring 1976.

42. Somers RL: *New ways to use the 1980 Abbreviated Injury Scale—Probability of Death Score (PODS),* Odense University Hospital, Odense, Denmark, 1982, Laboratory for Public Health and Health Economics, (internal report).

43. Taylor MS, Sacco WJ, Champion HR: On the power of a method for comparing survival of trauma patients to a standard survival curve, *Comput Biol Med* 16:1-6, 1986.

44. Teasdale G, Jennett B: Assessment of coma and impaired consciousness: a practical scale, *Lancet* 2:81, 1974.

45. Tepas JJ, Mollitt DL, Talbert JL et al: The Pediatric Trauma Score as a predictor of injury severity in the injured child, *J Pediatr Surg* 22:14, 1987.

46. Wesson DE, Williams JI, Spence LJ et al: Functional outcome in pediatric trauma, *J Trauma* 29:589-592, 1989.

47. Yager JY, Johnston B, Seshia SS: Coma scales in pediatric practice, *Am J Dis Child* 144:1088–1091, 1990.

60 System Assessment

Maureen S. McArdle and Gail F. Cooper

In order to discuss the primary tenets of pediatric trauma system assessment, it is important to understand issues concerning the development of systems of care and the role they play in the ongoing evaluation of system integrity and effectiveness.

Childhood injuries have been recognized for the past 40 years as the leading cause of childhood death.[1] However, only within the last 20 years have health officials focused on trauma as a major public health issue and only within the last 10 years have systems of care for pediatric trauma and critical care been actively discussed. In 1985 it was estimated that more than one million children and adolescents sustained injuries that required hospital care, 100,000 suffered some form of permanent psychological disability, and more than 25,000 died.[2] Efforts to improve injury outcome were focused on resuscitation and early definitive care. Unfortunately, the yearly cost of such care was approximately $14 billion, which suggested that changes in the approach to the care of injured children were necessary.[13]

During the last 10 years health care planners moved toward a "system of care" philosophy, which incorporates all regional health care resources in plans of care. This followed the eras of "survival of the fittest" in the 1960s and 1970s, when individuals were delivered to the nearest available facility by unskilled or poorly trained providers, and the 1970s and 1980s, which saw the identification of "centers" and increased training activities. This identification process provided excellent resources such as trauma centers, but there was no system for appropriate use. Although it may appear that the development of trauma systems followed on the coattails of Emergency Medical Service (EMS) development, the recognition of deficiencies in the treatment of the injured actually motivated national health activities in the area of emergency care.

In the 1950s and 1960s medical care providers, home from the battlefields of Korea and Vietnam, had returned with a renewed respect for the value of coordination of trauma services in attaining optimal outcome. In 1966 the National Academy of Sciences published a monumental report entitled *Accidental Death and Disability: The Neglected Disease of Modern Society.*[10] This document exposed the ineffective and inadequate nonsystematic approach to emergency medical treatment in the United States. In the same year, the Highway Safety Act,[11] followed in 1973 by the Emergency Medical Services Systems (EMSS) Act,[5] with amendments in 1976, provided federal grant programs that authorized the planning, initiation, and expansion of local and regional Emergency Medical Services Systems. Through the 1973 EMSS Act, Congress granted funds to localities based on level of service provided. Funds were made available for planning and implementing systems of care including 15 essential components for seven special-needs groups, including patients with trauma, burns, and spinal cord injuries.[8]

The 1973 congressional EMSS Act and its 1976 amendments set the stage for governmental responsibility in identification and coordination of emergency medical resources. The states had overall responsibility; however, many delegated the task to local authorities. Although the original idea was for a national-system approach, individual states or local authorities succeeded at diverse levels, and many failed. During the late 1970s and early 1980s groups such as the American College of Surgeons and the Colleges of Emergency Physicians and Pediatrics, spurred on by national injury data, voiced concern about availability and utilization of resources for critically injured children.

In 1985 *Injury in America,* published by the National Research Council and the Institute of Medicine, reemphasized that "*injury* was a public health problem whose toll is unacceptable." The study placed the percentage of years of potential life lost to injury at 40.8%.[6]

Following this report, and the 1988 *Injury Control* report by the same group, influential agencies such as the National Highway Traffic Safety Association, the Department of Transportation, the Centers for Disease Control, and national medical associations, reinforced by the success of state systems such as those in Maryland, Virginia, Oregon, and Pennsylvania, and county systems such as those in San Diego and Orange Counties in California, encouraged regions to develop a philosophy that incorporates all available trauma resources into a comprehensive system of care.

SYSTEM DEVELOPMENT AND EVALUATION

A system is a sequence of actions by, and interactions between, functional units that bring about the manufacture of a product or delivery of a service.[7] In pediatric trauma care, the product is the return of the injured child to health or optimal functional recovery.

The secondary evolution of trauma system development is the identification and coordination of specialized pediatric surgical and critical care resources for severely injured children. Although the trauma system development process began in the 1970s, the development of systems of care for severely injured children is a relatively new concept. It is now recognized that children, because of differences in anatomy, physiology, and disease entities, require specialized resources. The injured child has the potential to wreak havoc on the medical care delivery system. Care rendered by an unprepared and disorganized system can result in unnecessary, costly, and long-term treatment, permanent disability, or death.[12] Those responsible for assessment of needs and development of resource matching must have a clear understanding of necessary pediatric system components. This is essential for the formulation of measurable goals and objectives appropriate for system assessment.

In terms of level and scope of pediatric trauma care review, there are distinct differences between system evaluation and quality management. The level of system evaluation can vary from the complex organizational assessment of many variables to an indepth evaluation of one system component. Variables to be assessed may include resource allocation, patient access issues, and professional competence.[4] Thus, quality management, which is usually directed toward caregiver-patient activities, is merely one part of total system evaluation. System-focused evaluation has a much broader scope and may therefore be more time-consuming and costly.[9]

The systematic assessment of pediatric trauma care requires evaluation of all the interfaces of the continuum of care, from identification of the injured victim through medical care and on to recovery. This analysis incorporates all of the major emergency medical services' system components (Table 60-1). The basic evaluation format can be used during system phases: development, maintenance, improvement, and change.

Table 60-1 Emergency system components and phases of pediatric trauma care

Select emergency system components
Communications
Manpower and training
Transportation
Facilities and critical care resources
Data collection
Consumer information and education

Pediatric trauma care continuum phases
Prehospital phases
    Prevention opportunities
    System access
    First responder
    Dispatch
    Transport agencies
Hospital phase
    In-hospital institutional components
    Caregiver interfaces
Rehabilitation, long-term care, and home care
Reintroduction to school and community, and recovery resources

DEVELOPMENT PHASE ASSESSMENT

The desire to deliver quality pediatric trauma care coupled with appropriate tools to measure and interpret the care rendered provides the stimulus to drive system structure. It is therefore imperative in the developmental stage to provide for a structural framework that permits measurement of process and outcome. Collected data are measured against predetermined system expectations.

Within a pediatric trauma system, the structural framework for assessment must include examination and analysis of all components associated with care and treatment. System standards that outline expectations for optimal system performance must be formulated, and reliable data sources identified to monitor these standards. Much of the initial structure may be dictated by statutory authority, that is, state law, which provides the authority for implementation and management of programmatic and operational activities related to the trauma care system. Structural design and implementation should assure that the right patient goes to the right facility within the right time frame, and that the system continues to provide for postinjury needs. An effective system design takes into account population density and ethnic diversity, geographical issues as well as environmental, economic, and present resource utilization patterns. The structure should be further established by formulating locally accepted system standards for key operational and medical care issues.

These standards and criteria should address potential issues in each of the component areas, such as the following:

Authority for system implementation and coordination

Geographic boundaries for trauma service areas

Prehospital triage decisions

Interfacility transfer agreements

Minimum criteria for personnel training

Data collection needs

Format of periodic system and individual component evaluations

Consumer education responsibilities

Treatment standardization

Each developed standard or criterion should be written so that it is measurable and provides information pertinent to system evaluation.

Subsequent to development of structural assessment parameters, local system components can be identified and integrated. System policies should be developed and implemented, and appropriate contractual relationships should culminate in the development of a performance-based contract. This agreement should clearly articulate the minimum performance standards and system expectations of all parties. The importance of these contract agreements cannot be overemphasized. They become the basis for evaluation of caregivers and the institution or agency and provide a foundation for the establishment of an institutional quality surveillance program.

OUTCOME AND PROCESS SURVEILLANCE

Once the plan to measure efficacy of the structural components of a system is defined, performance measures in the area of care delivery must be reviewed. The appropriate utilization of system resources or *process* of use must be evaluated. In addition, the direct impact of this use on reduction of morbidity and mortality, *outcome,* must be scrutinized.

Each system component must develop and validate a means of performance measurement that results in comprehensive review of all key indicators of quality in the care of the pediatric trauma patient. This process will likely include prehospital and hospital-based quality management and research data; however, it should further include other patterns of utilization of care, such as nontrauma centers and clinics that might care for injured children.

Uniform information, gathered from trauma data bases and trauma registries, and through quality management activities, should be examined for outliers, which will represent select areas for in-depth study. At the present time, clinical *outcome* results are being used as a major quality indicator.

Clinical practice guidelines, where available, as well as peer review groups, should be used to determine appropriateness of care. It is important that the design of the data collection system, quality indicators, and interpretation of the data be accomplished by individuals skilled in this area, who also have appropriate authority to implement change when necessary.

The evaluation of "process" as a system assessment indicator is extremely important, particularly in pediatric trauma care delivery. Because of their resilience, children survive injuries of severe magnitude and may have remarkably good outcomes regardless of the appropriateness of care. Examination of the manner of utilization of resources and appropriateness of sequencing of care delivered is an important indicator of system efficacy. By developing clearly defined indicators of appropriate process throughout the continuum of care, reviewers will be able to identify deviations and reevaluate appropriateness of system objectives. These same process predictors are useful for review when patient outcome is not as expected.

SYSTEM IMPROVEMENT AND CHANGE

All assessment parameters involved in the care of the injured child can help in identifying areas for system improvement and, if necessary, system change. No matter how carefully a system is designed and monitored, there will be a certain percentage of poor outcomes or deviations in process in every system component. No true "system" of care can escape this reality. However, the real strength of a systems approach to pediatric trauma care is the ability to monitor, identify, and use unplanned outcomes as opportunities to improve system components or the structural system as a whole. By using the same careful consensus process, driven by reliable data, that developed the original system structure, the issues of improvement and change will be handled as a routine day-to-day task and will not cause system stress.

EXTERNAL REVIEW

A system's assessment process should be periodically validated by the use of outside consultants, either as individuals or through a formalized site-review process. Components of the trauma system will be scrutinized against predetermined standards or guidelines in an effort to assure system compliance and identify opportunities for further quality improvement.

Choice of process

The following are the types of review possible:

1. *Accreditation and certification.* Certified as to meeting certain agency standards at the time of review; frequently tied to reimburse-

ment (for example, the Joint Commission on the Accreditation of Health Care Organizations).

2. *Verification.* Review by association or organization that validates the meeting of the group's standards at the time of review (for example, the American College of Surgeons).

3. *Designation.* Granted by a governmental authority that requires the meeting, on a continuing basis, of standards usually tied to a contractual agreement to provide services.

Choice of team components

The choice of reviewers is between the following:

1. *Single discipline.* The reviewing consultants may be represented by a single discipline, generally medicine or surgery.

2. *Multidisciplinary.* The review team consists of members appropriate to each component and discipline to be examined. This is the best *systems* approach.

Areas of review

Areas of review should include but not be limited to

1. Determination that the system structure is consistent with county or national standards, state regulations, and system goals.

2. Review that ensures medical quality assurance activities that provide appropriate identification and effective correction of problems in trauma patient care. This includes appropriate medical education, counseling, and careful remonitoring activities.

3. Review of the degree of compliance with the system quality improvement model, such as recommended corrective action plans, correction of previously cited deficiencies; specifically, addressing areas that may indicate trends.

4. Assessment of physician and nurse coverage, training, credentials, and ongoing education. Performance is reviewed to assure facility continues to meet contract requirements.

5. Review that assures that system participants are maintaining a level of performance consistent with system goals.

MAINTAINING SYSTEM INTEGRITY

Perhaps the most difficult objective of pediatric trauma system assessment is the ongoing maintenance of system integrity. This requires constant reassessment of needs, resources, and system direction. Without continuing measurement, development, and planning for change, an active, functioning system may not be able to survive the period when the impetus that drove system development wanes and the "honeymoon" is over. This may come as early as the second year.

To maintain system integrity throughout this phase, and for the long term, there are several key elements that should be discussed on an ongoing basis. These are listed below.

Program flexibility

During the initial program development phase, various system configuration options should be discussed. It is important to ensure that the system has the flexibility to include or use other care configurations or plans. Do not devise a system so dependent on single components that alternate options to system design are not available. Options should be adaptable to changes in resource capabilities (increase or decrease), population shifts, and needs assessment changes.

Demonstration of program effectiveness

Ability to show that a system's goals for the care for injured children are met is essential to day-to-day, as well as long-term, maintenance of system integrity. This includes development of a reliable data system that provides comprehensive reports on key system components and quality indicators. In addition, conducting an evaluation of reimbursement issues cited by practitioners and other service providers, third-party and governmental payors will assist in identifying and evaluating cost-effective measures for system care.

It is important to have available specific data to support the ongoing need and effectiveness of the system and to identify directions for long-term goals. System components change on a continuing basis; however, this blueprint provides a guide for solid system direction.

Recruitment, retention, and ongoing education

The most likely groups to show "system fatigue" initially are the direct caregivers. However, system failures in many cases are due to loss of interest at governmental and hospital administrative levels. Throughout the life of the system there will be many changes in the total health care delivery system. These changes are forged by political and economic realities. Physicians, nurses, and prehospital providers, who are key to the system, may lose some of the initial "system start-up passion" just as the system begins to meet its goals. These practitioners may no longer feel a fervent need to be directly or actively involved in the system. This is particularly true of subspecialty groups, whose time commitment may be less than originally anticipated and who now may choose to move on to other less disruptive endeavors. Moreover, trauma medicine, in itself, may not be an attractive specialty for new caregivers, therefore diminishing the supply of resources as the system ages. Almost simultaneously, government officials, hospital boards, and hospital administrators may have moved on to the next identified political, community, or facility need. They may see the system running well and feel that it needs fewer resources, less attention, and lower capital expenditures.

As the system peaks in its effectiveness, the supporting and nurturing structure may recede. In the early stages of system planning, it is imperative that a long-term plan for system support during this period be developed. This should include the following components:

1. Development of a plan for continuous assessment of provider and system participant satisfaction that includes a forum for identifying system problem areas.
2. Provision for continuous evaluation of system effectiveness in both monetary and societal terms, measured against realistic system goals.
3. A comprehensive plan for ongoing recruitment and training at all system levels that provides continuing resources as fatigue occurs. These activities may occur at different intervals, given the differences in communities, but ongoing open communication with practitioners will help planners to anticipate needs in this area.

Dissemination and analysis of system data

A plan for timely dissemination of current system data and analysis of system improvement opportunities must be included. Systemwide data on focused topics should be shared and appropriately discussed with practitioners, system participants, the public, and third-party and governmental payors. Comparisons with presystem data on an ongoing basis are helpful in reminding all participants of the original system issues and goals and how they have been met. This may keep participants interested in a system survival.

Continuity of a consensus process

Continuity in the consensus process is pivotal in terms of day-to-day system maintenance and long-term system integrity. There must be a forum for issue discussion by all system principals. System planners must openly discuss all issues and continue to build system support by allowing interested principals to "buy into" the system by being an active force in system direction.

Fiscal independence

Another, and perhaps the most important, means of maintaining long-term system integrity is to develop fiscal independence. This is a most difficult task. However, ongoing development, implementation, and improvement in a pediatric trauma system is dependent upon it. It is important to work a plan through public-private partnerships, fostering an ongoing constituency whose goal is to find avenues of opportunity for fiscal stability. System integrity is dependent on provisions or incentives to system participants that provide funding for a well-coordinated, comprehensive system of pediatric trauma care.

SUMMARY

The goal of pediatric trauma system assessment is to improve all aspects of system resources and medical care through comprehensive systematic monitoring, reporting, and analysis of patient care activities. A solid system assessment process will ensure that each injured child reaps the benefits of all available resources that work together to provide the best possible outcome.

ACKNOWLEDGMENT. The authors wish to thank Melody Rodriguez for preparation and assistance with the manuscript.

REFERENCES

1. Alpert, Guyer B: Symposium on injuries and injury prevention (Foreword), *Pediat Clin North Am* 32:1-4, 1985.
2. Baber SP, O'Neill B, Karpf RS: *The injury fact book*, Lexington, Mass, 1984, Lexington Books.
3. Committee on Trauma Research, Commission on Life Sciences, National Research Council and Institute of Medicine, *Injury in America* and *injury control*, 1985 and 1988, The Committee.
4. Donebedian: *The definition of quality and approaches to its assessments*, Ann Arbor, Mich, 1980, Health Admin Press, p 21.
5. Emergency Medical Services System Act of 1973, Pub no 93-154, 1973.
6. Harris BH: Creating pediatric trauma systems, *J Pediatr Surg*, 24(2):1491-52, 1989.
7. Kritchevsky SB, Simmons BP: Continuous quality improvement, *JAMA*, 266(13):1817-1823.
8. McArdle M, Cooper G, Waldron J et al: Emergency medical services system: the San Diego experience, *Emerg Care Q* 6(1):35-48.
9. Mosleth R: A practical guide to multidisciplinary auditing, *Nursing Quality Assurance*, p 191-227.
10. National Academy of Sciences, Division of Medical Sciences: *Accidental death and disability: the neglected disease of modern society* U.S. Dept of Health, Education and Welfare, Public Health Service pub no 1071-A-13, Rockville, Md, 1966, The Academy.
11. National Safety Act of 1966, Public Law no 89-564, 1966.
12. Ramenofsky ML: Emergency medical services for children and pediatric trauma system components, *J Pediatr Surg* 24(2):153-5, 1989.
13. Rice DP et al: *Cost of injury in the United States: a report to Congress*, San Francisco Institute for Aging, University of California, San Francisco and Injury Prevention Center The Johns Hopkins University, 1989.

Performance Evaluation of Pediatric Intensive Care Units

Murray M. Pollack

Measurements of intensive care unit (ICU) performance have evolved to meet at least two important needs. The first is the assurance of appropriate quality of care. Quality assurance methods that emphasize outcomes have become necessary as researchers realized that process and outcome are poorly linked; the commonly used quality assurance methods that concentrate on process tend to evaluate efficiency. Therefore, intensive care outcome evaluations will be an important part of quality assurance. Second, the high cost of medical care has lead to a national cost-containment effort emphasizing cost reductions, especially in the treatment of patients who are "too healthy to benefit." Since ICUs are expensive hospital areas, utilization evaluations directed at this care area are logical.

SEVERITY OF ILLNESS

Measuring severity of illness is necessary for performance evaluations of both quality assurance and ICU costs. Conceptually, severity of illness can be considered a continuous variable with extremes of outcomes (e.g., survival, death) occurring at low and high values; the threshold value determining outcome is unknown and may vary from patient to patient. Because ICUs exist to monitor physiologic status and treat life-threatening physiologic dysfunction, physiologic status is the variable that unites essentially all ICU patients, even if they have substantial differences (e.g., diagnoses, ages). Clinical measurements of physiologic status are observable and, if taken in some combination, define severity of illness. This concept follows closely from the observation that mortality rates increase as the number of organ system failures increase. For example, in pediatric ICUs the mortality rates for one, two, three, and four or more organ system failures are approximately 1%, 10%, 50%, and 75%, respectively.[18]

Quantitative methods to measure severity of illness evolved because physicians' subjective opinions lack consistency, reliability, and accuracy. Physicians are generally poor prognosticators,[7] and their poor performance in accuracy of prediction is not surprising. The art of prognostication is infrequently taught, and even if it were taught, improvement of predictive performance is difficult.[17] For example, systematic performance checks are necessary to maximize learning based on experience, but few physicians are sufficiently disciplined to consistently check their own accuracy when uncommon events (e.g., deaths) are being predicted. In addition, they frequently disagree about the appropriateness of care, in part because their routine function in case reviews is evaluation of process, not of outcome. Even when simplified case synopses are reviewed by physicians, agreement concerning the appropriateness of outcome is relatively low.[17] The result of these problems is that more accurate predictions result from actuarial methods than from clinical assessments.[1]

Modern severity of illness methods relevant to critically ill patients measure physiologic status and relate this to mortality risk. In the early 1970s the methods were qualitative and indirect (for example, the Clinical Classification System). Other methods, such as the Therapeutic Intervention Scoring System (TISS), quantified amounts of monitoring and therapy. Therefore, TISS was objective but only indirectly assessed severity of illness. TISS assumes that physiologic instability will translate into increased monitoring and therapeutic interventions. However, many patients receive monitoring and therapeutic interventions because of the diagnosis, not physiologic instability. For example, the monitoring received by postoperative cardiovascular surgical patients is dictated as much by the operation as by postoperative physiologic status. In the 1980s investigators realized that physiologic status was a direct and relevant reflection of intensive care mortality risk. Measures of physiologic status provided investigators with important advances in understanding intensive care. The most relevant of these advances is the ability of physiologic scores to adjust mortality rates for severity of illness.[13]

The major pediatric mortality risk-assessment method applicable to the wide variety of pediatric

Table 61–1 The pediatric risk of mortality (PRISM) score

Variable scores	Age restrictions and ranges		
Systolic BP (mm Hg)	**Infants**		**Children**
2	130-160		150-200
2	55-65		65-75
6	>160		>200
6	40-54		50-64
7	<40		<50
Diastolic BP (mm Hg)		**All ages**	
6		>110	
Heart rate (beats/min)	**Infants**		**Children**
4	>160		>150
4	<90		<80
Respiratory rate (breaths/min)	**Infants**		**Children**
1	61-90		51-70
5	>90		>70
5	Apnea		Apnea
Pao_2/Fio_2*		**All ages**	
2		200-300	
3		<200	
$Paco_2$ (mm Hg)†		**All ages**	
1		51-65	
5		>65	
Glasgow Coma Scale score‡		**All ages**	
6		<8	
Pupillary reactions		**All ages**	
4		unequal or dilated	
10		fixed and dilated	
PT/PTT		**All ages**	
2		>1.5 × Control	
Total bilirubin (mg/dl)		**>1 month**	
6		>3.5	
Potassium (mEq/l)		**All ages**	
1		3.0-3.5	
1		6.5-7.5	
5		<3.0	
5		>7.5	

intensive care patients is the Pediatric Risk of Mortality (PRISM) score (Table 61-1),[8] which is a revision of the Physiologic Stability Index (PSI). The PSI was originally used subjective opinions of experts to develop a list of 36 variables and 76 variable ranges, each range weighted 1, 3, or 5, depending on the clinical significance of the abnormality.[19] Of special importance to pediatrics, unmeasured variables are assumed to be normal; therefore, extra tests are not required. The PSI was prospectively validated in our ICU by its relationship to mortality risk. As our data base expanded, we improved the PSI score using organ-system weighting derived with multivariate logistic tech-

Table 61–1 The pediatric risk of mortality (PRISM) score—cont'd

Variable scores	Age restrictions and ranges
Calcium (mg/dl)	**All ages**
2	7.0-8.0
2	12.0-15.0
6	<7.0
6	>15.0
Glucose (mm Hg)	**All ages**
4	40-60
4	250-400
8	<40
8	>400
Bicarbonate (mEq/l)§	**All ages**
3	<16
3	>32

Score only 1 abnormality/variable.

P (ICU death) = exp (R)/(1 + exp [R]) where R = .207*PRISM$_a$ − .005*age (in months) − .433*operative status − 4.782. Operative status = 1 if postoperative, 0 if not postoperative.

P (death within 24 hours) = exp (R)/(1 + exp [R]) where R = .160*PRISM$_a$ − 6.427 if only PRISM$_a$ is available *or* R = .154*PRISM$_t$ + .053*PRISM$_a$ − 6.791 if more than 1 PRISM score is available. PRISM$_t$ = most recent PRISM score. PRISM$_a$ = admission day PRISM score.

*Cannot be assessed in patients with intracardiac shunts or chronic respiratory insufficiency. Requires arterial blood sampling.

†May be assessed with capillary blood gases.

‡Assessed only if there is known or suspected central nervous system dysfunction. Cannot be assessed in patients during iatrogenic sedation, paralysis, anesthesia, etc. Scores <8 correspond to deep stupor or coma.

§Use measured values.

niques. The performance of the PSI was then prospectively tested on 1572 consecutive admissions to eight other ICUs.[13] The major hypothesis was that mortality rate differences among ICUs could be explained by differences in the distributions of severity of illness. We were able to prove this hypothesis even though there was a sixfold mortality rate difference. In all ICUs, as well as in the total data base, both the numbers and the distribution of outcomes predicted by the PSI were not different from expected with use of "goodness-of-fit" tests. In all, 131 ICU deaths were observed and 136.4 were predicted.

The PSI was revised by splitting our national data base of 2642 patients in two, half for score revision and half for validation of the revision. The resulting PRISM score has only 14 variables and 23 ranges of these variables.[8] The variables consist of cardiovascular vital signs, neurologic vital signs, and laboratory variables. All highly invasive variables, such as intracranial pressure and central venous pressure, have been eliminated. The ranges of abnormality are weighted by using a logistic scale according to their contribution to mortality risk. The most deviant variable recorded (usually found in laboratory reports or in the bedside cardiovascular and neurologic vital sign sheets) for the

admission day is used for scoring. As in the PSI, extra tests are not required or advised. The admission-day period used for scoring is a variable period of time of at least 8 hours that ends at an arbitrary, consistent time. If less than 8 hours of time is accumulated, that time period is included in the next 24-hour period. If the patient dies during the admission day, all data excluding the preterminal period are included. This variable admission-day time period functions well because survivors' physiologic dysfunction remains stable, whereas nonsurvivors' physiologic instability is high and become even higher during the period of interest. Mortality risks are calculated as indicated in Table 61-1.

Table 61-2 illustrates the performance of the PRISM score in six validating ICUs (1227 patients).[8] Overall, 105 deaths were observed and 103.9 deaths were predicted. The corresponding mortality rates are 8.6% observed and 8.5% predicted. The agreement between the observed and the predicted outcomes in mortality risk groups was statistically evaluated with chi-square goodness-of-fit tests and was excellent in each of the validating ICUs, both in major diagnostic categories based on the primary physiologic system of dysfunction (respiratory, cardiovascular, neurologic, and mis-

Table 61–2 Performance of the PRISM score in six validating ICUs*

Mortality risk categories	Survivors	Nonsurvivors
	Observed/expected	
0%-1%	418/418.6	3/2.4
1%-5%	512/511.0	11/12.0
5%-15%	129/131.1	15/12.6
15%-30%	31/31.1	8/7.9
>30%	32/31.0	68/69.0

Chi-square (5 degrees of freedom) = 0.80.
*Expected outcome numbers are the sum of the mortality risk probabilities for each patient in each category. Mortality risks are calculated as in Table 61-1.
From Pollack MM, Ruttimann UE, Getson PR. The pediatric risk of mortality (PRISM) score, *Crit Care Med* 16:1110, 1988.

cellaneous), and in the classification groups of operative and nonoperative patients. Both the PSI and PRISM have also been validated in national pediatric trauma patient samples. However, this does not indicate that the score can be applied with accurate mortality-risk predictions to all diagnostic categories. Oncology disorders and AIDS are diagnoses in which the general meaning of physiologic instability may be altered by the diagnosis.

A drawback to the PSI and PRISM scores is that they fail to assess the changing course of severity of illness during disease worsening or recovery. Therefore, predictors of short-term (<24 hr) mortality risk use sequential daily data to assess the changing aspects of disease and recovery. The Dynamic Risk Index (DRI) uses PSI scores, and the Dynamic Objective Risk Assessment (DORA) uses PRISM scores.[14,15] Perhaps most important, they demonstrate that predictors need not be confined to single measurements. Just as physicians revise their assessments of patient status, predictors can be developed that adjust predictions of outcome. The prediction equation for the DORA score is given in Table 61-1. Dynamic assessment of mortality risk is important for measurement of ICU efficiency.

OUTCOME-BASED QUANTITATIVE QUALITY ASSURANCE

The rigorous, multiinstitutional validation of PSI and PRISM scores is the backbone of their use in outcome-based, quantitative quality assurance. These same validation methods are available to individual hospitals and regions with commonly available computer technology and appropriate software. These methods are not designed to replace all other quality assurance tasks, such as evaluations of nosocomial infections, unplanned extubations, and the like. However, they are designed to provide objective, outcome-based quality assur-

ance, because they overcome the difficulties in using crude mortality rates.

Studies of critical care quality

Pediatric and adult studies demonstrate that quantitative quality assurance using objective predictors to compare observed and predicted numbers of outcomes can be successful. In a prospective regional pediatric critical-care quality study in Oregon and southwestern Washington, we examined the relationship between intensive care resources and the outcomes of patients with respiratory failure and head trauma.[10] Severity of illness–adjusted mortality rates in tertiary and nontertiary hospitals were determined with the use of admission-day PRISM scores, and care modalities were assessed daily. The crude mortality rate of tertiary patients was four times higher than that of nontertiary patients (23.4% versus 6.0%; $p < .0001$). In tertiary patients, the number of outcomes were accurately predicted by PRISM scores. However, for nontertiary patients, the number of the deaths were significantly different than predicted. The odds ratios of dying in a nontertiary versus a tertiary facility were about 1.1, 2.3, and 8 ($p < .05$) for mortality risk groups of under 5%, 5% to 30%, and over 30%. These mortality rate differences also corresponded to significant differences in the use of monitoring and therapeutic techniques. In another study of a single hospital, we compared severity of illness–adjusted mortality rates before and after a pediatric intensivist joined the hospital staff. The ICU mortality rate improved after the intensivist was added to the staff.[12]

Studies of adult ICUs and trauma centers also demonstrated the power of outcome-based, quantitative quality assurance. Knaus and colleagues found that the actual mortality rate was well predicted by the Acute Physiology and Chronic Health Evaluations (APACHE) II score in 11 of 13 hos-

Table 61–3 Use of the PRISM score in ICU trauma patients

Mortality risk categories	Survivors	Nonsurvivors
	Observed/expected	
0%-1%	83/82.5	0/0.5
1%-5%	45/45.0	1/1.0
5%-50%	17/17.3	5/4.6
50%-100%	3/1.9	10/11.1

Chi-square (4 degrees of freedom) = 1.216.
Z-score = 0.479.
From Klem SA, Pollack MM, Glass NL et al: Resource use, efficiency, and outcome prediction in pediatric intensive care of trauma patients, *J Trauma* 30:32-36, 1990.

pitals.[5] In 2 hospitals, however, APACHE II did not accurately predict mortality rates. In one hospital the mortality rate was better than expected, whereas in another it was worse than expected. In an *a posteriori* analysis, the authors related their findings to the organizational structure of care delivery in the ICUs. They concluded that the degree of coordination of care may significantly affect outcome. Trauma center studies also support the validity and importance of outcome-based, quantitative quality assurance. The most common methods used for assessment of severity of illness in trauma patients are the physiology-based scores, the Trauma Score (TS) and the Revised Trauma Score (RTS), and the anatomic index of injury, the Injury Severity Score (ISS). Trauma scores have been validated in one pediatric institution.[2] Using these methods, outcomes controlled for severity of illness were improved after regionalization of trauma care.[16]

Use of PRISM or PSI score

If an institution decides to use PRISM or PSI scores for quantitative quality assurance, the process follows the principles discussed above. First, a consecutive patient sample must be acquired. In addition to the guidelines given above, we recommend that the data collector not be involved in the patients' care. Each patient has an estimated mortality risk reflecting his or her PRISM score, age, and operative status (see Table 61-1). The observed number of survivors and deaths and the estimated numbers of survivors and deaths are calculated by summing the individual patients' mortality risks.

Statistical tests

The comparison of the observed ICU survivors and ICU deaths with the estimated numbers of ICU survivors and ICU deaths is tested in two ways. Table 61-3 illustrates the methods used for testing in trauma patients admitted to five pediatric ICUs.[4]

First, the Z-score as proposed by Flora is used.[3] This test is based on the Z statistic and tests the total number of outcomes, but not the distribution of outcomes (see below). A major advantage of the Z-score is that it can be used with a total sample of as few as five deaths. A second, more sensitive, method tests both the distribution of outcomes as well as the total numbers of outcomes. This follows the simple observation that a higher proportion of very sick patients die as opposed to the healthiest patients. If the patients are divided into mortality-risk groups based on the estimated mortality risk, then both the total number of outcomes as well as the distribution of outcomes can be tested by using a goodness-of-fit test based on the chi-square statistic.[6] In Tables 61-2 and 61-3, the samples are divided into different mortality risk categories because the cells of the goodness-of-fit categories should all have as many patients as possible. In practice, this involves trying to make divisions, with deaths in each mortality-risk category. For smaller samples in individual ICUs, we usually use the following groups: 0%-5%, 5%-30%, and more than 30%. Users of these methods will need to review the statistical methods in more detail.

Analysis of results

If the observed number and distribution of outcomes are similar to the predicted number and distribution of outcomes, then the performance of the institution is equivalent to that of those institutions validating the predictor in the multiinstitutional studies. If the performance of the institution is different than expected, an explanation must be sought. As with any test, physicians using this quality assurance methodology will need to understand its strengths and limitations, when pediatric ICUs might be incorrectly classified as delivering poor care (false-positive) or good care (false-negative), confounding variables, and peculiarities of the method. If the goodness-of-fit methodology is used, a specific mortality-risk interval can be targeted for in-depth chart reviews. The investigation of "extra" deaths detected by the mortality predictors may or may not indicate that unnecessary events have occurred. There are legitimate explanations for "extra" ICU deaths. For example, if the ICU patient population is skewed toward diagnostic groups that have not been extensively tested (e.g., bone marrow transplantation, oncology patients), then the scores may not be applicable. Subjective chart reviews may determine that the deaths were not unexpected. For example, a logical explanation for an underestimation of deaths in low severity-of-illness strata might be that many physiologically stable patients with terminal conditions were admitted.

It is also possible that a fewer-than-expected number of deaths will be detected. Of course, this could indicate that the care delivered in the ICU is better than that delivered in the other institutions validating the score. However, other explanations must also be sought. An important possibility is that resuscitative efforts prior to arrival in the ICU were less complete than those in other institutions. Therefore, some ICU admissions would have more *treatable* physiologic instability (and higher physiology scores) because of the less complete resuscitation. Improper use of the score may also explain the results. Data collectors who are also bedside caregivers might bias data by attempting to alter an observation on how sick the patient appears.

Users of these quality assurance methods should also be aware that the power to detect severity-of-illness outcomes different from those predicted is related to the size of the sample and, especially, to the number of deaths. The more deaths that are accumulated during a study, the greater the power to detect a statistical deviation from the expected. Preferably, at least 20 deaths should be accumulated, although small units with low mortality rates may accumulate fewer. In these circumstances, the power to detect a deviation from the expected will be reduced.

EVALUATING ICU EFFICIENCY

Numerous studies have documented that intensive care units are poorly utilized. Within the context of the costly nature of intensive care and the potential advantages of lax ICU admission requirements, increased local effort will be directed at documenting the current uses and abuses of intensive care utilization and improving ICU efficiency. Current methodology enables sophisticated evaluation of intensive care bed use. As in the previous section, evaluations of ICU utilization equivalent to those referenced in this section can be done with the current, widely available computer technology

Table 61–4 Unique ICU therapies

Cardiac arrest and/or countershock
Mechanical ventilation
Balloon tamponade of varices
Continuous arterial infusion
Acute cardiac pacing
Hemodialysis or peritoneal dialysis (unstable patient)
Induced hypothermia
Push or pressure activated blood transfusion for hypotension
G-suit
Emergency operative procedures (within 24 hours)
Lavage of acute gastrointestinal tract bleeding
Intubation
Continuous positive airway pressure
Blind intratracheal suctioning
Frequent infusions of blood products (> 20 cc/kg)
Vasoactive drug infusions
Continuous antiarrhythmic infusions
Emergency thoracenteses, pericardiocenteses, and paracenteses
Therapy for seizures or metabolic encephalopathy
Concentrated potassium infusion
Cardioversion for arrhythmias
Extracorporeal support systems

Modified from Pollack MM, Getson PR, Ruttimann UE et al: Efficiency of intensive care: a comparative analysis of eight pediatric intensive care units, *JAMA* 258:1481, 1987. Copyright 1987, American Medical Association.

and software. The time requirements are more extensive, however. Evaluations of ICU utilization generally take 10 to 15 minutes for every patient-day.

Evaluations of intensive care utilization require (1) a list of unique ICU therapies and (2) a method of assessing severity of illness. Unique therapies are those that are delivered only in the ICU, such as mechanical ventilation, vasoactive agent infusion, dialysis for unstable patients, and treatment of life-threatening arrhythmias (cardioversion, defibrillation, antiarrhythmic infusions). There are unique therapy lists for pediatric patients (Table 61-4).[9,11] In most studies, these therapies have been taken from the TISS score; however, individual ICUs can determine their own lists of unique ICU therapies. Monitoring modalities generally carried out in the intensive care unit (e.g., arterial catheters) should not be included as unique therapies. Monitoring philosophies differ widely. In the context of utilization review, monitoring that does not lead to a unique ICU therapy or detect a threshold value of severity of illness (see below), was probably not required.

The second requirement for evaluation of ICU utilization is a measure of severity of illness. Increasing physiologic instability correlates to increasing risk of requiring an active ICU therapy. We estimate the risk of requiring an active ICU therapy using the acute (< 24 hour) mortality risk measured with the DORA score (see above). An acute mortality risk of $< 1\%$ indicates a very low likelihood of requiring a unique therapy.

Using the preceding information, the following new terms can be defined (Table 61-5): *Monitor patients* are those who do not use a unique therapy during any portion of their ICU stay. *Low-risk, monitor patients* are monitor patients with daily mortality risks under 1% during every ICU day. *Potential early-discharge patients* are those who did use a unique ICU therapy or had an acute mortality risk over 1% during the early portion of their ICU stay, but whose last, consecutive days of ICU stay extend into a period identical to low-risk, monitor patients (no unique therapy and low risk).[11] Efficiency is defined, using days of care, as follows:

Efficiency = ([Total patient days of care] −
[days of low-risk, monitor patients] − [days of
potential early-discharge])/(total patient days of care).

Therefore, efficient utilization of ICUs requires that most patients are either at risk to need a unique therapy in the ICU or are receiving such a therapy.

Studies using these concepts indicate that there is a clear disparity among pediatric ICUs in the efficiency of their bed utilization.[11] In a study of eight pediatric ICUs, low-risk, monitor patients constituted between 16% and 58% of the patient populations, and these patients used from 5.4% to 34.5% of the total days of care. Potential early-discharge patients constituted from 12% to 29% of the patient populations, and their days of care ranged from 5.1% to 17.2% of the total days of care. Most important, efficiency ratings ranged from .89 to .55, with four ICUs having efficiency ratings greater than .8 and four having efficiency ratings of less than .8. This disparity in efficiency strongly indicates that costly pediatric ICU resources are being utilized with substantial differences among hospitals. Some pediatric ICUs are using their resources for many more patients who do not require their services (low-risk, monitor patients) or could be discharged sooner (potential early-discharge patients) without compromising care, than are other ICUs. If cost-containment initiatives are to make major impacts in pediatric ICUs, eliminating costly care for patients "too healthy to benefit," such as these patient groups, is a logical effort.

It is important to recognize that evaluations of

Table 61–5 New ICU cost containment definitions

Term	Definition
Unique ICU therapy	Therapy best accomplished in the ICU.
Monitor patient	Patient who did not receive a unique ICU therapy.
Low-risk	Risk of requiring a unique ICU therapy very low (e.g., acute [<24 hr] mortality risk is <1%).
Potential early-discharge patient	Patient who did receive a unique ICU therapy or was not at low-risk during the initial portion of the ICU stay, but whose ICU stay extended into a period of low-risk, monitor status on the last consecutive day(s) of ICU stay.
Efficiency	[(Total patient days of care) − (days of low-risk, monitor patients) − (days of potential early-discharge)]/ (total patient days of care).

inefficient users of intensive care services have not been designed to have direct clinical use. Physician decision making must incorporate many facts—about the patient's disease, the possibility of acute, life-threatening events, and the hospital's facilities and abilities outside the intensive care unit. However, evaluations of efficiency will enable intensive care units to compare their performances with those of other institutions. If institutions are functioning in a very inefficient manner, they may reevaluate their admission and discharge criteria, as well as other hospital services, to enable more efficient utilization of the ICU. If these units have too many low-risk, monitor patients, potential early-discharge patients, or low efficiency rates, creation of an intermediate care unit, emphasizing the services for which these patients were admitted to the ICU, may improve ICU utilization. This type of evaluation would be most beneficial prior to costly ICU bed expansion.

REFERENCES

1. Dawes RM, Faust D, Meehl PE: Clinical versus actuarial judgement, *Science* 243:1668-1674, 1989.
2. Eichelberger MR, Mangubat A, Sacco WS et al: Comparative outcomes of children and adults suffering blunt trauma, *J Trauma* 28:430, 1988.
3. Flora JD: A method for comparing survival of burn patients to a standard survival curve, *J Trauma* 18:701-705, 1978.

4. Klem SA, Pollack MM, Glass NL et al: Resource use, efficiency, and outcome prediction in pediatric intensive care of trauma patients, *J Trauma* 30:32-36, 1990.

5. Knaus WA, Draper EA, Wagner DP et al: An evaluation of outcome from intensive care in major medical centers, *Ann Intern Med* 104:410, 1986.

6. Lemeshow S, Hosmer DW: A review of goodness-of-fit statistics for use in the development of logistic regression models, *Am J Epidemiol* 115:92, 1982.

7. Perkins HS, Jonsen AR, Epstein WV: Providers as predictors: using outcome predictions in intensive care, *Crit Care Med* 14:105, 1986.

8. Pollack MM, Ruttimann UE, Getson PR: The pediatric risk of mortality (PRISM) score, *Crit Care Med* 16:1110, 1988.

9. Pollack MM, Ruttimann UE, Glass NL: Monitoring patients in pediatric intensive care, *Pediatrics* 76:719, 1985.

10. Pollack MM, Alexander SR, Clarke N et al: Comparison of tertiary and nontertiary intensive care: a statewide comparison, *Crit Care Med* 19, 1991.

11. Pollack MM, Getson PR, Ruttimann UE et al: Efficiency of intensive care: a comparative analysis of eight pediatric intensive care units, *JAMA* 258:1481, 1987.

12. Pollack MM, Katz RW, Ruttimann UE et al: Improving the outcome and efficiency of pediatric intensive care: the impact of an intensivist, *Crit Care Med* 16:11-17, 1988.

13. Pollack MM, Ruttimann UE, Getson PR et al: Accurate prediction of the outcome of pediatric intensive care: a new quantitative method, *N Engl J Med* 316:134, 1987.

14. Ruttimann UE, Pollack MM: Dynamic objective risk assessment (DORA) score, *Crit Care Med* 1991.

15. Ruttimann UE, Albert A, Pollack MM et al: Dynamic assessment of severity of illness in pediatric intensive care, *Crit Care Med* 14:214, 1986.

16. Shackford SR, Mackersie RC, Hoyt DB et al: Impact of a trauma system on outcome of severely injured patients, *Arch Surg* 122:523, 1987.

17. Tversky A, Kahneman D: Judgement under uncertainty: heuristics and biases, *Science* 185:1124, 1974.

18. Wilkinson JD, Pollack MM, Ruttimann UE et al: Outcome of pediatric patients with multiple organ system failure, *Crit Care Med* 14:271-274, 1986.

19. Yeh TS, Pollack MM, Ruttimann UE et al: Validation of a physiologic stability index for use in critically ill infants and children, *Pediatr Res* 18:445, 1984.

62 Legal Considerations

Melinda G. Murray and Amy R. Templeton

For the in-house hospital lawyer, who is exposed to every kind of medical malpractice claim, those arising out of care in the emergency room or trauma unit are the most troubling. This is so because the mistakes made in these areas are often understandable, under the circumstances, yet often difficult to defend. In fact, of the myriad legal issues that arise in trauma care and emergency medicine, the issue that looms largest is the threat of malpractice. Hospital trauma units and emergency rooms are increasingly fertile grounds for malpractice suits. The reason lies in the nature of trauma and emergency care and the types of situations and children who are treated.

1. The type of child seen in the trauma unit or emergency room ranges from one with the flu who lacks a primary care physician, to the motor vehicle crash victim with a critical head injury. Even in non-trauma cases, care is often complicated by the fact that a child's condition may change rapidly. Care for victims of the most severe trauma involves working with a multidisciplinary team of perhaps 10 to 15 people, including x-ray technicians, surgeons, anesthesiologists, nurses, respiratory therapists, and social workers. This makes communication essential, but difficult, in the press of time and in situations of inadequate staffing.

2. A physician can rarely spend much time with an emergency room patient. He or she therefore does not have the opportunity to develop the level of trust that fosters a strong physician-patient relationship that might survive a misdiagnosis or other kind of error.

3. The emergency room is the busiest unit in a hospital. In one metropolitan emergency room that logs more than 50,000 visits a year, the staff saw 278 patients in one 24-hour period—a record for that unit, but illustrative of the need for quick decision making. The sheer volume of children, coupled with the fact that many of these patients arrive between 5:00 PM and 5:00 AM, or when the number of attending physicians physically present is dramatically reduced, places great demands on emergency room personnel and poses substantial staffing challenges.

4. In severe trauma cases, every second counts. Physicians must make instantaneous decisions, often without the benefit of reflection or even an accurate or complete history. Furthermore, the information they receive may be by telephone, may be second- or third-hand, or may be delivered by a hysterical parent in a stream-of-consciousness explanation.

5. A parent's guilty conscience may be a factor in emergency room malpractice claims. Parents sometimes feel guilty because the "accident" was preventable, or because they should have brought the child into the hospital sooner or, as in abuse cases, because a parent actually contributed to or caused the injury.

6. Crowded conditions, long waits, and a triage system that does not treat children on a first-come, first-serve basis, breeds resentment and hostility on the part of children and parents. Sometimes children leave without actually seeing a physician, often with disastrous results.

7. Because the child is in a hospital equipped with state-of-the-art ancillary, high-tech services, expectations about treatment outcome are high. Thus, any failure to meet these expectations is a setup for a lawsuit.

MAJOR RISK MANAGEMENT ISSUES

Risk management issues in the trauma unit or emergency room fall into four main categories: (1) failure to diagnose or treat, (2) documentation errors, (3) communication problems, and (4) transport issues. Each of these is discussed below.

Failure to diagnose or treat

Failure to diagnose is the most common risk management issue in the emergency room. Indeed, our experience is that it may account for as many as 80% of emergency room claims. Given the number of children a trauma center sees annually, it is to be expected that a certain percentage of those will file suit for a missed diagnosis. Because of the high volume of children, and because the symptoms of a serious infection may mimic a garden-variety viral infection, or garden-variety symptoms may mask a serious disorder, an emergency room physician may miss the appendicitis, meningitis, epiglottitis, obstruction, or arrhythmia with unusual presenting symptoms. Usually, these mistakes are not costly because the child is either admitted or returns a day or so later with more severe complaints, at which time the correct diagnosis is made. The question in a subsequent lawsuit is, was there a failure to exercise the care of a reasonably competent trauma specialist or emergency room physician—not measured against the best diagnostician, but against the norm of emergency rooms or trauma centers?

The second element, one often forgotten by the patient, is whether he or she was damaged as a result of the missed or incorrect diagnosis. Not surprisingly, the cases in which hospitals have paid small amounts for missed diagnosis arise when the missed diagnosis results in no damage or simply in a delay in treatment (for example, failure to take an x-ray for a jaw fracture). A physician may completely miss the diagnosis of an appendicitis, but if there is no damage, there is no case. Damage may consist of a ruptured appendix, resulting in a prolonged hospitalization and the risk of future obstruction caused by adhesions. A savvy plaintiff's lawyer will have his or her expert say that the appendix had *not* ruptured as of the first visit, and that the 24- or 48-hour delay was the cause of the injury. In that context, it may be that by the second visit the appendix had not ruptured, but there had been additional delay in obtaining blood, providing intravenous fluids, obtaining a surgical consultation, and starting antibiotics, which may be crucial. Had the diagnosis been made on the first day, the preoperative delays may not have been an issue.

The importance of timing is illustrated by a recent jury trial involving a failure to diagnose meningitis. The patient was a 12-year-old child first seen with a 1-day history of aches and pain, fever, an episode of talking nonsense (but no persistent confusion), an episode of vomiting (but no diarrhea), and an episode of synocopy while in the hospital. A physical examination revealed a supple neck, and an orthostatic examination was equivocal. The child's temperature was 39.3° C. The emergency room physician considered meningitis, drew a blood culture, and began intravenous administration of fluids, because she thought the illness was more likely viral flu or hypovolemia. Laboratory results of blood tests showed a white blood cell count of 12,000 with 50 segs, 28 bands.

After 4 hours of hydration, the child said he felt better and was taking fluids. He was discharged 5 hours after coming to the emergency room, with instructions to drink fluids and to return if he felt worse. He returned to the emergency room 30 hours later with leg stiffness, nuchal rigidity, and ringing in his ears. The culture that had been drawn eventually revealed *Neisseria meningitis*. The child suffered profound hearing loss in one ear—normal in the middle range, with profound loss in the upper range and mild loss in the lower range. Despite expert testimony by a leading infectious disease expert that the child did not exhibit signs of meningitis on the first visit and that he could have gone on to suffer a hearing loss regardless of antibiotic treatment, the jury awarded the plaintiff $1,250,000.

This case also illustrates an important point about claims involving the emergency room: return visits to the emergency room greatly increase the risk of liability, owing to the expectation that a specialized staff and high-tech equipment will make the diagnosis. Furthermore, in contrast to those of some other specialties, such as cardiac surgery or neurosurgery, the medicine and liability issues involved in emergency room treatment can be grasped by a jury fairly readily.

This case also highlights the agonizing position of the physician in regard to every emergency room patient. It is impossible to admit every child, even though in the differential diagnosis process, serious illness requiring hospitalization is bound to be considered. Is it enough to say, "When in doubt, treat and admit," as plaintiffs' experts would have you believe? Of course, there are doubts with almost every emergency case. Given the scarcity of medical resources and concern about overutilization of these resources, such a practice makes no sense. Perhaps a better way to make these difficult decisions is to adopt a "sliding-scale" approach. That is, the greater the potential damage if the test or therapy is not performed, and the less intensive and less costly the test or therapy, the more necessary it is to perform or administer it. But no matter what approach is used, the element of professional judgment is determinative. The court instructs juries that a physician should not be held liable for exercising professional judgment.

Documentation errors

The other major category of risk management issues in the trauma center or emergency room is documentation, or lack thereof. From a plaintiff's and, frequently, a jury's perspective, if a physician does not document his or her good care, it did not happen. Documentation must be timely, accurate, thorough, and objective. The level of detail should reflect the fact that minutes and hours in the emergency room may be the equivalent of days in an inpatient unit.

Aside from deliberate alteration of a medical record, which could result in punitive damages, the absence of documentation is the most costly error in medical charts. In a recent case, a note in the chart of a 3-month-old who died of sudden infant death syndrome (SIDS) cost a hospital $85,000 ($25,000 to settle and $60,000 in fees for experts and attorneys). The resident who examined the child for a complaint of bleeding from the nose not only performed a complete physical examination, but then performed an endoscopy procedure. None of this was documented on the emergency room sheet. When the baby was returned to the hospital 12 hours later in full arrest and eventually died, the resident wrote an "addendum" documenting the complete examination. It was better than no note, but had the case gone to trial, it would have looked as if it were written because the child had died, not to document actual care. A less credible witness than the resident might have had a harder time convincing a lawyer or jury that the examination had actually been performed. As it was, the hospital still had to spend substantial monies that could have been saved had the note been written at the time the child was first seen. The moral of the story is good documentation prevents or minimizes lawsuits.

Communication problems

The third area of risk is miscommunication or lack of communication. Recognizing that a person or family in the emergency room is severely stressed goes a long way in establishing the kind of rapport that might prevent a lawsuit. Listening to the child, or to the person who brings the child to the emergency room, can also assist in reaching a diagnosis. For example, if the caregiver of a child with Down syndrome questions the use of a laryngoscopy because of the child's severe reflux problems, the physician should pay attention. If a patient's family states he has been seen by another service, such as cardiology, their statement should be credited and that service should be consulted when the child is seen in the emergency room with chest and abdominal pain. Likewise, if a mother brings in a 3-month-old on two consecutive nights at 3:00 AM, with the same symptoms, a physician should consider that as part of the clinical picture.

Conversely, a child or a family member known to a service or department as an unreliable historian should not necessarily be relied upon to give an accurate report of symptoms in an emergency. Consider the case of a 10-year-old girl who had been followed for a year after resection of an abdominal tumor. One Friday night, after a week of chemotherapy, she arrived at the hospital with colicky abdominal pain and vomiting. The emergency room physician performed a physical examination and found no positive symptoms of obstruction other than tenderness on deep palpation. The phy-

sician did not order an abdominal x-ray, but consulted with the oncologist on call. Their joint conclusion was that the child was suffering the ill effects of chemotherapy, and the child went home with her mother. The oncologist conscientiously contacted the child's mother three times over the weekend. The mother, who had originally brought her child in so late for tumor evaluation that the child looked pregnant, kept saying the child was no worse. Two days after the first visit she brought the child into the emergency room, dead on arrival. As soon as the physician saw her, he realized how seriously dehydrated the child was and how far off the mother had been in her reports. The diagnosis at autopsy was volvulus and primary peritonitis. At the time of this writing, the plaintiff had sued for 30 million dollars.

Listening and talking to the child can also assist in reducing a family's high expectations. In a survey done by I.A. Lewis in April 1990 for the *Los Angeles Times*, 43% of the responses placed concern as the foremost characteristic of a good physician, equal to ability. Children are most likely to express satisfaction when the doctor discovers and deals with the child's concerns and expectations, when his or her manner communicates concern, and when the doctor explains things in understandable terms. According to a study by Barbara Korsch at Children's Hospital of Los Angeles, gaps in physician-patient communications exist when there is a lack of friendliness or warmth on the part of the physician, the physician does not take into account the parents' concerns or expectations, or does not give a clear explanation of the illness.[1]

The need to listen also extends to the transfer setting, when the duty to inquire does not end simply because the person at the other end of the telephone is another hospital, nurse, or physician. It is common for the referring physician or institution not to tell the accepting institution how sick the child really is. In such a situation, the person who has the child and is assessing him would be primarily liable for negligence, but the accepting institution may be secondarily liable for not asking the right questions and for providing inadequately staffed transport.

A relevant example is the case of a 3-week-old who was being seen by a private pediatrician. The pediatrician had been concerned about the infant's weight loss for about a week. He had the baby in his office and called the hospital emergency room, asking that the baby be seen, and describing weight loss and listlessness. The pediatrician told the child's mother to take the baby by car to the emergency room. The baby and mother waited in the emergency room approximately 10 minutes without triage. The mother told the triage nurse that the baby was very sick and, when the nurse looked, the baby was blue and emaciated. The baby coded and died 40 minutes later of congenital adrenal hyperplasia. The mother blamed the hospital for not treating the baby more quickly, despite the fact that she and her child had spent only 10 minutes in the emergency room. The tape in the emergency room communication center confirmed the referring pediatrician's relatively low-key approach to the baby's condition. The question remained as to whether the accepting physician should have asked more questions and whether triage nurses should examine every child as soon as he or she comes into the emergency room.

Transport issues

Despite the prevalence of emergency helicopter transports, there are few guidelines or standards of care describing the type of equipment or level of personnel needed for various categories of patients, aside from those dealing with institutions setting up a trauma team. Until national standards are established, trauma centers that have their own transports should attempt to write guidelines for the number of personnel, the level of training, and the type of equipment that will be needed. For example, is a nurse experienced in intubation sufficient for the transport of a child with an unstable airway? Should the helicopter be equipped with monitors?

And what of the designated trauma center that uses helicopters or aircraft of other institutions in the system? How can it control the quality of these transport personnel? Whether a hospital arranges for or provides its own transport, it will be responsible for providing at least one Level I paramedic trained in airway management. In 1990 the parents of a 3-year-old who died in transit to a tertiary care center to be treated for epiglottitis obtained a $350,000 settlement from the transferring community hospital, its anesthesiologist, its CRNA, and the accepting hospital. A transport service not usually used by the accepting hospital had been called because the primary carrier was unavailable. The only personnel on board were a pilot and a paramedic with no experience in airway management. Apparently, the child's endotracheal tube dislodged as she was being loaded onto the helicopter. She did a barrel roll and vomited. Instead of being taken back to the operating room for reintubation, she was given another dose of fentanyl, the tube was "replaced," and the CRNA testified that he heard breathing sounds despite the clattering, whirring blades of the helicopter. Although the accepting hospital knew none of these facts, it was forced to pay a large portion of the settlement on the theory that, having undertaken to arrange

the transport, it was responsible for providing safe transport with properly trained personnel on board. Thus, it is the obligation of the institution that arranges transport to find out what it needs to know about a child's condition to determine the appropriate method of transport. The accepting institution should also tell the physicians at the transferring hospital how to prepare an unstable child for transport. In such cases, the trauma center is viewed as the expert and therefore must provide a high level of care.

OTHER LEGAL ISSUES

Physicians in the emergency room or trauma unit may face other difficult legal issues in addition to risk management and malpractice concerns. Consider the following situation: The telephone rings in the communication center of a regional trauma center in a major metropolitan area. A 15-year-old female has been shot in the abdomen on the school playground, possibly as a result of her involvement in a drug deal. The school has attempted to reach the girl's mother, but has not yet located her. The girl's father is unknown. It appears that the girl is pregnant and may be an intravenous drug abuser. She has no health insurance.

This situation presents trauma personnel with several important legal issues and questions: consent to treatment, a hospital's obligation to treat emergency patients regardless of whether they have insurance or can pay for treatment, obligation to report gunshot wounds, confidentiality concerning certain conditions such as pregnancy, and the risk to health care professionals of exposure to HIV.

The rest of this chapter addresses two of the issues raised in this situation—consent to treatment and duty to treat. Other legal issues, such as HIV exposure, organ donation, and disposal of dead bodies, are not unique to the emergency room or trauma unit and are therefore not included.

Consent to treatment

Most states have statutes that address consent to emergency medical and surgical treatment of children. Under these statutes, consent may be implied or presumed when it is not possible, owing to time constraints or the unavailability of parents, to obtain parental consent and when failure to treat would "substantially increase the risk to the minor's life, health, mental health, or welfare, or would unduly prolong suffering."[2] In addition, many hospitals have policies that allow a physician to treat an emergency patient with the concurrence of another physician. The focus, however, must be on the child's need for immediate medical intervention to prevent death, serious bodily impairment, or, at a minimum, great pain or suffering.

Failure to obtain proper consent may become an issue in a lawsuit if (1) the child's parents' religious or other beliefs prohibit a particular treatment (for example, a Jehovah's Witness's refusal to consent to a blood transfusion), (2) the procedure will result in long-term impairment (for example, amputation of a limb), or (3) the outcome is poor. Thus, the reasons for failing to obtain consent, attempts to contact the parent or guardian, and the nature of the threat to health, its immediacy and magnitude, should all be thoroughly documented in the chart.

Through case law or legislation, a majority of states have adopted, in addition to the "emergency" exception, an "emancipated minor" exception that allows a child who meets certain criteria (for example, is self-supporting, married, or serving in the armed forces) to consent to medical treatment. In addition, some states recognize a "mature minor" exception to the parental consent requirement that allows a minor to consent to treatment if he or she is capable of understanding the nature, extent, and consequences of the proposed treatment. Many states also allow minors to consent to certain health services related to pregnancy or its prevention or termination, substance abuse, mental health, or sexually transmitted diseases.

If a minor is treated in the emergency department under one of the above exceptions, the physician may still be faced with the dilemma of whether to inform the child's parents of the treatment. Some statutes that allow minors to be treated for certain conditions, such as sexually transmitted diseases, without parental consent prohibit a physician from notifying parents of such treatment without the child's consent. On the other hand, a physician may be required to report treatment of some of these conditions to public authorities (for instance, communicable diseases, child abuse, or gunshot or stab wounds).

Although obtaining proper consent is important, failure to obtain consent should not prevent the administration of proper medical treatment. Because of the potentially disastrous consequences, a physician is more likely to be sued for refusal to treat than for treating without proper consent. Thus, the better rule from a risk management, as well as medical, perspective is, when in doubt, treat, but document carefully the circumstances surrounding the absence of parental consent.

Duty to treat

Federal law (the so-called "antidumping" or COBRA [Consolidated Omnibus Budget Reconciliation Act] statute)[3] requires all hospital emergency rooms to treat and stabilize or arrange for an appropriate transfer of patients with an "emergency medical condition"[4] or who are in active labor, regardless of their ability to pay. The patient can be transferred only after he or she is stabilized. Certain hospitals, such as regional referral centers and trauma units, are required to accept all appropriate transfer patients who require specialized care as long as they have the capacity to treat the persons. For this reason, COBRA mandates may be of less concern for a specialized facility, such as a pediatric trauma unit, than for a community hospital.

Sanctions for violating the antidumping statute are severe, including revocation of a hospital's participation in the Medicare-Medicaid program and stiff fines. In 1989 the Office of the Inspector General (OIG) of Health and Human Services assessed a $20,000 fine against a Texas obstetrician for transferring a severely hypertensive pregnant woman to a distant hospital.[5] In addition, the Health Care Financing Administration (HCFA), the agency primarily responsible for enforcing COBRA, has issued several Notices of Termination threatening to terminate hospitals from the Medicare-Medicaid program unless they can refute the alleged COBRA violations and provide satisfactory assurance of future compliance.[6] Even if a hospital survives an investigation by HCFA or the OIG, the adverse publicity generated by a government inquiry can severely affect a hospital's public image and standing in the community.

Most of the COBRA cases to date involve elderly or pregnant patients, but the problem is obviously one with which a pediatric hospital should be concerned as well. A recent Maryland case illustrates the application of COBRA to pediatric facilities. A 3-year-old with a history of seizures was seen in the emergency room of a pediatric facility. Because the pediatric intensive care unit (PICU) at that facility was full, the hospital referred the child to a children's hospital located in another state approximately 60 miles away. But when, after a brief delay, a patient was moved out of the PICU to provide a bed for the 3-year-old, the child was admitted to the Maryland hospital. The family sued, claiming the hospital had a duty of care under COBRA to provide a bed for an emergency patient. The Maryland Court of Special Appeals held that the Maryland hospital had no obligation to admit the child when it could not provide an appropriate level of care, saying that a hospital cannot be placed in a position where the admission of an additional patient will jeopardize the care of existing patients.[7]

Some commentators believe that COBRA will produce an explosion of lawsuits.[8] But even without COBRA, a physician is vulnerable to a charge of abandonment in a malpractice action if he or she fails to stabilize a patient before discharging him. To avoid such liability, physicians should always provide written instructions to patients regarding follow-up care when appropriate to the diagnosis, and such instructions should, in simple but precise words, tell the family to come back if certain symptoms appear or persist, or other events occur. The legal guardian of a child patient should sign the instruction sheet, indicating that he or she has received the follow-up instructions and understands them.

Most hospitals have enacted policies to implement COBRA, including signs informing patients of their rights under COBRA, patient transfer-discharge forms and checklists, and other documentation requirements. Educational programs to acquaint emergency room personnel with these policies and requirements constitute an important factor in decreasing liability in this area.

CONCLUSION

The keys to avoiding liability in the emergency room or trauma unit are the same as in other units: maintain good communication with the child and parents, give good medical care, and document that care thoroughly and completely. Inability to obtain adequate background information and lack of time within which to formulate carefully reasoned treatment decisions place the emergency room physician at great risk. Thus, in the emergency department, more than in any other department, good communication (giving *and* receiving information) and careful documentation are essential.

REFERENCES

1. Korsch B, Gozzi E, Francis V: *Pediatrics* 42:855-869, 1968.
2. District of Columbia Municipal Regulations ¶ 600.4 (1988).
3. Consolidated Omnibus Budget Reconciliation Act (COBRA) of 1985, Pub No 99-272, § 9121, 100 Stat 164-67, § 1867 of the Social Security Act (codified as amended at 42 USCA § 1395dd).
4. "Emergency medical condition" is defined as an illness so severe that lack of treatment will put the patient's health in serious jeopardy or will seriously impair bodily functions or organs. 42 USCA § 1395dd(e)(1).
5. *Inspector General v Burditt,* No C-42 (HHS Departmental Appeals Board, Civil Remedies Div, July 28, 1989).
6. Krugh T: Is COBRA poised to strike? A critical analysis of medical COBRA, *J Health Hospital Law* 23(6):165, June 1990.
7. *Davis v Johns Hopkins Hospital,* 86 Md App 134, 585 A.2d 841, 849, 1991.
8. Krugh, *Supra.*

PART SEVENTEEN

National SAFE KIDS Campaign

63 National SAFE KIDS Campaign

Cure for the disease*

Herta B. Feely and Esha Bhatia

*If a disease were killing our children in the
proportions that accidents are, people would be
outraged and demand that this killer be stopped.*
C. EVERETT KOOP, M.D., CHAIRMAN, NATIONAL SAFE
KIDS CAMPAIGN

Injury is the leading cause of death among children in the United States. More children die each year from injuries than from all childhood diseases combined.[8] Injuries cause 44% of all deaths in children ages 1 to 4, and 52% of all deaths in children ages 5 to 14.[4] Each year, more than 8000 children aged 14 and below are killed and 50,000 are permanently disabled.[7] Annually, injuries result in 360,000 hospitalizations and 10,400,000 emergency room visits.[2] This year alone one in four children will suffer a preventable injury serious enough to require medical attention.† Childhood injury death rates in this country are significantly higher than those found in most other industrialized countries for all but those 5 to 9 years old.[6]

The National SAFE KIDS Campaign was launched in January 1988 to help reduce the number of children who are disabled or killed as a result of unintentional injury. This chapter presents the National SAFE KIDS Campaign as one case study of a cure for the disease of unintentional pediatric trauma. It discusses the Campaign's unique combination of national and grassroots efforts to reduce childhood injury, as well as some of the specific programs that the Campaign has developed and undertaken in the areas of bicycle-related, scald burn, residential fire, and motor vehicle injuries.

The National SAFE KIDS Campaign is the first and only *nationwide* childhood injury prevention program, focusing on unintentional injury to children from birth to 14 years. The Campaign began in 1988 as a 5-year effort and has evolved into an ongoing campaign to reduce unintentional childhood injury (Fig. 63-1). The Campaign was initiated by Children's National Medical Center in Washington, D.C., with major support from the Johnson & Johnson Family of Companies. The National Safety Council provided additional funding in the first year. Now funding is derived from a variety of sources, including the private and public sectors.

A nationwide survey[1] conducted in December 1987 demonstrated that parents had little awareness of the dangers of unintentional injury to children and that many injuries could be prevented. The National SAFE KIDS Campaign was developed with the aim of reaching children, parents, and caregivers in order to reduce the incidence of childhood unintentional injury. Although a number of excellent local and state injury prevention programs did exist, they were scattered, largely underfunded, and lacked broad national impact. At the federal level, injury prevention programs were also underfunded. Specifically, injuries lead to twice as many life years lost (36 years) as cancer (16 years) and three times the number lost to heart disease and

---

*For more information about the National SAFE KIDS Campaign, please write to the National SAFE KIDS Campaign, Children's National Medical Center, 111 Michigan Avenue N.W., Washington, D.C. 20010-2970.

†Based on the number of children treated for injuries yearly (12,636,000 in 1985 according to the National Center for Health Statistics) divided by the total number of children under 15 in the United States (51,290,339 according to the U.S. Summary General Population Characteristics, PC80-1-B1, U.S. Bureau of the Census).

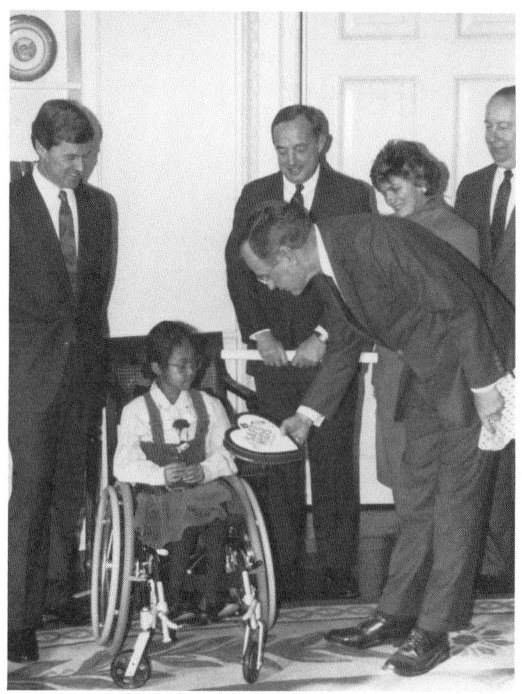

Figure 63–1 President Bush honors National SAFE KIDS Week, February 2-18, 1989. President Bush accepts a valentine from Kim Patterson, age 7, who was partially paralyzed in a car collision. To Patterson's right is Carl Spalding, president of Johnson & Johnson Dental Care Company. Standing behind President Bush are Dr. Martin R. Eichelberger, president of the National SAFE KIDS Campaign and director of trauma services at Children's National Medical Center; Herta B. Feely, the Campaign's executive director, and Donald L. Brown, president and CEO of Children's National Medical Center. (© by the National SAFE KIDS Campaign, 1991. Reprinted with permission.)

stroke (12 years). Yet, cancer research receives ten times more funding, and research on heart disease and stroke six times more federal funding than injury research.[5]

At the heart of the Campaign are State and Local Coalitions that share a common goal: to create safer homes and communities for children. There are now over 100 Local and State SAFE KIDS Coalitions in 40 states and the District of Columbia, and the number of Coalitions continues to grow. Each Coalition is comprised of local and state organizations and individuals working in communities to reduce childhood injury. In addition, the Campaign organized the National Coalition to Prevent Childhood Injury (NCPCI), consisting of more than 90 national organizations directly concerned with, or in contact with, children, parents, and caregivers. Member organizations include the American Academy of Pediatrics, the American Public Health As-

sociation, the Centers for Disease Control, the Boy Scouts of America, and the National PTA. NCPCI members help to identify local groups interested in launching and sustaining Local and State SAFE KIDS Coalitions. They also disseminate information on the Campaign and injury prevention strategies to their members.

The Campaign takes a multifaceted approach to injury prevention, incorporating coalition building, public policy, program development, and educational and media efforts. The Campaign's national office in Washington, D.C., coordinates national media efforts, advocates public policy, develops educational materials, and facilitates the development of Local and State Coalitions. The Campaign also produces comprehensive injury prevention strategies, secures financial donations and product discounts for the Coalitions, and provides training for and fosters communication and information sharing among the Coalitions.

The National SAFE KIDS Campaign focuses on five major unintentional injury risk areas for children: traffic injuries (motor vehicle—occupant, bicycle, and pedestrian), fire and burns, drownings, poisonings and chokings, and falls. The long-term goals of the Campaign are to work for change in adult and child behavior, in products, and in the environment to reduce the incidence of injury; to raise awareness among adults, especially parents and caregivers, that injuries are the leading health threat facing children today; to make childhood injury a public policy priority for federal, state, and local policymakers; and to change society's notion that "accidents" just happen, to the understanding that unintentional injuries are preventable through active (behavioral) and passive (environmental and legislative) interventions.

To meet its goals the National SAFE KIDS Campaign has five principal objectives:

1. Building long-term grassroots coalitions to implement childhood injury prevention strategies in states and communities nationwide
2. Focusing attention on and designing injury prevention strategies for children of low-income families, who, statistics show, are at highest risk for injuries
3. Collaborating with voluntary and governmental agencies to increase the level of monetary and other resources allocated to injury prevention programs and activities
4. Stimulating changes in environments, products, laws, and behaviors that will prevent injuries to children
5. Supporting and expanding on the 1990 and Year 2000 national health promotion and disease prevention objectives regarding unintentional childhood injury

These objectives are accomplished by working at the national and grassroots levels in four major areas: community-based childhood injury prevention coalitions, public policy, program development, and education and media, and by working to create partnerships with corporations in the fight to reduce childhood injury.

LOCAL AND STATE SAFE KIDS COALITIONS: COMMUNITY-BASED CHILDHOOD INJURY PREVENTION PROGRAMS

Local and State SAFE KIDS Coalitions are broad-based grassroots organizations working in their communities to reduce childhood injury. Each Coalition has a lead organization that commits a staff person to serve as coordinator and other resources necessary to build and sustain a unified approach to fight childhood injury. Lead organizations include children's and other hospitals, state and local health departments, state and local safety councils, and state and local chapters of other NCPCI member organizations.

Coalitions draw upon all segments of their communities—parents, children, medical and safety organizations, children's advocates, business leaders, teachers, enforcement agencies, elected officials, schools, civic groups, and the media—in order to change behavior, strengthen laws, and modify the environment to reduce childhood injury. Ongoing technical expertise is offered to the coalitions by the Campaign's Public Policy, Program, Media, and national Field departments.

Local and State SAFE KIDS Coalitions serve as primary vehicles for achieving community improvements in childhood injury prevention. The Coalitions work in several areas, including public policy, education, environmental change, and raising public awareness (Figs. 63-2 and 63-3). For example, some Coalitions have worked to improve their child safety-seat laws. In 1989 the Alabama SAFE KIDS Coalition successfully worked with the Alabama state legislature to raise the age of children who must be properly restrained while riding in an automobile from age 2 to age 5, thus extending coverage by the law to an additional 190,000 children. In Minnesota, the statewide SAFE KIDS Coalition responded to the deaths of several children by working toward the passage of a law regulating garage door openers. The new law, which went into effect on January 1, 1991, requires that all automatic garage door openers bought, sold, or installed in Minnesota meet a standard developed by the American National Standards Institute (ANSI). The law also stipulates that automatic door openers cannot be purchased or installed unless they incorporate a safety mechanism that

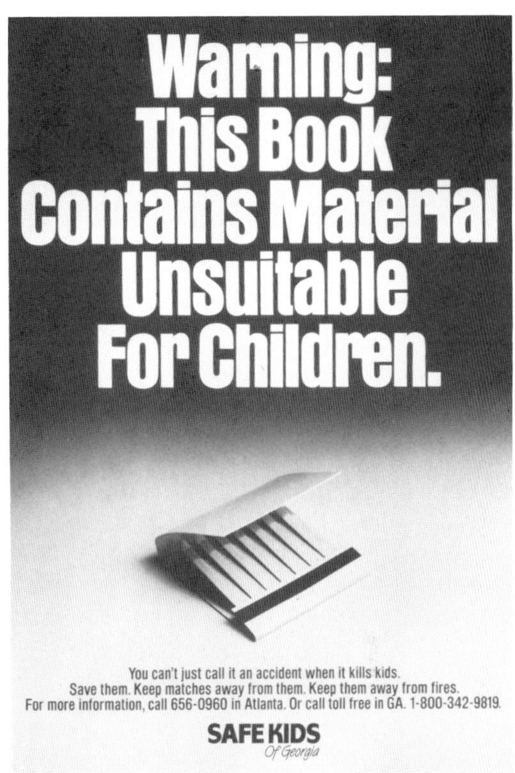

Figure 63–2 Print public service announcement produced by the Georgia SAFE KIDS Coalition. (© by the National SAFE KIDS Campaign, 1991. Reprinted with permission.)

automatically reverses the door within 2 seconds after it touches an object.

In addition, Coalitions in several communities have urged their local hospitals to ensure consistent use of E codes in hospital discharge summaries to aid in injury data collection.

Local and State SAFE KIDS Coalitions use several strategies to reach out to economically disadvantaged populations who are at greatest risk for unintentional childhood injury. First, Coalitions are encouraged to work closely with member organizations that have specific programs and resources designed to reach low-income populations. For example, many Coalitions have a state or local health department as their lead organization. These health departments often have staff members who focus on programs for the economically disadvantaged (such as WIC, AFDC, and Medicaid) and are also familiar with social service organizations with which Coalitions can work to reach these populations. Coalitions with health departments as the lead organization include Colorado, North Dakota, Virginia, North Carolina, and New Mexico (State SAFE KIDS Coalitions); Mobile and Montgomery, Alabama; Montgomery County, Maryland; and

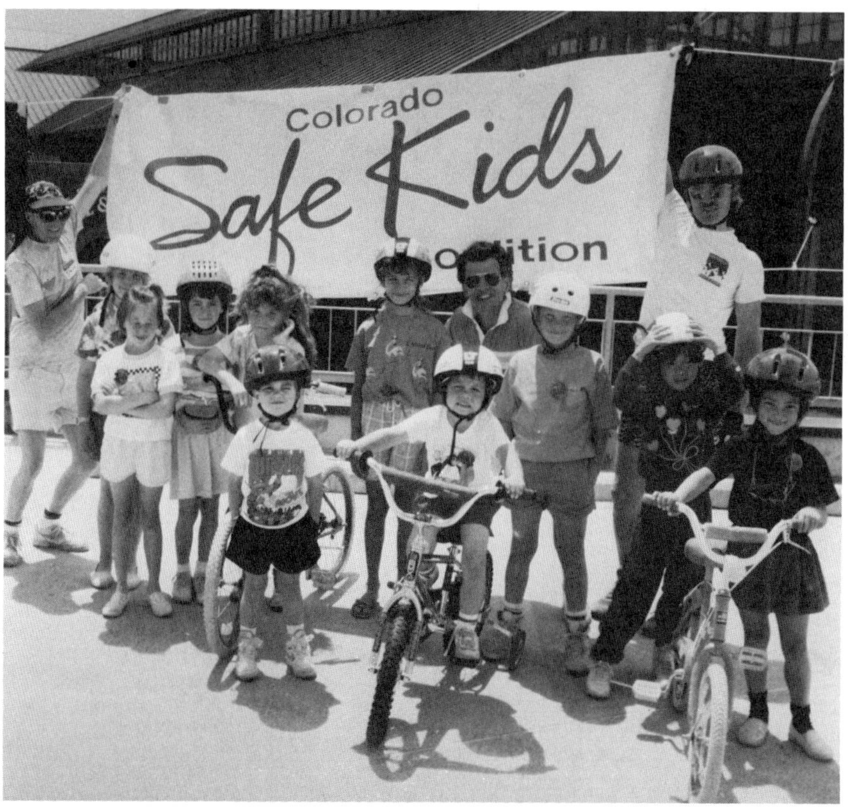

Figure 63–3 Even the smallest children wore helmets at the Colorado SAFE KIDS Coalition's Bicycle Jamboree. (© by the National SAFE KIDS Campaign, 1991. Reprinted with permission.)

Dalton, Savannah, and DeKalb, Georgia (Local SAFE KIDS Coalitions).

Second, Coalitions are encouraged to reach out in their communities and work with community groups that traditionally have had access to the target populations. These groups often have forums and scheduled meetings that Coalitions can use to make educational presentations and may provide a guaranteed audience that is more receptive to a message when it is sanctioned by the host organization. Most economically disadvantaged parents will not be reached through traditional community networks such as PTAs, civic clubs, and women's groups. Access will more likely be gained through other outlets, such as health care providers, ministries, and community and tenant organizations. These include group health organizations, Head Start and child-care centers, prenatal and postnatal clinics, and tenants' associations, unions, and Women, Infants, and Children (WIC) clinics.

Third, Coalitions are encouraged to reach out to economically disadvantaged populations through the appropriate local media. These might include Hispanic and black newspapers, cable television programs, and radio stations, as well as general media outlets.

National office support for Local and State SAFE KIDS Coalitions

The National SAFE KIDS Campaign staff provides Local and State SAFE KIDS Coalitions with multifaceted support, which ranges from phone consultations to written materials and on-site visits. With national support, the Coalitions collect data and information on childhood injury problems in their communities and implement targeted action plans to reduce the incidence of these injuries.

National support also includes the research and development of an annual childhood injury prevention strategy specifically tailored to meet the needs of the Coalitions, along with media and educational materials (audiovisual and print) in support of the injury risk area focus. The national office also works with the Coalitions to evaluate various components of each specific campaign. The Coalitions are also provided with information on safety products (for example, bicycle helmets, antiscald devices, smoke detectors) related to specific

Table 63-1 National SAFE KIDS CAMPAIGN publications

Leader's guide

A comprehensive guide to conducting grassroots injury prevention programs. Contains background material on the childhood injury issue and strategies for building and maintaining community-based injury prevention coalitions, developing partnerships with corporations and foundations, working with the media, influencing public policy, and evaluating injury prevention activities.

Bike helmet and bike safety strategy

A comprehensive guide to initiating a community-based bike helmet and bike safety awareness program. Contains guidelines for involving the community, reaching parents, caregivers, and kids, and evaluating the program, as well as a list of available resources.

Scald burn prevention strategy

A comprehensive guide for implementing a community-based scald burn prevention program. Provides guidelines for working to amend plumbing codes, conducting a project to retrofit housing with antiscald devices, educating parents and caregivers about scald burn prevention, raising public awareness through the media, and evaluating the program.

Project GET ALARMED: A residential fire strategy

A comprehensive guide for implementing a community-based residential fire detection program. Provides guidelines for promoting new or strengthening existing smoke-detector ordinances, conducting a smoke detector pick-up or installation project, educating parents and caregivers about the importance of the early detection of residential fires, raising public awareness through the media, and evaluating the program.

SAFE KIDS BUCKLE UP: A child occupant protection strategy

A comprehensive guide to implementing a multifaceted community-based child occupant protection program. Details the steps necessary to educate economically disadvantaged parents and caregivers about the need to increase use and reduce misuse of child safety seats and safety belts; increase economically disadvantaged families' access to child safety seats through discount and loan programs; strengthen existing child occupant protection laws and improve their enforcement; and raise public awareness through the media about: (1) the importance of increasing use and reducing misuse of child safety seats and safety belts; (2) the availability of seats through discount and loan programs; and (3) increased enforcement of child occupant protection laws.

Childhood injury prevention quarterly

A quarterly publication including case studies of injury prevention programs, interviews with leaders in the field, and synopses of articles from the injury prevention literature.

Campaign update

A bimonthly newsletter featuring SAFE KIDS activities and childhood injury prevention activities throughout the country.

---

injury interventions available to them, along with a quantity of the actual products. Ongoing technical assistance is provided to Coalitions implementing the strategy.

The national office designs and conducts periodic Coalition Coordinators' training conferences. These conferences are designed to provide in-depth training in the implementation of a newly developed injury prevention strategy, as well as to provide training in other areas, such as how to build and sustain community involvement, fundraising, data collection, and evaluation. In addition, the national office holds symposia and conferences designed to bring together Local and State SAFE KIDS Coalition Coordinators, NCPCI members,

and injury prevention specialists. The first symposium "Uniting America to Prevent Childhood Injury" was held in 1989. In May 1992, the Campaign sponsored "SAFE KIDS 2000," a national conference on childhood injury prevention.

The national staff also provides Coalitions with two free publications, *Campaign Update* and *Childhood Injury Prevention Quarterly* (Table 63-1). *Campaign Update,* issued every other month, updates the Coalitions on local, state, and national Campaign activities and on childhood injury prevention activities throughout the country. *Childhood Injury Prevention Quarterly,* published four times a year, is aimed at enhancing Coalition members' knowledge of injury prevention and improving their leadership skills. It includes case studies of injury prevention programs, interviews with leaders in the field, and synopses of articles from the injury prevention literature.

PUBLIC POLICY

The National SAFE KIDS Campaign's public policy efforts endeavor to influence the laws, regulations, and institutional policies that help to determine this country's safety agenda for children. The public policy goals and objectives are designed to coincide with the Campaign's long-term goal to make childhood injury prevention a public policy priority for federal, state, and local lawmakers and are developed in conjunction with the National Coalition to Prevent Childhood Injury. A public policy committee meets quarterly to draw on the expertise of NCPCI member organizations and elected officials at all levels. The Campaign urges public policy changes through the following suggestions.

1. Product manufacturers, regulatory agencies, and standards-setting bodies can help to establish tough mandatory safety standards for the design, production, and use of consumer products. For example, during its first year the Campaign (with other organizations) was able to secure the agreement of the Gas Appliance Manufacturers Association (GAMA) to preset all newly built water heaters at 125° F, reducing the probability of tap-water scald burns to children.

An important policy objective of the National SAFE KIDS Campaign has been the establishment of mandatory national bike-helmet standards for children and adults. There are currently no mandatory national standards for the manufacture of adult and child bicycle helmets, although two voluntary standards do exist. In May 1989, the Campaign and 34 members of the NCPCI petitioned the U.S. Consumer Product Safety Commission (CPSC) to establish mandatory safety standards for bicycle helmets. The petition outlined the deficiencies of current voluntary safety standards for helmets. Of primary concern was the lack of standardized testing procedures for adult and child helmets.

Following a recommendation from its staff, the Commission voted (2 to 1) to deny the petition on July 30, 1991. The Campaign has disputed the Commission's denial in letters to the commissioners and through newspaper editorials printed across the country. The Campaign plans to continue its pursuit of mandatory safety standards for bicycle helmets through legislative and regulatory processes.

At the request of the National SAFE KIDS Campaign and several members of the National Coalition to Prevent Childhood Injury, CPSC recently

voted to publish an advance notice of proposed rul making to address the hazards posed by balloons small balls, and marbles and to require warnin labels for toys and other products intended for chil dren ages 3 through 6. The Commission recentl granted a petition to issue mandatory regulation addressing the risks of strangulation presented b certain crib toys. The petition was also submitte by members of the NCPCI.

2. Legislators can enact laws mandating certai product safety standards or establishing require ments of public behavior (such as wearing se belts). They can also designate increased fundin for injury prevention research and programs. T focus national attention on the number of childre killed and severely disabled each year by uninten tional injuries, the Senate Subcommittee on Chil dren, Family, Drugs, and Alcoholism held hearing on childhood injury on February 9, 1989. Re quested by the Campaign, and with the support o the subcommittee chairman, Senator Christophe Dodd (D-Conn.), these hearings were designed t uncover areas where federal legislation could en hance injury prevention efforts in the United States Campaign Chairman Dr. C. Everett Koop and Pres ident Dr. Martin R. Eichelberger testified befor the subcommittee during the landmark hearings along with Commissioner Anne Graham of th U.S. Consumer Product Safety Commission an Dr. Mark Widome, a member of the Campaign' technical advisory board and chairman of th American Academy of Pediatrics Injury and Poiso Prevention Committee.

One example of injury prevention legislation en acted at the national level is the regulation of au tomatic residential garage door openers. The Con sumer Product Safety Improvement Act of 199(includes a provision requiring that each automati residential garage door opener manufactured on o after January 1, 1991, conform to the entrapmen protection standards developed by the America National Standards Institute. The provision sets national standard of protection from the risk o injury associated with automatic residential garag door openers that preempts any state law whos standards fall below those designated in the ne federal law. The law is similar to a more compre hensive law passed through the efforts of the Min nesota SAFE KIDS Coalition. The Campaign ac tively supported the passage of the federa legislation through a letter-writing campaign b State and Local SAFE KIDS Coalitions.

The National SAFE KIDS Campaign, in coop eration with members of the NCPCI, also helpe to secure the passage of the Trauma Care System Planning and Development Act of 1990. This bil provides matching funds to states for developing implementing, and monitoring statewide trauma-care system plans. The funds will be designated for rural areas that do not have access to emergency 911 phone services, basic life support services, or advanced life support services. The new law also requires the U.S. Department of Health and Human Services to develop a model trauma-care system plan and establish an Advisory Council on Trauma Care Systems to assess periodically the country's trauma care needs. In addition, a National Clearinghouse on Emergency Medical Services and Trauma Care will be established to collect, compile, and disseminate information and to provide technical assistance to states and local agencies.

The National SAFE KIDS Campaign has been extremely active in the area of bicycle safety legislation. Since enactment of the first bicycle helmet law in California in 1986, state and local interest in developing mandatory bicycle helmet legislation has grown rapidly across the country. The national office has taken an active role in helping interested State and Local SAFE KIDS Coalitions to introduce and support mandatory bike helmet legislation in Howard and Montgomery Counties, Maryland, in New Jersey, and in Pennsylvania. The Campaign's public policy staff has developed a legislation chart that is updated quarterly to track the current legislative efforts relating to bicycle helmets at both the state and local levels. In the fall of 1991, the Campaign also submitted model mandatory bicycle helmet legislation to the State Council of Governments for consideration by state legislatures around the country.

In an effort to reduce traffic-related injuries to children nationwide, the Campaign is supporting the development of comprehensive passenger safety-belt and motorcycle helmet laws in all fifty states. The Campaign is also seeking improved safety features in automobiles, including driver and passenger-side airbags, antilock brakes, adjustable safety belts, and strengthened child booster seats.

As part of the Campaign's efforts to prevent fire deaths and injuries to children, the public policy department has identified key states that possess weak or nonexistent smoke detector laws. After assessing the potential of these states to implement comprehensive smoke detector legislation, the Campaign will draw upon the resources of its State and Local SAFE KIDS Coalitions and NCPCI members to advocate for comprehensive statewide smoke detector laws. To coincide with this goal on a national level, Executive Director Herta B. Feely and Assistant Director William C. Kamela have testified at congressional hearings to discuss the tremendous number of fire deaths and injuries to children and to support the need for residential smoke detector laws in all fifty states.

As part of the public policy department's goal to increase funding for federal injury prevention programs, the Campaign's public policy director testified in support of a $50 million appropriation for the U.S. Consumer Product Safety Commission. The U.S. Senate Appropriations Committee on Veteran Affairs, Housing and Urban Development, and Independent Agencies held a public hearing on the agency's budget needs in 1990.

The Campaign also supported the passage of the Head Start Expansion and Quality Improvement Act of 1990. The Act is intended to increase the amount of money available to train Head Start teachers, leading to further promotion of health and safety issues within the Head Start curriculum. The bill was enacted during the 101st Congress.

3. Public health administrators and other public officials can set policy that raises the priority of injury prevention. Wisconsin's Lieutenant Governor Scott McCallum headed a trauma and injury prevention task force, created in response to Campaign Chairman Dr. C. Everett Koop's request that states set up governors' task forces on childhood injury prevention. In June 1990, the Wisconsin task force released its report on trauma and injury prevention. The report contains an introduction to childhood injury, 84 injury-specific recommendations for control and prevention activities, and a summary of the task force's activities. In addition, the Wisconsin Department of Health and Social Services announced a new grant program in September 1990 for injury prevention efforts in communities throughout the state.

4. Code officials can enact model building and plumbing code language for adoption by states and localities. The Campaign has developed model plumbing code language to reduce tap-water scalds to children in the bathtub. The Campaign's amendment to the plumbing codes requires that an anti-scald device be installed in bathtub and shower fixtures in all new construction to automatically shut the water down to a trickle whenever it reaches 120° F. The Campaign has testified in support of the amendment at hearings for each of the major plumbing code-making bodies and has sent letters to code change committee members.

The Campaign's public policy department has made substantial progress in amending these codes. Most of the national and regional code-making bodies have amended their plumbing codes to require the installation of pressure-balancing or thermostatic control valves in all new construction of bathtubs and showers. The adopted amendments also require a maximum limit of 120° F on hot water heaters.

These organizations have come a long way in addressing the problem of tap-water scalds to children. The Campaign is encouraged by their willingness to work together to develop a solution. However, there is still work to be done. Individual states and localities must now adopt the plumbing code language developed by the national and regional code-making bodies.

Several states and localities have already initiated code changes in their areas. For example, the Ohio Board of Building Standards approved an antiscald amendment to the Ohio Plumbing Code in July 1991. The Campaign's public policy director provided testimony at the March 1991 hearing in support of the code revision.

The New York State legislature has taken an alternate approach to reducing tap-water scalds in the bathtub. The legislature introduced a bill that incorporates the Campaign's model plumbing code language during the 1990-1991 sessions. With widespread support from New York's Local SAFE KIDS Coalitions, the bill's Senate and Assembly sponsors expect to enact the antiscald legislation by the end of the 1992 session.

PROGRAM DEVELOPMENT

The National SAFE KIDS Campaign develops comprehensive community-based programs to reduce the incidence of unintentional childhood injury. These programs are developed specifically to meet the needs of the Campaign's State and Local SAFE KIDS Coalitions. Each year a specific injury-risk area focus is chosen and a comprehensive program or "strategy" developed. Each strategy incorporates efforts in four areas corresponding to the four *E*s of injury control: enactment-enforcement, engineering (technologic change), education-media, and evaluation. National and local-state objectives are developed in each of the four areas for the national office and the Coalitions.

In the Campaign's first year the focus was on increasing public awareness of the childhood injury problem, using the theme "SAFE KIDS Are No Accident." In 1989 the focus was on bicycle safety, and the Campaign launched a Bike Helmet and Bike Safety Awareness Strategy. Every year, more than 350,000 children are injured in bike-related incidents and require emergency room care. In bicycle collisions with motor vehicles, 400 children under age 15 are killed and another 34,000 injured each year. Forty percent of all bike-related deaths involve children 14 years old and younger.

The education-media aspects of the Bike Helmet and Bike Safety Awareness Strategy focused on raising parents', caregivers', and children's awareness of the ways in which bicycle-related injuries happen and of how bicycle helmets are an extremely effective means of reducing these injuries—reducing 85% of the risk of head injury. The enactment-enforcement and engineering aspects initially focused on petitioning the U.S. Consumer Product Safety Commission to establish a mandatory standard for the manufacture of bicycle helmets to replace the two existing voluntary standards established by the Snell Memorial Foundation and the American National Standards Institute. The Campaign's national office has also been working with several Local and State SAFE KIDS Coalitions to promote passage of mandatory helmet laws. Another aspect of the bicycle campaign has involved working with helmet manufacturers to reduce the cost of bicycle helmets through discount programs. The evaluation aspect of this campaign centers on process, impact, and outcome evaluations of the strategy. Several Coalitions have provided the national office with pre- and postintervention data on helmet use, helmet sales, and the incidence of bicycle injuries. Helmet use was measured through school-based self-report surveys and observational studies. Helmet sales were tracked through bicycle helmet distributors and direct sales at local bicycle shops. Coalitions also tracked bicycle injuries through E codes in hospitals.

Because burns constitute the leading form of childhood injury in the home (each year, burns kill 1300 children and disable three times as many),[3] the Campaign developed a dual-focus burn prevention campaign, launched in 1990. The Campaign's burn prevention efforts have been targeted at economically disadvantaged populations. For its Scald Burn Prevention Strategy, the Campaign's objectives have centered on educating parents and caregivers about how to prevent scald burns to children (education-media), encouraging Local and State SAFE KIDS Coalitions to retrofit antiscald devices in the bathtub and shower fixtures in the homes of low-income families with young children (environmental change), working with manufacturers of plumbing devices to produce lower-cost antiscald devices (engineering), and advocating amendments to plumbing codes (enactment-enforcement). With the assistance of the national office, coalitions will also be working to evaluate the antiscald device retrofit project and scald-burn prevention educational presentations to low-income parents and caregivers (evaluation).

For Project GET ALARMED: A Residential Fire Detection Strategy, the Campaign has been working to educate parents and caregivers about the importance of working smoke detectors in the early detection of residential fires, and of developing and practicing escape plans (education-media) (Fig. 63-4). Coalitions continue to work toward passage or strengthening of community and state smoke detector ordinances, and the national office is pursuing federal smoke detector legislation in con-

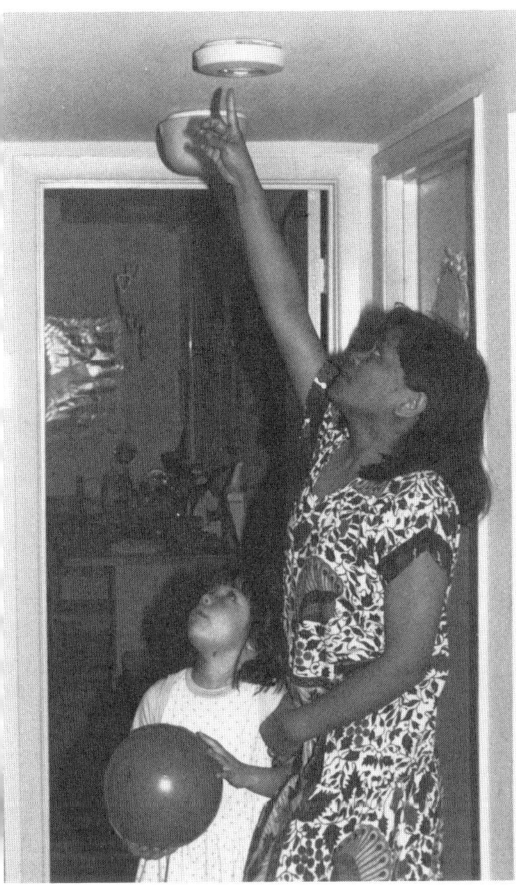

Figure 63–4 Project GET ALARMED: A Residential Fire Detection Strategy is aimed at increasing the number of working smoke detectors in the homes of low-income families with children under age 5. (© by the National SAFE KIDS Campaign, 1991. Reprinted with permission.)

junction with the Congressional Fire Caucus and the U.S. Fire Administration (enactment-enforcement). The Coalitions are also working with fire departments and other organizations to install smoke detectors in the homes of low-income families with young children (environment). The Campaign will be evaluating the effectiveness of educational presentations and smoke detector maintenance reminders (evaluation).

The SAFE KIDS BUCKLE UP: A Child Occupant Protection Strategy focuses on educating economically disadvantaged parents and caregivers about the need to increase use and reduce misuse of child safety seats and safety belts (education-media) (Fig. 63-5). Coalitions will be working to improve the access of low-income parents and caregivers to child safety seats through discount and loan programs (environment) and to strengthen existing child occupant protection laws and improve

their enforcement (enactment-enforcement). The Coalitions will also, with the assistance of the national office, evaluate their activities by conducting pre- and postimplementation observational surveys of child safety seat and safety belt use and misuse (evaluation).

These strategies are ongoing and will have new components developed for implementation each year. Coalitions may launch their own efforts in a specific risk area simultaneously with the national office, or when they feel it appropriate for them and their communities.

EDUCATION-MEDIA

The National SAFE KIDS Campaign uses a combination of education, at the national, state, and local levels, and awareness building through the media to change public perceptions about unintentional childhood injuries. The Campaign's educational efforts include the development of audiovisual and print materials to support Local and State SAFE KIDS Coalitions' educational activities as outlined in the strategies developed by the national office. These materials are often developed specifically for economically disadvantaged populations, which are considered to be most at risk for unintentional injuries.

The Campaign has also developed educational materials for the general public, such as a parents' magazine (available in English and Spanish) entitled *How to Protect Your Child from Injury,* which outlines safety measures that parents and caregivers can take in each of five major risk areas: traffic injuries, fire and burns, drownings, poisoning and choking, and falls. This magazine is supplemented by magazines for children focusing on bicycle and traffic safety and on fire safety.

The Campaign also works with health professionals to educate parents, caregivers, and children about injury prevention. The Campaign is currently working with 19 member organizations of the NCPCI in a professional outreach program to reduce bicycle-related injuries. The NCPCI members involved include the American Academy of Family Physicians, the American Academy of Pediatrics, the American College of Emergency Physicians, and the American Red Cross. In addition, the Campaign is currently working with national organizations concerned with the education of children to develop a school-based bicycle safety curriculum.

The Campaign's work with the media includes efforts to increase the general public's awareness of the problem, risk areas, resources, and injury-control activities through radio, television, and print exposure. The CBS, ABC, and CNN television networks have aired the National SAFE KIDS

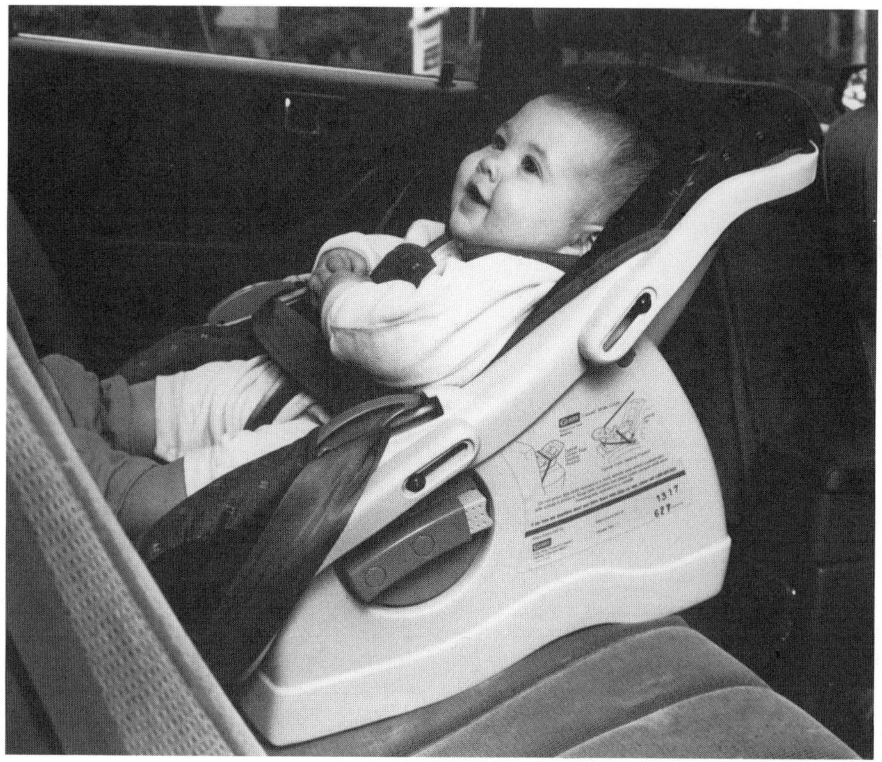

Figure 63–5 SAFE KIDS BUCKLE UP: A Child Occupant Protection Strategy was launched in February 1992. The Strategy focuses on increasing the use and reducing the misuse of child safety seats and safety belts. (© by the National SAFE KIDS Campaign, 1991. Reprinted with permission.)

Campaign's public service announcements about bicycle helmets, scald burn prevention, and residential fire detection. Articles have been placed in most national print media, including the Associated Press and UPI; the *New York Times*, the *Washington Post*, and the *Wall Street Journal; Parade, USA Today*, the "Mini Page," *U.S. News and World Report*, *Parenting*, *Essence*, *American Baby*, and *Ladies Home Journal* (Fig. 63-6).

During 1988, in just over 10 weeks, the Campaign generated more than 72,000 calls to its toll-free number requesting free safety information. Markie Post, co-star of NBC's top-rated "Night Court" and mother of a new baby girl, lent her support to the Campaign by participating in the production of videotapes, public service announcements, a satellite news conference, and Community SAFE KIDS Week kick-off activities. Malcolm Jamal Warner of the "Cosby Show" joined the festivities at the Campaign's February 1989 "Champions of SAFE KIDS" first annual awards dinner. In February 1989 "Mr. Belvedere" 's Rob Stone served as co-host of the awards dinner, and in March 1990 as Master of Ceremonies for the Campaign's second annual awards dinner. In May 1991 CBS News medical correspondent Dr. Bob Arnot was the master of ceremonies for the third annual "Champions of SAFE KIDS" awards dinner.

NATIONAL SAFE KIDS CAMPAIGN: PUBLIC-PRIVATE PARTNERSHIPS IN INJURY CONTROL

In addition to its efforts in the four areas outlined above, the National SAFE KIDS Campaign has been extremely active in creating partnerships between private industry and the public sector to help reduce the incidence of childhood injury. Those involved in the Campaign believe that childhood injury is a community-wide problem that requires a community-wide response. The Campaign therefore works to show national and local businesses that they have a role in the fight to reduce childhood injury. The Campaign works with companies with a reputation for excellence in industry, employee programs, and community relations, such as the Johnson & Johnson Family of Companies, the Campaign's founding sponsor. The National SAFE KIDS Campaign also works with companies recognized as number one in the manufacture of safety products, including Bell Bicycle, Inc., and BRK Electronics/First Alert.

Corporate support furthers the missions and

History of the Smoke Detector

The first "smoke detector" was a canary. In the late nineteenth century, canaries were used in factories to warn the workers about fires. The canaries were trained to trigger an alarm when they smelled smoke. This alarm alerted everyone to get out fast.

Today, millions of people have working smoke detectors in their homes. Since smoke detectors became available to everyone, fire deaths have dropped by one half. And, to think, if it weren't for a canary and some smart scientists, we might not have smoke detectors!

A smoke detector should be kept cleaned and tested at least once a month. Although almost 80 percent of American homes have at least one smoke detector, between one-third and one-half are not cleaned and don't work because of dead or missing batteries. So, make sure you test and clean your smoke detector.

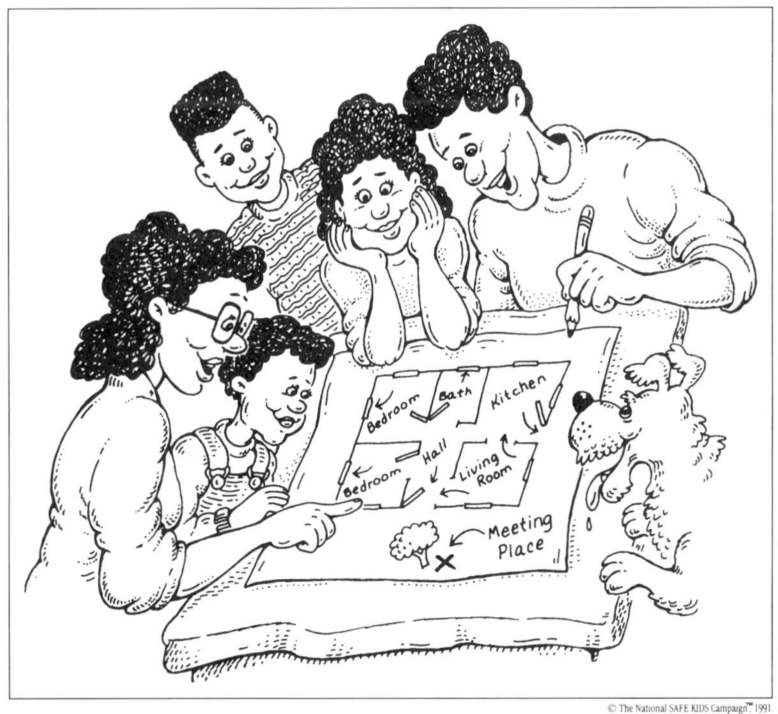

Figure 63–6 Illustrations developed for the Campaign's fire safety media kit targeted at children's magazines. (© by the National SAFE KIDS Campaign, 1991. Reprinted with permission.)

goals of childhood injury control by providing resources to conduct national and local educational, awareness building, public policy advocacy, and coalition-building activities. Businesses also serve as disseminators of safety information through employee networks and community outreach programs, provide employee volunteers to participate in Coalition activities, give visibility to community-based efforts through corporate-sponsored advertising, public service announcements, and special events, and create relationships between grassroots activists and corporate sales forces and retailers. Corporate sponsors themselves benefit from this partnership, which creates a positive corporate image with consumers, parents, children, and health care professionals, raises the visibility of the corporation in the community, provides useful information to employees, and may help to reduce health-care costs for businesses.

Childhood injury control can find a supportive partner in the business and corporate sector. By identifying common goals (reducing injuries, reducing health care costs, raising visibility of an important issue) and objectives (building awareness, targeting specific audiences, providing information), injury prevention activists and corporate sponsors can help to eliminate unnecessary risks from children's lives.

OUR CHILDREN'S TIME HAS COME

Children have moved to center stage on America's agenda for the 1990s. Failures in the past have made it clear that it is far better to invest in children now than to wait and pay the social cost later. Childhood injury prevention is one important aspect of creating the best possible future for the nation's children and, thus, for society. It is hard to say no to the National SAFE KIDS Campaign. In fact, everyone should be involved. Through the Campaign, there is a new direction in American life and culture. The National SAFE KIDS Campaign is leading the way into a new epoch in which childhood injury, like smallpox and polio, will no longer be a major problem in children's lives.

The National SAFE KIDS Campaign cannot win the fight alone. Readers are urged to join in the fight against the number one killer of children—preventable injury.

REFERENCES

1. Eichelberger MR, Gotschall CS, Feely HB et al: Parental attitudes and knowledge of child safety: a national survey, *Am J Dis Children* 144:714-720, 1990.
2. Gallagher SS, Finison K, Guyer B et al: The incidence of injuries among 87,000 Massachusetts children and adolescents: results of the 1980-81 statewide childhood injury prevention surveillance system, *AJPH* 74(1):1340-1347, 1984.
3. McLoughlin E, Crawford JD: Types of burn injuries, *Pediatr Clin N Am* 32(1):61-75, 1985.
4. National Committee for Injury Prevention and Control: Injury prevention: meeting the challenge, *Am J Prevent Med* 5(3s), 1989.
5. Rice DP, Mackenzie EJ, Jones AS et al: *The cost of injury in the United States: a report to Congress*, San Francisco, 1989, Institute for Health and Aging, University of California; Injury Prevention Center, Johns Hopkins University.
6. Secretary of Health and Human Services: *Childhood injury in the United States: a report to Congress*, Atlanta, 1989, U.S. Department of Health and Human Services, Public Health Service, Centers for Disease Control.
7. Waller AE, Baker SP, Szocka A: Childhood injury deaths, *AJPH* 79(3):310-315, 1989.
8. Waller AE, Baker SP, Szocka A: Childhood injury deaths: national analysis and geographic variation, *AJPH* 79(3):310-315, 1989.

Index

f indicates figure or illustration; t indicates table

A

Abbreviated injury scale (AIS), 642, 643
ABCs in life support phase of resuscitation, 145-151
Abdomen
    aerophagia and, 175
    anatomical differences in, 51
    biomechanics of injury to, 27, 28
    CT of, 238f
    gunshot wounds to, 337, 341f
    of infant and toddler, 151
    infections of, 290, 291
    prehospital care and, 110
    stab wounds to, 337
Abdominal injury
    algorithm for, 452f
    anesthesia for, 223
    assessment of, 453, 454
    blunt, mechanism of injury in, 235t
    as evidence of child abuse, 560
    indications for serious, 453t
    intentional versus unintentional, 561t
    mechanisms of, 451
    patterns of, 451-455
    penetrating, 337-340
    resuscitation and diagnosis of, 451-454
ABO blood group, 272, 273
Abscess, abdominal, 291
Acceptance phase in brain death, 317
Access
    to circulation, in life support phase, 148, 149
    to prehospital care, 102
    vascular, 187, 188, 199f
Accidental Death and Disability publication, 136
Accreditation, 652, 653
Acetazolamide, 210
Acetyl-CoA, 69
Acid burns, 585, 586
Acid indigestion, 480
Acid-base balance
    blood transfusion and, 277, 278
    in hypovolemic shock, 183
Acid-etch splint, 416f
Acidosis in cardiac arrest, 189, 190
ACTH; *see* Adrenocorticotropic hormone
Acute tubular necrosis (ATN), 80
Adherent PMN, 77f
Adolescence, 85
Adolescents, 57
    education and training in rehabilitation of, 133-135
    history of public health services for, 3-5
Adosterone, 63t
Adrenocorticotropic hormone (ACTH), 61-64
Adult respiratory distress syndrome (ARDS), 79, 172
    identification and treatment of, 176
Advanced Pediatric Life Support (APLS) course, 96, 138
Advanced Trauma Life Support (ATLS) course, 95
Advocacy, 122, 123
Aerophagia, 175
Afipia felis, 625
Age
    in child abuse, 558
    as factor in childhood injury, 17
    incidence of hemorrhagic lesions grouped by, 348f
    organ donation and, 319
    and outcome of head injury, 345, 346f
Agents of childhood injury, 17, 18
Air bag, 31

Air embolism 440, 441
Airway edema, 42
Airway injury, causes of, 427f
Airway management in head injury, 207
Airway obstruction, 145-147
Airways, 162-168
    anatomical differences in, 42, 43
    anatomy of, 162
    in burn injuries, 166t-168
    cricothyrotomy and, 166
    foreign body in, 173
    head injury and, 355
    in injuries to children, 26
    in life support phase of resuscitation, 145-147
    in maxillofacial injury, 395, 396
    obstruction of, 171
    opening, 103
    oral and nasopharyngeal, complications of, 164
    pathophysiology of, 61
    pediatric, anatomy of, 103
    penetrating injuries to neck and, 332
    prehospital care and, 102-105
AIS; *see* Abbreviated injury scale
Alanine, 70
Albumin, 183
    burn injuries and, 573, 575
    formula for calculating deficit of, 282
    normal blood laboratory value of in children, 602t
    nutritional assessment and, 281
Aldosterone, 64
Algorithm
    for abdominal injury, 452f
    for hypovolemic shock, 150f, 184f
    for pediatric trauma, 145-161
    for resuscitation, 610f
Alkali burns, 585
Allen's test, 634
Allograft, 580, 581f
Alopecia, 561t
Alpha receptors, 65
Alveolar bone, 411f
Alveolar fracture, 416
Ambulance equipment, 100t, 101
American Academy of Pediatrics, 4, 96
    dietary recommendations of, 594
    prevention of childhood injury and, 9
American Association of Critical-Care Nurses, 121
American Association of Poison Control Centers, 621t
American College of Surgeons, 647
    committee on trauma of, 136
American Public Health Association, 647
American Trauma Society, 121
Amicar; *see* aminocaproic acid
Amide linked local anesthetics, 305t
Amikacin, 288
Amino acids, 280
Aminocaproic acid in ocular trauma, 403
Aminoglycoside in open fracture therapy, 538
Aminophylline in treatment of anaphylactic reaction, 626
Amoxicillin, 462
Ampicillin, 288t
Amputated parts, 110
Amputation, 552-554
    compartment syndrome and, 550
    of digit, 620
    of fingertip, 619
    techniques in child versus adult, 552, 553
Amylase, serum, in pancreatic injury, 491, 492
Anal area, curvilinear incision over, 488f
Analgesia in management of intracranial pressure, 210